Estimated minimum sodium, chloride, and potassium requirements for healthy persons

Age	Weight (kg)	Sodium (mg)*†	Chloride (mg)*†	Potassium (mg)‡
Months				
0-5	4.5	120	180	500
6-11	8.9	200	300	700
Years				
1	11	225	350	1000
2-5	16	300	500	1400
6-9	25	400	600	1600
10-18	50	500	750	2000
>18§	70	500	750	2000

*No allowance has been included for large, prolonged losses from the skin through sweat.

†There is no evidence that higher intakes confer any additional health benefit.

‡Desirable intakes of potassium may considerably exceed these values (~13,500 mg for adults).

§No allowance has been included for growth. Values given for people under 18 years of age assume a growth rate corresponding to the 50th percentile reported by the National Center for Health Statistics and averaged for males and females.

Estimated safe and adequate daily dietary intakes (ESADDIs) of selected vitamins and minerals*

Category	Age (years)	Vitamins			Trace Elements†			
		Biotin (μg)	Pantothenic acid (mg)	Copper (mg)	Manganese (mg)	Fluoride (mg)	Chromium (μg)	Molybdenum (μg)
Infants	0-0.5	10	2	0.4-0.6	0.3-0.6	0.1-0.5	10-40	15-30
	0.5-1	15	3	0.6-0.7	0.6-1	0.2-1	20-60	20-40
Children and adolescents	1-3	20	3	0.7-1	1-1.5	0.5-1.5	20-80	25-50
	4-6	25	3-4	1-1.5	1.5-2	1-2.5	30-120	30-75
	7-10	30	4-5	1-2	2-3	1.5-2.5	50-200	50-150
	11+	30-100	4-7	1.5-2.5	2-5	1.5-2.5	50-200	75-250
Adults		30-100	4-7	1.5-3	2-5	1.5-4	50-200	75-250

*Because there is less information on which to base recommendations for allowances of minerals, these figures are not given in the main table of RDAs and are provided here in the form of ranges of recommended intakes.

†Since toxic levels for many trace elements may be reached with only several times usual intakes, the upper levels for the trace elements given in this table should not be habitually exceeded.

Perspectives In
NUTRITION

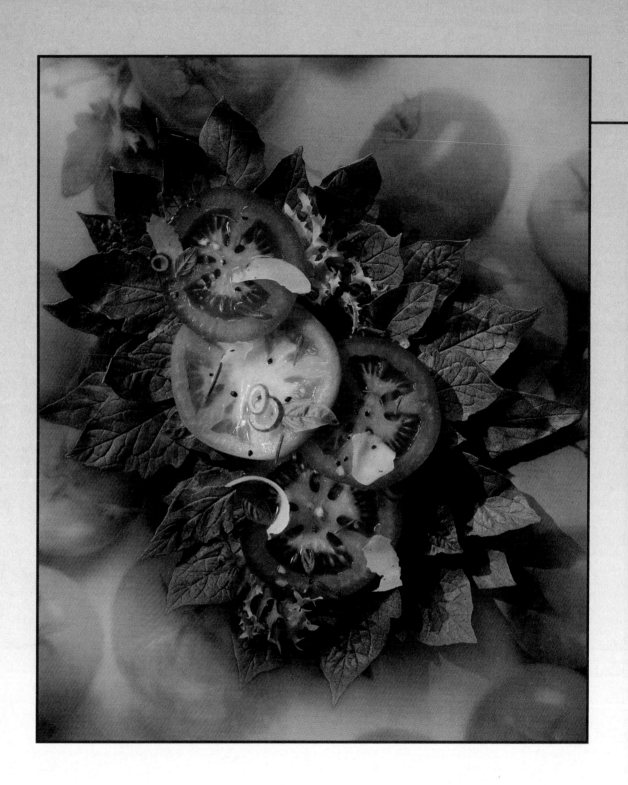

THIRD EDITION

PERSPECTIVES IN
NUTRITION

Gordon M. Wardlaw, Ph.D., R.D., L.D.
The Ohio State University

Paul M. Insel, Ph.D.
Stanford University

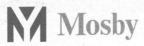

St. Louis Baltimore Boston Carlsbad Chicago Naples New York Philadelphia Portland
London Madrid Mexico City Singapore Sydney Tokyo Toronto Wiesbaden

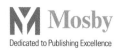
Mosby
Dedicated to Publishing Excellence

A Times Mirror Company

Publisher: James M. Smith
Senior Acquisitions Editor: Vicki Malinee
Managing Editor: Janet Russell Livingston
Senior Developmental Editor: Jean Babrick
Project Manager: Mark Spann
Production Editor: Melissa Martin
Designer: David Zielinski
Manufacturing Supervisor: Betty Richmond
Cover Photograph: © 1995 Greg Stroube

Printed in the United States of America
Composition by Graphic World
Color separation by Color Associates
Printing/binding by Von Hoffmann Press

Mosby–Year Book, Inc.
11830 Westline Industrial Drive
St. Louis, Missouri 63146

Library of Congress Cataloging in Publication Data

Wardlaw, Gordon M.
    Perspectives in nutrition / Gordon M. Wardlaw, Paul M. Insel.—
3rd ed.
        p.   cm.
    Includes bibliographical references and index.
    ISBN 0-8151-9072-7
    1. Nutrition. I. Insel, Paul M. II. Title.
QP141.W38   1995
613.2—dc20   95-39088
                                                               CIP

96 97 98 99 00 / 9 8 7 6 5 4 3 2 1

Reviewers

As with earlier editions of this textbook, our goal is to provide the most accurate, up-to-date, and useful introductory nutrition text available. We would like to recognize and thank the people whose direction and insight guided us through the three editions.

FOR THE THIRD EDITION:

Elizabeth Chu, M.S., R.D.
San Diego Mesa College

Diane Veale Jones, M.S., R.D.
College of Saint Benedict

Susan M. Krueger, M.S., R.D.
University of Wisconsin–Eau Claire

Stella Miller, M.A.
Mount San Antonio College

Dorice M. Narins, Ph.D.
Texas Woman's University

FOR THE SECOND EDITION:

Paul Abernathy, Ph.D.
Purdue University

Ellen Brennan, M.S.
San Antonio College

Charlotte Britto, M.S.
San Joaquin Delta College

Thomas Castonguay, Ph.D.
University of Maryland
(Chapter 8)

Veryan Cumberbatch, M.S., R.D.
University of Kentucky

Robert DiSilvestro, Ph.D.
The Ohio State University

Hazel Forsythe, Ph.D.
University of Kentucky

Art Gilbert, Ph.D.
University of California–Santa Barbara

Jeffrey Harris, D.H.Sc., M.P.H., R.D.
West Chester University

Susan Houston, M.S.
City College of San Francisco

Carol Johnston, Ph.D.
Arizona State University

Murray Kaplan, Ph.D.
Iowa State University
(Chapter 7)

Robert Lee, D.H.Sc., M.P.H., R.D.
Central Michigan University

Lisa McKee, Ph.D.
New Mexico State University

Christopher Melby, D.H.Sc., M.P.H.
Colorado State University

Nina Mercer, Ph.D.
University of Guelph

Carol Mitchell, Ph.D., R.D.
Memphis State University

Cathy Rozmus, D.S.N., R.N.
Columbia State Community College

Anne Shaw
U.S. Department of Agriculture
(Chapter 2)

LuAnn Soliah, Ph.D.
Baylor University

Carol L. Thomas, M.A.
San Joaquin Delta College

Adrienne White, Ph.D.
University of Maine

Gregory Williams, Ph.D.
California State University–Fullerton

FOR THE FIRST EDITION:

Richard Ahrens, Ph.D., R.D.
University of Maryland

Kathy Beerman, Ph.D.
Washington State University

Wen Chiu, Ph.D.
Shoreline Community College

Sylvia Gartung, B.S.
Michigan State University

Catherine Justice, Ph.D., R.D.
Purdue University

Michael Keenan, Ph.D.
Louisiana State University

RoseAnn Kutschke, Ph.D.
University of Texas–Austin

Joseph Leichter, Ph.D.
University of British Columbia

Ricki Lewis, Ph.D.
State University of New York–Albany

Sandra Mitchell, Ph.D., R.D.
California State University–Chico

Jean Peters, M.S.
Oregon State University

Harry Sitren, Ph.D.
University of Florida

Joanne Slavin, Ph.D., R.D.
University of Minnesota

Anne Smith, Ph.D., R.D.
The Ohio State University

Linda Vaughan, Ph.D., R.D.
Arizona State University

Contributors

A unique feature of this book is its collection of Expert Opinion commentaries. In addition, several authorities addressed specialized topics in Nutrition Perspective essays. We would like to thank the experts whose outstanding and insightful articles highlight this text.

Bruce Arnow, Ph.D.
Stanford University

Stephen Barrett, M.D.
Psychiatrist (retired)
    Consumer Advocate
Allentown, Pennsylvania

Linda J. Boyne, M.S., R.D., L.D.
The Ohio State University

Susan Calvert Finn, Ph.D., R.D.
Ross Laboratories
Columbus, Ohio

J. Mark Davis, Ph.D.
University of South Carolina

Adam Drewnowski, Ph.D.
University of Michigan

Constance J. Geiger, Ph.D., R.D.
Geiger & Associates
Salt Lake City, Utah

Helen A. Guthrie, Ph.D., R.D.
The Pennsylvania State University

John N. Hathcock, Ph.D.
Food and Drug Administration
Washington, D.C.

Marc Hellerstein, M.D., Ph.D.
University of California–Berkeley

David M. Klurfeld, Ph.D.
Wayne State University

Susan M. Krueger, M.S., R.D.
University of Wisconsin–Eau Claire

David Lamb, Ph.D.
The Ohio State University

Robert D. Langer, M.D., M.P.H.
University of California–San Diego

Jim Leklem, Ph.D.
Oregon State University

Judy Loper, Ph.D., R.D., L.D.
Central Ohio Nutrition Center
Columbus, Ohio

Denis M. Medeiros, Ph.D., R.D.
The Ohio State University

Mark Messina, Ph.D.
Nutrition Consultant
Port Townsend, Washington

Gregory D. Miller, Ph.D., F.A.C.N.
National Dairy Council
Chicago, Illinois

Forrest H. Nielsen, Ph.D.
Human Nutrition Research Center
Grand Forks, North Dakota

Ellyn Satter, M.S., R.D., A.C.S.W.
Family Therapy Center
Madison, Wisconsin

Daniel Steinberg, M.D., Ph.D.
University of California–San Diego

Preface to the Instructor

If you teach nutrition, you undoubtedly already find it a fascinating topic. However, nutrition can also be quite frustrating to teach. Claims and counter-claims abound regarding the need for certain constituents in our diets. Sodium is a good example. One group of researchers promotes a low-sodium diet for the general population as an effective preventive measure for hypertension. Other groups believe that normal blood pressure values can often be maintained despite the excess intakes of sodium common among Americans.

As authors, we too are aware of conflicting opinions in our field and thus draw on as many sources as possible in the continual updating of this textbook, now in its third edition. We have incorporated much new material, especially from the recently published supplements to the *American Journal of Clinical Nutrition* and the latest edition of *Modern Nutrition in Health and Disease,* edited by Shils, Olson, and Shike. We have also consulted a number of experts and continue to include their insights about the current state of nutrition research.

We believe that this textbook continues to differ significantly from all others in the field. Like other textbooks, it focuses on the latest research in nutrition, but goes further by documenting important research studies throughout the chapters, listing those references at the end of each chapter, and providing Expert Opinion boxes in each chapter to examine more closely the most controversial issues introduced in the text. In all, we strive to present many perspectives in current nutrition research so that you and your students can better understand and participate in debates about current nutrition issues.

Personalizing Nutrition

One prominent theme in nutrition research today is *individuality.* Not all of us, for example, find that saturated fat in our diets raises our blood cholesterol values above recommended standards. Each person responds individually, often idiosyncratically, to nutrients, and that is something we continually point out in this textbook.

As well, even at this basic level we do not assume that all nutrition students are alike. We repeatedly ask students to learn more about themselves and their health status and to use this new knowledge to improve their health. After reading this textbook, students will understand much more clearly how the nutrition information given on the evening news, on cereal box labels, in popular magazines, and by government agencies applies to them. They will become sophisticated consumers of both nutrients and nutrition information. They will understand that their knowledge of nutrition allows them to personalize information, rather than follow every guideline issued for an entire population. After all, a population by definition consists of individuals with varying genetic and cultural backgrounds, and these individuals have varying responses to diet.

In addition, we cover important questions that students often raise concerning ethnic diets, eating disorders, nutrient supplements, phytochemicals, vegetarianism, diets for athletes, food safety, and fad diets. We emphasize the importance of understanding one's food choices and changing one's diet as needed.

Audience

This book is designed for a diverse audience. It is most useful for students majoring in nutrition, the health sciences, home economics, nursing, physical education, and other health-related areas and for premedical and predental students. However, because the chapter organization and content are flexible, the book can be adapted to meet the needs of students of diverse backgrounds. Although it is not absolutely necessary, most students will find that having taken a course in biology or having an understanding of basic biological concepts provides a helpful background for taking the introductory nutrition course.

Organization

Although the book is most suitable for a semester-length course, it can also be used in a quarter-length course by omitting chapters or by skipping various sections. A useful feature of this text is that it is presented in six segments:

Part One: Nutrition Basics
Part Two: The Energy-Yielding Nutrients
Part Three: Energy Production and Energy Balance
Part Four: The Vitamins and Minerals
Part Five: Nutrition Applications in the Life Cycle
Part Six: Putting Nutrition Knowledge into Practice

This organization makes it easy to tailor the text to specific course needs.

New to This Edition

The third edition of *Perspectives in Nutrition* incorporates several new features designed to enhance student learning and understanding:

NEW CRITICAL THINKING QUESTIONS

Each chapter presents three scenarios that allow students to apply information they have learned to practical situations. These questions will help students put the information in the chapter into the perspective of daily life and, by doing so, will enhance learning. Answers are provided in the back of the book so that students can compare their thinking with that of the authors.

EXPANDED COVERAGE OF NUTRITION LABELING

Constance J. Geiger, Ph.D., R.D., a noted authority on food labeling issues and a consultant to the food industry, wrote the Nutrition Perspective in Chapter 2. This accurate and up-to-date essay reviews food labeling in detail. Then, in the remaining chapters of the book, sample labels are shown to reinforce the value of reading food labels and to help the student practice obtaining important information from this nutrition tool.

EXPANDED COVERAGE OF ETHNIC DIETS

The Nutrition Perspective in Chapter 18 takes a broad look at ethnic influences on the American diet. It also covers the recently proposed Mediterranean diet pyramid.

EXPANDED COVERAGE OF THE IMMUNE SYSTEM

The Nutrition Perspective in Chapter 15 explores the physiology of the immune system and the role of nutrients in its various functions. Previously the focus was primarily on nutrients, but we believe that students will benefit from a wider discussion of the biological intricacies of the system.

NEW NUTRITION FOCUS BOXES

Phytochemicals and other breaking topics are now discussed in these new sections in each chapter.

MANY NEW EXPERT OPINION BOXES

Nutrition experts discuss intense sweeteners, women and heart disease, chromium picolinate, and vitamin E supplements. One expert provides a personal look at the fight against hunger and poverty in the United States.

OVER 100 NEW FULL-COLOR ILLUSTRATIONS

New figures provide greater anatomical detail and effectively convey important nutrition concepts.

FOOD GUIDE PYRAMID ILLUSTRATIONS

Twenty-five colorful variations on the USDA Food Guide Pyramid illustrate the nutrient density of the various food groups.

Additional Features

We have organized this text in response to the needs of instructors and students:

GENERAL CONTENT AND CONTROVERSIAL TOPICS ARE WELL REFERENCED

Approximately 80% of the referenced material is from sources published since the last edition of this text, in 1993. As instructors, we demand the latest information to present to our students. Providing this up-to-date research will not only give students the most accurate picture of nutrition today but will also direct them to current materials for further study.

SEPARATE CHAPTERS ON ENERGY BALANCE, WEIGHT CONTROL, AND EATING DISORDERS

A thorough discussion is presented of these very controversial and current topics.

EMPHASIS ON NUTRIENT DENSITY

Discussions of nutrients are based on the most nutrient-dense sources of foods. Leading food sources in the U.S. diet are identified for each nutrient when those data are available.

EMPHASIS ON THE EXCHANGE SYSTEM

An outline of the 1995 version of the Exchange System is presented in Chapter 2 and can be used or omitted at your option. The use of the Exchange System is reinforced in Chapters 3 through 5 and in the Student Study Guide and Mosby's new NutriTrac software.

MINIMAL USE OF CHEMISTRY

An explanation of chemistry principles is presented in Appendix B to help students whose chemistry backgrounds are weak. We use some chemistry concepts to help students comprehend the nature of nutrient metabolism. Overall, this is kept to a minimum, and chemical structures are found primarily in the margins.

EMPHASIS ON BEHAVIOR-CHANGE STRATEGIES

Behavior-change strategies have been integrated into Chapter 9, Weight Control, to encourage students to plan diets that will enhance health maintenance. The strategies allow students to apply the foundations of the course to daily life. Once students are able to put the main nutrition concepts into perspective, they can set nutritional goals and change their diets accordingly.

SUMMARY TABLES

Some chapters contain large, detailed summary tables that include the major points made in the chapter. These tables are convenient capsules for reference.

Design

Choosing the illustrations for this textbook was quite exciting. Because we drew heavily on the biological and physiological expertise of our publisher, this textbook is far ahead of any in the field in depicting important biological and physiological phenomena, such as transport across cell membranes, emulsification, glucose regulation, digestion and absorption, cancer progression, and fetal development. The extensive three-dimensional graphic presentations in this book make nutrition and relevant physiological principles come alive for students.

In addition, we have used many sources to provide what we consider to be the best photographic program in any nutrition text. The many full-color photographs in this text were researched and selected to reflect a modern view of food presentation and food consumption, providing the student with the most outstanding and timely perspective in the nutrition arena today.

Humor has been used throughout the text to aid the learning process. *Perspectives in Nutrition* includes some of the best work of our nation's leading cartoonists. The cartoons make important nutrition points in a way that students will remember.

Pedagogy

The following extensive pedagogical features were designed not only to interest the student but also to continually reinforce the learning process:

NUTRITION AWARENESS INVENTORIES

These sets of true or false questions heighten students' awareness of chapter content. This feature also allows students to gauge how much they have learned. The answers are listed by chapter at the end of the book.

MARGIN NOTES

Margin notes throughout the book provide clinical examples, references to other chapters, clarification of ideas, and further details about key concepts.

MARGIN DEFINITIONS

Important terms are set in boldface type at first mention. More difficult terms are defined in the text's margins. All boldface terms appear in the glossary.

CONCEPT CHECK BOXES

Concept Checks summarize chapter content every few pages, reinforcing students' understanding of the material.

NUTRITION FOCUS BOXES

Each chapter contains one or two short essays, often on controversial topics in nutrition, such as fat replacements.

TAKE ACTION BOXES

These activity boxes at the end of each chapter let students put theory into practice. The suggested assignments are usually proactive and at times involve students in the kinds of activities that registered dietitians perform.

CRITICAL THINKING QUESTIONS

Each chapter contains three scenarios that ask students to apply information they have learned to practical situations. Answers are provided at the end of the book.

CHAPTER SUMMARY POINTS

The content of each chapter is summarized in seven to ten major points. This feature, together with the Concept Checks, will help students to review for examinations.

*Available to qualified adopters.

STUDY QUESTIONS

Ten questions at the end of each chapter encourage students to probe deeper into the chapter content, making connections and gaining new insights.

UP-TO-DATE REFERENCES

Each chapter contains approximately 30 current references, most published since 1993.

NUTRITION PERSPECTIVE BOXES

These essays at the end of each chapter extend the chapter content by adding more detailed and controversial material.

EXPERT OPINION BOXES

Each chapter contains an Expert Opinion commentary written by a noted researcher. In most cases, the expert has been recognized by the American Dietetic Association or the American Institute of Nutrition.

GLOSSARY

A comprehensive glossary of more than 500 key terms is included for the student's reference. The glossary contains pronunciation keys for many unfamiliar words.

Supplementary Materials

The latest supplementary materials are provided to both the student and the instructor to make better use of the text and the concepts presented in the course:

*INSTRUCTOR'S MANUAL AND TEST BANK

Prepared by Jan Goshert, M.S., R.D., this comprehensive teaching aid includes chapter summaries with suggestions for teaching difficult material; activities; suggested readings; nutrition assessments; source lists of supplementary materials; and a "survival" chapter, addressed to the novice instructor, that discusses class organization, scheduling, and problem areas such as cheating.

Extensively reviewed for clarity and accuracy, the test bank features approximately 2000 test items (multiple choice, short answer, true/false, and matching questions) coded for level of difficulty, type of knowledge being tested, and text page reference. The resource manual also includes 75 transparency masters of key illustrations.

STUDENT STUDY GUIDE

Prepared by Gordon M. Wardlaw, this student aid has been thoroughly reviewed by experienced instructors and developed in consultation with a learning theory expert. This comprehensive guide reinforces concepts presented in the text and integrates them with study activities, such as flash cards, to emphasize key concepts. It features vocabulary review and sample examinations structured to reflect the actual examinations students will face in the classroom.

*COMPUTERIZED TEST BANK

Instructors who adopt the text receive EsaTest, a computerized test bank package compatible with IBM and Macintosh microcomputers. This test-generation software combines a number of user-friendly aids, enabling the instructor to select, edit, delete, or add questions and construct and print tests and answer keys. EsaTest also offers EsaGrade, a convenient electronic gradebook.

*TRANSPARENCY ACETATES

One hundred and fifty full-color transparency acetates are provided in a binder. They feature key illustrations from the text, with large, easy-to-read labels.

MOSBY'S NutriTrac™ SOFTWARE

Available for Windows and Macintosh, this nutrient-analysis software allows you and your students to analyze diets easily, using an icon-based interface and on-screen help features. Foods for breakfast, lunch, dinner, and snacks may be selected from more than 2250 items in the database. Records may be kept for any number of days. The program can provide intake analyses for individual foods, meals, days, or for an entire intake period. Intake analyses can compare nutrient values to RDA or RNI values and to the USDA Food Guide Pyramid, and provide breakdowns of fat and calorie sources.

*ViewStudy™ PRESENTATION SOFTWARE

This CD-ROM, compatible with either Windows or Macintosh, contains key illustrations from the text. Images are arranged by chapter, and a slide show tool allows selection of prearranged images. Illustrations can also be printed full size for use as acetates and may be exported for use with other programs and applications, such as the computerized testbank.

*Available to qualified adopters.

Acknowledgments
TEXT DEVELOPMENT

The authors wish to thank Margaret Kessell, Ph.D., R.D., L.D., for reviewing each chapter and providing important insights from a teacher's perspective. We also want to thank Rebecca Liebes, M.S., Linda Boyne, M.S., R.D., Sally Smith, R.D., and Jeffrey Harris, D.H.Sc., R.D., for help in various stages of chapter revisions. Mattie Cossio, Ph.D., contributed Critical Thinking questions that will help students learn to apply concepts to everyday situations. All of these individuals contributed to the final product, and we are greatly indebted to them.

SPECIAL ACKNOWLEDGMENTS

We would like to thank our developmental editor, Jean Babrick, who nurtured and assisted us through every step of the revision. Janet Russell Livingston, Managing Editor, Vicki Malinee, Senior Acquisitions Editor, and Jim Smith, Vice President and Publisher, facilitated the difficult decisions that frequently arose. Jean Babrick researched most of the exceptional photographs. Melissa Martin, our production editor, provided excellent and careful production work. Ruth Steyn and Katherine Aiken did an outstanding job copyediting the manuscript.

This book began with a dream. Each new edition is fostered by the excitement that improvements bring and ends with the revision of an innovative textbook that we believe continues to set a standard for introductory nutrition textbooks.

Gordon M. Wardlaw
Paul M. Insel

# About the Authors

GORDON M. WARDLAW, Ph.D., R.D., L.D., teaches nutrition to students in the Division of Medical Dietetics, School of Allied Medical Professions, The Ohio State University. Dr. Wardlaw is the author of many articles that have appeared in prominent nutrition, biology, physiology, and biochemistry journals and was the 1985 recipient of the American Dietetic Association's Mary P. Huddleson award. Dr. Wardlaw is a full member of the prestigious American Institute of Nutrition and is certified as a Specialist in Human Nutrition by the American Board of Nutrition.

PAUL M. INSEL, Ph.D., is Clinical Associate Professor of Psychiatry and Behavioral Sciences at Stanford University. He has been the principal investigator of many NIH studies, is the senior author of a leading introductory health text, and is Editor in Chief of *Healthline* magazine.

Preface to the Student

Cholesterol, sports drinks, food labeling, bulimia nervosa, alternative sweeteners, vegetarianism, and *Salmonella* food-borne illness—we suspect you have heard about these topics. Which of them are important enough to be a consideration in your life or in the life of someone you know?

Americans pride themselves on their individuality. Nutritional advice should be given accordingly. For example, not all of us have high serum cholesterol and thus don't have a significant risk of premature development of heart disease. The need to tailor dietary advice to each person's individual nature is the basic approach of this book. First we give you a brief introduction to the study of nutrition and discuss how to be a knowledgeable consumer. With so much information floating around—both accurate and inaccurate—you should know how to make informed decisions about your nutritional well-being. Then we encourage you to learn the basic principles of nutrition and to discover how to apply the concepts in this book that pertain specifically to you.

The text discusses some of the most interesting and important elements of nutrition and food consumption to help you understand both how your body works and how your food choices affect your health.

Features

PLANNING A NEW WAY OF EATING

Early in the text we present many of the basic guidelines for planning a healthy diet, including a description of the USDA Food Guide Pyramid, in Chapter 2. Later, in Chapter 9, we show you the steps involved in setting nutritional goals and designing a diet plan to attain those goals.

UNDERSTANDING THE WORLD AROUND US

In a college environment, it is often difficult to envision how real the problem of world hunger is. Chapter 20 examines the problem of undernutrition and the conditions that create it. The chapter allows you to explore possible solutions that offer hope for the future of our world.

CHEMISTRY REVIEW

In Appendix B we discuss in detail the critical chemistry concepts you need to know for an introductory study of nutrition. This information will give you a better understanding of how nutrients work and how nutrition information applies to you.

Pedagogy

The third edition of *Perspectives in Nutrition* incorporates some important tools (called *pedagogy*) to help you learn nutrition. Following is a guide to those tools:

1. Each chapter begins with a Nutrition Awareness Inventory. This group of 15 true or false questions helps you determine how much you already know about the chapter content. Take this examination again when you finish the chapter, and you will see how much you've learned.
2. Throughout each chapter are boldfaced key terms. The more difficult terms are defined in the margin. All boldfaced terms appear with their definitions and pronunciations in the glossary at the end of the text.
3. The numerous tables throughout the text provide convenient capsules of information for reference.

4. At the end of each chapter is a Take Action box that focuses on major concepts in each chapter as they pertain to your own life. The activity may include looking more carefully at your diet, examining your family history, or applying information you've learned to friends or family.

5. The Concept Checks that follow the major sections within each chapter list the key points made in each section. If you don't understand the material in the Concept Check, you should reread the preceding section.

6. Each chapter ends with summary points that convey the main ideas in the chapter. We also include several study questions per chapter. Both of these elements provide an excellent review for examinations.

7. In the Expert Opinion boxes, experts in the field of nutrition and health outline information you need to understand regarding nutrition issues of our day. Consider these boxed discussions to be like "visiting speakers" who come into your classroom to talk about the latest research findings.

8. We provide you with detailed references to back up material presented in the chapter. The research cited is from the most current publications—approximately 80% has been published since 1993. If you are preparing a research paper for your class or would just like more information on specific topics, consult these sources.

9. Nutrition Focus boxes allow you to explore current topics that your instructor may not have time to cover but that may nevertheless be of interest to you.

10. Critical Thinking questions ask you to apply information as you learn it. This fosters understanding of the material.

11. Nutrition Perspective essays at the end of each chapter develop current topics in nutrition in greater detail than in the chapter. Topics include nutrition labeling, the effects of alcohol, nutrition and cancer, and heart disease.

A Student Study Guide and Mosby's NutriTrac software are available to you with *Perspectives in Nutrition*. These instructional aids are designed to help you learn the major concepts developed in each chapter and prepare for class examinations.

Student Study Guide

The valuable Student Study Guide, by Gordon M. Wardlaw, Ph.D., R.D., reinforces concepts presented in the text and integrates them with activities to facilitate learning. Sample examinations reflect the actual tests you will face in the classroom. Vocabulary reviews increase your knowledge of the terminology. Flash cards help you review the major concepts in the chapter and, in turn, test your understanding of these important concepts. Activities include fill-in tables, labeling, and matching terms. These activities follow the text discussion and are anchored with quotations and page citations from the text.

A Request to Professors and Students Who Use This Book

As you might imagine, it is difficult for two people to range across the vast areas of nutrition science, following all of the various controversies and new developments. We try our best but realize that sometimes we make mistakes and sometimes we miss a side of an argument that deserves attention. If as you read this book you find content that you question or believe warrants a more detailed or broader look, feel free to contact the senior author by mail, fax, or e-mail.

Gordon M. Wardlaw, Ph.D., R.D.
The Ohio State University
516H School of Allied Medical Professions
1583 Perry Street
Columbus, OH 43210
Fax: 614-292-0210
E-mail: gwardlaw@magnus.acs.ohio-state.edu

Contents

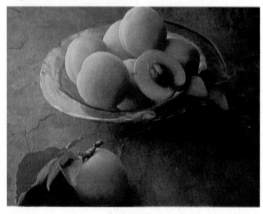

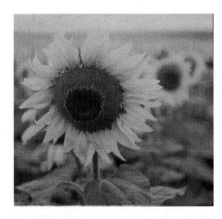

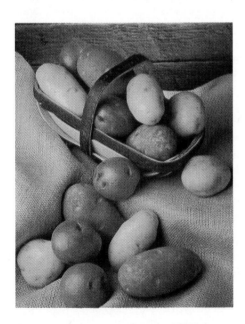

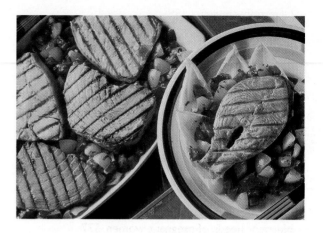

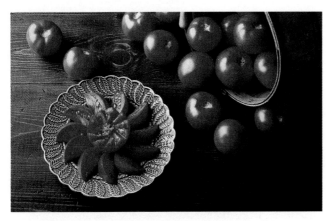

CHAPTER ONE

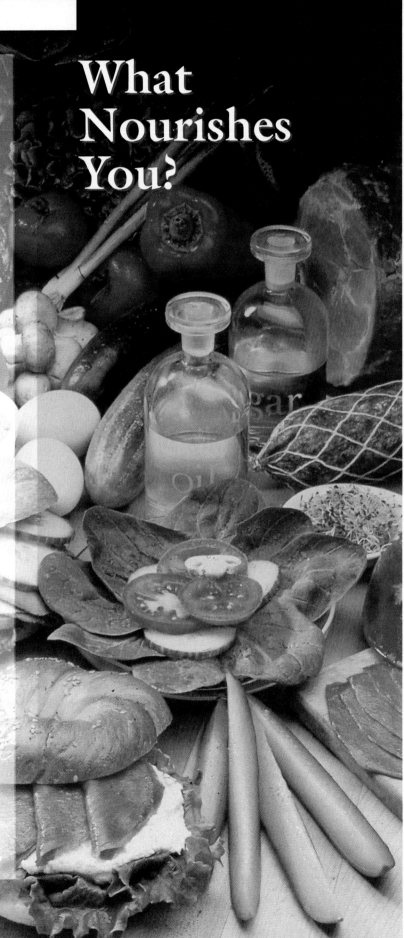

What Nourishes You?

We are continually bombarded with information about nutrition and health. Almost daily, the news media report new studies showing how our diets affect our well-being. The best-seller list usually contains at least one book about diet and health, and bookstores and libraries display row upon row of books telling us what to eat and what to avoid. This diverse mass of information often contains contradictory and confusing mixed messages. Worse, some diet "experts" promote unbalanced and gimmicky diets. These so-called experts try to exploit our desire for dietary shortcuts that promise health and beauty.

Turning to a more authoritative source, the 1988 Surgeon General's *Report on Nutrition and Health* re-minded us that "for the two out of three adult Americans who do not smoke and do not drink excessively, one personal choice seems to influence long-term health prospects more than any other: what we eat." The nutritional lifestyles of some Americans are out of balance with their physiology. And since we live longer than our ancestors, preventing the nutrition-related diseases that develop later in life is more important than in the past.

By changing our "problem" food habits, we can strive to bring the goal of a healthy life within reach. This is a primary theme not just in this chapter, but throughout this entire book.

NUTRITION AWARENESS INVENTORY

1. T F   Many foods are almost entirely water.
2. T F   Minerals can be changed into vitamins in the body.
3. T F   The terms *kilocalorie* and *calorie* can be used interchangeably; they refer to the same amount of food energy.
4. T F   Fats yield more energy per gram than carbohydrates.
5. T F   Vitamins directly provide energy to the body.
6. T F   Nutritional stores are reserve nutrients that the body can mobilize when needed.
7. T F   The body generally requires greater daily amounts of vitamins than minerals.
8. T F   One gram of water can provide 1 kilocalorie of energy when metabolized by the body.
9. T F   The chemical term *organic* is related to the concept of organic gardening.
10. T F   In reference to nutritional status, the terms *undernutrition* and *malnutrition* can be used interchangeably.
11. T F   Fatigue and ineffective control of body temperature may be evidence of advanced iron deficiency.
12. T F   In our society, problems related to overnutrition are more common than those associated with undernutrition.
13. T F   Taking vitamin and mineral supplements in any amount is considered a desirable practice.
14. T F   Alcoholic beverages are a major source of energy for some people.
15. T F   People's food choices are most often determined by their nutritional knowledge.

The Importance of Exploring Your Own Food Habits

In this opening chapter, you will be encouraged to explore your own food habits and to discover the underlying reasons for them. This is an important first step in your study of nutrition. Health authorities warn that what we eat can influence our prospects for long-term good health. People with nutritional lifestyles out of balance with their physiology are likely to have or eventually develop health problems.[3] Ironically, people often have good intuitions about healthy food choices but fail to act on them. Yet even small changes in behavior toward food can make big differences in achieving a long and vigorous life. The more you know about both nutrition and personal health risks, the better you can plan a diet to meet your nutritional needs.

A poor diet is a **risk factor** for the major **chronic** diseases that are the leading causes of adult death: **heart disease, stroke, hypertension, diabetes,** and some forms of **cancer.** Together, these disorders account for two thirds of all deaths in the United States.[18] In addition, **cirrhosis** of the liver, accidents, and suicides are associated with excessive alcohol consumption (Table 1-1). All of these consequences of modern living are partly an "affliction of affluence."

The great tragedy is that these diseases are often preventable. Government scientists have calculated that a poor diet combined with a lack of sufficient physical activity accounted for 300,000 fatal cases of heart disease, cancer, and diabetes in 1990. The combination of poor diet and lack of physical activity thus is indirectly the second leading cause of death.[18] An understanding of nutrition and the role it plays in your short-term and long-term health can significantly minimize your risks for these diseases.

heart disease A disease characterized by the deposition of fatty material in the blood vessels that serve the heart. These deposits restrict blood flow through the heart, which in turn can lead to heart damage and death.

diabetes A disease characterized by high blood sugar caused by inadequate insulin (a hormone) action. Although this disease is commonly referred to as "diabetes," its technical name is *diabetes mellitus*. There are several forms of this disease.

TABLE 1-1

Ten leading causes of death in the United States

Rank	Cause of death	Percent of total deaths
	All causes	100.0
1	Diseases of the heart*	29
2	Malignant neoplasms, including neoplasms of lymphatic and hematopoietic tissues (cancer)*	26
3	Cerebrovascular diseases (stroke)*	5
4	Chronic obstructive pulmonary diseases and allied conditions (lung diseases)	4
5	Accidents and adverse effects†	6
	Motor vehicle accidents	3
	All other accidents and adverse effects	3
6	Pneumonia and influenza	3
7	Diabetes*	2
8	Acquired immunodeficiency syndrome (AIDS)	2
9	Suicide†	2
10	Homicide and legal intervention†	2

From Centers for Disease Control and Prevention, *Morbidity and mortality weekly report,* December 16, 1994. Data are age-adjusted to the 1990 population.
*Causes of death in which diet plays a part.
†Causes of death in which excessive alcohol consumption plays a part.

What Is Nutrition?

The Council on Food and Nutrition of the American Medical Association defines **nutrition** as "the science of food, the nutrients and the substances therein, their action, interaction, and balance in relation to health and disease, and the process by which the organism ingests, digests, absorbs, transports, utilizes, and excretes food substances."

To begin your study of nutrition, we must start at the foundation—the **nutrients** themselves. We will first examine the nutrients and their functions in the body. This discussion sets the stage for understanding the Food Guide Pyramid, which is described in Chapter 2. Then, we will discuss how to assess a person's nutritional health and introduce the four components commonly used to evaluate a person's nutritional status. Next, we evaluate the "health" status of the American diet. Finally, we will describe the factors that influence our food habits.

nutrients Chemical substances in food that nourish the body by providing energy, building materials, and factors that regulate needed chemical reactions.

Classes and Sources of Nutrients

Food, water, and oxygen are life-giving and life-sustaining substances essential to human life. Food provides both energy and the materials needed to build and maintain all body cells.

It is important to distinguish between food and nutrients. Food is the source of nutrients. Nutrients are the nourishing substances in food that are essential for growth of the infant, development from childhood to adulthood, and the maintenance of body functions throughout life. In nutrition, an **essential nutrient** is one whose omission from the diet leads to a decline in certain aspects of human health, such as function of the nervous system. If the omitted nutrient is restored to the diet before permanent damage occurs, those aspects of human health hampered by its absence regain normal function. In other words, the lost aspects of health are recovered when the body receives the essential nutrient.

The nutrients in food can be organized into six classes (Table 1-2). The energy-yielding nutrients—carbohydrates, fats, and proteins—constitute the major portion of most food, as may water, another class. In contrast, vitamins and minerals constitute a minor portion of foods.

Some nutrients that perform life-sustaining functions can be produced by the body if they are missing from the diet. The essential nature of such nutrients sometimes is not clear cut. For example, the body requires a daily source of vitamin D, but the skin is capable of synthesizing its own vitamin D upon receiving sunlight. This reduces the daily need from dietary sources.

Glycogen
Storage form of carbohydrate in the body

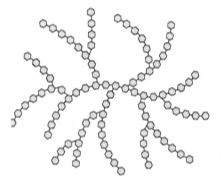

Each yellow circle represents one glucose molecule.

- - - - - - - - - - -

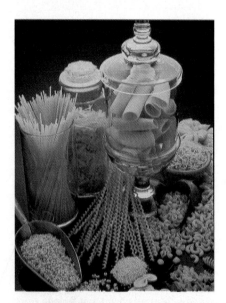

Carbohydrate is the nutrient most promoted for the American diet during the last two decades.

TABLE 1-2

Essential nutrients in the human diet and their classes*

Energy-yielding nutrients			
Carbohydrate	Fat (lipids)†	Protein (amino acids)	Water
Glucose‡ (or a carbohydrate that yields glucose)	Linoleic acid (omega-6) α-Linolenic acid (omega-3)	Histidine Isoleucine Leucine Lysine Methionine Phenylalanine Threonine Tryptophan Valine	Water

Vitamins		Minerals		
Water-soluble	Fat-soluble	Major	Trace	Questionable
Thiamin	A	Calcium	Chromium	Arsenic
Riboflavin	D§	Chloride	Copper	Boron
Niacin	E	Magnesium	Fluoride ‖	Cadmium
Pantothenic acid	K	Phosphorus	Iodide	Cobalt
Biotin		Potassium	Iron	Lithium
B-6		Sodium	Manganese	Nickel
B-12		Sulfur	Molybdenum	Silicon
Folate			Selenium	Tin
C			Zinc	

*This table includes nutrients that the current RDA publication lists for humans. Some disagreement exists over the questionable and other minerals not listed. Dietary fiber could be added to the list of essential substances, but it is not a nutrient (see Chapter 3).
†The lipids listed are needed only in slight amounts, about 2% of total energy needs (see Chapter 4).
‡In order to prevent ketosis and thus the muscle loss that would occur if protein was used to synthesize carbohydrate (see Chapter 3).
§Sunshine on the skin also allows the body to make vitamin D for itself (see Chapter 12).
‖Primarily for dental health (see Chapter 15).

CARBOHYDRATES

Carbohydrates are composed mainly of carbon, hydrogen, and oxygen. Carbohydrates provide a major source of fuel for the body. Small carbohydrate structures are called sugars or simple sugars. Table sugar (sucrose) is an example. Some simple sugars, such as **glucose,** link chemically to form large storage carbohydrates, called polysaccharides or complex carbohydrates. An example is the **starch** in potatoes.

Some sugars impart sweetness to many foods we eat. Aside from enjoying their taste, we need sugars and other carbohydrates in our diets primarily to satisfy the energy needs of body cells. Glucose, which the body can produce from most carbohydrates, is the primary source of energy in many cells. When not enough carbohydrate is eaten to supply sufficient glucose, the body is forced to make glucose from proteins. However, a typical diet contains more than enough carbohydrate to prevent this from happening.[14]

Digestion of some dietary starch intake begins in the mouth. The digestive process continues in the small intestine until starches and large sugars break down into single sugar molecules (such as glucose), which are absorbed into the bloodstream. However, the links between the sugar molecules in certain complex carbohydrates cannot be broken down by human digestive processes. These carbohydrates are part of what is called **dietary fiber.** Such dietary fiber passes through the small intestine undigested to provide bulk for the stool (feces), which is formed in the large intestine (colon). Chapter 3 focuses on carbohydrates.

LIPIDS

Lipids (mostly fats and oils) are composed mainly of carbon and hydrogen; they contain fewer oxygen atoms than carbohydrates. Because of this difference in composition, lipids yield more energy per gram than carbohydrates. (See Chapter 7 for the reason behind the high-energy yield of lipids.) Lipids are insoluble in water but dissolve in certain organic solvents (e.g., ether and benzene).

The basic structure of most lipids is the three-carbon glycerol molecule with a fatty acid attached to each of the three carbons. This form of lipid is called a **triglyceride.** Triglycerides are a key energy source for the body and the major form of fat in foods. They are also the major form for energy storage in the body.

In this book we will use the more familiar term, fats, or fats and oils, rather than lipids or triglycerides. Roughly speaking, fats are lipids that are solid at room temperature, and oils are lipids that are liquid at room temperature.

Fats are classified into two basic types—saturated and unsaturated—based on the chemical structure of their dominant fatty acids. This property determines whether a fat is solid or liquid at room temperature. Plant oils tend to contain many unsaturated fatty acids, which makes them liquid. Animal fats are often rich in saturated fatty acids, which makes them solid. Many foods contain both saturated and unsaturated fats.

Certain unsaturated fatty acids are essential nutrients. These key fatty acids that the body can't produce, called essential fatty acids, perform several important functions in the body: they help regulate blood pressure and play a role in the synthesis and repair of vital cell parts. Thus some fat is an important part of a diet.[14] However, we need only about 1 tablespoon of a common vegetable oil (such as corn oil found in supermarkets) each day to supply the essential fatty acids. The average American diet supplies about three times the amount of essential fatty acids needed daily.[14] Chapter 4 focuses on lipids.

PROTEINS

Like carbohydrates and fats, proteins are composed of carbon, oxygen, and hydrogen; in contrast to the other energy-yielding nutrients, all proteins also contain nitrogen. Proteins are the main structural building blocks of the body. For example, proteins constitute a major part of bone and muscle; they are also important components of blood, cell membranes, and the immune system.

Proteins are formed by the linking of **amino acids.** Twenty or so common amino acids are found in food; nine of these are essential nutrients for adults.[14] Chapter 5 focuses on proteins.

• • •

Three other classes of nutrients are vitamins, minerals, and water. Although **vitamins** and **minerals** are vital to good health, they are needed only in small amounts in the diet and provide no direct source of energy for the body.

VITAMINS

Vitamins exhibit a wide variety of chemical structures and can contain carbon, hydrogen, nitrogen, oxygen, phosphorus, sulfur, and other elements. The main function of vitamins is to enable many chemical reactions in the body to occur. Some of these reactions help release the energy trapped in carbohydrates, lipids, and proteins. Remember, however, that vitamins themselves provide no usable energy for the body.

Vitamins are divided into two groups: those that are fat soluble (vitamins A, D, E, and K) and those that are water soluble (vitamin C and the B vitamins). The two

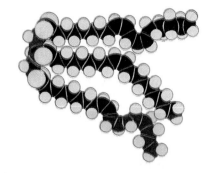

Triglyceride (fat)

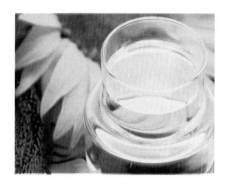

The black, blue, and yellow circles represent carbon, hydrogen, and oxygen, respectively, in the triglyceride molecule.

Protein
A structure of linked amino acids

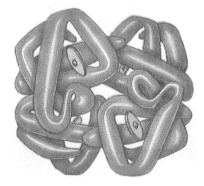

Hemoglobin, found in a red blood cell.

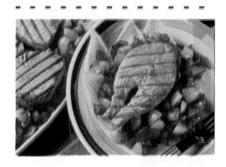

Animal sources supply about two thirds of protein intake for most Americans.

vitamins Compounds needed in very small amounts in the diet to help regulate and support chemical reactions in the body.

minerals Elements used in the body to promote chemical reactions and to form body structures.

- - - - - - - - - - - - - - - - -

Many basic chemistry concepts are reviewed in Appendix B. If you are unfamiliar with chemistry terms, you will find the review quite helpful. Appendix C reviews the metric system. If you are not familiar with the metric system—liters, grams, etc.—you will need to study this section carefully.

- - - - - - - - - - - - - - - - -

- - - - - - - - - - - - - - - - -

Provide energy
  carbohydrates
  proteins
  lipids (fats and oils)
Promote growth and development
  proteins
  lipids
  vitamins
  minerals
  water
Regulate body processes
  proteins
  lipids
  vitamins
  minerals
  water

- - - - - - - - - - - - - - - - -

metabolism Chemical processes in the body by which energy is provided in useful forms and vital activities are sustained.

groups of vitamins often act quite differently. For example, cooking destroys water-soluble vitamins much more readily than it does fat-soluble vitamins. Water-soluble vitamins are also excreted from the body much more readily than are fat-soluble vitamins. Thus the fat-soluble vitamins are much more likely to build up in excessive amounts in the body, which then can cause illness. The vitamins are the focus of Chapters 12 and 13.

MINERALS

The nutrients discussed so far are all **organic** compounds, whereas minerals are structurally very simple, **inorganic** substances, which exist as groups of one or more of the same atoms. These terms have nothing to do with organic gardening, but rather are based on simple chemistry concepts. Because of their simple structure, minerals are not destroyed during cooking, but can still be lost if they leak into the water used for cooking and then are discarded if that water is not consumed. Although minerals themselves yield no energy as such for the body, they are critical players in nervous system functioning, metabolic processes, water balance, and structural (e.g., skeletal) systems.

The amounts of the 20 or more essential minerals that are required in the diet for good health vary enormously. Thus they are divided into two groups: major minerals and trace minerals. The actual dietary requirement for some trace minerals has yet to be determined. Minerals are the focus of Chapters 14 and 15.

WATER

Although sometimes overlooked as a nutrient, water (chemically, H_2O) has numerous vital functions in the body. It acts as a **solvent** and lubricant, as a medium for transporting nutrients and waste, and as a medium for temperature regulation. For these reasons, and because the human body is approximately 60% water, we require about 2 liters (L)—equivalent to 2000 grams (g) or 8 cups—of fluid every day.

Water is not only available from the obvious sources, it is also the major component in some foods, such as many fruits and vegetables (e.g., lettuce, grapes, and melons). The body even makes some water as a by-product of **metabolism.** Water is examined in detail in Chapter 14.

Nutrient Composition of Diets and the Human Body

The quantities of the various nutrients that people consume vary widely, and the nutrient amounts present in different foods also vary a great deal. The total daily intake of protein, fat, and carbohydrate amounts to about 500 g. In contrast, the typical daily mineral intake totals about 20 g, and the daily vitamin intake totals less than 300 milligrams (mg). Although each day we require nearly a gram of some minerals, such as calcium and phosphorus, we need only a few milligrams or less of other minerals. For example, we need about 15 mg of zinc per day, which is just a few specks of the mineral.

Figure 1-1 contrasts the relative concentrations of all the major classes of nutrients in a lean man and a lean woman with the composition of both a cooked steak and a cooked stalk of broccoli. Note how the nutrient composition of the body differs from the nutritional profiles of the foods we eat. This is because growth, development, and later maintenance of the human body are directed by the genetic material inside the cell nucleus. This genetic blueprint determines how each cell uses the nutrients to perform body functions. These nutrients can come from a variety of sources. Cells are not concerned whether the amino acids available come from animal or plant sources. The carbohydrate glucose can come from sugars or starches. Thus, you aren't what you eat. Instead, what you eat provides cells with the ability to function as directed by the genetic material housed in the cell.

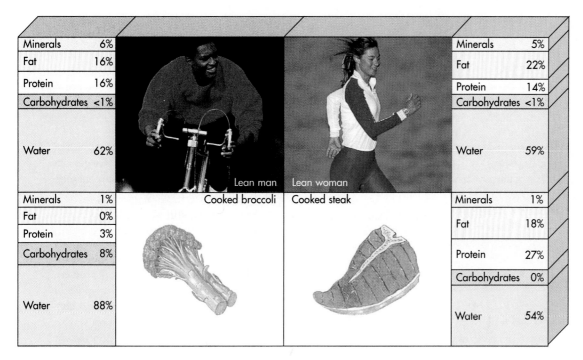

Minerals	6%
Fat	16%
Protein	16%
Carbohydrates	<1%
Water	62%

Lean man

Cooked broccoli

Minerals	1%
Fat	0%
Protein	3%
Carbohydrates	8%
Water	88%

Minerals	5%
Fat	22%
Protein	14%
Carbohydrates	<1%
Water	59%

Lean woman

Cooked steak

Minerals	1%
Fat	18%
Protein	27%
Carbohydrates	0%
Water	54%

Figure 1-1 You aren't what you eat! The proportions of nutrients in the human body do not match those found in typical foods—animal or vegetable.

Energy Content of Nutrients

We obtain the energy necessary to perform body functions and to do work from carbohydrates, fats, and proteins (and **alcohol** for some of us). Foods generally contain more than one form of these energy sources. Vegetable oil is one exception, as it is 100% fat. Energy is held in the chemical bonds of these energy-yielding compounds. Chapter 7 describes how that energy is released from these bonds and then used by body cells.

The energy in food is often measured in terms of calories. A calorie is the amount of heat it takes to raise the temperature of 1 g of water 1 degree **Celsius** (1° C, centigrade scale). Because a calorie is such a tiny measure of heat, food energy is more often expressed in terms of the **kilocalorie**, which equals 1000 calories. A *kilocalorie* is the amount of heat it takes to raise the temperature of 1000 g (1 L) of water 1° C. The term *kilocalorie* and its abbreviation *kcal* are used throughout this book. In everyday life, the word "calorie" is often used loosely to mean "kilocalorie." The values given on food labels in calories are actually in kilocalories. A suggested intake of 2000 calories on a food label is really 2000 kcal, or enough energy to raise the temperature of 2 million grams of water 1° C.

Carbohydrates, proteins, lipids, and alcohol provide the body with differing amounts of energy. Specifically, carbohydrates yield 4 kcal per gram (kcal/g), proteins yield 4 kcal/g, fats yield 9 kcal/g, and alcohol yields 7 kcal/g. These values have been adjusted for (1) **digestibility**; and (2) substances not available for energy use. Such substances include waxes and some fibrous parts of plants. The energy values are then rounded to whole numbers.

Knowing the quantities of the energy-yielding substances in a food, you can estimate the total energy in that food using these kcal values. For example, if a banana milk shake contains 45 g of carbohydrate, 7 g of protein, and 10 g of fat, it would provide 298 kcal ([45 × 4] + [7 × 4] + [10 × 9] = 298). If a banana-flavored rum drink contains 10 g of carbohydrate, 1 g of protein, 1 g of fat, and 15 g of alcohol, it would provide 158 kcal ([10 × 4] + [1 × 4] + [1 × 9] + [15 × 7] = 158).

You can also determine what portion of total energy intake is contributed by the various energy-yielding nutrients. Assume that one day you consume 290 g of car-

Text continued on p. 10.

alcohol Ethyl alcohol or ethanol (CH_3CH_2OH).

kilocalorie (kcal) The heat needed to raise the temperature of 1000 g (1 L) of water 1° Celsius.

In many scientific journals, the kilojoule (kJ), rather than the kilocalorie, is used to express the energy content of food. A kilojoule is the amount of work needed to move 1 kilogram for 1 meter with the force of 1 newton. Since heat and work are just two forms of energy, measurements expressed in terms of kilocalories (a heat measure) are interchangeable with measurements expressed in terms of kilojoules (a work measure): 1 kcal = 4.18 kJ.

digestibility Corresponds to the proportion of food substances eaten that can be broken down in the intestinal tract for absorption into the body.

Nutrition Focus

Genetics and Nutrition

The growth, development, and maintenance of cells, and ultimately of the entire organism, are directed by genes present in the cells. The genes contain the codes that control expression of individual traits, such as height or eye color, and susceptibility to many diseases. An individual's genetic risk for a given disease is an important factor, although often not the only factor, in determining whether he or she develops that disease.[23]

NUTRITIONAL DISEASES WITH A GENETIC LINK

Most chronic diseases in which nutrition plays a role are also influenced by genetics. The risks of developing heart disease, high blood pressure (hypertension), obesity, diabetes, cancer, and osteoporosis are influenced by interactions between genetic and nutritional factors.[14] Studies of families, including those with twins and adoptees, provide strong support for the effect of genetics in these disorders. In fact, family history is considered to be one of the important factors in the development of many serious diseases (Figure 1-2).[23]

Heart Disease

About one of every 500 people in the American population has a defective gene that greatly delays cholesterol removal from the bloodstream.[23] As you will learn in

Chapter 4, this genetic defect leads to an increased risk of developing heart disease at a young age. Diet changes can help these people, but medications, and possibly surgery, may be needed to address the problem.

Hypertension

An estimated 10% to 15% of the American population is very sensitive to salt intake. When these salt-sensitive individuals consume too much salt, their blood pressure climbs above the desirable range. The fact that more of these people are African-American than Caucasian suggests a genetic component.[23] At present, the only way to determine whether individuals with hypertension are salt sensitive is to place them on a salt-restricted diet and see if their blood pressure falls. Note also that many cases of hypertension are unrelated to salt sensitivity and are caused by other factors (see Chapter 14).

Obesity

Most obese Americans have at least one parent who is also obese. Findings from many human studies suggest that a variety of genes are involved in the regulation of body weight.[14] Little is known, however, about the specific nature of these genes in humans or how the actual changes in body metabolism (such as lower energy use at rest) are produced. Some individuals may be genetically

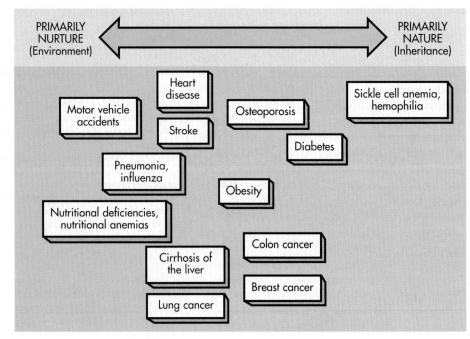

Figure 1-2 Common causes of death and illness in our population vary in their links to genetic and environmental influences. We must consider both influences as we study each disease.

predisposed to store body fat, but whether they actually do so depends on how much excess energy—above energy needs—they ultimately consume.

A common concept in nutrition is that **nurture**—how people live and the environmental factors that influence them—allows **nature**—each person's genetic potential—to be expressed. Although not everyone with a genetic tendency toward obesity develops this condition, they do have a higher lifetime risk than individuals without a genetic predisposition to obesity.

Diabetes

Both of the two common types of diabetes have genetic links, as revealed by family and twin studies.[14] Only sensitive and expensive testing can determine who is at risk. The form of diabetes involved in 90% of all cases also has a strong link to obesity. A genetic tendency for this major form of diabetes will be expressed once a person becomes obese, but often not before, again illustrating that nurture affects nature.

Cancer

A few types of cancer (e.g., colon cancer) have a strong genetic link, and genetics may play a role in others. Still, nutritional and other environmental factors also are important. Since obesity increases the risk of many forms of cancer, a diet high in energy and fat can be a risk factor.[14] And one third of all cancers result from smoking.[8] Again, genetics often is not enough—environment also contributes to the risk profile.

Osteoporosis

Bone mineral density, and hence bone strength, is similar in twins as well as in mothers and their daughters. The exact relative importance of genetic versus dietary factors is unknown. Nonetheless, children and adolescents need to consume sufficient calcium to build strong, dense bones, thus reducing the risk of problems, particularly osteoporosis in women, later in life.[14] Adults should then continue that practice. The porous bones that are a result of osteoporosis greatly increase the risk of fractures, especially in the wrist, spine, and hip. As discussed in Chapter 14, the risk of osteoporosis can be greatly reduced by a combination of medical and nutritional means if therapy is started at least by mid-life.

YOUR GENETIC PROFILE

From this discussion you can see that a family history of certain diseases raises your risk of developing those diseases. Recognizing your potential for developing a particular disease, you can avoid behavior that contributes to it. In general, the more of your relatives who had a genetically transmitted disease and the closer they are related to you, the greater your risk. One way to assess your risk is to put together a family tree of illnesses and deaths by compiling a few key facts on your primary relatives: siblings, parents, aunts and uncles, and grandparents.

Figure 1-3 shows an example of a family tree (also called a genogram). In this family, prostate cancer killed the man's father. This means that the son should be tested regularly for prostate cancer. His sisters should consider frequent mammograms because the mother died of breast cancer. Because heart disease and stroke are also common in the family, all the children should follow a lifestyle designed to minimize development of these diseases (see Chapter 4 for details). Colon cancer is also evident in the family, so careful screening throughout life is important. Finally, alcoholism seems to run in the family, which is true of many American families.[14] Whether nature or nurture is more important in the development of alcoholism is unclear. We discuss this question in Chapter 7.

GENE THERAPY

Scientists are currently developing therapies to correct some genetic disorders. An example is cystic fibrosis, which affects one of every 2500 newborns. The genetic defect, which must be inherited from both parents to cause the disease, typically leads to a buildup of sticky mucus in the lungs and respiratory tract, among other health problems. The accumulated mucus sets the stage for respiratory infections; generally, death from respiratory complications occurs before the age of 30.

Recently, scientists have inserted the correct gene into inactivated viruses and had patients inhale the viruses. Some of the inserted genes appear to enter the patients' lung cells and reduce the severity of the disease. Although this work is in its preliminary phase, experts believe that gene therapy will become a practical treatment within the lifetimes of many young patients with cystic fibrosis.

A similar approach has also been tested for one form of hemophilia. So far, gene therapy for this genetic disease has been tried only in dogs, but the results have been promising. As the genes involved with more diseases are identified, gene therapy will likely become more

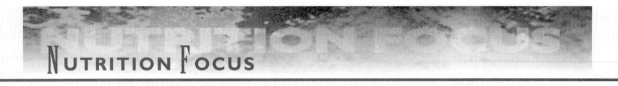

NUTRITION FOCUS

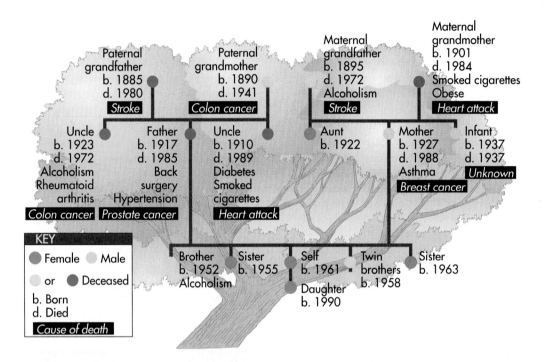

Figure 1-3 Example of a family tree. Create your own family tree, using the one here as a guide. Then show your tree to your physician to get a full picture of what the information means for your health.

common, but much more research is still needed for that to happen.

NUTRITIONAL IMPLICATIONS OF GENETIC RISK

Today in the United States, newborns are routinely tested for phenylketonuria, an inherited metabolic disease that leads to mental retardation and other problems if appropriate treatment is not given. Infants found to have this disorder are put on a special diet that reduces development of the disease (see Chapter 5 for details).

In contrast to infants with phenylketonuria, individuals with genetic predispositions for many other diseases do not always develop disease. In addition, because genetic background does influence disease risk, certain dietary guidelines are more beneficial for some people than for

others. For example, recommendations to consume more calcium or less salt are particularly important for individuals at genetic risk of developing diseases such as osteoporosis or hypertension.

It is not possible, given the resources presently allocated to medical care in America, to identify all people at genetic risk for the major chronic "killer" diseases. Thus many health authorities feel it is reasonable to give a general nutrition message to everyone, noting that some people will benefit from the advice much more than others. Throughout this book we will point out how you can personalize nutrition advice based on your genetic background. In this way, you can identify and avoid the "controllable" risk factors that would contribute to development of genetically linked diseases present in your family.

bohydrate, 60 g of fat, and 70 g of protein. This consumption yields a total of 1980 kcal ($[290 \times 4] + [60 \times 9] + [70 \times 4] = 1980$). The percentage of your total energy intake derived from each nutrient can then be determined:

% of kcal as carbohydrate = $(290 \times 4) \div 1980 = 0.586$ or 58.6%

% of kcal as fat = $(60 \times 9) \div 1980 = 0.273$ or 27.3%

% of kcal as protein = $(70 \times 4) \div 1980 = 0.141$ or 14.1%

CONCEPT CHECK

Food contains vital nutrients that are essential for good health: carbohydrates, lipids (fats and oils), proteins, vitamins, minerals, and water. Nutrients have three general functions in the body: (1) to provide materials for building and maintaining the body; (2) to act as regulators for key metabolic reactions; and (3) to participate in metabolic reactions that provide the energy necessary to sustain life. A common unit of measurement for this energy is the kilocalorie (kcal).

States of Nutritional Health

The body's nutritional health is determined by the sum of its **nutritional status** with respect to each needed nutrient. Three general categories of nutritional status are recognized: desirable nutrition, undernutrition, and overnutrition.

DESIRABLE NUTRITION

The nutritional status for a particular nutrient is desirable when body tissues have enough of the nutrient to support normal metabolic functions as well as surplus stores that can be mobilized in times of increased need.

UNDERNUTRITION

When nutrient intake does not meet nutrient needs, stores of nutrients soon become depleted by ongoing body use, some sooner than others. This results in undernutrition. The demand for these nutrients exists partly because the body is in a constant state of turnover. Cells lining the intestinal tract , for example, are replaced every 2–5 days, and red blood cells live only about 120 days. To support this turnover, body stores may be sufficient to compensate for an inadequate diet for a brief period of time, but serious problems can arise from an inadequate diet in the long run. Some women in the United States, for example, do not consume sufficient iron and eventually deplete their iron stores. Reduced biochemical functions and ultimately clinical signs and symptoms of an iron deficiency then can develop (Table 1-3).

Reduced Biochemical Functions

Once nutrient stores are depleted, a continuing nutritional deficit drains body tissues further. The body can only compensate to a certain point (see the discussion on homeostasis in Chapter 7). When tissue concentrations of an essential nutrient fall sufficiently low, the body's metabolic processes eventually slow down or even stop. This response results from a **biochemical lesion** that develops in response to the nutrient deficiency.[1] Diminished **enzyme** function often is the cause of the slowdown in biochemical function. This type of nutrient deficiency is termed **subclinical** because there are no outward signs or symptoms. At the subclinical stage for poor iron status, low concentrations of hemoglobin (a red blood cell protein) are found in the blood because synthesis of hemoglobin requires iron.

Clinical Signs and Symptoms

If a biochemical deficit becomes severe, clinical signs and symptoms eventually develop and become outwardly apparent. It is then possible to actually note **clinical lesions** in the body, perhaps in the skin, hair, nails, tongue, or eyes. At this stage of a nutritional deficiency, that vigorous glow that conveys good health also is lost. In the case of an iron deficiency, the complexion may become very pale, and the heart rate of an affected person can increase greatly during even moderate activity.

OVERNUTRITION

Prolonged consumption of more nutrients than the body needs can lead to **overnutrition.** In the short run, for instance a week or two, overnutrition may cause no

nutritional status The nutritional health of a person as determined by anthropometric measurements (height, weight, circumferences, and so on), biochemical measurements of nutrients or their by-products in blood and urine, a clinical (physical) examination, and a dietary analysis.

biochemical lesion An indication of reduced biochemical function (e.g., low concentrations of nutrient by-products or enzyme activities in the blood or urine) resulting from a nutritional deficiency.

enzyme A compound that speeds the rate of a chemical reaction but is not altered by the chemical reaction. Almost all enzymes are proteins.

- - - - - - - - - - - -

A sign is a feature visible on examination, such as flaky skin. A symptom is a change in body function that is not necessarily apparent to an examiner. An example is stomach pain.

- - - - - - - - - - - -

clinical lesion A sign seen on physical examination or a symptom perceived by the patient resulting from a nutritional deficiency.

overnutrition A state that results when nutrient intake exceeds the body's needs for a prolonged period.

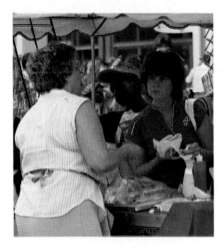

The major nutritional problems in the United States are caused by overnutrition.

TABLE 1-3

Categories of nutritional status with respect to iron*

General conditions	Condition with respect to iron
Overnutrition: nutrients consumed in excess of body needs (degree of toxicity varies for each nutrient).	Results in toxic damage to liver cells; may contribute to heart disease.
Desirable nutrition: nutrients consumed to support body functions and stores of nutrients for times of increased need.	Adequate liver stores of iron, adequate blood values for iron-related compounds.
Undernutrition: nutrient intake does not meet nutrient needs. Depleted tissue stores	Many changes in body functions are associated with a decline in iron status. Serum† ferritin, an iron-containing protein in the blood, drops below 12 nanograms per 100 ml (12 ng/100 ml).
Reduced biochemical function (biochemical lesion)	Hemoglobin, an iron-containing pigment in the red blood cells, drops below 11 g per 100 ml (11 g/100 ml).
Clinical signs and symptoms (clinical lesion)	Pale complexion; greatly increased heart rate during activity; "spooning" of the nails in a severe deficiency; poor body temperature regulation.

*This general scheme can apply to all nutrients. We have chosen iron because you are likely to be familiar with this nutrient.
†Serum is the liquid portion of blood present after the blood clots.

obesity A condition characterized by excess body fat, often defined in clinical settings as 20% above desirable body weight. See Chapter 8 for more details.

CRITICAL THINKING

Your friend Mary has been dieting and is consuming small amounts of foods. She's been taking extra doses of vitamins to compensate. What would you tell her about the hazards of taking extra vitamins?

signs or symptoms. But keep it up and some nutrients eventually may increase to toxic amounts, which can lead to serious disease. Iron overload, for example, can result in liver failure, and too much vitamin A can have negative effects. The most common type of overnutrition—excess intake of energy-yielding nutrients—is the principal cause of **obesity.**

At the beginning of the twentieth century, undernutrition was the main concern of nutrition scientists. Now, attention needs to be directed toward both undernutrition and overnutrition.[7] Today, the major nutritional problems in the United States and in most developed countries are the result of overnutrition, principally caused by excess intake of energy, saturated and total fat, and sodium.[3] Some people are especially susceptible to ill health when they consume too much saturated fat and sodium. Although excess energy intake has been possible for many people for centuries, overnutrition with other nutrients was uncommon in the past. Because of the increasing use of vitamin and mineral supplements in recent years, many forms of vitamin and mineral overnutrition have now become a concern.[14]

For most vitamins and minerals, the gap between desirable intake and overnutrition is wide.[1] Therefore, even if people take a typical multiple vitamin and mineral supplement daily, they probably won't receive a harmful amount of any nutrient. The gap between optimal intake and overnutrition is narrowest for vitamin A and vitamin D, as well as calcium, iron, and other minerals. In very high doses, vitamin B-6 and the vitamin niacin can cause health problems. It is important to remember that high doses of some vitamins and minerals are toxic to the body. If you take nutrient supplements, keep a close eye on your total vitamin and mineral intake both from food and from supplements (see Chapter 12 for further advice on use of nutrient supplements).

TABLE 1-4

Components of a nutritional assessment

Component	Example
Background histories	Medical history, including current diseases and past surgeries Medications history Social history (marital status; cooking facilities) Family history Economic status
Nutrition parameters	**A**nthropometric assessment: height, weight, skinfold thickness, arm muscle circumference, and other parameters **B**iochemical (laboratory) assessment of blood and urine: enzyme activities, concentrations of nutrients or their by-products **C**linical assessment (physical examination): general appearance of skin, eyes, and tongue, rapid hair loss, sense of touch, ability to walk **D**iet history: usual intake or record of previous days' meals

Nutritional Assessment

To find out how nutritionally fit you are, a nutritional assessment—either whole or in part—needs to be performed (Table 1-4).

ANALYZING BACKGROUND FACTORS

Since family history plays an important role in determining nutritional and health status, it must be carefully recorded and critically analyzed as part of a nutritional assessment.[23] Other related background components include (1) a medical history, especially for any disease states or treatments that could impede nutrient absorptive processes or ultimate use; and (2) socioeconomic history, to determine the ability to purchase and prepare appropriate foods needed to maintain health.

EVALUATING THE ABCDs

A thorough assessment of nutritional status, however, requires yet more information. Four components in combination add to the complete nutritional picture. **Anthropometric** measurements of height, weight, body skinfolds, and body circumferences are an excellent first line of attack. They are easy to obtain and generally reliable. However, an in-depth examination of nutritional health is impossible without the rather expensive process of **b**iochemical assessment. This involves the measurement of specific blood enzyme activities and of the concentrations of nutrients and nutrient by-products in the blood.

A **c**linical examination would follow, during which a health professional would search for any physical signs of diet-related diseases. Last, a **d**iet history, documenting at least the previous few days' intake, is an invaluable tool for insight into possible problem areas. Together these activities form the **ABCDs** of nutritional assessment: anthropometric measurements, biochemical assessment, clinical examination, and diet history.

RECOGNIZING THE LIMITATIONS OF NUTRITIONAL ASSESSMENT

A long time may elapse between the initial development of poor nutritional health and the first clinical evidence of a problem. For example, a diet high in animal fat often increases the serum **cholesterol** concentration without producing any clinical signs or symptoms for years. But when the blood vessels become sufficiently blocked by cholesterol and other materials, chest pain during physical activity may develop. This buildup of fatty substances also may eventually provoke a heart attack. Thus a person may be on the road to developing a serious disease but, be-

anthropometric Pertaining to the measurement of body weight and the lengths, circumferences, and thicknesses of parts of the body.

cholesterol A waxy lipid whose structure contains multiple chemical rings.

cause it progresses slowly, the effects won't be obvious until quite late—perhaps too late.

An example of this delay in serious consequences that is particularly relevant for adolescent females relates to calcium intake. A goal should be to build dense bones, especially during the years of adolescent growth and development, by consuming adequate calcium. Still, young women who consume well below the recommended amount of calcium often suffer no ill effects in their younger years. However, women whose bone-density values do not reach full potential during the years of growth are likely to face an increased risk for osteoporosis later in life.[14] This example highlights the idea that prolonged inadequate intake of certain nutrients can result in a subtle decline in health and performance that will initially be unnoticed.

Furthermore, clinical signs and symptoms of nutritional deficiencies are often not very specific. Typical signs to look for—diarrhea, an irregular walk, facial sores—have many different causes. It is often hard to decide whether the problem is caused by faulty nutrition or by some other medical disorder. Long lag times and vague signs and symptoms often make it difficult to establish a link between an individual's current diet and nutritional state.[1]

As you study nutrition and learn the importance of nutrients in foods, you may notice people who have very poor diets but show no outward clinical signs or symptoms of poor health. Nonetheless, their health is probably declining in subtle ways. A good example is the role of calcium in bone development just described. In addition, a chronically insufficient intake of vitamin C likely encourages development of cataracts in the eyes.[20] In addition, some studies show that heart disease is related to low intakes of vitamin B-6, folate, and vitamin B-12.[17] An insufficient intake of these vitamins leads to elevated blood concentrations of the substance homocysteine, which in turn probably promotes the development of heart disease.

Often it is not possible to separate the best nutritional state from one that is slightly jeopardized. We can usually distinguish between distinct **malnutrition** and good nutrition, but the gray area—the gradual slide from a "good" to a malnourished state caused by earlier significant undernutrition or overnutrition—is hard to detect. For example, a very sophisticated test is needed to detect elevated blood homocysteine. In the case of cataracts, clinical evidence of the disease is the first warning sign. This observation is not intended as a scare tactic, but rather to provide reasons why a careful evaluation of the adequacy of *your* diet is worth the effort.

malnutrition Failing health that results from long-standing dietary practices that do not coincide with nutritional needs.

CONCEPT CHECK

When the body has enough nutrients to function fully and contains stores to use in times of increased needs, it is in a desirable nutritional state. When nutrient intake fails to meet body needs, undernutrition develops. Poor body functioning and physical signs and symptoms of a nutrient deficiency eventually develop. Overnutrition—especially excess intake of energy, saturated and total fat, and sodium—can also lead to many problems. Eating a wisely planned diet can help you avoid both overnutrition and undernutrition.

Dietary Trends in the United States

As noted already, the major energy sources in human diets are carbohydrates, fats, and proteins. Alcoholic beverages also provide a large source of energy for some people; in fact, alcoholic beverages—generally also rich in carbohydrate—are the third leading contributor to energy intakes and supply about 11% of all dietary energy in the United States.[2] (The nutrient contents of alcoholic beverages are listed in Appendix A.) Exclusive of energy from alcohol, adults in the United States currently obtain about 16% of their energy intake as protein; 50% as carbohydrate; and 34% as fat.[5] These percentages vary slightly from year to year and from person to person.

Animal sources supply about two thirds of protein intake for most Americans; plant sources supply only about one third. In many other parts of the world, it is just the opposite: plant proteins—from rice, beans, corn, and other vegetables—dominate protein intake. About half the carbohydrate in American diets comes from simple sugars; the other half comes from starches (such as in pasta, bread, and potatoes). About 60% of our dietary fat comes from animal sources and 40% from vegetable sources.[2]

NATIONAL NUTRITIONAL SURVEYS

The federal government has sponsored large surveys to estimate the actual concentrations of nutrients in the U.S. food supply, as well as our nutrient intakes. The first such survey was the *Ten State Survey,* completed in the late 1960s. Because this focused mostly on low-income people in the participating states, it did not accurately assess the average nutrient intake of people in the United States. Therefore another study—the first National Health and Nutritional Examination Survey (NHANES I)—was conducted from 1971 to 1974; this was followed by NHANES II from 1976 to 1980. The NHANES surveys, which included a cross section of about 20,000 Americans, have collected data about food intakes; assessed heights, weights, and blood pressures; measured vitamin and mineral status in the blood; and examined other health parameters. Each time the NHANES survey is performed, more and more parameters are added. Results from NHANES III (1988 to 1991) are now becoming available.[5] The U.S. Department of Agriculture (USDA) also conducts, as it has since the beginning of this century, various other surveys that document the types of foods people eat, as part of National Food Consumption Surveys.[24]

Results from the NHANES and various food-consumption surveys show quite a diversity in our diets. Many Americans are meeting their nutrient needs; others are not. The studies suggest that some of us need to consume more foods that are rich in iron, calcium, vitamin A, various B vitamins, vitamin C, zinc, and dietary fiber.[14] Underconsumption of these nutrients occurs in part because many Americans do not consistently consume enough daily servings from all the major food groups: dairy; meat and alternative protein-rich plant sources; grains; fruits; and vegetables. Servings from the fruit, vegetable, and dairy sources are the most likely to be below recommended numbers on any given day.[11] In addition, some individuals, often because of cultural influences, consume excessive amounts of energy, saturated and total fat, alcohol, and sodium.[14]

AMERICAN ATTITUDES ABOUT DIET AND NUTRITION

Judging from the responses given in several recent surveys, most Americans are extremely concerned about good nutrition and are well aware of possible health hazards from excessive intakes of fat and **salt**.[12] About 90% of men and women surveyed say that they choose foods for health reasons and try to eat healthier foods often. Most survey respondents realize that there is a link between what they eat and their health, and they are concerned about the effect of their diet on weight control, physical fitness, general health maintenance, and disease prevention. For example, about 50% to 60% of adults "try a lot" to avoid consuming too much fat, 33% "try a little," and only 10% "don't try at all." In a survey of supermarket shoppers, published in 1991, two thirds said that they were eating healthier foods than they had 1 year earlier. These shoppers ranked nutrition second only to taste as the most important factor they consider when purchasing food—97% thought nutrition was a somewhat or very important factor in grocery-shopping decisions. Most shoppers (95%) were at least somewhat concerned about the nutritional content of foods; 56% of shoppers were very concerned about nutrition.[6]

A telephone survey of the dietary habits and attitudes of 1000 adult Americans representative of the U.S. population showed that 26% of the respondents felt that nutrition was important, that they were careful about what they ate, and that they were doing things right. Another 36% knew that they were not doing much to man-

salt Generally, compound of sodium and chloride in a 40:60 ratio by weight.

EXPERT OPINION

JUNK FOODS OR JUNK DIETS?

HELEN A. GUTHRIE, Ph.D., R.D.

Over the past few decades, the phrase "junk food" has invaded our vocabulary. To nutritionists, this term is misleading; it should be dropped from our vocabulary. There is no totally worthless food, any more than there is a perfect food that meets all of our nutritional needs. Obviously, some foods contribute different nutrients from others. But almost any food has some redeeming value under the right circumstances. The problem arises when foods that contribute a high proportion of our energy needs and limited amounts of our nutrient needs become so important in our diets that foods of higher nutritional value are excluded. It is equally possible to make an unbalanced selection from among the most sacred nutritious foods—for instance, milk or apples—and wind up with a diet overabundant in some nutrients yet deficient in others. In both cases, the result can be labeled a "junk diet."

SOME FOODS GO HAND-IN-HAND

In terms of nutrient density—roughly defined as the nutrients delivered per kilocalorie—foods with low values seldom carry much nutritional weight. For example, in some cakes and cookies, most of the energy comes from fat and sugar, and relatively little from nutrient-rich milk, flour, and eggs. However, if eating a cookie means that a child also drinks milk or fruit juice, we should look at the cookie-and-milk or cookie-and-beverage as a unit and judge the components together rather than condemn one and applaud the other. For an 8-year-old child, milk and one or two cookies makes a nutritious combination. Milk and five cookies, though, may create an imbalance between energy and nutrients and thus must be considered lower in nutrition.

Potato chips are another example of a food that can be valuable in the right context. Eaten alone, potato chips have sufficient vitamin C, vitamin B-6, and copper to make them a meaningful source of nutrients. Eaten with a sandwich, potato chips become part of a balanced meal. But if we eat so many potato chips that we're too full to eat dinner, we are misusing them. What about the salt, you ask? One ounce of potato chips provides about $\frac{1}{8}$ g of sodium—less than the amount in the bread in a sandwich and considerably less than the amount in two slices of bread with salted butter. Just because we see and taste the salt on potato chips doesn't mean they have more than those foods in which it is hidden.

For another example, consider pizza. All too frequently people see it as a junk food high in energy, cholesterol, and fat. But with essentially the same ingredients, pizza has nutritional merits comparable to a meat-and-cheese sandwich served with tomato, providing valuable amounts of protein, calcium, iron, and many vitamins.

CAN WE EAT TOO MUCH OF A GOOD THING?

How about the classically "healthful" foods like milk, chicken, orange juice, and oatmeal? Are they always desirable? Surprisingly, no. Milk, especially nonfat milk, has one of the most impressive nutrient profiles of any food. But it isn't perfect. Although high in calcium, protein, and riboflavin, it is low in iron and vitamin C. In con-

age their diets, but were not interested in changing because it would mean giving up their favorite foods and would take too much time. The remaining 38% believed that diet was fairly important, but only about half of them were doing as much as they thought they should do because most did not want to give up the foods they like and they thought that making changes would take too much time. Thus the unwillingness of some people to significantly change many of their nutritional practices is probably the major impediment to improving their diets—concern does not necessarily translate into change.[12]

Currently, many Americans are concerned about excessive consumption of several dietary components. About 60% are concerned about fat and cholesterol in

trast, oranges are high in vitamin C but low in iron, calcium, protein, and riboflavin. What does all this have to do with junk food? When a food doesn't meet an immediate nutritional need, its nutritional value is limited. After an adult has had two or three glasses of milk (which would meet many nutritional needs), additional milk becomes less and less useful. If the additional milk (which does not provide vitamin C) displaces a fruit juice that contains vitamin C, that milk becomes of limited nutritional value, or even worthless, except as a source of energy. In this context, the extra milk would be a "junk" food. Thus foods should not be judged in isolation, but in relation to the total diet and the individual's needs.

If all of our daily nutrient needs are met except for energy, technically we should be free to get the rest of our energy requirements from any food—even sugar, fat, or alcohol. In reality we recommend that the extra energy come from a food with a reasonable amount of other nutrients and one that does not create an imbalance among vitamins, minerals, or energy sources. In selecting food, moderation is a virtue. And so is avoidance of excess amounts of fat, sodium, and energy, all of which are essential in controlled amounts. Getting a maximum of 10% to 15% of our total daily energy intake from foods of limited nutritional value is reasonable—more than this can lead to nutritional problems.

COST PER NUTRIENT VARIES

In choosing nutritious foods, cost per nutrient is also important. Many parents feel good about giving their children toast with margarine and honey for breakfast but feel guilty if they serve a doughnut. Since both bread and doughnuts are made with enriched flour—to which by definition certain vitamins and minerals have been added—there is no appreciable difference in their overall nutrient content. Likewise, honey has no big advantage over jam, nor margarine over oil. In terms of cost, however, the doughnut is not as good a buy. Similar considerations hold for french-fried and baked potatoes. Nutritionally, a serving of french fries cooked in oil compares favorably with a baked potato served with a fat such as sour cream or butter. However, the cost per nutrient of commercially prepared french fries can be considerably higher than that of home-prepared baked potatoes.

THE BOTTOM LINE IS A HEALTHFUL, ENJOYABLE DIET

Nutritionists want people to eat appropriate amounts and combinations of nutrients to promote health, but they also want everyone to eat in a rational way, without feeling guilty about including a favorite food merely for pleasure. Special medical considerations aside, a healthful diet can include at least small amounts of any food you enjoy, as long as your overall diet is moderate in energy and is balanced to provide essential nutrients.

Dr. Guthrie is an endowed Professor Emerita of Nutrition at The Pennsylvania State University and is the editor of Nutrition Today.

their diets; 40%, about sodium; and 30%, about caffeine. Energy intake, sugar, and additives are of less concern. On a per-person basis, Americans consumed roughly 18 pounds of butter and 270 pounds of whole milk per year in the 1920s and 1930s, whereas today they consume less than 5 pounds of butter and 111 pounds of whole milk. Therefore, progress is being made in reducing key sources of fat and cholesterol in our diets.[19] But many of us need to do more to improve our diets, as we discuss in Chapter 2.

CONCEPT CHECK

The diets of many Americans could be improved by focusing on good food sources of iron, calcium, vitamin A, various B vitamins, vitamin C, zinc, and dietary fiber. In addition, some people should reduce their intake of energy, saturated and total fat, sodium, and alcoholic beverages.

Determinants of Our Food Preferences

The primary purpose of consuming food is to obtain nourishment. Chapter 8 describes the physiological factors that encourage us to seek and then eat food. But our relationship with food goes far beyond the animal instinct to eat. Food symbolizes much of what we think about ourselves. We bond with others and express goodwill around the dinner table. We enhance and maintain our social status by entertaining creatively or lavishly. We cope with stress and tension by eating or not eating. We influence others' behavior through our food practices. Some of us express religious beliefs or display our creative talents through food preparation and ceremonies.[16]

Food likes and dislikes are the most important determinants of what we eat. These preferences and food-related behavior are influenced by many factors (Figure 1-4). Taste and texture generally are the chief considerations in selecting foods; budget comes next.[4]

EARLY EXPERIENCES

Food preferences are learned early as social and cultural preferences. They are refined through interactions with parents and friends, social class, and the need for status.[16] Unfortunately for young children, adult caregivers may severely limit a child's experience with food. Adults may purchase only a small subset of available foods and may even consider many of these foods inappropriate for children. For example, at what age were you first introduced to okra, kiwis, lentils, spinach salad, or salmon?

Mere exposure to a variety of foods can help reduce the resistance to trying new foods. Young children tend to prefer foods that are sweet or familiar, but preschool-

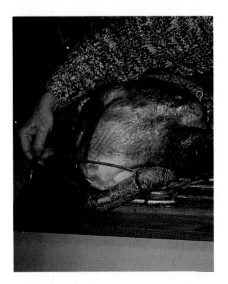

Holiday traditions help mold our food choices.

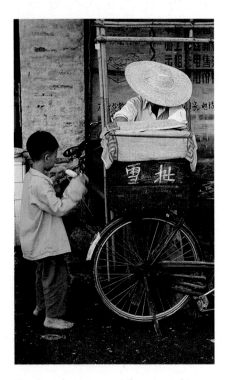

Food preferences are often rooted in childhood experiences. This Chinese child is buying ice cream from a street vendor.

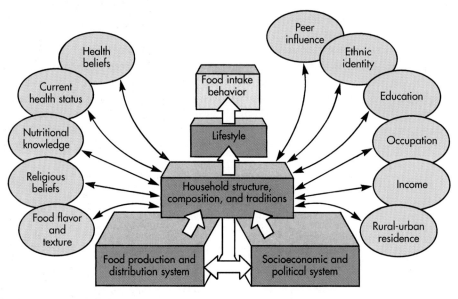

Figure 1-4 Food behavior can be influenced by many sources. Which are important in your life?

ers are often quite willing to try new foods. Caregivers need to provide the opportunity for experimentation. It may take many introductions, but the odds are in favor of final acceptance.[15]

Our built-in preferences are important, including universal enjoyment of sweet foods and dislike of bitter and sometimes spicy, burning ones. Bitter tastes often signal poisonous substances.[8] However, built-in responses can be modified through exposure and conditioning (i.e., learning). This allows some people—even entire cultures—to learn to enjoy very sour or hot, spicy foods, such as jalapeño peppers and fiery curries.

HABIT

Most of us eat foods from a core group consisting of only about 100 basic food items, which account for 75% of our total food intake. We may think we buy foods mainly based on their sensory appearance, freshness, safety, nutritional quality, healthfulness, convenience, and price. Those factors do figure in, but we still work within very narrow constraints, primarily dictated by the routines and habits surrounding the selection of foods. Many of us could use cooking classes to expand our nutritional horizons.

HEALTH CONCERNS

As we have seen already, good nutrition is an important influence on food purchases by many people. Those who focus on better nutrition are mainly well-educated middle-class professionals. This is the health-oriented and active lifestyle segment of the population whose tastes can set a trend.[4] Still, all of us should pay attention to nutritional health. In fact, increased health awareness among minority people is a major goal of current federal government health strategies.

In the past, sugar was the main diet concern; today, fat and cholesterol are in the limelight.[19] As a result, manufacturers are racing to the market with reduced-fat or nonfat items, including mayonnaise, salad dressings, cheeses, frozen desserts, luncheon meats, sausage, and butter sprinkles. In 1992 over 1200 new low-fat products were introduced into the American food supply. Currently about two thirds of the adult population in the United States consume low-fat or reduced-fat foods and beverages on any given day.[19]

Some of the most successful products recently introduced to U.S. markets are those with a healthy image, whether or not they actually contain healthful ingredients. Popular products have included fruit rolls and bars, bottled mineral water, low-fat granola bars, fruit juices, bulk frozen vegetables without sauce, and Oriental meals. Chicken intake since 1970 has been on the rise, while beef intake has fallen.

The recent movement toward better nutritional health began in the 1960s when the American Heart Association identified the fat-rich, cholesterol-rich diets in the United States as a major contributor to heart disease.[14] More recent research has shown that diet may be linked to 10% to 35% of all cancers. Some people have responded to these health risks by attempting to change their diets. Nevertheless, as stated earlier, taste and habit still profoundly dictate food choice. Recently, when people were asked why they did not include foods they knew were healthy parts of a diet (e.g., yellow vegetables, low-fat and nonfat milk, and whole-wheat bread), they said they didn't like them. Likewise, when asked why they didn't reduce intake of less healthy foods (e.g., whole milk, high-fat cheese, and fatty meat), respondents said they liked these foods too much.[12]

ADVERTISING

To capture consumers' interest, the food industry spends well over $6 billion annually on advertising and another $26 billion on packaging (another form of advertising)—a total of more than $32 billion (Table 1-5). Some of this advertising is helpful, as when it promotes the importance of calcium and fiber in our diets and encourages us to consume more low-fat and nonfat milk products, fruits, vegeta-

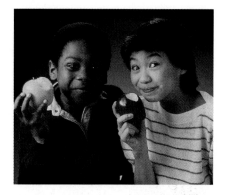

Healthy eating habits, such as including fruit in the diet, ideally start early in life.

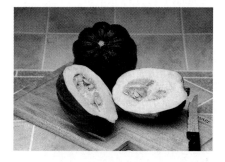

Yellow vegetables, such as acorn squash, are a healthy food choice.

TABLE 1-5

On a typical day in the United States ...

- 34 new restaurants open and 8 go out of business.
- 134 million people eat out, spending a total of $650 million. Of these people, 16 million eat at McDonald's. Note that McDonald's spends $500,000 per day to encourage this.
- Each person eats about 4 pounds of food. This includes 16 teaspoons of fat and 32 teaspoons of sugar.
- 40% of women and 25% of men are trying to lose weight. The average goal is 30 pounds.
- 50 million people have high blood pressure, with 65% realizing that they have the disease.
- 3 million pounds of yogurt is consumed.
- $1000 is spent by the National Cancer Institute to encourage us to consume at least 5 fruits/vegetables a day, while Kellogg spends over 100 times that much in advertising for Fruit Loops and Frosted Flakes.
- 100 million M&Ms are sold. 2 million Hershey's kisses and 17 million Tootsie Rolls are produced. This contributes to the 14 million pounds of candy eaten.
- 25 million hot dogs are eaten.
- 524 million Coca-Colas are consumed. To encourage this, Coca-Cola spends $500,000 per day on advertising.
- $3.5 million is spent on both tortilla chips and vitamin supplements, while $10.4 million is spent on potato chips.
- In total, $22 million is spent on snack foods, while $203 million is spent on low-calorie foods. $1.4 million is spent on laxatives.
- Children see approximately five beer and wine commercials on television. $3 million a day is spent to advertise beer, wine, and other liquors.
- $2 million is spent on baby food.

The United States has about 250 million people.

Modified from Heyman T: *On an average day,* New York, 1989, Fawcett Columbine, and other, more recent sources.

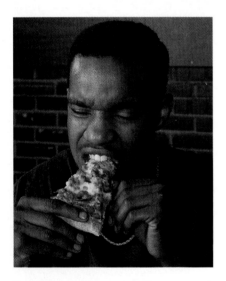

In 1994 a market research firm surveyed the eating habits of people in 2000 American households. The top meal choice was pizza, followed by ham sandwich, hot dog, peanut butter and jelly sandwich, steak, macaroni and cheese, turkey sandwich, cheese sandwich, hamburger on a bun, and spaghetti.

bles, and lean meats. The food industry, however, does not promote all foods equally: sellers tend to emphasize brand-name foods, especially highly sweetened cereals, cookies, cakes, and pastries, because they bring higher profits. Food manufacturers often pay for the best place in the supermarkets: at the end of the aisle and, depending on the product, at the child's or adult's eye level.

RESTAURANTS AND EATING OUT

Restaurants have long been a growth industry in America.[22] Nowadays about 45% of all food dollars are spent on meals outside the home. On weekdays, lunch is eaten out by 30% of all adults and dinner by 24%. Restaurant excursions are no longer a splurge but a real convenience for many people. Traveling sales representatives, students, truck drivers, and others regularly stop at quick-service (also called fast-food) restaurants. Drive-through restaurants are now a part of our culture, whereas 40 years ago they were much less common. Today, people drive through, wolf down 1200 kcal (about half their daily energy needs) via a burger, fries, and shake, and are on their way. Indeed, 8% of all food purchased in restaurants is consumed in the car.

Many restaurants, including quick-service restaurants, offer healthful alternatives to their energy-dense and high-salt foods. Yogurt has replaced ice cream in shakes, and low-fat hamburgers are offered in many restaurants. Salad bars are everywhere. Grilled chicken, fresh fruit, whole-grain muffins, and low-fat milk are widely available as well. Consumers must support this healthier fare by buying it if it is to succeed in a marketplace driven by profit.[13]

Still, the temptation to consume foods rich in fat and high in salt is often hard to resist when we eat out. The reality is that a cheeseburger, french fries, and a milk

FOR BETTER OR FOR WORSE / By Lynn Johnston

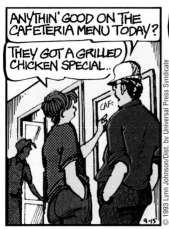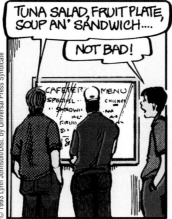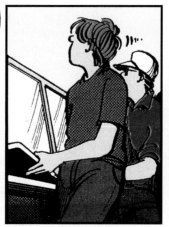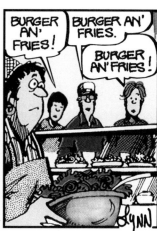

Figure 1-5 For Better Or For Worse

shake are more appealing than a well-stocked salad bar for many of us (Figure 1-5). Thus food chosen in a restaurant is generally poorer in nutritional quality than food eaten at or brought from home. Regular visitors to quick-service restaurants must be especially careful about their food choices if they want to have a healthy diet.

SOCIAL FACTORS

Many social changes in recent years have strongly affected the food marketplace, especially the large increases in the number of working women and single parents, both young and old. As a result of these and other factors, a general "time-famine" is emerging. Many people now turn to quick-service restaurants for meals on the run. Supermarkets also are competing for these restaurant customers, with already-prepared foods, microwavable entrees, and various other frozen foods being especially popular. Quick to meet the demand, food producers have increased the number of foods that require little or no preparation.[19] Almost 1000 new microwavable products were introduced in a recent year. Surveys show that one third to one half of consumers eat such foods regularly in order to save time. Sales of ready-to-eat and microwavable products marketed directly to children and weight-conscious adults are among the fastest-growing product segments.

Another social change with nutritional consequences is the advent of the pervasive shopping mall, which has created a new generation of "mall munchers." A diverse menu—ranging from ethnic foods to high-priced cookies—is offered in many malls.

As the age of the U.S. population has increased, so has the consumption of certain foods, such as shellfish, fresh vegetables, and alcoholic beverages. For the elderly, new health and nutrition problems often arise and compel changes in food habits (see Chapter 18).

Overall, in today's fast-paced world, many people are looking for ways to save time. Current estimates show that women want to spend only 30 minutes or less each day selecting and cooking food, and men want to spend only 15 minutes on such activities.[12] Not only do many people eat away from home, they also skip meals. In a recent survey of college students, more than half reported that they ate only two meals a day, eating many snacks to make up the difference. In families, approximately 30% of adults skip breakfast, which is the appropriate meal to replace the carbohydrate stores used during the night's sleep. Although skipping breakfast will save you a few minutes, you are likely to be less alert and less efficient than if you had eaten this meal. Thus you will most likely get much more accomplished during the day if you just take 20 minutes to relax and enjoy a nutritious breakfast.

CRITICAL THINKING

Tom loves to eat hamburgers, fries, and lots of pizza with double amounts of cheese. He rarely eats any vegetables and fruits, but instead snacks on cookies and ice cream. He insists that he has no problems with his health, that he's rarely ill, and that he doesn't see how his diet could cause him any health risks. How would you explain to Tom that despite his current good health, his diet could predispose him to future health problems?

It is also desirable to try to eat with others often. Meal time is a key social time of the day. The Japanese are ahead of us in recognizing that food's powers go beyond the realm of nutrition. Their national dietary guidelines, which like ours stress the importance of eating a variety of foods, maintaining healthy weight, and limiting fat in the diet, also advise people to make all activities pertaining to food and eating pleasurable.

ECONOMICS

Food habits also are influenced by the amount of money an individual or family has available for food purchases. As income increases, so do meals eaten away from home. More affluent people also tend to consume more vegetables, fruit, cheese, meat, fish, poultry, and fat, but they eat fewer dried beans and less rice. However, the relationship between income and overall food consumption is not as strong as you might expect, probably because food is relatively inexpensive in the United States. The average American spends only 12% of after-tax income for food: 7% for food at home and 5% for food away from home. Compare this to about 50% of income spent on food in China or India. Nevertheless, high meat prices have led to the use of beef as an ingredient rather than as a centerpiece in some households; chicken, turkey, and fish are used as alternatives.[19]

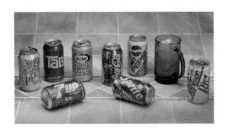
Soft drinks are more popular today than milk, although not as beneficial to a person's diet.

Improving Our Diets

Our cultural diversity, varied cuisines, and generally high nutritional status should be points of pride for Americans.[10] Today we can choose from a tremendous variety of food products, the result of continual innovation by food manufacturers. In 1993 alone, some 9200 new food products were introduced in the United States.[19]

The American food supply does not stand still, but is in a constant state of evolution. During the last hundred years, the United States has led the world in creating new food products (Table 1-6). From toaster pastries to microwave popcorn, the variety of food products in a typical supermarket is nearly limitless. Even astronauts in space have their unique food product: a plastic bag containing the nutritional equivalent of an entree, two side dishes, and a beverage, which is kneaded for several minutes and then squeezed into the mouth.

Today we are eating more breakfast cereals, pizza, pasta entrees, stir-fried meat and vegetables served on rice, salads, tacos, burritos, and fajitas than ever before. Sales of whole milk are down, while in the same time period sales of nonfat and 1% low-fat milk have increased.[19] Consumption of frozen vegetables, rather than canned vegetables, is also on the rise.

More than half the shoppers in a recent survey said they are eating more fruits and vegetables to contribute to healthful diets. Shoppers said they are also eating less meat (34%), fewer fats and oils (25%), and less sugar (19%), while eating more chicken (16%), dietary fiber (16%), and fish (14%).[12] Still, soft drinks are more popular than milk, although not as beneficial to the diet. Overall many of these recent diet changes are advantageous; some are not.

Today, Americans live longer than ever before and enjoy better general health. Many also have more money, more diverse food and lifestyle choices to consider, and more time to relax and enjoy life. The nutritional consequences of these trends are not fully known. Deaths from heart disease and strokes, for example, have dropped dramatically since the late 1960s, partly due to better medical care and diets. Still, if affluence leads to sedentary lifestyles and high intakes of fat, sodium, and alcohol, it can be a villain.[3] Because of better technology and greater choices, we can have a much better diet today than ever before—if we know what choices to make. Overall, we are doing well, but many of us can do better.[13] The goal here is to help you find your best path to good nutrition. Chapter 2 contains key information to aid you in that goal.

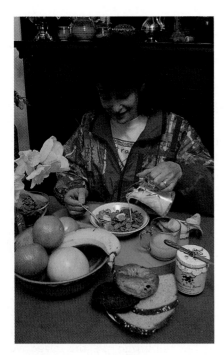
Most Americans enjoy a wide bounty of foods from which to choose.

TABLE 1-6

Years when common American foods were introduced

1875—Chocolate milk	1941—Cheerios
1876—Heinz ketchup	1944—Hawaiian Punch
1891—Fig Newtons	1946—Minute Rice, frozen orange
1896—Tootsie Roll	juice, instant coffee
1897—Jell-O	1950—Sugar Corn Pops
1897—Grape-Nuts	1952—Kellogg's Sugar Frosted Flakes
1898—Graham crackers	1953—Sugar Smacks, frozen pizza
1907—Hershey's Kisses	1956—Duncan Hines brownie mix
1912—Life Savers	1956—Jif peanut butter
1912—Oreos	1958—Tang
1916—All-Bran	1960—Instant potatoes
1921—Mounds, Wonder bread	1963—Tab
1923—Milky Way	1965—Shake 'n Bake
1923—Reese's Peanut Butter Cup	1966—Cool Whip
1927—Kool-Aid	1968—Pringles, Care Free sugarless
1928—Rice Krispies	gum
1930—Birds Eye frozen foods	1976—Country Time lemonade
1930—Snickers	1981—TCBY frozen yogurt
1932—3 Musketeers, Fritos corn chips	1984—Diet Coke (with aspartame)
1934—Ritz crackers, Bisquick	1986—Pop Secret microwave popcorn

Modified from Staten V: *Can you trust a tomato in January?* New York, 1993, Simon and Schuster, and other sources.

CONCEPT CHECK

Food choices are influenced mainly by taste and habit. Recently, factors such as health concerns, economics, convenience, and social structure are also becoming important dietary determinants. Good food habits developed and strengthened early in life provide many benefits in later years.

Summary

1. Nutrition is the study of the food substances vital for health and how the body uses these substances to promote and support growth, maintenance, and reproduction of cells.

2. Nutrients in foods fall into six classes: carbohydrates, lipids (mostly fats and oils), proteins, vitamins, minerals, and water. The first three, along with alcohol, provide energy for the body to use.

3. As nutritional health diminishes, nutrient stores in the body are depleted first. As stores are exhausted, biochemical reactions in the body eventually slow down. Finally, clinical evidence (signs and symptoms) develop.

4. The most common nutritional problems in the United States result from overnutrition, which includes overconsumption of energy, saturated and total fat, sodium, and sometimes certain vitamins and minerals.

5. The focus of nutrition planning should be food, not supplements. The use of foods to supply nutrient needs essentially eliminates the possibility of severe nutrient imbalances.

6. Genetic background influences a person's risk for developing many chronic diseases, such as obesity, heart disease, cancer, and diabetes. Evidence of these diseases in one's family should make a person more attentive to avoiding "controllable" risk factors for these diseases. These risk factors are discussed throughout this book.

7. Results from large nutrition surveys in the United States suggest that some of us need to concentrate on consuming foods that supply more vitamin A, certain B vitamins, calcium, iron, zinc, and dietary fiber.

8. The taste and texture of foods primarily influence our food choices. Several other factors also help determine food habits and choices: our upbringing, various social and cultural factors, our self-image and the image we want to project to others, economics, and concerns about health.

Study Questions

1. Describe how genetic tendencies and other risk factors interrelate in terms of developing one specific nutrition-related chronic disease.
2. Name three chronic diseases associated with nutrition and a few corresponding risk factors.
3. Identify a nutrition-related disease that develops over many years before clinical signs are evident. Why is there such a long lag time?
4. Outline the concept of energy content in foods. List the energy values for a gram of carbohydrate, fat, protein, and alcohol.
5. Wendy's Big Bacon Classic contains 44 g carbohydrate, 36 g fat, and 37 g protein. Calculate the percentage of energy derived from fat.
6. Describe the states of nutritional health associated with overnutrition, desirable nutrition, and undernutrition.
7. According to national nutrition surveys, which nutrients tend to be underconsumed by many adult Americans. Why is this the case?
8. Outline the ABCDs of a nutritional assessment; that is, the activities performed to assess an individual's nutritional status.
9. Describe how your own food preferences have been shaped by the following factors:
   a. exposure to foods at an early age
   b. advertising (what is the newest food you have tried?)
   c. eating out
   d. peer pressure
   e. economic resources

REFERENCES

1. Beaton GH: Criteria of an adequate diet. In Shils ME and others, editors: *Modern nutrition in health and disease,* ed 8, Philadelphia, 1994, Lea & Febiger.
2. Block G and others: Nutrient sources in the American diet, *American Journal of Epidemiology* 122:13, 1985.
3. Burkitt DP, Eaton SB: Putting the wrong fuel in the tank, *Nutrition* 5:189, 1989.
4. Callaway CW: The marriage of taste and health: a union whose time has come, *Nutrition Today,* May/June 1992, p 37.
5. Centers for Disease Control and Prevention: Daily dietary fat and total food energy intakes, NHANES III, *Journal of the American Medical Association* 271:1309, 1994.
6. Checking out the supermarket shopper, *Journal of the American Dietetic Association* 91: 1511, 1991.
7. Diet, nutrition, and prevention of chronic diseases—a report of the WHO study group on diet, nutrition, and prevention of noncommunicable diseases, *Nutrition Review* 49:291, 1991.
8. Falciglia GA, Norton PA: Evidence for a genetic influence on preference for some foods,

Journal of the American Dietetic Association 94:154, 1994.
9. Garn SM, Leonard WR: What did our ancestors eat? *Nutrition Review* 47:337, 1989.
10. Harper AE: The 1990 Atwater lecture: the science and the practice of nutrition: reflections and directions, *American Journal of Clinical Nutrition* 53:413, 1991.
11. Lofgren PA and others: Eating in America today, *Food and Nutrition News* 66:9, 1994.
12. McBean LD: Consumer attitudes and behavior regarding diet, nutrition, and health, *Dairy Council Digest* 65:31, 1994.
13. Morreale SJ, Schwartz WE: Helping Americans eat right, *Journal of the American Dietetic Association,* 95:305, 1995.
14. National Research Council–National Academy of Sciences: *Diet and health,* Washington DC, 1989, National Academy Press.
15. Pipes PL, Trahms CM: *Nutrition in infancy and childhood,* ed 5, St Louis, 1993, Mosby.
16. Rozin P: Acquisition of stable food preferences, *Nutrition Reviews* 48:106, 1990.
17. Selhub J and others: Vitamin status and intake as primary determinants of homocys-

teinemia in an elderly population, *Journal of the American Medical Association* 270:2693, 1993.
18. Siwek J: Ten steps to healthier patients in 1995, *American Family Physician* 51:33, 1995.
19. Stillings BR: Trends in foods, *Nutrition Today* 29:6, 1994.
20. Taylor A: Cataract: relationship between nutrition and oxidation, *Journal of the American College of Nutrition,* 12:138, 1993.
21. Thomas PR, Earl R: Creating the future of nutrition and food sciences, *Journal of the American Medical Association* 94:257, 1994.
22. Warshaw HS: America eats out: nutrition in the chain and family restaurant industry, *Journal of the American Dietetic Association* 93:17, 1993.
23. Williams RR: Diet, genes, early heart attacks, and high blood pressure. In Kotsonis FN, Mackey MA, editors: *Nutrition in the '90s,* New York, 1994, Dekker.
24. Wright HS and others: The 1987-88 nationwide food consumption survey, *Nutrition Today,* May/June 1991, p 21.

TAKE ACTION

Examine the factors that affect your eating habits

Choose one day of the week that is typical of your eating pattern. In the table below, list all foods and drinks you consumed for 1 day. In addition, write down the approximate amounts you ate in units like cups, ounces, teaspoons, and tablespoons. Check the food composition table in Appendix A for examples of appropriate serving units for different types of foods, such as meat, vegetables, etc. After completing this activity, you will use this list of foods for future activities.

After you record each food, drink, and serving size, indicate in the table why you chose to consume each item. Use the following symbols to indicate your reasons. Place the corresponding abbreviation in the space provided, indicating why you picked that particular food or drink.

TAST	Taste/texture	HUNG	Hunger
CONV	Convenience	FAM	Family/cultural
EMO	Emotions	PEER	Peers
AVA	Availability	NUTR	Nutritive value
ADV	Advertisement	$	Cost
WTCL	Weight Control	HLTH	Health

There can be more than one reason for choosing a particular food or drink.

Time	Minutes spent eating	M or S*	H†	Activity while eating	Place of eating	Food and quantity	Others present	Reason for food choice

*M or S: Meal or snack
†H: Degree of hunger (0 = none; 3 = maximum)

Application
Now ask yourself what your most frequent reason is for eating or drinking. To what degree is health a reason for your food choices? Should you make it a higher priority?

NUTRITION PERSPECTIVE

Determining Nutrient Needs by Scientific Research

The study of nutrient needs and nutrient metabolism relies on the scientific method, which is designed to detect and eliminate error. Scientists begin by observing physical phenomena. They conjecture and speculate about the causes of the phenomena and then suggest possible explanations or **hypotheses** about them (Figure 1-6). They then examine these possibilities using rigorous experimental tests to either support or refute them. If many lines of evidence support a hypothesis, it gains the status of a **theory.**

Science obliges us to view hypotheses and theories skeptically, avoiding hasty acceptance of them based on meager evidence and discarding those that fail to pass critical analysis. Nutrition science requires skeptical minds that critically evaluate all current ideas.[10] In other words, don't react to one research study by radically changing your life. When evaluating nutrition research, look for consistency of scientific results from different investigators, coupled with critical evaluation.

hypothesis An "educated guess" by a scientist to explain a phenomenon.

theory An explanation for a phenomenon that has many lines of evidence to support it.

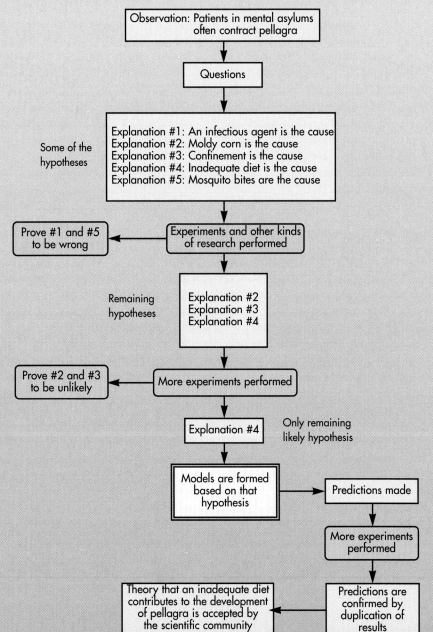

Figure 1-6 From question to theory—the process of science applied to nutrition. Only after careful and thorough analysis and repeated experimentation should a research finding influence our food choices, such as the need to consume the vitamin niacin to prevent development of pellagra.

Generating Hypotheses

Historical events have provided clues to important relationships in nutrition science. For example, in the fifteenth and sixteenth centuries, when Europeans left Europe to come to the Americas, many of them developed **scurvy** during the long sea voyages. This deficiency disease occurred because the sailors ate few fruits and vegetables and thus consumed very little vitamin C. Eventually British scientists discovered that lime juice prevented or cured scurvy. About 300 years later vitamin C was discovered. In the intervening years the British Navy, run by "Limeys," had a healthy work force and dominated the seas worldwide.

During World War II, the German army blockaded the Russian city of Leningrad, causing widespread semistarvation. Noting that lack of food was associated with increased infant **mortality,** scientists in North America eventually showed that food supplements given to poor women improved their chances of delivering a healthy baby.

Viewed from a historical perspective, humans appear capable of surviving on a diet consisting either mainly of meat or almost entirely of vegetables and fruit. The human species consumed a diet high in vegetable products and low in animal products for many thousands of years.[9] Early diets were about one third from animal sources and two thirds from plant sources, and they generally were higher in protein, lower in fat, and higher in dietary fiber than modern diets. This dietary pattern developed not because of nutritional reasons per se, but because of the foods that were available. These differences in human diets throughout history do not tell us which is better. Only closer scientific study can provide assessment of what constitutes a superior diet.

In a related approach to using historical observation, scientists establish nutritional hypotheses by studying the different dietary and disease patterns among various populations in today's world. If one group tends to develop a certain disease while another group does not, scientists can speculate about the role diet plays in this difference. The study of diseases in populations is called **epidemiology.**

In the 1920s, epidemiological studies suggested to Dr. Joseph Goldberger that **pellagra** was a dietary deficiency disease, rather than an infectious disease. He noticed that prisoners in jail—but not their jailers—suffered from pellagra. If pellagra were an **infectious disease,** both populations would be expected to suffer from it. As another example, Dr. Denis Burkitt noted in the 1970s that Africans had lower rates of intestinal problems than Americans. He speculated that the higher intake of dietary fiber by Africans compared with Americans might account for the difference in their intestinal health.

Epidemiological evidence, however, is not enough to establish the role of particular dietary components in various nutritional health problems. For instance, designed **experiments** were required to test hypotheses concerning the cause of pellagra and the effect of dietary fiber on intestinal health. During the 1920s, various foods were fed to patients in mental hospitals who suffered from pellagra. Yeast and high-protein foods were found to cure the disease, indicating that pellagra was caused by a deficiency of some nutrient present in these foods. Similarly, experiments in the 1970s showed that when people consuming typical (low) amounts of fiber increased their intake of dietary fiber, their intestinal health improved. Additional research eventually proved that pellagra is caused by deficiency of the vitamin niacin, but research on the importance of dietary fiber to health still continues.

Animal Experiments

When scientists cannot test their hypotheses by experiments with humans, they often use animals. Much of what we know about human nutritional needs and functions has been generated from animal experiments. Still, human experiments are the most convincing to scientists. In the 1930s, scientists showed that a pellagra-like disease seen in dogs, called blacktongue, was cured by nicotinic acid. But only when nicotinic acid actually cured the disease in humans were scientists convinced that nicotinic acid, later called niacin, was the critical dietary factor.

scurvy The deficiency disease that results after a few months of consuming a diet essentially free of vitamin C.

mortality A population's death rate. The term *morbidity* refers to the number of sick persons in a population

epidemiology The study of how disease rates vary among different population groups. For example, the rate of stomach cancer in Japan could be compared with that in Germany.

pellagra A disease characterized by inflammation of the skin, diarrhea, and eventual mental incapacity due to a dietary lack of the vitamin niacin.

infectious disease Any disease caused by invasion of the body by microorganisms, such as bacteria, fungi, or viruses.

experiment A test made to examine the validity of a hypothesis.

Today we know that low doses of the mineral fluoride can stimulate growth in rats. However, we still do not know whether this is true for humans because it is not practical to control the fluoride intake of humans accurately enough to answer the question. Thus there is speculation that fluoride might stimulate growth in humans, but real proof is lacking.

In addition, use of humans in certain types of experiments is considered unethical. For such studies, most people believe that the careful, humane use of animals is an ethical alternative to using human subjects. (Some people argue that animal experiments also are unethical.) For example, most people think it is reasonable to feed rats a low-copper diet to study the importance of this mineral in the formation of blood vessels. Almost universally, however, people would object to a similar study in infants.

The use of animal experiments to study the role of nutrition in certain human diseases depends on the availability of an **animal model**—a disease in laboratory animals that closely mimics a particular human disease. If no animal model is available and human experiments are ruled out, scientific knowledge often cannot advance beyond what can be learned from epidemiological studies.

animal model A disease in animals that duplicates human disease and thus can be used to understand more about the human disease.

Human Experiments

Various experimental approaches are used to test research hypotheses in humans, including case-control and double-blind studies.

CASE-CONTROL STUDY

In a case-control study, individuals who have the condition in question are compared with individuals who do not have the condition, but comparisons are made only between groups that are matched for other major characteristics (e.g., age and gender) not under study. This type of study is in effect a microscopic epidemiological study. It may identify factors, other than the condition in question, that differ between the two groups, thus providing researchers with clues about the cause or progression of the condition.

DOUBLE-BLIND STUDY

double-blind study An experimental design in which neither the subjects nor the researchers are aware of the subject's assignment (test or placebo) nor the outcome of the study until it is completed. An independent third party holds the code and the data until the study has been completed.

control group Participants in an experiment who are not given the treatment being tested.

An important approach for testing hypotheses is the **double-blind study**, in which a group of subjects—the experimental group—follows a specific protocol (e.g., eating a certain food) and a corresponding **control group** follows the normal pattern of living. People are randomly assigned to each group, as by the flip of a coin. Scientists then observe the experimental group over time to see if there is any effect that is not found in the control group. Sometimes subjects are used as their own control: first they are observed for a period of time, and then they are treated and their responses noted.

Two features of a double-blind study help reduce the introduction of bias (prejudice), which can easily affect the outcome of an experiment. First, neither the subjects nor the researchers know which subjects are in the experimental group and which are in the control group. Second, the expected effects of the experimental protocol are not disclosed until after the entire study is completed. This approach reduces the possibility that researchers may see the change they want to see in the subjects to prove a certain hypothesis, even though the change did not actually occur. This approach also reduces the chance that the subjects may begin to feel better, for example, simply because they are part of the experimental group.

placebo A fake medicine used to disguise the roles of participants in an experiment; if fake surgery is performed, it is called a *sham operation.*

The effect of mere suggestion is referred to as the "placebo effect." The Latin word *placebo* means "I shall please." The placebo effect cannot be accounted for on the basis of pharmacological or other direct physical action. Feeling better when the physician walks into the room is a common example of the placebo effect. In a double-blind experiment a **placebo** (fake medicine), such as a sugar pill, is often given to the control group to camouflage who is in what group and so eliminate the bias introduced by the placebo effect. Until the experiment is complete, an independent third party holds the code that identifies each participant and his or her treatment. Sometimes only a single-blind protocol is possible, in which either the subjects or the researchers are kept in the dark.

Drug studies lend themselves to double-blind protocols because it is often easy to substitute a placebo for the drug. However, food studies often cannot be placebo controlled. It is, for example, hard to disguise a diet high in fruits and vegetables from one devoid of them. However, in such a study, the experimenters should try to ensure that the results from blood assays or other measurements are not revealed until the end of the study. In addition, the results should be kept from the subjects until the end of the study. These precautions can eliminate much potential bias. The more bias that is controlled in an experiment, the more confidence we can have in the results.

Peer Review of Experimental Results

Once an experiment is complete, scientists summarize the findings and publish the results in a scientific journal. At the end of each chapter in this book, we list many reports describing important experiments that have been published in scientific journals. Generally, before articles are published in scientific journals, they are critically reviewed by other scientists familiar with the subject. The objective of this peer review is to ensure that only high-quality research findings are published. Results published in peer-reviewed journals, such as the *American Journal of Clinical Nutrition,* the *New England Journal of Medicine,* and the *Journal of The American Dietetic Association,* are much more reliable than those found in popular magazines or promoted on television talk shows. The information presented in such popular media usually has not been closely scrutinized by competent researchers for accuracy and scientific validity.

Follow-Up Studies

Finally, even if an acceptable protocol has been followed and the results of a study accepted by the scientific community, one experiment is not enough to prove a particular hypothesis or provide a basis for nutritional recommendations. Rather, the results obtained in one laboratory must be confirmed by experiments conducted in other laboratories. Only then can we really trust and use the results. We don't advise rushing to accept new ideas as fact or incorporating them into your health habits until they are proved by several lines of evidence (Figure 1-7). Overall, the best goal is still to have a varied diet and consume all foods in moderation.[10]

When you read accounts of scientific experiments, ask yourself: "Was a double-blind study protocol used? If a placebo could have been used, was it? During the experiment, were the researchers 'blinded' as much as possible as to who received the experimental treatment and the effects of that treatment?"

The American Dietetic Association has a toll-free hotline, staffed by registered dietitians, to answer consumers' food-related questions. Call (800) 366-1655, weekdays from 9 a.m. until 9 p.m. EST.

CATHY

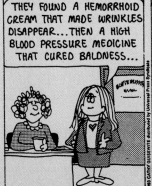 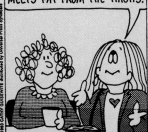 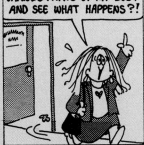 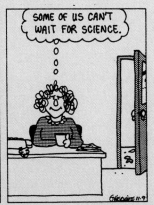

Figure 1-7 Cathy

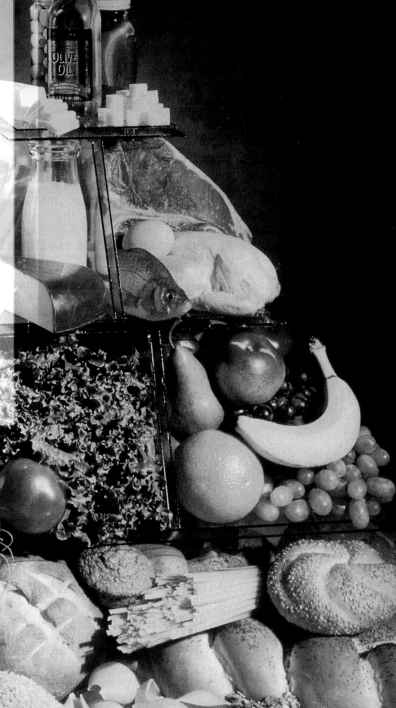

CHAPTER TWO

The Basis of a Healthy Diet

H ow many times have you heard wild claims about how healthful certain foods are for you? As consumers focus more and more on diet and disease, food manufacturers are asserting that their products have all sorts of health benefits. Supermarket shelves have begun to look like an 1800s medicine show.[12] "Take fish oil capsules to avoid a heart attack." "Eat more olive oil and oat bran to lower blood cholesterol." Hearing these claims, you would think that food manufacturers have solutions to all of our health problems.

Advertising aside, nutrient intake out of balance with nutrient needs is linked to many leading causes of death in the United States, including hypertension, heart disease, cancer, liver disease, and the major form of diabetes.[2,17] In this chapter we explore the components of a healthy diet—a diet that will minimize your risks of developing nutrition-related diseases. We want to provide you with a firm understanding of basic diet-planning concepts before you study the nutrients in detail.

justed downward for young children (see Chapter 17). Table 2-1 lists serving sizes and amounts for adults of various ages. The table also lists the major nutrients each food group supplies. Note the similarities and differences among the groups. The plan for an adult over age 24 essentially consists of the following:

- 2 servings from the milk, yogurt, and cheese group
- 2 to 3 servings from the meat, poultry, fish, dry beans, eggs, and nuts group (5 to 7 ounces total)
- 3 to 5 servings from the vegetable group
- 2 to 4 servings from the fruit group
- 6 to 11 servings from the bread, cereals, rice, and pasta group

For some population groups—children, teenagers, adults under age 25, and pregnant or lactating women—3 servings of the milk, yogurt, and cheese group are recommended. Foods from the final category, which includes fats, oils, and sweets, then could be eaten to help meet individual energy needs, but should not replace foods from other groups.

PLANNING MENUS WITH THE FOOD GUIDE PYRAMID

Table 2-2 illustrates a 1-day menu based on the Food Guide Pyramid. Remember the following points when using the Food Guide Pyramid to plan daily menus:

1. The guide does not apply to infant feeding nor to children under 2 years of age.

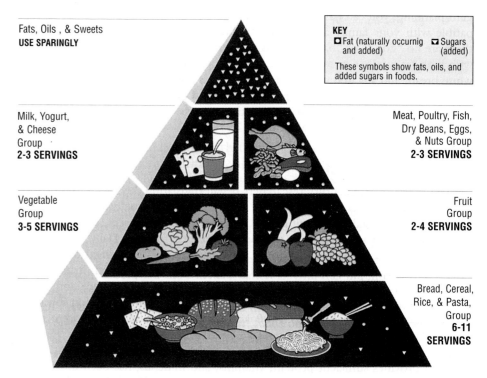

Figure 2-1 USDA's Food Guide Pyramid. This guide lists the food groups and the number of servings to consume from each group. Note that for children, teenagers, and adults under age 25, 3 servings should be chosen from the milk, yogurt, and cheese group. Once you have estimated your energy needs, recommended servings from the other groups with wider ranges are as follows:

Energy intake	1600 kcal	2200 kcal	2800 kcal
Bread group	6	9	11
Vegetable group	3	4	5
Fruit group	2	3	4
Meat group	2, for a total of 5 oz	2, for a total of 6 oz	3, for a total of 7 oz

2. No one food is absolutely essential to good nutrition. Each food is deficient in at least one essential nutrient.
3. No one food group provides all essential nutrients in adequate amounts. Each food group makes an important, distinctive contribution to nutritional intake.
4. Variety is the key to the success of the guide and is first guaranteed by choosing foods from all the groups. Furthermore, one should consume a variety of foods within each group.[1]
5. The foods within a group may vary widely with respect to nutrient and energy content. For example, the energy content of 3 ounces of baked potato is 98 kcal, whereas that of 3 ounces of potato chips is 470 kcal. Compare an orange and an apple with respect to vitamin C, using the food composition table in Appendix A.

Overall, the Food Guide Pyramid incorporates the foundations of a healthy diet: variety, balance, and moderation. The nutritional adequacy of diets planned using this tool, however, depends on selection of a variety of foods. In addition, to ensure enough vitamin E, vitamin B-6, magnesium, and zinc—nutrients sometimes low in diets based on this plan—consider the following advice:

1. Choose low-fat and nonfat items from the milk, yogurt, and cheese group. By reducing energy intake in this way, you can select more items from other food groups.
2. Be sure to include servings of vegetable proteins at least several times a week, as these are rich in minerals and dietary fiber.
3. For vegetables and fruits, try to include a dark green vegetable for vitamin A and a vitamin C–rich fruit, such as an orange, every day. Surveys show that only 25% of adults eat a green vegetable on any given day. Increased consumption of these foods is important because they contribute vitamins, minerals, and dietary fiber.
4. Choose whole-grain varieties of breads, cereals, rice, and pasta often, as they contribute dietary fiber. A daily serving of a whole-grain breakfast cereal is an excellent choice because the vitamins and minerals typically added to it, along with dietary fiber, help to fill in the potential gaps listed above.

By following the Food Guide Pyramid, it is possible to create daily diets containing as few as 1600 to 1800 kcal (see Table 2-2), sufficient for a sedentary adult or an elderly person. If 1600 to 1800 kcal represents too much food energy for you, your first option should be to become more active rather than to eat less. It is very difficult to obtain enough nutrients from a diet that supplies fewer than 1600 kcal/day. If you can't increase your energy output, you could make a special attempt to choose regularly some nutrient-fortified foods (e.g., breakfast cereals). As discussed in Chapter 12, nutrient supplements themselves are usually not needed for the average person, but certain people may benefit from this practice, such as pregnant women and elderly people with limited energy intakes. In addition, for those whose diets do not include meat or other animal products, the Nutrition Perspective on vegetarianism in Chapter 5 provides advice on adapting the Food Guide Pyramid to that dietary practice.

EVALUATING YOUR CURRENT DIET USING THE FOOD GUIDE PYRAMID

An average American diet, based on a recent survey of 2000 households, failed to meet the serving recommendations in the Food Guide Pyramid for all food groups. For example, the average diet included only 1 fruit serving (rather than the recommended 2 to 4 servings) and only 2 vegetable servings (rather than 3 to 5 servings). These were the most underrepresented groups. In contrast, the fats, oils, and sweets were well represented (average of 3.7 servings).[15]

Regularly comparing of your daily food intake with the Food Guide Pyramid recommendations is a relatively simple way to evaluate your overall diet. Strive to meet the recommendations. If that is not possible, identify the nutrients that are low

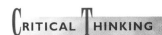

CRITICAL **T**HINKING

Joe is 66 years old and knows that he has to reduce his energy intake to about 1600 kcal. He doesn't see how he can possibly reduce his energy intake and still be healthy. How would you explain that this can indeed be accomplished?

TABLE 2-1

The Food Guide Pyramid—a summary

Food group

Milk, yogurt, and cheese

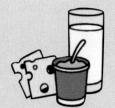

Meat, poultry, fish, dry beans, eggs, and nuts

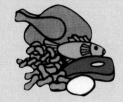

Fruits

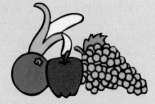

Vegetables

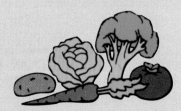

Bread, cereal, rice, and pasta

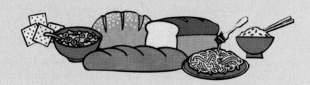

Fats, oils, and sweets

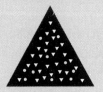

*Consuming the minimum number of servings from each food group provides about 1600 to 1800 kcal. Most adults must consume at least this much energy to meet their RDAs for nutrients, depending on use of nutrient-fortified foods and nutrient supplements.
†May be reduced for child servings.
‡≥25 years of age.
**Primarily in plant protein sources.
§Only in animal foods.

Number of servings*	Major contributions	Foods and individual serving sizes†
2 (adult‡) 3 (children, teens, young adults, and pregnant or lactating women)	Calcium Carbohydrate Protein Riboflavin Vitamin D Magnesium Zinc	1 cup milk 1½ oz cheese 2 oz processed cheese 1 cup yogurt 2 cups cottage cheese 1 cup custard/pudding 1½ cups ice cream
2-3	Protein Thiamin Riboflavin Niacin Vitamin B-6 Folate** Vitamin B-12§ Magnesium** Iron Zinc	2-3 oz cooked meat, poultry, or fish 1-1½ cups cooked dry beans 4 tbsp peanut butter 2 eggs ½-1 cup nuts
2-4	Carbohydrate Vitamin C Folate Magnesium Potassium Dietary fiber	¼ cup dried fruit ½ cup cooked fruit ¾ cup juice 1 whole piece of fruit 1 melon wedge
3-5	Carbohydrate Vitamin A Vitamin C Folate Magnesium Potassium Dietary fiber	½ cup raw or cooked vegetables 1 cup raw leafy vegetables ¾ cup vegetable juice
6-11	Carbohydrate Thiamin Riboflavin‖ Niacin Folate¶ Magnesium¶ Iron‖¶ Zinc¶ Dietary fiber¶	1 slice of bread 1 oz ready-to-eat cereal ½-¾ cup cooked cereal, rice, or pasta ½ hamburger roll, bagel, or English muffin 3-4 plain crackers
		Foods from this category should not replace any from the other groups. Amounts consumed should be determined by individual energy needs.

‖If enriched.
¶Whole grains especially.
To quickly estimate serving sizes, use the following equivalents:

A thumb = 1 oz of cheese	A fist = 1 cup
A thumb tip = 1 tsp	A handful = 1 or 2 oz of a snack food
Palm of a hand = 3 oz	

TABLE 2-2

Putting the Food Guide Pyramid into practice

Meal	Servings/food group*
Breakfast	
1 peeled orange	1 fruit
1½ cups Cheerios	2 bread
with ½ cup 1% milk	½ milk
1 slice raisin toast	1 bread
with 1 tsp margarine	1 fat/sweet
Optional: coffee or tea	
Lunch	
Ham sandwich	
2 slices whole-wheat bread	2 bread
2 oz ham	1 meat
2 tsp mustard	
1 Apple	1 fruit
2 oatmeal-raisin cookies (small)	2 fat/sweet
Optional: diet soda	
3 PM study break	
1 whole bagel	2 bread
1 tbsp peanut butter	¼ meat
½ cup 1% milk	½ milk
Dinner	
Lettuce salad	
1 cup Romaine lettuce	1 vegetable
½ cup sliced tomatoes	1 vegetable
1 tblsp Thousand Island dressing	1 fat/sweet
½ grated carrot	½ vegetable
3 oz broiled salmon	1 meat
½ cup rice	1 bread
¾ cup green beans	1 vegetable
with 1 tsp margarine	1 fat/sweet
Optional: coffee or tea	
Late-night snack	
1 cup low-fat fruit yogurt	1 milk
Nutrient breakdown:	
1800 kcal	
Carbohydrate 55% of kilocalories	
Protein 20% of kilocalories	
Fat 25% of kilocalories	

Meets RDA/ESADDI values for all vitamins and minerals for a 25-year-old adult. For adolescents and adults under age 25, add one additional serving from the milk, yogurt, and cheese group.
*Names of food groups abbreviated as follows: milk = milk, yogurt, and cheese group; meat = meat, poultry, fish, dry beans, eggs, and nuts group; bread = bread, cereal, rice, and pasta group; fat/sweet = fats, oils, and sweets category.

in your diet based on the nutrients found in each food group (see Table 2-1). For example, if you under-consume the milk, yogurt, and cheese group, your calcium intake most likely is too low. After completing the Take Action activity at the end of this chapter, you will be able to determine more accurately which nutrients are too low in your current diet, and by how much. Armed with this knowledge, find foods that you do enjoy that supply those nutrients, such as calcium-fortified orange juice. Customizing the Food Guide Pyramid to accommodate your own food habits may seem a daunting task now, but it is not difficult once you gain some additional nutrition knowledge.

CONCEPT CHECK

Variety, balance, and moderation are the foundations of a healthy diet. The Food Guide Pyramid translates these foundations and general needs for carbohydrate, protein, fat, vitamins, and minerals into the recommended number of daily servings from each of five major food groups, and it is a convenient and valuable tool for planning daily menus.

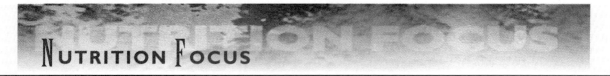

NUTRITION FOCUS

A FOUNTAIN OF YOUTH?

Although most of us wish for a long life, we do not like to think of ourselves as suffering poor health when we are old. And rightly so! We can truly enjoy a long life only if we are productive and free of illness. Rather than suffer the ravages of heart disease, stroke, diabetes, osteoporosis, and other chronic diseases from the age of 50 or 60 years until death, we should strive to be as free from disease as possible and to enjoy vitality even in the last years of life. Greater physical well-being contributes to our mental and social well-being.

Aging is a natural process: your body cells age no matter what health practices you follow. But to a considerable extent you can determine how quickly you age throughout your adult years. As we saw in Chapter 1, genetic background is very important in determining your

risk of nutrition-related diseases; nonetheless, you also have some control over it. How you act now is important to your later health. Successful aging is a result of wise choices. Age quickly or age slowly—you have some choice in the matter.

The best way to promote your health and prevent chronic diseases in the future is to observe the following guidelines:

• Eat a healthful diet—a varied diet that maintains a healthy weight should be a priority (Figure 2-2). The Food Guide Pyramid is a great place to start. Choose moderate portion sizes and pay particular attention to serving sizes of high-fat foods.

• Drink plenty of fluids—because the body is composed mostly of water, which is lost in perspiration and

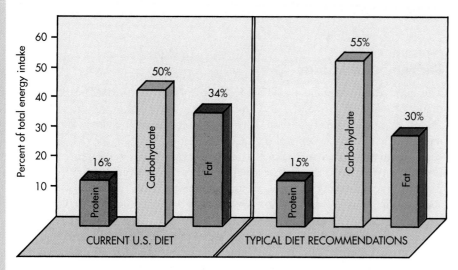

Figure 2-2 Is our current diet in our best interests? Many nutrition scientists, after evaluating the relationship between diet and health, have concluded that many Americans should eat more carbohydrate-rich foods and fewer fat-rich foods. For carbohydrate-rich foods, many of the choices should be good sources of dietary fiber and, ideally, low in simple sugars.

Nutrition Focus

urinewater should continually be replaced. Aim to drink 6 to 8 glasses of water and other beverages daily.

- Exercise—spend at least 30 minutes a day in a combination of brisk walking, jogging, swimming, stair climbing, and other activities that stimulate the cardiovascular system. See Chapter 10 for other options. But by all means, become and remain active.
- Don't smoke—lung cancer, caused primarily by smoking cigarettes, is the only form of cancer for which yearly rates still increase. About half of regular cigarette smokers die as a direct result of smoking. In addition, a recent British study showed that smokers eat fewer fruits and vegetables and more saturated fat and sugar than nonsmokers. Currently, about 25% of adults smoke, with low-income people more inclined to smoke than those with higher incomes. Slightly more men smoke than women.
- Limit alcohol intake—don't drink more than 1 oz of alcohol per day on a regular basis. Women are cautioned to cut even that amount in half because they are more likely than men to develop cirrhosis of the liver with the same intake of alcohol. One 12-oz beer, a 5-oz glass of wine, or a mixed drink supplies about $\frac{1}{2}$ oz (15 g) of alcohol. African-Americans are especially sensitive to the effects of alcohol on blood pressure. Furthermore, all women must avoid alcohol during pregnancy because it can harm the fetus, causing fetal alcohol syndrome (see Chapter 16 for a discussion of this disease).
- Get adequate sleep—establish a regular schedule to allow for an average of 7 to 8 hours of sleep a night. If

you have difficulty sleeping, look for factors that may be interfering, such as noise, stress, caffeine-containing products, lack of exercise, and late-night eating.

- Limit stress or adjust to the causes of stress—practice better time management, relax, listen to music, have a massage, and exercise regularly. Do your favorite things to reduce stress. In addition, maintaining self-esteem and interpersonal relationships contributes to limiting stress and reinforces wellness.
- Consult health-care professionals on a regular basis— early diagnosis is especially important for controlling the damaging effects of many diseases.

Your key to optimal health is to discover how to maintain your best physical, mental, psychological, and social states. There is no general formula for achieving this ideal. Each of us must juggle and balance personal goals with the opportunities and obstacles we encounter. Proper diet is not the only thing to consider. As we have discussed, other behavior is also critical. Taking responsibility for yourself is central to achieving long-term health. As individuals, we can do a lot to improve our health by establishing good health behavior.

Focusing on disease prevention may not allow you to live longer—because heredity, accidents, and other things are outside your control—but you'll probably live a healthier life.

It is especially important for current and future health-care professionals to develop and follow a plan that emphasizes wellness for themselves. By taking this initiative, they act as positive models for others.

Dietary Guidelines

The Food Guide Pyramid was designed to help meet nutritional needs for carbohydrate, protein, fat, vitamins, and minerals. However, most of the major chronic "killer" diseases in America, such as heart disease, cancer, and alcoholism, are not primarily associated with deficiencies of these nutrients.[17] Nor are deficiency diseases, such as scurvy (vitamin C deficiency) and pellagra (niacin deficiency), still common. For many Americans, the primary dietary culprit is an over-consumption of one or more of the following: energy, saturated and total fat, cholesterol, alcohol, and sodium (salt). Under-consumption of calcium, iron, folate, zinc, or dietary fiber is also a problem for some people.[17]

In response to concerns regarding disease patterns in the United States, a Senate Select Committee developed **Dietary Goals** for the United States. The first Dietary Goals were published and then quickly revised in 1977 (Appendix D). In response to criticisms that the Dietary Goals were not supported by sufficient scientific data, the USDA and Department of Health and Human Services (DHHS)

Dietary Goals Specific goals for nutrient intakes set in 1977 by a committee of the U.S. Senate.

published more general **Dietary Guidelines** in 1980, with slight revisions in 1985, 1990, and 1995.[18] The latest version of these guidelines is summarized as follows:

1. Eat a variety of foods.
2. Balance your food intake with physical activity; maintain or improve your weight.
3. Choose a diet with plenty of grain products, vegetables, and fruits.
4. Choose a diet low in fat, saturated fat, and cholesterol.
5. Choose a diet moderate in sugars.
6. Choose a diet moderate in salt and sodium.
7. If you drink alcoholic beverages, do so in moderation.

Dietary Guidelines General goals for nutrient intake and diet composition now set by the USDA and DHHS.

To interpret these general guidelines, consider the following points. Use the Food Guide Pyramid to obtain variety in your diet. Chaper 8 describes how to determine a desirable weight based on your current health status. A shortcut method is as follows: for women, 100 pounds plus 5 pounds for each inch over 60 inches in height; for men, 106 pounds plus 6 pounds for each inch over 60 inches. Most health authorities advise that total fat intake should be 30% or less of energy intake, and intake of saturated fat should be 10% or less of energy intake. Finally, a moderate alcohol intake consists of 2 or fewer servings of 12 ounces of beer, 5 oz of wine, or 1½ ounces of distilled spirits (80 proof) per day. Women are advised to limit alcohol to generally no more than 1 serving a day, as discussed in the Nutrition Focus.

The Dietary Guidelines refer to total intake over a day or week, not to a single meal or certain foods. Note also that the guidelines make no reference to protein intake. Rather, they seek to guide us away from the American bias toward high-fat meat and high-fat dairy products to lower-fat versions of these foods in order to moderate overall fat intake.

PRACTICAL USE OF THE DIETARY GUIDELINES

The Dietary Guidelines are published in the pamphlet *Nutrition and Your Health: Dietary Guidelines for Americans.*[18] The first guideline—eat a variety of foods—tries to ensure adequate vitamin and mineral intake. The other guidelines are intended to reduce the risk of obesity, hypertension, heart disease, diabetes, and alcoholism. The recommendations are not difficult to implement (Table 2-3). In addition, this overall diet approach is not inordinately expensive, as some people suspect. Fruits, vegetables, and low-fat and nonfat milk are no more costly than the chips, cookies, and soft drinks they should in part replace.

TABLE 2-3

Advice for applying the dietary guidelines to practical situations

You usually eat this:	Reconsider and eat this:
White bread	Whole-wheat bread (less nutrients lost in refinement/processing)
Sugared breakfast cereal	Low-sugar cereal (use the kilocalories you save for a side dish of fruit)
Cheeseburger and french fries	Hamburger (hold the mayonnaise) and baked beans (for less fat and cholesterol, and the benefits of plant proteins)
Potato salad at the salad bar	Three-bean salad
Doughnut, chips, salty snack foods	Bran muffin or bagel (no cream cheese)
Soft drinks	Diet soft drinks (save the kilocalories for more nutritious foods)
Boiled vegetables	Steamed vegetables (for more nutrient retention)
Canned vegetables	Frozen vegetables (less nutrients lost in processing)
Fried meats	Broiled meats (watch the fat drain away)
Fatty meats, like ribs	Lean meats, like ground round; also, eat chicken and fish often
Whole milk and ice cream	1% or nonfat milk and sherbet or frozen yogurt (to reduce saturated fat intake)
Mayonnaise or sour cream salad dressing	Oil and vinegar dressings, or diet varieties (to save kilocalories)
Cookies for a snack	Popcorn (air popped with minimal margarine)
Heavily salted foods	Foods flavored primarily with herbs, spices, and lemon juice

In Chapter 18 we will discuss diet recommendations for adults issued by other scientific groups. In essence, the current recommendations of the American Heart Association, U.S. Surgeon General, National Academy of Sciences, American Cancer Society, Canadian Ministries of Health (see Appendix E), and World Health Organization are consistent with the spirit of the Dietary Guidelines.[3,17] All of these groups encourage people to modify their eating behavior in ways that are both healthful and pleasurable.

Overall, we should combine concepts from the Food Guide Pyramid and the Dietary Guidelines. If your current diet diverges radically from what these plans recommend, try to make some appropriate changes (Table 2-4). There is no "optimal" diet.[10] Instead there are numerous healthful diets (Figure 2-3). The healthy eating habits that result from implementing the Food Guide Pyramid and Dietary Guidelines can pay you lifelong dividends in good health.[17]

LIMITATIONS OF THE DIETARY GUIDELINES

Some nutritionists are uneasy about the Dietary Guidelines. They think the plan is too general because it does not acknowledge that different individuals may need to strive for different dietary objectives. As we explain in later chapters, some individuals' health may be significantly affected by saturated fats, while others' is not; one person's health may be affected by a generous intake of sodium, while another's may not. As individuals, we vary in our tendencies to develop elevated serum cholesterol, hypertension, obesity, cancer, and other health problems that are linked to diet.[10] Genetic background is one key reason for the variation, as explained in Chapter 1. In addition, controversy exists over the harmfulness of sugar.

Even though the Food Guide Pyramid and the Dietary Guidelines provide

TABLE 2-4

What can we expect from a healthy diet?

Eating enough essential nutrients and meeting energy needs help prevent:
    Birth defects and low birth weight in pregnancy
    Poor growth and poor resistance to disease in infancy and childhood
    Poor resistance to disease in adult years
    Deficiency diseases, such as cretinism (lack of the mineral iodide), scurvy (lack of vitamin C), and anemia (lack of the mineral iron, the vitamin folate, or other nutrients)
Eating enough of the mineral calcium helps:
    Build bone mass in childhood and adolescent years
    Prevent some adult bone loss, especially in elderly years
Obtaining adequate intake of the mineral fluoride and minimizing sugar intake help prevent:
    Dental caries (decay)
Eating enough dietary fiber helps prevent:
    Digestive problems, such as constipation and possibly some forms of intestinal cancer
Eating enough vitamin A and related carotenoids in plants may help reduce:
    Susceptibility to some cancers
Moderating energy intake helps prevent:
    Obesity and related diseases, such as the major type of diabetes, hypertension, cancer, and premature heart disease
Limiting intake of the mineral sodium helps prevent:
    Hypertension and related diseases of the heart and kidney in susceptible people
Moderating intake of saturated fat and cholesterol helps prevent:
    Premature heart disease
Moderating use of vitamin and mineral supplements prevents:
    Most chances for nutrient toxicities

general rather than individual-specific diet recommendations, they are relevant and valuable for the vast majority of people.[5,23] In later chapters, we will see how to tailor diet planning for individuals with various specific needs and characteristics.

CONCEPT CHECK

Dietary guidelines have been set by a variety of private and government organizations. These guidelines are designed to reduce the risk of developing obesity, hypertension, diabetes, heart disease, and alcoholism. To do so, they first recommend eating a variety of foods, ideally by following the Food Guide Pyramid. They also recommend limiting energy intake to match energy output and moderating total fat, saturated fat, salt, sugar, and alcohol intake, while focusing more on fruits, vegetables, and grain products in daily diet planning.

Recommended Dietary Allowances (RDAs)

To evaluate a diet pattern based on the Food Guide Pyramid, we first need to know how frequently each nutrient should be consumed and how much represents a sufficient amount. People have puzzled over these questions for years. In fact, a major nutrition crisis arose when many men were rejected from military service during World War II because they had been adversely affected by inadequate diets earlier in their lives. In response to this health problem, the first Food and Nutrition Board was formed in 1940. Assigned the task of establishing dietary standards that could be used to evaluate nutritional intakes of large population groups and to provide guidelines for planning agriculture production, this board developed the first **Recommended Dietary Allowances (RDAs),** published in 1941.

PROCESS FOR SETTING NUTRIENT RDAs

Because the original RDAs were based on limited scientific information, they have been revised as new information became available. Generally the RDAs are revised every 4 to 5 years. To establish a new RDA or to reevaluate an existing one, the Food and Nutrition Board follows a four-step process[8]:

1. Determines the average physiological **requirement** for a nutrient for a given population group and the **variability** in the requirement among members of the group based on published scientific studies. Population groups are typically defined by gender and age, and sometimes by other characteristics.
2. Increases the average requirement by amounts sufficient to meet the needs of nearly all members of the given population. This usually means increasing the av-

Recommended Dietary Allowances (RDAs)   Recommended intakes of nutrients that meet the needs of almost all healthy people of similar age and gender. RDAs are established by the Food and Nutrition Board of the National Academy of Sciences.

requirement   The amount of a nutrient required by one person to maintain health. This varies among individuals. No one knows his or her true requirements for various nutrients.

variability   Differences in parameter, such as a nutrient requirement, among individuals within a population group.

FRANK & ERNEST ® by Bob Thaves

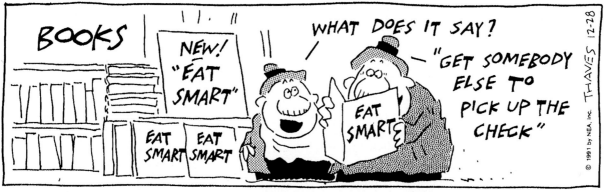

Figure 2-3 Frank & Ernest.

HOW TO FIND RELIABLE NUTRITION INFORMATION

SUSAN CALVERT FINN, Ph.D., R.D.

Here in America, as we prepare to enter the twenty-first century, you can roam the information highway on your computer. You can scan a dazzling variety of CD-ROMs. You can receive information via fax or, of course, on television, on the radio, and through the "old-fashioned" channels of communication—newspapers, magazines, books, and conversation.

But proliferation of information doesn't mean increased accuracy or consistency, particularly in nutrition. Almost daily, Americans are asked to judge the reliability of reports, studies, and news releases that often seem contradictory. We are told that our diets should contain low fat, no fat, some fat. We've been advised to drink wine and to avoid wine. The virtues of antioxidants, vitamins, and minerals are extolled and refuted. We've witnessed the Great Olive Oil and the Great Oat Bran debates. "Experts" advise gimmicks and gadgets, pills and potions. As the traveling medicine men of the nineteenth century liked to say, whatever is being sold is good for what ails you.

UNRELIABLE NUTRITION INFORMATION

The reason for the explosion of nutrition information is relatively simple: everyone wants to be healthy, and everyone wants to have a long and productive life. Consequently, health and nutrition are a multibillion dollar business. And where the dollar stakes are high, there are always unscrupulous players.

In November 1994, *USA Today* reported a Gallup survey revealing that 56% of Americans get their nutrition information from the media, 32% from physicians, and 31% from family or friends. These numbers indicate that more than two thirds of us are getting nutrition information from sources who may be untrained or unqualified. No wonder there is confusion.

Another survey, by Ira Milner, R.D., published in the May/June 1994 issue of *Nutrition Forum,* reported alarming news. Milner found that in 32 states "consumers had less than a fifty-fifty chance of finding a reliable 'nutritionist'" through the yellow pages of the phone book. The study further stated that "of the 618 entrants listed under the heading 'Nutritionists,' 358 (58%) [had] either spurious or suspicious [qualifications]. Sixty-three percent of the ads and boxed listings under this heading were for bogus nutritionists. . ." These "experts" had degrees from correspondence schools or diploma mills or were using invalid regimens and diagnostic methods.

SOUND NUTRITION INFORMATION

With all of these pitfalls, where and how do you find legitimate experts—true professionals who offer valid diagnoses and prescribe safe and effective nutrition programs? A number of avenues are available. If you have access to an accredited university, you may be able to obtain current and authoritative information from faculty members, particularly those who teach nutrition, dietetics, health, or medicine. Similarly, many hospital dietetics departments can be valuable references.

Most public, private, and school libraries stock nutrition books by experts on topics you are researching. But be aware that appearing in print does not necessarily make information credible. With all sources, it is essential to authenticate the background and training of the practitioner before accepting the material. A string of initials after a name does not automatically mean that the person is qualified. As we saw in Ira Milner's survey, a putative college degree is no guarantee of expertise or reliability. Even a legitimate degree may be misleading: a Ph.D. in mathematics, for example, is irrelevant to nutrition.

It also is important to look out for danger signals, which include an overemphasis on "magic" pills or "unique" apparatuses; heavy reliance on testimonials from people you don't know and who may not even exist; departure from established and legitimate medical practices; performance of strange procedures, such as hair analysis or eye color tests; and sale of vitamins or other items in the office.

The usual consumer warning is appropriate: if it sounds too good to be true, be cautious. If you have questions or doubts you can't resolve, check with recognized authorities or with organizations such as the American Dietetic Association (ADA) or the National Council Against Health Fraud (Figure 2-4).

THE REGISTERED DIETITIAN

The most dependable source for up-to-date, accurate nutrition data is a registered dietitian (R.D.). Registered dietitians are health-care professionals who are rigorously trained in a single specialty—nutrition science. Their goal is to promote health and fight illness by fostering the practice of proper nutrition. Through the ADA, R.D.s are the most reliable disseminators of educational and informational material on food and nutrition.*

An R.D. analyzes each patient's situation, taking into account such factors as medical history, lifestyle, and eating habits, and tailors specific regimens to meet those unique needs. Because R.D.s do not make medical diagnoses, the patient is encouraged to consult a physician regularly.

What is it about registered dietitians that makes them so qualified? A registered dietitian has a bachelor's degree in food and nutrition from an accredited university, has had thorough and extensive professional practice under expert supervision, and has passed a comprehensive examination. There are over 65,000 registered dietitians in the United States, and they can be identified by the letters *R.D.* after their names.

More than half of all states license dietitians. Unfortunately, in the other states anyone with no training, experience, license, or specific qualifications can call himself or herself a dietitian or nutritionist. But only a person who meets the qualifications listed above can use the designation "registered dietitian," which indicates that the practitioner is a trained, reputable expert who is educated in nutrition science and has both practical and theoretical experience.

As you seek nutrition information, you would do well to follow these guidelines. Keep in mind that availability doesn't mean accuracy, and abundance doesn't mean reliability. A good measure of common sense, sound research, and thorough verification of references and credentials will ensure that you have chosen an accurate and reliable source of information. Most health-care professionals are readily available and willing to answer questions or provide information. The benefits you will receive are well worth the extra effort required to secure their advice.

Dr. Finn is the Director of Nutrition Services for Ross Laboratories, a leading research facility and manufacturer of scientifically formulated nutritional products. She is past president of the American Dietetic Association and co-author of The Real Life Nutrition Book *(Penguin Books, 1992).*

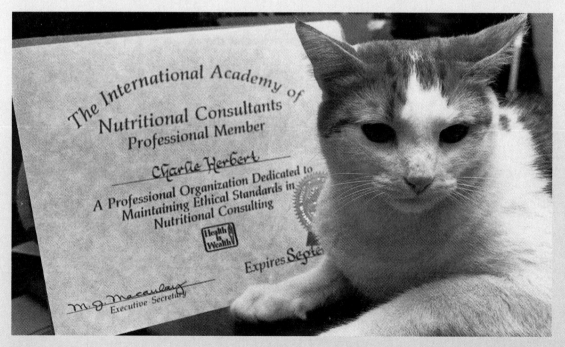

Figure 2-4 Consumers need to be wary of people with credentials from "diploma mills." Charlie Herbert (the cat) is a nutrition consultant, according to the diploma purchased by his owner. Seek out a true nutrition professional for dietary advice—a registered dietitian (R.D.).

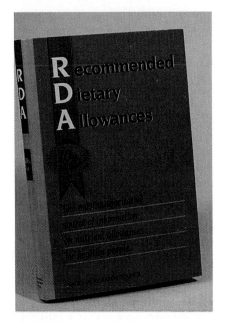

Figure 2-5 The 1989 RDAs are contained in a publication that incorporates much supporting evidence and discussion of the various nutrient recommendations made by the Food and Nutrition Board of the National Academy of Sciences.

erage requirement by approximately 30% to 50%. Thus, if the average requirement for a vitamin is 20 mg/day, the RDA may be 28 mg/day, or 40% higher than the average value.

3. Increases the RDA to account for inefficient use of the nutrient once consumed. This inefficiency could result from limited absorption, poor conversion of an inactive to an active form, or other causes.

4. Uses scientific judgment to interpret and establish allowances when information about requirements is limited. In other words, the members of the Food and Nutrition Board need to use their scientific judgment in lieu of specific scientific data in certain cases.

The RDAs for protein and various vitamins and minerals have been set for males and females in various age groups, as well as for pregnant and lactating women. These values are listed on the inside cover of this book. Note that the RDAs are based on the assumption that we meet our nutrient needs from a diet containing a variety of foods, which also meets our energy needs.[8] This proviso is important because RDAs have been developed for only 19 of approximately 40 important nutrients—not counting essential amino acids in proteins. Not enough is known about many nutrients for the Food and Nutrition Board to establish an RDA. However, all essential nutrients should be part of the diet, and the RDAs can serve as a guide for meeting these nutritional needs (Figure 2-5).

USES OF THE RDAs

One common misconception is that the *D* in RDA stands for daily. It does not; it stands for *dietary*. It is not necessary to consume the RDA for each nutrient every day. Think instead of averaging the RDAs for vitamins and minerals over a week's time. No nutrient need be consumed every day. A typical adult can survive for a few days to a week on a diet free of water, for months without any vitamin A, and for about 1 to 3 years on a diet without vitamin B-12. Notice also that the *R* in RDA stands for *recommended*, not *required*.

Because the RDAs are based on average requirements increased to account for variability in the population and for inefficient use, they are by definition generous allowances. The RDAs are set high enough so that healthy people are not expected to show any improvement in health if they consume more than RDA amounts.[8] In other words, the RDAs generally confer any possible benefit that may be achieved from the nutrients obtainable in a typical diet. Potential positive effects from nutrient intakes well above what can be obtained from food are medical or pharmacological in nature. The RDAs do not address these uses of nutrients, although they show efficacy in clinical practice in a limited number of diseases. We will discuss this topic further in Chapters 4, 12, and 13.

A key goal of developing and using RDAs is to protect Americans from receiving either too much or too little of needed nutrients; the RDA guidelines provide good protection against both possibilities. Too often, people think that if a little of something is good, a lot must be better.[12] This can lead to toxicity with some nutrients.

Thus the RDAs are estimates of the amount of each nutrient that should be consumed by healthy people to meet their nutritional needs. The word *healthy* needs emphasis. The RDAs are only applicable to people who are not taking medications or suffering from diseases that increase nutrient needs, are not experiencing temperature extremes, and do not participate in long, strenuous physical activity.[8]

Because of the way they are set, RDAs are most relevant to nutritional activities involving population groups, not individuals. Activities in which the RDAs are valuable and correctly used include the following:

• Planning and obtaining food supplies for population groups, such as schools, college dormitories, hospitals, and health-care facilities

• Establishing standards for food assistance programs, such as the USDA Thrifty Food Plan

• Evaluating dietary survey data, such as NHANES, and other scientific research

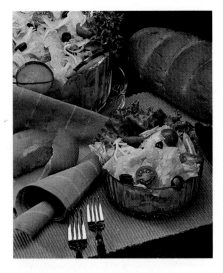

Meet Recommended Dietary Allowances with foods, not supplements.

- Developing food and nutrition information and education programs, such as those provided by federal food assistance programs
- Establishing food-labeling standards, such as the Daily Values that appear as part of the Nutrition Facts panel on food labels
- Regulating food fortification, such as setting standard fortification policies for enriched bread, milk, and infant formulas
- Developing new or modified food products, such as rations used by soldiers in military combat and by astronauts in space

A CLOSE LOOK AT THE RDAs, USING PROTEIN AS AN EXAMPLE

The RDA for protein is 0.8 g per kilogram of desirable body weight per day for an adult. This intake should provide more than enough protein to maintain an adult in a state of protein **equilibrium,** which exists when daily protein intake and daily protein losses are equal. Based on the protein RDA, a man weighing 70 kg should consume 50 to 60 g of protein daily (0.8 × 70 kg = 56). For this calculation to yield a realistic intake value, the protein RDA must provide enough protein to meet body losses and to maintain the limited protein stores in the body (Figure 2-6). Thus the overall economy of protein in the body should remain stable.

In setting the protein intakes for children, the RDA must provide enough protein to meet daily losses and maintain possible stores, plus some extra protein to accommodate growth and storage in new tissue that is built each day. The protein RDAs for children thus attempt to promote a **positive balance.** Equilibrium is not good enough because children need to lay down new tissue protein. Children should regularly consume a greater amount of protein than they lose. The same is true for pregnant women and for people recovering from significant injury or illness.

Because the RDAs are generous and are based on average nutrient requirements for population groups, many people meet their individual nutrient needs when they eat less than the various RDAs.[11] For example, if you estimate the amount of protein you consume in a week, take a daily average, compare it with the RDA, and discover that your intake is close to the RDA, fine. You are most likely consuming sufficient protein to meet your needs. However, if you take in much less protein than

equilibrium A state in which nutrient intake equals nutrient losses, so that the body maintains a stable condition.

- - - - - - - - - - - -

Different methods are used for determining needs for various other nutrients. One alternative approach is to consume a diet that causes depletion of stores of a specific nutrient and then determine how much of that nutrient is required to regain adequate nutrient status.

- - - - - - - - - - - -

positive balance A state in which intake of a nutrient exceeds losses, causing a net gain of the nutrient in the body. This occurs when tissue protein is gained during growth. The opposite is negative balance, when losses exceed intake, as in cases of starvation.

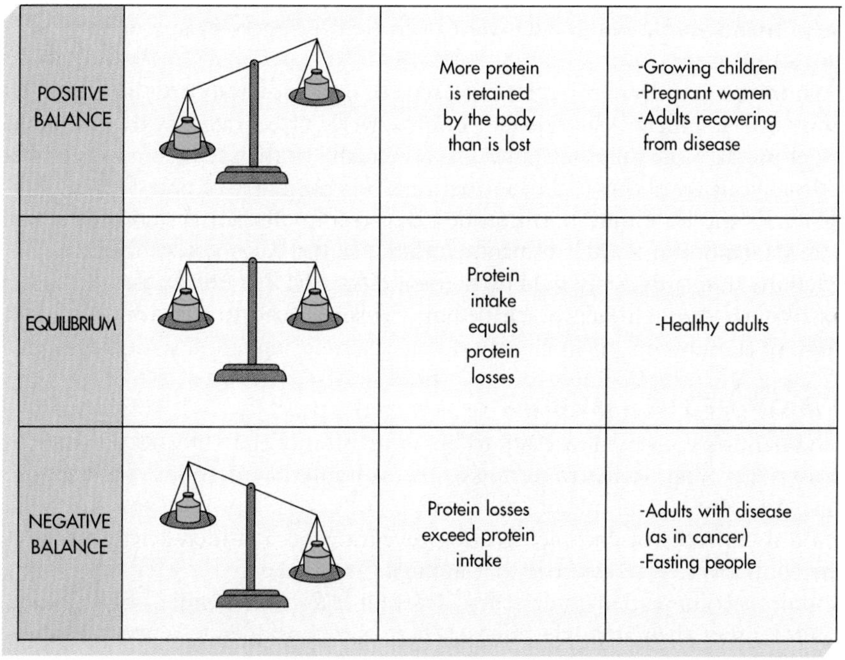

POSITIVE BALANCE	More protein is retained by the body than is lost	-Growing children -Pregnant women -Adults recovering from disease
EQUILIBRIUM	Protein intake equals protein losses	-Healthy adults
NEGATIVE BALANCE	Protein losses exceed protein intake	-Adults with disease (as in cancer) -Fasting people

Figure 2-6 Nutrient balance, using protein as an example. The concepts of positive balance, equilibrium, and negative balance apply to the health status of a person with respect to all nutrients.

the RDA suggests, you do not know whether you are eating enough protein for your individual needs. It is likely you need less than the RDA.[8] But the farther you stray from an RDA, the greater your risk for nutritional deficiency. Based on statistical theory, when you are consuming less than 50% of an RDA, it is likely that you are not consuming enough of that nutrient.

As we saw in Chapter 1, signs and symptoms of nutritional deficiencies may be subtle and develop slowly. Although your diet may be inadequate, you may show no telltale signs, such as insufficient bone strength from a chronic calcium deficiency, for a long time. No "smoke detector" will sound an alarm. For this reason, even though your individual nutrient needs may be less than the RDAs, it is best to eat a diet that meets this standard for your age and gender, rather than run the risk of developing health problems from an inadequate nutrient intake.

RDAs FOR ENERGY NEEDS

RDAs for nutrients are set high enough to meet the needs of almost all healthy people. In contrast, the Food and Nutrition Board sets the RDAs for energy at the average needs for various age groups (see inside cover). Note that no extra amount is added for human variability, as is done for nutrient RDAs.[8] Unlike most vitamins and minerals, excess energy consumed (above energy needs) is not excreted. Thus, to promote weight maintenance, a more conservative standard must be set for energy needs than for nutrient needs. The board also warns that the energy RDA is only a rough estimate, because energy needs depend on energy use. For most adults, obtaining and maintaining a desirable weight is the best yardstick of energy balance—energy intake matching energy output.

Other Nutrient Standards Set by the Food and Nutrition Board

In addition to the RDAs, the Food and Nutrition Board sets two other types of numerical standards for certain nutrients.

Estimated Safe and Adequate Daily Dietary Intakes (ESADDIs) have been established for several nutrients, including copper, biotin, and chromium (see inside cover). The board determined that insufficient data were available to set RDAs for these nutrients, but enough data were available to suggest a range for a reasonable intake for groups.[8]

Minimum requirements, the third type of numerical standard, have been set for sodium, potassium, and chloride (see inside cover). These values represent minimum nutrient needs. Note that these amounts are much less than typical intakes of sodium or chloride but are about equal to Americans' typical intake of potassium.[8]

To date, the Food and Nutrition Board has set no numerical standards for carbohydrates, fats, boron, nickel, and some other essential nutrients. Nonetheless, if you meet all the standards established by the board (i.e., RDAs, ESADDIs, and minimum requirements) through diet, not with nutrient supplements, then you should obtain enough of all nutrients, including those for which no numerical standards exist.

REVISION OF THE 1989 RDAs

When scientists convened in 1993 to begin revision of the 1989 RDAs, they began discussing new approaches to setting RDAs. Among the questions raised are the following [4,14,16]:

- Should concepts of chronic disease prevention be considered when developing the allowances, such as those for vitamins C and E?
- Should recommended intakes for different ages and genders be expressed as ranges rather than as single values? There was considerable support for presenting the revised RDAs as ranges of intake—such as likely deficient, RDA, and upper safe amount—rather than as a single value, as is currently done.
- Should separate RDAs be set for elderly people? Currently there is a category for age 51 and older for each gender.

Estimated Safe and Adequate Daily Dietary Intakes (ESADDIs) Nutrient intake recommendations first made in 1980 by the Food and Nutrition Board for certain nutrients for which not enough information is available to establish RDAs. The recommendations specify an intake range, rather than a single value, for each nutrient.

- Should RDAs for carbohydrate, total fat, and dietary fiber be set?

Work is continuing on the revision. Ask your professor whether new information is available.

World Nutrient Standards

Many countries have set numerical standards for various nutrients. These nutrient recommendations are set by different groups of scientists and may differ slightly from country to country. This is illustrated by Table 2-5, which compares some recent energy and nutrient standards developed in the United States, the United Kingdom, Canada, and Japan, as well as those published by the Food and Agriculture Organization and the World Health Organization (FAO/WHO) of the United Nations. Some of the variation in nutrient standards can be explained by differences in protein intake in different populations worldwide, which can lead to varying vitamin and mineral needs. The Canadian standards, called Recommended Nutrient Intakes (RNIs), are shown in more detail in Appendix E.

CONCEPT CHECK

Recommended Dietary Allowances represent the nutrient needs of groups, not of individuals. RDAs are established for specific age and gender categories. No one knows his or her own nutritional requirements; the best general rule is that the farther you stray from the RDAs for your age and gender, the greater your chance of having a nutritional deficiency.

TABLE 2-5

Dietary standards for adult males and adult females (over 24 years of age): United States (1989), United Kingdom (1991), Canada (1990), Japan (1991), and FAO/WHO (1957-1989)

Classification	Energy (kcal)	Protein (g)	Calcium (mg)	Iron (mg)	Vitamin A (RE†)	Thiamin (mg)	Riboflavin (mg)	Vitamin C (mg)
United States								
Female (63 kg, 1.63 m)	2200	50	800	15	800	1.1	1.3	60
Male (79 kg, 1.76 m)	2900	63	800	10	1000	1.5	1.7	60
United Kingdom								
Female	1940	45	700	15	600	0.8	1.1	40
Male	2550	56	700	9	700	1.0	1.3	40
Canada								
Female (59 kg)	1900	51	700	13	800	0.8	1.0	30*
Male (74 kg)	2700	64	800	9	1000	1.1	1.4	40*
Japan								
Female (low activity)	1800	60	600	12	400	0.7	1.0	50
Male (low activity)	2250	70	600	10	400	0.9	1.2	50
FAO/WHO								
Female (65 kg)	2300	49	400-500	14-28	500	0.9	1.3	30
Male (75 kg)	2900	56	400-500	5-9	600	1.2	1.8	30

*Nonsmoker; smoker, 50% higher
†Retinal Equivalents
Modified from Shils ME and others, editors: *Modern nutrition in health and disease*, ed 8, Philadelphia, 1994, Lea & Febiger.

Daily Values: The Standards for Food Labeling

The RDAs are not used in food labeling, since they are age and gender specific. We can't have different packages for men and women or for teens and adults. The Food and Drug Administration (FDA) has developed a set of generic standards, called **Daily Values,** that are used to express the nutrient content of foods for the Nutrition Facts panel on food labels. The content of a particular nutrient is listed on labels as a percentage of its Daily Value.[13]

The Daily Values are based on two sets of dietary standards. The first, **Reference Daily Intakes (RDIs),** replaced the term *U.S. Recommended Daily Allowances* (US RDAs) as a label reference value for vitamins and minerals. The second, **Daily Reference Values (DRVs),** are standards for protein and for various dietary components that have no RDA (e.g., total fat, cholesterol, and dietary fiber). These two terms—Reference Daily Intakes and Daily Reference Values—do not appear on labels. To make label reading less confusing for consumers, the term Daily Value is used to represent the combination of these two sets of dietary standards.[13]

REFERENCE DAILY INTAKES (RDIs)

Reference Daily Intakes (RDIs) make up the majority of the Daily Values. The RDIs were determined by the FDA using a compilation of the RDA values published in 1968.[13] Essentially, RDIs were set as the highest RDA values within specific age categories. For example, consider iron: in 1968 the RDA for adult men was 10 mg/day, and that for adult women and adolescents was 18 mg/day. The iron RDI for adults is the higher value: 18 mg/day. Table 2-6 lists RDI values for people over 4 years of age.

Four versions of the RDIs exist, one for each of the following groups: (1) people over 4 years of age, (2) infants less than 1 year of age, (3) children 1 to 4 years

Daily Values A set of standard nutrient-intake values developed by the FDA and used as a reference for expressing nutrient content on nutrition labels. The Daily Values include two types of standards—RDIs and DRVs.

Reference Daily Intakes (RDIs) Nutrient-intake standards set by the FDA based on the 1968 RDAs for various vitamins and minerals. RDIs have been set for four categories of people: infants, toddlers, people over 4 years of age, and pregnant or lactating women. Generally, the highest RDA value in each category is used as the RDI. The RDIs constitute part of the Daily Values used in food labeling.

Daily Reference Values (DRVs) Nutrient-intake standards established for protein and for some other dietary components lacking an RDA including fat, saturated fat, cholesterol, carbohydrate, dietary fiber, sodium, and potassium. The DRVs for cholesterol, sodium, and potassium are constant; those for the other nutrients increase as energy intake increases. The DRVs constitute part of the Daily Values used in food labeling.

TABLE 2-6

Comparison of Reference Daily Intakes (RDIs) with 1989 RDAs*

Nutrient	Unit of measure	RDI for people over 4 years of age	RDA (or ESADDI) Males 19 years old	RDA (or ESADDI) Females 19 years old
Vitamin A	Retinol Equivalents	1000	1000	800
Vitamin D	International Units	400	400	400
Vitamin E	"	30	10	8
Vitamin C	milligrams	60	60	60
Folate	"	0.4	0.200	0.180
Thiamin	"	1.5	1.5	1.1
Riboflavin	"	1.7	1.7	1.3
Niacin	"	20	19	15
Vitamin B-6	"	2	2	1.6
Vitamin B-12	micrograms	6	2	2
Biotin	milligrams	0.3	0.03-0.1	0.03-0.1
Pantothenic acid	"	10	4-7	4-7
Calcium	grams	1	1.2	1.2
Phosphorus	"	1	1.2	1.2
Iodide	micrograms	150	150	150
Iron	milligrams	18	10	15
Magnesium	"	400	350	280
Copper	"	2	1.5-3.0	1.5-3.0
Zinc	"	15	15	12

*RDI values are based on the 1968 RDAs and constitute the Daily Values used as reference standards for food labeling. Note that the RDIs for many nutrients are higher than the most recent RDAs.

of age (toddlers), and (4) pregnant and lactating (breastfeeding) women. Most nutrition labels that list Daily Values use the version of the RDIs for people over 4 years of age as the reference value for expressing nutrient content. Labels for infant formulas use Daily Values based on the infant RDIs; those for "junior" baby foods use Daily Values based on the "toddler" RDIs; and those for vitamin supplements designed for pregnant women use Daily Values based on the RDIs designed for pregnant and lactating women.

As shown in Table 2-6, the RDI values currently in use, which are based on the 1968 RDAs, generally are slightly higher than 1989 RDAs. An example is the above-mentioned adult RDI for iron. Even though the highest RDA value for iron—that for adult women—was 15 mg/day in 1989, the RDI still uses the earlier value of 18 mg/day of iron for all adults. Therefore, when you read a cereal label that claims a serving provides 25% of the Daily Value for a vitamin or mineral, you can be sure that it will provide at least 25% of the RDA for your age and gender, if the nutrient has an RDA. This is especially true for vitamin E, vitamin B-12, and folate because current RDAs are lower than those of 1968. Your individual need, if it is different from the Daily Value, will probably be lower. An exception is calcium for the age group 11 to 24 years; the RDI and, hence, Daily Value is 200 mg lower than the current RDA.

Although many scientists support revision of the RDIs based on the 1989 RDAs, some scientists and the vitamin industry in general oppose revision, which would reduce many RDIs.[19] Some opponents believe that the public generally under-consumes some of the nutrients covered (e.g., vitamin E). Since the amounts of nutrients added to "fortified" foods, such as breakfast cereals, are related to the RDI values, reduction of these values might have health consequences for some consumers. Revision of the RDIs also would reduce the market for the vitamins and minerals used in fortification, with unfavorable economic consequences for supplement manufacturers. It is unclear which group's interests and opinion will prevail.

DAILY REFERENCE VALUES (DRVs)

The Daily Values for some food constituents are based on Daily Reference Values (DRVs) rather than RDIs. Except for the protein DRV, which is based on RDA values, the other DRVs cover certain dietary components that have no true RDA: total fat, saturated fatty acids, cholesterol, carbohydrate, fiber, sodium, and potassium (Table 2-7). The DRVs are intended to help consumers evaluate their food choices by comparing their actual intakes of these food constituents with desirable (or maximum) intakes.[20]

Standards set for nutrients that have RDAs, called RDIs

Standards set for many nutrients that do not have RDAs, called DRVs

Daily Values consist of RDI and DRV standards for use in the Nutrition Facts panel of food labels

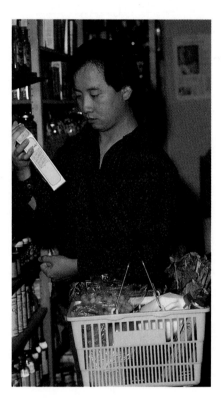

Nutrient content in foods is expressed on the nutrition label in terms of Daily Values.

TABLE 2-7

Daily Reference Values (DRVs)*

Food component	Unit of measure	DRV (2000 kcal intake)	DRV (2500 kcal intake)
Fat	grams	<65	<80
Saturated fatty acids	grams	<20	<25
Protein	grams	50	65
Cholesterol	milligrams	<300	<300
Carbohydrate	grams	300	375
Fiber	grams	25	30
Sodium	milligrams	<2400	<2400
Potassium	milligrams	3500	3500

*DRVs based on an energy intake of 2000 kcal constitute the Daily Values used as reference standards for food labeling. The DRVs for some nutrients (e.g., total fat) increase as energy intake increases.

Daily Values in Perspective

The Nutrition Facts panel on the label of a food product lists various components of the food as a percentage of their Daily Values. Except for the special products mentioned already, the Daily Values used are for people over 4 years of age. Suppose, for example, that 1 serving of a macaroni and cheese product contains 15% of the Daily Value for iron. Since the Daily Value for iron is 18 mg, this product contains about 3 mg of iron per serving (18 mg $\times$ 0.15 = 2.7 mg). The Nutrition Perspective at the end of this chapter describes nutrition labels on foods in detail.

Nutrient Density

As we've seen already, the RDAs are used for planning and evaluating complete diets of groups of individuals. However, these nutrient standards aren't useful for assessing the nutritional quality of an individual food. For this purpose, the concept of **nutrient density** has gained acceptance in recent years.

To determine the nutrient density of a food, simply compare its vitamin or mineral content with the number of kilocalories it provides. The higher a food's nutrient density, the better it is as a nutrient source. Comparing the nutrient density of different foods is an easy way to estimate their relative nutritional quality. Generally, nutrient density is assessed with respect to individual nutrients. For example, many fruits and vegetables have a high content of vitamin C compared with their energy content: that is, they are nutrient-dense foods for vitamin C.

Menu planning focuses on the total diet—not on selection of one critical food as key to an adequate diet. Nonetheless, nutrient-dense foods—such as skim and low-fat milk, lean meats, beans, oranges, carrots, broccoli, whole-wheat bread, and whole-grain breakfast cereals—do help balance less nutrient-dense foods—such as cookies and potato chips—that many people like to eat. The latter are often called empty-calorie foods because they tend to supply energy as sugar and/or fat, but few other nutrients.

nutrient density The ratio formed by dividing a food's contribution to nutrient needs by its contribution to energy needs. When the contribution to nutrient needs exceeds its energy contribution, the food is considered to have a favorable nutrient density.

CRITICAL THINKING

Your classmate John is having trouble understanding the concept of nutrient density. How would you show him that nonfat (skim) milk is more "nutrient dense" than whole milk?

CONCEPT CHECK

Daily Values are currently used as a benchmark for representing the nutrient content of foods on nutrition labels. Nutrient content is expressed as percentages of the Daily Values, which in turn are based on Reference Daily Intakes (RDIs) or Daily Reference Values (DRVs). The RDIs for vitamins and minerals constitute the majority of Daily Values; the current RDIs are based on the 1968 RDAs. The DRVs have been set for protein and for some nutrients that don't have an RDA, such as fat, cholesterol, and dietary fiber. To decrease confusion, the Daily Value is the only term that appears on food labels. Nutrient density is a measure of the nutrient contributions made by each food compared with its total energy content. Nutrient-dense foods supply much of one or many nutrients while providing a modest amount of energy.

The Exchange System: Another Menu-Planning Tool

The **Exchange System** is a valuable tool for quickly estimating the energy, protein, carbohydrate, and fat content of a food or meal. Although learning to use the Exchange System is a bit tedious, much like learning a foreign language, it greatly simplifies menu planning. The Exchange System organizes many details of the nutrient composition of foods into a manageable framework. By using the Exchange System, you can plan daily menus without having to look up or memorize the nutrient values of numerous foods. So the time you spend now becoming familiar with the Exchange System will pay dividends in the future. In the Exchange System, individual foods are placed into three broad groups: carbohydrate, meat and meat substitutes, and fat. Within these groups are lists that contain foods of similar macronutrient composition: various types of milk; fruit; vegetables; starch; other carbohydrates;

Exchange System A system for classifying foods into numerous lists based on their macronutrient composition and establishing serving sizes so that 1 serving of each food on a list contains the same amount of carbohydrate, protein, fat, and energy (kilocalories).

- - - - - - - - - -

The Exchange System arranges foods based on nutrient composition, not origin.

- - - - - - - - - -

various types of meat and meat substitutes; and fat. These lists are designed so that when the proper serving size is observed, each food on a list provides about the same amount of carbohydrate, protein, fat, and energy. This equality allows the exchange of foods on each list. Hence the term *Exchange System.*

The Exchange System was originally developed for planning diabetic diets. Diabetes is easier to control if the person's diet has about the same composition day after day. If a certain number of **"exchanges"** from each of the various lists is eaten each day, that regularity is easier to achieve. However, because the Exchange System provides a quick way to estimate the energy, carbohydrate, protein, and fat content in any food or meal, it is a valuable menu-planning tool.

exchange The serving size of a food on a specific exchange list.

BECOMING FAMILIAR WITH THE EXCHANGE SYSTEM

To use the Exchange System, you must know which foods are on each list and the serving sizes for each food.

Table 2-8 gives the serving sizes for foods on each exchange list, as well as the carbohydrate, protein, fat, and energy content per exchange. Note that the meat and milk lists are divided into subclasses that vary in fat content and hence in the number of kilocalories they provide. Foods on the meat and fat lists contain essentially no carbohydrate; those on the fruit and fat lists lack appreciable amounts of protein; and those on the vegetable, fruit, and other carbohydrates lists contain no fat. You need to study Table 2-8 to become familiar with the sizes of the exchanges (i.e., serving sizes) on each list and the amounts of carbohydrate, protein, fat, and energy per exchange.

Before you can turn a group of exchanges into a daily meal plan, you must be aware of which foods are on each exchange list (Figure 2-7). The entire U.S. Exchange System is presented in Appendix F, which you should consult frequently while exploring the system to discover its various peculiarities. For example, the starch list includes not only bread, dry cereal, cooked cereal, rice, and pasta, but also baked beans, corn on the cob, and potatoes. These foods are not identical to those composing the bread, cereal, rice, and pasta group in the Food Guide Pyramid. The

TABLE 2-8

Nutrient composition of Exchange System lists (1995 edition)

Groups/lists	Household measures*	Carbohydrate (g)	Protein (g)	Fat (g)	Energy (kcal)
Carbohydrate group					
Starch	1 slice, ¾ cup raw, or ½ cup cooked	15	3	1 or less†	80
Fruit	1 small/medium piece	15	—	—	60
Milk	1 cup				
Skim/very low-fat		12	8	0–3†	90
Low-fat		12	8	5	120
Whole		12	8	8	150
Other carbohydrates	Varies	15	Varies	Varies	Varies
Vegetables	1 cup raw or ½ cup cooked	5	2	—	25
Meat and meat substitutes group	1 oz				
Very lean		—	7	0–1	35
Lean		—	7	3	55
Medium-fat		—	7	5	75
High-fat		—	7	8	100
Fat group	1 tsp	—	—	5	45

The American Diabetes Association and American Dietetic Association: *Exchange lists for meal planning,* 1995.
*Just an estimate. See exchange lists for actual amounts.
†Calculated as 1 g for purposes of energy contribution.

Starch exchange choices

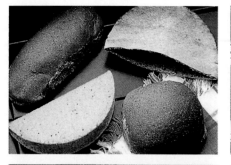

Meat and meat substitutes exchange choices

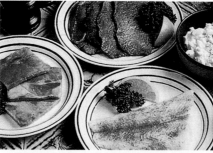

Vegetable exchange choices

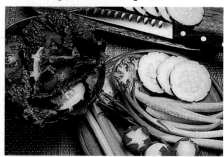

Fruit exchange choices

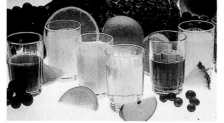

Milk exchange choices

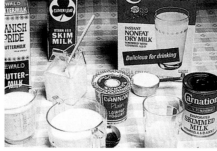

Fat exchange choices

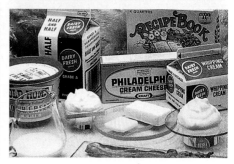

Figure 2-7 Foods arranged according to the Exchange System lists.

Exchange System is not concerned with the origin of a food, whether animal or vegetable. It is primarily concerned with the macronutrients carbohydrate, protein, and fat in each food on a specific list. For example, the carbohydrate composition of potatoes resembles that of bread more than that of broccoli, although potatoes are vegetables.

The very lean–meat list contains the white meat of chicken and turkey (without skin), water-packed tuna, shrimp, nonfat cottage cheese, and fat-free cheese. The lean-meat list contains round steak, lean ham, veal, the dark meat of chicken and turkey (without skin), fish, cottage cheese, and low-fat luncheon meat. The medium-fat meat list contains T-bone steak, pork loin roast, lamb rib roast, any fried fish, mozzarella cheese, and eggs. The high-fat meat list contains ribs, sausage, most luncheon meats (full fat), cheddar cheese, and peanut butter. Note that several foods on the meat and meat substitutes list are not meats, again demonstrating that origin is not important in classifying foods in the Exchange System.

The vegetable list contains most vegetables, but some starchy vegetables are on the starch list. Most vegetables, such as cabbage, celery, mushrooms, lettuce, and zucchini, can be considered "free foods"; their minimal energy contribution need not count in the calculations when they are eaten in moderation (1 to 2 servings per meal or snack). The fruit list contains fruits and fruit juices. The list of other carbohydrates includes jam, angelfood cake, fat-free frozen yogurt, and foods such as frosted cake that count as both other carbohydrate exchanges and fat exchanges.

The milk exchange list contains milk, plain yogurt, and buttermilk. The amount of fat in a product determines whether the serving is skim/very low fat, low fat, or whole.

The fat list contains margarine, mayonnaise, nuts and seeds, salad oils, olives, and full-fat sour cream and cream cheese. Bacon is listed as a fat, rather than as a high-fat meat.

Free foods, other than a moderate intake of most vegetables, include bouillon, diet soda, coffee, tea, dill pickles, and vinegar, as well as herbs and spices.

USING THE EXCHANGE SYSTEM TO DEVELOP DAILY MENUS

Now let's use the Exchange System to plan a 1-day menu. We will target an energy content of 2000 kcal, with 55% coming from carbohydrates (1100 kcal), 15% from

TABLE 2-9

Possible exchange patterns that yield 55% of energy as carbohydrate; 30% as fat; and 15% as protein for energy intakes ≥2000 kcal

kcal/day	1200*	1600*	2000	2400	2800	3200	3600
Exchange list							
Milk (low fat)	2	2	2	2	2	2	2
Vegetable	3	3	3	4	4	4	4
Fruit	3	4	5	6	8	9	9
Starch	4	7	10	12	14	16	19
Meat (medium fat)	4	4	3	5	6	7	8
Fat	2	4	8	8	9	11	14

This is just one set of options. More meat could be included if less milk is used, for example.
*Energy intakes of 1200 and 1600 kcal contain 19% of energy as protein and less carbohydrate to allow for greater flexibility in diet planning.

TABLE 2-10

Sample 1-day menu based on the Exchange System plan*

Breakfast
1 low-fat milk exchange	1 cup 2% milk (put some on cereal)
2 fruit exchanges	1 cup orange juice
2 starch exchanges	¾ cup cold cereal, 1 piece whole-wheat toast
1 fat exchange	1 tsp margarine on toast

Lunch
4 starch exchanges	2 slices whole-wheat bread, 16 animal cookies
4 fat exchanges	2 slices bacon, 2 tsp mayonnaise
1 vegetable exchange	1 sliced tomato
2 fruit exchanges	1 banana (9 inches)
1 low-fat milk exchange	1 cup 2% milk

Dinner
3 medium-fat meat exchanges	3 oz broiled T-bone steak (no bone)
2 starch exchanges	1 medium baked potato
1 fat exchange	1 tsp margarine
2 vegetable exchanges	1 cup broccoli
1 fruit exchange	1 kiwi fruit
	Coffee (if desired)

Snack
2 starch exchanges	1 bagel
2 fat exchanges	2 tbsp regular cream cheese

*The target plan was a 2000 kcal energy intake, with 55% from carbohydrate, 15% from protein, and 30% from fat. Computer analysis indicated that this menu yielded 2037 kcal, with 55% from carbohydrate, 16% from protein, and 29% from fat—in close agreement with the targeted goals.

protein (300 kcal), and 30% from fat (600 kcal). This can be translated into 2 low-fat milk exchanges, 3 vegetable exchanges, 5 fruit exchanges, 10 starch exchanges, 3 medium-fat meat exchanges, and 8 fat exchanges (Table 2-9). Note that this is only one of many possible combinations; the Exchange System offers great flexibility.

Table 2-10 arbitrarily separates these exchanges into breakfast, lunch, dinner, and a snack. Breakfast includes 1 low-fat milk exchange, 2 fruit exchanges, 2 starch exchanges, and 1 fat exchange. This total corresponds to ¾ cup of cold cereal, 1 cup of 2% milk, 1 slice of bread with 1 teaspoon margarine, and 1 cup of orange juice.

Lunch consists of 4 fat exchanges, 4 starch exchanges, 1 vegetable exchange, 1 low-fat milk exchange, and 2 fruit exchanges. This translates into 2 slices of bacon with 2 teaspoons mayonnaise on two slices of bread, with tomato. In other words, a

TAKE ACTION

Does your diet meet the RDAs and Food Guide Pyramid recommendations?

Complete either part I or part II. Then complete parts III, IV, and V. (For help in following the instructions for this activity, see the sample assessment in Appendix G.)

- -

Part I
Manual RDA Analysis

A. Take the information from the 1-day food-intake record you completed in Chapter 1 and record it on the blank form provided in Appendix E or by your instructor. Be sure to record the food or drink ingested and the amount (e.g., weight) consumed. NOTE: Your instructor may require you to keep the food record for more than 1 day.

B. Review the 1989 RDAs on the inside cover of the book and choose the appropriate recommendations for your gender and age. Write the appropriate value for each nutrient on the line on the form labeled "Your RDA." NOTE: The values for sodium and potassium from the table on the inside cover of the book are labeled, "Estimated Sodium, Chloride, and Potassium Requirements of Healthy Persons."

C. Look up the foods and drinks that you listed on the form in the food composition table, Appendix A. Record on the form the amounts of each nutrient and the kilocalories present in them, based on the serving size and the number of servings you ate. For example, if you drank 2 cups of milk and the serving size listed in Appendix A is 1 cup, double all nutrient values as you record them. If the food is not listed, choose a substitute, such as cola for rootbeer.

D. For each food and drink, add the amounts in each column and record the results on the line labeled "Totals."

E. Compare the totals to your RDAs. Divide the total for each nutrient by the specific RDA or minimum requirement and multiply that by 100. Record the result on the line labeled "% of Your RDA."

F. Keep this assessment for use in subsequent activities in other chapters.

Part II
Computer RDA Analysis

A. Obtain copies of the computer software from your instructor. Load the software into the computer.

B. Choose RDAs based on your age and gender.

C. Enter the information from the 1-day food intake record you kept in Chapter 1. Be sure to enter each food and drink, and the specific amount you ate.

D. This software program will give you the following results:
   1. the appropriate 1989 RDA value for each nutrient
   2. the total amount of each nutrient and the kilocalories consumed for the day
   3. the percentage of the 1989 RDA for each nutrient that you consumed

E. Keep this assessment for use in subsequent activities in other chapters.

Part III
Evaluation of Nutrient Intakes as a Percentage of RDAs

Remember that you don't necessarily need to consume 100% of the 1989 RDA values. A general standard is at least 70% averaged over 5 to 8 days. It would be best not to exceed 500% to avoid potential toxic effects.

A. For which nutrients did your intakes fall below 70% of the 1989 RDAs?

B. Did you exceed the minimum requirements for sodium? To what degree?

C. For which nutrients did you exceed the RDA by greater than 500% (5 times greater)?

D. What dietary changes could you make to correct or improve your dietary profile? If you're not sure, future chapters will help guide your decisions.

Part IV
Food Guide Pyramid

Based on the same food-intake record used in Part I or II, place each food item in the appropriate group of the Food Guide Pyramid in the chart below. That is, for each food item indicate how many servings it contributes to each group based on the amount you ate (see Table 2-1 for serving sizes). Note that many of your food choices may contribute to more than one group. For example, toast with margarine contributes to two catagories: (1) the breads, cereals, rice, and pasta group; and (2) fats, oils, and sweets. After entering all the values, add the number of servings consumed in each group. Finally, compare your total in each food group with the recommended number of servings shown in Figure 2-1. Enter a minus sign (−) if your total falls below the recommendation or a plus sign (+) if it equals or exceeds the recommendation.

TAKE ACTION

Complete either part I or part II. Then perform parts III, IV and V. (For help in following the instructions for this activity, see the sample assessment in Appendix G.)

Indicate the number of servings that each food represents.							
Food or beverage	Amount eaten	Milk, yogurt, and cheese	Meat, poultry, fish, dry beans, eggs, and nuts	Fruit	Vegetable	Bread, cereal, rice, and pasta	Fats, oils, and sweets

Part V

Further Diet Evaluation

Do the weaknesses, if any, suggested in your nutrient analysis (see Part III), correspond to missing servings in the Food Guide Pyramid chart? If so, consider changing your food choices based on the Food Guide Pyramid to help improve your nutrient profile. Finally, indicate whether your day's diet did or did not conform to the following items in the Dietary Guidelines:

	YES	NO
• Eat a variety of foods.	_____	_____
• Choose a diet with plenty of grain products, vegetables, and fruits.	_____	_____
• Choose a diet low in fat, saturated fat, and cholesterol.	_____	_____
• Choose a diet moderate in sugars.	_____	_____
• Choose a diet moderate in salt and sodium.	_____	_____
• Drink alcoholic beverages in moderation, if at all.	_____	_____

If your diet comes up short on any of these evaluations, we hope you will be motivated to take appropriate action to improve your eating patterns.

What's on the Label?

CONSTANCE J. GEIGER, Ph.D., R.D.

Today, people are very interested in nutrition and health. Increased consumer interest in health has resulted in greater availability of foods containing less energy (kilocalories), sodium, and fat and more dietary fiber than in the past. Consumers also have more nutrition information than ever before, thanks to expanded food labeling mandated by the federal government. What can a food label tell you and how can it help you learn about nutrition?

For the most part, foods packaged and sold in any American supermarket are labeled with the product name, the name and address of the manufacturer, the amount of product in the package, and the ingredients, which are listed in descending order by weight if the food contains more than one ingredient. Almost all foods must be so labeled except fresh fruits, vegetables, fish, meat, and poultry.

In the United States, FDA regulates the mandatory labeling of processed foods, except those containing meat and poultry, and the voluntary labeling of fresh fruits, vegetables, and fish. USDA's Food Safety and Inspection Service (FSIS) regulates the mandatory labeling of processed meat and poultry products (e.g., sausage pizza) and the voluntary labeling of fresh meat and poultry. Labeling of alcoholic beverages is regulated by the Bureau of Alcohol, Tobacco, and Firearms (ATF). The Federal Trade Commission (FTC) regulates the advertising of products and has authority to take action against unsubstantiated claims.

In 1990 FDA began a three-step approach for updating the nutrition label, and in November 1990 the Nutrition Labeling and Education Act (NLEA) became law. This act mandated nutrition labeling of almost all processed foods and urged voluntary nutrition labeling of fresh produce, fish, meat, and poultry. To ensure uniformity, FDA and FSIS issued parallel implementing regulations, which are now in place. The NLEA affected the entire nutrition label. The advantages of the new approach to food labeling are many:

- Consumers can easily determine which foods are healthful, since almost all labels now include a Nutrition Facts panel.
- The % Daily Values listed on the label show consumers how a particular food fits into their daily nutrition needs.
- Serving sizes are more realistic, are expressed in common household and metric units of measure, and are more consistent across product lines.
- Important information (e.g., fat, saturated fat, cholesterol, and sodium content) is highlighted.
- Descriptive terms for nutrient content, such as "low fat" and "light," can be used only if the product meets strict definitions set by FDA.
- Health claims must be supported by scientific findings approved by FDA. An example is the claim that calcium helps prevent osteoporosis.
- Ingredient labeling is now required on all foods having more than one ingredient. Fuller disclosure of ingredients is required, such as the inclusion of the protein source in protein hydrolysates.

Because of the new regulations, consumers can learn more about the foods they eat and have more confidence in what they read on the label. Let's look at these specific changes in more detail.

Nutrition Labels Are Required on Most Food Products

Nutrition labels are mandatory on nearly all packaged foods and processed meat products (e.g., chili and hot dogs). Supermarkets may voluntarily provide information on raw, single-ingredient meat, poultry, fish, fruit, and vegetable products. This information often appears as large posters in the appropriate sections of a store. Nutrition information also may be provided in brochures and videos and on the fresh product itself. Even though providing nutrition information about fresh foods is currently voluntary, if less than 60% of supermarkets comply with the new voluntary regulations, both FDA and FSIS will consider making the program mandatory.

Key Label Tips
- You can believe the claims on the package.
- You can easily compare products, because serving sizes are comparable for similar foods.
- The % Daily Value shows if a product is high or low in a nutrient.
- By consulting the Daily Values, you can determine how much (or how little) of the major nutrients you should eat on a daily basis.

FDA requires restaurants to follow labeling rules whenever health claims about restaurant foods or their nutrient content are presented on nonmenu items, such as posters, signs, or placards. FDA recently proposed that these regulations should also apply to listings of nutrient content and health claims made on menus. For example, under the proposed rule, an entreé described as "low fat" on a restaurant menu would have to meet the FDA definition of this term, similar to the requirements for individual food products. Restaurant operators would be required to demonstrate a "reasonable basis" for making a nutritional claim (e.g., recipe analysis using a recognized nutrition database), and they would have to inform customers how much of a claimed nutrient is present in a food or entreé.

Labels Provide Detailed Nutrition Information

A typical food label is shown in Figure 2-8. Mandatory food components must be listed on the Nutrition Facts panel, whereas listing of other (voluntary) components is optional. The order in which components must appear on the label is shown below, with mandatory components underlined:

- <u>Total kilocalories</u> (listed as calories)
- <u>Kilocalories from fat</u>
- Kilocalories from saturated fat
- <u>Total fat</u>
- <u>Saturated fat</u>
- Polyunsaturated fat
- Monounsaturated fat
- <u>Cholesterol</u>
- <u>Sodium</u>
- Potassium
- <u>Total carbohydrate</u>
- <u>Dietary fiber</u>
- Soluble fiber
- Insoluble fiber
- <u>Sugars</u> (includes both added and naturally occurring sugars)
- Sugar alcohols (e.g., the sugar substitutes xylitol, mannitol, and sorbitol)
- Other carbohydrate (the difference between total carbohydrate and the sum of dietary fiber, sugars, and sugar alcohol if declared)
- <u>Protein</u>
- <u>Vitamin A</u>
- Percentage of vitamin A present as beta-carotene
- <u>Vitamin C</u>
- <u>Calcium</u>
- <u>Iron</u>
- Other essential vitamins and minerals (thiamin, riboflavin, and niacin are not mandatory items, as deficiencies of these nutrients are rarely seen. They may, however, be listed voluntarily).

If a claim is made about any of the optional components, or if a food is fortified or enriched with any of them, nutrition information for these components becomes mandatory.

An optional footnote for packages of any size is the number of kilocalories per gram of fat (9), carbohydrate (4), and protein (4).

SERVING SIZE IS UNIFORM WITHIN A FOOD CLASS

Serving sizes are defined by regulation and required for nutrition labeling. FDA has established over 139 serving-size categories, called Reference Amounts Customarily Consumed Per Eating Occasion (i.e., 1 serving). The FSIS has defined about 45 additional categories for

The nutrition label uses the term *calorie* for energy values, but *kilocalorie* values are actually listed. We will use kilocalories in discussing labeling to be consistent throughout the book. Note that by convention the capitalized term *Calorie* is equivalent to kilocalorie when used to express energy content.

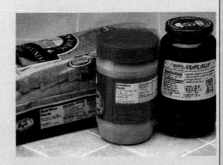

The food labels on these three products can be combined to indicate nutrient intake for a meal—a peanut butter and jelly sandwich.

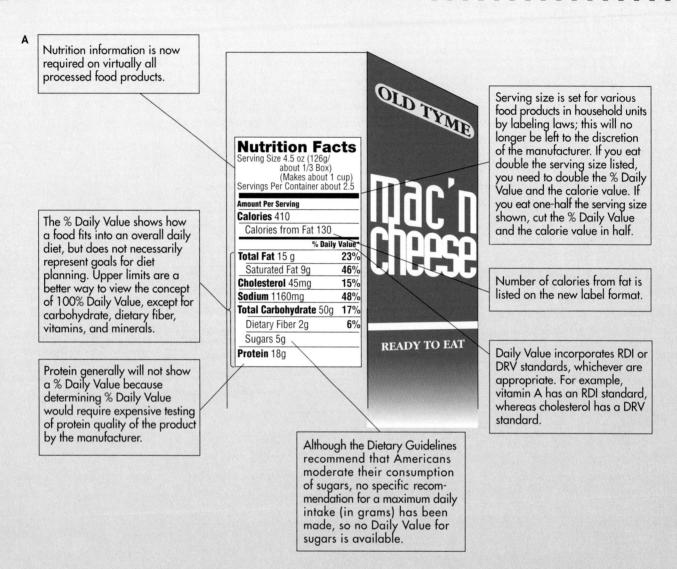

A

Nutrition information is now required on virtually all processed food products.

Nutrition Facts
Serving Size 4.5 oz (126g/ about 1/3 Box)
(Makes about 1 cup)
Servings Per Container about 2.5

Amount Per Serving

Calories 410

Calories from Fat 130

% Daily Value*

Total Fat 15 g	**23%**
Saturated Fat 9g	**46%**
Cholesterol 45mg	**15%**
Sodium 1160mg	**48%**
Total Carbohydrate 50g	**17%**
Dietary Fiber 2g	**6%**
Sugars 5g	
Protein 18g	

OLD TYME

mac'n cheese

READY TO EAT

Serving size is set for various food products in household units by labeling laws; this will no longer be left to the discretion of the manufacturer. If you eat double the serving size listed, you need to double the % Daily Value and the calorie value. If you eat one-half the serving size shown, cut the % Daily Value and the calorie value in half.

The % Daily Value shows how a food fits into an overall daily diet, but does not necessarily represent goals for diet planning. Upper limits are a better way to view the concept of 100% Daily Value, except for carbohydrate, dietary fiber, vitamins, and minerals.

Number of calories from fat is listed on the new label format.

Protein generally will not show a % Daily Value because determining % Daily Value would require expensive testing of protein quality of the product by the manufacturer.

Daily Value incorporates RDI or DRV standards, whichever are appropriate. For example, vitamin A has an RDI standard, whereas cholesterol has a DRV standard.

Although the Dietary Guidelines recommend that Americans moderate their consumption of sugars, no specific recommendation for a maximum daily intake (in grams) has been made, so no Daily Value for sugars is available.

Figure 2-8 The Nutrition Facts panel on a current food label. The box is broken into two parts: **A** is the top and **B** is the bottom. The % Daily Value listed on the label is the percentage of the generally accepted amount of a nutrient needed daily that is present in 1 serving of the product. You can use the % Daily Values to compare your diet with current nutrition recommendations for certain diet components. Let's consider dietary fiber and total fat. We'll assume you consume 2000 kcal/day, which is the energy intake corresponding to the % Daily Values listed on labels. If the total % Daily Value for dietary fiber in all the foods you eat in one day adds up to 100%, your diet meets the recommendations for fiber. Likewise, if the total % Daily Value for fat in all the foods you eat in one day adds up to 100% or less, your diet meets the recommendations for fat. The recommended intakes of saturated fat, total fat, and dietary fiber are related to total energy intake. However, by adjusting for this, you can use the same method to evaluate your diet even if your energy intake is more or less than the standard 2000 kcal. For example, if you consume only 1600 kcal/day, the total % Daily Value for each one of these dietary components can add up to 80%, since $1600 \div 2000 = 0.8$ or 80%. If you eat 2800 kcal, your total % Daily Value for each of these components in all the foods you eat in one day can add up to 140%, since $2,800 \div 2,000 = 1.4$ or 140%. However, the % Daily Values for cholesterol and sodium are not adjusted for differences in energy intake.

meat and poultry products. Most Reference Amounts are in metric measures, such as 85 g for waffles or 240 ml for juices. However, the Reference Amounts must be translated into a statement using common household measures, such as cups, items, and ounces, on labels. This makes it easier for consumers to interpret serving-size information.

B

Vitamin A 10% • Vitamin C 0%
Calcium 30% • Iron 15%

Percent Daily Values are based on a 2,000 calorie diet. Your daily values may be higher or lower depending on your calorie needs:

	Calories:	2,000	2,500
Total Fat	Less than	65g	80g
Sat Fat	Less than	20g	25g
Cholest	Less than	300mg	300mg
Sodium	Less than	2,400mg	2,400mg
Total Carb		300g	375g
Fiber		25g	30g

Calories per gram:
Fat 9 • Carbohydrate 4 • Protein 4

INGREDIENTS: WATER, ENRICHED MACARONI (ENRICHED FLOUR [NIACIN, FERROUS SULFATE (IRON), THIAMINE MONONITRATE AND RIBOFLAVIN], EGG WHITE), FLOUR, CHEDDAR CHEESE (MILK, CHEESE CULTURE, SALT, ENZYME), SPICES, MARGARINE (PARTIALLY HYDROGENATED SOYBEAN OIL, WATER, SOY LECITHIN, MONO- AND DIGLYCERIDES, BETA CAROTENE FOR COLOR, VITAMIN A PALMITATE), AND MALTODEXTRIN.

GOOD SOURCE OF CALCIUM SEE SIDE PANEL FOR NUTRITION INFORMATION

Some Daily Value standards, such as grams of total fat, increase as energy intake increases. The % Daily Values on the label are based on a 2000 kcal diet.

Labels on larger packages may list the number of calories per gram of fat, carbohydrate, and protein.

Ingredients, listed in descending order by weight, will appear here or in another place on the package. The sources of some ingredients, such as certain flavorings, will be stated by name to help people better identify ingredients that they avoid for health, religious, or other reasons.

Absolute and comparative claims, as well as health claims, can appear on the front panel or on the sides of the package. All must follow legal definitions.

For example, the Reference Amount for cookies is 30 g. The serving size listed on a package of cookies is the number of cookies that comes closest to meeting that Reference Amount. Since the approximate weight of an Oreo cookie is 15 g, two Oreos constitute 1 serving. The Reference Amount for snack foods is 30 g, which is equivalent to 13 or 14 tortilla chips.

Most Nutrient Amounts Are Expressed as % Daily Values

The actual amount of each listed component present in a serving size is indicated on the label. The amounts of most components also are expressed as percentages of their Daily Value (% Daily Value). As explained earlier, the Daily Values consist of the Recommended Dietary Intakes (RDIs) for vitamins and minerals and the Daily Recommended Values (DRVs) for other nutrients, including protein, fat, and carbohydrates (see Tables 2-6 and 2-7). The Daily

Values are general standards reflecting the recommended amounts of each nutrient that should be present in the total diet.

On many labels, the bottom portion of the Nutrition Facts panel lists the Daily Values for selected dietary components, such as fat, cholesterol, and total carbohydrate. The values for both a 2000 kcal and 2500 kcal diet are given. However, the % Daily Values listed in the top portion are based on an intake of 2000 kcal/day.

You can use the Daily Values to help monitor your intake of certain nutrients. For example, the label for the macaroni and cheese product shown in Figure 2-8 indicates that 1 serving (1 cup) of this product provides 23% of the Daily Value for fat (65 g), or 14 g of fat (0.23 × 65 = 14). The Daily Value for fat of 65 g was set to provide 30% of the energy content of a 2000 kcal diet, the maximum recommended contribution from fat:

$$\frac{(0.30 \times 2000\ kcal)}{9\ kcal/gram\ of\ fat} = 67\ grams$$

The calculated value of 67 is rounded to 65 for simplicity. Now, suppose that the first fat-containing food you eat one day is 1 serving of this macaroni and cheese product. You then would have 51 g of fat (65 − 14) to use for other food choices during the rest of the day, or 78% of the Daily Value allotment (51 ÷ 65 = 0.78 or 78%).

Since the Daily Value for fat is related to total energy intake, this calculation yields a different result for an energy intake of 2500 kcal. At that energy intake, the fat allotment is 80 g. Thus the total fat in 1 serving of the macaroni and cheese would provide 18% of the Daily Value, leaving 83% of the daily allotment for other food choices during the rest of the day.

Nutrient-Content Claims Must Follow Strict Legal Guidelines

Food companies may use descriptive terms like "low fat" or "sugar free" to help guide food choices, but such terms must meet strictly defined government standards. For example, if a food is labeled as "low calorie," the product must contain 40 kcal or less per Reference Amount. In the past, the nutrient-content claims on labels did not have legal definitions. For example, the term "light" or "lite" could mean light in color, weight, or energy. Now there are uniform definitions for all such terms used (Table 2-11).

Nutrient-content claims are either absolute or comparative claims. The absolute claims include terms such as "free," "low," "good source," and "high." The comparative claims include terms such as "reduced," "light" or "lite," "less," "fewer," "more," "lean," and "extra lean." These terms or their allowed synonyms usually appear on the front label, although manufacturers may place them on other parts of the label, too.

Figure 2-9 shows examples of both types of nutrient claims for salad dressing. The absolute claim "low fat" refers to the absolute amount of fat in the dressing. The comparative claims "light" and "reduced fat" compare the amount of fat in a nutritionally altered salad dressing with a regular salad dressing. A comparative claim is accompanied by an explanatory statement such as "40% less fat than our regular salad dressing. Fat lowered from 14 g to 8 g per serving."

LIMITED HEALTH CLAIMS ARE PERMITTED

In 1984, the Kellogg Company, in conjunction with The National Cancer Institute, printed a health claim on its "high-fiber" cereals stating that fiber may help prevent certain forms of cancer. This type of label message was not allowed at the time and caused a heated debate among nutrition scientists. After reviewing hundreds of comments on the proposed rule allowing health claims, FDA has decided to permit them with certain restrictions.

Currently, FDA limits the use of health messages to specific areas in which there is significant scientific agreement concerning a relationship between a nutrient, food, or food constituent and a chronic disease. The allowed claims may show a link between the following:
- A diet with enough calcium **and** a reduced risk of osteoporosis
- A diet low in total fat **and** a reduced risk of some cancers
- A diet low in saturated fat and cholesterol **and** a reduced risk of heart disease

TABLE 2-11

Definitions for comparative and absolute nutrient claims on food labels

Sugar
- *Sugar Free:* less than 0.5 grams (g) per serving.
- *No added sugar; Without added sugar; No sugar added:*
  - No sugars added during processing or packing, including ingredients that contain sugars (for example, fruit juices, applesauce, or jam).
  - Processing does not increase the sugar content above the amount naturally present in the ingredients. (A functionally insignificant increase in sugars is acceptable for processes used for purposes other than increasing sugar content.)
  - The food that it resembles and for which it substitutes normally contains added sugars.
  - If the food doesn't meet the requirements for a low- or reduced-calorie food, the product bears a statement that the food is not low-calorie or calorie-reduced and directs consumers' attention to the nutrition panel for further information on sugars and calorie content.
- *Reduced sugar:* At least 25% less sugar per serving than reference food.

Calories
- *Calorie free:* Fewer than 5 kcal per serving.
- *Low calorie:* 40 kcal or less per serving and, if the serving is 30 g or less, or 2 tablespoons or less, per 50 g of the food.
- *Reduced or fewer calories:* At least 25% fewer kcal per serving than reference food.

Fiber
- *High fiber:* 5 g or more per serving. (Foods making high-fiber claims must meet the definition for low fat, or the level of total fat must appear next to the high-fiber claim.)
- *Food source of fiber:* 2.5 to 4.9 g per serving.
- *More or added fiber:* At least 2.5 g more per serving than reference food.

Fat
- *Fat free:* Less than 0.5 g of fat per serving.
- *Saturated fat free:* Less than 0.5 g per serving, and the level of trans fatty acids does not exceed 0.5 g per serving.
- *Low fat:* 3 g or less per serving and, if

the serving is 30 g or less, or 2 tablespoons or less, per 50 g of the food.
- *Low saturated fat:* 1 g or less per serving and not more than 15% of kcal from saturated fatty acids.
- *Reduced or less fat:* At least 25% less per serving than reference food.
- *Reduced or less saturated fat:* At least 25% less per serving than reference food.

Cholesterol
- *Cholesterol free:* Less than 2 mg of cholesterol and 2 g or less of saturated fat per serving.
- *Low cholesterol:* 20 mg or less cholesterol and 2 g or less of saturated fat per serving, and if the serving is 30 g or less, or 2 tablespoons or less, per 50 g of the food.
- *Reduced or less cholesterol:* At least 25% less cholesterol and 2 g or less of saturated fat per serving than reference food.

Sodium
- *Sodium free:* Less than 5 mg per serving.
- *Very low sodium:* 35 mg or less per serving and, if the serving is 30 g or less, or 2 tablespoons or less, per 50 g of the food.
- *Low sodium:* 140 mg or less per serving and, if the serving is 30 g or less, or 2 tablespoons or less, per 50 g of the food.
- *Light in sodium:* At least 50% less per serving than reference food.
- *Reduced or less sodium:* At least 25% less per serving than reference food.

Other terms:
- *Fortified/Enriched:* Vitamins and/or minerals have been added to the product in amounts in excess of at least 10% of that normally present in reference product.
- *Healthy:* An individual food that is low fat and low saturated fat and has no more than 360 to 480 mg of sodium or 60 mg of cholesterol per serving can be labeled "healthy" if it provides at least 10% of vitamin A, vitamin C, protein, calcium, iron, or dietary fiber. Meal-type products, such as frozen entrées and multi-course frozen dinners, must provide 10% of two or three of these nutrients, depending on the type and size of the meal.

- *Light or Lite:* The descriptor "light" or "lite" can mean two things: first, that a nutritionally altered product contains one-third fewer kilocalories or half the fat of the reference food (if the food derives 50% or more of its kilocalories from fat, the reduction must be 50% of the fat); and second, that the sodium content of a low-calorie, low-fat food has been reduced by 50%.

  In addition, "light in sodium" may be used for foods in which the sodium content has been reduced by at least 50%. The term "light" may still be used to describe such properties as texture and color, as long as the label explains the intent; for example, "light brown sugar" and "light and fluffy."
- *Diet:* A food may be labeled with terms such as "diet," "dietetic," "artificially sweetened," or "sweetened with nonnutritive sweetener" only if the claim is not false or misleading. The food can also be labeled "low calorie" or "reduced calorie."
- *Good source:* "Good source" means that a food contains 10% to 19% of the Daily Value for a particular nutrient.
- *High:* "High" means that a food contains 20% or more of the Daily Value for a particular nutrient.
- *Organic:* FDA has deferred rulemaking regarding the use of the term "organic" until USDA has adopted appropriate regulations. At that time, FDA will determine whether any regulations governing the term "organic" are necessary.
- *Natural:* The food must be free of food colors, synthetic flavors, or any other synthetic substance.

The following terms apply only to meat and poultry products regulated by USDA.
- *Extra lean:* The product has less than 5 g of fat, 2 g of saturated fat, and 95 mg of cholesterol per reference amount (or 100 g of an individual food).
- *Lean:* The product contains less than 10 g of fat, 4.5 g of saturated fat, and 95 mg of cholesterol per reference amount (or 100 g of an individual food).

Many definitions are from FDA's *Dictionary of Terms*, as established in conjunction with the 1990 NLEA.

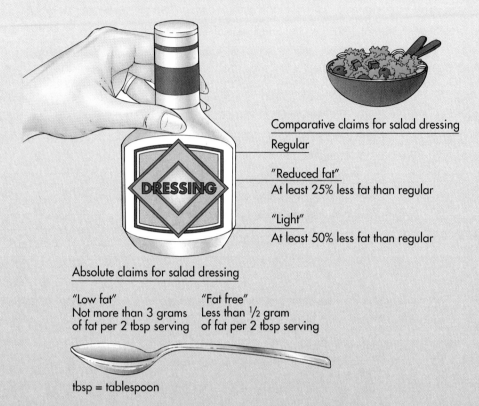

Comparative claims for salad dressing
Regular

"Reduced fat"
At least 25% less fat than regular

"Light"
At least 50% less fat than regular

Absolute claims for salad dressing

"Low fat"
Not more than 3 grams
of fat per 2 tbsp serving

"Fat free"
Less than ½ gram
of fat per 2 tbsp serving

tbsp = tablespoon

Figure 2-9 Comparative versus absolute nutrient claims. You can rely on these nutrient claims to guide food choices. These claims on food labels must follow the legal constraints listed in Table 2-11.

- A diet rich in dietary fiber–containing grain products, fruits, and vegetables **and** a reduced risk of some cancers
- A diet rich in fruits, vegetables, and grain products that contain fiber **and** a reduced risk of heart disease
- A diet low in sodium **and** a reduced risk of high blood pressure
- A diet rich in fruits and vegetables **and** a reduced risk of some cancers
- A diet adequate in folate **and** a reduced risk of neural tube defects (a type of birth defect)

A "may" or "might" qualifier must be used in the statement. Then before a health claim can be made for a food product, it must meet two general requirements. First, the food must be a "good source" (prior to fortification) of dietary fiber, protein, vitamin A, vitamin C, calcium, or iron. Second, a single serving of the food product cannot contain more than 13 g fat, 4 g saturated fat, 60 mg cholesterol, or 480 mg sodium. If a food exceeds any *one* of these amounts, no health claim can be made for it regardless of its other nutritional qualities. For example, even though whole milk is high in calcium, its label can't make the health claim about calcium and osteoporosis because whole milk contains 5 g of saturated fat per serving.

In addition, the product must meet the specific criteria for absolute and comparative claims for the nutrients about which a health claim is made. For example, a health claim regarding fat and cancer can be made only if the product contains 3 g or less of fat per serving, which is the standard for low-fat foods.

The primary danger with health claims is that not all the facts may be presented in some cases. For example, claims about dietary fiber often omit some adverse facts, such as that too much wheat bran fiber can lead to decreased absorption of iron, zinc, and calcium, as well as to intestinal problems, such as gas. A more complete statement is that too much— as well as too little—dietary fiber can be harmful (see Chapter 3 for more details).

Some Foods Don't Have to Be Labeled

Several categories of food are exempt from mandatory labeling, although they can carry voluntary nutrition information. However, if an exempt food carries a health or nutrient-content claim, then it must also have a label meeting all current requirements. Among the foods exempt from nutrition labeling are

- foods served for immediate consumption, such as that served in hospital cafeterias and on airplanes and that sold by food service vendors (e.g., mall cookie counters, sidewalk vendors, and vending machines)
- ready-to-eat foods that are not for immediate consumption but are prepared primarily on site (e.g., bakery, deli, and candy store items)
- foods shipped in bulk, as long as they are for sale in that form to consumers;
- medical foods, such as those used to address the nutritional needs of patients with certain diseases
- plain coffee and tea, some spices, and other foods that contain no significant amounts of any nutrients
- foods produced by small businesses or packaged in small containers

Labels on foods for children under 2 years of age (except for infant formula) do not carry information about kilocalories from fat to prevent parents from wrongly assuming that infants and toddlers should restrict their fat intake. Fat is important during these years to ensure adequate growth and development. The only % Daily Values required are those for protein, vitamins, and minerals (see Chapter 17 for details and for an example of a label).

Special Regulations Apply to Protein Labeling

Because protein deficiency is not a public health concern in the United States, declaration of the % Daily Value for protein is not mandatory on foods for people over 4 years of age. If the % Daily Value is given on a label, FDA requires that the product be analyzed for protein quality. Because this procedure is expensive and time consuming, many companies opt not to list a % Daily Value for protein. However, labels on foods for infants or children under 4 years of age must include the % Daily Value for protein, as must the labels on any food carrying a claim about protein content.

You Can Use Food Labels to Improve Your Diet

The new mandatory food labels, which are found on almost all processed food products, and the labels voluntarily placed on many fresh foods allow you to make informed food choices that are part of a healthy diet. Now a quick glance can tell you the nutrient content of your frozen dessert, candy bar, cookie, or other foods whose labels provided no nutrition information in the past (Figure 2-10). You can use the % Daily Value to compare food products

For more information, you can call the Food Labeling Education Information Center at 301-504-5719.

CATHY

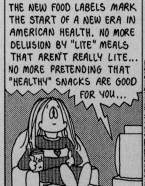 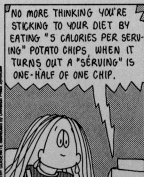 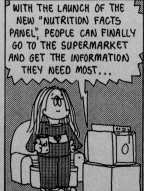 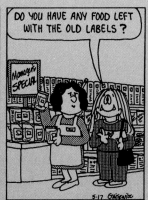

Figure 2-10 Cathy.

and to see if a food has a little or a lot of a nutrient. The % Daily Values let you gauge about how much you should consume each day. You can now rely on nutrient-content claims like "fat-free," because there are strict definitions for use of such claims. Use claims such as "high" and "good source" as signals to include foods with fiber and vitamins and minerals. "Free" and "low" claims help you moderate your intake of fat, saturated fat, and cholesterol. Health claims provide general dietary guidance about diet and prevention of chronic diseases. Use them to make wise choices among foods. Overall, the food label is an important tool to help you choose a healthful diet that supports the Food Guide Pyramid and the Dietary Guidelines.

Dr. Geiger is president of Geiger & Associates and is an adjunct research assistant professor at the University of Utah, both in Salt Lake City, Utah. Her company specializes in food labeling, health communications, and government affairs consulting for the food industry, health profession associations, and food trade organizations.

CHAPTER THREE

Carbohydrates

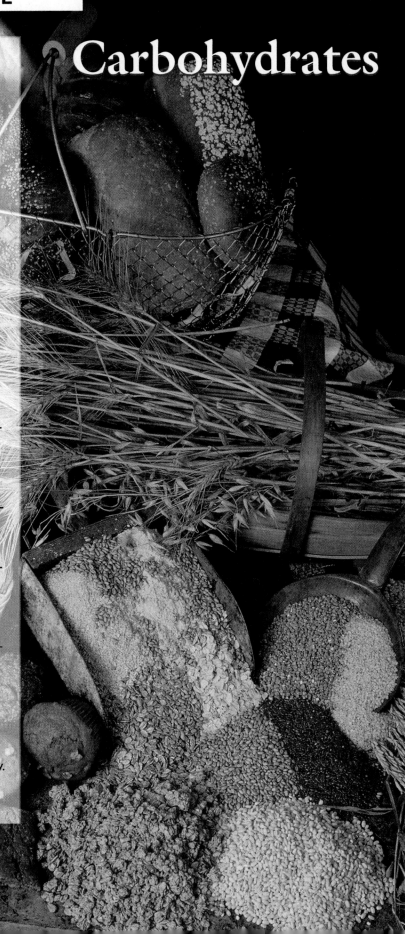

You have now studied what we eat, why we choose to eat certain foods, and the basic tools used to plan diets. The next three chapters examine the energy-yielding nutrients—carbohydrates, proteins, and fats. Learning about them will give you an advantage over the average consumer. Most people know that potatoes contain carbohydrates and steak contains fat and protein, but few people understand what these terms actually mean.

Because carbohydrates should be the major source of energy in your diet, they are an ideal topic with which to begin a detailed discussion of the macronutrients, substances needed in amounts of many grams per day. It is important to study carbohydrates in detail because this nutrient is often misunderstood. Some people think certain carbohydrates cause diabetes—they do not.[5,6] Others think certain carbohydrates can cause hyperactivity in children— again, they do not.[25] In fact, carbohydrates, especially the complex varieties, have been the nutrient most promoted by nutritionists during the last 20 years. The link between fat— especially animal fat—and heart disease should prompt us all to switch our focus away from high-fat foods toward more high-carbohydrate foods.[15] It is unfortunate that affluence tends to drive us the other way.

NUTRITION AWARENESS INVENTORY

Answer these 15 statements about carbo-hydrates to test your current knowledge. If you think the statement is true or mostly true, circle T. If you think the statement is false or mostly false, circle F. Use the scoring key at the end of the book to compute your total score. Repeat this test after you have read this chapter, and compare your results.

1. **T F** Common table sugar is more technically referred to as *sucrose*.
2. **T F** Plants store carbohydrates as starch.
3. **T F** Carbohydrates are necessarily fattening.
4. **T F** The primary role of carbohydrates is to supply energy to body cells.
5. **T F** Fiber and "roughage" mean the same thing.
6. **T F** The RDA for carbohydrates is 50 to 100 g/day.
7. **T F** The human body uses dietary fiber mainly as a source of energy.
8. **T F** Sugars play a role in promoting dental caries.
9. **T F** Protein can be converted to carbohydrate in the body.
10. **T F** Wheat bread is a good source of dietary fiber.
11. **T F** No desirable total sugar intake has been firmly established, but some people may consume too much sugar.
12. **T F** It is not safe to feed honey to infants.
13. **T F** Diabetes is a medical problem associated with low blood glucose.
14. **T F** Sugars cause hyperactivity in children, which can lead to juvenile delinquency.
15. **T F** Africans develop fewer intestinal disorders than Americans.

sugar A simple carbohydrate with the chemical composition $(CH_2O)_n$. Most sugars form ringed structures when in solution.

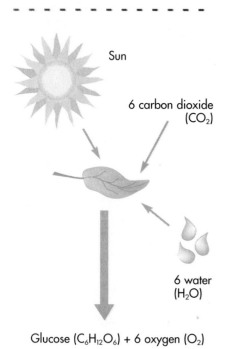

Sun

6 carbon dioxide (CO_2)

6 water (H_2O)

Glucose ($C_6H_{12}O_6$) + 6 oxygen (O_2)
Glucose is stored in the leaf, but can also undergo further metabolism

Structures and Functions of Simple Carbohydrates

The carbohydrate cellulose, which forms part of the structure of many plants, is the most abundant single biochemical compound on earth. Another carbohydrate, chitin, is probably second. It forms part of the structure of many insects and crustaceans, such as lobsters. And as we noted in the chapter overview, carbohydrates should also be the overwhelming source of energy in the diets of most adults.[15]

Most forms of carbohydrates are composed of carbon, hydrogen, and oxygen in the ratio of 1:2:1, respectively. The general formula is $(CH_2O)_n$, where *n* represents the number of times the ratio is repeated. The empirical formula for glucose is $C_6H_{12}O_6$, or $(CH_2O)_6$. The simpler forms of carbohydrates are called **sugars** and often take the form of single or double sugars, called **monosaccharides** and **disaccharides,** respectively. The more complex forms of carbohydrates are typically either **starches** or **dietary fibers.**[16]

Plants use carbon dioxide, water, and energy (from the sun) to produce the carbohydrates we eat.

MONOSACCHARIDES: GLUCOSE, FRUCTOSE, AND GALACTOSE

The common monosaccharides (*mono* meaning "one" and *saccharide* meaning "sugar") are glucose, fructose, and galactose. Glucose is the principal monosaccharide in the body. Other names for glucose are *dextrose* and *blood sugar.* In Figure 3-1, the chemical structure of the D-isomer of glucose is shown in both its linear and ring forms. Glucose exists in the body in the ring form. Because the body can metabolize only the D-isomer of glucose, the L-isomer might be useful as an alternative sweetener, an enticing possibility. (The concept of isomers is reviewed in Appendix B.)

Glucose, a six-carbon monosaccharide, is called a **hexose** (*hex* meaning "six," for six carbons; *ose* is the standard word ending for carbohydrates). The six-member ring formed by glucose includes an oxygen atom.

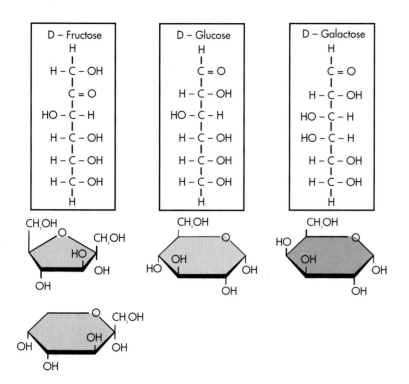

Figure 3-1 Structures of the D-isomer of the six-carbon monosaccharides—fructose, glucose, and galactose—shown in the linear form and in the ring form (predominant form when in solution).

Fructose is a structural isomer of glucose, and although it is a hexose, it can form either a five- or six-member ring (Figure 3-1). Fructose, also called levulose, is found in:

- fruit
- honey (about half fructose, half glucose)
- **high-fructose corn syrup,** which is used in the production of soft drinks, frozen desserts, and confections. The presence of fructose in these products makes it a major sugar in our diets. In most American diets, fructose accounts for about 8% to 10% of total energy intake.

Fructose, after absorption by the small intestine and transport to the liver, is almost all metabolized to glucose. Some fructose is converted to **glycogen, lactic acid,** or fat, depending on the metabolic state of the individual.[22] Synthesis of lactic acid and fat is stimulated by fructose intakes that are two or more times typical intakes.

Galactose is the last major monosaccharide of nutritional importance. Comparison of the structure of this simple sugar with that of glucose shows that the two structures are identical except that the hydrogen (–H) and the hydroxyl group (–OH) on carbon-4 are reversed (Figure 3-1).[16] Galactose is not usually found free in nature in large quantities, but rather combines with glucose to form a disaccharide called **lactose.** Lactose is present in milk and other dairy products. Once absorbed into the body, galactose is converted into glucose, which is used to provide energy or is built into *glycogen.*[16]

Now is a good time to begin emphasizing a key concept in nutrition: the difference between *intake* of a substance and the body's *use* of that substance. The body often does not use all nutrients as such. Some of these substances are broken down and later reassembled into the same or a different substance when and where necessary. For example, galactose in the diet is metabolized to glucose or glycogen. When later required, as in the mammary gland of the lactating female, galactose is resynthesized, using a wide variety of potential carbon atom sources.

A common misconception is that honey contains vitamins and minerals. You can prove to yourself that honey is no more nutritious than sucrose by consulting Appendix A. Only the sweetener molasses, a by-product of sucrose production, contains any appreciable amount of minerals. However, our consumption of molasses is very low.

high-fructose corn syrup A corn syrup that has been manufactured to contain between 40% and 90% fructose.

glycogen A carbohydrate made of multiple units of glucose with a highly branched structure; sometimes known as *animal starch.* It is the storage form of glucose in humans and is synthesized (and stored) in the liver and muscles.

lactic acid A three-carbon acid, also called lactate, that is formed during anaerobic cell metabolism; a partial breakdown product of glucose.

ribose A five-carbon sugar found in genetic material, specifically RNA.

Another monosaccharide found in nature is **ribose,** a five-carbon sugar (or pentose; *penta* means "five"). This is present in a cell's genetic material. Very little ribose is present in our diet; we produce this sugar from other foods we eat.[16] Finally, a few sugar alcohols are present in foods and will be discussed in the section on nutritive sweeteners in foods. Currently, the major sugar alcohols used in the manufacture of edible products are **sorbitol** and **mannitol.**[3]

Once you are familiar with the chemical forms of the sugars, it is much easier to understand how they are interrelated, combined, digested, metabolized, and synthesized.

DISACCHARIDES: MALTOSE, SUCROSE, AND LACTOSE

disaccharides A class of sugars formed by the chemical bonding of two monosaccharides.

glycosidic bond The covalent bond formed between two monosaccharides when a water molecule is lost.

alpha (α) bond A type of glycosidic bond that can be digested by human intestinal enzymes; drawn as c⌞o⌟c .

beta (β) bond A type of glycosidic bond that cannot be broken by human intestinal enzymes during digestion when it is part of a long chain of glucose molecules; drawn as c⌜o⌝c .

Disaccharides (*di* means "two") are formed when two monosaccharides combine in a so-called condensation reaction. In the reaction, a water molecule is released and a **glycosidic bond** forms between the two monosaccharides. The three most common disaccharides found in nature are **maltose, sucrose,** and **lactose** (Figure 3-2).[16]

A glycosidic bond is represented in general as C–O–C. Two forms of this bond exist in nature, called **alpha (α)** and **beta (β),** and are depicted slightly differently. As shown in Figure 3-2, maltose and sucrose contain the alpha form, while lactose contains the beta form. Many complex carbohydrates contain glucose molecules linked by glycosidic bonds. Humans can digest such carbohydrates only if the glucose molecules are linked by alpha glycosidic bonds. This topic will be covered later when we discuss dietary fiber.

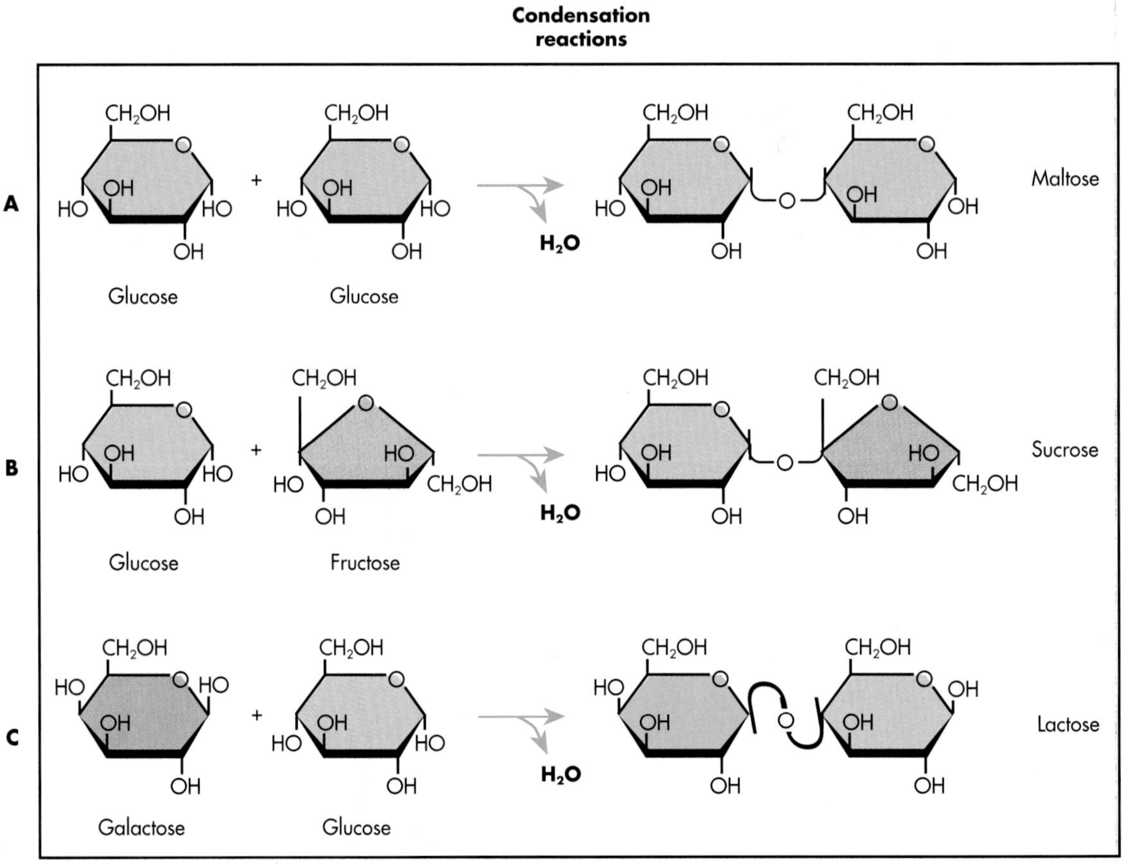

Figure 3-2 Condensation between two monosaccharides forms a disaccharide. **A,** Maltose is made from two glucose molecules and is formed in germinating grains. **B,** Sucrose, or common table sugar, is made from glucose and fructose. **C,** Lactose, or milk sugar, is made from glucose and galactose. Note that lactose contains a type of glycosidic bond (β) different from that of maltose and sucrose (α), a property that can make lactose difficult to digest for individuals who show a relative or total lack of the enzyme lactase.

Maltose consists of two glucose molecules joined by an alpha bond. It is of nutritional interest primarily because it is a chemical intermediate in alcohol production in the beer and liquor industry. In the production of alcoholic beverages, complex carbohydrates (e.g., starches) in various cereal grains are first converted to simpler carbohydrates by enzymes present in the grains. The end products of this step—maltose, glucose, and other simple sugars—are then mixed with yeast cells in the absence of oxygen. The yeast cells convert most of the sugars to ethanol and carbon dioxide, a process termed **fermentation.** Little maltose remains in the final product. Although few food products or beverages contain maltose, digestion of starch—a common dietary component—in the mouth and small intestine yields maltose during the digestive process (Figure 3-3).

Sucrose, our common table sugar, is composed of glucose and fructose linked via an alpha bond. Significant amounts of sucrose are found only in plants, such as sugar cane, sugar beets, honey, and maple syrup.[3] The sucrose from these sources may be purified to various degrees. Brown, white, and powdered sugars are common forms of sucrose sold in grocery stores.

Lactose, the primary sugar in milk and milk products, consists of glucose joined to galactose via a beta bond. As we discuss in the Nutrition Focus, many people are unable to digest large amounts of lactose. This can cause intestinal gas, bloating, cramping, and discomfort as the unabsorbed lactose is metabolized into acids and gases by bacteria in the large intestine.[17]

maltose Glucose bonded to glucose.

sucrose Fructose bonded to glucose; table sugar.

lactose A sugar composed of glucose linked to another sugar called galactose.

fermentation The conversion, without the use of oxygen, of carbohydrates to alcohols, acids, and carbon dioxide.

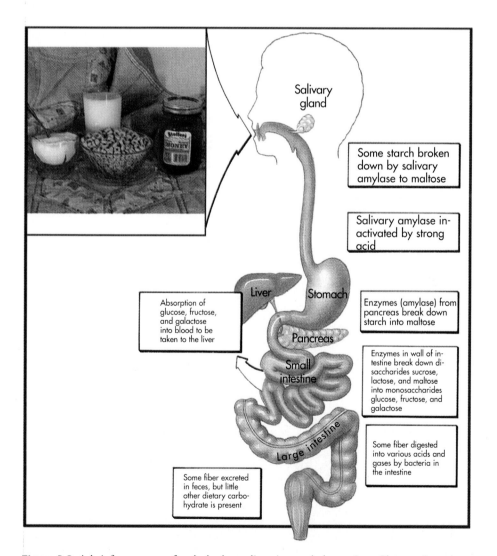

Salivary gland

Some starch broken down by salivary amylase to maltose

Salivary amylase inactivated by strong acid

Liver   Stomach

Pancreas

Small intestine

Large intestine

Absorption of glucose, fructose, and galactose into blood to be taken to the liver

Enzymes (amylase) from pancreas break down starch into maltose

Enzymes in wall of intestine break down disaccharides sucrose, lactose, and maltose into monosaccharides glucose, fructose, and galactose

Some fiber digested into various acids and gases by bacteria in the intestine

Some fiber excreted in feces, but little other dietary carbohydrate is present

Figure 3-3 A brief summary of carbohydrate digestion and absorption. Chapter 6 covers this topic in detail.

You are likely to encounter many different words referring to monosaccharides and disaccharides or products containing these simple sugars. Note that all of the terms listed in Table 3-1 are names for sugars either naturally present in food products or added during their manufacture.

CONCEPT CHECK

Monosaccharides are single sugars. Important monosaccharides from a nutritional standpoint are glucose, fructose, and galactose. Disaccharides are double sugars. The major disaccharides in the diet are sucrose (glucose bonded to fructose), maltose (glucose bonded to glucose), and lactose (glucose bonded to galactose). Once absorbed into the body, most of these carbohydrates are ultimately transformed into glucose by the liver.

Functions of Glucose and Other Sugars in the Body

The functions of glucose in the body start with energy production, but that is only the beginning. Since the other sugars can generally be converted to glucose, and more complex carbohydrates (e.g., starches) are broken down to yield glucose, the functions described here apply to most carbohydrates.

SUPPLYING ENERGY

The main function of glucose is to supply energy to body cells. Certain tissues, such as the red blood cells and most parts of the brain, derive almost all of their energy from glucose. In fact, except when the diet contains almost no carbohydrates, the brain and nervous system use mostly glucose for fuel. Glucose can also fuel muscle cells and other body cells, but many of these cells usually use fat to meet energy needs.[16]

SPARING PROTEIN FROM USE AS AN ENERGY SOURCE

Glucose is protein sparing. That is, dietary protein can be used to make body tissues and to perform other vital processes only when carbohydrate intake yields enough glucose for body needs. Therefore, if you do not consume enough carbohydrate to yield that glucose, your body is forced to make it from other nutrients, such as proteins. This process is termed **gluconeogenesis,** which means "production of new glucose." The hormone cortisol stimulates this process, and the liver and kidneys perform most of the gluconeogenesis in the body.[16]

The source of most of this new glucose must be protein because fats generally cannot be converted into glucose. Amino acids from proteins in the muscles, heart, liver, kidneys, and other vital organs supply the carbons needed to make this glucose.[16] If the process continues for weeks, these organs can become partially weakened. Generally, Americans consume adequate sources of protein, so sparing protein is not an essential function of carbohydrate in the diet under such conditions. It does

gluconeogenesis The production of new glucose by metabolic pathways in the cell. Amino acids derived from protein usually provide the carbons for this glucose.

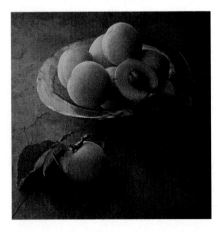

Fruits contain sugars, such as fructose.

TABLE 3-1

Names of sugars used in foods			
Sugar	Invert sugar	Honey	Maple syrup
Sucrose	Glucose	Corn syrup or	Dextrin
Brown sugar	Sorbitol	sweeteners	Dextrose
Confectioner's	Levulose	High-fructose corn	Fructose
sugar (pow-	Polydextrose	syrup	Maltose
dered sugar)	Lactose	Molasses	Caramel
Turbinado sugar	Mannitol	Date sugar	Fruit sugar

NUTRITION FOCUS

LACTOSE INTOLERANCE

The inability to digest lactose results from a reduction in activity of the enzyme **lactase.** This enzyme, which is embedded within the surface of intestinal cells, splits the disaccharide lactose into glucose and galactose. These monosaccharides are absorbed from the small intestine into the bloodstream, but lactose is not. When lactase activity is low, lactose travels unaltered into the large intestine, where resident bacteria metabolize it into acids and gases, causing intestinal gas, bloating, cramping, and discomfort.[17] (See Chapter 6 for more details on carbohydrate digestion.)

Primary lactose intolerance is common in Asians, Hispanics, Native Americans, people of Mediterranean descent, African-Americans, and some other ethnic races. In this case, the loss of lactase activity is not due to another disease per se, hence its designation as a **primary disease.** Some individuals may be born with little or no lactase, but more commonly the lactase levels decline with age, starting at about 2 years of age. Even though lactose intolerance is more prevalent in some ethnic groups than others, between 30 and 60 million Americans and up to 75% of adults worldwide experience a large decrease in their ability to synthesize lactase as they age. Thus they are unable to tolerate large amounts of milk products, since much of the lactose in these products tends to remain undigested.

Secondary lactose intolerance by definition develops as a result of another disease, as is true of **secondary diseases.** Most cases are caused by intestinal bacterial infections. The inability to digest lactose also may result from the use of certain medications, especially anti-cancer drugs. Both infection and some drugs can inhibit the growth of the rapidly reproducing cells that line the gastrointestinal tract and produce lactase.

Clinically, lactose intolerance can be diagnosed from a history of gas and bloating after milk consumption. This history can then be confirmed by having the person consume 50 g of lactose, which is equal to 1 L (4 cups) of milk. If blood glucose does not rise much after consuming the lactose, lactose maldigestion is the likely cause. Some clinicians prefer to use 12.5 g of lactose, a more realistic amount for the test dose. Other, more technical procedures are available to confirm the diagnosis of lactose intolerance.

An individual who is sensitive to even small amounts of lactose must become an avid label reader in order to avoid products with ingredients such as milk, milk solids, casein, and whey. Some medications contain lactose as binders or fillers. Moderate lactose intolerance, however, is more common than nearly complete intolerance. Most people who are moderately intolerant quickly learn by trial and error how much lactose they can tolerate and easily adjust the amount of dairy products in their diet. Such people need not avoid all milk and milk products; nor is this recommended because these foods are very good sources of calcium, riboflavin, potassium, and magnesium. Although these four nutrients are present in other food groups, many people don't eat much of these alternative sources. Obtaining enough of these nutrients is much easier if milk and milk products are included in the diet.

Several options are available to moderately lactose-intolerant individuals who prefer to continue using milk products. First, they can consume small portions of milk products and take them with other foods; this often works because they are able to digest some lactose, but not large amounts at one time. Also, fat in a meal slows digestion, leaving more time for lactase action. Secondly, they can eat cheese. Much lactose is lost when milk is made into cheese. Finally, they can consume yogurt. The bacteria that make yogurt provide their own lactase activity. Thus, if the yogurt contains active bacteria cultures, the lactose present is essentially digested by the yogurt. Freezing destroys the bacteria's activity, so frozen yogurt—as currently manufactured—may have little remaining lactase activity. In general, the foods tolerated best by lactose-intolerant individuals are hard cheeses and regular yogurt. However, sweetened yogurt typically may have as many as 240 kcal/serving, approximately three times more energy than a glass of skim milk, making it a high-calorie option. Supermarkets also sell low-fat, aspartame-sweetened, fruit-flavored yogurts with as few as 120 kcal/serving (8 oz).

During the past few years, manufacturers have been producing low-lactose milk by treating regular milk with lactase isolated from yeast. The added lactase breaks down most of the lactose into glucose and galactose, yielding a milk that causes few symptoms in most moderately intolerant people. Compared with regular milk, low-lactose milk tastes sweeter, because of its higher concentration of glucose, which is three to four times sweeter than lactose. Low-lactose milk can be made at home by adding a commercially available lactase preparation to reg-

NUTRITION FOCUS

ular milk. Lactase pills are also available and can be used at mealtimes. Few people actually need to use enzyme-treated milk or lactase pills because their intolerance is moderate. Minor changes in diet suffice, even for people who feel they are quite sensitive to lactose. For those who nevertheless wish to consume less lactose, these products allow greater versatility in the diet. Several options, then, are available to lactose-intolerant people, only one of which is abandoning milk products. People with severe lactase deficiency who avoid all dairy products should seek other sources of calcium (see Chapter 14).

become important in some low-kilocalorie diets and in starvation. (Chapters 5 and 20 discuss specific effects of starvation and famine.)

The life-threatening wasting of protein that occurs during long-term fasting (or starvation) has prompted companies that produce products used for rapid weight loss, like Optifast, to include 30 to 120 g of carbohydrate in the formula. This significantly decreases protein breakdown and thus helps protect vital tissues and organs, including the heart, during rapid weight loss.

PREVENTING KETOSIS

An adequate intake of carbohydrates—glucose, other sugars, or both—is necessary for the complete metabolism of fats to carbon dioxide (CO_2) and water (H_2O) in the body. A low carbohydrate intake, with the resulting decline in release of the hormone **insulin,** leads to incomplete breakdown of fatty acids in the liver's metabolic pathways and to formation of **ketones**—acetoacetic acid and its derivatives.[16] The liver is the major organ that produces these ketones. In Chapter 7 we will discuss in detail ketone metabolism and situations that lead to extensive production of ketones.

For now, remember that you need to eat at least 50 to 100 g of carbohydrates per day to ensure complete fat metabolism, thus avoiding high accumulation of ketones in the blood and other tissues, a condition called **ketosis.** This intake of 50 to 100 g per day prevents the body weakness that usually results from an insufficient carbohydrate intake. Note that normally we eat at least twice that much carbohydrate, on average about 200 to 300 g/day.

In starvation, people do not consume enough carbohydrate, so ketones soon appear in the blood. Again, this is the normal metabolic response to a fuel shortage.[16] Part of the brain and other tissues can use these ketones for fuel. In fact, the use of ketones by the brain and other organs, such as the heart, is an important adaptive mechanism for survival during starvation; it reduces body protein breakdown by about one third. If part of the brain could not use ketones, the body would be forced to produce much more glucose from protein to support the brain's energy needs. The resulting self-cannibalization would rapidly break down the muscles, heart, and other organs, severely limiting the body's ability to tolerate starvation. Thus a starving person could not survive very long if the brain could not use ketones for energy.

In untreated **insulin-dependent diabetes,** excessive production of ketones can occur, partly because there is not enough insulin to allow for normal glucose metabolism.[6] In such patients, the resulting ketosis can cause numerous complications (see Nutrition Perspective for further discussion of diabetes).

IMPARTING FLAVOR AND SWEETNESS TO FOODS

From birth, humans respond to sugars with a smile. Receptors for tasting sweetness are located on the tip of the tongue. These receptors recognize a variety of sugars

insulin A hormone produced by the beta cells of the pancreas. Insulin increases the synthesis of glycogen in the liver and the movement of glucose from the bloodstream into muscle and adipose cells, among other processes.

ketones Incomplete breakdown products of fat, containing three or four carbons. These contain a chemical group called a ketone, hence the name. An example is acetoacetic acid.

ketosis The condition of having high levels of ketones in the bloodstream and tissues.

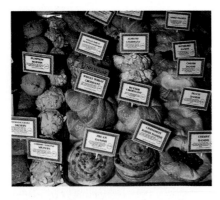

Many foods we enjoy are sweet and should be eaten only in moderation.

TABLE 3-2

The sweetness of sugars and alternative sweeteners

Type of sweetener	Relative sweetness* (sucrose = 1)	Typical sources
Sugars		
Lactose	0.2	Dairy products
Maltose	0.4	Sprouted seeds
Glucose	0.7	Corn syrup
Sucrose	1	Table sugar, most sweets
Invert sugar†	1.3	Some candies, honey
Fructose	1.2-1.8	Fruit, honey, some soft drinks
Sugar alcohols		
Sorbitol	0.6	Dietetic candies, sugarless gum
Mannitol	0.7	Dietetic candies
Xylitol	0.9	Sugarless gum
Alternative sweeteners		
Cyclamate	30	Not currently in use in the United States
Aspartame	200	Diet soft drinks, diet fruit drinks, sugarless gum, powdered diet sweetener
Acesulfame	200	Sugarless gum, diet drink mixes, powdered diet sweeteners, puddings, gelatin desserts
Saccharin (sodium salt)	300	Diet soft drinks

From the American Dietetic Association, 1993.
*On a per gram basis.
†Sucrose broken down into glucose and fructose.

and even some noncarbohydrate substances. The sugars vary in sweetness: on a per gram basis, for example, fructose is almost twice as sweet as sucrose under either acid or cold conditions; sucrose is 30% sweeter than glucose; and lactose is less than half as sweet as sucrose (Table 3-2).[3]

Sugars improve the palatability of many foods and thus enhance diets in general. For example, a small amount of sucrose on a grapefruit improves the taste of this sour fruit. Moderation in using sugars is recommended, but there is no need to believe that sugars are to be avoided altogether.[3]

CONCEPT CHECK

Carbohydrates provide glucose for the energy needs of red blood cells and parts of the brain and nervous system. Eating less than 50 to 100 g of carbohydrates per day forces the liver and kidneys to make glucose (via gluconeogenesis), using carbons from amino acids. These amino acids are derived from the breakdown of proteins in body organs. An inadequate carbohydrate intake also inhibits efficient fat metabolism by the liver, which in turn can lead to ketosis. Sugars also improve the flavor of many foods and so can be part of a diet when used in moderation.

Regulation of Blood Glucose

You now know the form and functions of simple carbohydrates and understand that one of the most important functions of glucose is to supply energy. The next ques-

hyperglycemia High blood glucose, above 140 mg/100 ml of blood.

hypoglycemia Low blood glucose, below 40 to 50 mg/100 ml of blood.

adipose (fat) cells Fat-storing cells.

glucagon A hormone, made by the alpha cells of the pancreas, that stimulates the breakdown of glycogen to glucose in the liver, thus raising blood glucose. It also performs other functions.

epinephrine A hormone (also known as adrenaline) that is released by the adrenal gland. The related hormone norepinephrine is released from various nerve endings in the body. Both hormones increase glycogen breakdown in the liver, among other functions.

cortisol A hormone, made by the adrenal glands, that stimulates production of glucose from amino acids, among other functions.

tion then becomes, how is this essential energy source regulated in the bloodstream?

Under normal circumstances, blood glucose usually varies between about 70 and 115 mg/100 ml of blood in the fasting state, which is normally established a few hours after a meal is eaten. If blood glucose rises above 170 mg/100 ml, glucose begins to spill over into the urine.[16] This leads to hunger and thirst, and eventually to weight loss. If blood glucose falls below 40 to 50 mg/100 ml, a person begins to feel nervous, irritable, and hungry, and may develop a headache. Having high blood glucose is called **hyperglycemia.** Having low blood glucose is called **hypoglycemia.**[23]

The liver is the main organ for controlling the amount of glucose that is eventually found in the bloodstream. Since it is the first organ to screen the sugars absorbed from the small intestine, the liver serves as guard, helping to control the amount of glucose that enters the bloodstream after a meal (Figure 3-3).

The pancreas is another important site of blood glucose control. Small amounts of the hormone insulin are released by the pancreas as soon as a person starts to eat. Once much of the dietary glucose enters the bloodstream, the pancreas releases large amounts of insulin. Insulin affects blood glucose in a variety of ways. It promotes increased glycogen synthesis and thus glucose storage in the liver, as well as increased glucose uptake by muscle cells, **adipose (fat) cells,** and many other cells. Both of these actions of insulin lower blood glucose and help return it to the normal fasting range within a few hours after a person eats.[16] In addition, insulin reduces gluconeogenesis by the liver.

Other hormones counteract the effects of insulin. When a person has not eaten carbohydrates for some time, blood glucose begins to fall below the normal fasting range. It can be restored by the hormone **glucagon,** which is also released from the pancreas. This hormone prompts the breakdown of glycogen in the liver, resulting in release of glucose to the bloodstream.[16] Glucagon also enhances gluconeogenesis. In these ways glucagon helps restore blood glucose to normal concentrations (Figure 3-4).

At the same time, the hormones **epinephrine** (adrenaline) and norepinephrine are released from the adrenal glands and nearby nerve endings. These hormones trigger breakdown of glycogen in the liver; the resulting glucose is released into the bloodstream. These hormones are responsible for the "fight or flight" reaction. They are released in large amounts in response to a perceived threat, such as a car approaching head-on. The resulting rapid flood of glucose into the bloodstream promotes quick mental and physical reactions. Other hormones, such as **cortisol** and growth hormone, also help to regulate blood glucose (Table 3-3).

In essence, the actions of insulin on blood glucose are balanced by the actions of glucagon, epinephrine, norepinephrine, cortisol, and other hormones.[20] If hormonal balance is not maintained, such as during over- or under-production of insulin or glucagon, major changes in blood glucose concentrations occur. The Nutrition Perspective provides examples of these phenomena.

Before we move on, let's step back and look at one of the intricacies of our body's metabolism. To maintain blood glucose within an acceptable range the body relies on a complex regulatory system. This provides a safeguard against extreme hyperglycemia or hypoglycemia if one control mechanism fails. Suppose instead there were only one mechanism for controlling blood glucose, such as a nerve connection between the brain and pancreas that when appropriately stimulated caused release of pancreatic hormones. Damage to this nerve would prevent hormone release, causing extreme fluctuations in blood glucose, with dire physiological consequences. In fact, a disturbance in one of the body's control mechanisms—such as hormonal release from the pancreas—can greatly influence blood glucose levels, but it doesn't knock out all of the other regulatory systems. The liver and adrenal glands still act to provide moderate regulation of blood glucose. This example of checks and balances is typical of how the body maintains blood and other tissue concentrations of its key constituents within fairly narrow ranges. This tendency of the

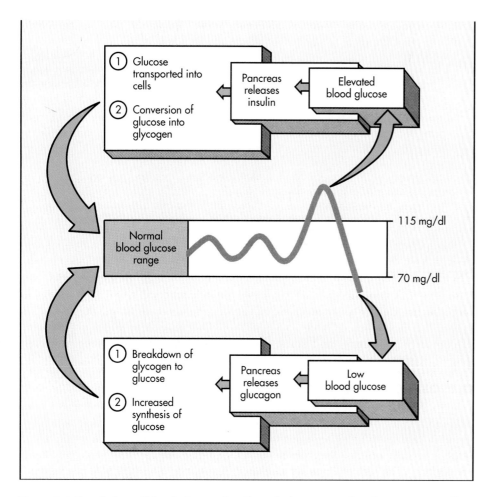

Figure 3-4 Regulation of blood glucose. Insulin and glucagon are key factors in controlling blood glucose. Other hormones, such as epinephrine, norepinephrine, cortisol, and growth hormone, also contribute to blood glucose regulation.

TABLE 3-3

Role of various hormones in the regulation of blood glucose[20]

Hormone	Source	Target organ or tissue	Overall effect on organ or tissue	Effect on blood glucose
Insulin	Pancreas	Liver; muscle; adipose tissue	Increases glucose uptake by muscles and adipose tissue; increases glycogen synthesis; suppresses gluconeogenesis	Decrease
Glucagon	Pancreas	Liver	Increases glycogen breakdown, with release of glucose by the liver; increases gluconeogenesis	Increase
Epinephrine and norepinephrine	Adrenal glands and nerve endings	Liver; muscle	Increase glycogen breakdown, with release of glucose by the liver; increase gluconeogenesis	Increase
Cortisol	Adrenal glands	Liver; muscle	Increases gluconeogenesis by the liver; decreases glucose use by muscles and other organs	Increase
Growth hormone	Adrenal glands	Liver; muscle; adipose tissue	Decreases glucose uptake by muscles; increases fat mobilization and utilization; increases glucose output by the liver	Increase

body to maintain a stable internal environment is called *homeostasis* (see the Nutrition Focus in Chapter 7 for a detailed discussion of homeostasis).

CONCEPT CHECK

Fasting blood glucose is maintained within the very narrow range of about 70 to 115 mg/100 ml of blood. When blood glucose rises after a meal, the hormone insulin restores normal concentrations, partly by increasing glucose uptake by muscle and adipose tissue. When blood glucose falls during periods of little or no food consumption, glucagon, epinephrine, and other hormones increase the liver's release of glucose into the bloodstream to restore normal concentrations. Whether a person has just eaten or has fasted overnight, hormonal activity and the action of the liver together strive to maintain blood glucose within a very narrow range.

Structures and Functions of Complex Carbohydrates

Carbohydrates containing more than two monosaccharide units are classified as **oligosaccharides** or **polysaccharides,** depending on how large they are. The polysaccharides, often referred to as *complex carbohydrates,* include some that are digestible (e.g., **starch**) and some that are largely indigestible, such as dietary fiber.[4]

OLIGOSACCHARIDES: RAFFINOSE AND STACHYOSE

Oligosaccharides contain three to ten single sugar units (*oligo* means scant). Two oligosaccharides of nutritional importance are **raffinose** and **stachyose,** which are found in beans and other legumes.[16] These are constructed of typical monosaccharides chemically bonded together in such a way that our digestive enzymes cannot break them apart. Thus when we consume beans and other legumes, the raffinose and stachyose are still undigested upon reaching the large intestine. There, bacteria metabolize them, producing gas and other by-products.

Recently, stores have begun selling an enzyme preparation (Beano) that prevents the unpleasant side effects of intestinal gas if consumed right before a meal. Once consumed, the enzyme preparation breaks down many of the indigestible oligosaccharides in legumes and other vegetables in the gastrointestinal tract before they reach the large intestine. This allows for the absorption of their monosaccharide components in the small intestine, as is the case for digestible carbohydrates. We discuss the use of this product in more detail in Chapter 5.

DIGESTIBLE POLYSACCHARIDES: STARCH AND GLYCOGEN

Polysaccharides are polymers containing many monosaccharide units, up to 3000 or more.[16] Most polysaccharides of nutritional importance are synthesized from glucose, as when vegetables turn glucose into starch during maturation. This makes peas and corn sweetest when they are young. Starch, the major digestible polysaccharide in our diet, is the storage form of carbohydrate in plants. There are two types of plant starch—**amylose** and **amylopectin**—both of which are a source of energy for plants and animals.

Both amylose and amylopectin are glucose polymers containing many glucose units linked by alpha glycosidic bonds. Recall that these alpha bonds can be broken by human digestive enzymes. The primary difference between the two types of starch is that amylose is a straight-chain polymer, whereas amylopectin is a highly branched polymer. The linking alpha bonds at the branch points in amylopectin also extend from the sixth carbon in the glucose unit rather than from the fourth carbon, as in the straight-chain portions of amylopectin, or amylose. Despite this difference, the body can digest both types of starch. Cooking increases the digestibility of these starches by making them more soluble in water and thus more available for attack by digestive enzymes.

oligosaccharides Carbohydrates containing three to ten monosaccharide units.

polysaccharides Carbohydrates containing many glucose units, up to 3000 or more.

raffinose An indigestible oligosaccharide made of three monosaccharides (galactose-glucose-fructose).

stachyose An indigestible oligosaccharide made of four monosaccharides (galactose-galactose-glucose-fructose).

amylose A straight-chain type of starch composed of glucose units.

amylopectin A branched chain type of starch composed of glucose units.

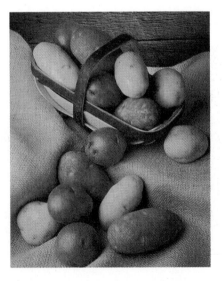

Potatoes are rich in plant starch.

Amylose and amylopectin are found in potatoes, beans, breads, pasta, rice, and other starchy products, typically in a ratio of about 1:4. The branches in amylopectin allow it to form a very stable starch gel, enabling it to retain water and resist water seepage. Food manufacturers commonly use starches rich in amylopectin in sauces and gravies for frozen foods because they remain stable over a wide temperature range. Manufacturers may also use processes to bond the starch molecules to one another, further increasing their stability. This product, called **modified food starch,** is used in baby foods, salad dressings, and instant puddings.[3]

Glycogen, the storage form of carbohydrate in humans and other animals, is a glucose polymer with alpha bonds and numerous branches. No glycogen is found in meat, however, because it is used up during slaughter and later storage. Overall, the structure of glycogen is similar to that of amylopectin, but the branching patterns are more complicated (Figure 3-5). Enzymes that break down glycogen in cells act only at the ends of the glucose chains. The more numerous the branches of a molecule, the more sites (ends) are available for enzyme action.[16] Because glycogen is so highly branched, it is quickly broken down by the body cells in which it is stored. Therefore it is an ideal form for carbohydrate storage in the body. In other words, when the body needs an immediate source of blood glucose, the many branches of glycogen provide multiple points at which a glucose molecule can be broken off, rather than waiting for each glucose molecule in a single chain to be released sequentially.

The liver and muscles are the major storage sites for glycogen.[16] Enzymatic breakdown of glycogen first yields glucose-phosphate molecules. The liver contains the enzyme that converts this glucose-phosphate to glucose, which can then enter the bloodstream, but muscles lack this enzyme. Thus, as we saw already, liver glycogen plays a role in regulation of blood glucose. Although muscle glycogen isn't converted to blood glucose, it does supply glucose for muscle use, especially during high-intensity and endurance physical activity. (See Chapter 10 for a discussion of carbohydrate use during physical activity.)

INDIGESTIBLE POLYSACCHARIDES: DIETARY FIBER

Folklore surrounding dietary fiber has been a part of American culture since the 1800s. In the 1820s and 1830s, a minister named Sylvester Graham traveled up and down the East Coast extolling the virtues of fiber. He left us a legacy—the graham cracker. However, today's graham cracker bears little resemblance to the whole-grain product he promoted. The next wave of fiber frenzy crested in the mid-1870s with Dr. John Harvey Kellogg and his brother William, of breakfast cereal fame. Dr.

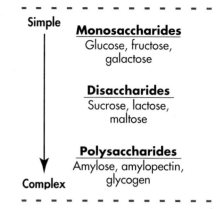

Simple

Monosaccharides
Glucose, fructose, galactose

Disaccharides
Sucrose, lactose, maltose

Polysaccharides
Amylose, amylopectin, glycogen

Complex

modified food starch A product consisting of chemically linked starch molecules that is more stable than normal, unmodified starches.

dietary fiber Substances in food (essentially from plants) that cannot be broken down by the normal digestive processes in the stomach and small intestine. These substances add bulk to the feces. Some are metabolized by bacteria in the large intestine.

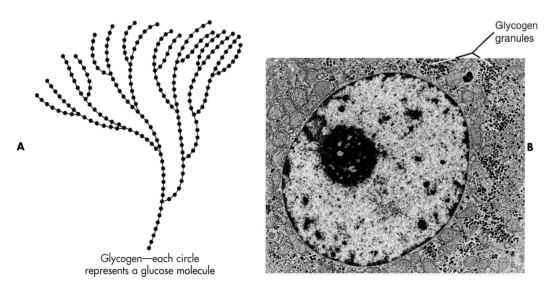

Glycogen granules

A

B

Glycogen—each circle represents a glucose molecule

Figure 3-5 **A,** Glycogen structure. **B,** Glycogen stores as found in the cell.

Kellogg became the first person to earn a million dollars from "health foods." One of his patients was Charles W. Post, who followed the Kelloggs' lead and started the Post Toasted Cornflakes Company. In 1901 alone, Post netted one million dollars from his Grape Nuts cereal and other products. As we will see, present-day scientific evidence supports this early promotion of fiber as part of a total diet.[4]

Insoluble and Soluble Forms of Dietary Fiber

In terms of their chemical composition, dietary fibers are composed primarily of the polysaccharides **cellulose, hemicellulose, pectin, gum,** and **mucilage.** The only noncarbohydrate components of dietary fibers are **lignins,** which are complex alcohol derivatives (Table 3-4). All forms of dietary fiber come from plants and are not digested in the human stomach or small intestine.[11]

Cellulose is a straight-chain glucose polymer similar to amylose; but unlike amylose, which contains alpha bonds, the glucose units in cellulose are linked by beta bonds. As we noted earlier, glucose molecules joined by beta bonds are not broken down by human digestive enzymes. Thus cellulose is not digestible by humans and is classified as a dietary fiber, not a starch. Because the long glucose chains of cellulose are linear, they can pack closely together, forming fibrous structures of great strength. Overall, cellulose, hemicelluloses, and lignins form the structural part of the plant. A cotton ball is pure cellulose. Bran fiber is rich in hemicelluloses. Since bran layers form the outer covering of all grains, **whole grains** are good sources of this dietary fiber.[21] The woody fibers in broccoli are partly lignins. As a class, these dietary fibers generally do not dissolve in water and thus are called **insoluble fibers.**

Pectins, gums, and mucilages are found inside and around plant cells. They help "glue" plant cells together. These dietary fibers either dissolve or swell when put into water and thus are called **soluble fibers.**[22] Some forms of hemicellulose also fall into this soluble-fiber category. Soluble fibers such as gum arabic, guar gum, locust bean gum, and various pectins are present in numerous food products, especially salad dressings, inexpensive ice creams, jams, and jellies. Other rich sources of soluble fibers include fruits and vegetables in general, soybean fiber, rice bran, and **psyllium** seeds (found in many commercial fiber laxatives).[21]

One workable definition of dietary fiber is "the foodstuffs that remain undigested as they enter the large intestine." There is really no common property that characterizes dietary fibers except their ability to resist digestion in the small intestine. Since some dietary fibers—especially the soluble fibers—are digested by bacteria in the large intestine, it is not accurate to say that dietary fiber is the carbohydrate found in the feces.[11]

whole grains Grains containing the entire seed of the plant, including the bran, germ, and endosperm (starchy interior).

insoluble fibers Fibers that mostly do not dissolve in water and are not metabolized by bacteria in the large intestine. These include cellulose, some hemicelluloses, and lignins.

soluble fibers Fibers that either dissolve or swell in water and are metabolized (fermented) by bacteria in the large intestine. These include pectins, gums, and mucilages.

psyllium A mostly soluble type of dietary fiber found in the seeds of the plantain plant.

- - - - - - - - - - - - - -

Many people think of wheat bran as pure fiber, but it is actually a mixture of several dietary fibers. It also contains some protein, fat, and trace minerals, as is true for all fiber sources. The age of a plant may also influence its fiber composition; for example, young carrots contain very little lignin, whereas old carrots may contain 10% to 20% of this material.

- - - - - - - - - - - - - -

TABLE 3-4

Classification of dietary fibers

Type	Component(s)	Examples	Physiological effects	Major food sources
Insoluble				
Noncarbohydrate	Lignins	Wheat bran	Under study	All plants
Carbohydrate	Cellulose	Wheat products	Increases fecal bulk	All plants
	Hemicelluloses	Brown rice	Decreases intestinal transit time	Wheat, rye, rice, vegetables
Soluble				
Carbohydrate	Pectins, gums, mucilages, some hemicelluloses	Apples Bananas Citrus fruits Carrots Barley Oats Kidney beans	Delays gastric emptying; slows glucose absorption; can lower serum cholesterol	Citrus fruits, oat products, beans

Bacteria in the large intestine metabolize soluble dietary fibers into products such as short-chain fatty acids (e.g., acetic acid, butyric acid, and propionic acid) and gases. These acids, especially butyric acid, provide fuel for the cells in the large intestine and enhance their health. All these products can also be absorbed into the bloodstream. As a result of bacterial metabolism, soluble dietary fibers yield about 3 kcal/g on average, although the actual value is still in question. When intake of dietary fiber is high, its breakdown by bacteria can cause certain gases, such as methane (CH_4) and hydrogen (H_2), to increase in the breath, but this is not harmful. Because of the potential for breakdown in the large intestine of some forms of dietary fiber, soluble fibers are also defined as those that are fermentable in the large intestine, while insoluble fibers are defined as those that are nonfermentable.

An outmoded term used for dietary fiber is **crude fiber.** This term arose during the early 1900s to reflect the amount of indigestible foodstuff present in animal feed. The animal feed was boiled for 1 hour in acid and for another hour in an alkaline solution. The remains of that chemical digestion was called crude fiber; it consisted mostly of cellulose and lignins. All other types of fiber were destroyed by the chemical action. Food composition tables may still report dietary fiber values in terms of crude fiber. These values often bear little resemblance to dietary fiber values because crude fiber no longer contains many fiber components. This point is important. When nutrition scientists talk about fiber, they are referring to dietary fiber, not crude fiber. Other outmoded terms for dietary fiber include *roughage* and *bulk*.

Health Benefits of Dietary Fiber

Dietary fiber supplies mass to the feces, making elimination much easier. When enough fiber is consumed, the stool will be large and soft because many types of plant fibers attract water. The larger size stimulates the intestinal muscles, which aids elimination. Consequently, less pressure is necessary to expel the stool.[11]

When too little dietary fiber is eaten, the opposite can occur: the stool may be small and hard. Constipation may result, which can force one to exert excessive pressure in the large intestine during defecation. This high pressure can force parts of the large intestine wall out from between the surrounding bands of muscle, forming small pouches called **diverticula.**[2] A person can have many diverticula (Figure 3-6). **Hemorrhoids** may also result from excessive straining during defecation (see Chapter 6).[11]

Diverticula are asymptomatic in about 80% of affected people; that is, they are not noticeable. The asymptomatic form of this disease is called **diverticulosis.** If the diverticula become filled with food particles, such as hulls and seeds, bacteria can metabolize these food particles into acids and gases. The acids and gases irritate the diverticula and may eventually cause them to become inflamed, a condition known as **diverticulitis.** Antibiotics may be administered to lessen the bacterial action, and intake of dietary fiber should be reduced to limit further bacterial activity. Once the inflammation subsides, a high-fiber diet (but free of seeds and hulls) is started to ease stool elimination and reduce the risk of a future attack.[23]

Although diverticula occur in about 50% of elderly persons in Western countries, they are rare in Third World countries. The major reason for this difference probably is the much lower intake of dietary fiber in Western countries compared with that in the Third World.[4]

Additional health benefits can accrue from consumption of dietary fiber. A diet high in fiber aids weight control and reduces the risk of developing obesity. The bulky nature of high-fiber foods fills us up without yielding much energy. High-fat foods tend to do just the opposite, contributing to obesity. Increasing intake of foods rich in dietary fiber is one strategy for remaining satisfied after a meal even if the fat content in a diet is low.[4]

When consumed in large amounts, soluble dietary fiber somewhat slows glucose absorption from the small intestine. This effect can be helpful in treatment of diabetes (see the Nutrition Perspective). A high intake of soluble dietary fiber also inhibits cholesterol absorption from the small intestine, thereby reducing serum cho-

crude fiber What remains of dietary fiber after acid and alkaline treatment. This primarily consists of cellulose and lignin.

diverticula Pouches that protrude through the exterior wall of the large intestine.

hemorrhoid A pronounced swelling of a large vein, particularly veins found in the anal region.

diverticulosis The condition of having many diverticula in the large intestine.

CRITICAL THINKING

Your grandfather has diverticulosis. At a holiday party, he insists on eating nuts and seeds even though you tell him that doing so is not good for his condition. He ignores your warning and 2 days later tells you that he has abdominal cramps and a fever. How would you explain his symptoms?

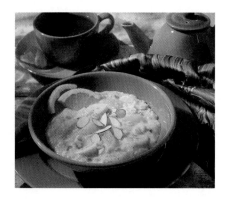

Oatmeal is a rich source of soluble fiber.

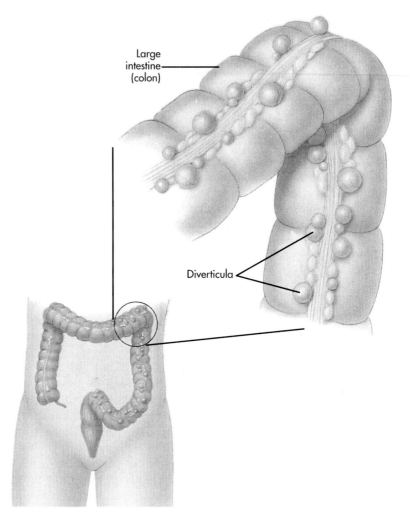

Figure 3-6 Diverticula in the colon. A low-fiber diet increases the risk of developing diverticula.

CRITICAL THINKING

Celia decides to go on a diet and buys over-the-counter pills. You look at the ingredients and note that the pills contain *psyllium*, a word you recognize from the nutrition course you're taking. What advice can you give Celia about the wisdom of using these diet pills?

lesterol. The short-chain fatty acids resulting from bacterial degradation of soluble fiber also probably reduce cholesterol synthesis in the liver once these fatty acids are absorbed and enter the liver. In addition, the reduced glucose absorption that occurs with diets high in soluble fiber is linked to a decrease in insulin release. Since insulin stimulates cholesterol synthesis in the liver, this reduction in insulin may contribute to the ability of soluble dietary fiber to lower serum cholesterol. All of these potential mechanisms for lowering serum cholesterol are still under study.

To be useful in treating diabetes or elevated serum cholesterol, however, soluble dietary fiber must be consumed in considerable quantity. For example, oat bran affects serum cholesterol levels only at daily intakes of 40 to 60 g or above, which is more than half a cup. Other rich sources of soluble fiber include fruits, vegetables, legumes (cooked dry beans), soybeans, and psyllium seeds.[21]

Dietary fiber may also play a key role in preventing cancer of the large intestine, commonly called colon cancer (*colon* is another name for the large intestine). Colon cancer ranks among the top three lethal cancers in the United States.[1] Many epidemiological and case-control studies have shown an association between colon cancer and diets low in whole grains, fruits, and vegetables—all good sources of dietary fiber—and, conversely, diets high in fat, meat, and excess energy content.[22] Many other factors are also involved in development of the disease, such as genetic background.

We currently know little about how dietary fiber might affect colon cancer development. There is good reason for suggesting that potential carcinogens in the intestinal contents are (1) diluted by fluid attracted to the fiber; (2) bound to the fiber; and (3) more rapidly excreted, since dietary fiber speeds passage of a meal through the intestinal tract. Colon cancer has been prevented in laboratory animals by adding fiber to the diet. Cellulose, hemicelluloses, and lignins have the major protective role.[21]

In human studies, dietary fiber from fruits and vegetables has tended to be most protective against colon cancer. This finding suggests that increased consumption of vitamin C and carotenoids from fruits and vegetables, or simply the reduction in meat and fat intake when a high-fiber diet is instituted, may exert the main protective effect, rather than dietary fiber alone. Currently, foods, rather than nutritional supplements, are regarded as the best source of this preventive effect of dietary fiber. In a recent 4-year trial, consumption of vitamin E, vitamin C, and beta carotene supplements by people who had already had one occurrence of colon cancer was shown to be ineffective in reducing subsequent colon cancer risk.[13] Critics of the study suggest that 4 years is an insufficient treatment period to demonstrate the possible protective effects of supplements. Another supplement trial, extending over 10 years, will be completed soon; the results of this study should clarify the role, if any, of supplements in protecting against colon cancer.

A low calcium intake is also implicated in colon cancer risk. We cover the reasons for this in Chapter 14. Finally, inactivity is also a risk factor for colon cancer. Regular physical activity aids bowel regularity, likely reducing contact of the colon with cancer-causing substances.

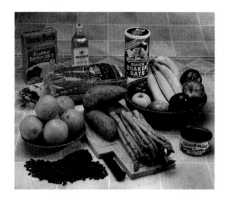

These foods are all good sources of dietary fiber.

CONCEPT CHECK

Amylose, amylopectin, and glycogen are all storage forms of glucose, called polysaccharides. Amylose and amylopectin combine in varying proportions to form food starch, such as that found in potatoes and bread. Glycogen is a storage form of glucose in humans. Liver glycogen yields a ready source of blood glucose.

Dietary fiber is essentially the portion of ingested food that remains undigested as it enters the large intestine. Fiber components include cellulose, hemicelluloses, lignins, pectins, gums, and mucilages. There are two general classes of dietary fiber: insoluble and soluble. Insoluble fibers are mostly made up of cellulose, hemicelluloses, and lignins. Soluble fibers are made up mostly of pectins, gums, and mucilages. Both insoluble and soluble fibers are resistant to human digestive enzymes, but bacteria in the large intestine can break down soluble fibers.

Dietary fiber forms a vital part of the diet by adding mass to the stool, which eases elimination. Soluble fibers can also be useful for controlling blood glucose in patients with diabetes and in lowering serum cholesterol. Whole grains, vegetables, beans, and fruits are excellent sources of dietary fiber. An ample intake of dietary fiber is promoted as a tool in the prevention of colon cancer.

Recommended Carbohydrate Intakes

No RDA for carbohydrates has been established. As discussed before, it is important to consume at least 50 to 100 g of carbohydrates per day to prevent ketosis. Remember, this is just the minimum; additional carbohydrate intake continues to spare protein and helps meet energy needs (Figure 3-7).

It is easy to consume 50 g of carbohydrates. Just three pieces of fruit or three slices of bread or a little more than three cups of milk will suffice. In fact, it is difficult to follow a diet that will produce ketosis. Again, the average American eats 200 to 300 g of carbohydrates per day. The top five contributors of carbohydrates to American diets are white breads, sugared soft drinks, baked goods, table sugar, and milk.

In the United States carbohydrates supply about 50% of dietary energy intake for adults. Worldwide, however, carbohydrates account for about 70% of all energy

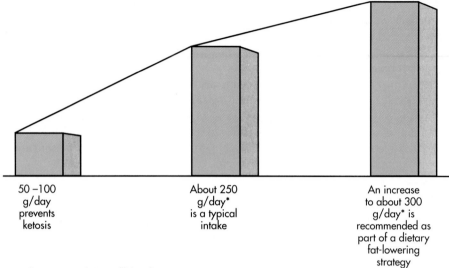

50 –100
g/day
prevents
ketosis

About 250
g/day*
is a typical
intake

An increase
to about 300
g/day* is
recommended as
part of a dietary
fat-lowering
strategy

*Based on 48% and 55% of kilocalories,
respectively, for a 2200 kcal diet

Figure 3-7 The dietary carbohydrate continuum. Relatively little dietary carbohydrate is needed to prevent ketosis. Experts advise higher intakes, especially of complex carbohydrates, so that we can reduce our fat intake while still consuming enough energy.

consumed. In some countries, carbohydrates account for up to 80% of the energy consumed.

Nutrition experts recommend that we include more starch and fiber in our diets. A reasonable goal is about 45% of energy intake from starch, with total carbohydrates accounting for about 55% to 60% of total energy intake. As carbohydrate intake increases—by eating more foods from the bottom part of the Food Guide Pyramid—fat intake should automatically decrease, as long as added fat is kept to a minimum and foods are prepared and served without additional fat.

As for dietary fiber, a reasonable intake is 20 to 35 g/day (10 to 13 g/1000 kcal). Average intake in the United States is closer to 16 g/day. Thus most of us should increase our dietary fiber intake. A fiber intake of 20 to 35 g should prevent much of the diverticulosis that typically develops in people in Western countries.[2] Eating a high-fiber cereal for breakfast is one easy way to increase dietary fiber intake (Figure 3-8). Whole-food sources like cereals, not bran supplements, are preferable because foods provide a broader variety of nutrients. This is especially true for many natural high-fiber foods—whole grains, fruits, vegetables, and beans.[21]

Table 3-5 lists a diet containing 25 to 30 g of dietary fiber but only 1750 kcal. This is an easy diet to follow to meet fiber recommendations if you like whole-wheat bread, fruits, and beans (Figure 3-9). Table 3-6 lists general tips on increasing dietary fiber intake.

Note that manufacturers list enriched white (refined) flour as wheat flour on food labels. Most people think that if "wheat bread" is on the label, they are buying a whole-wheat product. Not so. If the label does not list "whole-wheat flour" first, then the product is not primarily a whole-wheat bread, and thus will not contain as much dietary fiber as it could. Careful reading of labels is important in the search for more dietary fiber—look especially for whole grains.

Keep in mind, however, that any nutrient can lead to health problems when consumed in excess, including carbohydrate and dietary fiber. High carbohydrate, high fiber, and low fat does not mean zero kilocalories. Carbohydrates help moderate energy intake in comparison to fats, but the contribution of high-carbohydrate foods to total energy intake still has to be accounted for. However, Americans are becoming fatter generally not because they are eating too much bread and pasta, but because there is an epidemic of physical inactivity and high-fat diets. Still, variety,

Nutrition Facts

Serving Size 1 cup (55g/2.0 oz.)
Servings Per Container 10

Amount Per Serving	Cereal	Cereal with ½ Cup Vitamins A & D Skim Milk
Calories	170	210
Calories from Fat	10	10
	% Daily Value**	
Total Fat 1.0g*	2%	2%
Sat. Fat 0g	0%	0%
Cholesterol 0mg	0%	0%
Sodium 300mg	13%	15%
Potassium 340mg	10%	16%
Total Carbohydrate 43g	14%	16%
Dietary Fiber 7g	28%	28%
Sugars 17g		
Other Carbohydrate 19g		
Protein 4g		
Vitamin A	15%	20%
Vitamin C	0%	2%
Calcium	2%	15%
Iron	45%	45%
Vitamin D	10%	25%
Thiamin	25%	30%
Riboflavin	25%	35%
Niacin	25%	25%
Vitamin B$_6$	25%	25%
Folate	25%	25%
Vitamin B$_{12}$	25%	35%
Phosphorus	20%	30%
Magnesium	20%	25%
Zinc	25%	25%
Copper	15%	15%

*Amount in cereal. One half cup skim milk contributes an additional 40 calories, 65mg sodium, 6g total carbohydrate (6g sugars), and 4g protein.
**Percent Daily Values are based on a 2,000 calorie diet. Your daily values may be higher or lower depending on your calorie needs:

	Calories:	2,000	2,500
Total Fat	Less than	65g	80g
Sat Fat	Less than	20g	25g
Cholesterol	Less than	300mg	300mg
Sodium	Less than	2,400mg	2,400mg
Potassium		3,500mg	3,500mg
Total Carbohydrate		300g	375g
Dietary Fiber		25g	30g

Calories per gram:
Fat 9 • Carbohydrate 4 • Protein 4

Ingredients: Wheat bran with other parts of wheat, raisins, sugar, corn syrup, salt, malt flavoring,

Vitamins and Minerals: iron, niacinamide, zinc oxide, pyridoxine hydrochloride (vitamin B$_6$), riboflavin (vitamin B$_2$), vitamin A palmitate, thiamin hydrochloride (vitamin B$_1$), folic acid, vitamin B$_{12}$, and vitamin D.

Nutrition Facts

Serving Size 1 cup (30g)
Servings Per Container about 13

Amount Per Serving	Lucky Charms	with ½ cup skim Milk
Calories	120	160
Calories from Fat	10	15
	% Daily Value**	
Total Fat 1g*	2%	2%
Saturated Fat 0g	0%	1%
Cholesterol 0mg	0%	1%
Sodium 200mg	8%	11%
Potassium 55mg	2%	7%
Total Carbohydrate 25g	8%	10%
Dietary Fiber 1g	6%	6%
Sugars 13g		
Other Carbohydrate 11g		
Protein 2g		
Vitamin A	25%	30%
Vitamin C	25%	25%
Calcium	2%	15%
Iron	25%	25%
Vitamin D	10%	25%
Thiamin	25%	30%
Riboflavin	25%	35%
Niacin	25%	25%
Vitamin B$_6$	25%	25%
Folate	25%	25%

*Amount in Cereal. A serving of cereal plus skim milk provides 1.5g fat, <5mg cholesterol, 260mg sodium, 260mg potassium, 31g carbohydrate (19g sugar) and 6g protein.
**Percent Daily Values are based on a 2,000 calorie diet. Your daily values may be higher or lower depending on your calorie needs:

	Calories:	2,000	2,500
Total Fat	Less than	65g	80g
Sat Fat	Less than	20g	25g
Cholesterol	Less than	300mg	300mg
Sodium	Less than	2,400mg	2,400mg
Potassium		3,500mg	3,500mg
Total Carbohydrate		300g	375g
Dietary Fiber		25g	30g

INGREDIENTS: WHOLE OAT FLOUR (INCLUDES THE OAT BRAN), MARSHMALLOW BITS (SUGAR, MODIFIED CORN STARCH, CORN SYRUP, DEXTROSE, GELATIN, RED 40, YELLOW 5 & 6, BLUES 1 & 2 AND OTHER COLOR ADDED, ARTIFICIAL FLAVOR), SUGAR, CORN SYRUP, WHEAT STARCH, SALT, COLOR ADDED, CALCIUM CARBONATE, TRISODIUM PHOSPHATE, VITAMIN C (SODIUM ASCORBATE), A B VITAMIN (NIACIN), IRON (A MINERAL NUTRIENT), VITAMIN B$_6$ (PYRIDOXINE HYDROCHLORIDE), VITAMIN A (PALMITATE), VITAMIN B$_2$ (RIBOFLAVIN), VITAMIN B$_1$ (THIAMIN MONONITRATE), ARTIFICIAL FLAVOR, A B VITAMIN (FOLIC ACID), VITAMIN D, VITAMIN E (MIXED TOCOPHEROLS) ADDED TO PROTECT FRESHNESS.

Figure 3-8 Reading the Nutrition Facts panel on food labels helps us choose more nutritious foods. Based on the information from these nutrition labels, which cereal is the better choice for breakfast? Consider the amount of dietary fiber in each cereal. Did the ingredients lists give you any clues? Remember that ingredients are always listed in descending order by weight on a label.

TABLE 3-5

Sample 1750 kcal menu containing 25 to 30 g of fiber*†

Menu	Fiber content (grams)	Exchanges	Carbohydrate content (grams) based on the Exchange System
Breakfast			
1 cup orange juice	—	2 fruit	30
¾ cup Wheaties	3	1 starch	15
½ cup 2% milk	—	½ very-low-fat milk	6
1 slice whole-wheat toast	1.5	1 starch	15
1 tsp margarine	—	1 fat	0
Coffee	—	Free	0
Lunch			
2 oz lean ham	—	2 lean meat	0
2 slices whole-wheat bread	3	2 starch	30
2 tsp mayonnaise	—	2 fat	0
¼ cup lettuce	0.2	1 vegetable	0
⅓ cup cooked white beans	4.8	1 starch	15
1 pear (with skin)	4	1 fruit	15
½ cup 1% milk	—	½ skim/very-low-fat milk	6
Snack			
1 carrot (as carrot sticks)	2.2	1 vegetable	5
Dinner			
3 oz broiled chicken (no skin)	—	3 very lean meat	0
1 baked potato (large, with skin)	4.8	2 starch	30
1½ tsp margarine	—	1½ fat	0
1 cup cooked green beans	2.2	2 vegetable	10
½ tsp margarine	—	½ fat	0
1 cup 1% milk	—	1 skim/very-low-fat milk	12
1 apple (with peel)	3.7	1 fruit	15
Snack			
1 raisin bagel	1.2	2 starch	30
Total	30.6 grams		Total 234 grams

*The overall diet pattern is based on the Food Guide Pyramid
†Carbohydrate, 60% of kilocalories; protein, 20% of kilocalories; fat, 20% of kilocalories.

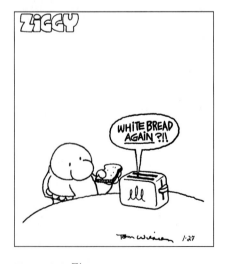

ZIGGY

WHITE BREAD AGAIN ?!!

Figure 3-9 Ziggy.

balance, and moderation are the watchwords when it comes to carbohydrate intake, despite the emphasis we place on a generous carbohydrate intake in this chapter. Let's consider this issue in more detail, particularly the intake of simple sugars, which are often maligned as being unhealthy.

MODERATE INTAKES OF SIMPLE SUGARS

Many people think it is not healthy to consume simple sugars. True, simple sugars by themselves have very low nutrient densities. In other words, sugary foods may supply few, if any, vitamins, minerals, or proteins compared with the amount of energy they supply. However, if you can afford to consume some extra food energy, there is nothing wrong with eating sugars. Simple sugars become a problem primarily when substituted for more nutritious foods.[3] In that case, deficiencies of vitamins and other important nutrients may occur.

TABLE 3-6

Increasing dietary fiber intake is not hard to do		
Try this:	**Instead of this:**	**Dietary fiber bonus (grams)**
Whole-wheat bread, 1 slice	White bread, 1 slice	1.5
Brown rice, ½ cup	White rice, ½ cup	0.5
Baked potato with skin, 1 medium	Mashed potatoes, ½ cup	1.5
Unpeeled apple (or applesauce made with unpeeled apples), 1 medium	Regular applesauce, ½ cup	1.5
Orange segments, 1 orange	Orange juice, 1 cup	1
Whole-grain cereal (hot or ready-to-eat), 1 cup	Sweetened cereal, 1 cup	2.5
Popcorn (lightly seasoned with butter or salt, if at all), 3 cups	Potato chips, 12	1
Bean dip, ¼ cup	Sour cream dip, ¼ cup	1.5
Kidney beans on salad, 2 tbsp	Bacon bits on salad, 2 tbsp	3
Fruit juice, 1 cup	Coffee or tea, 1 cup	1.5
Salad, 2 cups	French fries, 12	1

Nutritionists suggest that simple sugars should provide no more than 10% to 15% of total energy intake daily.[3] This moderate intake, which corresponds to a maximum of about 75 g (or 15 tcaspoons) of simple sugars, allows for inclusion of a considerable amount of complex carbohydrates in the diet. On average, Americans eat about 80 g of simple sugars daily, not including the lactose in dairy products. This average sugar intake corresponds to about 18% of total energy intake[3]; many people, no doubt, consume much more than this amount. Intake of simple sugars by young children, for example, can exceed 50% of total energy intake. Table 3-7 suggests ways to reduce intake of simple sugars if that is necessary. Table 3-8 lists the amount of sugar in many popular sweetened foods.

Most of the simple sugar that we eat has been added to foods and beverages during processing and manufacturing. The rest of the sugar in our diets is present naturally in foods such as fruits or comes from the sugar bowl.[3] During food processing, the simple-sugar content is often increased. The more processed the food, generally the higher the simple-sugar content. An apple contains no added sugars, canned apples in heavy syrup contain 10 to 15 g (2 to 3 teaspoons) of added sugars, and ⅙ of a 9-inch apple pie contains 30 g (6 teaspoons) of added sugars.

Overall, consumption of table sugar (sucrose) has dropped during the last 10 years, but consumption of corn sweeteners has increased dramatically. Corn sweeteners are cheaper and easier to transport than other forms of sugar used in food manufacturing and processing.[3]

HEALTH EFFECTS OF SIMPLE SUGARS

Some people claim that simple sugars cause heart disease, diabetes, hyperactivity, juvenile delinquency, obesity, and other problems. Little or no credible research supports these allegations. A systematic cause-and-effect relationship between these conditions and consumption of sugars—specifically sucrose—has not been established. There is a widespread notion that high sugar intake by children causes hyperactivity, typically part of the syndrome called *attention deficit hyperactive disorder (ADHD)* described in Chapter 17. Some researchers claim that sucrose creates an excited—even antisocial—state, which may lead to violence and disruptive behavior. However, most researchers find that sucrose itself is not the villain, and indeed may have the opposite effect.[25] A high-carbohydrate meal, for example, calms many chil-

We have mentioned several times that milk and some dairy products contain the milk sugar lactose. This should in no way be construed to mean that milk is a food to avoid in order to limit simple-sugar consumption. In fact, low-fat and nonfat dairy products have an overall high nutrient density and would be one of the last sources of sugars to limit.

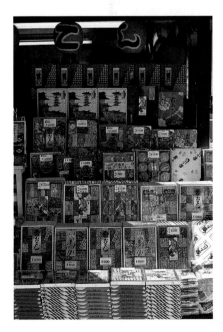

Candy and other sucrose-rich foods are part of diets worldwide, as shown in this photo from Japan.

TABLE 3-7

Suggestions for reducing simple sugar intake

At the supermarket

- Read ingredients labels. Identify all the added sugars in a product. Select items lower in total sugar when possible.
- Buy fresh fruits or fruits packed in water, juice, or light syrup rather than those packed in heavy syrup.
- Buy fewer foods that are high in sugar, such as prepared baked goods, candies, sugared cereals, sweet desserts, soft drinks, and fruit-flavored punches. Substitute vanilla wafers, graham crackers, bagels, English muffins, and diet soft drinks, for example.
- Buy reduced-fat microwave popcorn to replace candy for snacks.

In the kitchen

- Reduce the sugar in foods prepared at home. Try new recipes or adjust your own. Start by reducing the sugar gradually until you've decreased it by one third or more.
- Experiment with spices, such as cinnamon, cardamom, coriander, nutmeg, ginger, and mace to enhance the flavor of foods.
- Use home-prepared items (with less sugar) instead of commercially prepared ones that are higher in sugar, when possible.

At the table

- Use less of all sugars. This includes white and brown sugars, honey, molasses, and syrups.
- Choose fewer foods high in sugar, such as prepared baked goods, candies, and sweet desserts.
- Reach for fresh fruit instead of a sweet for dessert or when you want a snack.
- Add less sugar to foods—coffee, tea, cereal, or fruit. Get used to using half as much; then see if you can cut back even more.
- Cut back on the number of sugared soft drinks and punches you drink. Substitute water, fruit juice, or diet soft drinks.

Modified from USDA Home and Garden Bulletin No. 232-5, 1986.

dren and induces sleep; this effect may be linked to changes in the synthesis of certain neurotransmitters in the brain (see Chapter 5 for more details). If there is a villain, it is probably the excitement or tension in situations in which high-sucrose foods are served, such as at birthday parties and on Halloween. Any improvement in behavior that is observed when a child is put on a relatively sugar-free diet is probably because of the extra attention he or she receives, not the reduction in the intake of sugars.

Many reputable scientific groups have reviewed the current research concerning the health effects of the typical sugars in American diets. In general, these groups have given simple sugars a clean bill of health except for the tendency of many sugars to cause **dental caries.**[18] Caries are formed when sugars and other carbohydrates are metabolized into acids by bacteria that live in the mouth (Figure 3-10). The main bacterium is *Streptococcus mutans*. The acid produced by *Streptococcus mutans* dissolves the tooth enamel and underlying structure. These bacteria lodge themselves in fissures in the teeth. Dentists now apply sealants to heavily fissured areas of certain teeth as a preventive measure. Bacteria also use the sugars to make plaque, a sticky substance that both adheres bacteria to teeth and diminishes the acid-neutralizing effect of saliva.

The worst offenders in terms of dental caries are sticky or gummy foods high in sugars, such as caramel, because they stick to the teeth and supply the bacteria with a long-lived carbohydrate source. Since the bacteria need time to produce enough acid to erode the teeth, such foods provide the sugars needed throughout that time

dental caries Erosion in the surface of a tooth caused by acids made by bacteria as they metabolize sugars.

TABLE 3-8

Some sources of sugars

Food	Serving	Teaspoons of sugar	Food	Serving	Teaspoons of sugar
Beverages			**Jellies and Jams**		
Cola drinks	1 (12 oz bottle or glass)	7	Apple butter	1 tbsp	1
			Jelly	1 tbsp	4-6
Ginger ale	1 (12 oz bottle)	10	Orange marmalade	1 tbsp	4-6
Orangeade	1 (8 oz glass)	5	Peach butter	1 tbsp	1
Root beer	1 (10 oz bottle)	4½	Strawberry jam	1 tbsp	4
Seven-Up	1 (12 oz bottle)	7½	**Candies**		
Cakes and cookies			Average milk chocolate bar (e.g., Hershey's)	1 (1½ oz)	2½
Angelfood cake	1 (4 oz piece)	7	Chewing gum	1 stick	½
Applesauce cake	1 (4 oz piece)	5½	Fudge	1 oz square	4½
Banana bread	1 (2 oz piece)	2	Gum drop	1	2
Cheesecake	1 (4 oz piece)	2	Hard candy	4 oz	20
Chocolate cake (plain)	1 (4 oz piece)	6	Lifesavers	1	½
Chocolate cake (iced)	1 (4 oz piece)	10	Peanut brittle	1	3½
Coffee cake	1 (4 oz piece)	4½	**Canned fruits and juices**		
Cupcake (iced)	1	6			
Fruit cake	1 (4 oz piece)	5	Canned apricots	4 halves/1 tbsp syrup	3½
Jelly roll	1 (2 oz piece)	2½	Canned fruit juices, sweetened	½ cup	2
Orange cake	1 (4 oz piece)	4	Canned peaches	2 halves & 1 tbsp syrup	3½
Pound cake	1 (4 oz piece)	5			
Sponge cake	1 (1 oz piece)	2	Fruit salad	½ cup	3½
Strawberry shortcake	1 serving	4	Fruit syrup	2 tbsp	2½
Brownie (unfrosted)	1 (¾ oz)	3	Stewed fruits	½ cup	2
Chocolate cookie	1	1½			
Fig newton	1	5			
Dairy products			**Breakfast cereals***		
Ice cream	⅓ pint (3½ oz)	3½	Cheerios	1 oz	⅕
Ice cream bar	1	1-7 accord. to size	Special K	1 oz	⅔
			Total	1 oz	⅔
Ice cream cone	1	3½	Quaker 100% Natural	1 oz	2
Ice cream soda	1	5	Sugar Frosted Flakes	1 oz	2
Ice cream sundae	1	7	Sugar Smacks	1 oz	3
Malted milkshake	1 (10 oz glass)	5	Raisin Bran	1 oz	1½
Frozen yogurt	3 oz	3	Cracklin' Oat Bran	1 oz	1½
			Fruit Loops	1 oz	2½
			Cap'n Krunch	1 oz	2½
			Rice Krispies	1 oz	⅔

*As served; no sugar added by the consumer.

frame. These long-lived carbohydrates are termed **cariogenic** (*cario* means "cavity").[18] Although liquid sugar sources (e.g., fruit juices) are not as potent at causing dental caries as sticky or gummy foods, they still warrant consideration. Snacking regularly on sugary foods is also likely to cause caries because it gives the bacteria on the teeth a steady source of carbohydrate from which to continually make acid. Sugared gum chewed between meals is a prime example of a poor dental habit.

Sugar-containing foods are not the only foods that allow acid production by the bacteria in the mouth. If starch-containing foods (e.g., saltines and bread) are held in the mouth a long time, they can be acted on by enzymes in the mouth that break down the starch to sugars; bacteria can then produce acid from these sugars. Overall, the sugar and starch content of a food and its retentive ability largely determine its cariogenicity.[18]

It is important to recognize the benefits and risks of certain recommendations made by those who offer nutrition advice. There are very few simple answers. For example, raisins contain vitamins and minerals and are recommended as a good snack for the preschool-age child. But what about the cariogenic nature of raisins? Does that make raisins a poor snack choice? The answer is yes only for those who are particularly susceptible to dental caries, especially in conjunction with poor dental hygiene.

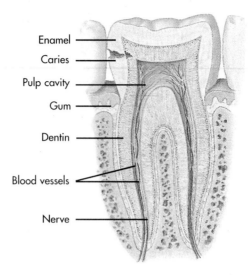

Enamel

Caries

Pulp cavity

Gum

Dentin

Blood vessels

Nerve

Figure 3-10 Dental decay. Bacteria can collect in various areas on a tooth. Bacteria metabolize simple sugars into acids, which can dissolve tooth enamel, leading to cavities. If the caries process progresses and enters the pulp cavity, damage to the nerve may occur. The bacteria also produce plaque to adhere themselves to the tooth's surface.

CRITICAL THINKING

John and Mike are identical twins who like the same games, sports, and foods. However, John likes to chew sugar-free gum and Mike doesn't. At their last dental visit, John had no cavities, but Mike had two. Mike wants to know why John, who chews gum after eating, doesn't have cavities and he does. How would you explain this to him?

cariogenic Literally "caries-producing"; a substance, often carbohydrate-rich (such as caramel), that promotes dental caries.

phytobezoars Pellets of dietary fiber, characteristically found in the stomach.

During the past 20 years, the incidence of dental caries in the United States has decreased by 30%, while consumption of simple sugars has remained about constant. This decline is primarily attributable to the addition of fluoride to drinking water. When teeth develop in the presence of this mineral, they become much more resistant to acid (see Chapter 15). Partly because of this, the number of caries-free children increased from 37% in 1980 to 50% in 1988.[18] Fluoride in toothpaste also contributes to dental health because it promotes remineralization of damaged teeth and inhibits the metabolism and growth of bacteria on the teeth.

Research has also indicated that certain foods—such as cheese, peanuts, and sugar-free chewing gum—can actually help reduce the amount of acid on teeth.[18] In addition, rinsing the mouth after meals and snacks reduces the acidity level in the mouth. Certainly, good nutrition, habits that do not present an overwhelming challenge to oral health, and routine visits to the dentist all contribute to improved dental health.

PROBLEMS WITH HIGH-FIBER DIETS

Very high intakes of dietary fiber—for example, 60 g/day—can pose some health risks and so require close physican supervision if employed. A high dietary fiber intake requires a high water intake. Not consuming enough water with the fiber can leave the stool very hard and make it difficult and painful to eliminate. Large amounts of dietary fiber may also bind important minerals, such as calcium, zinc, and iron.[11]

High-fiber diets often contribute to intestinal gas and occasionally to the production of fiber balls, called **phytobezoars,** in the stomach. These have been found in diabetic people and in elderly people who consume large amounts of dietary fiber. Phytobezoars can lead to blockage of intestinal flow.[11] Dietary fiber may also contribute to blockages in the intestine when intake is high and sufficient fluid is not consumed. Finally, large amounts of dietary fiber may add such an excess of bulk to a child's diet that energy intake is reduced; dietary fiber fills the stomach before food intake meets energy needs.

CONCEPT CHECK

Americans eat about 80 g of simple sugars each day, not including the lactose in dairy products. Most of these sugars are added to foods and beverages in manufacturing. The rest occurs naturally in foods or is added from the sugar bowl. To reduce consumption of sugars, one must reduce consumption of items with added sugars, such as some baked goods, sweetened beverages, and presweetened breakfast cereals. This is one practice that can help reduce development of dental caries. Diets providing more than 20 to 35 g of fiber daily should be followed only under a physician's guidance, since they can cause certain health problems, especially in people with diabetes, the elderly, and young children.

Carbohydrate Content of Foods

In the Exchange System, the milk exchanges each yield 12 g of carbohydrates; one starch exchange, one other carbohydrates exchange, and one fruit exchange each yield 15 g of carbohydrates; and one vegetable exchange yields 5 g of carbohydrates (see Table 2-8).

The foods that yield the highest percentage of energy from carbohydrates are table sugar, honey, jam, jelly, fruit, and plain baked potatoes. These foods are nutrient dense for carbohydrate; that is, carbohydrates deliver much of their food energy. Corn flakes, rice, bread, and noodles all contain at least 75% of energy as carbohydrates. Foods with moderate amounts of carbohydrate energy are peas, broccoli, oatmeal, dry beans and other legumes, cream pies, french fries, and skim milk. In these foods the carbohydrate content is diluted either by protein, as in the case of skim milk, or by fat, as in the case of a cream pie.

Chocolate, potato chips, and whole milk contain 30% to 40% of energy as carbohydrates. Again, the energy supplied from the carbohydrate content of these foods is overwhelmed by either their fat content or their protein content. Foods with essentially no carbohydrates include beef, chicken, fish, vegetable oils, butter, and margarine.

Figure 3-11 shows that, in planning a high-carbohydrate diet, you need to emphasize potatoes, grains, pasta, fruits, and vegetables. On the other hand, you can't create a diet high in carbohydrate energy from chocolate, potato chips, and french fries because these foods contain too much fat. The percentage of energy from carbohydrate is more important than the total amount of carbohydrate in a food when planning a high-carbohydrate diet.

Food Sweeteners

The various substances that impart sweetness to foods fall into two broad classes: nutritive sweeteners, which can be metabolized to yield energy, and alternative sweeteners, which provide no food energy. As shown in Table 3-2, the alternative sweeteners are much sweeter on a per-gram basis than the nutritive sweeteners.[3]

NUTRITIVE SWEETENERS

Both sugars and sugar alcohols provide energy along with sweetness. Sugars are found in many different food products, whereas sugar alcohols have rather limited uses.

Sugars

All of the monosaccharides (glucose, fructose, and galactose) and disaccharides (sucrose, lactose, and maltose) that we discussed earlier are designated *nutritive sweeteners*. The taste and sweetness of sucrose makes it the tried-and-true sweetener—the benchmark against which all other sweeteners are measured. A relatively new sweet-

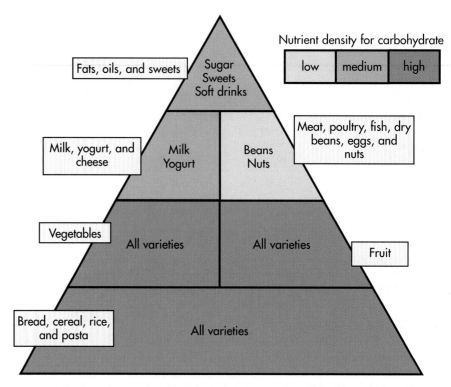

Figure 3-11 Sources of carbohydrates in foods from the Food Guide Pyramid. The bread, cereal, rice, and pasta group, fruit group, vegetable group, and milk, yogurt and cheese group contain many foods rich in carbohydrate. The other groups contain only a few foods rich in carbohydrate. The background color of each group indicates the average nutrient density for carbohydrate in that group.

ener is high-fructose corn syrup, which is 40% to 90% fructose. High-fructose corn syrup is made by treating cornstarch with acid and enzymes. This treatment breaks down much of the starch into glucose. Then some to almost all of the glucose is converted by enzymes into fructose.[3] The final syrup is usually as sweet as sucrose. Its major advantage is that it is cheaper than sucrose. Also, it doesn't form crystals, and it has better freezing properties. High-fructose corn syrups are used in soft drinks, candies, jam, jelly, other fruit products, and desserts.

In addition to sucrose and high-fructose corn syrup, brown sugar, turbinado sugar, honey, maple syrup, and other sugars are also added to foods. No raw (unrefined) sugars can be sold in the United States because FDA considers them unfit for human consumption. Turbinado sugar, a partially refined version of raw sucrose, can be sold and has a slight molasses flavor. Brown sugar is essentially sucrose containing some molasses; either the molasses is not totally removed from the sucrose during processing or it is added to the sucrose crystals.

Maple syrup is made by boiling down and concentrating the sap that runs during the spring in sugar maple trees. Most pancake syrup sold in supermarkets is not pure maple syrup, which is quite expensive. Instead, it is primarily corn syrup and high-fructose corn syrup.

Honey is a product of plant nectar that has been altered by bee enzymes. The enzymes break down much of the nectar's sucrose into fructose and glucose. As we noted earlier, honey offers essentially the same nutritional value as other simple sugars—a source of energy and little else. However, honey is not safe to feed to infants because it can contain spores of the bacterium *Clostridium botulinum*. These spores can become the bacteria that cause fatal food-borne illness. Honey does not pose the same threat to adults because the acidic environment of an adult's stomach inhibits the growth of the bacteria. An infant's stomach, however, does not produce much acid, making infants susceptible to the threat that this bacterium poses.

Sugar alcohols

The sugar alcohols sorbitol, mannitol, and **xylitol** are also used as nutritive sweeteners. They are absorbed or metabolized to glucose more slowly than simple sugars.[16] Because sugar alcohols contribute energy and affect blood glucose, they are of little or no advantage in diabetic diets. Nonetheless, many products containing these sugar alcohols are marketed to people with diabetes.

Sorbitol is used in sugarless gum, breath mints, and candy. It yields energy but is not readily metabolized by bacteria in the mouth. Thus sorbitol does not promote dental caries nearly so readily as simple sugars like sucrose. Another sugar alcohol, xylitol, is no longer widely used in the United States, partly because of past safety concerns, although its use in food processing is still legal. It is widely used in Canada and in Scandinavian countries. Any of these sugar alcohols consumed in excess has a tendency to remain in the intestine unabsorbed and so can cause diarrhea, especially in children who chew large amounts of sugarless gum (see Chapter 17).

ALTERNATIVE SWEETENERS

Often called artificial sweeteners, alternative sweeteners include **saccharin,** cyclamate, **aspartame,** and **acesulfame.**[12] From 1971 to 1991, Americans nearly quintupled their intake of low-calorie sweeteners, from 5 pounds per person to 24 pounds. During the same period, consumption of nutritive sweeteners rose 14%. Alternative sweeteners yield little or no energy when consumed in amounts typically used in food products. Only three are available in the United States: saccharin, aspartame, and acesulfame. Cyclamate was banned for use in the United States in 1970, although it has never been conclusively proved to cause health problems when used appropriately. Cyclamate is used in Canada as a sweetener in medicines and as a table-top sweetener.

Saccharin

The oldest alternative sweetener, saccharin, was first produced in 1879 and is currently approved for use in more than 90 countries. High doses of saccharin promote development of bladder cancer in laboratory animals, especially in animals in the second generation after exposure. Arguments continue concerning the magnitude of the cancer risk associated with the saccharin intakes typical of humans,[3] as population studies of humans have failed to show a link to any form of cancer.

In 1977, FDA attempted to ban saccharin because of this link to cancer. Many users protested because it left them with no other low-energy sweetener. The others mentioned above either were not yet available or, as in the case of cyclamate, had also been banned. Although aware of the association between saccharin and cancer, some people still wanted to use it. Responding to public pressure, Congress prevented FDA from banning saccharin, and in 1991 FDA decided to give up on any further attempts to do so. The agency requires only that a cancer warning label accompany any product containing saccharin.

Aspartame

In 1981 a new alternative sweetener, aspartame, became available. Its trade name is NutraSweet when added to foods and Equal when sold as a powder. Aspartame is in widespread use throughout the world. It has been approved for use by more than 90 countries, and its use has been endorsed by the World Health Organization, the American Medical Association, the American Diabetes Association, and the American Academy of Pediatrics Committee on Nutrition.[3]

The components of aspartame are the amino acids phenylalanine and aspartic acid, along with methanol. Recall that amino acids are the building blocks of proteins, so aspartame is more of a protein than a carbohydrate. Aspartame yields 4 kcal/g, but it is 180 to 200 times sweeter than sucrose. Thus only a small amount of aspartame is needed to obtain the desired sweetness, so the amount of energy added is insignificant unless the product is abused. Today aspartame is used in beverages, gelatin desserts, chewing gum, and many other foods. Its use in toppings

MADE IN U.S.A. WM. WRIGLEY JR. COMPANY, CHICAGO, IL 60611©1991 MADE OF: SORBITOL, GUM BASE, MANNITOL, GLYCEROL, HYDROGENATED GLUCOSE SYRUP, XYLITOL, ARTIFICIAL AND NATURAL FLAVORS, ASPARTAME, RED 40, YELLOW 6 AND BHT (TO MAINTAIN FRESHNESS). PHENYLKETONURICS: CONTAINS PHENYLALANINE. *NUTRASWEET IS A REGISTERED TRADEMARK OF THE NUTRASWEET CO.

Wrigley's
Extra

Sugar alcohols can be found in sugarless gum. Note that aspartame is also used to sweeten this product.

saccharin An alternate sweetener that yields no energy to the body; it is 500 times sweeter than sucrose.

aspartame An alternate sweetener made from two amino acids and methanol; it is 200 times sweeter than sucrose.

acesulfame An alternate sweetener that yields no energy to the body; it is 200 times sweeter than sucrose.

EXPERT OPINION

THE VALUE OF INTENSE SWEETENERS

ADAM DREWNOWSKI, Ph.D.

Recent reports that the use of intense sweeteners results in increased hunger and greater food consumption have led many consumers to question the value of low-energy foods and beverages in weight control. The so-called "sweetener paradox" implies that providing sweetness without kilocalories, far from helping to control body weight, might actually lead to overeating and thus to weight gain. According to this view, drinking a diet soda rather than mineral water could be the first step on the road to obesity and eating disorders.

SWEETENER PARADOX NOT SUPPORTED

The conclusion that intense sweeteners have a paradoxical effect on appetite was based on only two published studies. The first, a brief letter in the journal *The Lancet,* reported that drinking a sweet aspartame solution as opposed to plain water suppressed preferences for the sweet taste of sucrose (implying a reduction in appetite), but briefly increased the reported motivation to eat. The second study reported that the consumption of a single small portion of a saccharin-sweetened yogurt as opposed to plain yogurt increased appetite and stimulated food consumption for more

than 12 hours afterward.

Both studies implied that consumption of sweetened foods, as opposed to plain foods of equal energy value, promoted appetite and stimulated eating. However, neither claim was confirmed by other scientists. Most later studies reported that the use of diet soft drinks, compared with plain water, did not lead to increased hunger ratings, at least as measured up to 2 hours afterward. Other studies found that the use of sweetened versus plain preloads (that is foods eaten before a meal) did not lead to increased food consumption at the next meal. There was no evidence that intense sweeteners promoted hunger or resulted in greater food consumption. In addition, there was no evidence at all that the use of intense sweeteners would lead to weight gain.

ENERGY COMPENSATION WITH SWEETENERS

One important issue remains unresolved. The studies cited above showed that adding aspartame to plain foods or beverages of equal energy value did not increase hunger or stimulate food consumption. Yet the most common use of intense sweeteners is as noncaloric substitutes for sugars. Although the sweet taste of

foods and beverages is preserved, their energy content is sometimes greatly reduced by the use of intense sweeteners.

Some scientists have argued that regular and diet beverages have exactly the same effects on hunger and satiety, measured shortly afterward. Yet intense sweeteners are not appetite suppressants. Even if the effects of an energy deficit are not immediately apparent, they will become obvious later. The question is whether energy savings that can be realized by the use of intense sweeteners will result in increased hunger and increased food consumption at the next meal. If such savings are simply followed by compensatory eating, with no net reduction in daily energy intake, then we might have good reason to question the value of intense sweeteners in weight control.

To date, published studies on the effects of intense sweeteners on appetite and food consumption have variously reported perfect energy compensation, partial compensation, or no compensation at all. However, such studies have used a variety of subject populations and study designs. In the most frequently used study design, the consumption of a single sweet preload was followed shortly by a single test meal or snack. The sweet

and fillings in precooked bakery goods and cookies has recently been approved by FDA. Aspartame does not cause tooth decay. Like other proteins, however, aspartame is damaged when heated for a long time and thus cannot be widely used in products requiring cooking.

To date, about 7000 complaints have been filed with FDA by people claiming to have had adverse reactions to aspartame: headaches, dizziness, seizures, nausea, and other side effects. It is important for people who are sensitive to aspartame to avoid it. But the percentage of sensitive people is likely to be extremely small. The preload was generally a beverage, although some studies made use of foods such as Jello, pudding, cereal, or soft, creamy white cheese. The difference in energy between low-energy and high-energy preloads was usually less than 200 kcal.

The few studies that reported perfect compensation were generally conducted with 2- to 5-year-old children or normal-weight, nondieting young men. In one longer-term residential study, the energy content of lunch was reduced by 400 kcal for 3 days, largely by substituting aspartame for sugar. The subjects, seven young men, made up the energy deficit on every day of the study, and their daily energy intakes remained constant.

In contrast, studies conducted with 9- to 10-year-old children or with lean women and overweight women showed that energy compensation either was only partial or was absent altogether. In one study, a 400 kcal deficit at breakfast led to slightly higher (111 kcal) energy intakes at lunch, with no further compensation thereafter. Another study, conducted with lean women and obese women, found no compensation for the amount of energy consumed at breakfast. The subjects who consumed lower-energy breakfasts had lower total energy intakes at the end of the day.

It appears that nondieters in a state of energy need (e.g., children and young men) are best able to compensate for energy deficits. There is also preliminary evidence that overweight dieters, especially mature adults, are least likely to compensate for the missing energy. Since these groups are the most frequent users of diet products, including both intense sweeteners and fat replacements, further studies should be directed at these segments of the population.

DIETING AND SWEETENERS

The effect of intense sweeteners on weight control practices of the American public is difficult to assess, since there are no data on how many people might become overweight if low-calorie foods were not available. Intense sweeteners have replaced sugars in many foods that are the major sources of carbohydrate calories in the typical American diet. Furthermore, noncaloric soft drinks are widely used by dieters, not all of whom are obese, and are widely regarded as a valuable tool in weight control. However, hard data are extremely limited. One study of diet practices of 19- to 50-year-old women, based on the 1985 Continuing Survey of Food Intakes of Individuals (CSFII), showed that the use of intense sweeteners was associated with a drop in energy intake from 1670 to 1505 kcal per day.

One point deserves special mention. The few long-term studies of the effects of intense sweeteners on weight control have tended to focus on the amount of weight lost as the chief measure of success. Yet intense sweeteners may be most useful in promoting compliance with a low-calorie diet, which typically restricts the consumption of both sugars and fats. Prolonged dieting often leads to bingeing, and many dieters have blamed eating binges involving sweet desserts as the main reason for noncompliance and for diet failure. Thus the availability of good-tasting low-energy foods may promote long-term adherence to a weight-reducing diet. In this case, the value of intense sweeteners will be measured in consumer satisfaction and improved quality of life.

Dr. Drewnowski is a professor of Community Health Programs and the director of the Program in Human Nutrition at the University of Michigan School of Public Health. He has conducted many studies on taste preferences for sweet and high-fat foods and on the usefulness of low-energy foods in weight reduction.

relatively small number of complaints about aspartame, considering its wide use in food products, means that most people can use it. In addition, careful double-blind studies cast doubt on whether it causes headaches[19] and suggest that it generally does not stimulate later food intake either.[9]

Aspartame's phenylalanine content has concerned some people. Blood concentrations of this amino acid may increase significantly if aspartame is not consumed with the other amino acids normally found in protein foods. This problem can be easily avoided by consuming aspartame with protein foods. Some people are con-

CONTAINS: CARBONATED WATER, ORANGE JUICE, CITRIC ACID, NUTRASWEET* BRAND OF ASPARTAME**, POTASSIUM BENZOATE (A PRESERVATIVE), CITRUS PECTIN, POTASSIUM CITRATE, CAFFEINE, MALTODEXTRIN, GUM ARABIC, NATURAL FLAVORS, BROMINATED VEGETABLE OIL, YELLOW #5 AND ERYTHORBIC ACID (TO PROTECT FLAVOR).
*NUTRASWEET® AND THE NUTRASWEET SYMBOL ARE REGISTERED TRADEMARKS OF THE NUTRASWEET COMPANY.
PHENYLKETONURICS: CONTAINS PHENYLALANINE.

Note the warning for people with PKU that this diet soft drink with aspartame contains phenylalanine.

phenylketonuria (PKU) A disease in which the liver has a limited ability to metabolize the amino acid phenylalanine into the amino acid tyrosine.

cerned about aspartame's methanol content. However, the amount of methanol in a soft drink sweetened with aspartame is no more than that found in a cup of fruit or vegetable juice.

Overall, the scientific community agrees that aspartame is safe to use in moderation. The acceptable daily intake set by FDA is 50 mg/kg of body weight per day. This is equivalent to about 17 cans of diet soft drink for an adult. Aspartame appears to be safe for pregnant women and children, but some scientists suggest cautious use by these groups, especially in young children, who need ample food energy to grow.

One final note about aspartame. Persons with a rare disease called **phenylketonuria (PKU)**, which interferes with metabolism of phenylalanine, should avoid aspartame because of its high phenylalanine content.[3] (We discuss PKU further in Chapter 5.)

Acesulfame

The newest alternative sweetener in the United States, acesulfame (Sunette), was approved by FDA in July 1988. It is approved for use in more than 40 countries and has been in use in Europe since 1983. Acesulfame is 200 times sweeter than sucrose.[3] It contributes no energy to the diet because it is not digested by the body. Acesulfame also does not cause dental caries.

Unlike aspartame, acesulfame can be used in baking because it does not lose its sweetness when heated. In the United States, acesulfame is currently approved for use in chewing gum, powdered drink mixes, gelatins, puddings, and nondairy creamers, but additional uses may soon be approved. Because acesulfame was initially approved much more quickly than other alternative sweeteners, some nutrition professionals still have doubts about the wisdom of its widespread use.

Other Alternative Sweeteners

Research continues on new forms of alternative sweeteners. Three are awaiting FDA approval:

- Alitame, which is formed from two amino acids and another small nitrogen group, is 2000 times sweeter than sucrose.
- Sucralose, which is made by substituting three chlorine atoms for three hydroxyl groups (–OH) on sucrose, is 400 to 800 times sweeter than sucrose and is approved for use in Canada.
- D-Tagatose, a compound derived from lactose, has the same sweetness as sucrose, but yields only half the energy.

Overall, alternative sweeteners enable people with diabetes to enjoy the flavor of sweetness while controlling sugars in their diets; they also provide noncaloric or very low-kilocalorie sugar substitutes for persons trying to lose weight. Thus alternative sweeteners provide people who want to reduce their intake of sugars with another tasteful option.[3] In the future there likely will be more use of blends of the alternative sweeteners, such as aspartame and acesulfame. Improved flavor (more like sucrose) and greater sweetness from the various possible combinations can result. These blends are commonly used in Europe.

CONCEPT CHECK

Foods that are essentially all carbohydrate are sugars, jam, jelly, fruit, and plain baked potatoes. Grains and vegetables are also rich sources of carbohydrate. Most simple sugars are added to foods and beverages during manufacturing or are added from the sugar bowl. To reduce your intake of simple sugars, eat fewer items that contain a lot of added sugar, such as some baked goods, certain beverages, and some breakfast cereals. Simple sugars contribute to dental caries and provide few vitamins and minerals, if any. Three major alternative sweeteners are available in America today—saccharin, aspartame, and acesulfame. These can aid in the goal of reducing simple-sugar intake.

Summary

1. The common monosaccharides are glucose, fructose, and galactose. Once these are absorbed from the small intestine and delivered to the liver, much of the fructose and galactose is converted to glucose.

2. The major disaccharides are sucrose (glucose plus fructose), maltose (glucose plus glucose), and lactose (glucose plus galactose). When digested, these yield their component monosaccharides. The ability to digest lactose often diminishes with age. People in some ethnic groups have an especially limited ability to digest lactose. This condition develops early in childhood and is referred to as *lactose intolerance.*

3. Carbohydrates provide energy, protect against wasteful breakdown of body protein, prevent ketosis, and impart flavor and sweetness to foods. Although no RDA for carbohydrate has been set, a daily intake of at least 50 to 100 g is required to prevent ketosis. If carbohydrate intake is inadequate to supply the body's needs, protein is broken down to provide glucose (gluconeogenesis) for energy needs. However, the price is loss of body protein, ketosis, and eventually a general body weakening. For this reason, low-carbohydrate diets are not recommended for extended periods.

4. Several hormones play a role in regulating blood glucose so that it remains within a fairly narrow range. Insulin and glycogen, both released from the pancreas, have opposite effects: insulin removes excess glucose from the bloodstream and deposits it in the tissues, as well as stimulates glycogen synthesis; glucagon increases blood glucose when it is low by stimulating breakdown of glycogen and synthesis of glucose from protein. Epinephrine, norepinephrine, and cortisol also increase blood glucose.

5. One major group of polysaccharides consists of storage forms of glucose: starches in plants and glycogen in humans. In these polymers, the multiple glucose units are linked by alpha glycosidic bonds, which can be broken by human enzymes, releasing the glucose units. The main plant starches—straight-chain amylose and branched-chain amylopectin—are digested by enzymes in the mouth and small intestine. In humans, glycogen is synthesized in the liver and muscle tissue. Liver glycogen is readily broken down to glucose, which can enter the bloodstream. Breakdown of muscle glycogen yields glucose-phosphate; this compound is not released into the bloodstream but is a ready source of energy for muscle.

6. Dietary fiber is composed primarily of the polysaccharides cellulose, hemicellulose, pectin, gum, and mucilage, as well as the noncarbohydrate lignins. These substances are not broken down by human digestive enzymes. However, soluble dietary fibers are metabolized by bacteria in the large intestine. Dietary fiber provides mass to the feces, thus easing elimination, and an adequate intake of dietary fiber likely reduces colon cancer risk. In high doses, certain fibers can help control blood glucose in diabetic people and also lower serum cholesterol.

7. Diets high in complex carbohydrates are encouraged as a replacement for high-fat diets. A goal of at least 45% of energy as complex carbohydrates is a good one, with about 55% to 60% of total energy coming from carbohydrates in general. Foods to consume are potatoes, whole-grain cereal products, pasta, legumes, fruits, and vegetables. Alternative sweeteners, such as aspartame and acesulfame, aid in reducing intake of simple sugars. Moderating sugar intake, especially between meals, in turn reduces the risk of dental caries.

Study Questions

1. Outline the basic steps in blood glucose regulation, including the roles of insulin and glucagon.
2. What are the three major disaccharides? Describe how each plays a part in the human diet.
3. How do amylose, amylopectin, and glycogen differ from one another? Why can this be important metabolically and in food processing?
4. What are the important roles that dietary fiber plays in the diet?
5. What, if any, are the proven ill effects of sugars in the diet?
6. How is high-fructose corn syrup made? Why is its use in food products increasing?
7. Briefly describe the chemical structure, sweetness, and food uses of alternative sweeteners.

Continued.

After reading the Nutrition Perspective, answer the following questions:

8. How does insulin-dependent diabetes differ from non–insulin-dependent diabetes in cause and treatment?

9. What treatment is recommended for the common form of hypoglycemia?

REFERENCES

1. Alcorn JM: Colorectal cancer prevention: a primary care approach, *Geriatrics* 47:24, 1992.

2. Aldoor WH and others: A prospective study of diet and the risk of symptomatic diverticular disease in men, *American Journal of Clinical Nutrition* 60:757, 1994.

3. American Dietetic Association Reports: Position of the American Dietetic Association: use of nutritive and non-nutritive sweeteners, *Journal of the American Dietetic Association* 93:816, 1993.

4. Anderson JW and others: Health benefits and practical aspects of high-fiber diets, *American Journal of Clinical Nutrition* 59:1242S, 1994.

5. Atkinson MA, Maclaren WK: The pathogenesis of insulin-dependent diabetes mellitus, *New England Journal of Medicine* 331:1428, 1994.

6. Clark CM, Lee DA: Prevention and treatment of the complications of diabetes mellitus, *New England Journal of Medicine* 332:1210, 1995.

7. Coulston AM: Nutrition considerations in the control of diabetes mellitus, *Nutrition Today,* Jan/Feb 1994, p 6.

8. DCCT Research Group: Nutrition interventions for intensive therapy in the diabetes control and complications trial, *Journal of the American Dietetic Association* 93:768, 1993.

9. Drewnowski A: Intense sweeteners and the control of appetite, *Nutrition Reviews* 53:1, 1995.

10. Garg A and others: Effects of varying carbohydrate content of diet in patients with non-insulin-dependent diabetes mellitus, *Journal of the American Medical Association* 271:1421, 1994.

11. Gray DS: The clinical uses of dietary fiber, *American Family Physician* 51:419, 1995.

12. Greeley A: Not only sugar is sweet, *FDA Consumer,* April 1992, p 17.

13. Greenberg ER and others: A clinical trial of antioxidant vitamins to prevent colorectal adenoma, *New England Journal of Medicine* 331:141, 1994.

14. Jenkins DDA, Jenkins AL: Glycemic index and diabetes, *Journal of the American College of Nutrition* 13:541, 1994.

15. Jequier E: Carbohydrates as a source of energy, *American Journal of Clinical Nutrition* 59:682S, 1994.

16. Mayes PA: Carbohydrates of physiologic significance and integration of metabolism and provision of tissue fuels. In Murray RK and others, editors: *Harper's biochemistry,* ed 23, East Norwalk, Conn, 1993, Appleton & Lange.

17. McBean LD: Managing lactose intolerance, *Dairy Council Digest* 65:7, 1994.

18. McBean LD: Diet and dental caries: an overview, *Dairy Council Digest* 65:1, 1994.

19. Schiffman SS and others: Aspartame and susceptibility to headache, *New England Journal of Medicine* 317:1181, 1987.

20. Service FJ: Hypoglycemic disorders, *New England Journal of Medicine* 332:1144, 1995.

21. Slavin JL: Whole grains and health: separating the wheat from the chaff, *Nutrition Today* 29:6, 1994.

22. Swanson JE and others: Metabolic effects of dietary fructose in healthy subjects, *Perspectives in Applied Nutrition* 1:22, 1993.

23. Tierney LM and others: *Current diagnosis and treatment,* Norwalk, Conn, 1995, Appleton & Lange.

24. Tinker LF and others: Commentary and translation: 1994 nutrition recommendations for diabetes, *Journal of the American Dietetic Association* 94:507, 1994.

25. Wolraich ML and others: Effects of diets high in sucrose or aspartame on the behavior and cognitive performance of children, *New England Journal of Medicine* 330:301, 1994.

TAKE ACTION

> **How does your diet rate for carbohydrate and dietary fiber?**
> *Let's reevaluate the nutritional assessment you completed at the end of Chapter 2. Here are your tasks:*

1. Look at your analysis and find the total number of grams of carbohydrate you ate.

   TOTAL GRAMS OF CARBOHYDRATE _____
   A. Did you consume more than the minimum amount to avoid ketosis, 50 to 100 g?
   B. Now calculate the percentage of energy in your diet from carbohydrate. You will need the total grams of carbohydrate from your assessment as well as the total kilocalories you ate. Use this formula to calculate it:

   $$\frac{\text{Total grams of carbohydrate} \times 4}{\text{Total kilocalories consumed}} \times 100 = \% \text{ of energy intake from carbohydrate}$$

   ANSWER: _____

   Was 55% or more of your total energy intake from carbohydrate? Yes _____ No _____
   If not, list several ways you could increase your carbohydrate intake.

   _____

   _____

   _____

2. Look again at the list of foods you ate, including the amounts, and determine the total amount of dietary fiber you consumed. If you have a computer analysis of your diet, your dietary fiber intake is listed in the printout. Otherwise, look up the dietary fiber content of each food you ate in the food composition table in Appendix A; then calculate your total intake, taking into account the amount of each food you ate.

   TOTAL AMOUNT OF DIETARY FIBER CONSUMED _____grams
   A. Did you eat the 20 to 35 g suggested in this chapter?
   B. If not, what could you do to increase your dietary fiber intake? What foods could you substitute for some of the foods you ate?

   _____

   _____

   _____

   _____

3. Finally, use Table 3-7 to see if you can reduce your intake of sugars, especially if you need to watch your total energy intake to maintain an appropriate weight. What three foods might you in fact limit in the future?

   _____

   _____

   _____

When Blood Glucose Regulation Fails

Improper regulation of blood glucose results in either hyperglycemia (high blood glucose) or hypoglycemia (low blood glucose). High blood glucose is most commonly associated with diabetes (technically *diabetes mellitus*), a disease that affects about 14 million Americans. Low blood glucose is a much rarer condition.

Diabetes Mellitus

insulin-dependent diabetes A form of diabetes in which the person with the disease is prone to ketosis and requires insulin therapy.

non–insulin-dependent diabetes A form of diabetes in which ketosis is not commonly seen. Insulin therapy can be used but is often not required. This form of the disease is often associated with obesity.

There are two major forms of diabetes: **insulin-dependent diabetes** (also called *type I* or *juvenile-onset diabetes*) and **non–insulin-dependent diabetes** (also called *type II* or *adult-onset diabetes*).[6]

INSULIN-DEPENDENT DIABETES

The insulin-dependent form often begins in late childhood, around the age of 8 to 12 years, but can occur at any age. The disease runs in certain families, indicating a clear genetic link. The symptoms of the disease are abnormally high blood glucose after eating and the tendency to develop ketosis.

The onset of insulin-dependent diabetes is generally associated with decreased release of insulin from the pancreas. As insulin in the blood declines, blood glucose increases, especially after eating. When blood glucose exceeds the kidney's threshold, excess glucose spills over into the urine. Hence the term diabetes mellitus, which means "flow of much urine" (*diabetes*) that is "sweet" (*mellitus*). Figure 3-12 shows a typical glucose tolerance curve observed in a patient with this form of diabetes, following a test load of 50 g (10 teaspoons) of glucose.

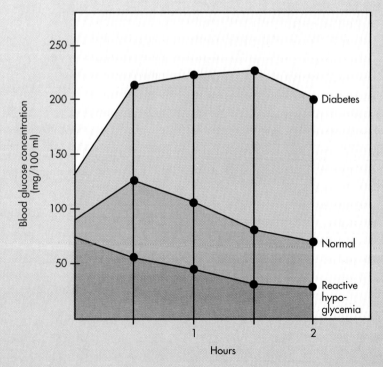

Figure 3-12 Glucose tolerance test. These are typical responses seen after consumption of 50 g (10 teaspoons) of glucose by a healthy person and by a person with uncontrolled diabetes mellitus or reactive hypoglycemia. Blood glucose concentration is determined during fasting and then at regular intervals after the person consumes the glucose test load.[16] The depiction of reactive hypoglycemia is theoretical; the actual existence of this syndrome is in question. In any case, true hypoglycemia is rare.[20]

An exciting new finding regarding the cause of insulin-dependent diabetes may help physicans to treat this disease, or even prevent its onset in the future. At least some cases of insulin-dependent diabetes begin with an immunological disorder that causes destruction of the insulin-producing beta cells in the pancreas.[5] Most likely a virus or protein foreign to the body sets off the destruction. Cow's milk is suspected of supplying such a protein, so its introduction before 1 year of age is not advised (see Chapter 17). In response to the destruction, the affected beta cells release other proteins that stimulate a more furious attack. Eventually the pancreas loses its ability to synthesize insulin, and the clinical stage of the disease begins. For this reason, early treatment to stop the immune-linked destruction may be important.[5] Research on this is continuing.

Currently, insulin-dependent diabetes is treated primarily by insulin therapy, either with injections one to six times a day or with an insulin pump. The pump dispenses insulin at a steady rate into the body, with greater amounts delivered after each meal. Dietary measures include three regular meals and one or more snacks (including one at bedtime) having a precise carbohydrate:protein:fat ratio to maximize insulin action and minimize swings in blood glucose concentrations.[7] The diet should be rich in complex carbohydrates, include ample dietary fiber, and supply an amount of energy in balance with energy needs.[4] If a high carbohydrate intake raises serum triglyceride and cholesterol concentrations beyond desired ranges, carbohydrate intake can be reduced and replaced with unsaturated fat.[10] This change tends to reduce serum triglycerides and cholesterol. We discuss how to implement such a diet in Chapter 4. Moderate consumption of sugars with meals is fine as long as blood glucose regulation is preserved and the sugars replace other carbohydrates in the meal.[8]

In normal individuals, the insulin output decreases as glucose is cleared from the bloodstream after a meal. Because this does not necessarily occur in diabetic people who are taking insulin, consumption of meals at regular intervals is especially important for them. If they do not eat often enough, the injected insulin can cause severe hypoglycemia, since it acts on whatever little glucose is available.

The hormone imbalances that occur in people with untreated diabetes lead to mobilization of body fat, which floods into liver cells. Ketosis is the result because the fat is mostly converted to ketones. Ketone concentration can rise excessively in the blood, eventually forcing ketones into the urine. These ketones pull sodium and potassium ions with them. This series of events can contribute to a chain reaction that eventually leads to dehydration, ion imbalance, coma, and even death, especially in patients with poorly controlled insulin-dependent diabetes.[23]

Other complications of diabetes can be degenerative conditions, such as blindness, heart disease, kidney disease, and numbness from nerve damage; all are caused by poor blood glucose regulation. These degenerative health problems arise in part from microscopic changes that occur in small blood vessels, namely the capillaries. Nerves can also deteriorate, resulting in many changes that decrease proper nerve stimulation. When this occurs in the intestinal tract, intermittent diarrhea and constipation result. Because of nerve deterioration in the extremities, many people with diabetes lose the sensation of pain associated with injuries or infections. Not having as much pain, they often delay treatment of hand or foot problems. This delay, combined with a rich environment for bacterial growth (bacteria thrive on glucose) sets the stage for complications in the extremities. High blood glucose also contributes to a rapid build-up of fats in blood vessel walls, which eventually chokes off the blood supply to nearby organs. See Chapter 4 for details on this latter process, called **atherosclerosis.**

Current research shows that the development of blood vessel and nerve complications of diabetes can be slowed with aggressive treatment directed at keeping blood glucose within the normal range.[6] The therapy poses some risks of its own, such as hypoglycemia, so it must be implemented under close supervision of a physician.

A person with diabetes generally must work closely with a physician to make the correct alterations in diet and medications and to perform physical activity safely. Physical ac-

Researchers are currently investigating methods of replacing destroyed beta cells with functional ones from human cadavers. Once isolated and injected into a diabetic patient, they can lodge in the liver and produce insulin. See the July 1995 issue of *Scientific American* for a review of this exciting area of research.

atherosclerosis A build-up of mostly fatty material (plaque) in the arteries, including those surrounding the heart.

tivity can enhance glucose uptake by muscles, which in turn can lower blood glucose. This outcome is beneficial, but people with diabetes need to be aware of their own blood glucose response to physical activity and compensate appropriately.

NON–INSULIN-DEPENDENT DIABETES

Non–insulin-dependent diabetes usually begins after age 20. This is the most common type of diabetes, accounting for about 90% of the cases diagnosed in the United States. The number of people affected is on the rise, because of widespread inactivity and obesity in our population. This type of diabetes is also genetically linked, but the initial problem is not with the beta cells of the pancreas, but instead with the insulin receptors on the cell surfaces of certain body tissues, especially muscle tissues. In this case, blood glucose is not readily transferred into cells, so the patient develops hyperglycemia as a result of the glucose's remaining in the bloodstream. The pancreas attempts to increase insulin output to compensate, but there is a limit to its ability to do this. So rather than insufficient insulin production, there is an abundance of insulin, particularly during the onset of the disease. As the disease develops, pancreatic function can fail, leading to reduced insulin output.[23]

Many cases of non–insulin-dependent diabetes are associated with obesity, but the hyperglycemia is not directly caused by the obesity. In fact, some lean people also develop this type of diabetes. Obesity associated with oversized fat cells simply increases the risk for insulin resistance by the body.

Non–insulin-dependent diabetes linked to obesity often disappears if the obesity is corrected. Achieving a desirable weight should be a primary goal of treatment, but even limited weight loss can lead to better blood glucose regulation. Oral medications that increase the ability of the pancreas to produce insulin are often prescribed. Sometimes it may be necessary to provide insulin injections because nothing else is able to control the disease. Regular physical activity also helps the muscles to take up more glucose. And regular meal patterns, with an emphasis on control of energy intake, consumption of complex carbohydrates, and ample dietary fiber, is important therapy. Moderate intake of sugars is fine with meals, but again these must be substituted for other carbohydrates, not simply added to the meal plan. Distributing carbohydrates throughout the day is also important, as this helps minimize the high and low swings in blood glucose concentrations.[24]

People with non–insulin-dependent diabetes who have high serum triglycerides should moderate their carbohydrate intake and increase their intake of unsaturated fat and dietary fiber, as we noted earlier for people with insulin-dependent diabetes.[10]

Although many cases of non–insulin-dependent diabetes can be relieved by reducing excess fat stores, many people are not able to lose weight. They remain affected with diabetes and may experience the degenerative complications seen in the insulin-dependent form of the disease. Ketosis, however, is not usually seen in this form of diabetes.

THE GLYCEMIC INDEX: A TOOL FOR PLANNING DIABETIC DIETS

Research concerning the body's response to various carbohydrates has led to development of a clinical tool known as the *glycemic index*.[14] This index compares the total amount of glucose appearing in the blood after eating a specific food with the total amount of glucose appearing in the blood after eating the same amount of carbohydrate in the form of white bread or glucose.

Several factors must be considered when predicting the glycemic index of a food, including its dietary fiber content, digestion rate, and total fat content. Foods containing much soluble fiber (e.g., oatmeal) are digested slowly and thus produce a slow increase in blood glucose after eating. In contrast, foods such as potatoes are digested quickly, producing a rapid increase in blood glucose after eating. If a diabetic person eats many foods having low glycemic indices, then each meal in the entire diet can contribute to blood glucose regulation.[14]

The glycemic index for common foods

100	Glucose, white bread
90	Whole-wheat bread, shredded wheat cereal, raisins
80	Rice, oatmeal, potatoes
70	Bananas, All-Bran cereal
60	Oranges, baked beans, spaghetti
50	Yogurt, apple
40	Nonfat (skim) milk, peach

Hypoglycemia

As we noted earlier, diabetic people who are taking insulin sometimes have hypoglycemia if they don't eat frequently enough. Hypoglycemia can also develop in nondiabetic individuals. The two common forms of nondiabetic hypoglycemia are termed *reactive* and *fasting*.[23]

Reactive hypoglycemia is described as irritability, nervousness, headache, sweating, and confusion 2 to 4 hours after eating a meal, especially a meal high in simple sugars (Figure 3-12). The cause of reactive hypoglycemia is unclear, but it may be over-production of insulin by the pancreas in response to rising blood glucose.[19] Some researchers are unwilling even to acknowledge the existence of reactive hypoglycemia, pointing out that the symptoms are more likely tied to recent intense exercise, psychological stress, medication use, or alcohol consumption.[20] **Fasting hypoglycemia** usually is caused by pancreatic cancer, which may lead to excessive insulin secretion. In this case, blood glucose falls to low concentrations after fasting for about 8 hours to 1 day. This form of hypoglycemia is rare.[20]

The diagnosis of hypoglycemia requires the simultaneous presence of low blood glucose and the typical hypoglycemic symptoms. Blood glucose of 40 to 50 mg/100 ml is suggestive, but just having low blood glucose after eating is not enough evidence to make the diagnosis of hypoglycemia. Although many people think they have hypoglycemia, few actually do.[20]

The popular press and television talk shows have popularized hypoglycemia, relating it to a variety of symptoms that most everyone has at one time or another. No clear evidence, however, has conclusively linked hypoglycemia to the difficulties popularly attributed to it: depression, chronic fatigue, allergies, nervous breakdowns, alcoholism, juvenile delinquency, childhood behavior problems, drug addiction, or inadequate sexual performance. Most people complaining of fatigue, shakiness, occasional heavy sweats, and emotional instability do not have documentable hypoglycemia. Also, for most people in good health, eating simple sugars does not induce hypoglycemia. Unless a metabolic disorder is present, the body generally can respond adequately to an intake of simple sugars and complex carbohydrates.

It is normal for healthy people to have some hypoglycemic symptoms, such as irritability, headache, and shakiness, if they have not eaten for a prolonged period of time. Although not diagnostic of hypoglycemia, if you sometimes have symptoms of hypoglycemia, the standard nutrition therapy is one we all could follow. You need to eat regular meals, make sure you have some protein and fat in each meal, and eat complex carbohydrates with ample soluble fiber.[23] Avoid meals or snacks that contain little more than simple carbohydrates. If symptoms continue, try small protein-containing snacks between meals. Fat, protein, and soluble fiber in the diet tend to moderate swings in blood glucose.[8]

reactive hypoglycemia Low blood glucose that follows a meal high in simple sugars, with corresponding symptoms of irritability, headache, nervousness, sweating, and confusion; also called *postprandial hypoglycemia*.

fasting hypoglycemia Low blood glucose that follows about a day of fasting.

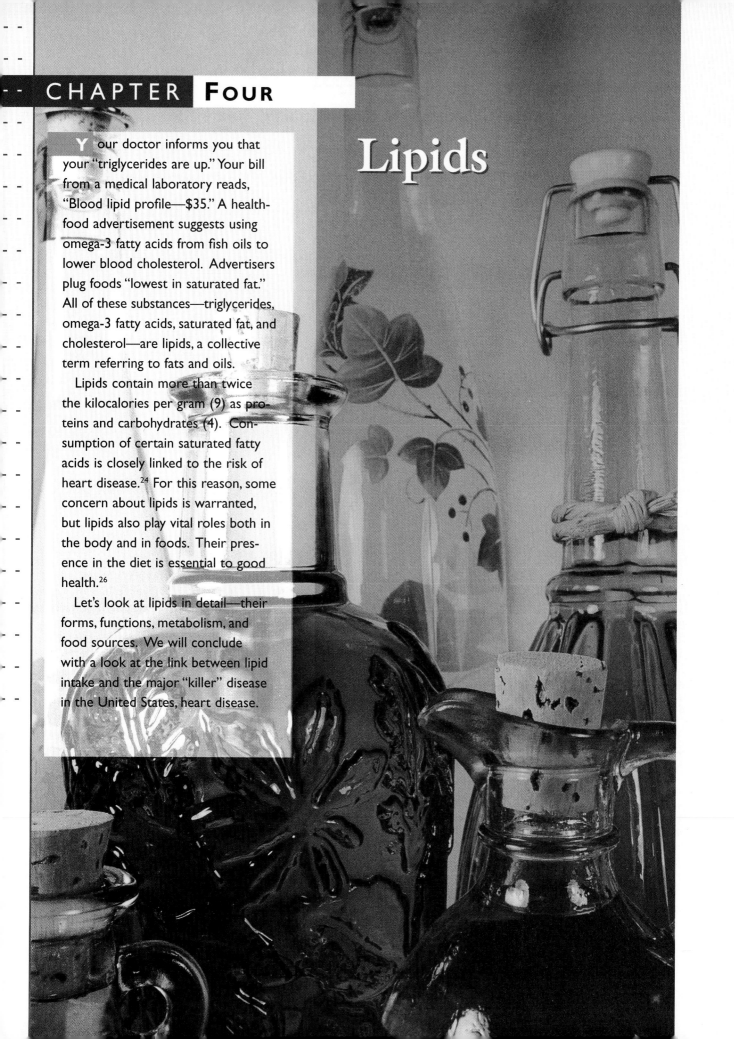

CHAPTER FOUR

Lipids

Your doctor informs you that your "triglycerides are up." Your bill from a medical laboratory reads, "Blood lipid profile—$35." A health-food advertisement suggests using omega-3 fatty acids from fish oils to lower blood cholesterol. Advertisers plug foods "lowest in saturated fat." All of these substances—triglycerides, omega-3 fatty acids, saturated fat, and cholesterol—are lipids, a collective term referring to fats and oils.

Lipids contain more than twice the kilocalories per gram (9) as proteins and carbohydrates (4). Consumption of certain saturated fatty acids is closely linked to the risk of heart disease.[24] For this reason, some concern about lipids is warranted, but lipids also play vital roles both in the body and in foods. Their presence in the diet is essential to good health.[26]

Let's look at lipids in detail—their forms, functions, metabolism, and food sources. We will conclude with a look at the link between lipid intake and the major "killer" disease in the United States, heart disease.

NUTRITION AWARENESS INVENTORY

Answer these 15 statements about lipids to test your current knowledge. If you think a statement is true or mostly true, circle T. If you think the statement is false or mostly false, circle F. Use the scoring key at the end of the book to compute your total score. Repeat this test after you have read the chapter, and compare your results.

1. **T F** Lipids containing mostly polyunsaturated fatty acids are liquid at room temperature.
2. **T F** Lipids yield more energy (kilocalories) per gram than either carbohydrates or proteins.
3. **T F** Total serum cholesterol is the most important blood test in assessing risk for a heart attack.
4. **T F** Cholesterol is found only in food constituents of purely animal origin.
5. **T F** Animal fat is the major dietary component that raises serum cholesterol concentrations.
6. **T F** Triglycerides are the main form of fat found in foods.
7. **T F** Fat is an essential part of human diets.
8. **T F** Hydrogenation makes vegetable oils more solid at room temperature.
9. **T F** Fresh fruits and vegetables are essentially fat free.
10. **T F** Antioxidants help protect foods from becoming rancid.
11. **T F** The small intestine absorbs some vitamins better when dietary fat is present.
12. **T F** A serum cholesterol measurement is unnecessary for persons under the age of 40.
13. **T F** Butter and margarine contain about the same amount of fat.
14. **T F** Deep fat–fried foods purchased in quick-service restaurants are likely to be rich in trans fatty acids.
15. **T F** The effect of dietary cholesterol on heart disease can be ignored in most people.

Lipids: Common Properties and Main Types

Lipids that are solid at room temperature commonly are called *fats;* those that are liquid are called *oils.* Referring to them both as *lipids* simplifies the terminology and makes a food's temperature irrelevant. Otherwise, butter becomes an oil after being placed near a hot stove and a solid fat when refrigerated.

Although lipids form a diverse group, they share two main characteristics: (1) they all dissolve in organic solvents, such as chloroform, benzene, and ether; and (2) they are not readily soluble in water.[20] Think of an oil and vinegar salad dressing. The oil is not soluble in the water-based vinegar; upon standing, the two separate into distinct layers, with oil on top and vinegar on the bottom. Lipids as a class also have a lower ratio of oxygen to carbon compared with carbohydrates, proteins, or alcohols. Otherwise various lipids have few other common properties.

Triglycerides are the most common type of lipid found in the body and in foods. Each triglyceride molecule consists of a glycerol with three fatty acids attached to it. **Phospholipids** and **sterols** are also classified as lipids, although their structures can be quite different from the structure of triglycerides (Figure 4-1).[20] We describe all these lipid compounds in this chapter.

When we discuss lipid chemistry or metabolism, we will use the term *lipid* or a more specific term, such as **serum triglycerides.** When we discuss lipids in foods, we will use the term *fats,* or *fats and oils.* This usage is common today in health-care settings.

Fatty Acids

Fatty acids are found in most lipids in the body and in the lipids in food. Their basic structure is a long chain of carbons bonded together, which in turn are bonded

---

triglycerides The major form of lipid in the body and in food. It is composed of glycerol with three fatty acids attached by ester bonds.

serum The portion of blood that remains after (1) blood is allowed to clot; and (2) the red and white blood cells are removed by centrifugation.

- - - - - - - - - - - -

The reference standard for measuring and expressing blood lipid concentrations is the *serum concentration.* Although *blood cholesterol* is a common term, the value actually refers to the concentration in the serum portion of the blood. When we refer to specific cutoff values for various blood lipids in health and disease, we will indicate that these are for serum concentrations.

- - - - - - - - - - - -

fatty acid A hydrocarbon found in lipids containing a carboxyl (acid group) ($-\overset{\displaystyle O}{\overset{\|}{C}}-$ OH) at one end and a methyl group ($-CH_3$) at the other.

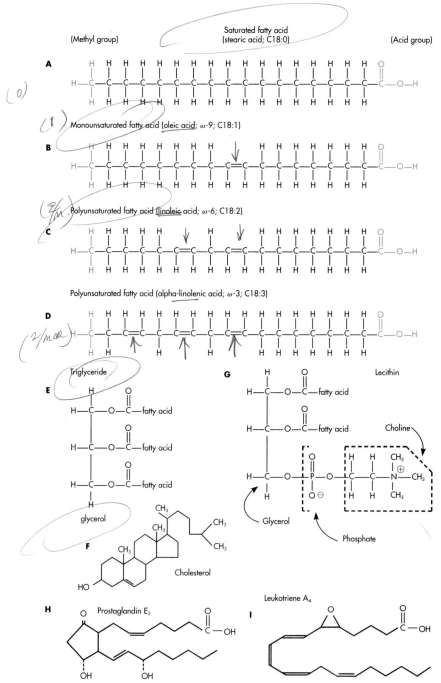

Figure 4-1 The families of lipids and some key metabolic products (the eicosanoids). For simplicity's sake the last three structures have most of the carbons and hydrogens deleted. Wherever there is a corner, it represents a carbon with two hydrogens, since a carbon atom must form four bonds for a stable structure. Note also the shorthand notation used to describe fatty acids. The first number indicates the number of carbons; the second number lists the number of double bonds. Thus stearic acid (structure A) is C18:0.

to numerous hydrogens. At one end of the molecule, designated the *alpha end,* is an acid (specifically a carboxyl) group. At the other end, called the *omega end,* is a methyl group (Figure 4-1A). In the Greek alphabet, *alpha* is the first letter and *omega* is the last.

If all bonds between the carbons are single bonds, a fatty acid is classified as **saturated.** In other words, all the carbons are saturated with hydrogens, like a sponge saturated with water. Animal fats are often rich sources of saturated fatty acids.

saturated fatty acid A fatty acid with no carbon-carbon double bonds.

monounsaturated fatty acid A fatty acid containing one carbon-carbon double bond.

polyunsaturated fatty acid A fatty acid containing two or more carbon-carbon double bonds.

omega-3 (ω-3) fatty acid Unsaturated fatty acid with the first double bond located on the third carbon atom from the methyl end (–CH_3) of the molecule.

omega-6 (ω-6) fatty acid Unsaturated fatty acid with the first double bond located on the sixth carbon atom from the methyl end (–CH_3) of the molecule.

alpha-linolenic acid An essential omega-3 fatty acid with 18 carbons and three double bonds.

linoleic acid An essential omega-6 fatty acid with 18 carbons and two double bonds.

oleic acid An omega-9 fatty acid with 18 carbons and one double bond.

If a fatty acid has one carbon-carbon double bond, it is **monounsaturated** (Figure 4-1B). Canola and olive oils have a high percentage of fatty acids with only one carbon-carbon double bond, and so are designated *monounsaturated* oils.

If two or more bonds between the carbons are double bonds, the fatty acid is **polyunsaturated** (Figure 4-1C,D). Corn, soybean, and safflower oils are rich sources of polyunsaturated fatty acids and so are designated *polyunsaturated oils* (Figure 4-2). Note, however, that dietary lipids contain a mixture of various saturated and unsaturated fatty acids (Figure 4-2). A lipid is classified as a saturated, monounsaturated, or polyunsaturated fat or oil, based on the nature of the fatty acids present in the greatest concentration.

The actual location of the carbon-carbon double bonds in the carbon chain of a polyunsaturated fatty acid makes a big difference in how the body metabolizes it.[26] If the first double bond is located three carbons from the methyl (omega) end of the fatty acid, it is an **omega-3 (ω-3) fatty acid** (Figure 4-1D). If the first double bond is located six carbons from the methyl end of the fatty acid, it is an **omega-6 (ω-6) fatty acid** (Figure 4-1C). Following the same scheme, an omega-9 fatty acid has the first double bond nine carbons from the methyl end of the fatty acid. In foods, **alpha-linolenic acid** is the major omega-3 fatty acid; **linoleic acid** is the major omega-6 fatty acid; and **oleic acid** is the major omega-9 fatty acid.

ESSENTIAL FATTY ACIDS

Cells in the human body can produce carbon-carbon double bonds in a fatty acid only after the ninth carbon numbered from the methyl end. In other words, human cells do not have the capacity to place double bonds between the ninth carbon and the methyl end. For this reason, we can obtain the omega-3 or omega-6 fatty acids only by ingesting them as part of our diets.[26]

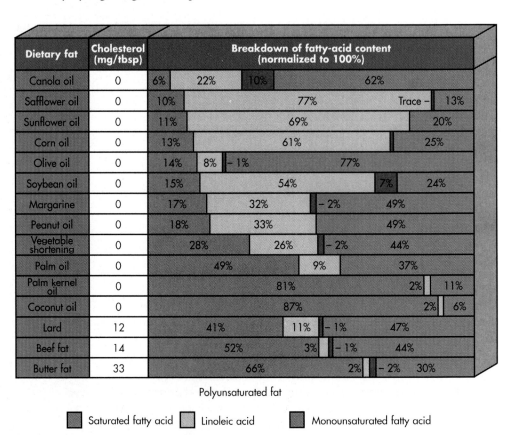

Dietary fat	Cholesterol (mg/tbsp)	Breakdown of fatty-acid content (normalized to 100%)
Canola oil	0	6% 22% 10% 62%
Safflower oil	0	10% 77% Trace 13%
Sunflower oil	0	11% 69% 20%
Corn oil	0	13% 61% 25%
Olive oil	0	14% 8% 1% 77%
Soybean oil	0	15% 54% 7% 24%
Margarine	0	17% 32% 2% 49%
Peanut oil	0	18% 33% 49%
Vegetable shortening	0	28% 26% 2% 44%
Palm oil	0	49% 9% 37%
Palm kernel oil	0	81% 2% 11%
Coconut oil	0	87% 2% 6%
Lard	12	41% 11% 1% 47%
Beef fat	14	52% 3% 1% 44%
Butter fat	33	66% 2% 2% 30%

Polyunsaturated fat

■ Saturated fatty acid   □ Linoleic acid   ■ Monounsaturated fatty acid

■ Alpha-linolenic acid

Figure 4-2 Comparison of dietary lipids in terms of saturated fatty acids, the most common unsaturated fatty acids, and cholesterol content.

Omega-3 and omega-6 fatty acids form parts of vital body structures, perform important roles in immune system function and vision, help form cell membranes, and produce hormonelike compounds called **eicosanoids** (Figure 4-1H,I).[3] So we must consume these fatty acids to maintain good health.

Because of their essential role in a diet, the omega-3 and omega-6 polyunsaturated fatty acids alpha-linolenic acid and linoleic acid, respectively, are called **essential fatty acids.** The 1989 RDA publication states that adults need to consume about 1% to 2% of their total energy intake from linoleic acid; current consumption is about 7%. Up to 10% of energy intake from a combination of linoleic acid plus alpha-linolenic acid is a safe upper amount. Since common plant seed oils—corn, soybean, cottonseed, sunflower, and safflower oils—generally contain over 50% of their fatty acids as polyunsaturated fatty acids, plant oils should supply about 4% of our total energy intake. On a 2500 kcal diet, this corresponds to 1 tablespoon of highly polyunsaturated vegetable oil per day consumed as part of usual food intake. Salad dressing is the common vehicle for incorporating essential fatty acids into our diets.

The 1989 RDA publication states that in the future an allowance for omega-3 fatty acids should be considered. Leading researchers support this idea.[26] Currently Canada is the only national government to establish dietary guidelines for omega-3 fatty acids. The Canadian recommendation is a dietary ratio of 4:1 omega-6 to omega-3 fatty acids. The current ratio in American diets is about 10:1. Many scientists today suggest that we have a regular intake of alpha-linolenic acid or one of its related omega-3 fatty acids, **eicosapentaenoic acid (EPA)** and **docosahexaenoic acid (DHA).** This would almost certainly require weekly consumption of fatty fish, such as salmon, tuna, or sardines, or regular intake of canola or soybean oil. All are good sources of omega-3 fatty acids. Omega-3 fatty acids will be explored further in the next few pages.

CONCEPT CHECK

Lipids are a group of compounds that dissolve in organic solvents but do not dissolve readily in water. They include fatty acids, triglycerides, phospholipids, and sterols. Fatty acids differ from each other mainly in the number and location of the double bonds between carbons in the carbon chain. Saturated fatty acids contain no carbon-carbon double bonds; that is, they are fully saturated with hydrogens. Monounsaturated fatty acids contain one carbon-carbon double bond, and polyunsaturated fatty acids contain two or more carbon-carbon double bonds. If a double bond first occurs at the third carbon from the methyl ($-CH_3$) end of the carbon chain, the fatty acid is an omega-3 fatty acid. If a double bond first occurs at the sixth carbon, it is an omega-6 fatty acid. Because humans can't synthesize omega-3 and omega-6 fatty acids, which perform vital functions in the body, they are designated *essential fatty acids,* indicating that they must be included in the diet.

METABOLISM AND THE ROLE OF ESSENTIAL FATTY ACIDS IN THE BODY

Omega-3 and omega-6 fatty acids are further metabolized by cells as part of the ultimate synthesis of some of the biologically active substances that cells produce. Once linoleic acid is in a cell, it can be lengthened to 20 carbons and can undergo desaturation, in which two more carbon-carbon double bonds are added, yielding **arachidonic acid.**[20] Alpha-linolenic acid can be elongated to 20 carbons and have two carbon-carbon double bonds added to form EPA.[18] In some instances, arachidonic acid and EPA are made even longer by having more carbons added, such as when EPA is metabolized to DHA.[26] The rate at which all these reactions take place and their significance depend on the type of human cell in which it occurs. As a direct dietary source, EPA and DHA are especially concentrated in cold-water fishes.[3]

eicosanoids Hormonelike compounds synthesized from polyunsaturated fatty acids, such as arachidonic acid. Within this class of compounds are prostaglandins, thromboxanes, and leukotrienes.

CRITICAL THINKING

Advertisements often claim that fats are bad. Your classmate Mike asks, "If fats are so bad for us, why do we need to have any in our diets?" How would you answer him?

essential fatty acids Fatty acids that must be supplied by the diet to maintain health. Currently only linoleic acid and alpha-linolenic acid are classified as essential.

eicosapentaenoic acid (EPA) An omega-3 fatty acid with 20 carbons and five carbon-carbon double bonds. It is present in large amounts in fish oils and is also synthesized in the body from alpha-linolenic acid.

docosahexaenoic acid (DHA) An omega-3 fatty acid with 22 carbons and six carbon-carbon double bonds. It is present in large amounts in fish oils and also is synthesized in the body from alpha-linolenic acid.

arachidonic acid An omega-6 fatty acid with 20 carbons and four carbon-carbon double bonds.

prostaglandins A group of eicosanoids that produce diverse hormonelike effects in the body.

prostacyclin A potent inhibitor of blood clotting made by the blood vessel walls; an eicosanoid.

thromboxane A stimulant of blood clotting made in certain blood cells; an eicosanoid.

leukotrienes A group of eicosanoids that are involved in inflammatory and hypersensitivity reactions, such as asthma.

- - - - - - - - - - - - -
Aspirin has diverse effects on the body—from lowering body temperature and inhibiting blood clotting to easing muscle pain—because it blocks the synthesis of certain eicosanoids. Physicians commonly prescribe small amounts of aspirin taken on a regular basis for patients at high risk of heart attack. This practice inhibits formation of blood clots.
- - - - - - - - - - - - -

hemorrhagic stroke Damage to part of the brain resulting from rupture of a blood vessel and subsequent bleeding within or over the internal surface of the brain.

The long-chain, highly polyunsaturated fatty acids, including arachidonic acid and EPA, can be metabolized further to form the group of biologically active compounds called eicosanoids. These hormonelike compounds include the **prostaglandins, prostacyclins, thromboxanes,** and **leukotrienes**[20] (Figure 4-1H,I). As mentioned earlier, eicosanoids are important and potent regulators of vital body functions, such as blood pressure, childbirth, blood clotting, immune responses, inflammatory responses, and stomach secretions.[3] In essence, the eicosanoids act as hormones but do so in the vicinity in which they arise, rather than traveling via the blood to their site of action, as is the case for true hormones.

Fish oils: Rich sources of EPA and DHA

Fish oils—rich in EPA and DHA—reduce the tendency for blood to clot.[3] They do so by changing the nature of eicosanoid synthesis in the body. An important class of prostaglandins and thromboxanes is usually made from arachidonic acid, an omega-6 fatty acid. Since fish oils contain a lot of the omega-3 fatty acids (EPA and DHA), cells of people who eat a lot of fish have a greater tendency to synthesize eicosanoids with EPA and DHA, instead of almost exclusively using arachidonic acid. In effect, EPA and DHA compete with arachidonic acid for the same metabolic pathways.[3] When they are highly concentrated in a cell, EPA and DHA win more often.

Now when cells use these different starting compounds, they synthesize different types of eicosanoids. Arachidonic acid yields one class of prostaglandins and thromboxanes, while EPA and DHA yield another class of prostaglandins and thromboxanes. The subtle differences in structure between the two forms of these compounds yield key differences in function. For example, many of the eicosanoids made from arachidonic acid (omega-6) increase blood clotting, while those made from EPA and DHA (omega-3) primarily decrease it. The net effect is that diets high in arachidonic acid increase the tendency for blood to clot, while diets high in EPA and DHA do not.[3]

As we discuss in the Nutrition Perspective, the lower the tendency for blood to clot, the lower the risk of heart attack. This relationship suggests that omega-3 fatty acids, especially EPA and DHA, reduce the risk of heart attack. Some evidence supports this conclusion.[26] For example, Greenland Eskimos obtain 40% of their energy intake from omega-3 fatty acids, as they eat many fish, whale, seal, and walrus products. These Eskimos have one tenth the risk of heart attacks of Danes, who consume much less fish and other marine foods. Other studies show that people who eat fish just twice a week (240 g or 8 ounces of total weekly intake) also run lower risks for heart disease than people who rarely eat fish.

As we noted already, alpha-linolenic acid and linoleic acid are classified as essential nutrients, which must be present in the diet to sustain good health. However, conversion of alpha-linolenic acid (omega-3) to EPA and DHA appears to be relatively inefficient, especially in people who consume the usual amounts of linoleic acid, which slows the conversion process. Because of the important biological effects of the eicosanoids made from EPA and DHA, some scientists believe that these long-chain omega-3 fatty acids should also be considered essential nutrients.[26]

Although Eskimos who eat a lot of fish have a lower risk for heart attack than Danes, they have a higher risk for **hemorrhagic stroke**, probably because their blood does not readily clot. Thus, significantly altering the tendency of blood to clot is a double-edged sword. Because of this possibility, the safest way to take advantage of this research is simply to eat fish regularly, about twice a week.[13] Among the fish with the highest omega-3 fatty acid content are Atlantic and Pacific herring; sardines, Atlantic halibut and salmon; lake trout; coho, pink, and king salmon; blue fish; albacore tuna; and Atlantic mackerel (see Appendix H).

No major health organization, including the American Heart Association, recommends consuming fish oil capsules without a physician's advice and close supervision. The potential for seriously increasing bleeding tendencies by altering the types of eicosanoids formed is only one possible result from use of fish oil capsules.[3]

Because eicosanoids have significant and wide-ranging effects besides blood clotting, altering their production can have profound consequences on health. This caution regarding fish oil capsules should not be confused, however, with the suggestion that we regularly include some fish in our diets.[13]

Essential Fatty Acid Deficiency

Unless enough essential fatty acids are consumed, profound physiological consequences result. In infants, the skin becomes flaky and itchy, sores may develop on the scalp, diarrhea and other symptoms such as infections often are seen, and growth and wound healing may be retarded. In adults, skin disorders and anemia develop. These signs of deficiency have been seen in people fed **intravenous** solutions containing little or no fat for long periods of time and in infants receiving formulas low in fat. However, since we need only about 1 tablespoon of polyunsaturated plant oil a day to meet essential fatty acid needs, even a low-fat diet, if it follows the Food Guide Pyramid, will provide enough essential fatty acids if fish is also eaten about twice a week.

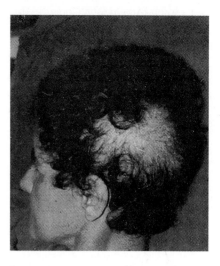

Essential fatty acid deficiency produces changes in the skin, resulting in hair loss

intravenous Introduced directly into the bloodstream.

CONCEPT CHECK

The hormonelike eicosanoids are produced by body cells from both omega-3 and omega-6 fatty acids. However, the biological effects of eicosanoids synthesized from the two types of precursors differ markedly. In general, eicosanoids made from omega-3 fatty acids tend to decrease blood clotting, blood pressure, and inflammatory responses in the body. In the future, dietary guidelines for intake of omega-3 fatty acids may be set in the United States, as is currently done in Canada. Presently the recommendation to eat fish about twice a week is a good guide for obtaining omega-3 fatty acids.

FUNCTIONS AND USES OF FATTY ACIDS IN FOODS

Like the fatty acids in the body, the fatty acids in foods are present primarily in the form of triglycerides. The degree of saturation and the chain length of the fatty acids in the triglycerides found in foods are important determinants of the properties of food fats.

As we saw already, many food fats contain a mixture of saturated and unsaturated fatty acids. Generally, lipids with a high content of saturated fatty acids are more solid than lipids with a high content of unsaturated fatty acids. This difference arises from a key difference in the shape of these molecules. Saturated fatty acids are linear, allowing them to pack tightly together.[20] In contrast, unsaturated fatty acids have a kinked shape and thus pack together only loosely. The loose organization of unsaturated fats is more easily disrupted by heat than is the more ordered organization of saturated fats. Thus fats high in unsaturated fatty acids melt at a lower temperature than fats high in saturated fatty acids (especially long-chain ones). In fact, most unsaturated food fats are liquid at room temperature and are commonly referred to as oils.

The chain length of the saturated fats in foods also affects their melting temperature. Fats rich in **long-chain** saturated **fatty acids** (12 carbons or more), such as animal fats, are solid at room temperature. **Medium-chain** saturated **fatty acids** (6 to 10 carbons), such as those found in coconut oil, can produce liquid oils at room temperature. The shorter chain length overrides the effect of the high degree of saturation. **Short-chain** saturated **fatty acids** (2 to 4 carbons) form oils at room temperature. Food sources of short-chain saturated fatty acids include dairy fats (see Appendix H).

Hydrogenation of Fatty Acids

Vegetable oils containing polyunsaturated fatty acids can be converted into solid margarines and shortenings by a process called **hydrogenation,** which increases the satu-

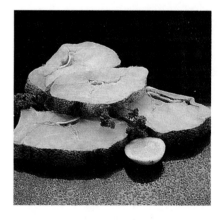

Eating fish about twice a week makes a healthy contribution to a diet.

long-chain fatty acids Fatty acids that contain 12 or more carbon atoms.

medium-chain fatty acids Fatty acids that contain 6 to 10 carbon atoms.

short-chain fatty acids Fatty acids that contain fewer than 6 carbon atoms.

hydrogenation Addition of hydrogen to a carbon-carbon double bond, producing a single bond. Because hydrogenation of unsaturated fatty acids in a vegetable oil increases its hardness, this process is used to convert liquid oils into more solid fats, which are used in making margarine and shortening. Trans fatty acids are produced during hydrogenation of vegetable oils.

trans fatty acid An isomeric form of an unsaturated fatty acid, usually a monounsaturated one when found in food, in which the hydrogens on both carbons forming the double bond lie on opposite sides of that bond.

oxidizing agents Compounds (e.g., oxygen) that capture electrons, thereby removing them from other compounds, which then are said to be "oxidized." Oxidation of double bonds in unsaturated fatty acids often causes them to be broken, yielding smaller and more aromatic products.

rancid Having an unpleasant flavor or odor.

ration of the product. In this process, hydrogens are added at many of the carbon-carbon double bonds of the fatty acids, turning them into single bonds (Figure 4-3). It also produces some **trans fatty acids.**[34] (We discuss these by-products of hydrogenation in a Nutrition Focus in this chapter.) Both changes increase hardness. Generally, the harder the product—stick margarine compared with tub margarine—the more hydrogenation has occurred and the higher the trans fatty acid content.

Hydrogenated fats are easier to use than vegetable oils in some aspects of food production, such as in making pastries and cakes. Manufacturers also prefer to use solid shortening for the production of many crackers and snack products. As public pressure has persuaded manufacturers to eliminate the tropical oils rich in saturated fat (palm, palm kernel, and coconut) from food processing, partially hydrogenated soybean oil has become the major replacement.[34] During the next few days, study food labels and notice how many chips, snack products, and crackers contain a "partially hydrogenated vegetable oil."

Rancidity

The carbon-carbon double bonds in polyunsaturated fatty acids are easily broken by ultraviolet light, heat, and various **oxidizing agents,** forming **rancid** products. You may have noted a disagreeable odor and sour, stale taste in old potato chips and other products. The altered taste and smell come from the shorter and more aromatic products that result from the breakdown of polyunsaturated fatty acids.

Even though rancid oils are potentially toxic, their unappealing taste and vile odor discourage people from eating enough to pose a threat. However, rancidity reduces a product's shelf life and is therefore costly to the manufacturer.

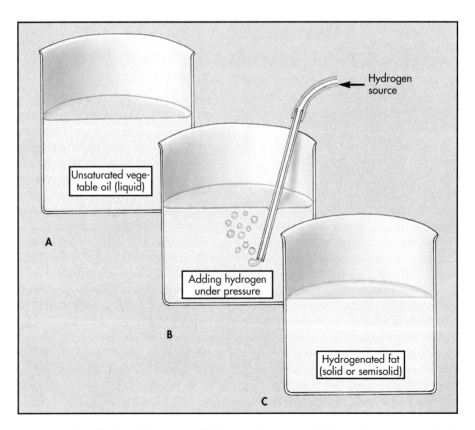

Figure 4-3 How liquid oils become solid fats. **A,** Unsaturated fatty acids are present in liquid form. **B,** Hydrogens are added (hydrogenation), changing some carbon-carbon double bonds to single bonds and producing some trans fatty acids. **C,** The completed hydrogenated product, which is likely to be used in margarine, shortenings, or deep fat frying.

Some naturally occurring **antioxidants** prevent oxidizing agents from breaking carbon-carbon double bonds. These natural protectors against rancidity include vitamin E found in plant oils, as well as vitamin C and various carotenoids found in fruits and vegetables.

Food manufacturers have several options for reducing rancidity and the consequent deterioration of their products. In some cases, they can use hydrogenated or partially hydrogenated vegetable oils rather than polyunsaturated vegetable oils. They can also add **BHA** or **BHT,** which are synthetic antioxidants. Look for these food additives in salad dressings, breakfast cereals, cake mixes, and other products that contain fat. Manufacturers also tightly seal their products from the atmosphere and use other methods to reduce the presence of oxygen inside packages.

CONCEPT CHECK

At room temperature, fats rich in saturated fatty acids tend to form solid fats, and fats rich in polyunsaturated and monounsaturated fatty acids tend to form liquid oils. During hydrogenation of unsaturated fatty acids, hydrogen is added to carbon-carbon double bonds to produce single bonds; some trans fatty acids are also created. Hydrogenation changes vegetable oil to solid fat. The carbon-carbon double bonds in polyunsaturated fatty acids are easily broken, yielding products responsible for rancidity. The presence of antioxidants, such as vitamin E in oils, naturally protects unsaturated fatty acids against oxidative destruction. Manufacturers can use partially hydrogenated oils and add synthetic antioxidants to reduce the likelihood of rancidity.

Triglycerides

Very few fatty acids exist in a free form in the body or in foods. Some free fatty acids are bound to the blood protein albumin as they are transferred from storage in adipose cells to the liver, muscles, and other sites. Each albumin molecule can carry up to 10 fatty acids. However, about 95% of all fatty acids, both in the body and in food, are in the form of triglycerides.[20] Thus body fat, butter, and corn oil all consist primarily of triglycerides.

As we noted earlier, triglyceride molecules contain a "backbone" of the three-carbon alcohol **glycerol.** A fatty acid is attached to each of the three hydroxyl groups (–OH) of glycerol. Three water molecules are released in the process of bonding three fatty acids to glycerol (Figure 4-5).[20] Note that triacylglyceride is the chemical name of the molecule, as *acyl* refers to a fatty acid that has lost its hydroxyl group, and a hydroxyl group is lost when each fatty acid attaches to glycerol.

Although triglycerides are most common, monoglycerides (composed of glycerol with only one attached fatty acid) and diglycerides (composed of glycerol with two attached fatty acids) also occur. In all of these compounds the bonds between glycerol and each fatty acid are called *ester bonds*. The process of chemically attaching fatty acids to glycerol is called **esterification.** The release of fatty acids from glycerol is called *deesterification*.

Free fatty acids, monoglycerides, and glycerol—but not triglycerides—can cross cell membranes. During digestion, enzymes break down the triglycerides in the foods to free fatty acids and monoglycerides; only a small portion of dietary triglycerides is broken down completely to free fatty acids and glycerol. After the free fatty acids, monoglycerides, and any free glycerol enter the intestinal cells, most of these components are rebuilt into new triglycerides (Figure 4-6).[20] The reattachment of fatty acids to glycerol is called *reesterification*. Every time a triglyceride enters or leaves a cell, it must also be deesterified; after entering a cell, the free fatty acids are reesterified into triglycerides. Thus the body continually breaks down and rebuilds triglycerides.

antioxidant A compound that prevents the oxidation of substances in food or the body, particularly lipids. Antioxidants are especially important in preventing oxidation of polyunsaturated lipids in cell membranes. By donating electrons to electron-seeking compounds, antioxidants reduce the ability of electron-seeking compounds (oxidizing agents) to break down unsaturated fatty acids and other cell components. Vitamin E is a natural antioxidant that cells use for protection.

BHA and BHT Butylated hydroxyanisol and butylated hydroxytoluene—two common synthetic antioxidants added to foods to prevent rancidity.

glycerol A three-carbon alcohol containing three hydroxyl groups (OH) that forms the "backbone" of triglycerides.

esterification The process of attaching fatty acids to a glycerol molecule, creating an ester bond and releasing water. Removing a fatty acid is called deesterification; reattaching a fatty acid is called reesterification.

NUTRITION FOCUS

CIS AND TRANS FATTY ACIDS

Monounsaturated and polyunsaturated fatty acids can exist in two isomeric forms—**cis** and **trans.** Isomers share the same chemical formula but have different chemical structures. The *cis* form has the hydrogen atoms on the same side of the carbon-carbon double bond. The *trans* form has the hydrogen atoms on opposite sides of the carbon-carbon double bond (Figure 4-4). Plant-derived foods contain cis fatty acids. Milk fat contains a few trans fatty acids, which are formed by bacterial conversion of cis to trans fatty acids in the cow's multiple stomachs (rumen). However, meat does not contain many trans fatty acids. The greatest contributors of trans fatty acids to human diets are margarine and partially hydrogenated vegetable shortenings; manufacture of these products involves hydrogenation, which yields trans fatty acids as by-products. Partially hydrogenated vegetable shortenings are used in many food products and in deep-fat frying.[34]

EFFECTS OF TRANS FATTY ACIDS

As you can see in Figure 4-4, the *cis* bond causes the fatty acid backbone to bend, whereas the *trans* bond allows the

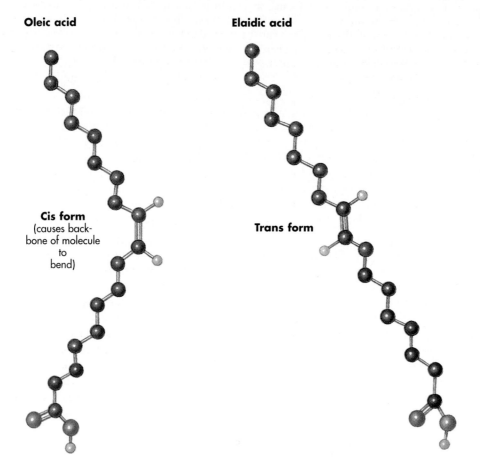

Oleic acid

Elaidic acid

Cis form
(causes backbone of molecule to bend)

Trans form

Figure 4-4 *Cis* and *trans* isomers of fatty acids. Cis fatty acids are more common in foods than trans fatty acids. The latter are primarily found in foods containing hydrogenated fats, notably stick margarine, shortening, and deep fat–fried foods.

backbone to remain straighter. The presence of trans fatty acids, rather than cis fatty acids, in cell membranes makes the membranes stiffer. This stiffness then may reduce the function of cell-membrane receptors that clear cholesterol from the bloodstream. This may be the mechanism whereby both trans fatty acids and saturated fatty acids raise serum cholesterol.[36]

Some scientists believe that trans fatty acid intake in the general public is not linked to a significantly increased risk for any major chronic disease, notably heart disease and cancer, probably because most of us eat so little trans fatty acid, about 8 to 13 g/day. Use of margarine—a major source of trans fatty acids in our food—has increased during the last 40 years while heart disease deaths have declined and cancer deaths, except for lung cancer, have remained steady for the last few decades.

Other researchers, however, have estimated that trans fatty acid intake may be causing more than 30,000 of the approximately 500,000 deaths from heart attack each year. Furthermore, the number of cases of nonfatal heart disease may be even larger.[34] Intakes of two to four times the usual intake do raise serum cholesterol when these replace unsaturated fats in the diet.[36] For people who eat a large number of commercially prepared foods and quick-service foods, this effect may be significant, since trans fatty acid intake can reach 30 g/day or more. Trans fatty acids also show no essential fatty acid activity and may inhibit essential fatty acid metabolism.[26]

In recent years many quick-service restaurants have switched from using beef fat (tallow) to using partially hydrogenated vegetable shortenings in an effort to reduce the saturated fat in their menus. Inadvertently this has increased the trans fatty acid content of some of their products, thus increasing the potential for high intakes of trans fatty acids by some customers.[34]

Currently the trans fatty acid content of foods is not listed as such on food labels. Rather, it is included with monounsaturated fat, since trans fatty acids are primarily monounsaturated in composition. Because trans fatty acids are "hidden" on labels, consumers are not aware of their presence. Thus today's food labels don't inform consumers about the true trans fatty acid content of products.

LIMITING DIETARY TRANS FATTY ACID INTAKE

It is easy to limit trans fatty acid intake if one chooses to do so. First, use little or no stick margarine or shortening; substitute softer, tub margarine and vegetable oils that list vegetable oil or water as the first ingredient (currently some diet tub margarines tout their low trans fatty acid content). Second, minimize consumption of deep fat–fried foods, since hydrogenated fat was probably used in the fryer. Foods to avoid include french fries, doughnuts, potato skins, and any deep fat–fried meat, fish, or poultry. As an alternative, a typical hamburger sandwich, bowl of chili, and soft drink or milk in a quick-service restaurant contain minimal trans fatty acids and still make a satisfying meal. Finally, limit intake of high-fat baked foods, such as pastries.

An additional consideration is use of nondairy creamers. Initially these may appear to be a healthful substitute for cream, which is rich in saturated fatty acids. However, many nondairy creamers are rich in hydrogenated vegetable oils, and thus are rich in trans fatty acids. Low-fat or nonfat milk is a better choice than liquid or dry nondairy creamer when trying to reduce trans fatty acid intake.

Overall, intakes of trans fatty acids will remain low if one eats limited amounts of high-fat food (e.g., chips, cakes, cookies), adds little extra fat such as stick margarine to foods, and avoids especially concentrated sources, such as deep fat–fried foods.

The recent introduction of many fat-reduced products also will likely further diminish the intake of all fats, including trans fatty acids, over the next few years. Many nutrition scientists agree that the most important consideration for Americans is to reduce overall fat intake, with a focus on fat-rich foods in general and on saturated fatty acids in particular. They feel that following this advice obviates any need for alarm regarding trans fatty acids in foods, since this practice will likely result in a minimal intake of trans fatty acids as well.

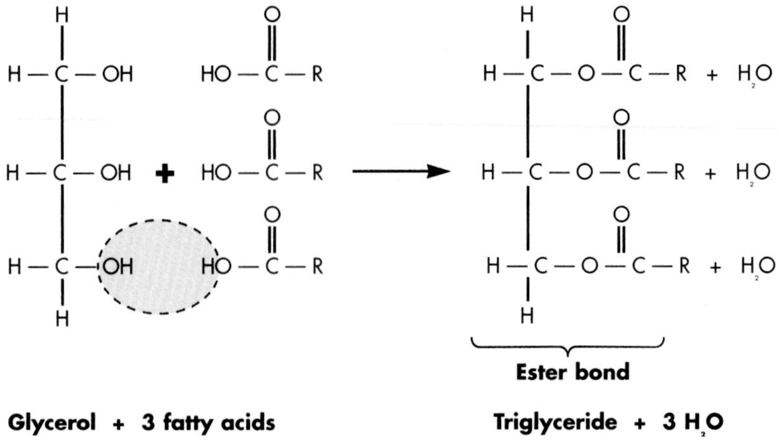

Glycerol + 3 fatty acids   **Triglyceride + 3 H₂O**

Figure 4-5 Forming a triglyceride via esterification. This process yields water as a by-product as ester bonds are formed. The *R* represents the fatty acids.

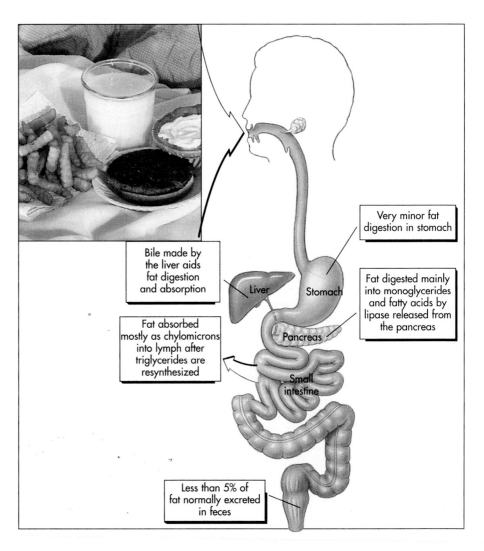

Figure 4-6 A summary of fat digestion and absorption. Chapter 6 covers this process in detail.

FUNCTIONS OF TRIGLYCERIDES IN THE BODY

Here we describe several of the numerous important functions of triglycerides in the body.

Storing Energy and Supplying It to Tissues

Triglycerides are the main chemical form of stored energy in the body. The ability to store triglyceride is essentially unlimited, since storage sites, adipose cells, can increase about 50 times in weight. If the amount of triglyceride to be stored exceeds the ability of the cells to expand, whether during infancy or adulthood, the body will form new adipose cells.

When we store triglyceride in adipose cells, we store little else. Adipose cells are about 80% lipid and only 20% water and protein.[20] In contrast, if we stored energy as protein in muscle tissue, we would also need to store large amounts of water, since muscle is about 73% water. The same is true for energy stored as glycogen. About 2.6 g of water are stored along with every gram of glycogen. A 3-day supply of energy as glycogen would weigh about 14 pounds (6 kg). Think of the consequences if we stored energy as muscle tissue or glycogen—for most of us, body weight would greatly increase because of the excess water we would need to carry.

Another advantage to storing triglycerides for energy is their energy density. Recall that triglycerides yield over twice as much energy per gram as proteins and carbohydrates. In addition, triglycerides are chemically very stable, so that they are not likely to react with other cell constituents, making them a safe form for storing energy.[20]

Free fatty acids released from triglycerides make up the main fuel for muscles at rest and during light activity. In endurance exercise the muscles utilize a lot of carbohydrate in addition to fatty acids (see Chapter 10 for a detailed account of fuel use in exercise). Mostly, however, muscles derive energy from fatty acids. Other body tissues also use fatty acids for energy—about half of the energy used by the entire body at rest and during light activity is derived from fatty acids. For the entire body, use of fatty acids by muscles is balanced by glucose use in the brain, other nervous tissue, and red blood cells.[20]

Protecting and Insulating the Body

A layer of adipose tissue—composed mostly of triglycerides—protects and insulates the body, especially the breasts and kidneys. Women typically have more adipose tissue in the hips, buttocks, and lower abdomen than men. The preservation of the species depends on the protection of the reproductive organs by adipose tissue. In this way the ovaries and uterus are protected in women, whereas a testicular fat pad protects the testes in men.

We usually don't notice the important insulating function of adipose tissue because we wear clothes, but it is quite apparent in animals. Polar bears, whales, and other animals that live in cold climates build thick layers of adipose tissue to insulate themselves against their cold environment. This tissue also represents stored energy for winter.

People with the disease **anorexia nervosa** often lose 25% or more of their body weight, resulting in a body-fat percentage that is dangerously low. We can never be totally fat free, because fat is an essential part of all cells. However, a person with anorexia nervosa may get as lean as is biologically possible. If body fat falls below 5% of total body weight, harmful side effects occur, especially in women (see Chapter 11). In response to this extreme thinness, the person often develops **lanugo**, which is downy hair all over the body. These hairs stand erect, trapping air around them. The air acts as insulation and represents an adjustment for the missing layer of adipose tissue usually present under the skin. Lanugo also normally insulates a growing **fetus** before its layer of adipose tissue is produced late in pregnancy.

Aiding Intestinal Absorption of Fat-Soluble Vitamins

Triglycerides and other lipids in foods carry fat-soluble vitamins to the small intestine and in doing so aid in absorption of these nutrients. If the small intestine is dis-

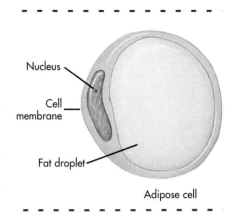

Nucleus

Cell membrane

Fat droplet

Adipose cell

anorexia nervosa An eating disorder involving a psychological loss of appetite and self-starvation, caused in part by a distorted body image and various social pressures often associated with puberty.

lanugo Downlike hair that appears after much body fat is lost because of semi-starvation. As the hair stands erect and traps air, it acts as insulation, replacing that supplied by body fat.

fetus A developing human in utero from 8 weeks after conception until birth.

- - - - - - - - - - - -

Unabsorbed fatty acids can bind minerals, such as calcium and magnesium, and draw them into the stool for elimination. This can harm mineral status (see Chapter 14).

- - - - - - - - - - - -

satiety A state in which there is no desire to eat; a feeling of satisfaction.

CRITICAL THINKING

In a class discussion, the topic of "diets" comes up. One of the most frustrating feelings dieters have, the students remark, is "being hungry all the time." Many dieters not only reduce their energy intake but also eliminate much of the fat from their diets. As a nutrition student, you suggest that some fat should be included in meals even while on a weight-reduction diet. How would you justify this advice?

lecithins A group of phospholipids containing two fatty acids, a phosphate group, and a choline molecule. Lecithins are a group of compounds, since they can differ based on the types of fatty acids found on each lecithin molecule.

eased, dietary fat may not be properly digested and absorbed. In this situation, much fat passes through the small intestine and enters the large intestine. The fat-soluble vitamins bound to unabsorbed fat also are carried into the large intestine, bypassing their absorption sites in the small intestine.

People with cystic fibrosis often absorb fat poorly and are at risk for deficiencies of fat-soluble vitamins, especially vitamin K. People who use mineral oil as a laxative close to mealtimes are also at risk, since humans cannot digest or absorb mineral oil. The undigested mineral oil, which itself is a mixture of liquid petroleum hydrocarbons, carries fat-soluble vitamins into the large intestine, where they are eliminated in the stool. This can make mineral oil a poor choice for a laxative, especially when taken near mealtimes.

TRIGLYCERIDES IN THE DIET: SATIETY AND FLAVOR

The composition of a meal helps determine the rate of stomach emptying, which is linked to various hormonal responses (see Chapter 6). Because dietary fat causes the stomach to empty more slowly than either carbohydrate or protein, it imparts **satiety,** that is, a satisfied feeling after eating.

Many people who want to reduce body weight know that fats are energy dense. They find that the easiest way to cut energy intake is to cut out much of the fat in their diet. However, if dieters reduce fat intake too much, they lose its satiety value and get hungry more quickly. Thus, reducing fat intake below about 20% of total energy intake can actually be self-defeating, unless high-fiber foods are added to contribute bulk, which also makes us feel full (see Chapter 8 for further discussion).

Triglycerides and other lipid components in foods provide important textures and carry flavors. The most tender cuts of meat are high in fat, visible as the marbling of meat. Low-fat meats, such as flank steak or brisket, require special preparation techniques, such as marinating or slow, moist cooking, to ensure tenderness. Many flavoring compounds are fat soluble: their essences dissolve in fat, and the fat carries them to the sensory cells in the mouth that discriminate taste and smell. Perhaps you have used an oil flavoring in baking or in making candy. Heating spices in oil intensifies the flavors of an Indian curry or Mexican dish far more than simply adding them at the table. We thus associate flavorful foods with high-fat foods for good reason.[19]

CONCEPT CHECK

Triglyceride is the major form of fat in the body and in food. Triglycerides in the body are used to store and supply energy, to protect and insulate body organs, and to aid in absorption of fat-soluble vitamins. Thus some fat is needed in the body to maintain good health. Triglycerides also contribute to satiety from a meal and add flavor and texture to foods.

Phospholipids

Many phospholipids, including the **lecithins,** consist of a glycerol backbone with one or two attached fatty acids, plus a different structure that includes a phosphate group attached to the other hydroxyl group(s). Lecithins and similar phospholipids thus not only look like triglycerides, but in fact originate from triglycerides (Figure 4-1). Lecithins are important components of all cell membranes and participate in fat digestion in the small intestine.[20] Egg yolks contain lecithins in abundance, as do liver, wheat germ, and peanuts.

Many other types of phospholipids exist in the body, such as sphingomyelins and cerebrosides, both of which are found in the brain and other nerve tissue. Even though lecithins and other phospholipids are necessary components of body tissues, we don't have to consume phospholipids as such because the body can make them when and where it is necessary. For this reason, phospholipids receive less attention than other lipids from nutritionists. In addition, phospholipid intake is not linked to any major disease state.

Cell membranes are composed primarily of phospholipids. A cell membrane looks much like a sea of phospholipids with protein "islands" (Figure 4-7). Among their many roles, the proteins form receptors for hormones, function as enzymes, and act as transporters for essential nutrients.[20] Some cholesterol is also present in the membrane. Notice also the carbohydrates on the surface of the receptor proteins. A function of this carbohydrate is to help an incoming molecule identify the protein receptor on the cell surface.

Many phospholipids function as emulsifiers, which are compounds that promote the breakup of fat into small particles and stabilize their suspension in a water (aqueous) environment. To see how phospholipids function as emulsifiers, look again at Figure 4-1. The charged end of a lecithin molecule attracts water, while the other fatty acid ends attract lipids. The long hydrocarbon chains in fatty acids show no net positive or negative charge; they are **nonpolar,** as electrons are distributed uniformly. Triglycerides also are nonpolar and so are attracted to fatty acids. In contrast, the phosphate group and nitrogen-containing choline of the lecithin molecule are charged; they are **polar,** as electrons are distributed nonuniformly. Water is also polar. The slightly negative-charged oxygen and the two slightly positive-charged hydrogens create poles, similar to magnetic poles. Since water is attracted to the charges on lecithin, this part of lecithin is called **hydrophilic,** which means "loving water." The parts with fatty acids are called **hydrophobic,** since they don't attract (they fear) water.

When an emulsifier is mixed with oil and water in the proper proportions, it forms **micelles,** spherical structures in which the hydrophobic parts of the emulsifier molecules are oriented toward the interior and the hydrophilic parts toward the exterior (Figure 4-8). Oil is attracted to the hydrophobic interior of the micelles, and water is attracted to the hydrophilic exterior. The mixture produced has tiny oil droplets surrounded by thin shells of water. In an emulsified solution there are millions of these tiny oil droplets, all separated from one another by shells of water.

The complete digestion and absorption of fat requires emulsification of dietary fats in the small intestine (Chapter 6 provides a full account of this process). Lecithins and **bile acids** are produced by the liver and secreted into the small in-

nonpolar Referring to a compound with no charges present.

polar Referring to a compound with distinct positive and negative charges, which act like the poles of a magnet.

hydrophilic Attracts water (literally means "water loving").

hydrophobic Repels water (literally means "water fearing").

micelles Water-soluble spherical structures formed by emulsifier molecules in which the hydrophobic parts of the molecules face inward and the hydrophilic parts face outward. Lipids enclosed within micelles do not separate out into an oily layer as they normally do when mixed with water.

bile acids Emulsifiers synthesized by the liver and released by the gallbladder during digestion.

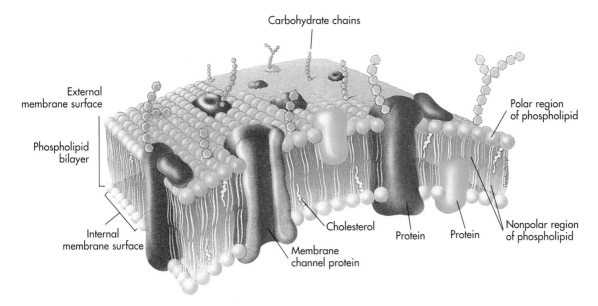

Figure 4-7 A cell membrane. This membrane is composed of protein islands within a sea of lipids. The lipids are mostly phospholipids, with some cholesterol present. Carbohydrate chains are attached to the outside of the cell membrane.

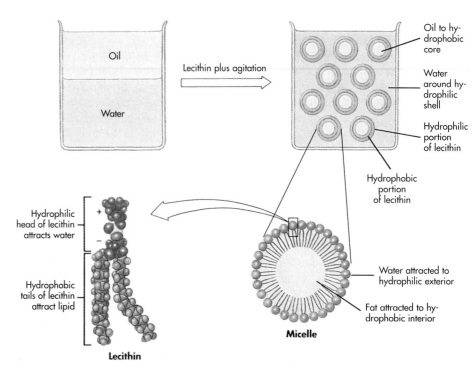

Figure 4-8 Emulsification and emulsifiers. Emulsifiers organize oil and water into micelles—droplets of oil surrounded by shells of water. The emulsifier molecules form a bridge between the oil and water molecules, isolating one from the other. In the micelle, oil enters the central core, while water surrounds the core. The emulsifier molecules are sandwiched between the two. Micelle formation is a key step in digestion of dietary fat and is important in the manufacture of certain food products, such as mayonnaise and cakes.

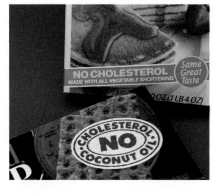

Manufacturers offer a variety of low-cholesterol foods.

sterol A compound containing a multi-ring (steroid) structure and a hydroxyl group (–OH).

acetic acid A two-compound fatty acid that is used in the synthesis of lipids.

$$CH_3 - \overset{\overset{\textstyle O}{\|}}{C} - OH$$

testine via the gallbladder to emulsify dietary fats (Figure 4-8). These two substances—one a phospholipid and the other a **sterol**—are the body's main emulsifiers.

Food manufacturers add emulsifiers in the preparation of many food products. For example, lecithins and polysorbate 60, another emulsifier, are added to salad dressings to keep the vegetable oil suspended in water. Eggs added to cake batters likewise emulsify the fat with the milk. Monoglycerides and diglycerides also are good emulsifiers and are sometimes used in cake mixes and salad dressings for that reason. Over the next few days, examine the ingredients list on the labels of salad dressings and cake mixes. See how many emulsifiers are listed.

Sterols

Sterols, another type of lipid, consist of a multi-ring (steroid) structure and at least one hydroxyl group (–OH).[20] The most familiar sterol is cholesterol (Figure 4-1F). Cholesterol does not look like a triglyceride, but since it dissolves in organic solvents, it is a lipid. The main building block for synthesis of cholesterol in the body is acetyl-CoA, a derivative of **acetic acid,** the smallest fatty acid. Synthesis of longer fatty acids, triglycerides, and phospholipids also makes use of acetyl-CoA.[20]

Cholesterol is found only in animal-derived food constituents we eat (Table 4-1). Each day the liver makes at least 1000 mg of cholesterol, which circulates through the body by way of the bloodstream to meet the body's needs. Every type of human cell studied to date makes cholesterol, which is essential to the structure and function of cells, especially the cell membrane. We consume an average of 200 to 400 mg of cholesterol per day, with men generally consuming the higher amount. We make cholesterol whether we eat it or not, but when following diets very low in cholesterol, we make even more than usual. Some plants have related sterols, such as ergosterol, that can form a type of vitamin D. However, the plant-based foods we eat do not contain cholesterol unless animal products have been added.

Manufacturers who advertise peanut butter, vegetable shortening, margarine, and vegetable oil as containing "no cholesterol" are taking advantage of consumer naivete. Of course peanut butter and margarine have no cholesterol—no purely plant food we eat contains this lipid.[20]

Cholesterol forms part of some important hormones, such as the **corticosteroids,** the estrogens, testosterone, and a form of the active vitamin D hormones, namely **calcitriol.**[20] Cholesterol is also the precursor of bile acids, which are needed for fat digestion. Cholesterol is an essential structural component of membranes and the outer layer of particles that transport lipids in the blood, as we discuss in the next section. Table 4-1 shows that the cholesterol content of the heart, egg (embryonic stage of life), liver, kidney, and brain is quite high, reflecting the critical role of cholesterol in these organs. Because infants and toddlers are forming new tissue, especially in the brain, their intake of this and other dietary lipids should not be greatly restricted.

Cholesterol does not have a unique role in food, as do some of the other lipids, nor is it an essential part of an adult's diet. It just happens that many of us like foods that naturally contain cholesterol, such as eggs and meat.

CONCEPT CHECK

Phospholipids are important components of cell membranes. Because they have both hydrophilic and hydrophobic parts, phospholipids are effective emulsifiers—compounds that can suspend fat in water. Emulsification of fat improves digestion. Phospholipids also help carry lipid particles in the blood. Cholesterol is a precursor for numerous hormones and bile acids and is incorporated into cell membranes and particles that transport lipids in the bloodstream. Cholesterol in the diet comes from animal-derived foods. Adults have no dietary requirement for cholesterol, as body cells can produce it from simple carbon structures.

corticosteroid A steroid produced by the adrenal gland; an example is cortisol.

calcitriol An active hormone form of vitamin D that contains a derivative of cholesterol as part of its structure.

Cholesterol

Testosterone

TABLE 4-1

Cholesterol content of common measurements of selected foods (in ascending order)

Food	Amount	Cholesterol in milligrams	Food	Amount	Cholesterol in milligrams
Milk, skim	1 cup	4	Oysters, salmon	3 oz	40
Mayonnaise	1 tbsp	10	Clams, halibut, tuna	3 oz	55
Butter	1 pat	11	Chicken, turkey (light meat)	3 oz	70
Lard	1 tbsp	12	Beef,* pork*	3 oz	75
Cottage cheese	½ cup	15	Lamb, crab	3 oz	85
Low-fat milk (2%)	1 cup	22	Shrimp, lobster	3 oz	90-110
Half and half	¼ cup	23	Heart, beef	3 oz	165
Hot dog*	1	29	Egg (egg yolk)*	1 each	210
Ice cream, ≈10% fat	½ cup	30	Liver, beef	3 oz	410
Cheese, cheddar	1 oz	30	Kidney	3 oz	540
Whole milk	1 cup	34	Brains	3 oz	2640

*Leading contributors of cholesterol to the U.S. diet.

Transport of Lipids in the Bloodstream

The blood, the main medium for moving materials around in the body, is a water-based substance. Since lipids and water don't mix, the body must employ ingenious mechanisms for transporting lipids in the bloodstream.

CARRYING LIPIDS FROM DIETARY SOURCES

Once dietary fat is digested and then absorbed into the cells of the small intestine, triglycerides are re-formed. They are then packaged into **lipoprotein** particles—large droplets of lipid surrounded by a thin shell of protein, cholesterol, and phospholipid (Figure 4-9). The lipoprotein particles produced by intestinal cells are called **chylomicrons**.[20] The shell around a chylomicron allows the lipid it is carrying to float freely in the water-based blood. Some of the proteins present, namely **apolipoproteins,** also help other cells identify this particle as a chylomicron.

The chylomicron structure, in essence, emulsifies dietary fats before they enter the bloodstream. This process resembles the action of lecithins and bile acids in the small intestine when they emulsify dietary fats during digestion. The difference is that in digestion, a layer of bile acids—rather than of protein, cholesterol, and phospholipid—surrounds the lipid droplets.

Once assembled in intestinal cells, chylomicrons enter the lymphatic system and travel to the thoracic duct, which is located along the spinal column. This duct opens into a large vein in the neck called the subclavian vein. Chylomicrons enter the general circulation at that point.

Chylomicrons in the bloodstream are acted on by **lipoprotein lipase,** an enzyme attached to the outside surface of blood vessel cells. Lipoprotein lipase deesterifies (breaks down) the triglycerides in chylomicrons into free fatty acids and glycerol.[20] Much of the free glycerol travels via the blood to cells in the liver or kidney, where it can be made into glucose. Muscle, adipose, and other cells in the vicinity of lipoprotein lipase activity absorb most of the free fatty acids. The absorbed fatty acids may be used immediately to provide energy, or they may be reesterified into triglycerides, using glycerol molecules derived from glucose metabolism. Muscle cells tend to use absorbed fatty acids to provide energy, whereas adipose cells tend to reesterify and store fatty acids as triglycerides.

Once lipoprotein lipase has removed most of the triglycerides from a chylomicron, the remnant, which contains mostly cholesterol and protein, is taken up by the liver and metabolized (Figure 4-10).[20]

After eating a meal, the whole process of clearing chylomicrons from the blood takes about 2 hours or more. After 14 hours of fasting, they should be totally absent from the bloodstream. People should fast for 14 hours before having certain blood tests to assure that chylomicrons, whose presence could affect the results, have been cleared.

CARRYING LIPIDS FROM NONDIETARY SOURCES

When we consume more energy than immediately needed, some of the proteins and carbohydrates are degraded by the liver and the resulting carbons and hydrogens are used to make new triglycerides and cholesterol. Alcohol intake also contributes to this process. In other words, if total energy intake exceeds energy expenditure, the liver can convert the extra proteins and carbohydrates (and alcohol as well) into body fat. The liver is the major lipid-producing (**lipogenic**) organ in the body.[20] In contrast, adipose tissue primarily stores rather than makes lipid.

Critical Role of the Liver

The liver must resolve the same problem faced by the small intestine: equip lipids so they can travel in the water component of the blood. So when the liver cells synthesize cholesterol or triglycerides, they also coat the lipids with a protein, cholesterol, and phospholipid shell, forming a lipoprotein analogous to intestinal chylomicrons. The liver's version of a chylomicron is called a **very-low-density lipoprotein (VLDL)**.[20]

---

lipoprotein Any particle found in the blood containing a core of lipids with a shell of protein, phospholipid, and cholesterol. The outer shell around a lipoprotein allows the lipid it is carrying to float freely in the water-based blood.

chylomicron The lipoprotein assembled in intestinal cells that carries dietary lipid absorbed from the small intestine in the bloodstream.

apolipoprotein A protein attached to the surface of a lipoprotein or embedded in its outer shell. Apolipoproteins can help enzymes function, act as a lipid-transfer protein, or assist in the binding of a lipoprotein to a cell-surface receptor.

lipoprotein lipase An enzyme attached to blood vessel cells that breaks down triglycerides carried by lipoproteins (especially chylomicrons) into free fatty acids and glycerol.

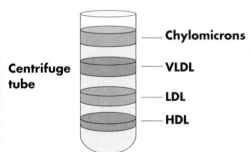

Centrifuge tube — Chylomicrons — VLDL — LDL — HDL

One way to actually measure the amount of chylomicrons, VLDLs, LDLs, and HDLs is to centrifuge the serum at high speed for about 24 hours. The lipoproteins settle out in the centrifuge tube based on their density, with chylomicrons at the top and HDLs at the bottom.

very-low-density lipoprotein (VLDL) The lipoprotein created in the liver that carries cholesterol and lipids newly synthesized by the liver.

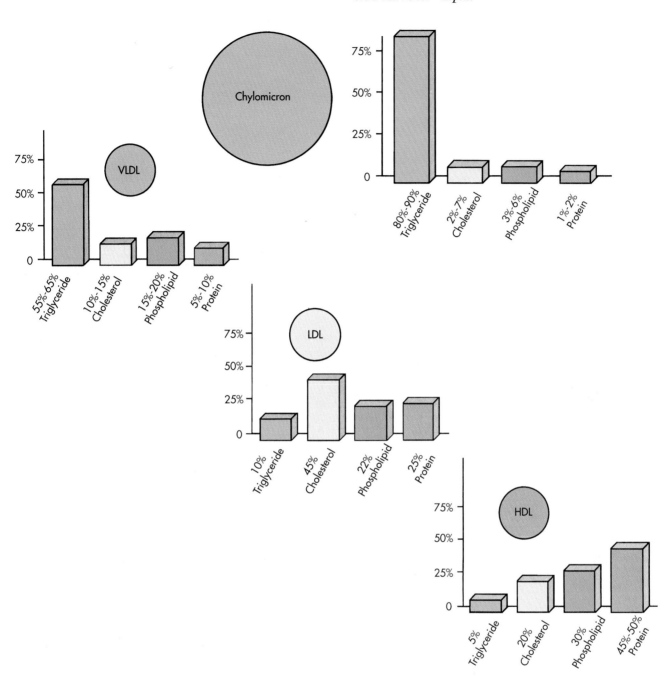

Figure 4-9 The structure and composition of lipoproteins. This lipoprotein structure allows fats to circulate in the bloodstream.

After VLDLs leave the liver and enter the general circulation, lipoprotein lipase deesterifies some of their triglycerides, just as this enzyme acts on chylomicrons. As a result, the VLDLs become more dense (i.e., no longer a *very-low*-density lipoprotein), because the lipids lost are less dense than water. The remnant of each VLDL is termed an **intermediate-density lipoprotein (IDL).** About two thirds of the IDLs are taken up by the liver. Lipoprotein lipase acts further on the rest of the IDLs, converting them to **low-density lipoproteins (LDLs).** Because LDLs have even less lipid than IDLs, they are even more dense. Note that each LDL still contains all the cholesterol present in the VLDL from which it originated. Thus LDLs have a much higher ratio of cholesterol to triglycerides than do VLDLs and IDLs; that is, they are enriched with cholesterol.[20]

intermediate-density lipoprotein (IDL) The product formed after much of the triglyceride in a very-low-density lipoprotein (VLDL) is removed.

low-density lipoprotein (LDL) The cholesterol-rich lipoprotein product resulting from breakdown of triglyceride in intermediate-density lipoprotein (IDL). Elevated serum LDL is strongly linked to heart disease.

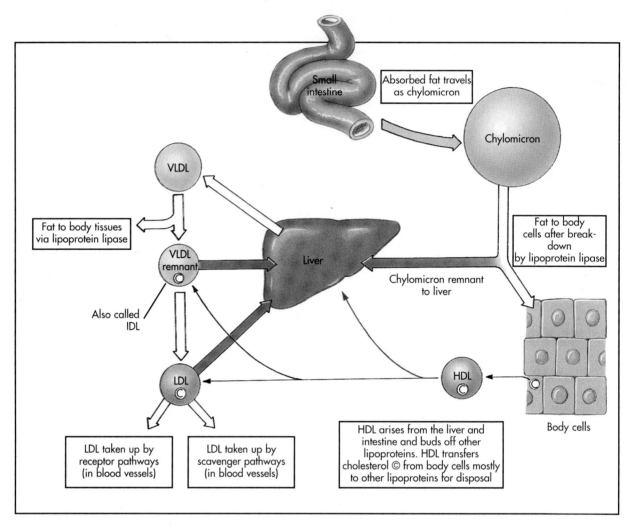

Figure 4-10 Lipoprotein interactions. Chylomicrons carry absorbed fat to body cells. VLDL carries fat synthesized in the liver to body cells. LDL arises from VLDL and carries mostly cholesterol to cells. HDL arises from body cells, mostly in the liver and intestine, as well as from particles that bud off the other lipoproteins. HDL carries cholesterol from cells to other lipoproteins and to the liver for excretion.

Low-density lipoproteins traveling in the bloodstream are destined for cells that have specific LDL receptors in the cell membrane.[20] After an LDL binds to a receptor, it is taken up by the cell; the particle is then broken down, and its components—protein and cholesterol—are released within the cell. By this process, called the **receptor pathway for cholesterol uptake,** cells absorb some of the building blocks necessary for cell growth and development.

Because the liver contains about 50% to 75% of the body's LDL receptors, this organ is crucial for the regulation of serum cholesterol. Various types of genetic defects lead to a reduction in the number of LDL receptors per liver cell or to their complete absence; other defects result in receptors that take up LDL inefficiently. All of these genetic defects reduce the liver's ability to remove LDL from the bloodstream, causing an elevation in serum cholesterol.[35]

A second process, called the **scavenger pathway for cholesterol uptake,** can also remove LDLs from the circulation. This pathway is carried out by certain "scavenger" white blood cells that tend to leave the bloodstream and bury themselves in blood vessels. When these cells detect high concentrations of circulating LDLs in their vicinity, they engulf and digest the LDLs, especially once these have become oxidized.[27] The process does not involve the typical LDL receptors per se, but a receptor highly specific for oxidized LDL. This process of LDL uptake pro-

receptor pathway for cholesterol uptake A process by which LDL is bound by cell receptors and incorporated into the cell.

scavenger pathway for cholesterol uptake A process by which LDL is taken up by scavenger cells embedded in the blood vessels.

ceeds more rapidly as the serum LDL concentration increases, especially when it exceeds a range of 130 to 160 mg/dl. Once within scavenger cells, the oxidized LDLs are prevented from reentering the bloodstream. Consuming fruits and vegetables rich in natural antioxidants, such as vitamin C, vitamin E, and various carotenoids, may inhibit LDL oxidation. Use of nutrient supplements to do the same thing is controversial. This topic is discussed further in the Expert Opinion section in Chapter 12.

To review, as the blood LDL concentration rises, much LDL is oxidized within the vicinity of the scavenger cells and is then taken up by scavenger cells in blood vessels. This oxidized LDL becomes trapped within the cells. Then, as the LDL is degraded, cholesterol is released. Repetition of this scavenger process over many years leads to accumulation of cholesterol in the vessel wall, and **plaque** develops (Figure 4-14 in the Nutrition Perspective illustrates this process). This plaque, which is probably first deposited to repair injuries in a vessel lining, eventually mixes with protein and is then covered with a cap of muscle cells and calcium. The injuries that start plaque formation can be caused by smoking, diabetes, high blood pressure, and LDL itself. Viral and bacterial infections also are implicated. Eventually, deposition of fat and cholesterol in the arteries leads to **atherosclerosis,** a precipitating factor in many heart attacks.[27]

A final critical participant in this whole process of lipid transport—**high-density lipoprotein (HDL)**—is produced by the liver and intestine. Some HDL also buds off other lipoproteins in the bloodstream. As HDLs roam the bloodstream, they pick up cholesterol from dying cells and other sources and transfer it primarily to other lipoproteins for transport back to the liver for excretion (Figure 4-10). Some HDLs interact directly with liver cells as well.[6] This process is called **reverse transport of cholesterol.** Another beneficial function of HDL is that it may block oxidation of LDL. Serum HDL ≥60 mg/dl reduces the risk of developing heart disease, whereas serum HDL ≤35 mg/dl increases the risk. Women tend to have the higher values, especially before **menopause**, while the lower values are more commonly seen in men. The Nutrition Perspective in this chapter covers in detail the role of serum lipids as they relate to heart disease.

CONCEPT CHECK

The bloodstream carries absorbed dietary fat as chylomicrons. Lipid synthesized by the liver is carried in the bloodstream as very-low-density lipoprotein (VLDL). Once a VLDL has most triglycerides removed, it eventually becomes low-density lipoprotein (LDL), which is enriched in cholesterol. LDL is picked up by body cells, especially liver cells. High-density lipoprotein (HDL) picks up cholesterol from cells and transports it primarily to other lipoproteins for eventual transport back to the liver. HDL may also decrease LDL oxidation, thereby reducing LDL uptake into atherosclerotic plaque. Elevated serum LDL is one major risk factor associated with heart disease, as is low serum HDL.

Recommendations for Fat Intake

There is no RDA for fat. To obtain the essential fatty acids, adults should consume about 4% of energy from plant oils incorporated into foods and eat fish about twice a week. Recall that it takes only about 1 tablespoon of oil per day to meet linoleic acid needs and that polyunsaturated fatty acids currently supply about 7% of energy content of the average American diet. An upper limit of 10% of energy intake as polyunsaturated fatty acids is often recommended, in part because the breakdown (oxidation) of those present in lipoproteins is linked to increased cholesterol deposition in the arteries, as we just covered. This breakdown may also increase cancer risk. Depression of immune function is also suspected to be caused by an excessive intake of polyunsaturated fats.

plaque A cholesterol-rich substance deposited in the blood vessels; it contains various white blood cells, smooth muscle cells, cholesterol and other lipids, and eventually calcium. Sometimes called *atherosclerotic plaque* to distinguish it from bacterial plaque, which forms on teeth.

high-density lipoprotein (HDL) Lipoprotein, synthesized in part by the liver and small intestine, that picks up cholesterol from dying cells and other sources and transfers it to the other lipoproteins in the bloodstream, as well as directly to the liver. Low HDL increases the risk for heart disease.

reverse transport of cholesterol The process by which cholesterol is picked up by HDL and transferred to other lipoproteins or to the liver for disposal.

- - - - - - - - - - - - -

Note that in the clinical laboratory the amount of cholesterol in the HDL fraction of blood lipids is what is determined, rather than the amount of HDL itself. The same holds true for LDL. Thus it is more correct to refer to HDL cholesterol and LDL cholesterol. To simplify the discussion, we sometimes just use the terms LDL and HDL.

- - - - - - - - - - - - -

menopause The cessation of menses in women, usually beginning at about 50 years of age.

WOMEN AND HEART DISEASE

ROBERT D. LANGER, M.D., M.P.H.

Many women harbor the potentially deadly misconception that they are immune to heart disease. Nothing could be further from the truth. Cardiovascular disease is the cause of death in 45% of American women, and heart disease alone kills 34%. These fractions are actually lower in men, 39% and 32%, respectively. Twelve times more women die from cardiovascular diseases than die from breast cancer. Some health-care professionals perpetuate this myth. Studies using videotaped patient interviews have shown that doctors were twice as likely to consider heart disease in a man than in a woman when both described identical symptoms of chest pain and had the same historical profile other than sex.

The myth that women do not get heart disease probably arose from the fact that men typically develop heart problems earlier in life. An epidemic of premature death from heart disease in U.S. men became obvious about 60 years ago. Early research on heart disease focused on men, setting a precedent that was broken only with a new generation of studies beginning in the 1980s. The peak gender difference in heart disease rates occurs at about age 40, when men are 4.5 times more likely to be affected than women. This 10-year advantage gradually declines to about 5 years at age 70. It is probably no coincidence that the female advantage in heart disease protection begins to narrow near the age of menopause. Reduced levels of female hormones are most likely responsible for this increase in risk.

Once heart disease is recognized, the course is often worse in women than men. Some researchers speculate that this is because of delayed diagnosis, so that women have more advanced disease when it is finally recognized. Others attribute these findings to smaller blood vessels in women, which may be less resilient with injury and more difficult to repair with current techniques, such as bypass surgery or balloon angioplasty.

Heart disease is also more difficult to diagnose in women. The electrocardiogram (ECG) is a relatively inexact test in both sexes. Still, it is less useful in women than men because of interference from breast tissue. The exercise electrocardiogram (treadmill test) is also less accurate in women than in men. Estimates vary, but reports suggest that treadmill tests may be only about half as good at finding heart disease in women compared with men. Angiography, the definitive test for heart disease, requires that a tube be threaded through the blood vessels. This procedure is technically more difficult in women because their blood vessels are smaller, and complication rates are higher, so it is used more sparingly in women than in men.

HEART DISEASE RISK FACTORS

Cigarette smoking, high blood pressure, high serum cholesterol, diabetes, and lack of exercise are major risk factors for heart disease in women and men. Smoking is responsible for far more heart attacks than cases of lung cancer. It dramatically increases heart disease risk in women. Women aged 30 to 44 years old who smoke three packs of cigarettes per day have ten times the risk of heart disease of nonsmokers in the same age range. Smoking continues to elevate heart attack risk even at the oldest ages.

The interpretation of high serum cholesterol is somewhat different in women than in men. High-density lipoprotein (HDL) cholesterol, the protective part of total serum cholesterol, typically accounts for a greater fraction of total serum cholesterol in women than in men. Low-density lipoprotein (LDL) cholesterol, the dangerous part, tends to be lower in women. Casual screening for elevated total serum cholesterol in women can be misleading. Before acting on an elevated serum cholesterol, women should also have HDL checked.

Diabetes is a particularly important risk factor in women. Studies have shown that, at the same degree of glucose intolerance, women have about twice the risk of heart disease compared with men. Uncontrolled high blood pressure increases heart disease to a similar degree in both sexes.

Researchers remain divided on the question of whether exercise is protective against heart disease in its own right, or works by favorably influencing the other major risk factors. Regardless of the mechanism, it is associated with lower rates of heart disease at any age. In a recent study our research group found that it was especially protective after age 75. Women 75 years old and older who said they exercised three or more times per week were 70% less likely to die over a 5-year period than women who didn't exercise this much.

FEMALE HORMONES

Female hormones, especially estrogen, are generally associated with healthy risk factor profiles for heart disease. Still, the effects of female hormones on heart disease risk are complex and not fully understood. The change in hormone concentrations associated with menopause has been implicated as the reason for increased heart disease in postmenopausal women. A further inference is that the premenopausal hormone milieu is protective.

But there are inconsistencies in this picture. Use of oral contraceptives (OCs) has been associated with an increase in cardiovascular events. While this risk is less with the newer low-dose formulations, it remains

higher in users than in nonusers of OCs. It is possible that this seeming reversal of the protection associated with female hormones is because of the more potent chemicals used in OCs, which have effects that overlap those of male hormones. The combination of cigarette smoking and OC use is particularly dangerous. Although it is often said that this combination is not a problem until age 30, the relative risk is probably increased at any age. In one large study, women aged 25 to 49 who took OCs and smoked up to 2.5 packs per day had four times the risk of heart attack compared with those who did not take OCs nor smoke. The risk soared to 39 times for OC users who smoked more than 2.5 packs per day. This risk also increases with age, so that OC users who smoke are at greatest risk after 40.

After menopause, estrogen replacement may be protective against heart disease. More than 20 studies have found a reduction in cardiovascular disease risk averaging about 50% in postmenopausal women who take estrogen compared with women who do not. Unfortunately, these studies are not definitive, since they didn't account for likely differences between women who use or don't use hormones. Also, nearly all of these studies looked at estrogens without concurrent use of progestins, the most common pattern of hormone use until the mid-1970s.

Since the early 1980s the standard of practice has been to use combined estrogen and progestin therapy, to minimize possible complications with the lining of the uterus. Progestins antagonize many of the known beneficial effects of estrogen on at least some heart disease risk factors. For example, while estrogen tends to lower LDL and raise HDL, progestin moderates or reverses this effect.

Studies are now under way to see if hormone replacement after menopause, including combined estrogen and progestin, actually prevents future heart disease. Results will be a long time coming, though, since heart disease takes years to develop. Researchers conducting the major study on this subject, the Women's Health Initiative, sponsored by the National Institutes of Health, began enrolling 163,000 women in 1993 (25,000 for the test of hormones and heart disease alone) and expect to have results in 2006.

Dr. Langer is an assistant professor in the Division of Epidemiology and the Department of Family and Preventive Medicine at the University of California–San Diego. He is a principal investigator in the ongoing Women's Health Initiative, sponsored by the NIH.

- - - - - - - - - - - - - -

Recommendations for fat intake are stated as a percentage of total energy intake—usually 20% or 30%. This chart shows how many grams of fat per day are allowed with diets ranging from 1000 to 3900 kcal.

Energy intake (kcal)	Fat intake (g) 30% of energy	20% of energy
1000	33	22
1200	40	27
1500	50	33
1800	60	40
2100	70	47
2400	80	53
2700	90	60
3000	100	67
3600	120	80
3900	130	87

- - - - - - - - - - - - - -

Dietary fat supplies about 34% of total energy intake by Americans. Vegetable and animal foods each supply about half of the fat. Major sources of fat in the U.S. diet include animal flesh, whole milk, pastries, cheese, margarine, and mayonnaise.

Because many Americans are at risk for developing heart disease, the American Heart Association (AHA) promotes dietary changes aimed at reducing this risk (Table 4-2). Many health agencies agree with the AHA recommendation that total fat intake should not exceed 30% of total energy intake, with a ratio of about 10:10:10 for saturated to monounsaturated to polyunsaturated fatty acids.[24] The intake of saturated fats currently averages about 12% of energy intake. Table 4-3 shows a diet that follows the basic AHA guidelines. Current research shows that our palates adapt to a lower fat intake over time, and so we miss it less.[19] Reducing fat intake also allows us to include more healthful foods—fruits, vegetables, and whole grains—in our diets. A good start for this type of diet is a low-fat breakfast: a high-fiber cereal, low-fat or nonfat milk, and fruit juice is one option.

For people who have elevated LDL even when following the guideline of 30% of energy intake from fat, the AHA recommends a more stringent diet that includes no more than 20% of total energy from fat. Some cancer researchers also advocate such a diet for adults in general (see Chapter 13). To achieve this goal, fat intake must be strictly limited (Table 4-3). The advice and counsel of a registered dietitian is helpful in planning such diets.

The National Cholesterol Education Program, established in 1985 in the United States, recommends reducing saturated fatty acids to 7% of total energy intake if elevated LDL does not respond to 10% of energy intake.[24] In other words, the lower the saturated fat intake the better. Cholesterol intake in this case should be limited to 300 mg/day, with a reduction to 200 mg/day if serum LDL remains elevated when following a fat-restricted diet containing the higher amount of cholesterol. Recall that adults consume an average of about 200 to 400 mg of cholesterol per day, with men generally consuming the higher amount. By encouraging a reduction in total fat, saturated fat, and cholesterol intake, all of these suggestions are in line with the Dietary Guidelines discussed in Chapter 2. Recall, however, that the latter two suggestions are most important for people with elevated serum LDL.

TABLE 4-2

Dietary guidelines for healthy American adults
A statement for physicians and health professionals by the Nutrition Committee, American Heart Association (AHA)*

1. Total fat intake should be less than 30% of energy intake.
2. Saturated fat intake should be less than 10% of energy intake.
3. Polyunsaturated fat intake should not exceed 10% of energy intake.
4. Cholesterol intake should not exceed 300 mg/day.
5. Carbohydrate intake should constitute 50% or more of energy intake, with emphasis on complex carbohydrates.
6. Protein intake should provide the remainder of the energy intake.
7. Sodium intake should not exceed 3 g/day.
8. Alcohol consumption should not exceed 1 to 2 oz of ethanol per day. Two ounces of 100-proof whiskey, 10 oz of wine, and 24 oz of beer each contain about 1 oz of ethanol.
9. Total energy intake should be sufficient to maintain the individual's recommended body weight.
10. A wide variety of foods should be consumed.

From: *Circulation* 77:721A, 1988.
*Chapter 2 listed the Dietary Guidelines for Americans. Chapter 18 reviews these guidelines in the context of adult health. "Moderate fat intake" is a common general health message for adults, notwithstanding who issues the report.

Fat Content of Foods

Table 4-3 provides an example of the amount of fat in foods in a day's menu. In the Exchange System, foods from both the vegetable and fruit lists are essentially fat free. On the milk list, the amount of fat per cup varies with food choice: skim/very-low-fat milk has a trace (1-3 g); low-fat milk has 5 g; and whole milk has 8 g. Most exchanges from both the starch and other carbohydrates lists contain only small amounts of fat, so this is ignored. However, read the label carefully, as some gourmet breads, snack crackers, and cereals can surprise you! On the meat list, the amount of fat per ounce also varies with food choice: very lean meat has a trace (0-1 g); lean meat has 3 g; medium-fat meat has 5 g; and high-fat meat has 8 g. Foods on the fat list have 5 g of fat per serving.

The foods with the highest nutrient density for fat are salad oils, butter, margarine, and mayonnaise (Figure 4-11). All contain about 100% of energy as fat. Many fat-reduced margarines have been introduced, with water replacing some of the fat. Typical margarines are 80% fat by weight (11 g/tablespoon). Some fat-reduced margarines are as low as 30% fat by weight (4 g/tablespoon). The extra water added to these margarines can cause texture and volume changes when used in recipes. Cookbooks can provide guidance for appropriate use for these products by suggesting alterations in recipes to compensate. You may be surprised to note that

TABLE 4-3

Daily menus containing 2000 kcal and various percentages of fat

	30% of energy as fat		20% of energy as fat
Breakfast	Teaspoons of fat		Teaspoons of fat
Orange juice, 1 cup	0	Same	0
Shredded wheat, ¾ cup	⅕	Same	⅕
Bagel, toasted	⅕	Same	⅕
Margarine, 2 tsp	1¾	Margarine, 1 tsp	⅞
1% milk, 1 cup	½	Nonfat milk, 1 cup	¹⁄₁₀
Lunch			
Whole-wheat bread, 2 slices	½	Same	½
Roast beef, lean, 2 oz	1	Ham, broiled, 2 oz	½
Mayonnaise, 2 tsp	1½	Mayonnaise, 1 tsp	¾
Lettuce	0	Same	0
Tomato, sliced	0	Same	0
Animal crackers, 8	⅕	Same	⅕
Snack			
Apple	⅙	Same	⅙
Dinner			
Pork chop, broiled, 3 oz	2⅓	Halibut, broiled, 3 oz	⅔
Pasta, 1½ cup	⅔	Pasta, 2½ cups	1
Margarine, 2 tsp	1¾	Margarine, 1 tsp	⅞
Broccoli, ½ cup	0	Same	0
1% milk, 1 cup	½	Nonfat milk, 1 cup	¹⁄₁₀
		Banana	¹⁄₁₀
Snack			
Raisins, 2 tbsp	0	Raisins, ¼ cup	0
Popcorn, air-popped, 6 cups	½	Same	½
With 2 tsp margarine	1¾	With 1 tsp margarine	⅞
TOTALS	14½		7½

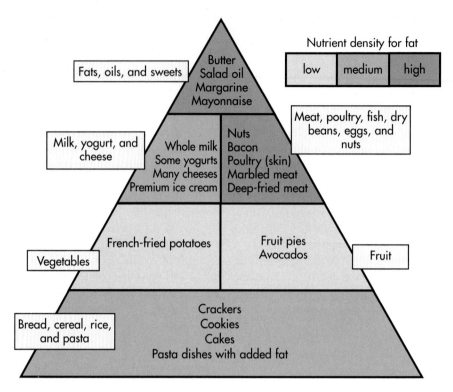

Figure 4-11 Sources of fats in foods from the Food Guide Pyramid. The fruit group and vegetable group are generally low in fat. In the other groups, both high-fat and low-fat choices are available. Careful label reading can lead a person along the low-fat path. In general, any type of frying adds significant amounts of fat to a product, as with french-fried potatoes and fried chicken. The background color of each group indicates the average nutrient density for fat in that food group.

some margarines are even advertised as being fat-free. Close inspection of the label shows that these products are made up of monoglycerides and diglycerides. These are not considered to be fats for labeling purposes, as they are not triglycerides, but of course they are still fats.

Walnuts, bologna, avocados, and bacon have about 80% fat. Peanut butter and cheddar cheese have about 75%. Marbled steak and hamburgers (ground chuck) have about 60%, and chocolate bars, ice cream, doughnuts, and whole milk have about 50% of energy as fat. Eggs, pumpkin pie, and cupcakes have 35%, as do lean cuts of meat, such as top round (and ground round) and sirloin. Bread contains about 15% of energy as fat. Corn flakes, sugar, and skim milk have essentially no fat. Careful label reading is necessary to determine the true fat content of a food—these are only rough guidelines.

Animal fats, which contain about 40% to 60% of total fat as saturated fatty acids, are the chief contributor of saturated fatty acids to the U.S. diet. Saturated fatty acids with 12, 14, and 16 carbons (lauric acid, myristic acid, and palmitic acid, respectively) are the primary contributors to elevated LDL in humans. Of these, the 14-carbon myristic acid is mainly responsible for elevating LDL. Dairy fats are rich sources of myristic acid. The 16-carbon palmitic acid does the same primarily when there is much cholesterol in the diet (>200 to 300 mg/day) and serum cholesterol is elevated.[29] In contrast, stearic acid, the saturated fatty acid with 18 carbons, does not raise LDL[10]; it constitutes about 20% of the saturated fat in meats. The saturated fatty acids with 12, 14, or 16 carbons generally constitute about 25% to 50% of the total fat in animal foods. Overall, dairy fats and meat are rich in those fatty acids that raise LDL. In some plant oils, these saturated fatty acids also make up a notable percentage of the total fat: for example, cottonseed oil (27%) and coconut oil (89%).

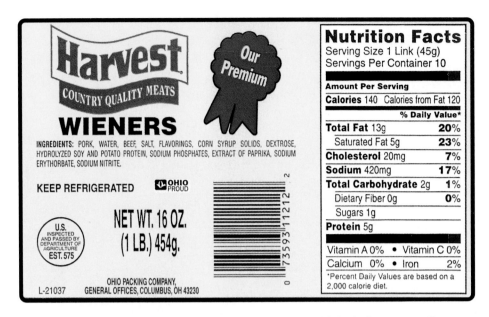

Figure 4-1 Reading labels helps locate hidden fat. Who would think that wieners (hot dogs) can contain 85% of food energy as fat? Looking at the hot dog itself does not suggest that almost all its food energy comes from fat, but the label shows otherwise.

Plant oils contain mostly unsaturated fatty acids, ranging from 73% to 94% of total fat, excluding palm kernel and coconut oils. Canola oil, olive oil, and peanut oil contain moderate to high amounts of total fat as monounsaturated fatty acids (49% to 77%). Some animal fats are also good sources of monounsaturated fatty acids (30% to 47%) (Figure 4-2). Corn, cottonseed, sunflower, soybean, and safflower oils contain mostly polyunsaturated fatty acids (54% to 77%) in terms of total fat. These plant oils supply the majority of the linoleic acid and alpha-linolenic acid in the U.S. food supply. Note that plant oils vary in their content of polyunsaturated fatty acids. Oils that are similar in appearance still may vary significantly in fatty acid composition.

REDUCING FAT AND SATURATED-FAT INTAKE

Some fat in food is obvious: butter on bread, mayonnaise in potato salad, and marbling in raw meat. Fat is less obvious in other foods, such as whole milk, pastries, cookies, cake, cheese, hot dogs, crackers, french fries, and ice cream (Figure 4-12). To reduce your fat intake, you must recognize and control hidden fats, along with the more obvious sources. Use food labels to learn more about the fat content of the food you eat. Table 2-11 lists the definitions for various fat descriptors on food labels, such as "low fat," "reduced fat," and "fat free." Remember that when there is no food label to inspect, moderating portion size is a good way to keep fat intake down. Tables 4-4 and 4-5 list many ways you can avoid eating too much total fat and saturated fat.

USING FAT-REDUCED FOODS WISELY

In recent years, fat-reduced versions of numerous food products have been introduced. The fat content of these alternatives ranges from 0 in fat-free Fig Newtons to about 75% of the original fat content in other products. However, the total energy content of most fat-reduced products is not substantially lower than that of their conventional versions (Table 4-6). Generally, when fat is removed from a product, something must be added, commonly carbohydrate, in its place. Overall, it is very difficult to reduce both the fat and carbohydrate content of a product at the same time.

For this reason, many fat-reduced fat products (e.g., cakes, cookies, and yogurt) are still very energy dense. Don't be fooled into thinking you can eat more of such

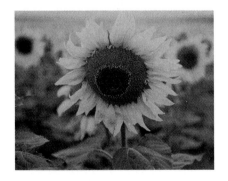

Plant oils should supply about 4% of our total energy intake.

TABLE 4-4

Tips for avoiding too much fat and saturated fat

1. Steam, boil, or bake vegetables. For a change, stir-fry in a small amount of vegetable oil. Consider buying an insert for a pot so you can easily steam your vegetables.
2. Season vegetables with herbs and spices rather than with sauces, butter, or margarine.
3. Try lemon juice on salad or use limited amounts of oil-based salad dressing.
4. To reduce saturated fat, use tub margarine instead of butter or stick margarine in baked products. When possible, use vegetable oil instead of either of these solid fats or hydrogenated shortenings.
5. Limit baked goods made with large amounts of fat, especially saturated fats: croissants, doughnuts, muffins, biscuits, and butter rolls.
6. Try whole-grain flours to enhance flavors when baking goods with less fat. Use applesauce and other fruit purees in place of fat.
7. Replace whole milk with skim or low-fat milk in puddings, soups, and baked products and for use as a beverage.
8. Substitute plain low-fat yogurt, blender-whipped low-fat cottage cheese, or buttermilk in recipes that call for sour cream or mayonnaise.
9. Choose lean cuts of meat. Limit bacon, ribs, and meatloaf.
10. Trim fat from meat before and after cooking.
11. Roast, bake, or broil meat, poultry, and fish so that fat drains away as the food cooks.
12. Remove skin from poultry before cooking. This eliminates the temptation to eat it along with the meat.
13. Use a nonstick pan for cooking so that added fat will be unnecessary; use a vegetable spray for frying.
14. Chill meat or poultry broth until the fat solidifies. Spoon off the fat before using the broth.
15. Eat a vegetarian main dish at least once a week. Include fish (cooked without much added fat) in the diet two times or more a week.
16. Choose ice milk, low-fat frozen yogurt, sorbet, and popsicles as substitutes for ice cream.
17. Try angelfood cake, fig bars, and ginger snaps as substitutes for commercial baked goods high in saturated fat.
18. Limit high-fat cheese intake.
19. Read labels on commercially prepared foods to find out what type of fat or how much saturated fat they contain.
20. Use jam, jelly, or marmalade on bread and toast instead of butter or margarine.
21. Buy whole-grain breads and rolls. They have more flavor and do not need butter or margarine to taste good. The dietary fiber present is an added bonus.
22. Think about the balance of fats in your menu. If your meal contains whole milk, cheese, ice cream, a higher-fat meat, or poultry with skin, use margarine and unsaturated vegetable oils for your spreads and dressings. Small amounts of butter, sour cream, or cream cheese can be included if other menu items are low in saturated fat.

products without necessarily increasing your total energy intake. By using common sense and consuming moderate-size portions, however, you can take advantage of fat-reduced products to help lower your fat intake without increasing your energy intake. Remember also that fruits and vegetables are naturally low in fat and deserve as much or more attention in diet planning as fat-reduced products.

TABLE 4-5

Tips for avoiding too much fat and saturated fat when dining out

APPETIZERS

Best bets:	Vegetable juice, bouillon, fresh fruit, celery, radishes	**Avoid:**	Deep-fried vegetables, creamed soup

MEAT/POULTRY/FISH

Best bets:	Roasted, baked, broiled—trim off excess fat	**Avoid:**	Fried, sauteed, breaded; gravy, ribs, fatty luncheon meat

EGGS (you may wish to limit as well to reduce cholesterol intake)

Best bets:	Poached, boiled; egg whites	**Avoid:**	Fried

POTATOES/RICE/PASTA

Best bets:	Mashed, baked, boiled, steamed	**Avoid:**	Home fried, french fried, creamed, escalloped

VEGETABLES

Best bets:	Steamed, stewed, boiled	**Avoid:**	Creamed, fried, sauteed

BREADS

Best bets:	Plain bread, toast, dinner rolls, or muffins	**Avoid:**	Sweet rolls, coffee cake, croissants, biscuits

FATS

Best bets:	Limited amounts of soft margarine, reduced-calorie salad dressing, low-fat yogurt, low-fat cheese	**Avoid:**	Gravy, cream sauce, fried foods, heavy-based dressings, sour cream, whole-milk cheese

DESSERTS

Best bets:	Fresh fruit, nonfat frozen yogurt, sorbet, angelfood cake, new fat-free cake products; split a dessert with a friend	**Avoid:**	Pastries, custard, ice cream

BEVERAGES

Best bets:	Water, coffee, tea, low-fat or nonfat milk, soft drinks	**Avoid:**	Milk shakes, whole milk

TABLE 4-6

Energy and fat content of original and fat-reduced forms of some food products

Food product	Amount/serving	Energy (kcal)	Fat (g)
Nabisco Chips Ahoy! Cookies			
Original	1 each/11 g	53	3
Reduced fat	1 each/11 g	50	2
Nabisco Fig Newtons			
Original	1 each/16 g	55	1
Fat free	1 each/15 g	50	0
Hostess Cupcakes			
Original	1 each/46 g	170	5
Low-fat Cupcake Lights	1 each/40 g	120	2
Hostess Twinkies			
Original	1 each/41 g	140	4
Low-fat Twinkie Lights	1 each/40 g	120	2
Nabisco Ritz Crackers			
Original	5 each/16 g	80	4
Reduced fat	5 each/16 g	70	3
Nabisco Triscuit Wafers			
Original	5 each/23 g	100	4
Reduced fat	5 each/22 g	85	2
Sunshine Cheez-It Snack Crackers			
Original	10 each/11 g	60	3
Reduced fat	10 each/10 g	50	2
Kraft Miracle Whip Salad Dressing			
Original	1 tbsp/14 g	70	7
Light	1 tbsp/15 g	40	3
Nestle Crunch Vanilla Ice Cream Bars			
Original	1 bar/60 g	200	14
Reduced fat	1 bar/50 g	130	7
Breyer's Natural Vanilla Ice Cream			
Original	½ cup/70 g	150	8
Premium Light	½ cup/68 g	130	5
Pringles Original Potato Chips			
Original	10 each/20 g	114	8
Right Crisps Original (reduced fat)	10 each/18 g	88	4
Betty Crocker Creamy Deluxe Chocolate Frosting			
Original	2 tbsp/36 g	140	6
Low fat	2 tbsp/36 g	120	1
Kraft Ranch Dressing			
Original	2 tbsp/29 g	170	18
Deliciously Right (reduced fat)	2 tbsp/30 g	110	11
Oscar Meyer Bologna			
Original	1 slice/28 g	90	8
Light	1 slice/28 g	50	4
Land O' Lakes Sweet Cream Salted Butter			
Original	1 tbsp/14 g	100	11
Light	1 tbsp/14 g	50	6
Cool Whip Whipped Topping			
Original	2 tbsp/8 g	25	2
Lite	2 tbsp/8 g	20	1
Kraft Singles American Cheese			
Original	1 slice/21 g	70	5
⅓ less fat	1 slice/21 g	50	3

NUTRITION FOCUS

FAT REPLACEMENTS

Currently five different types of fat replacements are available or awaiting FDA approval. Addition of these substances during manufacture yields products that to varying degrees satisfy consumers' desire for fat-reduced products that are tasty (Figure 4-13).[1]

WATER, STARCH DERIVATIVES, AND GUMS

The first and simplest fat replacement is water. Addition of water yields a product, such as diet margarine, with less fat per serving than the normal product. Starch derivatives that bind water form a second type of fat replacement. Derivatives commonly used by food manufacturers include cellulose, N-Oil, Paselli SA2, Sta-Slim, Maltrin, Stellar, Slendid, and Oatrim. These substances have been used in a variety of foods, including luncheon meats, salad

dressings, frozen desserts, table spreads, dips, baked goods, and candies. Gums extracted from plants can also be used to replace fat. They thicken a product and replace some of the body that fat provided. Diet salad dressings have gums added for this reason.

PROTEIN-DERIVED FAT REPLACEMENTS (SIMPLESSE)

The newest type of fat replacement on the market consists of proteins that have been treated to produce microscopic, mistlike protein globules. Both egg and milk proteins can be used. When these substances replace fat in a food product, they feel like fat in the mouth, although the product does not contain any fatty acids. Simplesse is a currently used fat replacement of this type. Since it contains protein, Simplesse yields some energy—but only about 1.3 kcal/g, much less than the 9 kcal/g supplied by regular fats. Simplesse has this low energy value primarily for two reasons: proteins contain only 4 kcal/g, and it has quite a high water content.

Simplesse is used primarily in frozen desserts. It reduces energy content by about one half and fat content to a negligible amount in these products. However, these products tend to develop a grainy texture upon refreezing. This is one reason for their limited acceptance to date. Simplesse can also replace fat in mayonnaise, salad dressing, yogurt, sour cream, cheese, and other dairy products. Because high temperatures alter the structure of Simplesse so much that it no longer resembles fat, it cannot be used for cooking or frying. However, people who are allergic to milk or egg proteins should not consume Simplesse. With extensive use, Simplesse could help reduce total fat intake.

ENGINEERED FATS

The final form of fat replacement is the engineered fat. This type of product is synthesized in the laboratory from various food constituents. The experimental product Olestra is a good example. It is made by chemically linking fatty acids to sucrose (table sugar). The resulting product cannot be digested by either human digestive enzymes or bacteria that live in the intestine. Therefore Olestra yields no energy to the body. As it leaves the body, it can even pull cholesterol-containing substances into the intestine, thereby lowering serum LDL.

GRIN & BEAR IT   **By Wagner**

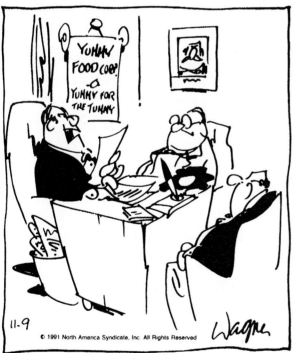

© 1991 North America Syndicate, Inc. All Rights Reserved

Reprinted with permission of North America Syndicate, Inc.

"Figby Foods has reduced its fat content by another gram! This is war, gentlemen!"

Figure 4-13 Grin & Bear It.

NUTRITION FOCUS

Olestra is quite a versatile ingredient. It can replace much of the fat in salad dressings and cakes and can be used for frying in food manufacturing. But some problems are associated with Olestra use. It tends to bind the fat-soluble vitamins A and E, thus reducing absorption. To compensate for this effect, the manufacturer has proposed adding more vitamins A and E to Olestra. Some years ago FDA would not permit the use of mineral oil in foods as a no-calorie fat, because it bound up fat-soluble vitamins. For this and other reasons, it is unclear whether Olestra will be approved by FDA.

Food manufacturers are working on other types of engineered fats that either wholly or partially escape absorption by the body. Examples include Caprenin, produced by Procter & Gamble company. This triglyceride product contains two medium-chain fatty acids and a long-chain (22-carbon) saturated fatty acid, called behenic acid. Because of its length and saturation, behenic acid is solid even at body temperature and therefore is difficult to absorb from the small intestine. Studies show the fat yields only about 5 kcal/g to the body, mostly because of the limited absorption of the behenic acid. Caprenin is currently used in reduced-calorie confections. Another example is Salatrim, which yields only about 4 to 6 kcal/g. It is generally composed of stearic acid, which the body absorbs poorly, and short-chain fatty acids. This product has yet to enter our food supply.

FAT REPLACEMENTS IN PERSPECTIVE

So far, fat replacements have had little impact on the American diet, partly because the currently approved forms either are not very versatile or have not been used extensively by manufacturers. In addition, fat replacements are of little use in the foods that contribute the most fat to our diets—hamburgers, hot dogs, whole milk, doughnuts and cake products, and beef steaks and roasts, to name some key players. We consumers must decide to limit these sources; the replacements currently can't help us much.

The main benefit of fat replacements will be in helping people cut some fat from their diets, most importantly saturated fat and cholesterol. The reduction in energy intake will probably be less impressive because studies show that people tend to make up the lost energy by increasing their intake of other foods or by eating more of fat-reduced foods than the corresponding conventional foods.

We will always need balanced eating habits and moderation in food choice. A diet rich in fruits, vegetables, whole grains, and lean animal products still deserves the most attention. Use of fat replacements in popular foods Americans are unwilling to relinquish, such as ice cream, could reduce intake of saturated fat and cholesterol. But we won't know the true impact of fat replacements on American diets until either more are approved, as in the case of Olestra, or the available ones become more widely used. For now they are of limited significance.[1]

Olestra, a sucrose polyester (with the maximum number of fatty acids attached)

CONCEPT CHECK

There is no RDA for fat. We need about 4% of total energy intake from plant oils to obtain the needed essential fatty acids. Eating fish about twice a week is also advised to supply omega-3 fatty acids. Many health-related agencies recommend a diet containing no more than 30% of energy intake as fat, with no more than 10% of energy intake as saturated fat. The current American diet contains about 34% of energy content as fat, with about 12% of energy content as saturated fat. Fat-dense foods—those with more than 60% of total energy as fat—include plant oils, butter, margarine, mayonnaise, walnuts, bacon, avocados, peanut butter, cheddar cheese, steak, and hamburger.

Summary

1. Lipids are a group of relatively oxygen-poor compounds, compared with carbohydrates and proteins, that also dissolve in organic solvents, such as chloroform, benzene, and ether. Saturated fatty acids contain no carbon-carbon double bonds, monounsaturated fatty acids contain one carbon-carbon double bond, and polyunsaturated fatty acids contain two or more carbon-carbon double bonds in the carbon chain.

2. In omega-3 polyunsaturated fatty acids, the first of the carbon-carbon double bonds is located three carbons from the methyl end of the carbon chain. In omega-6 polyunsaturated fatty acids, the first carbon-carbon double bond counting from the methyl end occurs at the sixth carbon. Both omega-3 and omega-6 fatty acids are essential fatty acids, which must be included in the diet to maintain health.

3. Body cells can synthesize hormone compounds called eicosanoids from both omega-3 and omega-6 fatty acids. The eicosanoids produced from omega-3 fatty acids tend to reduce blood clotting, blood pressure, and inflammatory responses in the body. Those produced from omega-6 fatty acids tend to increase blood clotting.

4. Triglycerides containing lots of saturated fatty acids tend to be solid at room temperature, while those containing lots of polyunsaturated fatty acids are usually liquid at room temperature. Hydrogenation is the process of converting carbon-carbon double bonds into single bonds by adding hydrogen at the point of unsaturation. Hydrogenation of fatty acids in vegetable oils changes the oils to solid fats and helps reduce rancidity, which results from breakdown of fatty acids. Hydrogenation also increases the trans fatty acid content.

5. Triglyceride is the major form of fat in both food and the body. It allows for efficient energy storage, protects certain organs, transports fat-soluble vitamins, and helps insulate the body. Triglyceride also adds flavor and texture to foods and increases satiety after meals. Phospholipids are derivatives of the triglycerides. Phospholipids are important parts of cell membranes, and some act as efficient emulsifiers.

6. Cholesterol forms vital biological compounds, such as hormones, parts of cell membranes, and bile acids. Cells in the body make cholesterol whether we eat it or not. It is not a necessary part of an adult's diet.

7. Lipids are carried in the bloodstream by various lipoproteins, which are particles consisting of a central triglyceride core encased in a shell of protein, cholesterol, and phospholipid. Chylomicrons are released from intestinal cells and carry lipids arising from dietary intake. Very-low-density lipoprotein (VLDL) and low-density lipoprotein (LDL) carry lipids synthesized in the liver from excess carbohydrate and protein, as well as alcohol. High-density lipoprotein (HDL) picks up cholesterol from cells and acts in transporting it back to the liver.

8. In the serum portion of the blood, elevated LDL and low HDL are strong predictors of the risk for heart disease.

9. There is no RDA for fat. We need about 4% of total energy intake from plant oils to obtain the needed essential fatty acids. Fish is a good source of omega-3 fatty acids.

10. The typical American diet contains about 34% of total energy as fat. Many health agencies and scientific groups suggest reducing fat intake to no more than 30% of energy intake. Some health experts advocate an even further reduction to 20% of energy intake, but such a diet is generally difficult to plan and follow without some initial professional guidance. Fat-reduced products aid in the goal of reducing fat intake, but they must be eaten in moderate amounts to maintain control of total energy intake.

Study Questions

1. Describe the chemical structures of saturated and polyunsaturated fatty acids and their different effects in both food and the human body.

2. Relate the need for omega-3 fatty acids in the diet to the recommendation to consume fish at least two times per week.

3. Describe the structures, origins, and roles of the four major blood lipoproteins.

4. What are the recommendations of health-care professionals regarding fat intake? What does this mean in terms of actual food choices?

5. What are two important functions of fat in food? How are these different from the general functions of lipids in the human body?

6. What are the significance of and three possible uses for the new fat-reduced foods?

7. Does the total cholesterol concentration in the bloodstream tell the whole story with respect to heart disease risk?

Read the Nutrition Perspective before answering the following questions:

8. List five risk factors for the development of premature heart disease.

9. What actually brings on a myocardial infarction? What dietary practices are thought to help precipitate this event?

10. When are medications most effective in preventing heart disease, and how in general do the various classes of medications operate to reduce risk?

REFERENCES

1. Adler T: Designer fats, *Science News* 145:296, 1994.
2. Anonymous: Dietary flavonoids and risk of coronary heart disease, *Nutrition Reviews* 52:59, 1994.
3. Berdanier CD: ω-3 fatty acids: panacea? *Nutrition Today* 29:28, 1994.
4. Denke MA and others: Short-term dietary calcium fortification increases fecal saturated fat content and reduces serum lipids in men, *Journal of Nutrition* 123:1047, 1993.
5. Dreon DM and others: Low-density lipoprotein subclass patterns and lipoprotein response to a reduced-fat diet in men, *FASEB Journal* 8:121, 1994.
6. Fraser GE: Diet and coronary heart disease: beyond dietary fats and low-density-lipoprotein cholesterol, *American Journal of Clinical Nutrition* 59:1117S, 1994.
7. Fuhrman B and others: Consumption of red wine with meals reduces the susceptibility of human plasma and low-density lipoprotein to triple peroxidation, *American Journal of Clinical Nutrition* 61:549, 1995.
8. Gaziano JM and others: Moderate alcohol intake, increased levels of high-density lipoprotein and its subfractions, and decreased risk of myocardial infarction, *New England Journal of Medicine* 329:1829, 1993.
9. Glore SR and others: Soluble fiber and serum lipids: a literature review, *Journal of the American Dietetic Association* 94:425, 1994.
10. Grundy SM: Influence of stearic acid on cholesterol metabolism relative to other long-chain fatty acids, *American Journal of Clinical Nutrition* (suppl) 60:986S, 1994.
11. Halliwell B: Oxidation of low-density lipoproteins: questions of initiation, propagation, and the effect of antioxidants, *American Journal of Clinical Nutrition* 61(suppl):670S, 1995.
12. Herbert V: Iron worsens high-cholesterol-related coronary artery disease, *American Journal of Clinical Nutrition* 60:299, 1994.

13. Katan M: Fish and heart disease, *New England Journal of Medicine* 332:1024, 1995.
14. Klatsky AL: Cardiovascular effects of alcohol, *Scientific American Science & Medicine* March/April 1995, p 28.
15. Krumholz HM and others: Lack of association between cholesterol and coronary heart disease mortality and morbidity and all-cause mortality in persons older than 70 years, *Journal of the American Medical Association* 272:1335, 1994.
16. Law MR and others: Assessing possible hazards of reducing serum cholesterol, *British Medical Journal* 308:373, 1994.
17. Levine GN and others: Cholesterol reduction in cardiovascular disease, *New England Journal of Medicine* 332:512, 1995.
18. Mantzioris E and others: Dietary substitution with α-linolenic acid-rich vegetable oil increases eicosapentaenoic acid concentrations in tissues, *American Journal of Clinical Nutrition* 59:1304, 1994.
19. Mattes RD: Fat preference and adherence to a reduced-fat diet, *American Journal of Clinical Nutrition* 57:373, 1993.
20. Murray RK and others: *Harper's biochemistry,* ed 22, Norwalk, Conn, 1993, Appleton & Lange.
21. Pancharuniti N and others: Plasma homocyst(e)ine, folate, and vitamin B-12 concentrations and risk for early-onset coronary artery disease, *American Journal of Clinical Nutrition* 59:940, 1994.
22. Potter SM and others: Depression of plasma cholesterol in men by consumption of baked products containing soy protein, *American Journal of Clinical Nutrition* 58:501, 1993.
23. Proulx WR, Weaver CM: Ironing out heart disease, *Nutrition Today* 30:16, 1995.
24. Schaefer EJ and others: Lipoproteins, nutrition, aging, and atherosclerosis, *American Journal of Clinical Nutrition* 61(suppl):726S, 1995.

25. Schaefer EJ and others: Lipoprotein(a) levels and risk of coronary heart disease in men, *Journal of the American Medical Association* 271:999, 1994.
26. Simopoulos AP and others: The 1st Congress of the International Society for the Study of Fatty Acids and Lipids (ISSFAL): fatty acids and lipids from cell biology to human disease, *Nutrition Today* 29:24, 1994.
27. Slyper AH, Chir B: Low-density lipoprotein density and atherosclerosis, *Journal of the American Medical Association* 272:305, 1994.
28. Superko HR, Krauss RM: Coronary artery disease regression, *Circulation* 90:1056, 1994.
29. Sundram K and others: Dietary palmitic acid results in lower serum cholesterol than does a lauric-myristic acid combination in normolipemic humans, *American Journal of Clinical Nutrition* 59:841, 1994.
30. Thompson SG and others: Hemostatic factors and the risk of myocardial infarction or sudden death in patients with angina pectoris, *New England Journal of Medicine* 332:635, 1995.
31. Urgert R and others: Effect of cafestol and kahweol from coffee grounds on serum lipids and serum liver enzymes in humans, *American Journal of Clinical Nutrition* 61:149, 1995.
32. U.S. Public Health Service: Cholesterol screening in adults, *American Family Physician* 51:129, 1995.
33. Warshafsky S and others: Effect of garlic on total serum cholesterol: meta-analysis, *Annals of Internal Medicine* 119:599, 1993.
34. Willet WC, Ascherio A: Trans fatty acids: are the effects only marginal? *American Journal of Public Health* 84:722, 1994.
35. Williams RR: Diet, genes, early heart attacks, and high blood pressure. In Kotsonis FN, Mackey MA, editors: *Nutrition in the 90s,* New York, 1994, Dekker.
36. Zock PL and others: Dietary trans fatty acids and lipoprotein cholesterol, *American Journal of Clinical Nutrition* 61:617, 1995.

TAKE ACTION

Is your fat and cholesterol intake too high?

How do your food practices compare with general guidelines suggested for fat, saturated fat, and cholesterol intake? Refer to the nutritional assessment you completed at the end of Chapter 2, and compare it with the guidelines listed below, issued by the American Heart Association and the National Cholesterol Education Program:

- Limit or reduce total fat intake to 30% or less of total energy intake.
- Reduce saturated fat intake to 7% to 10% of energy intake or less.
- Limit cholesterol to 200 to 300 mg/day.

To compare your nutritional assessment with these guidelines, first fill in the values for your intakes of the following:

TOTAL ENERGY: _____

TOTAL FAT: _____

SATURATED FAT: _____

CHOLESTEROL: _____

Now complete the following steps:

1. Multiply your total grams of fat by 9 (kcal/g of fat). Then divide the result by your total energy intake. Next multiply this number by 100. This will give you the % of energy you consumed from fat.

   % OF ENERGY FROM FAT _____

   IS IT 30% OR LESS OF TOTAL ENERGY?   YES _____   NO _____

2. Multiply your grams of saturated fat by 9 (kcal/g of fat). Divide the result by your total energy intake. Now multiply this number by 100. This will give you the % of energy you consumed from saturated fat.

   % OF ENERGY FROM SATURATED FAT _____

   IS IT 10% OF ENERGY OR LESS?   YES _____   NO _____

3. Look at your milligrams of cholesterol.

   IS YOUR INTAKE LESS THAN 300 MG?   YES _____   NO _____

4. Look back at the foods you ate and notice the foods that contributed the most fat, saturated fat, and cholesterol. If you didn't meet one or more of the guidelines and had elevated serum LDL, how could you change what you ate that day to improve your diet?

5. Now take the next step. Do you know your serum HDL and LDL values? If not, have them checked soon. All adults should know whether these values are in the abnormal ranges.

6. Finally, fill in the following assessment of your risk for developing premature heart disease. Decide today how you could modify your diet and lifestyle, if necessary, to reduce your risk.

Do you have . . .	YES	NO
a history of smoking?	_____	_____
high blood pressure?	_____	_____
high serum LDL?	_____	_____
low serum HDL?	_____	_____
diabetes?	_____	_____
a history of physical inactivity?	_____	_____
a family history of premature heart disease?	_____	_____
a history of obesity?	_____	_____

Other factors also could be considered, but this provides a good start for assessing your risk.

Heart Disease

A heart attack can strike with the sudden force of a sledgehammer, with pain radiating up the neck or down the arm. It can also sneak up at night, masquerading as indigestion, with slight pain or pressure in the chest.

Heart disease—more precisely termed *cardiovascular disease*—is the major killer of Americans. Each year about 500,000 people die of heart disease in the United States, about 60% more than die of cancer. The figure rises to almost 1 million if we include strokes and other circulatory diseases in the more global term cardiovascular disease. The overall male-to-female ratio for heart disease is about 2:1. Still, heart disease eventually kills more women than any other disease—twice as many as cancer.[32]

For each person in America who dies of heart disease, 10 more (over 6 million people) have symptoms of heart disease. In addition, about twice the number who die, 1.5 million, suffer heart attacks each year, accounting for about $47 billion in health-care costs.

Worldwide, the highest incidence of heart attacks in men—915 per 100,000—is found in Finland. For women, Scotland posts the high—256 per 100,000. The lowest rate for men of 76 per 100,000 is found in China; for women, the lowest rate of 30 per 100,000 is found in Spain. In the United States, the heart-attack incidence per 100,000 is about 500 for men and 140 for women.

Development of Heart Disease

The symptoms of heart disease develop over many years and often do not become obvious until old age. Nonetheless, autopsies of young adults under 20 years of age have shown that many of them have atherosclerotic plaque in their arteries. This finding indicates that plaque buildup can begin in childhood and continue throughout life, although it usually goes undetected for quite some time.[17]

Preventing premature heart disease—that which appears before age 70 to 80—deserves everyone's consideration. Although we all die, one key to a better life is to prevent premature death and live in good health until essentially the entire body wears out, the heart included. Heart attacks at ages 40 through 60 are closely linked to the risk factors discussed later. Most people at risk can greatly improve their chance to avoid premature heart disease by making some long-term lifestyle changes.[24] (See Chapter 18 for further discussion of the premature appearance of disease and how to prevent it.)

Heart disease and strokes are associated with inadequate blood circulation in the heart and brain. Blood supplies the heart muscle and brain—and other body organs—with oxygen and nutrients. When blood flow via the coronary arteries surrounding the heart is interrupted, the heart muscle can be damaged. A heart attack, or **myocardial infarction,** may result (Figure 4-14). This may cause the heart to beat irregularly or to stop altogether. If blood flow to parts of the brain is interrupted long enough, part of the brain dies, causing a cerebrovascular accident, or **stroke.** When a stroke causes loss of muscle control, death may occur.

More than 95% of all heart attacks are caused by blood clots that stop blood flow to the heart or brain. Clots form more readily where atherosclerotic plaque has built up in the arteries that serve the heart (coronary arteries) or brain (carotid arteries). Actually, the most dangerous lesions aren't the large, advanced ones, but smaller, unstable lesions covered by a small fibrous cap.[17] In essence, heart attacks are caused not by total blockage of the coronary arteries by plaque, but by disruption of a partial blockage, leading to clot formation. Because aspirin in small doses reduces blood clotting, it is often used under a physician's guidance to treat people at risk for heart attack, especially if one has already occurred.

As we mentioned in this chapter, plaque is probably first deposited to repair injuries in a vessel lining.[17] The *athero* in "atherosclerosis" comes from the Greek and means "gruel or paste." Hypertension, diabetes, LDL, and smoking are some of many agents that likely lead to injury, which in turn starts the repair process. Current research also implicates certain bacteria and viruses in vessel injury. This process of damage repair is part of the initiation

myocardial infarction Death of part of the heart muscle.

Heart disease involves the coronary arteries and thus is frequently termed *coronary heart disease (CHD)* or *coronary artery disease (CAD).*

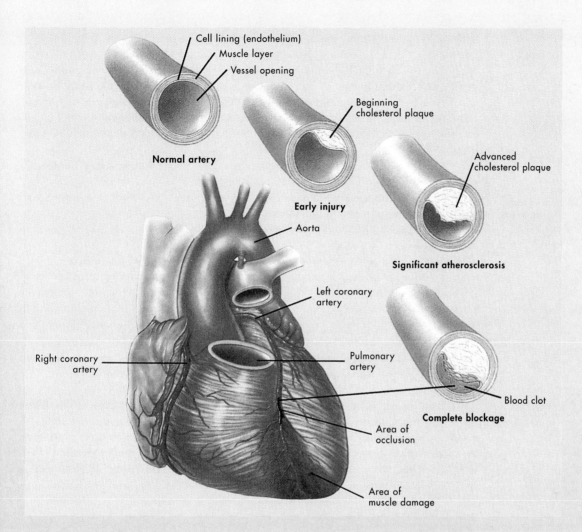

Figure 4-14 The road to a heart attack. Injury to an artery wall begins the process. This is followed by a progressive build-up of plaque in the artery walls. The heart attack represents the terminal phase of the process. Blockage of the left coronary artery by a blood clot is evident. The heart muscle that is served by the portion of the coronary artery beyond the point of blockage lacks oxygen and nutrients and is damaged and may die. This can lead to a significant drop in heart function and often total heart failure. Current research suggests that the smaller, early plaques cause most heart attacks as they break up and in turn stimulate blood clotting.

phase of atherosclerosis. The rate of further plaque deposition in the next phase, called the progression phase, partly depends on the amount of LDL in the blood. The plaque thickens as layers of cholesterol (part of LDL), protein, smooth muscle, and calcium are deposited. Arteries harden and narrow as plaque builds up, making them less elastic and thus unable to expand to accommodate alterations in blood pressures.

Affected arteries become further damaged as blood pumps through them and pressure increases. Finally, in the terminal phase, a clot or spasm in a plaque-clogged artery leads to a myocardial infarction or cerebrovascular accident.[30] The risk for progressing to this terminal phase increases during the few hours after people who have already developed significant atherosclerosis eat a fat-rich meal or perform strenuous work (e.g., snow shoveling), and during the early morning hours as they awaken.[6]

Risk Factors for Heart Disease

Many of us are free of the risk factors that contribute to rapid development of atherosclerosis and premature heart disease. If so, the advice of health experts is to simply consume a balanced diet, perform regular physical activity, and reevaluate risk factors every 5 years.[24]

People who face the highest risk for premature heart disease have one or another rare genetic defect that substantially blocks clearance of chylomicrons from the blood, reduces LDL uptake by the liver, or limits synthesis of HDL.[35] Other medical conditions, such as certain forms of liver and kidney disease, low thyroid hormone concentrations, and use of certain medications to treat hypertension, can increase LDL, and thus increase the risk for heart disease.[32]

For most people, however, the most likely risk factors for premature heart disease are the following[24]:

- Total serum cholesterol >200 mg/dl, especially when it is ≥240 mg/dl and coupled with serum LDL cholesterol >130 to 160 mg/dl
- Serum HDL cholesterol <35 mg/dl, especially when the ratio of total serum cholesterol to HDL cholesterol is >4.5:1
- Age: men > 45 years; women ≥ 55 years, if not following estrogen replacement therapy
- Family history of premature heart disease
- Smoking
- Hypertension
- Diabetes

Clearly, many of these risk factors are strongly linked to diet and lifestyle choices. Physical inactivity and obesity (especially fat accumulation around the waist) also are significant risk factors. Researchers also are currently trying to unravel and quantify numerous other factors that are possibly linked to premature heart disease (Table 4-7) .

The more of these risk factors you have, the greater your chances of ultimately developing heart disease. However, common sense suggests that we should initially focus on the three most common contributors: smoking, hypertension, and high LDL. By minimizing these three risk factors, along with following the Food Guide Pyramid and staying physically active, you will most likely reduce the other, less common controllable risk factors as well.

SMOKING

Chemicals in smoke alter blood vessels, enabling plaque to build up faster. Smoking greatly contributes to the ultimate expression of a person's genetically linked risk for heart disease. Smoking also makes blood more likely to clot.

HYPERTENSION

If your **systolic blood pressure** is over 140 (millimeters of mercury) or your **diastolic blood pressure** is 90 or more, you have hypertension. (We cover treatment of high blood pressure in Chapter 14.)

HIGH LDL

A total serum cholesterol >200 mg/dl is widely touted in the popular press as the key value for predicting heart disease risk. In fact, much more important serum lipid values are LDL (>130 to 160 mg/dl), HDL (<35 mg/dl), and the ratio of total cholesterol to HDL cholesterol (>4.5:1). As explained in the chapter, LDL cholesterol is the main contributor to plaque formation, whereas HDL helps dispose of cholesterol and may decrease oxidation of LDL as well.

If a high total serum cholesterol, >200 mg/dl, is primarily due to high HDL (especially >60 mg/dl), the risk of heart disease is not increased and may even be lower than average. Thus to assess heart disease risk, both total serum cholesterol and HDL cholesterol need to be considered along with family history and other contributing factors. It is not uncommon for premenopausal women to have a relatively high total serum cholesterol because of high HDL, as noted in the Expert Opinion section. Unfortunately, men with elevated total serum cholesterol usually also have elevated LDL, and the ratio of total cholesterol to HDL cholesterol is above 4.5:1.

The National Institutes of Health encourages all people over age 20 to have their total serum cholesterol and HDL measured. Children over 2 years of age with a family history of

---

Most commonly LDL cholesterol is not actually measured but is calculated using the following equation: LDL cholesterol = total cholesterol − HDL cholesterol − (triglycerides/5). Typical LDL cut-off values are the following:
- about 100 mg/dl is ideal
- >130 mg/dl is borderline
- >160 mg/dl is high

systolic blood pressure The pressure in arterial blood vessels associated with the pumping of blood from the heart.

diastolic blood pressure The pressure in arterial blood vessels found when the heart is between beats.

CRITICAL THINKING

As part of his annual health checkup, Juan has a blood sample drawn for measurement of cholesterol values. The results of the test indicate that his total cholesterol is 210 mg/dl, HDL cholesterol is 65 mg/dl, and triglycerides are 100 mg/dl. Juan has read that total cholesterol should be less than 200 mg/dl to minimize cardiovascular problems. However, he is happy with the results of the blood test. How would Juan explain his satisfaction to his parents?

TABLE 4-7

Possible factors related to heart disease that are currently under evaluation by researchers

Factor	Probable mechanism
LDL particle size[5]	Small LDL particles appear to enter atherosclerotic lesions more readily than larger LDL particles. Genetics influences the size of LDL made by each of us.
Lipoprotein patterns that develop after eating (postprandial)[17]	Remnants of chylomicron and VLDL metabolism appear to contribute to atherosclerosis and blood clotting, especially after a high-fat meal is consumed.
Homocysteine[21]	Homocysteine, which is toxic to cells of the blood vessel walls, increases when there is an inadequate intake of vitamin B-6, folate, or vitamin B-12.
Certain forms of apolipoproteins[17]	Certain apolipoproteins of the E class delay lipoprotein clearance from the bloodstream, thus enhancing atherosclerosis. On the other hand, certain apolipoproteins of the A class are associated with a significant reduction in heart disease risk.
Elevated serum triglyceride[24]	Values greater than 150 to 200 mg/dl are not desirable and may contribute to atherosclerosis, linked to the lipoproteins that carry the triglyceride.
Loneliness and stress	Social isolation and stress have been linked to an increased risk of myocardial infarction, especially if heart disease is already present. Increased blood clotting is one likely mechanism.
Coffee[31]	Boiled coffee, as served in Scandinavia, is associated with increased LDL, linked to specific compounds in the coffee bean. These in turn may influence liver metabolism of lipoproteins. Coffee prepared by other methods (filter) has a similar, but smaller, effect.
Excess iron intake	Iron likely speeds oxidation of LDL, which makes LDL more atherogenic. The degree to which this takes place in the body is a subject of debate.[23] The effect is especially prominent in people with elevated LDL.[12]
Nonnutrient substances in plants (see Chapter 12)[2]	Quercetin, found in plants, and related substances found in tea may reduce oxidation of LDL, and thus reduce atherosclerosis development.
Garlic[33]	Garlic (1 clove per day) has been shown in some studies to lower LDL, probably by affecting cholesterol metabolism in the liver.
Nitrous oxide[6]	Nitrous oxide is made by cells and causes muscles controlling the arteries to relax. The amino acid arginine is used to produce nitrous oxide; plants are rich sources of arginine in comparison with animal products.
Abdominal fat storage[17]	Abdominal fat leads to elevated insulin values, which in turn increase blood lipoproteins.
Various blood-clotting factors[30]	People with high concentrations of various clotting factors in their blood show higher risks of heart attack.
Dietary calcium intake[4]	Some studies show a fall in LDL when calcium intake increases from about 400 mg/day to 2000 mg/day. At the higher intake, calcium is likely binding fatty acids in the intestine, in turn reducing fat absorption.
Tocotrienols	These compounds in the vitamin E class likely reduce cholesterol synthesis in the liver.
Soy compounds[22]	Phytosterols and dietary fiber present in soy products likely reduce cholesterol absorption from the intestine, while the protein present may affect cholesterol metabolism in the body.
Pharmacologic intake of antioxidants	Work is ongoing to see if intake of antioxidants well above that generally available from a diet reduces heart disease. Current protocols use about 10 to 25 times or more the RDA for vitamin E and 5 to 10 times the RDA for vitamin C (see Chapter 12 for details).
Lipoprotein(a)[25]	Lipoprotein(a) appears to lead to atherosclerosis and increased blood clotting. It consists of LDL with a large protein attached that is related to a blood clotting factor. The blood concentration of this lipoprotein generally isn't altered by diet changes.
Syndrome X	Syndrome X, which includes high insulin values, hypertension, high serum triglycerides, and low serum HDL, is linked to increased heart disease risk.
Red wine[7]	Phenolic substances in red wine may act as antioxidants and in turn reduce LDL oxidation.

heart disease deserve similar scrutiny. Heart disease experts also recommend having the serum triglyceride concentration measured, as this is used to calculate LDL. If you don't know your various cholesterol values and ratio, you don't know your risk of developing premature heart disease. Keep in mind that you can do many things to prevent heart disease, but first you must recognize your risk factors.[17]

Lowering LDL by Diet Changes

If someone discovers that his or her LDL is high, the first step is to consult a physician. Some diseases (e.g., a form of kidney disease) raise LDL, and treating the disease may remedy the LDL problem as well.[32] If no such disease is present, diet change is advised.

Nutrition experts recommend several approaches for lowering LDL. Because changes that work for one person may be ineffective for another, LDL and HDL should be rechecked a month or so after any of the changes discussed here are implemented.

REDUCING DIETARY SATURATED FAT AND CHOLESTEROL

Reducing saturated-fat intake can lower elevated LDL. Although high total cholesterol in the blood indicates that an individual is at risk for heart disease, the most potent dietary factor associated with high LDL is overconsumption of saturated fat, not of cholesterol.

Almost everyone who minimizes saturated-fat intake can lower elevated LDL by about 10% to 20%, especially if the person has been eating lots of foods that are high in saturated fats. About 10% of the population has trouble decreasing LDL by dietary means. Genetic defects are one reason. On the other hand, about 10% can expect an even bigger drop in LDL.

About 30% of the population who eats a diet low in saturated fat finds that reducing dietary cholesterol lowers LDL even more. Some people can eat six eggs a day for a month without having their fasting serum cholesterol value increase, likely because of a genetic propensity of the liver to compensate by making less cholesterol. Still, most authorities encourage limiting cholesterol intake to less than 300 mg/day, partly to keep the cholesterol content of the chylomicrons that arise right after eating as low as possible. Deposition of cholesterol from circulating chylomicrons probably contributes to atherosclerosis.[17] In addition, as we noted in this chapter, the tendency for palmitic acid—one of the main saturated fatty acids in our diets—to raise LDL is especially prominent when dietary cholesterol intake exceeds 200 to 300 mg/day and total serum cholesterol is elevated. These factors likely reduce the activity of LDL receptors in the liver. Thus at lower cholesterol intakes, LDL receptors are more efficient in removing cholesterol from the bloodstream.[29]

High intakes of saturated fat also affect the liver's ability to clear LDL from the bloodstream, in turn leading to increased LDL.[10] One explanation for this effect is that the saturated-fat content of liver cells is increased at higher intakes, causing membrane "stiffness." This stiffness in turn is thought to reduce the activity of LDL receptors. Moreover, at high fat intakes total energy consumption is likely to be more than needed; in this situation, the liver forms lipids and releases lipoprotein into the bloodstream.

The contribution of dietary saturated fat to elevated LDL can be minimized by eating no more than 7% to 10% of total energy as saturated fats. Finding substitutes for foods rich in animal fat, such as butter, shortening, and other hydrogenated (solid) fats, is a must (Tables 4-2 and 4-3 and Figure 4-11). Routinely reading food labels is also important, as saturated fats are often hidden in foods (Figure 4-12).

Many people think they need to eliminate beef from their diets to moderate their saturated-fat intake. That is not necessary if they choose the right cuts of beef and cook them appropriately, especially trimming the fat off before cooking. If loin or round is part of its name, the cut is relatively low in fat. Also, an occasional meal high in saturated fats won't increase LDL over the long run as long as it is balanced by subsequent meals low in saturated fats.

Only animal and fish products contain cholesterol (Table 4-1). Although egg whites contain no cholesterol, a single egg yolk contains about 210 mg of cholesterol. Thus to meet recommendation for cholesterol intake of no more than 300 mg/day, intake of egg yolks must be watched carefully and limited to no more than four per week. A reduction to 200 mg/day would essentially mean not consuming egg yolks as such except occasionally. Many egg-containing foods (e.g., pancakes, French toast, cookies, and cakes) can be prepared using egg whites rather than whole eggs. Cholesterol-free egg substitutes are also available in the grocery store. Most of these are egg whites colored yellow, to which a small amount of fat has been added to improve the flavor. Trimming the fat before and after cooking a 3- to 4-ounce serving of chicken, beef, or pork leaves roughly one third to one half the cholesterol content

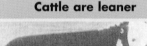

Cattle are leaner

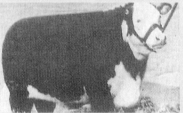

1950s steer

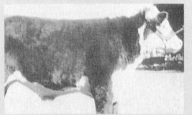

1990s steer

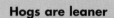

Hogs are leaner

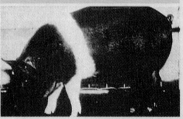

1940s hog

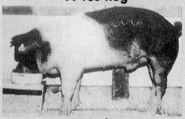

1990s hog

Many manufacturers and food producers are trying to devise products that are lower in fat, particularly in saturated fat. During the past several decades, beef and hog producers have altered breeding and feeding practices to increase muscle mass and decrease body fat.

of an egg. A 10-ounce portion of meat can contain 260 mg of cholesterol, slightly more than in one egg. If meats have a reputation for being high in cholesterol, it is mainly because of an overly generous portion size.

INCREASING MONOUNSATURATED AND POLYUNSATURATED FATS

Until recently, polyunsaturated fatty acids, but not monounsaturated fatty acids, were recommended as a substitute for saturated fatty acids in the diet to lower LDL. However, recent studies show that both monounsaturated and polyunsaturated fatty acids have this effect.[10] In fact, monounsaturated fatty acids may be more beneficial, since LDLs containing these fatty acids are less likely to be oxidized. Recall that oxidized LDL probably contributes more to plaque formation in the arteries than does LDL itself.[11]

However, aside from moving to Crete or some other Mediterranean country where monounsaturated fat–rich olive oil is a major part of the diet, it would be difficult for a typical American to take advantage of this research on monounsaturated fats. Foods and meals rich in monounsaturated fats are not widely available in the United States, nor are they a big part of our cuisine. If a person does much of his or her own cooking, using canola oil, canola oil blended with other vegetable oils, and olive oil on a regular basis will increase intake of monounsaturated fats. A further emphasis on monounsaturated fat would probably require the counsel of a registered dietitian to design a specific meal pattern.

The Nutrition Perspective in Chapter 18 reviews the monounsaturated fat–rich Mediterranean diet in detail.

INCREASING DIETARY FIBER

Another dietary means for reducing LDL is increasing intake of soluble fibers as we discussed in Chapter 3. Although large amounts of fiber must be eaten to have a significant effect on LDL, any amount helps—and has other health benefits as well. Diets with an overall fiber content of 25 to 50 g/day, especially those that emphasize soluble fiber, are most effective in lowering LDL. Most people would have to change their diets extensively to achieve high intakes of soluble fiber. Moreover, dietary fiber intake above 35 g/day may cause binding of dietary minerals, a potentially deleterious side effect. A person should consult a physician if considering a very high-fiber diet. Therefore we think it is easier and safer to reduce LDL by cutting down on saturated fat and cholesterol intake and focusing on regular consumption of high-fiber foods—fruits, vegetables, dry beans, and whole grains—rather than by increasing soluble-fiber intake dramatically.

Diets high in soluble fiber probably work by binding cholesterol and bile in the small intestine and carrying them into the large intestine for elimination.[9] Removing bile from the body forces the liver to pull more cholesterol out of the bloodstream to make new bile. This action resembles that of some medications that lower LDL. Other mechanisms have also been suggested to account for the LDL-lowering effect of soluble fibers. For example, fermentation of soluble fiber by bacteria in the large intestine produces short-chain fatty acids, which may directly reduce cholesterol synthesis by the liver.[9]

Despite the hoopla by some manufacturers about the ability of oat bran to lower LDL, it clearly is no "magic bullet." You would have to eat about a cup a day to reap a substantial LDL-lowering effect; an oat bran muffin alone won't do much.

Raising HDL: A More Difficult Task

Scientists believe that raising HDL may be just as important as lowering LDL in reducing the risk of premature heart disease. Physical activity is one way to raise HDL. Exercising for at least 45 minutes four times a week can raise serum HDL by about 5 mg/dl. Sedentary people in particular should focus on increasing physical activity. Losing excess weight (especially around the waist) and avoiding smoking also help to maintain or raise HDL.

In addition, eating regularly (three balanced meals daily), matching the amount of energy eaten with that expended, and eating less total fat often raise HDL because these practices lower serum triglycerides. Low serum triglycerides often are associated with higher HDL. The reason for this is not clear. Nevertheless, the goal is to keep fasting serum triglycerides below 150 to 200 mg/dl. Certain medications also act to lower serum triglycerides, thereby indirectly increasing HDL.

Consumption of 4 alcoholic drinks per day is also associated with higher HDL levels and reduced blood clotting—two factors that reduce the risk of heart attack.[8] However, this much alcohol has too many negative side effects to be used as a prescription to raise HDL. The Dietary Guidelines indicate that most people can consume 1 to 2 drinks daily (no more) without negative health consequences. But for people at risk of alcoholism, any alcohol may be too much (see discussion in Chapter 7).

It is unfortunate that raising HDL is difficult. Lowering LDL is much easier. And sometimes as LDL falls, so does HDL. This often occurs with very low-fat diets. However, if serum LDL ends up about 100 mg/dl, the low HDL is not of much concern. Researchers note that people in rural Asia who eat low-fat diets generally have low LDL and HDL, but they also show low risks for premature heart disease.

LDL-LOWERING MEDICATIONS

Medications are a last resort for treating high LDL or low HDL; most are expensive and all have troublesome side effects. But sometimes diet changes do not reduce LDL enough, especially in people with strong genetic tendencies toward heart disease. Current medications to lower LDL work in one of two ways. One group inhibits the liver from synthesizing some lipoproteins. These medications include the vitamin nicotinic acid, lovastatin, probucol, and gemfibrozil.[24] Nicotinic acid and gemfibrozil are also notable for raising HDL. The side effects of these medications, however, necessitate a physician's careful supervision. The other group of medications includes cholestyramine and colestipol; they bind bile in the small intestine and lead to its elimination, forcing the liver to synthesize new bile. The liver removes LDL from the blood to do this. All these medications work better when a proper diet is followed; they do not substitute for recommended diet changes.

A controversy currently rages about the use of medications and significant diet changes to combat heart disease. The vast majority of researchers in the heart disease arena agree that diet changes and medications (if needed) to lower elevated LDL, ideally to around 100 mg/dl, are especially important for people who already show evidence of heart disease.[24] The current debate concerns how aggressive treatment should be for people who have high LDL but exhibit no symptoms of heart disease and have no other risk factors. Still, mortality from all causes, including that resulting from heart disease, is reduced when treatment to lower elevated LDL in people at high risk for heart disease is followed for a few years or more. And new research even shows that plaque regresses in arteries when high LDL is aggressively treated with (1) surgery on the intestinal tract that reduces bile acid uptake; (2) LDL-lowering diet plus medications; or (3) even diet alone, although the diet used was very low in fat and contained essentially no cholesterol.[28] We discuss the type of diet used—a vegan diet— in the next chapter. It is suspected that these aggressive therapies to lower LDL stabilize the development of atherosclerotic plaque, thereby lowering the risk of rupture and, in turn, myocardial infarction caused by clot formation.

Some research has suggested that low serum cholesterol itself poses certain risks. These studies indicate that people with total serum cholesterol less than 160 mg/dl have an increased risk of dying of cerebral hemorrhage (a type of stroke) and certain types of cancer. But closer inspection reveals that low serum cholesterol itself isn't the likely culprit. In most cases these people have some underlying medical condition, such as a stomach or liver disorder, that lowers serum cholesterol and increases the risk of death.[16]

In summary, individuals with elevated LDL, in consultation with their physicians, are best suited to determine their desire and ability to make lifestyle changes, supplemented by medications (if necessary) to lower heart disease risk. Some physicians also recommend caution about initiating aggressive LDL-lowering treatment in persons over 65 to 70 years of age because of concern about the safety and cost effectiveness of such interventions in older people (see Chapter 18).[15]

General Strategy for Reducing Heart Disease Risk

Table 4-8 outlines the most effective general strategy for lowering LDL and thus reducing the risk of heart attack.

The bottom line is actually quite simple. Remove as much saturated fat from the diet as possible while moderating total fat and cholesterol intake. To do this, a person should select foods that are lower in total fat and especially in saturated fat. That means eating fewer high-fat foods of animal origin, such as marbled meat, eggs, and whole-milk dairy products, while eating more plant foods, such as fruits, vegetables, and whole grains.

A diet with 30% total energy from fat is an appropriate goal for children age 2 or older. But parents shouldn't go overboard limiting fat intake because children need to consume about 30% of total energy as fat to grow properly. Experts do not recommend fat-restricted diets in children under the age of 2 (see Chapter 17).

TABLE 4-8

General diet-related strategy for reducing the risk of premature heart disease and heart attack[12,14,24]

Action	Rationale
Follow the Food Guide Pyramid, consuming less total fat, especially saturated fat, and less cholesterol.	This supplies vitamins and minerals associated with reduced risk of heart disease, such as vitamins B-6 and B-12, folate, and calcium. The key focus is on reducing intake of animal fat and hydrogenated fat (especially deep fat–fried foods) where possible.
Eat plenty of fruits, vegetables, and whole grains. Include some soy and garlic on a regular basis.	The dietary fiber, antioxidants, and other phytochemical substances present in these foods can contribute to lower heart disease risk.
Eat regularly spaced meals, not one or two large ones.	The frequency of meals helps determine fasting serum triglycerides. Studies show increasing meal frequency (from three to nine meals per day or so) can even help reduce LDL.
Lose weight, ideally to attain a desirable body weight (see Chapter 8).	This especially helps reduce serum triglycerides (if elevated), lowers high blood pressure, and can increase HDL, especially if the fat was lost from the abdominal region.
Eat fish about twice a week.	This provides EPA and DHA to reduce blood clotting and thus lessens the risk of heart attack. Regular use of aspirin for people at high risk of a heart attack (under a physician's scrutiny) is promoted for the same reason.
Consume moderate amounts of alcohol if you can control this practice.	Consumption of red wine in particular has been noted to reduce heart disease risk, but it is speculated that small doses of any form of alcohol may do the same. A reduction in blood clotting is thought to be one mechanism.
Moderate coffee intake.	An intake of more than 5 to 6 cups of regular coffee a day has been linked in some studies to an increased risk of heart attack in men and women, and can raise LDL.
Use iron supplements with caution.	Although this point is still being debated, some experts recommend that iron supplements not be consumed unless medically needed because this may increase LDL oxidation. People who have an iron storage disease need to pay careful attention to this warning (see Chapter 15).[12] With regard to dietary iron intake, the **heme iron** found in animal products is most highly linked to the risk of heart attack, rather than the iron found in plants or added to enriched grains (see Chapter 15).

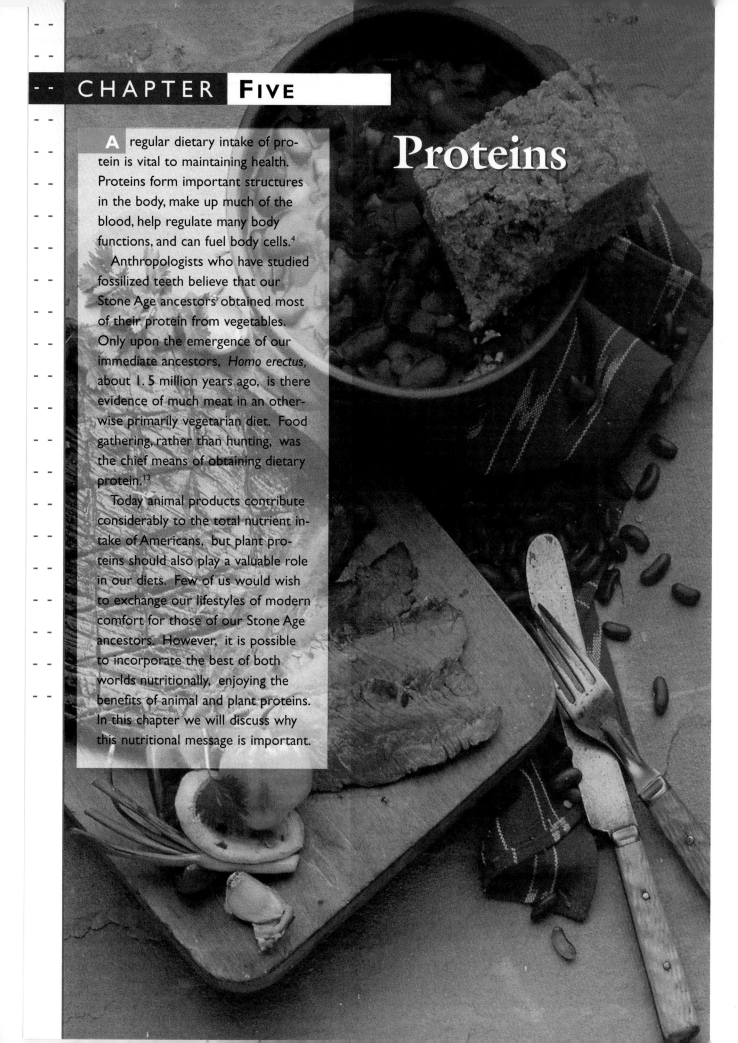

CHAPTER FIVE

Proteins

A regular dietary intake of protein is vital to maintaining health. Proteins form important structures in the body, make up much of the blood, help regulate many body functions, and can fuel body cells.[4]

Anthropologists who have studied fossilized teeth believe that our Stone Age ancestors obtained most of their protein from vegetables. Only upon the emergence of our immediate ancestors, *Homo erectus,* about 1.5 million years ago, is there evidence of much meat in an otherwise primarily vegetarian diet. Food gathering, rather than hunting, was the chief means of obtaining dietary protein.[13]

Today animal products contribute considerably to the total nutrient intake of Americans, but plant proteins should also play a valuable role in our diets. Few of us would wish to exchange our lifestyles of modern comfort for those of our Stone Age ancestors. However, it is possible to incorporate the best of both worlds nutritionally, enjoying the benefits of animal and plant proteins. In this chapter we will discuss why this nutritional message is important.

If the R portion of the amino acid is anything other than a hydrogen, the amino acid has four different groups attached to it. You may recall from basic chemistry that a carbon with four different groups attached to it can exist as one of two isomer forms, in this case D and L. In nature, almost all amino acids occur in the L form. However, we can metabolize some D isomer forms by converting them in the body to L forms. (Appendix B reviews the concept of isomerism.)

The key part of the amino acid is the amino group. It is the distinguishing feature of amino acids. Cells produce carbon backbones, commonly called carbon skeletons, and then add amino groups from other amino acids to synthesize 11 of the 20 amino acids the body needs. In the case of the other nine amino acids, body cells either cannot make the needed carbon skeleton, cannot put an amino group on the carbon skeleton, or just cannot do the whole process fast enough to meet body needs. The amino acids that body cells cannot synthesize are called **essential (indispensable) amino acids** and must be consumed in the diet (Table 5-1). The 11 amino acids the body can make are called **nonessential (dispensable) amino acids.** Note that both essential and nonessential amino acids are present in foods that contain protein.[4]

All amino acids are necessary for proper body function. Only the essential amino acids, however, must be derived from the diet. If we don't consume enough essential amino acids in our food, the rate of protein synthesis slows progressively until protein breakdown exceeds protein synthesis. Poor health can result. In contrast, nonessential amino acids can be omitted from the diet without consequence.

Two amino acids—cysteine and tyrosine—are synthesized in the body from methionine and phenylalanine, respectively. Both methionine and phenylalanine are essential amino acids. Cysteine and tyrosine must be made from their essential amino acid counterparts unless they are consumed in the diet. If cysteine and tyrosine are consumed, the body can synthesize protein from them directly. Thus consumption of cysteine and tyrosine then frees the essential amino acids methionine and phenylalanine for protein synthesis. Therefore cysteine and tyrosine are classed as semiessential (conditionally indispensable) amino acids.[12] Dietary methionine need is reduced about 50% if ample cysteine is consumed.

essential (indispensable) amino acids The amino acids that cannot be synthesized in sufficient amounts by humans and must, therefore, be included in the diet; there are nine essential amino acids.

nonessential (dispensable) amino acids Amino acids that can be readily synthesized by the body. There are 11 types of nonessential amino acids in foods.

- - - - - - - - - - - -
Because two cysteine molecules can bind to form a new amino acid called *cystine,* the number of nonessential amino acids is sometimes listed as 12. If this form of cysteine is not counted as a unique form, then there are 11 nonessential amino acids. We do not count cystine, and thus use the figure of 20 amino acids in foods—9 essential and 11 nonessential.
- - - - - - - - - - - -

TABLE 5-1

Classification of amino acids

Essential amino acids	Nonessential amino acids
Histidine	Alanine
Isoleucine	Arginine§
Leucine	Asparagine
Lysine‡	Aspartic acid
Methionine†	Cysteine (cystine)*
Phenylalanine	Glutamic acid
Threonine	Glutamine‖
Tryptophan	Glycine
Valine	Proline
	Serine
	Tyrosine*

*These amino acids are also classified as semiessential.
†The limiting amino acid in legumes and vegetables. One should also consume legumes with grains, nuts, and seeds during the same day to supply complete protein for the diet if no animal protein is eaten.
‡A limiting amino acid in grains, nuts, and seeds. One should also consume grains with legumes during the same day to supply complete protein for the diet if no animal protein is eaten.
§Synthesized at rates inadequate to support growth of chidren and thus is considered essential during growth.
‖Currently hypothesized to be essential to the diet in some states of traumatic injury, especially regarding maintenance of GI tract function, and thus is often supplemented in specialized formulas used with hospitalized patients.[24]

TRANSAMINATION AND DEAMINATION

A common metabolic process for synthesizing nonessential amino acids is called **transamination.**[20] This process requires vitamin B-6. Figure 5-2 illustrates transamination: pyruvic acid accepts the amino group ($-NH_2$) from the amino acid glutamic acid and becomes the amino acid alanine. In the process, glutamic acid becomes a carbon skeleton, called alpha-ketoglutaric acid.

Some amino acids, such as glutamic acid, can simply lose their amino group without transferring it to another carbon skeleton. This process is called **deamination.**[20] The amino group, in the form of ammonia, is incorporated into urea in the liver. The urea is then transferred through the bloodstream to the kidneys and is mostly excreted in the urine (Figure 5-3). Once an amino acid breaks down to its carbon skeleton, the carbon skeleton can be used for fuel or synthesized into other compounds, such as fatty acids (see Chapter 7).[4]

There is extensive recycling of amino acids in the body. Each cell contains a pool of amino acids—available for a limited time and in limited quantity—yielded from dietary intake, body synthesis, and amino acid recycling.[12] If the pool of amino acids becomes too large, excess amino acids are used for energy, glucose, or fat production. Figure 5-3 can help you understand how the amino acid pool diminishes from inadequate dietary protein intake. Additional amino acids must then come from the breakdown of cellular protein. This leads to the breakdown of essential body tissue. This is why essential amino acids need to be replaced by the diet.[4]

Overall, the two main functions of proteins in our diets are: (1) to provide the nine essential amino acids needed for protein synthesis; and (2) to provide amino nitrogen needed to synthesize missing nonessential amino acids. Enough protein must be consumed to serve these two functions.

PUTTING ESSENTIAL AMINO ACIDS INTO PERSPECTIVE

As noted before, amino acids are the building blocks of proteins. Eating a balanced diet can supply both the essential and nonessential amino acids (or building blocks needed for the latter) to maintain good health. Let's now look in more detail at this concept of essential amino acids, especially in relation to nonessential amino acids.

Some amino acids that are normally nonessential may become an essential part of the diet of a person whose health is compromised. One example is arginine, which is essential for children born preterm. Another example is glutamine, which may become essential for adults experiencing traumatic injury, especially involving the gastrointestinal tract.

transamination The transfer of an amine group from an amino acid to a carbon skeleton to form a new amino acid.

deamination The removal of an amine group from an amino acid.

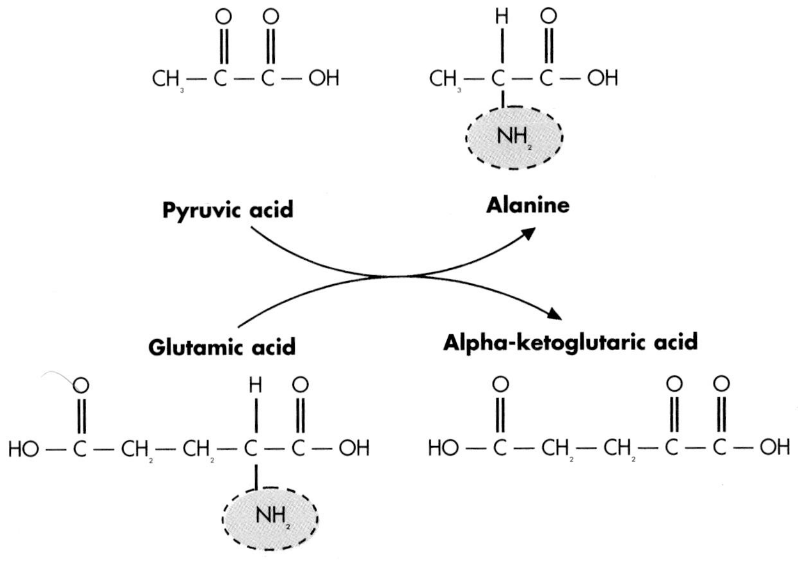

Figure 5-2 Transamination. This pathway allows cells to synthesize nonessential amino acids. In this example, pyruvic acid gains an amino group to form the amino acid alanine.

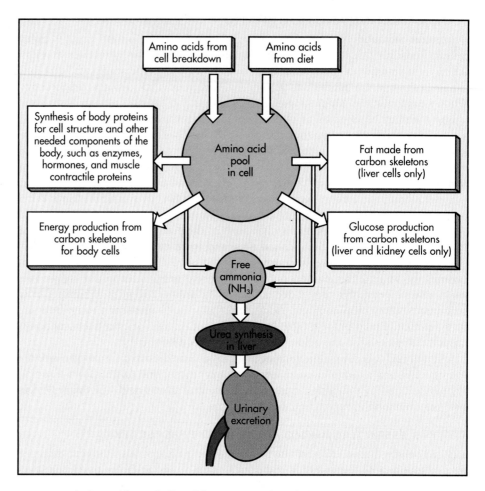

Figure 5-3 Amino acid metabolism. The amino acid pool shown is supplied both by the release of amino acids from the breakdown of old cells and by amino acids from protein in the diet. Each cell builds new protein from amino acids that are available from this pool. Should the pool become too large, the amino acids become a source of energy or are converted to either glucose or body fat.

Physiological Aspects

The disease phenylketonuria (PKU) illustrates the concept of essential and nonessential amino acids. Phenylalanine is an essential amino acid. Tyrosine is a nonessential amino acid because phenylalanine can be converted into tyrosine. However, the liver of a person with PKU lacks sufficient enzyme activity to make the conversion efficiently. This impairment of enzyme activity can vary from mild to severe. Two problems result from the lack of this enzyme: (1) phenylalanine cannot be degraded sufficiently when present in excess; and (2) tyrosine is not synthesized from phenylalanine. Tyrosine becomes an essential amino acid because it must now come from the diet.[4]

The diet of a person with PKU must be carefully designed to contain enough phenylalanine for protein synthesis—because it is an essential amino acid—but not an excess. Dairy products especially have to be limited in the diet because they are among the many protein-rich foods that contain significant amounts of phenylalanine. The inability to readily metabolize excess phenylalanine to tyrosine can lead to a build-up of abnormal products from alternative routes of phenylalanine metabolism. These products are thought to cause the severe mental retardation seen in untreated PKU cases.[20]

Dietary Considerations

Animal proteins and plant proteins can differ greatly in their amino acid compositions. Animal proteins, except gelatin, contain ample amounts of all essential amino acids. (Gelatin lacks the sulfur-containing amino acids, and the heat and acid processing it undergoes, destroys tryptophan.) Plant proteins are always relatively low in one or more of the essential amino acids (Table 5-2).

In essence, human tissue composition resembles animal tissue far more than it does plant tissue. Thus proteins from animal sources are used more efficiently to support human growth and maintenance because they closely match the human pattern of essential amino acids. In turn, animal proteins, except gelatin, are considered **high-quality proteins** (often called complete proteins). They can support body growth and maintenance because they contain all of the essential amino acids in sufficient amounts and in a pattern that closely matches human needs. Plant proteins are considered **low-quality proteins** (often called incomplete proteins).[12] This means that proteins from a single plant variety cannot easily support body growth and maintenance because each protein lacks adequate amounts of one or more essential amino acids. One then must eat more low-quality protein than high-quality protein to eventually meet essential amino acid needs.

If your diet does not provide an appropriate balance of all nine essential amino acids, protein synthesis will soon stop when any one essential amino acid is depleted. Considering body needs in comparison with a food or a diet, the amino acid in shortest supply in relation to need is called the **limiting amino acid.** When protein synthesis stops because one type of essential amino acid has been used up, the "all-or-none law" applies: if all nine essential amino acids are not available to synthesize needed protein, the ones present cannot be used at that time and will be wasted.[12]

For example, assume the letters of the alphabet represent the 20 different amino acids we eat. If A represents an essential amino acid, we would need four of these to synthesize the hypothetical protein ALABAMA. If the body had an L, B, and M, but only 3 A's, the "synthesis" of ALABAMA would be impossible. "A" would then represent the limiting amino acid.

Most Americans consume an assortment of protein-rich foods in amounts sufficient to easily obtain enough of all nine essential amino acids. That is, Americans eat a high-quality (complete) protein diet.[12]

Worldwide, most adults who eat sufficient protein consume enough essential amino acids to obtain a high-quality protein diet, even if the various protein sources in the diet individually are of low quality. The combination of low-quality proteins eaten generally makes up for deficiencies in essential amino acids in each separate protein. When two or more proteins combine to compensate for deficiencies in essential amino acid content in each individual protein, the proteins are called **complementary proteins** (Table 5-2).[1] Varied diets generally provide high-quality protein, since a complementary protein pattern results.[12]

Complementing proteins need not be consumed at the same meal by adults. It is reasonable for adults to achieve amino acid needs over the course of a day, since there is temporary storage of essential amino acids in skeletal muscle pools.[26] Overall, healthy adults should have little concern about balancing foods to yield the proteins needed to obtain all nine essential amino acids. Thus, although both the "all-or-none law" and the concept of the limiting amino acid are interesting, they can be overemphasized when typical eating patterns are considered. Adults also need only about 15% of their total protein requirement to be supplied by essential amino acids.[26] Typical diets supply an average of 50% of protein as essential amino acids.

Infants and preschool children, on the other hand, need approximately 35% of their protein requirements to come from essential amino acids.[26] So food for young children must be carefully planned to include enough of all nine essential amino acids.[4] If infants consume enough breast milk or commercial formula to meet protein requirements, essential amino acid needs will be met. For growing children,

high-quality proteins Dietary proteins that contain ample amounts of all nine essential amino acids.

low-quality proteins Dietary proteins that lack an ample amount of one or more amino acids essential for human protein needs.

limiting amino acid The essential amino acid in lowest concentration in a food or diet relative to body needs.

complementary proteins Two food proteins that make up for each other's lack of a specific essential amino acid, such that together they yield complete protein.

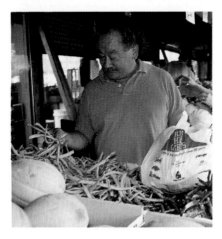

Amino acids in vegetables are best used when a combination of sources is consumed.

TABLE 5-2

Limiting amino acids in plant foods

Food	Limiting amino acids	Good plant source of the limiting amino acids*	Traditional uses where the proteins complement each other
Soybeans and other legumes	Methionine	Grains, nuts, and seeds	Tofu (soybean curd) and rice
Grains	Lysine, threonine	Legumes	Rice and red beans, lentils, curry, and rice
Nuts and seeds	Lysine	Legumes	Soybeans and ground sesame seeds (miso); peanuts, rice, and black-eyed and green peas; and sunflower seeds
Vegetables	Methionine	Grains, nuts, and seeds	Green beans and almonds
Corn	Tryptophan, lysine	Legumes	Corn tortillas and pinto beans

As you might suspect from the information in this table, the amino acids most likely to be low in a diet are lysine, methionine, threonine, and tryptophan. If a diet is low in an amino acid, we recommend finding a good food source to supply it. Forget about amino acid supplements—they can lead to problems, as we discuss later in this chapter.

*Animal products in the diet serve the same purpose, such as when fish is consumed with rice.

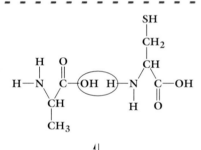

peptide bond A chemical bond formed by the reaction of an amino group from one amino acid with a carboxyl group from another amino acid, splitting off a water molecule; the main bond that links amino acids in a polypeptide chain.

complementary amino acids should be consumed in each individual meal or within two subsequent meals. A major health risk for children occurs in famine situations in which only one type of grain is available, increasing the probability that one or more of the nine essential amino acids may be lacking in the total diet.[19] We discuss this further in a later section in the chapter.

CONCEPT CHECK

Twenty amino acids important to the body exist in food. A healthy body synthesizes 11 of these—nonessential (dispensable) amino acids. The other nine—essential (indispensable) amino acids—must be consumed. Foods that contain all nine essential amino acids in about the proportion needed by the body provide high-quality protein, whereas proteins that provide a low quantity of one or more essential amino acids are lower in quality. When different low-quality protein foods are eaten together in a meal, their amino acids often complement each other, providing a high-quality protein meal.

PROTEINS—AMINO ACIDS JOINED TOGETHER

One way of classifying proteins is based on the number of amino acids present. Two amino acids chemically bonded together form a dipeptide, and three amino acids form a tripeptide. An oligopeptide has more than 3 but less than 50 amino acids. A **polypeptide** has 50 to 100 amino acids, and a protein has a minimum of 100 amino acids.[20] Most foods contain just proteins. However, specialized feeding supplements used in hospitals often contain various peptides.

Amino acids are joined by a strong, covalent **peptide bond.** An amino group ($-NH_2$) reacts with a carboxyl group ($-\overset{O}{\underset{}{C}}-OH$), and a water molecule is split off in an enzyme-catalyzed reaction. The body can synthesize many different proteins by joining the 20 different types of amino acids with peptide bonds. Imagine the number of combinations that can be made using multiple amounts of the 20 amino acids, especially considering the great lengths of many proteins.

A peptide bond can be broken—water is returned to the molecule during a process called hydrolysis. Acids, enzymes, or other agents can break peptide bonds.

STAGES OF PROTEIN ORGANIZATION

The structural elements of proteins are commonly described as primary, secondary, and tertiary.[20]

Sequence—primary structure

The sequence of amino acids in a protein dictates the structure of the protein. This is often called a protein's primary structure. The sequence of the amino acids eventually yields a specific three-dimensional shape, which in turn determines the function of the protein.[20]

Interactions between adjacent amino acids—secondary structure

The chain of amino acids in a protein is not a long, straight string but rather becomes a three-dimensional structure. The ultimate shape results from the folding, twisting, and turning of the amino acids linked in the sequence. The location of an amino acid may allow a fold or twist to occur at a certain spot. For example, a fold may occur at a very small amino acid, such as glycine or alanine. In contrast, a fold is unlikely to occur in a location where there is a very large amino acid. The folded shape may then be stabilized by hydrogen bonds and disulfide bonds (S–S), as well as by other forces. These forces that stabilize the shape are referred to as *secondary structure* and are best thought of as interactions that occur between amino acids near each other in the protein chain.[20]

Configuration—tertiary and quaternary structure

The R groups (side chains) on amino acids have special characteristics that may attract or repel other amino acids in the chain. This is another reason why amino acid sequence determines a protein's final shape. Some amino acids are hydrophilic or hydrophobic (remember those definitions from Chapter 4). The hydrophilic amino acids will mostly remain on the outside of a large protein molecule, while the hydrophobic amino acids will mostly be hidden on the inside.[20]

The final configuration proteins assume is a globular (spherical) or coiled (fiber-like) shape and is often called the tertiary structure, to reflect the three-dimensional nature of the protein stabilized by noncovalent forces.[20] Occasionally two or more separate protein units interact to form an even larger new protein form termed *quaternary structure* (Figure 5-4). This organization becomes significant when it is important to have a protein active only at certain times. A protein may be active when the units are joined but inactive when the units are separate.[20]

> Sulfur-containing amino acids stabilize many compounds, such as the hormone insulin. Sulfur groups can bond (–S–S–), creating a bridge between two protein strands or two parts of the same strand. This stabilizes the structure of the molecule and can be regarded as a part of secondary structure.

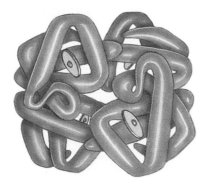

FIGURE 5-4 Protein organization. Proteins often form a coiled shape, as shown by this drawing of the blood protein hemoglobin. This shape is dictated by the sequence of amino acids in the protein chain. To give you an idea of its size, each teaspoon (5 ml) of blood contains about 10^{18} hemoglobin molecules (one billion is 10^9).[20]

Sickle-cell disease (also called sickle-cell anemia) illustrates the importance of the correct sequence of amino acids to allow for a protein's function. African-Americans and people of Mediterranean descent are especially prone to this genetic disease, which affects about 1 in 400 African-American infants. The major problem leading to sickle-cell disease is an altered formation of the protein chains in hemoglobin, a red blood cell protein. Only one incorrect amino acid is present in each of two of the four protein chains. Specifically, the amino acid valine is exchanged for the amino acid glutamic acid. However, this small error profoundly changes the structure of hemoglobin; it can no longer assume the proper shape needed to carry oxygen efficiently within the red blood cell. The red blood cells then form a crescent rather than a circular shape (Figure 5-5). The resulting illness can lead to episodes of infection, severe bone and joint pain, abdominal pain, headache, convulsions, and paralysis.[22] This demonstrates how critical even a minor error in the primary structure of a protein can be.

How does this error in the formation of hemoglobin happen? It results from a defect in the person's genetic blueprint, DNA, which is inherited from his or her parents. Defective DNA can lead to an incorrect amino acid's being built into the sequence of body proteins.[20]

DENATURATION OF PROTEINS

denature To alter a protein's three-dimensional form, usually by treatment with heat, acid or alkaline solutions, or agitation.

Treatment with acid or alkaline substances, heat, or agitation can severely alter the three-dimensional shape of a protein, leaving the protein in an unfolded, or **denatured,** state. Once denatured, a protein loses its biological activity. For example, once an egg is cracked into a hot frying pan and solidifies, it can no longer produce a chicken. (The same is true for a beaten egg.) Once the bacteria in yogurt have synthesized enough acid and enzymes to precipitate the milk protein casein, the protein can never be resuspended in water.

The body uses this characteristic of protein denaturation to its advantage. When foods reach the stomach, stomach acid denatures some bacteria, plant hormones, many active enzymes, and other forms of proteins in the food. This activity renders foods safer to eat, since disrupting a protein's three-dimensional shape often effectively prevents it from performing its normal physiological function.[20] Denaturation also contributes to the digestive process.

Recall that we need proteins in the diet to supply essential amino acids—we do not need the active proteins themselves. We can build all the proteins we need from amino acids.

A 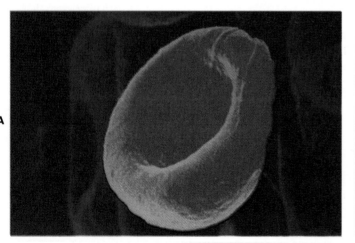 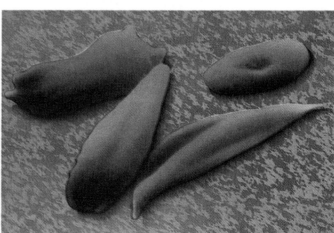 B

Figure 5-5 The effects of sickle-cell disease on red blood cells. **A,** Normal red blood cell. **B,** Blood of a person with sickle cell disease. Note the abnormal crescent (sicklelike) shape of the red blood cell near the center.

Concept Check

Proper sequencing of the amino acids that make up a protein ensures that each amino acid in the protein will be inserted in the correct position in relation to the other amino acids when the folds and twists form. It may help to view the protein structure as first being stabilized by attractions formed among amino acids located close together. A more complex structure then may be created by attractions among amino acids located far apart in the sequence of amino acids. Only appropriately positioned amino acids can chemically bond properly so that the correct folded shape—whether coiled or globular—forms. Destruction of the structure or shape of a protein by acid or alkaline conditions, heat, or other factors unfolds—denatures—the protein, yielding an inactive form.

Functions of Proteins

Proteins function in the body as enzymes, structural units, transport systems in the blood, immune constituents, regulatory factors, and mobility components (contractile proteins).[4] In order to use dietary protein efficiently for these purposes, we must also consume enough energy to meet energy needs. Otherwise, the amino acids in dietary protein will be used mostly for energy needs, rather than for synthetic purposes.

PRODUCING VITAL BODY CONSTITUENTS

Proteins form structural components in the body—muscle contractile tissue, connective tissue, and the support network (protein matrix) inside bones. Measurements of the amount of certain structural proteins in the body, such as the circumference of the upper arm muscle, can be used to estimate body protein status in health and disease. In addition, blood-clotting factors, blood transport proteins, lipoproteins, and visual pigments contain protein.[4]

Each cell membrane contains protein. In fact, as discussed in Chapter 4, a cell membrane is essentially composed of islands of protein in a sea of lipids. Some cell membrane proteins act as receptors for absorption of nutrients into the cell. Others act as receptor sites for some hormones or as pumps to help maintain ion balance inside and outside a cell.[20]

Most of these vital body proteins are in a constant state of breakdown, rebuilding, and repair, especially in the intestine and bone marrow. Most of the protein breakdown products, namely amino acids, can be reused, and thus add to the pool of amino acids available for future protein synthesis (see Figure 5-3).[4] However, some amino acids and other protein breakdown products are not reused. They are lost rather than recycled. If a person habitually fails to eat enough protein to replace this loss, the protein rebuilding and repairing process slows. Thus for body growth and maintenance, amino acids must be supplied constantly from food. Otherwise, skeletal muscles, heart, liver, blood proteins, and other organs decrease in size or amount. Only the brain resists breakdown.[19]

MAINTAINING FLUID BALANCE

The blood proteins, albumin and globulin, help maintain fluid balance in the body. Blood pressure in the arteries acts to force the blood fluid (serum) out of the blood vessels and into the **capillary beds.** The fluid then spills out into the **extracellular spaces** to provide nutrients to cells (Figure 5-6). Proteins in the bloodstream can counteract this effect of blood pressure because they are too large to move out of the capillary beds into the tissues and because they attract fluid. This causes most of the fluid to remain in the blood vessels.[20]

The ability of blood proteins, simply by their presence, to attract and retain fluid in the bloodstream arises from their **osmotic potential** (see Chapter 14 for a full discussion of osmosis). In essence, the blood proteins exert an attraction, also called

Critical Thinking

Samantha's mother's blood concentration of urea is high. From a nutritional point of view, what might this indicate?

capillary bed Minute vessels one cell thick that create a junction between arterial and venous circulation. It is here that gas and nutrient exchange occurs between body cells and the bloodstream.

extracellular space The space between cells.

Arterial end of
capillary bed

Venous end of
capillary bed

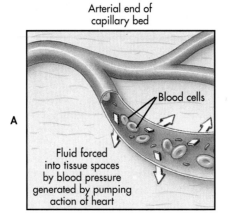

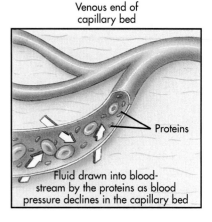

A

Blood cells

Proteins

Fluid forced
into tissue spaces
by blood pressure
generated by pumping
action of heart

Fluid drawn into blood-
stream by the proteins as blood
pressure declines in the capillary bed

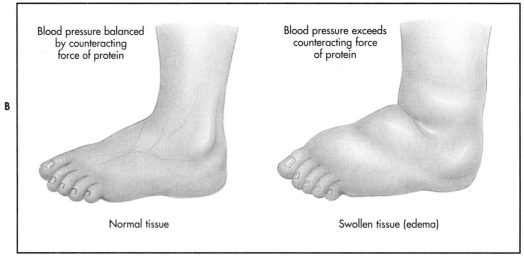

B

Blood pressure balanced
by counteracting
force of protein

Blood pressure exceeds
counteracting force
of protein

Normal tissue

Swollen tissue (edema)

FIGURE 5-6 Blood proteins in relation to fluid balance. **A,** Blood proteins are important for maintaining the body's fluid balance. **B,** Without sufficient protein in the bloodstream, edema develops.

osmotic potential The tendency to attract water across a semipermeable membrane, usually to dilute some constituent in a fluid.

oncotic force The osmotic potential exerted by proteins in the bloodstream.

edema The build-up of excess fluid in extracellular spaces.

oncotic force, on the fluid in the bloodstream that counters the force of blood pressure.

If a person doesn't eat enough protein, eventually the amount of protein in the bloodstream decreases. Blood pressure can then force excessive fluid out of the blood vessels and into the extracellular spaces because there is no strong counteracting force to oppose it. As more and more fluid pools in the extracellular spaces, clinical **edema** results.[19] Other conditions, such as heart failure, kidney disease, liver disease, and pregnancy, can also lead to edema. Thus the cause of the edema needs to be investigated. An initial step is to measure the concentration of blood protein, such as albumin, to see if it is adequate.

Children with protein malnutrition often show severe edema.[19] If they are fed protein along with the other nutrients needed for good health, their bodies can make more blood proteins. The fluid is then attracted back into bloodstream, and the edema disappears. We will discuss this in detail, along with other effects of protein deficiency, later in this chapter.

CONTRIBUTING TO ACID-BASE BALANCE

The concentration of hydrogen ions in the bloodstream determines the acid-base balance (pH) of the blood. Proteins help regulate the amount of free hydrogen ions by readily accepting or donating hydrogen ions.[20] This regulation helps to keep the blood pH fairly constant and slightly alkaline (pH 7.35 to 7.45). Compounds that act to keep pH within a narrow range are called **buffers.** Blood proteins are important buffers in the body.

FORMING HORMONES AND ENZYMES

Many hormones, such as the thyroid hormones triiodothyronine (T_3) and thyroxine (T_4), are derivatives of amino acids; insulin is a polypeptide. These and other hormones that are classified as proteins perform many important regulatory functions in the body, such as controlling metabolic rate and facilitating glucose uptake from the bloodstream into cells.[20]

Many hormone medicines from the protein class, such as insulin, must be injected. If taken orally, insulin would be destroyed; the stomach and small intestine would digest the hormone, dismantling it into amino acids as they do with foods. The digestive tract is unable to distinguish between a protein that is being taken for medication and one that is being consumed for nutrients.

Almost all enzymes are proteins (a few are composed of nucleic acids).[20] Enzymes are organic compounds that catalyze (speed) chemical reactions. Occasionally a cell lacks the correct DNA structure for instructions on how to make needed enzymes. For example, the cells of an infant who suffers from the disease **galactosemia** cannot make the enzyme needed to metabolize the single sugar galactose. If the infant is not put on a galactose-free diet soon after birth, its growth and mental development will be depressed. This case demonstrates the crucial roles that enzymes, and thus proteins, play in body function.

CONTRIBUTING TO IMMUNE FUNCTION

Proteins compose key parts of the cells used by the immune system (Figure 5-7). Also, the **antibodies** produced by one type of immune cell (β-lymphocytes) are proteins.[4] These antibodies can bind to foreign proteins in the body, an important step in removing invaders from the body (see Chapter 15 for a description of how the immune system works). Without sufficient dietary protein, the immune system lacks the cells and other tools needed to function properly. Thus immune incompetence—**anergy**—and a protein-deficient diet often appear together. Anergy can turn measles into a fatal disease for a malnourished child.[19] It also can encourage unusual infections, such as widespread yeast *(Candida)* growth in the mouth and throat of a hospitalized adult. This yeast can more easily reproduce and spread when an immune system does not function well.

FORMING GLUCOSE

In Chapter 3 we noted that the body must maintain a fairly constant concentration of glucose in the bloodstream to supply energy for red blood cells and nerve tissue. The brain uses about 35% of the resting body's energy requirement, and it gets most of that energy from glucose. If a diet does not contain enough carbohydrate to supply the glucose, the liver, and to a lesser extent the kidneys, is forced to metabolize amino acids to make the glucose (Figure 5-3). Many types of amino acids can be used for this purpose. Recall that the metabolic process of turning amino acids into glucose is called gluconeogenesis.[4]

Some gluconeogenesis is normal; for example, it occurs if you skip breakfast when you haven't eaten since 7 o'clock the night before. Taken to the extreme, however, constant gluconeogenesis causes much of the muscle wasting that occurs in starvation.[19]

PROVIDING ENERGY

Proteins supply about 2% to 5% of the energy the body uses (see Chapter 10 for information about the use of amino acids for energy during exercise). Most cells use primarily carbohydrates and fats for energy. Proteins and carbohydrates contain the

buffers Compounds that can take up or release hydrogen ions to maintain a certain range of pH values in a solution.

- - - - - - - - - - - - -

Neurotransmitters, made by nerve endings, are often derivatives of amino acids. This is true for dopamine (synthesized from tyrosine), epinephrine (synthesized from tyrosine), and serotonin (synthesized from tryptophan). The way in which diet influences the synthesis of some of these neurotransmitters is currently under study. For example, high-carbohydrate meals can induce sleepiness as a result of increased serotonin synthesis in the brain. The mechanism involves the effect of insulin on amino acid balance in the blood. The net result is an increase in tryptophan in the blood, and in turn more serotonin synthesis by the brain. Serotonin induces a sense of sleepiness and calm.[7]

- - - - - - - - - - - - -

antibody A protein that prevents infections by inactivating foreign proteins found in the body.

anergy Lack of an immune response to foreign compounds entering the body.

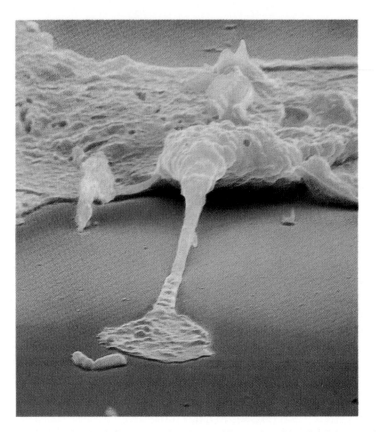

Figure 5-7 Going in for the kill. Ever vigilant, a patrolling white blood cell (macrophage) attacks a bacterium. Adequate protein in the diet aids immune system responses like this one.[4]

same amount of usable energy, 4 kcal/g. However, proteins are a very inefficient source of energy, considering the amount of metabolism and processing the liver and kidneys must perform to use this energy source. The monetary cost of protein-rich foods is also a consideration.

CONCEPT CHECK

Proteins form vital body constituents, such as muscle, connective tissue, blood transport proteins, enzymes, hormones, and immune bodies. Many key body processes, such as acid-base balance, fluid balance, and immune function, rely on proteins. Proteins can also provide fuel for the body and carbons for the synthesis of glucose.

Evaluation of Protein Quality

Protein quality refers to the ability of a food protein to support body growth and maintenance. Methods exist to both measure and estimate protein quality. We will discuss the more important approaches. Keep in mind, however, that the concept of protein quality applies only under conditions in which the amount of protein consumed is equal to or less than the amount of protein required to meet the need for essential amino acids. When protein intake exceeds this amount, efficiency of protein use declines, regardless of the balance of amino acids present. This occurs even with the highest quality proteins because, after the need for essential amino acids has been met, the remaining essential and nonessential amino acids cannot be stored in significant amounts on a long-term basis and will primarily be degraded and used as a source of energy.[12]

BIOLOGICAL VALUE

The **biological value (BV) of a protein** is a measure of how efficiently food protein can be turned into body tissues. If a food possesses enough of all nine essential amino acids, it should allow a person to efficiently incorporate the food protein into body proteins. The biological value of a food, then, depends on how closely its amino acid pattern reflects the amino acid pattern in body tissues. The better the match, the more completely food protein turns into body protein.[4]

$$BV = \frac{\text{nitrogen retained}}{\text{nitrogen absorbed}} = \frac{\text{dietary nitrogen} - (\text{urinary nitrogen} + \text{fecal nitrogen})}{\text{dietary nitrogen} - \text{fecal nitrogen}}$$

We actually measure protein retention by measuring nitrogen retention. Nitrogen itself is easier to measure than protein, and all amino acids contain nitrogen. Both humans and laboratory animals are used to generate data for determining biological value of food proteins.

If the amino acid pattern in a food is quite unlike tissue amino acid patterns, many amino acids in the food will not become body protein. They simply become "leftovers." Their nitrogen groups are removed and excreted in the urine as urea. The remaining carbon skeleton is converted to either glucose or fat or is used to meet energy needs (Figure 5-3). Since the nitrogen is not retained, the ratio of retained nitrogen to absorbed nitrogen, and the consequent biological value, is small.[4]

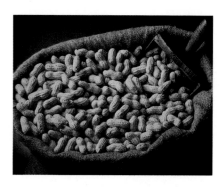

Eaten alone, as a sole source of protein, peanuts have a low biological value. This value is enhanced if other food sources of protein, such as wheat protein or animal protein, accompany the peanuts.

Egg-white protein has the highest biological value of any single food protein. Milk and meat proteins also have high biological values. This makes sense because humans and other animals have similar tissue amino acid compositions. Because plant amino acid patterns differ greatly from those of humans, corn has only a moderate biological value of 70; it is high enough to support body maintenance, but not growth. Peanuts consumed as the only source of protein show a low biological value of about 40.

As with essential amino acids, the importance of the biological value of a single food can be overemphasized. It is the biological value of an entire meal that must be considered. Rarely does a meal yield a low biological value overall, even if only plant foods are eaten. The amino acids in the peanuts and bread of a peanut butter and jelly sandwich combine to yield complete protein. In other words, the two proteins complement each other. Given a variety of foods in a meal, different amino acids usually combine to yield complete protein. This results in a good overall amino acid pattern and hence a high biological value for the meal.[1]

Biological value is a very important consideration in treating some kidney and liver diseases. These organs must help metabolize and dispose of extra amino acids, especially their nitrogen groups. In treating these diseases, it is desirable to have as much dietary protein as possible synthesized into body tissues, with as few amino acids left over to burden the already elevated blood urea ($H_2N-\overset{\overset{\text{O}}{\|}}{C}-NH_2$) or ammonia ($NH_3$) levels. Egg or milk proteins, then, are the sources of choice.[4] These provide high biological value, in turn allowing protein synthesis to occur without generating large amounts of unused amino acids.

PROTEIN EFFICIENCY RATIO

The **protein efficiency ratio (PER)** is another means of measuring a food's protein quality. FDA uses this method to set standards for labeling of foods intended for infants. The PER compares the amount of weight (in grams) gained by a growing rat after 10 days or more of eating a standard amount of protein (9.09% of its energy intake) from a single protein source to the grams of protein consumed.[4]

$$PER = \frac{\text{weight gained during a given period (grams)}}{\text{protein intake during that period (grams)}}$$

The PER of a food reflects its biological value, since both basically measure protein retention by body tissues. Plant proteins, because of their incomplete nature, yield low PER values, while the values of animal proteins are higher. However, as with biological value, the low PER values for individual plant proteins are often of little consequence. Usually we eat many foods—not just one—at a meal. The PER of a peanut butter sandwich is higher than that of either the bread or peanut butter alone. Why?

CHEMICAL SCORE OF PROTEINS

chemical score A ratio comparing the essential amino acid content of the protein in a food with the essential amino acid content in a reference protein, such as one established by the Food and Agriculture Organization of the United Nations; the lowest ratio for any essential amino acid in the protein becomes its chemical score.

Protein quality of a food can be estimated by its chemical score. To calculate a food's **chemical score,** the amount of each essential amino acid provided by a gram of the food's protein is divided by an "ideal" amount for that essential amino acid per gram of food protein. The "ideal" protein pattern is based on the minimal amount (in milligrams) of each of the nine essential amino acids that is needed per gram of food protein.

$$\text{chemical score} = \frac{\text{milligrams of essential amino acid per gram of test protein} \times 100}{\text{milligrams of essential amino acid per gram of the "ideal" protein}}$$

The lowest amino acid ratio calculated for any essential amino acid is the chemical score. Various "ideal" patterns are available. The pattern set by the Food and Agriculture Organization (FAO) of the United Nations for preschool children is often used. It is designed to represent the amino acid content in human tissue proteins. Note that, because children need a greater percentage of protein as essential amino acids than do adults, applying the children's standard to adults underestimates the chemical score value for adults.[4]

For an example of a chemical score calculation, assume that the "ideal" lysine level in a diet is 5.1% or 5.1 mg/100 mg of total protein. Wheat protein is most deficient in lysine, with a concentration of 2.4% of total protein. The chemical score for wheat is:

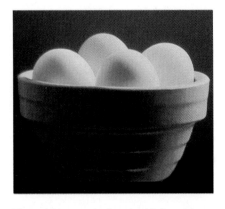

Egg white protein has the highest biological value of any single food protein.

$$\frac{2.4}{5.1} = 0.47, \text{ or } 47\% \text{ of needs}$$

The chemical score is quite similar in concept to biological value, since both are based on meeting the body's need for the right balance of essential amino acids. The main advantage of the chemical score method is that it can easily be determined because of the availability of instruments able to measure the amino acid content of a food. There are two disadvantages of using the chemical score for protein evaluation: (1) it does not consider digestibility; and (2) it does not take into account whether toxic substances, such as those present in some root crops and tubers, are also present in the source of the food protein. Feeding the protein to animals, as is done for a biological value or PER determination, indicates both.

PROTEIN DIGESTIBILITY CORRECTED AMINO ACID SCORE (PDCAAS)

Protein Digestibility Corrected Amino Acid Score (PDCAAS) A measure of protein quality that has recently been accepted by FDA. This replaces PER evaluations for foods intended for children over 4 years of age and for nonpregnant adults. The PDCAAS of a protein is based on its chemical score multiplied by digestibility.

An additional measure of protein quality that has recently been accepted by FDA is the **Protein Digestibility Corrected Amino Acid Score (PDCAAS).** This replaces PER evaluations for foods intended for children over 1 year of age and for nonpregnant adults.[14] To calculate the PDCAAS of a protein, its chemical score is determined. This chemical score varies from 0 to 1. The example of wheat (see above) would be expressed as 0.47. The score is then multiplied by the digestibility of the protein (generally 0.8 to 1.0), in turn yielding the PDCAAS. The PDCAAS for wheat would be about 0.47 × 0.90, which equals about 0.40. The maximum value is 1.0, which is the value of milk, eggs, and soy protein.[14] A protein totally lacking any of the nine essential amino acids will have a PDCAAS of 0, since its chemical score is 0.

For labeling purposes, protein content, listed as % Daily Value, is reduced when the PDCAAS is less than 1. For example, if the protein content of ½ cup of spaghetti is 3 g, only 1.2 g will be counted when calculating % Daily Value, since the PDCAAS of wheat is 0.40 (3 g × 0.40 = 1.2).[14] Recall from Chapter 2 that a manufacturer may choose not to list the % Daily Value for protein on food products intended for older children and adults. Only the gram amount of protein need be listed, and this latter figure is not adjusted for PDCAAS. FDA allows the calculation of % Daily Value to be omitted for two reasons: (1) it is expensive for the manufacturer to determine PDCAAS; and (2) protein is generally abundant in the American diet.

Again, keep in mind that we usually eat meals, not single foods, as protein sources. The concepts of PDCAAS and PER as related to food labels are important. And biological value is useful in designing diets for sick people. Chemical score is useful in evaluating individual proteins for famine relief and in determining the effects of processing on food proteins. However, if you eat enough protein from a variety of foods, you will meet your essential amino acid needs.[12]

CONCEPT CHECK

Protein quality can be measured by determining a food's biological value. This essentially represents the body's ability to retain the food protein absorbed. Protein quality can also be measured by a food's ability to support weight gain in a young growing rat: this measurement is the protein efficiency ratio. To simply estimate protein quality, the essential amino acid composition of the protein can be compared with a reference protein. A chemical score can then be calculated that indicates how well the food protein matches body tissue needs. This value multiplied by the digestibility of the protein yields the Protein Digestibility Corrected Amino Acid Score (PDCAAS). The protein quality values of individual foods are important, but the protein quality of a total meal is more important.

The Recommended Dietary Allowance for Protein

How much protein (actually, how much of each essential amino acid) do we need to consume each day? If a person is not growing, he or she simply needs to eat enough protein to match daily losses from the urine, feces, skin, hair, nails, and so on. In short, the person needs to balance protein intake with protein losses. This maintains the body in protein equilibrium.[4]

When either growing or recovering from an illness, the body needs to achieve a positive protein balance to supply the resources needed for producing new tissues. Consequently, protein intake must exceed daily losses. Extra protein intake is not sufficient, however; this positive balance also requires an appropriate hormonal state. The hormones insulin, growth hormone, and testosterone all promote positive protein balance and allow the body to build extra tissues.[4]

During starvation or illness, protein losses from the body often exceed intake, and the body enters a state of negative protein balance. Hormones that promote this state are cortisol and thyroid hormone (Figure 5-8). They both increase muscle tissue breakdown.[20]

To measure the balance between protein gain and loss by the body, we actually calculate nitrogen balance; only the nitrogen from proteins is excreted to any degree by the body. Nitrogen makes up about 16% of the weight of a protein. So nitrogen intake or output divided by 0.16 yields a rough estimate of protein intake or output. We can also multiply by the reciprocal of 0.16, which is 6.25:

$$\text{nitrogen (grams)} \times 6.25 = \text{protein (grams)}$$

In a healthy person, the amount of dietary protein needed to maintain protein (nitrogen) balance can be determined by increasing protein intake until it just equals protein loss. Energy needs must be met so that amino acids are not diverted for energy use. Any protein intake above that needed for protein equilibrium will lead to an equal output. To estimate the requirement, however, we actually need to determine the least amount of protein intake that still allows intake to equal output. An optimal protein intake should yield a balance in the rate of protein synthesis and breakdown. Too little protein in the diet will slow protein synthesis and may not allow it to keep up with breakdown.[12]

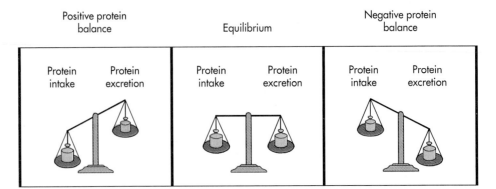

Positive protein balance   Equilibrium   Negative protein balance

Situations in which protein balance is positive:

Growth
Pregnancy
Recovery stage after illness
Athletic training*
Increased secretion of hormones, such as insulin, growth hormone, and testosterone

Situations in which protein balance is negative:

Inadequate intake of protein (fasting, intestinal tract diseases)
Inadequate energy intake
Conditions such as fevers, burns, and infections
Bed rest (for several days)
Deficiency of essential amino acids
Increased protein loss (as in some kidney diseases)
Increased secretion of certain hormones, such as thyroid hormone and cortisol

*Only when additional lean body mass is being gained. Nevertheless, the athlete is probably already eating enough protein to support this extra protein synthesis; protein supplements are not needed.

Figure 5-8 Protein balance in practical terms.

RDA calculations

$$\frac{154 \text{ pounds}}{2.2 \text{ pounds/kg}} = 70 \text{ kg}$$

$$70 \text{ kg} \times \frac{0.8 \text{ g protein}}{\text{kg body weight}} = 56 \text{ g protein}$$

Edward Smith, a British physician, studied energy and protein metabolism and in 1862 concluded that a physically active man needs 80 g of protein daily. During the next 40 years, other estimates of protein needs, based on records of protein amounts consumed by healthy working men, ranged up to 150 g/day. A controversy developed in the early 1900s after Russell Chittenden, an American chemist, concluded from studies on himself, his colleagues, and students at Yale University that only 35 to 45 g of protein was required daily for healthy adults.

Today the best estimate for the amount of protein required for nearly all adults is 0.8 g of protein per kilogram of desirable body weight. This is half the amount needed during infancy.[4] (We discuss specific values for infants and children in Chapter 17 and the concept of desirable weight in Chapter 8.) Desirable weight is used as a baseline because excess fat storage doesn't increase protein needs much. This recommended amount works out to a daily intake of about 56 g of protein for a 70 kg (154 pound) man and about 44 g of protein for a 55 kg (120 pound) woman. Approximate protein needs, based on the 1989 RDA publication, are listed in the inside cover of this textbook.

An RDA is an allowance, not a requirement. Though some people require less protein than the RDA, it is easy to consume the amount of protein suggested each day to meet body needs (Table 5-3). American men typically consume about 105 g of protein daily, whereas women typically consume 65 g daily.[21] Most Americans eat many high-protein foods. It is in fact difficult for the average adult to keep protein intake at RDA guidelines unless very little meat, poultry, and fish are eaten. Meeting energy needs by adults essentially guarantees that protein needs will be met.

We have noted that excess protein cannot be stored. The nitrogen group is removed, and the carbon skeleton is converted to glucose or fat and then either stored or used for energy needs (Figure 5-3).

TABLE 5-3

The protein content of a 1400 kcal diet and a 2400 kcal diet*

1200 kcal diet	Protein (g)	2400 kcal diet	Protein (g)
Breakfast			
Nonfat milk, 1 cup	8	2% milk, 1 cup	8
Cheerios, ¾ cup	3	Cheerios, ¾ cup	3
Orange	—	Eggs, soft-boiled, 2	12
		Orange	—
Lunch			
Whole-wheat bread, 2 slices	7	Whole-wheat bread, 2 slices	7
Chicken breast, 2 oz	18	Chicken breast, 2 oz	18
Mayonnaise, 1 tsp	—	Provolone cheese, 2 oz	13
Tomato slices, 2	—	Tomato slices, 2	—
Carrot sticks, 1 cup	1	Mayonnaise, 1 tsp	—
Fig	0.5	Oatmeal-raisin cookies, 2	2
Diet soda	—	Figs, 2	1
		Diet soda	—
Dinner			
Mixed green salad, ½ cup	—	Mixed green salad, ½ cup	—
Italian dressing, 2 tsp	—	Italian dressing, 2 tsp	—
Beef tenderloin, 2 oz	18	Beef tenderloin, 4 oz	36
Spinach pasta, 1 cup, with garlic butter, 1 tsp	7	Spinach pasta, 1 cup, with garlic butter, 1 tsp	7
Zucchini, ½ cup, sautéed in oil, 1 tsp	0.5	Zucchini, ½ cup, sauteed in oil, 1 tsp	0.5
Nonfat milk, 1 cup	8	Carrot sticks, ½ cup	1
Bagel, toasted, ½	4	**Snack**	
Jam, 2 tsp	—	2% milk, 1 cup	8
		Bagel, toasted	7
		Jam, 2 tsp	—
TOTAL	75 g	Fruited yogurt, 1 cup	10
			133

*This table illustrates how little energy need be consumed while still meeting the RDA for protein. It also shows how much protein we eat when we consume typical energy intakes.

Mental stress, physical labor, and routine weekend sports activities do not require an increase in the protein RDA. To support training needs of endurance athletes, substantial gains in muscle tissue in highly trained athletes, or a large muscle mass formerly acquired, increasing the allowance up to 1.5 times the RDA might be considered. But there is no demonstrated advantage in exceeding 1.5 g of protein per kilogram of desirable body weight per day. Many Americans, especially men, eat that much protein already.[21] Protein intakes above usual adult intakes are rarely needed for athletes. In addition, there is usually no reason for athletes to take either protein or individual amino acid supplements. All of us, athletes included, can meet our protein needs using basic foods.

Surveys show that only elderly women as a group fail to eat enough protein to meet the RDA, and the discrepancy is very slight.[21] The elderly also may have slightly higher protein needs than those set by the RDA. Some researchers advocate up to 1.25 g of protein per kg of desirable body weight. If elderly people eat inadequate amounts of protein, which they may do because their energy intake is so low, they can suffer loss in muscle mass.

ARE AMERICANS' HIGH PROTEIN INTAKES HARMFUL?

The question is often asked whether the high protein intake of adults in America is harmful. The extra vitamin B-6, iron, and zinc that accompany protein foods are of-

Infants' diets must not contain excess protein because their kidneys have difficulty excreting the excess urea and minerals remaining after protein metabolism. Thus regular cow's milk must not be used by itself for feeding young infants—it is too high in protein and other nutrients (see Chapter 17 for details).

osteoporosis A bone disease characterized by decreased bone density, which
develops primarily after menopause in
women.

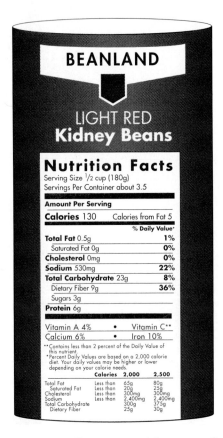

Figure 5-9 Legumes are rich sources of
protein. One-half cup meets about 10%
of daily protein needs, and at a "cost"
of only about 5% of energy needs. The
addition of dietary fiber to the diet is an
added bonus.[8]

CRITICAL THINKING

Leon, a vegetarian, has heard of the "all-
or-none law" of protein synthesis but
doesn't understand how this law applies
to protein synthesis in the body. He
asks you, "How important is this nutritional concept for diet planning?" How
would you answer his question?

ten beneficial, but research in the 1970s suggested that a diet high in animal protein
increased calcium loss in the urine. This concerned researchers, who thought that
protein caused calcium to leach out of the bones. Animal proteins were singled out
because they are rich in sulfur-containing amino acids, and the acidic nature of these
amino acids tends to draw calcium out of the body in order to neutralize the acid.[13]
Populations in areas of the world where animal protein intake is high also show the
highest rates of **osteoporosis,** but this is associated with other factors as well, such
as inadequate calcium intake and exercise, excessive alcohol intake, and smoking.

The RDA for calcium is set high to compensate for the calcium loss induced by
the high protein intake of Americans. Also, follow-up studies showed that if extra
phosphorus is consumed with animal proteins, urinary calcium does not increase so
much. Animal foods are excellent sources of both protein and phosphorus. In addition, women are at highest risk of osteoporosis, and their protein intakes are generally only moderately above RDA guidelines. Thus typical American protein intakes
of women probably don't significantly contribute to the risk of osteoporosis, as long
as the RDA for calcium is met, but amounts greatly in excess of the RDA may do so.

A high red meat intake is linked to colon cancer in population studies.[10] This link
could be attributable to the protein or fat in the food products or to substances that
form during cooking of red meat at high temperatures. Excessive fat intake associated with diets rich in red meat, or low dietary fiber intake, may also be contributing factors. More research on this topic is needed before red meat can be singled
out as a causative factor.

There is also some concern that a high protein intake may unduly burden the
kidneys to excrete the resulting excess nitrogen (mostly as urea) into the urine.
Low-protein diets marginally slow the decline in kidney function in humans if begun early in the course of developing kidney disease,[17] and laboratory animal studies show that protein intakes that just meet nutritional needs preserve kidney function over time better than high-protein diets. Preserving kidney function is especially important for people with diabetes and for people who show signs of kidney
disease, such as excess urea in the blood, or who have only one functioning kidney.
High-protein diets are discouraged in these cases.[17] For people without diabetes or
kidney disease, the risk of suffering kidney failure is very low, and thus the risk of a
high-protein diet contributing to kidney disease in later life is also low.

Overall, the caution against high protein intake issued by the National Academy
of Sciences in their 1989 *Diet and Health Report* deserves consideration. The panel
recommended that not more than twice the RDA for protein be consumed on a
regular basis. Reducing intake to approximately RDA amounts may benefit some of
us, as pointed out above, but the research is still too incomplete to permit a firm
conclusion.

THE IMPORTANCE OF PLANT PROTEINS

Vegetable proteins deserve more attention.[8] These proteins, in proportion to the
amount of energy they supply, provide much magnesium, soluble fiber, and other
important nutrients. Whenever the USDA has rated foods according to the best
protein buy, dry beans have always been at or near the top of the list. Furthermore,
vegetable proteins contain no cholesterol and are naturally low in saturated fat and
high in dietary fiber (Figure 5-9).

As we discovered in Chapter 2, one to two servings of plant proteins per day is
consistent with the recommendations of the Food Guide Pyramid. Presently, plant
proteins are not very popular in America, except for peanut butter, baked beans, and
refried beans. They deserve a second look.

When one first adds plant proteins, such as beans, to the diet, they may cause intestinal gas. Split peas, limas, and lentils are less likely to do so then the others, so
start with them. Taking them in small servings at first and giving the gastrointestinal tract a few weeks to adjust, helps.

Another way to reduce the tendency for beans to produce intestinal gas is in the
method in which they are cooked. Dry beans should be cooked in boiling water for

3 minutes to soften them. Then the heat should be turned off and the beans left covered to soak for a few hours, during which much of the indigestable sugars will leach into the water. The water should then be poured off and the beans further cooked in fresh water as desired. This practice leads to some vitamin loss, but does not affect protein or dietary fiber content. For canned beans, draining and rinsing with water is an excellent way of producing beans with lower undigestable sugars content.

Many people have no trouble digesting beans and other legumes, but it's best to be cautious. As we discussed in Chapter 3, an enzyme preparation called Beano is also available to ease gas symptoms. Taken right before a meal in tablet or liquid form in the dose suggested on the package, it helps break down the undigestable carbohydrates in beans that contribute to intestinal gas. Beano is made from mold, so persons sensitive to molds may react allergically and should avoid it or use with caution. For more information or free samples, contact the manufacturer (800-257-8650).

CONCEPT CHECK

The Recommended Dietary Allowance of protein for adults is 0.8 g of protein per kg of desirable body weight. For a 70 kg (156 pound) person, this means 56 g of protein per day. The average American man consumes about 105 g of protein per day, and the average woman consumes about 65 g of protein per day. Thus typical American protein intakes are more than ample to meet protein needs, except for some elderly women.

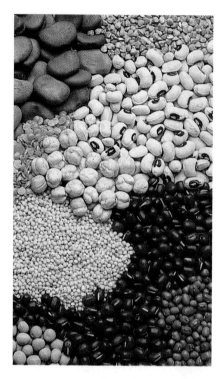

Legumes can meet the body's need for protein, as well as supply other nutrients.

Proteins in Foods

The Exchange System provides an easy means of estimating the protein content of a food. The fruit and fat lists contain no protein; the vegetable list yields 2 g of protein; the starch list yields 3 g of protein; the meat list yields 7 g of protein; and the milk list yields 8 g of protein.

The most nutrient-dense source of protein is water-packed tuna, which has over 80% of energy as protein. Of the typical foods we eat, those with more than 20% of energy as protein are animal foods. They are also the major sources of protein in the American diet; over 65% of our protein comes from animal sources (Figure 5-10). In the United States, meat, poultry, and fish consumption amounts to about 145 pounds (weight without bones) per person per year. Worldwide, 35% of protein comes from animal sources. In Africa and East Asia, about 20% of the protein eaten comes from animals.

The amino acids most likely to be low in a diet are lysine, methionine, threonine, and tryptophan. Table 5-2 lists plant foods that are characteristically low in these amino acids, although new strains of high-lysine and high-tryptophan corn are now available, as well as other improved grains. These strains yield better protein quality.

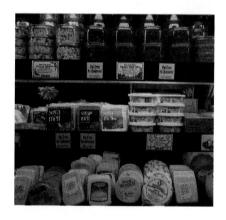

Both animal and vegetable products contribute to protein nutriture.

POTENTIAL FOR AMINO ACID TOXICITY

The amino acids most likely to be toxic when consumed in large amounts are methionine and tyrosine. The potential for amino acid imbalances and toxicities is too great to recommend that any be taken individually as supplements.[4]

As a case in point, recently an unexpected increase in cases of eosinophilia-myalgia syndrome has been reported. The condition leads to marked changes in the blood, severe muscle and joint pain, swelling in the limbs, skin rash, and occasionally fever, which can run as high as 105° F. Deaths have been reported. Through careful detective work, it was found that many of these cases were associated with the consumption of the amino acid, L-tryptophan.[15] Eventually, it was discovered that this may have been the result of a contaminant introduced into the tryptophan

It is always wise to weigh the documented benefits against the risks when self-prescribing nutrient supplements, including amino acids.

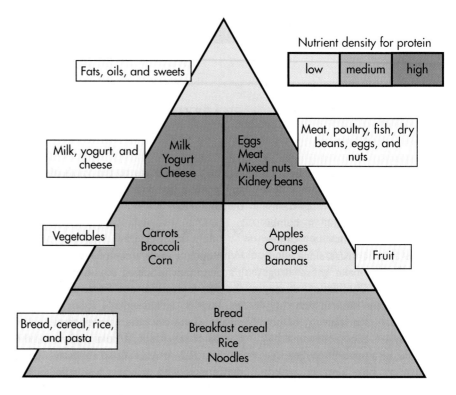

Figure 5-10 Sources of protein in foods from the Food Guide Pyramid. The fruit group, vegetable group, and fats, oils, and sweets group contain few foods rich in protein. The background color of each group indicates the average nutrient density for protein in that group.

supplement, but there is some suspicion that tryptophan shares some of the blame. In response to this outbreak of eosinophilia-myalgia syndrome, FDA ordered a recall of all L-tryptophan supplements.[15]

People were using L-tryptophan supplements for a variety of problems, including insomnia, premenstrual syndrome, depression, and attention deficiencies in children. FDA had not approved its use for any of these problems.

The risk associated with taking L-tryptophan supplements is not the main point here. Amino acid supplements are not necessary, because everyone's protein needs, including those of athletes, can be easily met through diet (see Chapter 10). There are no significant amounts of free amino acids in our food, nor is there any dietary need for, or unique dietary value from, consuming free amino acids.[15]

Protein Deficiency Conditions

In nonindustrialized areas of the world, people often eat diets low in energy and protein. Such diets retard growth and increase susceptibility to disease. A person who eats too little protein and energy food can develop symptoms of undernutrition, usually called **protein-energy malnutrition (PEM)** but also referred to as protein-calorie malnutrition (PCM).[19] Although the number of people who have PEM is difficult to determine because of the inaccessibility of some areas of occurrence and because of variation in interpretation of definitions, the World Health Organization (WHO) estimates that at least 500 million children worldwide suffer from PEM. Common factors that contribute to PEM, especially in young children, are listed in Table 5-4.

In the United States and other industrialized countries, PEM exists in hospitalized patients, where it may be secondary to other conditions, such as AIDS, pulmonary disease, malabsorption syndromes, kidney and liver ailments, cancer, and anorexia nervosa.

protein-energy malnutrition (PEM) A condition resulting from insufficient consumption of energy and protein. The deficiency eventually results in body wasting and an increased susceptibility to infections.

TABLE 5-4

Factors contributing to protein-energy malnutrition in young children[19]

1. Younger children's relative needs for protein and energy (per kilogram of body weight) are greater than those of older family members.
2. Diets that are of low energy density (often high in fiber and unappealing), low in protein, and not fed frequently enough.
3. Not enough food for the family as a result of poverty, inequity, and insufficient land to farm; and inappropriate food distribution within the family.
4. Infections (viral, bacterial, and parasitic) may cause lack of appetite, reduced food intake, diarrhea, or poor nutrient absorption and utilization, or may result in nutrient losses.
5. Famine caused by droughts, natural disasters, wars, and civil disturbances.
6. Inappropriate formula preparation and weaning practices; inappropriate use of infant formula in place of breastfeeding in poor families or in areas with an unsanitary water supply.

It is difficult to tell whether a person with a mild form of PEM is suffering primarily from an inadequate intake of energy, protein, or both. As the disease progresses, and depending in part on the age of onset, the symptoms are primarily those of general starvation (**marasmus**) or those of not meeting protein needs in the face of high requirements (**kwashiorkor**). Similarities can be seen in the disorders (Figure 5-11).[19]

KWASHIORKOR

Kwashiorkor is a word from Ghana that means "the disease that the first child gets when the new child comes." From birth, an infant is usually breast-fed. By the time the child reaches 1 to 1.5 years, his or her mother is probably pregnant or has already given birth again, and breast-feeding is no longer possible for the first child.[19] This child's diet abruptly changes from nutritious breast milk to native starchy roots and gruels. These foods have low protein densities compared with total energy. The foods are also often so bulky and full of plant fibers that it is difficult for the child to eat enough of them to meet energy needs. The child may also have infections and parasites, which acutely raise energy and protein needs. So energy needs of these children are met marginally, at best, and their protein needs are not met, especially when needs are greatly increased by infections and marginal energy intakes. Usually many vitamin and mineral needs are also far from being met. Famine victims who eat starchy roots, such as cassava (tapioca), face similar problems.

The major symptoms of kwashiorkor are apathy, listlessness, failure to grow and gain weight, and withdrawal from the environment. These symptoms complicate other diseases present and can make conditions such as measles, a disease that normally makes a healthy child ill for only a week or so, severely debilitating and even fatal. Further signs and symptoms of the disease are changes in hair color, potassium deficiency, flaky skin, fatty infiltration in the liver, reduced muscle mass, and massive edema in the abdomen and legs. The presence of edema in a child who has some subcutaneous fat still present is the hallmark of kwashiorkor (see Figure 5-11).[19] In addition, these children hardly move. If you pick them up, they don't cry. When you hold them, you feel the plumpness of edema, not muscle and fat tissue.

We can explain many of the symptoms of kwashiorkor based on what we know about proteins. Proteins play important roles in fluid balance, lipoprotein transport, immune function, and production of tissues such as skin and hair. We should not expect children with an insufficient protein intake to grow and mature normally. And they don't!

If a child with kwashiorkor is helped in time—if infections are treated and the child is fed a diet ample in protein, energy, and other essential nutrients—the disease process reverses. The child begins to grow again and may even show no signs

marasmus A disease that results from consuming a grossly insufficient amount of protein and energy; one of the diseases classed as protein-energy malnutrition. Victims will have little or no fat stores, little muscle mass, and poor strength. Death from infections is common.

kwashiorkor A disease occurring primarily in young children who have an existing disease and consume a marginal amount of energy and considerably insufficient protein in the face of high needs. The child generally suffers from infections and exhibits edema, poor growth, weakness, and an increased susceptibility to further illness.

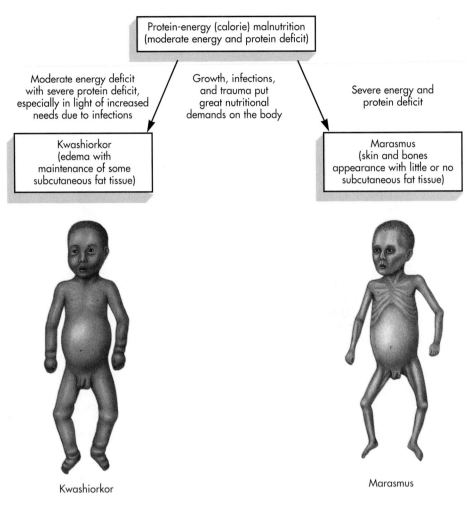

FIGURE 5-11 A schema for classifying undernutrition. The presence of subcutaneous fat (directly underneath the skin) is a diagnostic key.[19]

of his or her previous condition, except perhaps shortness of stature. Unfortunately, by the time many of these children reach a hospital or care center, they already have severe infections. In spite of the best care, they still die. Or, if they survive, they return home only to repeat the cycle.

MARASMUS

Marasmus typically occurs as an infant slowly starves to death. It is caused by consumption of greatly insufficient amounts of protein, energy, and other nu-trients. The condition is also commonly referred to as *protein-energy malnutrition,* especially when experienced by older children and adults. The word *marasmus* means "to waste away." Victims have the "skin and bones" appearance you see on posters from relief agencies (See Figure 5-11).[19] Little or no subcutaneous fat is present.

Marasmus commonly develops in infants who either are not breast-fed or have stopped breast-feeding in the early months. Often the weaning formula used is improperly prepared because of unsafe water and because the parents cannot afford sufficient formula for the child's needs. The latter problem may lead the parents to dilute the formula to provide more feedings, not realizing that all this does is provide more water for the infant.

Marasmus in infants commonly occurs in the large cities of poverty-stricken countries. In the cities, it is often necessary to bottle-feed because the infant must be cared for by others when the mother is working or away from home. When people are poor and sanitation is lacking, bottle-feeding often leads to marasmus.[19] An infant with marasmus requires large amounts of energy and protein—like a preterm infant—and unless the child receives them, full recovery from the disease may never occur. Most brain growth takes place between conception and the child's first birthday. In fact, the brain is growing at its highest rate at birth. If the diet does not support brain growth during the first months of life, the brain may not grow to its full adult size. This reduced or retarded brain growth may lead to diminished intellectual function.

Both kwashiorkor and marasmus wreak havoc on infants and children; mortality rates in poorer countries are often 10 to 20 times higher than in the United States. This high mortality rate in part encourages the high birth rate in poorer countries; if a mother wants four children to survive, she had better have ten. The overload of babies makes infant mortality much more likely. The problem is further fueled by politics and war. Better food availability and sanitation would improve the health of many children worldwide. Chapter 20 looks at the issue of undernutrition worldwide in more detail.

KWASHIORKOR AND MARASMUS MALNUTRITION IN THE HOSPITAL

Kwashiorkor can result when a hospitalized patient is fed glucose intravenously for many days, such as when a slow recovery from surgery prevents normal food consumption. Or a person may feel too sick to eat, in spite of the increased nutrient needs caused by his or her disease. Intravenous glucose feeding meets energy needs to some extent but provides no protein. As a result, the person develops edema, and often the immune function is diminished, leaving the patient at great risk for infections. One of the best markers for kwashiorkor is a person's serum albumin. When the value falls below 3.5 g/100 ml, the person is at risk. By the time serum albumin falls to 2.2 g/100 ml, the person is at a very high risk for infections and disease.

Studies have demonstrated that a hospital patient with low body weight, low serum albumin, and a low white blood cell (especially lymphocyte) count is at four to six times greater risk of complications and death than a patient with normal values for those three factors. In the last 15 years, nutrition support teams have been formed in hospitals. One of their missions is to ensure that patients receive enough oral or balanced intravenous nutrition to meet their needs for energy, protein, carbohydrate, and other nutrients.

Marasmus occurs in a hospitalized patient who simply does not receive enough energy and other nutrients. This can be caused by anorexia nervosa, cancer, AIDS, and some intestinal disorders. The person either does not eat enough food or does not absorb enough nutrients from the intestinal tract to meet nutritional needs. Muscle, vital organ tissue, and fat stores waste away, and the person eventually looks like "skin and bones." Death from starvation or heart failure can result. A hospitalized person may also have mixed kwashiorkor-marasmus. This is characterized by edema in a person with greatly diminished fat stores.

Concept Check

If a person regularly consumes a marginal amount of energy and insufficient protein, protein-energy malnutrition (PEM) develops. The person with kwashiorkor, a severe form of this disease, has decreased immune function, edema, weakness, and increased susceptibility to infections. Young children are especially susceptible to kwashiorkor after weaning, especially if they have infections that increase their nutritional needs. Marasmus is another severe form of PEM. This condition results when people, especially infants, continually receive too little food, notably not enough protein or energy. Symptoms that develop include muscle wasting, absence of fat stores, and weakness. Both an adequate diet and treatment of infections or other diseases must be offered if health is to be restored in cases of kwashiorkor and marasmus. This is true in an adult suffering from cancer or AIDS and in an infant suffering from famine; the symptoms of both kwashiorkor and marasmus are seen in these situations.

Summary

1. Amino acids are the building blocks of protein. They contain nitrogen in the form of an amino group. Of the 20 different amino acids found in food, 9 are essential in the diet and 11 can be synthesized by the body if amino groups from extra amino acids are available.

2. High-quality protein foods contain all nine essential amino acids in sufficient quantity for protein synthesis. This is typical of animal foods. Low-quality protein foods lack good supplies of one or more of the essential amino acids. This is typical of plant foods. Two plant foods can be combined to complement each other's amino acid deficiencies, in turn providing a high-quality protein meal.

3. Individual amino acids chemically bond to form proteins. The order (sequence) of the amino acids in the polypeptide chain is important. This order determines the ultimate form and thus the function of the protein. The three-dimensional shape that the protein eventually forms is dictated by the sequence. This structure can be unfolded—denatured—by treatment with heat, acid or alkaline solutions, and other processes. A denatured protein can no longer perform its intended biological activity.

4. Proteins form essential body constituents, such as muscle contractile tissue, connective tissue, transport proteins, visual pigments, enzymes, hormones, and immune bodies. Proteins also provide a source of carbon atoms that can be synthesized into glucose.

5. Protein quality can be measured by determining the extent to which the body can retain the nitrogen contained in the protein absorbed. This ratio of nitrogen retention to nitrogen absorption is called *biological value*. The ability of a food to support the growth of rats is also a measure of protein quality and is known as the *protein-efficiency ratio*. In addition, the balance of essential amino acids in a food can be compared to an ideal pattern. The comparison to the ideal pattern is referred to as the *chemical score*, which predicts the ability of the body to retain in tissues the food protein eaten. When multiplied by the degree of digestibility, the chemical score yields the Protein Digestibility Corrected Amino Acid Score (PDCAAS).

6. The RDA for protein for adults is 0.8 g per kg of desirable body weight. For a 70 kg (156 pound) person, this corresponds to 56 g of protein per day. The average American man consumes about 105 g of protein per day; women consume closer to 65 g of protein per day. Thus American diets generally supply ample protein.

7. Animal proteins are the most nutrient-dense sources of protein. Plant foods generally contain less than 20% of their energy as protein, in contrast to water-packed tuna, which contains over 80% of its energy as protein. Still, plant proteins can provide ample protein to a diet if they are consumed as part of a varied diet.

8. Protein- and energy-deficiency conditions include kwashiorkor and marasmus. These two diseases are difficult to separate and result either from marginal energy intake and insufficient protein intake (kwashiorkor) or from an inadequate intake of both protein and energy (marasmus). Infections, which increase nutritional needs, can tip the balance between health and illness, especially when the diet is limited to a few high-carbohydrate, low-protein foods. Variations of these diseases appear in some hospitalized Americans.

Study Questions

1. Discuss the relative importance of essential and nonessential amino acids in the diet. Why is it important for essential amino acids lost from the body to be replaced in the diet?

2. What are four of the functions of proteins? How does the structure of a protein relate to its functions?

3. What factors can denature proteins?

4. Why is the quality of a protein important? What foods provide high-quality protein?

5. What would be the health-related benefit of preventing protein-energy malnutrition in children worldwide?

6. What characteristics of a vegetarian diet could improve the American diet?

7. What hormones promote gluconeogenesis, and when does gluconeogenesis occur?

8. What are the possible long-term effects of an inadequate intake of dietary protein on children between ages 6 months and 4 years?

9. What foods would you include to provide a diet that has ample protein from both plant and animal sources but is moderate in fat?

REFERENCES

1. ADA Reports: Position of the American Dietetic Association: vegetarian diets, *Journal of the American Dietetic Association* 93:1317, 1993.
2. Christensen HN: Amino acid nutrition: a two-step absorptive process, *Nutrition Reviews* 51:95, 1993.
3. Craig WJ: Iron status of vegetarians, *American Journal of Clinical Nutrition* 59:1233S, 1994.
4. Crim MC, Munro HN: Protein and amino acids. In Shils ME and others, editors: *Modern nutrition in health and disease*, Philadelpia, 1994, Lea & Febiger.
5. Dwyer JT: Vegetarian eating patterns, *American Journal of Clinical Nutrition* 59:1255S, 1994.
6. Farley D: Vegetarian diets, *FDA Consumer*, p 21, May 1992.
7. Fernstrom JD: Dietary amino acids and brain function, *Journal of the American Dietetic Association* 94:71, 1994.
8. Geil PB, Anderson JW: Nutrition and health implications of dry beans: a review, *Journal of the American College of Nutrition*, 13:549, 1994.
9. Gibson RS: Content and bioavailability of trace elements in vegetarian diets, *American Journal of Clinical Nutrition* 59:1223S, 1994.
10. Giovannuci E and others: Intake of fat, meat, and fiber in relation to colon cancer in men, *Cancer Research* 54:2390, 1994.
11. Haddad EH: Development of a vegetarian food guide, *American Journal of Clinical Nutrition* 59:1248S, 1994.
12. Harper AE, Yoshimura NY: Protein quality, amino acid balance, utilization, and evaluation of diets containing amino acids as therapeutic agents, *Nutrition* 9:460, 1993.
13. Heaney RP: Protein intake and calcium economy, *Journal of the American Diabetes Association*, 93:1259, 1993.
14. Henley EC, Kuster JM: Protein quality evaluation by protein digestibility-corrected amino acid scoring, *Food Technology*, April 1994, p 74.
15. Herbert V: l-tryptophan, *Nutrition Today*, p 27, March/April 1992.
16. Herbert V: Staging vitamin B-12 (cobalamin) status in vegetarians, *American Journal of Clinical Nutrition* 59:1213S, 1994.
17. Klahr S and others: The effects of dietary protein restriction and blood-pressure control on the progression of chronic renal disease, *New England Journal of Medicine* 330:877, 1994.
18. Lamberg-Allardt C and others: Low serum 25-hydroxyvitamin D concentrations and secondary hyperparathyroidism in middle-aged white strict vegetarians, *American Journal of Clinical Nutrition* 58:684, 1993.
19. Latham MC: Protein-energy malnutrition. In Brown ML, editor: *Present knowledge in nutrition*, Washington, DC, 1990, International Life Sciences Institute-Nutrition Foundation.
20. Lehninger AL and others, *Principles of biochemistry*, ed 2, New York, 1993.
21. McDowell MA and others: Energy and macronutrient intakes of persons ages 2 months and over in the United States, *Advance Data*, number 225, October 24, 1994, Centers for Disease Control, USDHS.
22. Samuels-Reid JH: Common problems in sickle cell disease, *American Family Physician* 49:1477, 1994.
23. Weaver CM, Plawecki KL: Dietary calcium: adequacy of a vegetarian diet, *American Journal of Clinical Nutrition* 59:1238S5, 1994.
24. Wernerman J, Hammarqvist F: Clinical experiences with glutamine supplementation, *Nutrition* 10:176, 1994.
25. Whorton JC: Historical development of vegetarianism, *American Journal of Clinical Nutrition* 59:1103S, 1994.
26. Young VR, Pellett PL: Plant proteins in relation to human protein and amino acid nutrition, *American Journal of Clinical Nutrition* 59:1203S, 1994.

TAKE ACTION

How much protein do you eat?

How much protein do you eat in a typical day? Look at the nutrition assessment you completed at the end of Chapter 2. Review it closely. Find the figure indicating the amount of protein you consumed during your 1-day record. Write it in the space below:

- -

Total protein

_____

Let's compare this to your RDA for protein. Find your desirable weight in pounds from the height-weight table listed on the inside cover of this book. Choose a mid-range value. Divide it by 2.2. This will give you your desirable weight in kilograms. Next multiply that by 0.8 g/kg of body weight. This will indicate your RDA for protein. Write it in the space below:

RDA for protein

_____

How does your consumption compare to your RDA?

_____

If you consumed either more or less than the RDA, what foods could you add, omit, or eat more of or less of? (Look at the foods you ate.)

_____

Was most of your protein from animal or plant sources?

_____

is milk, which is omitted from the vegan diet. Vitamin D can be obtained through regular sun exposure and fortified margarine. Otherwise, a supplement containing vitamin D should be considered (see Chapter 12).[18]

The vegan should find a reliable source of vitamin B-12, such as fortified soybean milk or special yeast grown on media rich in vitamin B-12. Vitamin B-12 occurs naturally only in animal foods; plants can contain soil or microbial contamination that provides at most a trace amount of vitamin B-12. Because the body can store enough vitamin B-12 for about 4 years, it takes a long time for a deficiency to develop after animal foods are removed from the diet. If a deficiency develops, nerves can be damaged irreversibly and brain function can decrease. Evidence of a vitamin B-12 deficiency has been noted in vegetarian mothers and their infants. The human milk produced by the vegetarian mothers was low in vitamin B-12. The earliest sign of a vitamin B-12 deficiency is mental dysfunction. Therefore vegans need to be careful to prevent a vitamin B-12 deficiency (see Chapter 13).[16]

To obtain calcium, the vegan can drink fortified soybean milk or fortified orange juice, consume calcium-rich tofu (check the label), or consume other calcium-fortified foods, such as certain breakfast cereals and snacks.[23] Green leafy vegetables and nuts also contain calcium, but the calcium is either not well absorbed or not very plentiful. Calcium supplements are another option (see Chapter 14).

For iron, the vegan can consume whole grains, dried fruits and nuts, and legumes. The iron in these foods is not absorbed as well as that found in animal foods, but a good source of vitamin C taken with these foods enhances iron absorption. Thus an excellent strategy is to consume vitamin C with every meal that contains adequate iron-rich plant foods.[3]

The vegan can find zinc in whole grains, nuts, and legumes, but phytic acid in whole grains limits zinc absorption. Grains are most nutritious when leavened, as in bread, because this process reduces the influence of phytic acid.[9]

Of all these nutrients, calcium is the most difficult to consume in sufficient quantities. Special diet planning is required.[23]

Veganism during childhood can pose problems. The sheer bulk of a plant-based diet may make it difficult for a child to eat foods that supply enough energy to permit dietary protein to be used for synthesis of body proteins, rather than used for energy needs. Vegan children need concentrated sources of energy to avoid this problem.[1] Examples include fortified soybean milk, nuts, dried fruits, avocados, cookies made with vegetable oils or tub margarine, and fruit juices.

Soy milk, soy yogurt, and soy cheese are excellent choices for vegan children (and vegan adults). When fortified with calcium and vitamin B-12, these substitutes can provide many of the key nutrients found in milk.

Finding excellent zinc sources is important in planning vegan diets for infants and children.[9] Overall, both infancy and childhood are life stages in which vegetarianism is appropriate, but it must be implemented with knowledge and professional guidance.[1]

TABLE 5-6

Nutrients likely to be marginal in the diet of a total vegetarian (vegan)	
Nutrient	**Plant sources**
Vitamin D	Fortified margarine, fortified breakfast cereal
Riboflavin	Whole and enriched grains, leafy vegetables, mushrooms, beans, nuts, seeds
Vitamin B-12	Fortified breakfast cereal, fortified yeast, fortified soy milk
Iron	Whole grains, prune juice, dried fruits, beans, nuts, seeds, leafy vegetables
Calcium	Fortified soy milk, tofu, almonds, dry beans, leafy vegetables, some fortified breakfast cereals, flour, certain brands of orange juice, and certain snacks
Zinc	Whole grains, wheat germ, beans, nuts, seeds

The terminus of the larg[...]
to the anus. These final secti[...]
pare the feces for eliminatio[...]

The liver, pancreas, and [...]
cal part of it.[6] The liver prov[...]
is stored in the gallbladder t[...]
bladder and connects with t[...]
other products from the pa[...]
num for digestion.

GASTROINTESTINAL C[...]

A **sphincter** is a circular m[...]
to regulate passage or flow [...]
ters, which respond to stil[...]
and pressure that builds up [...]

The flow of food throi[...]
esophageal sphincters. The [...]
sphincter due to its proxir[...]
contents into the esophag[...]
tions in the esophagus, wh[...]

In the oral cavity, saliva is secreted [...]
food is ingested. The food is then ch[...]
and broken down, and digestion of [...]
carbohydrates begins before the fo[...]
is swallowed.

Liver produces and secretes 1 to 6 [...]
(250–1000 ml) of bile per day. Thi[...]
is secreted into the duodenum via tl[...]
gallbladder.

Pancreatic juice contains a wide vc[...]
of digestive enzymes that are secre[...]
into the duodenum. These enzyme[...]
include trypsin, which digests prot[...]
amylase, which digests starch; and [...]
which digests fats. Enzymes on the [...]
border of the small intestine help t[...]
complete digestion.

Gallbladder stores and concentra[...]

Large intestine receives food resic[...]
small intestine; absorbs water an[...]
minerals; forms, stores, and help[...]
feces.

Rectum stores feces and expels [...]
via the anus.

Figure 6-3 Physiology c[...]
low digestion and subse[...]

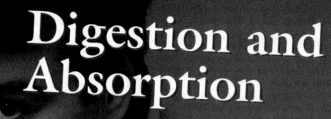

Digestion and Absorption

Merely ingesting foods doesn't nourish you. Only after the nutrients contained in the foods have been released and then absorbed can they be taken up by the bloodstream and distributed to all of your body's cells.[6] The major organs involved in this process are the gastrointestinal tract, pancreas, liver, and gallbladder.

We can take our digestion and absorption system for granted because most of the processes involved are autonomic; that is, they control themselves. We don't decide when the pancreas secretes digestive enzymes into the small intestine, what the liver does with absorbed glucose, or how quickly food is propelled through the intestinal tract. Hormones, hormone-like compounds, and nerves control these functions.[6] The only two voluntary responses are deciding how well to chew food and when to eliminate the fecal remains. Thus while you go about your daily routine—playing tennis, working in a laboratory, walking from class to class, or eating lunch—many digestive reactions and functions occur automatically in your gastrointestinal tract. Let's examine these processes.

CRITICAL THINKING

James has a cold and doesn't ha
appetite. He says that he can't
guish the flavors of the foods h
they all taste the same. How ca
explain this?

- - - - - - - - -

At autopsy, the small intestine
relax, allowing the jejunum and
to lengthen to about 11 feet (3
each. The small intestine is th
23 feet (7.1 m) long, a figure o
in textbooks.

- - - - - - - - -

GI tract flow

Mouth
↓
Esophagus
↓
Stomach—4-cup (1 L) capaci
mains about 2 to 3 hours. Hig
take the longest time to emp
↓
Small intestine—duodenum (
long), jejunum (4 feet long), i
long)—about 10 feet (3.1 m)
length; food remains about 3
↓
Large intestine (colon)—cec
ing colon, transverse colon, c
colon, sigmoid colon—3 1/2
in total length; food can rem
hours.

- - - - - - - - -

NUTRITION FOCUS

BODY SYSTEMS USED IN DIGESTION AND ABSORPTION

The body is composed of millions of **cells.** Each is a self-contained, living entity (see Chapter 7 for a drawing of a typical cell). Cells of the same type bond together using intercellular substances to form **tissues,** such as bone, cartilage, muscle, and nerve. Often two or more tissues combine in a particular way to form more complex **organs,** such as skin, kidneys, and the liver. At still higher levels of coordination, several organs can cooperate for a common purpose to form an **organ system,** such as the respiratory system or digestive system. The human body is a coordinated unit of many such organ systems.[6]

Every cell in the human body performs a specialized job. A cell's master plan for work and for the necessary machinery to do that work is all encoded into the cell's genetic material, the **DNA** (deoxyribonucleic acid). The DNA acts as a blueprint for synthesizing specific proteins, often enzymes, required to perform specific tasks. Even though most cells in an organism contain the same DNA information, cells throughout the body are programmed differently. As the embryo forms, different parts of the DNA become active in different cell types. For example, the intestinal cells make digestive enzymes; in the bone marrow, cells that make the oxygen-carrying protein hemoglobin become active.

Chemical reactions occur all the time in every living cell. Synthesis of new substances is balanced by the breaking down of older ones. For this turnover to occur, cells require a continuous supply of energy. Most cells need oxygen to extract this energy from nutrients for cell use. Cells also need water, the medium in which they live. They further need building blocks, especially the materials they can't make themselves—the essential nutrients supplied from food. All these substances enable the tissues, composed of individual cells, to function properly.

An adequate supply of all nutrients to body cells is the result of a healthful diet. But to ensure optimal use of these nutrients by cells, the following systems, in addition to the digestive system, must work efficiently.

CIRCULATORY SYSTEM

The blood follows two general routes. It circulates between the right side of the heart and the lungs (the pulmonary circuit) and between the left side of the heart and all other body parts (the systemic circuit) (Figure 6-7). The heart is a muscular pump that normally contracts and relaxes 50 to 90 times a minute while the body is at rest.

This continuous pumping action keeps blood moving through the body.[6]

The circulatory system distributes nutrients from digestion and oxygen from the air we breathe to all body cells. All blood goes to the lungs to pick up oxygen and release carbon dioxide. The oxygenated blood returns to the heart to be pumped to all other body tissues. In the capillaries, cells exchange nutrients and waste with the blood—cells empty their waste products into the blood and take nutrients from it. Capillaries, networks of tiny blood vessels, serve every region of the body via individual capillary beds one cell thick. Nutrients, gases, and other substances can pass through capillary cells both into and out of other body cells.[6]

The lymphatic system of circulatory vessels serves the body by carrying lymph, the clear fluid formed between cells (see Figure 6-7). This fluid filters into tiny lymphatic vessels, which compose a one-way network that funnels lymph from all over the body into two large lymphatic vessels that empty into major veins returning to the heart.[6]

Lymphatic vessels that serve the small intestine have an important role in nutrition. These vessels pick up and transport the majority of products released from fat absorption—those substances too large to enter the bloodstream directly. The lymphatic vessels from the intestine drain into a large duct, called the thoracic duct, that stretches from the abdomen to the neck. This duct connects with the bloodstream through a vein near the neck. In this way the majority of absorbed fat-soluble products eventually enter the bloodstream.[13] Other parts of the lymphatic system play a key role in the immune system.

EXCRETORY SYSTEM

The kidneys, digestive tract, skin, and lungs all remove wastes from the body. The primary function of the kidneys is to regulate the **extracellular fluid** composition in the body. This is accomplished by the formation of urine. For example, as blood passes through the kidneys, body wastes such as urea are removed for excretion. Excess water-soluble nutrients and other substances are also filtered and excreted in this manner. So, if the body already has enough vitamin C, for example, the kidneys filter the extra amount out of the blood and redirect it into the urine. The skin excretes body wastes through the pores along with perspiration. The lungs remove the car-

Digestion and Absorption

M erely ingesting foods doesn't nourish you. Only after the nutrients contained in the foods have been released and then absorbed can they be taken up by the bloodstream and distributed to all of your body's cells.[6] The major organs involved in this process are the gastrointestinal tract, pancreas, liver, and gallbladder.

We can take our digestion and absorption system for granted because most of the processes involved are autonomic; that is, they control themselves. We don't decide when the pancreas secretes digestive enzymes into the small intestine, what the liver does with absorbed glucose, or how quickly food is propelled through the intestinal tract. Hormones, hormone-like compounds, and nerves control these functions.[6] The only two voluntary responses are deciding how well to chew food and when to eliminate the fecal remains. Thus while you go about your daily routine—playing tennis, working in a laboratory, walking from class to class, or eating lunch— many digestive reactions and functions occur automatically in your gastrointestinal tract. Let's examine these processes.

NUTRITION AWARENESS INVENTORY

Answer these 15 statements about digestion and absorption to test your knowledge. If you think the statement is true
or mostly true, circle T. If you think the
statement is false or mostly false, circle F.
Use the scoring key at the end of the
book to compute your total score. Repeat
this test after you have read this chapter,
and compare your results.

1. **T F** The process of digestion always begins in the mouth.
2. **T F** Nutrients that are absorbed directly into the bloodstream from the digestive tract go immediately to the liver.
3. **T F** The small intestine is more than 8 feet (2.5 meters) long.
4. **T F** Mucus kills most bacteria that enter the stomach.
5. **T F** The colon is another name for the large intestine.
6. **T F** Fruit and meat will not be digested fully if they are eaten together.
7. **T F** Many stomach enzymes work less efficiently in the small intestine.
8. **T F** The interior lining of the small intestine is protected from ulcer development by a thick layer of mucus.
9. **T F** Bile is required if the foods within the digestive tract are to be fully digested.
10. **T F** The liver, gallbladder, and pancreas are all organs through which foods must pass during digestion.
11. **T F** A significant portion of the nutrients we consume is absorbed in the large intestine.
12. **T F** The absorption of glucose requires energy, whereas fat absorption does not.
13. **T F** Peristalsis uses coordinated muscle action.
14. **T F** Malabsorption of some foods results in gas production by bacteria in the large intestine.
15. **T F** The entire gastrointestinal tract normally contains a large and thriving population of bacteria.

The Physiology of Digestion

The **gastrointestinal (GI) tract** is a long tube stretching from the mouth to the anus. This tube, also known as the *alimentary canal,* is in one sense "outside" the body. It is partitioned from the body in such a way that nutrients must pass through its walls in order to be absorbed into the bloodstream. Just eating a food is not enough—most nutrients must be **digested** and all nutrients must be absorbed to be of use to body cells.[6] Disease may hamper digestion and/or absorption, denying the body use of dietary nutrients.[24]

The GI tract is a complex system that performs a variety of physiological functions: movement (motility), secretion, digestion, absorption, elimination, and nutrient production.[6] (*Nutrient production* refers to the synthesis of vitamins by bacteria that live in the intestine.) Most of these processes are under autonomic control; that is, they are involuntary. Almost all functions involved in digestion and absorption are controlled by **hormones,** hormonelike compounds, and nerves.[13]

The most important aspects of GI tract physiology from a nutritional viewpoint are discussed in this chapter. A more detailed discussion of all the organs and processes involved can be found in a physiology textbook.

THE FLOW OF DIGESTION

Let's begin by reviewing the major parts of the body used in digestion. In the mouth, glands produce **saliva** (Figure 6-1). Saliva contains enzymes that break down carbohydrates to simple sugars, and **mucus** that lubricates the foods (Table 6-1).[8] Chewing divides solid food into smaller, more manageable pieces, which increases the surface area of the food, allowing more efficient digestive action by enzymes.

gastrointestinal (GI) tract Comprises the main sites in the body used in digestion and absorption of nutrients. The tract consists of the mouth, esophagus, stomach, small intestine, large intestine, rectum, and anus.

digestion The process by which large ingested molecules are mechanically and chemically broken down to produce smaller molecules that can be absorbed across the wall of the GI tract.

hormone A compound with a specific site of synthesis that, when secreted into the bloodstream, controls the function of cells in its target organ or organs. Hormones can be either amino acidlike (epinephrine), proteinlike (insulin), or fatlike (estrogen).

saliva A watery fluid produced by the salivary glands in the mouth; it contains lubricants, enzymes, and other substances.

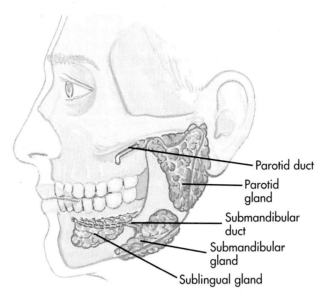

Figure 6-1 Location of the salivary glands. These glands produce saliva to aid in swallowing and digesting food.

TABLE 6-1

Important secretions of the digestive tract

Secretion	Site of production	Purpose
Saliva	Mouth	Contributes to starch digestion, lubrication
Mucus	Mouth, stomach, small intestine, large intestine	Protects cells, lubricates
Enzymes	Mouth, stomach, small intestine, pancreas	Promote digestion of food into molecules small enough for absorption from the GI tract
Acid	Stomach	Promotes digestion of protein, among other functions
Bile	Liver (stored in gallbladder)	Suspends fat in water to aid fat digestion in the small intestine
Bicarbonate	Pancreas	Neutralizes stomach acid in the small intestine

mucus A thick fluid secreted by glands throughout the body. It contains a compound that has both a carbohydrate and a protein nature. It acts as both a lubricant and a means of protection for cells.

Saliva also contains **lysozyme,** a set of enzymes that kill bacteria by rupturing "foreign" cell membranes.[6]

The tongue contains taste receptors for sweet, salty, sour, and bitter tastes. The sweet and salt receptors are near the tip of the tongue, while the sour and bitter receptors are near the base.[6] A fifth taste sensation called **umami** has been proposed. This taste sensation is elicited by monosodium glutamate. Brothy, meaty, and savory are examples of umami sensations. Monosodium glutamate is often added to Chinese and Japanese foods to enhance the umami flavor.

The sensation of flavor is augmented by input from the approximately 6 million **olfactory receptor cells** in the nose. These receptors can detect hundreds of thousands of different molecules.[20] Overall, flavor is a complex combination of taste, olfaction, physical sensations from certain chemicals in foods (such as in chili pep-

lysozyme A set of enzyme substances produced by a variety of cells in the body that can destroy bacteria by rupturing their cell membranes.

umami A brothy, meaty, savory flavor in some foods. Monosodium glutamate (MSG) enhances this flavor when added to foods.

CRITICAL THINKING

James has a cold and doesn't have much appetite. He says that he can't distinguish the flavors of the foods he eats—they all taste the same. How can you explain this?

- - - - - - - - - - - - -

At autopsy, the small intestine muscles relax, allowing the jejunum and the ileum to lengthen to about 11 feet (3.4 m) each. The small intestine is then about 23 feet (7.1 m) long, a figure often cited in textbooks.

- - - - - - - - - - - - -

- - - - - - - - - - - - -

GI tract flow

Mouth
↓
Esophagus
↓
Stomach—4-cup (1 L) capacity. Food remains about 2 to 3 hours. High-fat meals take the longest time to empty.
↓
Small intestine—duodenum (10 inches long), jejunum (4 feet long), ileum (5 feet long)—about 10 feet (3.1 m) in total length; food remains about 3 to 10 hours.
↓
Large intestine (colon)—cecum, ascending colon, transverse colon, descending colon, sigmoid colon—3 1/2 feet (1.1 m) in total length; food can remain up to 72 hours.

- - - - - - - - - - - - -

pers), and textural sensations. Flavor is also affected by human genetic variability in both taste and olfactory sensations.[6]

A variety of diseases and drugs, as well as the effects of aging, can alter the sense of taste. Adding spices and flavorings to foods can enhance the pleasure of eating in these cases.[12]

The mouth and stomach are connected by the esophagus. At its entrance is a valvelike flap of tissue, the epiglottis, that prevents food from being lodged in the trachea (windpipe). When food is swallowed it lands on the epiglottis, which then covers the larynx (the opening of the trachea). Breathing automatically stops. These involuntary responses ensure that swallowed food travels only down the esophagus, aided by muscle contractions of the esophagus and by gravity (Figure 6-2).[6]

As food exits the esophagus, it passes through the diaphragm, which separates the abdominal and thoracic cavities of the body, and enters the stomach. The stomach is essentially a holding tank, with a capacity of about 4 cups (1 L). The stomach continues the digestive process by secreting acid and enzymes and slowly mixing them into the food. The resulting soupy mass of food and secretions is called **chyme**.[6] The chyme is usually ready to leave the stomach within 2 to 4 hours after food is eaten. The more solid the chyme, the longer it takes to leave the stomach, and chyme that is high in fat generally takes longer than chyme that contains much carbohydrate.

The stomach empties into the small intestine, which is coiled below it in the abdomen (Figure 6-3). The small intestine is divided into three sections: the first part, the duodenum, is about 10 inches long (0.3 meters [m]); the middle segment, the jejunum, is about 4 feet long (1.3 m); and the last section, the ileum, is about 5 feet long (. 6 m). The small intestine is considered small because of its narrow diameter (1 inch ⌊2.5 cm⌋). Most digestion is completed in the duodenum and upper jejunum, with the help of enzymes made by intestinal cells and the pancreas.[13]

Muscular contractions in the small intestine constantly mix the food with digestive fluids, enhancing digestion. A meal remains in the small intestine about 3 to 10 hours.

The small intestine empties into the large intestine, or colon. This organ is about 3½ feet long (1.1 m) and is separated into five sections: the cecum, ascending colon, transverse colon, descending colon, and sigmoid colon. Bacteria in the large intestine digest some plant fiber; little other digestion occurs in this organ.[5] However, there is no need for it—about 95% of total digestion occurs in the small intestine. Food that reaches the large intestine is mostly indigestible. This residue remains in the large intestine for about 24 to 72 hours before elimination from the body as **feces**.

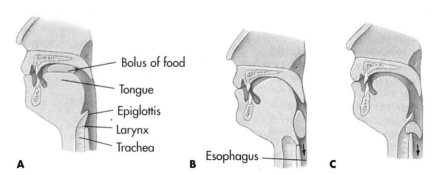

Figure 6-2 The process of swallowing. **A,** During swallowing, food cannot normally enter the trachea because the epiglottis closes over the larynx. **B,** The arrow shows that this allows food to proceed down the esophagus. **C,** When a person chokes, food becomes lodged in the trachea, blocking air flow to the lungs. The food should have gone down the esophagus.

The terminus of the large intestine is attached to the rectum, which is connected to the anus. These final sections of the GI tract work with the large intestine to prepare the feces for elimination.

The liver, pancreas, and gallbladder work with the GI tract but are not a physical part of it.[6] The liver provides **bile,** which aids in fat digestion and absorption and is stored in the gallbladder until needed. The common bile duct leads from the gallbladder and connects with the pancreatic duct, which allows digestive enzymes and other products from the pancreas to be mixed with bile before entering the duodenum for digestion.

GASTROINTESTINAL CONTROL VALVES: SPHINCTERS

A **sphincter** is a circular muscle arrangement (as in the mouth) that acts as a valve to regulate passage or flow of material. The intestinal tract includes several sphincters, which respond to stimuli from nerves, hormones, hormonelike compounds, and pressure that builds up around them.[6]

The flow of food through the esophagus is controlled by the upper and lower esophageal sphincters. The lower esophageal sphincter (also known as the *cardiac sphincter* due to its proximity to the heart) prevents backflow (reflux) of stomach contents into the esophagus. It generally opens only in response to muscle contractions in the esophagus, which propel ingested food down to the stomach. The lower

feces Substances discharged from the bowel during defecation, including undigested food residue, dead GI tract cells, mucus, bacteria, and other waste material. Another term for feces is *stool.*

bile A substance made in the liver and stored in the gallbladder; it is released into the small intestine to aid fat absorption by emulsifying fat into micelles.

sphincter A muscular valve that aids in controlling the flow of food in the GI tract.

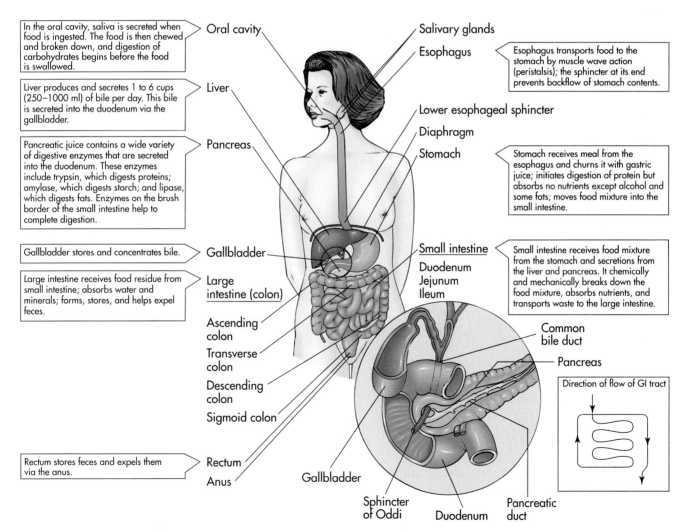

Figure 6-3 Physiology of the GI tract. Many organs cooperate in a regulated fashion to allow digestion and subsequent absorption of nutrients.

heartburn Pain caused by stomach acid backing up into the esophagus and irritating the tissue in that organ.

ulcer Erosion of the tissue lining in either the stomach (gastric ulcer) or upper small intestine (duodenal ulcer). The general condition in either area is often termed a *peptic ulcer*.

cholecystokinin (CCK) A hormone that stimulates enzyme release from the pancreas and bile release from the gallbladder.

laxative A medication or other substance that stimulates evacuation of the intestinal tract.

peristalsis A coordinated muscular contraction that propels food down the GI tract.

mass movement A peristaltic wave that simultaneously coordinates contraction over a large area of the large intestine. Mass movements propel material from one portion of the large intestine to another and from the large intestine into the rectum.

segmentation Contractions of the circular muscles in the intestines that lead to dividing and mixing of the intestinal contents. This action aids digestion and absorption of nutrients.

esophageal sphincter should otherwise remain closed, as the stomach contents are highly acidic. If stomach acid comes in contact with the esophagus, it can cause a pain known as **heartburn.** Coffee, alcohol, and nicotine can weaken the hormonally induced tension of the lower esophageal sphincter and cause heartburn in some susceptible people (see the Nutrition Perspective).[6]

The pyloric sphincter, located at the junction of the stomach and first part of the small intestine (duodenum), controls the movement of the stomach contents into the small intestine. Under hormonal and nervous system control, the pyloric sphincter allows only a few milliliters (about a teaspoon) of stomach contents at a time to squirt into the small intestine. This rate allows bicarbonate ions (HCO_3-) from the pancreas to efficiently neutralize the hydrogen ions (H^+) coming from the stomach acid. This neutralization is critical to reduce the risk of acid erosion of the small intestine. Such erosion might produce an **ulcer** (see the Nutrition Perspective). The pyloric sphincter also prevents backflow of intestinal contents into the stomach, to protect the stomach lining from bile in the intestinal contents.[13]

The sphincter of Oddi is at the end of the common bile duct. When the hormone **cholecystokinin (CCK)** stimulates the gallbladder to contract during digestion, the sphincter of Oddi relaxes and allows the contents of the gallbladder to flow down the common bile duct and enter the duodenum.

The ileocecal valve forms the terminus of the small intestine and opens in response to the presence of intestinal contents in its vicinity. Otherwise the sphincter remains closed to prevent the contents of the large intestine from backing up into the small intestine. In this way bacteria from the large intestine are prevented from invading and colonizing the small intestine.[6] The small intestine must have a relatively low concentration of bacteria because bacteria can compete for nutrients, absorbing them before the host body can. These bacteria also tend to break down bile, interfering with both the digestion of dietary fat and the recycling of bile from the GI tract back to the liver (see later section on enterohepatic circulation). Bile not recycled then enters the large intestine and acts as a powerful **laxative,** often producing diarrhea.[4]

At the terminus of the large intestine are two anal sphincters, one under voluntary control. Once toilet-trained, a child can determine when to relax the sphincter and when to keep it constricted.

Thus sphincters along the intestinal tract perform important functions. Without them we would suffer more heartburn, ulcers, and diarrhea.

GASTROINTESTINAL MUSCULARITY: MIXING AND PROPULSION

Food is propelled down the GI tract by a process called **peristalsis.** Watching a snake swallow its prey graphically illustrates the process. Peristalsis consists of a coordinated squeezing and shortening of the GI tract (Figure 6-4).[6] This begins in the esophagus in the form of two waves of muscle action closely following each other. In the stomach, peristaltic waves create a mixing and grinding action as often as three times per minute during digestion. The stomach wall is composed of three opposing muscle layers (circular, diagonal, and longitudinal), which in combination enable the stomach to contract in enough directions to fully mix food with gastric juices. This is seen especially in the terminal portion of the stomach (Figure 6-5).

The most prominent peristalsis occurs in the small intestine, where contractions occur about every 4 to 5 seconds. One group of muscles forms a circular pattern around the GI tract (Figure 6-5).[6] These muscles constrict behind and relax in front of ingested food, moving it down the intestinal tract. Contraction of lengthwise muscles shortens the tract at the same time. The large intestine has very sluggish peristalsis, employing occasional **mass movements** to help eliminate the feces.

Adding to the action of peristalsis is another process that occurs in the intestines called **segmentation** (see Figure 6-4).[6] Segmentation occurs when muscle contractions cause an alternate forward-and-backward mixing movement within a specific region of the GI tract, in which the intestinal contents show little net movement.

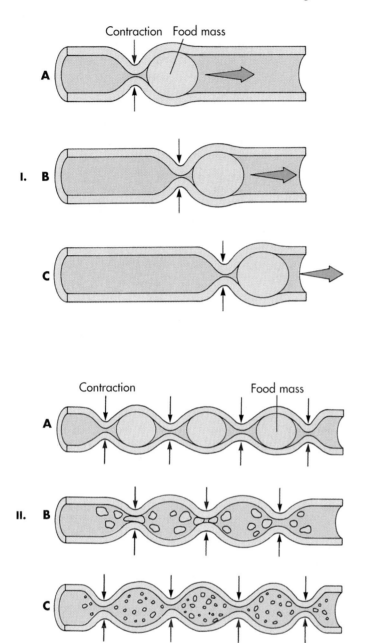

Figure 6-4 Peristalsis and segmentation. I. **Peristalsis.** Peristalsis is a progressive movement, propelling material along the GI tract. **A,** A ring of contraction occurs where the GI wall is stretched, passing the food mass forward. **B,** The moving food mass triggers a ring of contraction in the next region, which pushes the food mass even farther along. **C,** The ring of contraction moves like a wave along the GI tract, pushing the food mass forward.

II. **Segmentation.** Segmentation is the back-and-forth action that breaks apart chunks of the food mass and mixes in digestive juices. **A,** Ringlike regions of contraction occur at intervals along the GI tract. **B,** Previously contracted regions relax and adjacent regions contract, effectively "chopping" the contents of each segment into smaller chunks. **C,** Contracted regions continue to alternate back and forth, chopping and mixing the contents of the GI tract.

The circular muscles are primarily involved. Such movement helps to mechanically break down food particles and mix in digestive juices. Segmentation also brings digested food into contact with the intestinal wall to facilitate absorption. Peristalsis and segmentation can occur alternately.

Enzymes in Digestion

Enzymes are important in digestion. They speed up digestion by catalyzing chemical reactions, bringing certain molecules close together and then creating a favorable environment for the intended reaction. The enzyme lowers the amount of energy needed for the reaction to proceed (Figure 6-6). Individual enzymes usually act only on a specific substance; for example, enzymes that recognize table sugar (sucrose) ignore milk sugar (lactose).[13]

- - - - - - - - - - - -
Enzyme nomenclature is often quite simple. The prefix of the enzyme name usually indicates the target; the suffix is then *-ase*. For example, lipase is the enzyme that digests certain lipids.
- - - - - - - - - - - -

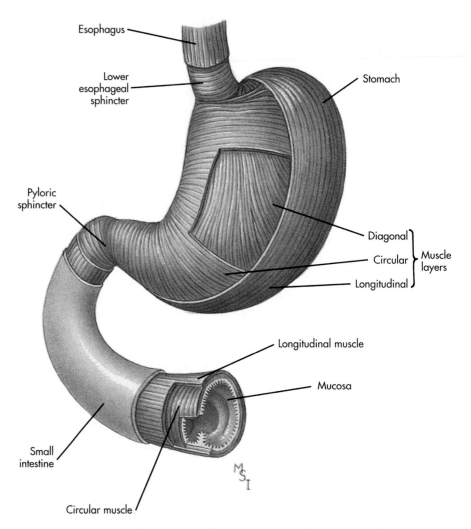

Figure 6-5 Muscularity of the GI tract. The arrangement of muscles in different directions is a key to the function of both the stomach and intestinal tract.

The activities of the enzymes used in digestion must be controlled. Enzymes must be readily activated when needed and inactivated when their job is complete. Enzymes are not always able to distinguish proteins, carbohydrates, and fats in food from the same materials that exist as components of body tissues. In essence, it is possible for a digestive tract to digest itself. To minimize this risk, the digestive tract has mechanisms to vary enzyme activation. Enzyme activation is usually dependent on pH. Digestive enzymes that work in the acid environment of the stomach do not work well in the alkaline environment of the small intestine. In addition, the body produces some enzymes as **zymogens,** inactive molecules that require the removal of some minor part of the chemical structure in order to work. The zymogen is converted into an active enzyme at the appropriate time.[13]

A few digestive enzymes are made by the mouth and stomach. Most are synthesized by the pancreas and small intestine (Table 6-2). The pancreas is capable of responding to changes in nutrient intake with appropriate changes in enzyme production.[21] Increased protein intake leads to increased protein digestive capability. This is likely linked to the ability of the hormone cholecystokinin (CCK) to increase the synthesis of protein-digesting enzymes by the pancreas. Diets high in fat and low in carbohydrate lead to an increase in fat-digesting enzymes and a decrease in starch-digesting enzymes. These latter adaptations may be directed by the products of lipid and carbohydrate digestion.

zymogen An inactive form of an enzyme that requires the removal of some minor part of its structure in order to function. The zymogen is converted into an active enzyme at the appropriate time, such as when released into the stomach or small intestine.

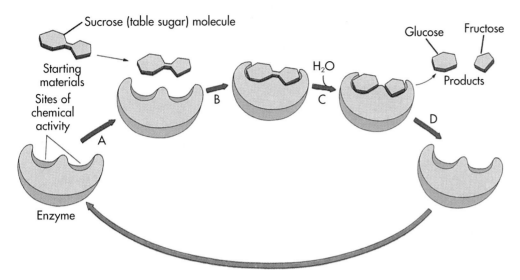

Figure 6-6 A model of enzyme action. With some enzymes, the reaction can go both ways. Sometimes energy in the form of ATP is needed to allow the enzyme to push the reaction in the forward direction.

When either the small intestine or the pancreas is diseased, inadequate quantities of important digestive enzymes may be produced. This scarcity can result in incomplete digestion and very limited absorption. In such cases, nutrients in the undigested food travel into the large intestine rather than being absorbed into the bloodstream. In the large intestine the undigested food is metabolized into acids and gases by bacteria. The resultant feces appear foamy and greasy due to trapped gases and the presence of undigested fat. Intestinal malabsorption often causes a distended abdomen due to intestinal gas.[24] Whenever digestion and absorption are hampered, the body pays a price. Insufficient enzyme production or insufficient time to complete enzyme action is often the cause of these problems.

People who have pancreatic disease may not produce sufficient enzymes for digestion. In cystic fibrosis, excess production of mucus may block release of enzymes from the pancreas. This results in malabsorption of nutrients and associated discomfort. An affected person can consume replacement enzymes with meals. Some forms are coated to protect against destruction by stomach acid.[24]

TABLE 6-2

Summary of digestive enzymes[13]

Secretion origin	Enzyme	Substrate	Major end products
Salivary glands	Salivary amylase	Starch, glycogen	Maltose and dextrins
Stomach glands	Pepsin	Protein	Peptides, peptones
	Gastric lipase	Short-chain triglycerides, medium-chain triglycerides	Fatty acids, monoglycerides
Pancreas	Trypsin	Protein, peptides	Polypeptides, smaller peptides
	Chymotrypsin	Protein, peptides	Same as trypsin, but more coagulating power for milk protein
	Carboxypeptidase	Polypeptides	Smaller peptides, free amino acids
	Pancreatic amylase	Starch, glycogen, dextrins	Maltose
	Lipase	Triglycerides	Monoglycerides, free fatty acids
Intestinal wall	Aminopeptidase	Peptides	Amino acids, smaller peptides
	Maltase	Maltose	Glucose
	Sucrase	Sucrose	Glucose, fructose
	Lactase	Lactose	Glucose, galactose
	Enterokinase	Trypsinogen	Trypsin

NUTRITION FOCUS

BODY SYSTEMS USED IN DIGESTION AND ABSORPTION

The body is composed of millions of **cells.** Each is a self-contained, living entity (see Chapter 7 for a drawing of a typical cell). Cells of the same type bond together using intercellular substances to form **tissues,** such as bone, cartilage, muscle, and nerve. Often two or more tissues combine in a particular way to form more complex **organs,** such as skin, kidneys, and the liver. At still higher levels of coordination, several organs can cooperate for a common purpose to form an **organ system,** such as the respiratory system or digestive system. The human body is a coordinated unit of many such organ systems.[6]

Every cell in the human body performs a specialized job. A cell's master plan for work and for the necessary machinery to do that work is all encoded into the cell's genetic material, the **DNA** (deoxyribonucleic acid). The DNA acts as a blueprint for synthesizing specific proteins, often enzymes, required to perform specific tasks. Even though most cells in an organism contain the same DNA information, cells throughout the body are programmed differently. As the embryo forms, different parts of the DNA become active in different cell types. For example, the intestinal cells make digestive enzymes; in the bone marrow, cells that make the oxygen-carrying protein hemoglobin become active.

Chemical reactions occur all the time in every living cell. Synthesis of new substances is balanced by the breaking down of older ones. For this turnover to occur, cells require a continuous supply of energy. Most cells need oxygen to extract this energy from nutrients for cell use. Cells also need water, the medium in which they live. They further need building blocks, especially the materials they can't make themselves—the essential nutrients supplied from food. All these substances enable the tissues, composed of individual cells, to function properly.

An adequate supply of all nutrients to body cells is the result of a healthful diet. But to ensure optimal use of these nutrients by cells, the following systems, in addition to the digestive system, must work efficiently.

CIRCULATORY SYSTEM

The blood follows two general routes. It circulates between the right side of the heart and the lungs (the pulmonary circuit) and between the left side of the heart and all other body parts (the systemic circuit) (Figure 6-7). The heart is a muscular pump that normally contracts and relaxes 50 to 90 times a minute while the body is at rest.

This continuous pumping action keeps blood moving through the body.[6]

The circulatory system distributes nutrients from digestion and oxygen from the air we breathe to all body cells. All blood goes to the lungs to pick up oxygen and release carbon dioxide. The oxygenated blood returns to the heart to be pumped to all other body tissues. In the capillaries, cells exchange nutrients and waste with the blood—cells empty their waste products into the blood and take nutrients from it. Capillaries, networks of tiny blood vessels, serve every region of the body via individual capillary beds one cell thick. Nutrients, gases, and other substances can pass through capillary cells both into and out of other body cells.[6]

The lymphatic system of circulatory vessels serves the body by carrying lymph, the clear fluid formed between cells (see Figure 6-7). This fluid filters into tiny lymphatic vessels, which compose a one-way network that funnels lymph from all over the body into two large lymphatic vessels that empty into major veins returning to the heart.[6]

Lymphatic vessels that serve the small intestine have an important role in nutrition. These vessels pick up and transport the majority of products released from fat absorption—those substances too large to enter the bloodstream directly. The lymphatic vessels from the intestine drain into a large duct, called the thoracic duct, that stretches from the abdomen to the neck. This duct connects with the bloodstream through a vein near the neck. In this way the majority of absorbed fat-soluble products eventually enter the bloodstream.[13] Other parts of the lymphatic system play a key role in the immune system.

EXCRETORY SYSTEM

The kidneys, digestive tract, skin, and lungs all remove wastes from the body. The primary function of the kidneys is to regulate the **extracellular fluid** composition in the body. This is accomplished by the formation of urine. For example, as blood passes through the kidneys, body wastes such as urea are removed for excretion. Excess water-soluble nutrients and other substances are also filtered and excreted in this manner. So, if the body already has enough vitamin C, for example, the kidneys filter the extra amount out of the blood and redirect it into the urine. The skin excretes body wastes through the pores along with perspiration. The lungs remove the car-

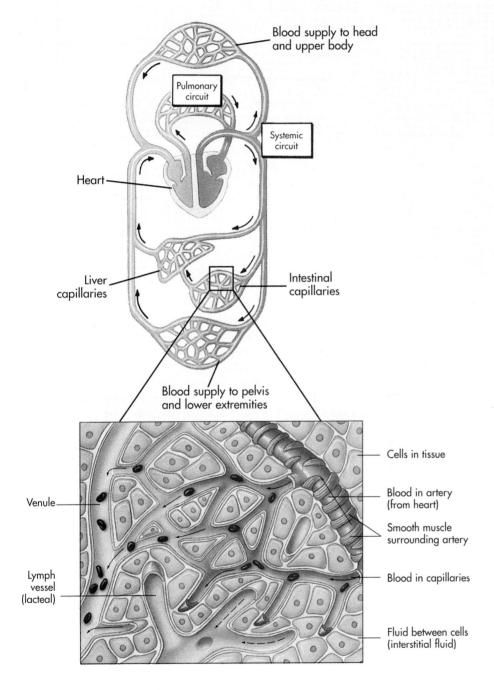

Blood supply to head and upper body

Pulmonary circuit

Systemic circuit

Heart

Liver capillaries

Intestinal capillaries

Blood supply to pelvis and lower extremities

Venule

Lymph vessel (lacteal)

Cells in tissue

Blood in artery (from heart)

Smooth muscle surrounding artery

Blood in capillaries

Fluid between cells (interstitial fluid)

Figure 6-7 Blood circulation throughout the body. This represents the route blood takes through the two circuits that begin and end at the heart. The red color indicates blood that is richer in oxygen; blue is for blood carrying more carbon dioxide. Oxygen and nutrients are exchanged for carbon dioxide and waste products in the capillaries, the points at which the arteries and veins merge. The box at the bottom shows a close-up of a capillary bed in the small intestine, including the location of the lymphatic vessels. Lymph vessels in the intestine are also called *lacteals*.

NUTRITION FOCUS

bon dioxide produced during metabolism of carbohydrates, fats, and proteins and exhale it into the air.

STORAGE SYSTEM

The human body must maintain reserves of nutrients; otherwise we would need to eat continuously. Storage capacity varies for each nutrient. Most fat is stored at sites designed specifically for this purpose—adipose tissue. Short-term storage of glucose occurs in muscles and in the liver, as glycogen, and as glucose in blood. Many vitamins and minerals are stored in the liver.[6] Other nutrient stores are found in individual cells.

During a period of dietary deficiency some nutrients are obtained by breaking down tissues that contain high concentrations of nutrients. Calcium is removed from bone, and protein is taken from muscle. Since neither bones nor muscles are meant to act as nutrient reserves, nutrient losses in cases of dietary deficiency can harm these tissues.

CONTROL SYSTEMS

The endocrine (hormone) and nervous systems form two control mechanisms that greatly influence nutrient use in the body.[6] The hormone insulin helps regulate blood glucose, and thyroid hormones help regulate the body's metabolic rate. Nerves influence acid secretion in the stomach and regulate GI tract muscle action. The senses of sight, hearing, touch, smell, and taste all use nerve pathways to communicate information—the availability of food or the need for it, for example—to the brain.

CONCEPT CHECK

The gastrointestinal (GI) tract includes the mouth, esophagus, stomach, small intestine, large intestine (colon), rectum, and anus. Associated with the GI tract are the salivary glands, liver, gallbladder, and pancreas. Together these organs perform the digestion and absorption needed to extract nutrients from food and deliver them to the bloodstream. In the GI tract, a coordinated muscular activity called peristalsis propels food from the esophagus to the anus. Segmentation in the intestines divides and mixes the contents, aiding digestion and absorption. Enzymes produced by cells in the mouth, stomach, pancreas, and small intestine digest the food to free nutrients for absorption. The time from ingestion of food to the eventual elimination of the feces from the body is usually about 1 to 3 days.

Digestion—Nutrient by Nutrient

A good way to study digestion is to track a single food from the time it enters the mouth until its components are absorbed into the blood or eliminated in the feces. We use banana bread as an example. Nutrients in the banana bread are digested at different sites along the GI tract and by different means (Figure 6-8). Enzymes do the work, while nerves, hormones, and hormonelike substances control the process.[13]

Digestion actually begins before we start to eat. Cooking food can be viewed as a first step in digestion. Cooking unfolds (denatures) proteins and softens tough connective tissue in meat and fibers in plants such as broccoli. When starchy plant material is heated, the starch granules soak up water and swell, rupturing the plant cell wall. This makes the starches, and plant material in general, much easier to digest and absorb. Cooking also makes food easier to chew, swallow, and break down during later digestion and absorption. As you will see in Chapter 19, cooking also makes many foods, such as meats, fish, and poultry, much safer to eat.

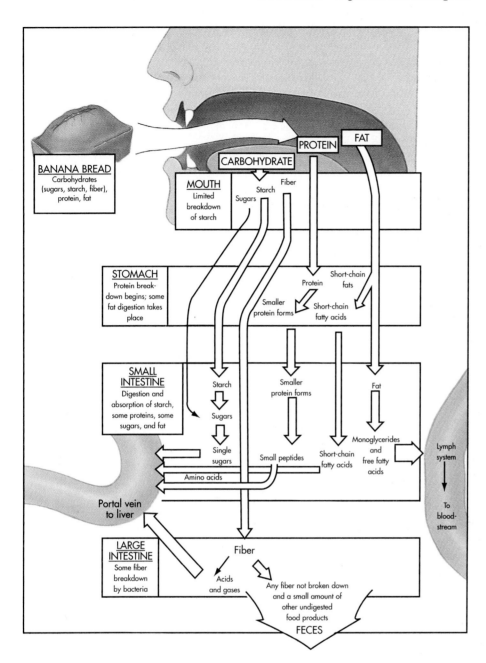

Figure 6-8 Digestion in practical terms. Many enzymes contribute to the digestion of foods, as seen in this example of banana bread. Absorption occurs via the blood and the lymphatic system. Sugars, amino acids, short- and medium-chain fatty acids (the latter not depicted), and most vitamins enter the bloodstream. Long-chain fatty acids re-form into triglycerides and enter the lymphatic system in the form of chylomicrons.

PROTEIN DIGESTION

The digestion of protein begins in the stomach. When the egg and milk proteins in the banana bread are denatured by stomach acid, **pepsin,** a major enzyme for proteins, goes to work (Table 6-2). Pepsin attacks all proteins and breaks them down into shorter units, called **peptones.** Pepsin does not completely separate proteins into amino acids because it can break only a few of the many peptide bonds found in these large molecules.[13]

Pepsin is secreted as pepsinogen, its inactive zymogen form, by the chief cells of the stomach. These cells, along with acid-forming cells (called *parietal cells*) and mucus-forming cells (called *goblet cells*), lie in gastric pits in the stomach (Figure 6-9). If pepsin were not stored as an inactive enzyme, it would digest the stomach glands while waiting to be secreted from the pits. This is one way the stomach prevents **autodigestion** (digesting itself). Once pepsinogen enters the stomach's acidic environment (pH between 1 and 2), part of the enzyme is split off, forming the active enzyme pepsin.[6]

pepsin A protein-digesting enzyme produced by the stomach.

peptones Partial breakdown products of proteins.

autodigestion Literally, "self-digestion." The stomach limits autodigestion by covering itself with a thick layer of mucus and producing enzymes and acid only when needed for digestion of food.

gastrin A hormone that stimulates enzyme and acid secretion by the stomach.

The release of pepsin is controlled by the hormone **gastrin** (Table 6-3). Thinking about food or chewing food stimulates the vagus nerve, which "primes" the stomach for the forthcoming meal by stimulating special gastrin-producing cells in the terminus of the stomach. Gastrin signals the chief cells to begin producing pepsinogen.[6] Now stomach enzymes will be ready to go to work when the meal arrives. Pepsin is present in the stomach only when food enters or is about to reach the stomach because gastrin is released only at such times. This is another means of preventing autodigestion.

Gastrin also strongly stimulates the stomach's parietal cells to produce acid. In addition, stomach distention (stretching due to the presence of food) and a by-product of protein digestion called **histamine** also stimulate the parietal cells. When stimulated, the parietal cells produce hydrochloric acid (HCl) from water, carbon dioxide, and chloride ions (see Figure 6-9).[6] Hydrochloric acid activates pepsin, improves the absorption of iron and calcium, keeps the stomach essentially bacteria free, and inactivates plant and animal hormones that might otherwise have undesirable effects in the body. The parietal cells also produce intrinsic factor, a compound needed for vitamin B-12 absorption.

histamine A breakdown product of the amino acid histidine that stimulates acid secretion by the stomach.

Since gastrin is released only when we eat or think about eating, acid production follows this same pattern. Furthermore, as the stomach's pH approaches 2, gastrin release stops as an additional protection against autodigestion.[6] The final barrier against autodigestion is the thick layer of mucus the stomach secretes. The mucus lines the inside of the stomach, protecting it from the acid and pepsin produced for digestion.

Protein Digestion Continues in the Small Intestine

The partially digested proteins move with the rest of the nutrients and other substances in the banana bread from the stomach into the duodenum, the first part of the small intestine. The acidic mixture is squirted a few milliliters at a time through the pyloric sphincter, which separates the stomach from the duodenum. The more liquid parts of the chyme leave first; the more solid parts exit later. As soon as chyme squirts into the duodenum, bicarbonate ions (HCO_3^-) synthesized in the pancreas are delivered through the common bile duct to the duodenum to neutralize the acid. This process is coordinated by the hormone **secretin**, which is made in the walls of the upper portion of the small intestine.[13] Acid entering the duodenum causes secretin release. Secretin causes the pancreas to release bicarbonate ions and causes a reduction in stomach peristalsis (motility).

secretin A hormone that causes bicarbonate ion release from the pancreas.

We noted earlier that the pyloric sphincter is under hormonal and nervous system control. Specifically, proteins and fats in the chyme stimulate the release of the

TABLE 6-3

Hormones that regulate the digestive tract[13]

Hormone	Origin	Stimulus to secretion	Action
Gastrin	Pyloric region of the stomach and upper duodenum	Food and other substances in the stomach, especially proteins, caffeine, spices, alcohol; nerve input	Stimulates flow of stomach enzymes and acid; stimulates contraction of lower esophageal sphincter; slows gastric emptying
Gastric inhibitory peptide	Duodenum, jejunum	Fats, protein	Inhibits secretion of stomach acid and enzymes; slows gastric emptying
Cholecystokinin (CCK)	Duodenum, jejunum	Food, especially fat and protein in duodenum	Causes contraction of gallbladder and flow of bile to duodenum; causes secretion of enzyme-rich pancreatic juice and bicarbonate-rich pancreatic fluid; slows gastric emptying
Secretin	Duodenum, jejunum	Acid chyme; peptones	Causes secretion of bicarbonate-rich pancreatic fluid and slows gastric emptying

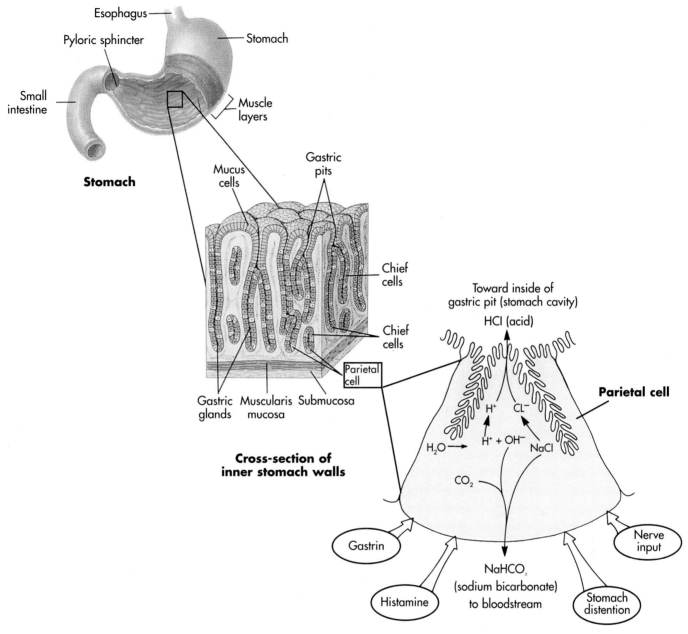

Figure 6-9 Physiology of the stomach. Below the parietal cell are noted factors that stimulate acid secretion in the stomach. The reactants for acid production are water, carbon dioxide, and sodium chloride. The product is hydrochloric acid (HCl).

hormone **gastric inhibitory peptide (GIP)** from the walls of the upper portion of the small intestine.[6] GIP slows the release of stomach contents into the small intestine (Table 6-3). In addition, the hormones secretin, gastrin, and cholecystokinin (CCK) help keep the stomach from overwhelming the small intestine with acid chyme by slowing the emptying process. This helps explain why fats in a meal cause a feeling of fullness: the chyme remains in the stomach longer, so we feel full longer. Adding to this hormonal input are receptors in the duodenum that monitor the

gastric inhibitory peptide (GIP) A hormone that slows gastric motility and stimulates insulin release from the pancreas.

concentration of the chyme. A high concentration of substances slows gastric emptying, easing the load placed on the intestine at one time.[21]

The pH of the neutralized chyme is approximately 5 to 7, rather than 2 to 3. If the acid chyme is not neutralized, it digests the wall of the duodenum, eventually leading to an ulcer. Unlike the stomach, the small intestine is not protected by a thick layer of mucus because the small intestine must absorb most of the products of digestion, and absorption cannot occur through a thick layer of mucus. The stomach absorbs only small amounts of alcohol and certain fats; thus a thick layer of mucus poses no problem. The duodenum is protected instead by rapid neutralization of acid chyme and constant shedding of its cell lining.[6]

Once in the small intestine, the peptones (and any fats accompanying them) trigger the release of the hormone cholecystokinin (CCK) from the walls of the small intestine. CCK, in turn, travels through the bloodstream to its target organs, the pancreas and gallbladder.

The pancreas is responsible for the production and storage of many digestive enzymes. Among these are the protein-splitting enzymes **trypsin,** chymotrypsin, and carboxypeptidase, which are released into the small intestine in their zymogen forms.[13] On their arrival, the intestinal enzyme enterokinase cleaves the tail portion of trypsinogen to form trypsin. The activated trypsin cleaves the tail portions of both chymotrypsin and carboxypeptidase, as well as cleaves the tail portion off of other trypsinogens, creating more of itself.

Together these digestive enzymes divide the peptones into short **peptides** and amino acids. Eventual digestion of all peptides into amino acids occurs inside the absorptive cells of the small intestine.[1]

FAT DIGESTION

The stomach produces gastric **lipase,** an enzyme that digests fat (*gastric* refers to the stomach). This enzyme acts primarily on triglycerides containing short- and medium-chain fatty acids, such as those found in butter fat. The digestion occurs only in the stomach because gastric lipase requires an acidic environment to function. The action of gastric lipase, however, is usually dwarfed by the action of pancreatic lipase in the small intestine.[13] Triglycerides containing long-chain fatty acids, such as those found in common vegetable oils, must generally wait for intestinal digestion.

Thus the digestion of fat from the vegetable oil, milk, and other ingredients in the banana bread primarily takes place in the small intestine. The hormone CCK, which releases enzymes for protein digestion, simultaneously releases lipase from the pancreas for fat digestion. In the small intestine, this pancreatic lipase digests the triglycerides into smaller products, monoglycerides and fatty acids.[13]

Pancreatic lipase enters the small intestine through the common bile duct in a concentration many times greater than needed. This "overkill" makes fat digestion very rapid and thorough in the right circumstances. These circumstances include the release of **colipase** from the pancreas to aid in lipase enzyme action. Bile from the gallbladder is also important. Released in response to CCK, bile helps to emulsify the fatty substances in the small intestine, in the same way a dishwashing detergent breaks up oil spots in dishwater. This increases the surface area for lipase action, facilitating fat digestion. Bile also organizes the digestive products of lipase action into micelles (see Chapter 4 for a review). This improves fat absorption because the digestive products of fat are transported mostly as micelles to the intestinal wall to begin fat uptake.[13]

CARBOHYDRATE DIGESTION

Digestion of starches, mostly from the flour in the banana bread, begins as these mix with saliva during chewing. Saliva contains an enzyme called salivary **amylase.** This enzyme is capable ultimately of breaking down starch into maltose (two glucose units bonded together). During this digestion many small units of simple sugars

trypsin A protein-digesting enzyme secreted by the pancreas to act in the small intestine.

peptide A few amino acids chemically bonded together (often two to four).

lipase Fat-digesting enzymes; gastric lipase is produced by the stomach, pancreatic lipase is produced by the pancreas.

colipase A protein secreted by the pancreas that changes the shape of pancreatic lipase, facilitating its action.

amylase Starch-digesting enzymes from the salivary glands or pancreas.

called **dextrins** are first formed; these then yield maltose.[13] You can observe this starch breakdown while chewing a saltine cracker, which becomes sweeter during prolonged chewing as some starch is converted to sugars.

Once food moves down the esophagus into the stomach, the acid environment halts further salivary amylase action and starch digestion. Salivary amylase is relatively unimportant, however, because pancreatic amylase in the small intestine finishes needed amylase action (see Table 6-2).[13]

When carbohydrates move into the intestine, the pancreas releases its amylase to continue the digestion of starches through the dextrin phase into maltose. The carbohydrates from the banana bread are now present as monosaccharides (glucose and fructose) and disaccharides (maltose, lactose, and sucrose). Eventually all the disaccharides are digested to monosaccharides by specialized enzymes called *disaccharidases.* These enzymes are synthesized by, and attached to, the cells of the small intestine.[13] Maltose is acted on by maltase to produce two glucose molecules. Sucrose (table sugar) is acted on by sucrase to produce glucose and fructose. Lactose (milk sugar) is acted on by lactase to produce glucose and galactose. The single sugars are the only form of carbohydrates that can be absorbed (see Figure 6-8).

It is important to remember that enzymes essential to carbohydrate digestion originate both from the pancreas and from cells of the intestinal wall. Intestinal disease can interfere with the production of enzymes formed in the intestinal wall. Such conditions may interfere with the efficient digestion of the sugars maltose, lactose, and sucrose. If these carbohydrates are not fully digested, they are not absorbed. Instead, when they reach the large intestine, the resident bacteria use the sugars to produce acids and gases, causing abdominal discomfort. People recovering from intestinal disorders, such as diarrhea or bacterial infection, may need to avoid lactose for a few weeks because of temporary lactose intolerance. In two weeks the small intestine begins producing enough lactase to permit lactose digestion (see Chapter 3).[24]

Hormones—A Key to Orchestrating Digestion

Four hormones regulate the GI tract: gastrin, secretin, cholecystokinin, and gastric inhibitory peptide (see Table 6-3).[13] The term *hormone* comes from the Greek for "to stir or excite." To be a true hormone, a regulatory compound must have a specific synthesis site from which it enters the bloodstream to reach target cells. At first the behavior of gastrin may seem confusing; its site of synthesis and its target organ are both the stomach, but it enters the bloodstream before acting.

Many hormonelike compounds, such as vasoactive intestinal peptide, bombesin, substance P, and somatostatin, control important aspects of GI function.[13] These compounds diffuse from cells or nerve endings to nearby cells. Many hormonelike compounds are found in the intestine and the brain. When a person thinks about eating or prepares to eat, the whole GI tract begins to prime itself for action. Hormonelike substances participate in this process. The cells that synthesize these hormones and hormonelike compounds are scattered throughout the GI tract.

Digestion—A Recap

The response of the digestive tract to ingested food is directly related to the nutritional makeup and amount of the food. Foods generally contain a mixture of macronutrients as well as vitamins and minerals; therefore multiple enzymatic responses to the contents of the small intestine are the rule. The contention of the authors of some fad diet books that ingestion of certain combinations of foods, such as meats and fruits together, hinders the absorptive process does not make sense in light of both what we know about gastrointestinal physiology and our collective experiences of eating various combinations of foods.

dextrins Partial breakdown products of starch that contain few to many glucose molecules. These appear as starch is digested into many units of maltose by salivary and pancreatic amylase.

CONCEPT CHECK

Digestion is the process by which foods are broken down into smaller, simpler forms. It begins with cooking, as heat and moisture unfold proteins, swell starch granules, and soften tough fibrous tissue. Enzymes produced in the mouth begin to digest starch. The stomach primarily digests protein, producing breakdown products called *peptones*. The small intestine is the major site for all digestion. There, peptones separate into small peptides and amino acids, carbohydrates yield single sugars, and triglycerides form monoglycerides and free fatty acids. Enzymes used for digestion in the small intestine come from the pancreas and from the cells lining the intestinal wall. Fat digestion is aided by bile, which is produced by the liver and released by the gallbladder.

The Physiology of Absorption

absorption The process by which nutrient molecules are absorbed by the GI tract and enter the bloodstream.

Most nutrient **absorption** occurs in the small intestine; the stomach and large intestine participate to a minor extent. The small intestine can absorb about 95% of the food energy it receives in the form of protein, carbohydrate, fat, and alcohol.[6] Only water, small amounts of alcohol, and certain types of fats are absorbed to a significant extent by the stomach. Some minerals, water, and short-chain fatty acids (produced by bacterial action) are absorbed in the large intestine.[15]

The extent and efficiency of absorption in the small intestine are linked to its incredible surface area. The wall of the small intestine is folded, and within the folds are fingerlike villi projections (Figure 6-10). The "fingers" trap nutrients between each other to enhance absorption. Each villus "finger" is made up of numerous **absorptive cells** (enterocytes). Each of these cells has a brush border, or microvilli, cap covered with hairlike projections called **glycocalyx.** Intestinal enzymes are often found on the glycocalyx. All these folds, fingers, and indentations in the small intestine increase its surface area 600 times beyond that of a simple tube.[6]

absorptive cells A class of cells, also called *enterocytes,* that cover the surface of the villi (fingerlike projections in the small intestine) and participate in nutrient absorption.

glycocalyx Hairlike projections that cover the microvilli of the absorptive cells.

ABSORPTIVE CELLS

The absorptive cells of the small intestine lie side by side with goblet cells, which produce mucus, and endocrine cells, which produce hormones and hormonelike substances. All these cells form a principal part of the intestinal **mucosa.** The absorptive cells are produced in open-ended pits (called *crypts*) buried deep in the mucosa of the small intestine and migrate from the crypts to the tips of the villi. As the cells migrate, they mature, and their absorptive efficiency increases. By the time they reach the tips of the villi, however, they have been partially degraded by digestive enzymes and are ready to be sloughed off. Newly formed absorptive cells constantly migrate from the crypts to replace dying ones.[11]

mucosa Mucous membrane consisting of cells and supporting connective tissue. In the digestive tract there is also a layer of smooth muscle supporting the mucosa. Mucosa lines cavities that open to the outside of the body, such as the stomach and intestine, and generally contains glands that secrete mucus.

The journey from the crypt to the top of the villi takes 2 to 5 days for each absorptive cell.[6] Thus these cells have a very short life span, which probably serves as an important adaptive mechanism. Absorptive cells face a harsh environment of enzymes, bacteria, and various toxins found in the small intestine. Contact with alcohol also damages absorptive cells. Therefore constant formation of new intestinal lining becomes a biological necessity.

Since cell production requires a variety of nutrients, groups of cells undergoing constant replacement have a correspondingly enhanced need for nutrients. For this reason the small intestine rapidly deteriorates during a nutrient deficiency or in semistarvation. In addition, the products of digestion and the hormones associated with the digestive process have a direct growth-promoting action on the cells of the small intestine. The absorptive cells in the small intestine are healthier when GI tract hormones and digestive products are present.[5]

- - - - - - - - - - - - -

One cancer treatment uses medication (chemotherapy) to prevent rapid cell growth. This can stop tumor cells from growing. However, chemotherapy also affects body cells that normally have a rapid turnover, such as the absorptive cells of the intestinal villi. Because the cells of the villi are affected, people on these medications usually develop diarrhea as a side effect.[23]

- - - - - - - - - - - - -

If a disease causes the villi to lie down, the surface area in the small intestine decreases and malabsorption results. This happens in celiac disease (also called *gluten-*

Organization of the small intestine

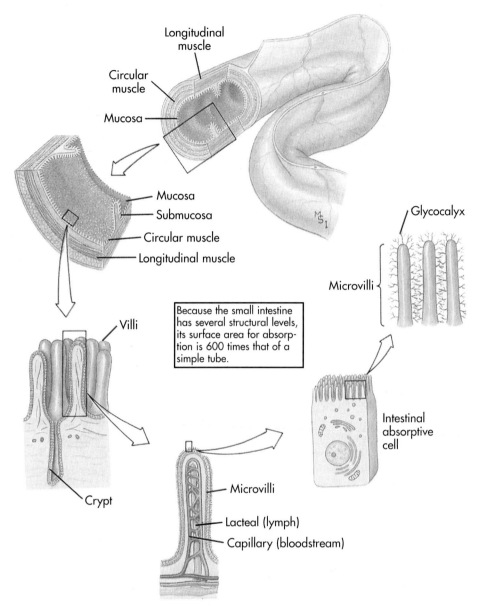

Figure 6-10 Organization of the small intestine. The small intestine has several structural levels that increase the surface area for absorption up to 600 times that of a simple tube.

induced enteropathy). This disease is caused by an allergic response to a protein called *gluten*, found in wheat, rye, oats, barley, and buckwheat.[19] To prevent attacks, any foods derived from these grains must be avoided.

TYPES OF ABSORPTION

The small intestine uses four basic types of **absorptive** processes: **passive, facilitated, active,** and **endocytosis (phagocytosis/pinocytosis)** (Figure 6-11).[6] Passive absorption occurs when nutrients enter absorptive cells without a carrier or energy expenditure. For this to happen, the wall of the intestine must be permeable to the nutrient, and the nutrient must be present in a higher concentration in the intestinal **lumen** than in the absorptive cells. The difference in concentration drives passive absorption. Water, most fats, and some minerals are passively absorbed.

passive absorption Absorption that requires permeability of the substance through the wall of the small intestine and a concentration gradient higher in the intestinal contents than in the absorptive cell.

facilitated absorption Absorption in which a carrier shuttles substances into the absorptive cell but no energy is expended. A concentration gradient higher in the intestinal contents than in the absorptive cell drives the absorption.

active absorption Absorption using a carrier and expending ATP energy. In this way the absorptive cell can absorb nutrients, such as glucose, against a concentration gradient.

EXPERT OPINION

GASTROQUACKERY

STEPHEN BARRETT, M.D.

The importance of "regularity" to overall health has been greatly overestimated for thousands of years. Ancient Egyptians associated feces with decay and used enemas and laxatives liberally. In more recent times, this concern has been embodied in the concept of "autointoxication" and has been promoted by warnings against "irregularity."

The theory of "autointoxication" states that stagnation of the large intestine (colon) causes toxins to form that are absorbed and poison the body. Some proponents depict the large intestine as a "sewage system" that becomes a "cesspool" if neglected. Other proponents state that constipation causes hardened feces to accumulate for months (or even years) on the walls of the large intestine and block the large intestine from absorbing or eliminating properly. This, they say, causes food to remain undigested and wastes from the blood to be reabsorbed by the body.

Around the turn of the twentieth century many physicians accepted the concept of autointoxication, but it was abandoned during the 1930s after scientific observations proved it wrong. Among other things, direct observation of the large intestine during surgical procedures found no evidence that hardened feces accumulate on the intestinal walls.

Today we know that most of the digestive process takes place in the small intestine, from which nutrients are absorbed into the body. The remaining mixture of food and undigested particles then enters the large intestine, which can be compared to a 40-inch-long hollow tube. Its principal functions are to transport food wastes from the small intestine to the rectum for elimination and to absorb minerals and water. Careful observations have shown that the bowel habits of healthy individuals can vary greatly. Although most people have a movement daily, some have several movements each

day, while others can go several days or even longer with no adverse effects.

Despite these facts, some chiropractors, naturopaths, and assorted food faddists claim that "death begins in the colon" and that "90% of all diseases are caused by improperly working bowels." The practices they recommend include fasting, periodic "cleansing" of the intestines, and colonic irrigation. Fasting is said to "purify" the body. "Cleansing" can be accomplished with a variety of "natural" laxative products. Colonic irrigation is performed by passing a rubber tube through the rectum for a distance of up to 20 or even 30 inches. Warm water—often 20 gallons or more—is pumped in and out through the tube, a few pints at a time, to wash out the contents of the large intestine. (An ordinary enema uses about a quart of fluid.) Some practitioners add herbs, coffee, enzymes, wheat or grass extract, or other substances to the enema solution.

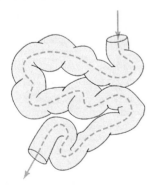

Lumen: The inside of a tube, such as the inside cavity of the GI tract.

Facilitative absorption uses a carrier molecule to shuttle the nutrients from the lumen of the small intestine into the absorptive cells, but no energy is expended. Again, a concentration difference drives the reaction. Facilitative absorption takes place for the simple sugar fructose; the nature of the carrier molecule is in question.[18]

Active absorption uses a carrier, and the process requires energy. The single sugars glucose and galactose, amino acids, and other nutrients are actively absorbed. Adenosine triphosphate (ATP) is the energy source (see Chapter 7 for a discussion of ATP). Using this energy, absorptive cells can take up a substance in low concentration in the intestinal contents and move it into the cell, where the concentration is higher. Since the bloodstream constantly bathes the absorptive cells, their relative concentration of glucose is higher than that of the intestinal contents. Therefore the ability to absorb against a concentration gradient is critical.

A second type of active absorption involves the processes of endocytosis: phagocytosis (literally, "cell eating") and pinocytosis (literally, "cell drinking"). In endocytosis an absorptive cell engulfs compounds or liquids indenting its cell mem-

The danger of these practices depends on how much they are used and whether they are substituted for necessary medical care. Whereas a 1-day fast is likely to be harmless (though useless), prolonged fasting can be fatal. "Cleansing" is unlikely to be physically harmful, but the products involved can be expensive. Colonic irrigation, which also can be expensive, has considerable potential for harm. The process can be very uncomfortable, since the presence of the tube can induce severe cramps and pain. If the equipment is not adequately sterilized between treatments, germs from one person's large intestine can be transmitted to others. Several outbreaks of serious infection have been reported, including one in which contaminated equipment caused amebiasis in 13 people, six of whom died following bowel perforation. Cases of heart failure (from excessive fluid absorption into the bloodstream) and electrolyte imbalance have also been reported.

The popular diet book *Fit for Life* (1986) is based on the notion that when certain foods are eaten together they "rot," poisoning the system and making the person fat. To avoid this, the authors recommend that fats, carbohydrates, and protein foods be eaten at separate meals, emphasizing fruits and vegetables because foods high in water content can "wash the toxic waste from the inside of the body" instead of "clogging" the body. These ideas are utter nonsense.

Although laxative advertisements warn against "irregularity," constipation should be defined not by the frequency of movements but by the hardness of the feces. Ordinary constipation usually can be remedied by increasing the fiber content of the diet, drinking adequate amounts of water, and engaging in regular exercise. If the bowel is basically normal, dietary fiber increases the bulk of the feces, softens it, and speeds transit. Defecating soon after the urge is

felt can also be helpful because if urges are ignored, the rectum may eventually stop signaling when defecation is needed. Stimulant laxatives (such as cascara or castor oil) can damage the nerve cells in the colon wall, decreasing the force of contractions and increasing the tendency toward constipation. Thus people who take strong laxatives whenever they "miss a movement" may wind up unable to move their bowels without them. A medical doctor should be consulted if constipation persists or represents a significant change in bowel pattern.

Dr. Barrett, a retired psychiatrist, is a board member of the National Council Against Health Fraud. His 37 books include Health Schemes, Scams, and Frauds *(Consumer Reports Books, 1990) and the college textbook* Consumer Health—A Guide to Intelligent Decisions, *edition 5 (Mosby, 1993).*

brane. When particles or fluids move into the indentation, the cell surrounds them.[6] An infant's absorption of antibodies from the mother's milk occurs this way.

PORTAL AND LYMPHATIC CIRCULATION

The villi in the intestine are drained by two different circulation systems, portal and lymphatic (see Figure 6-7). The nutrients follow one of these systems based on solubility in either (1) water or (2) organic solvents. The nutrients that are soluble in water (proteins, carbohydrates, short- and medium-chain fatty acids, B vitamins, and vitamin C) are carried in the blood.[13] Blood leaves the heart through arteries, travels to the intestine, and eventually travels in capillary beds inside the villi. The blood exits the capillary beds and collects in the large **portal vein,** which leads directly to the liver. This direct path enables the liver to process absorbed nutrients before they enter the general circulation. Blood flow used for portal absorption accounts for 30% of the heart's total output.

Nutrient intake also directly influences nutrient absorption. For example, vitamin C in a meal increases iron absorption in the same meal as it changes elemental iron into a more absorbable state (Fe^{2+}).

portal vein Capillaries from the intestine and stomach drain into a large portal vein that leads to the liver.

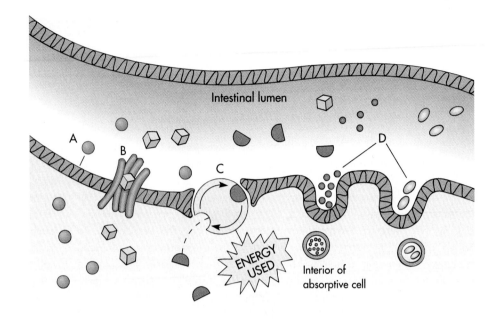

Figure 6-11 Nutrient absorption uses four basic types of absorptive processes:
A, Passive absorption involves simple diffusion of substances across the cell membrane of absorptive cells. No energy is expended, as the substances follow a favorable concentration gradient (from high to low concentration). Water and fats are absorbed in this manner.
B, Facilitated absorption uses a carrier or other process to aid in absorption of specific substances, such as fructose. No energy is expended; the process is simply aided by the carrier.
C, Active absorption (transport) uses a carrier and energy. The use of energy allows the absorptive cell to absorb nutrients against their concentration gradient (from low to high concentration). Glucose undergoes active absorption.
D, Endocytosis. Pinocytosis—"cell drinking"—involves cells taking in liquids by forming an indentation in the cell membrane and then surrounding the liquid, with eventual incorporation into the cell. Phagocytosis—"cell eating"—involves cellular uptake of substances, including whole particles, in a manner analogous to pinocytosis.

lymphatic system A system of vessels that can accept large or fat-soluble particles, such as chylomicrons, and eventually pass them into the bloodstream.

The **lymphatic system** also drains the villi. The lymphatic vessels carry particles that are either fat soluble (long-chain fatty acids and the fat-soluble vitamins A, D, E, and K) or too large to pass through the capillaries into the bloodstream (large proteins that escape from the bloodstream and chylomicrons that form after the absorption of fat).[13] Substances are squeezed through the spongelike vessels of the lymphatic system by muscular activity. As mentioned earlier, the lymphatic vessels from the intestine drain into the thoracic duct, which stretches from the abdomen to the neck. This duct is connected to the bloodstream via a large vein near the neck, the left subclavian vein.

ENTEROHEPATIC CIRCULATION

During meals bile circulates through the liver to the gallbladder, through the small intestine into the portal vein, and then returns to the liver about twice. This recycling is called **enterohepatic circulation.** Approximately 98% of the bile is recycled; only 1% to 2% is removed from the body by elimination in the feces.[13]

enterohepatic circulation A continual recycling of compounds between the small intestine and the liver; bile acids are one example of a recycled compound.

As discussed in Chapter 4, one way to reduce elevated serum cholesterol is to consume resins that bind bile and draw its constituents into the feces. This treatment reduces bile's enterohepatic circulation, forcing the liver to make new bile rather than use recycled bile. The building block for bile synthesis is cholesterol, which the liver removes from the bloodstream to make new bile, thus reducing serum cholesterol.

CONCEPT CHECK

The small intestine is the major site for nutrient absorption. Numerous folds and fingerlike projections increase the surface area 600 times that of a simple tube. This provides a large area for nutrient absorption. Absorptive cells have a life span of 2 to 5 days, so the lining of the small intestine is constantly being renewed. These cells perform passive absorption, promoted by a concentration gradient; facilitative absorption, promoted by a concentration gradient plus a carrier; and active absorption, which uses energy in addition to a carrier to work against a concentration gradient. Absorptive cells also engulf compounds and liquids via endocytosis (phagocytosis/pinocytosis). The products of absorption, if water soluble, pass into the portal vein and enter the liver. The products of fat digestion mostly enter the lymphatic system. Some participants in digestion, such as bile, are reabsorbed after use in the small intestine and returned to the liver, to be sent back again to the small intestine during another round of digestion. This circulation is called *enterohepatic circulation*.

Some cancer cells also travel through the lymph. When cancer is found in the body during surgery, the surgeon examines the lymph nodes closest to the site of the cancer to see if it has traveled from the original site to other sites in the body. If cancer cells are found in the lymph nodes, they have probably already spread to other organs in the body.[23]

Absorption—Nutrient by Nutrient

Absorption of all types of energy-yielding nutrients occurs simultaneously. We separate the absorption of each here for simplicity.

PROTEIN ABSORPTION

Small peptides and amino acids—breakdown products of the egg and milk protein in the banana bread—are actively absorbed into the cells of the small intestine (Figure 6-12).[13] Few whole proteins are absorbed. The small peptides are eventually broken down to individual amino acids inside the absorptive cells. The amino acids travel via the portal vein to the liver, where they are combined into protein, converted to glucose or fat, used for energy needs, or released into the bloodstream.

FAT ABSORPTION

Most of the products of fat digestion—from the vegetable oil and milk fat in the banana bread—are fatty acids and monoglycerides. These are passively absorbed into the absorptive cells. The carbon chain length of fatty acids and monoglycerides affects the manner of their absorption. If a fatty acid is a short- or medium-chain variety (less than 12 carbon atoms), it is water soluble and probably travels through the portal vein to the liver. If the fatty acid is a long-chain variety (12 or more carbon atoms), it is re-formed into a triglyceride molecule and transported via the lymphatic system (Figure 6-13).[13]

The stomach is capable of limited absorption of short-chain fatty acids. These are present mainly as a result of the action of gastric lipase on foods (like butter or milk fat) that contain high amounts of short-chain fatty acids.

The major by-products of lipid digestion are long-chain free fatty acids and monoglycerides. These products of fat digestion are absorbed from micelles formed during fat digestion and resynthesized into new triglycerides in the villi.[13] The triglycerides are then combined with cholesterol, protein, phospholipid, and other substances and covered with a protein coat. This collective structure of fat and protein is termed a *lipoprotein*, or as in this specific case, a *chylomicron*. This chylomicron is what enters the lymphatic system and eventually the bloodstream to carry most of the absorbed fat from the banana bread to target tissues.

Cholesterol in foods often comes with an attached fatty acid. Enzymes from the pancreas break off this fatty acid, yielding the cholesterol itself, about 60% of which is absorbed.[13]

CRITICAL THINKING

The medical history of a young girl with undernutrition shows that she had three quarters of her small intestine removed after she was injured in a car accident. Explain how this accounts for her undernutrition even though her chart shows that she eats well.

CARBOHYDRATE ABSORPTION

In the banana bread, sugars occur naturally in the fruit, are added as table sugar, and are formed as by-products of starch digestion in the mouth and small intestine.

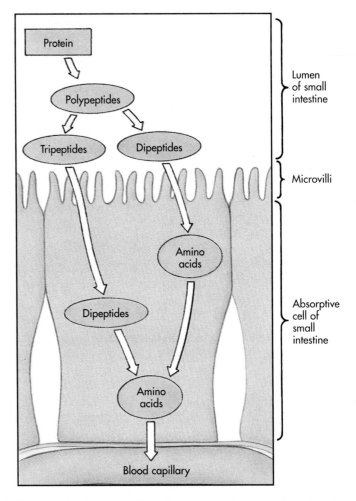

Figure 6-12 Final protein digestion. This takes place in the absorptive cells of the small intestine. In a sodium-dependent, energy-requiring process much like glucose absorption, all of the end products of protein digestion are broken down at the microvilli surface and within the absorptive cell to amino acids. These are sent to the bloodstream.

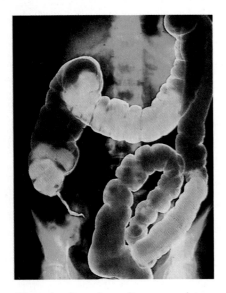

The colon has a large diameter and no villi.

Fructose is taken up by the absorptive cells via facilitative absorption.[18] Glucose and galactose (its close relative) are actively pumped into the absorptive cells of the villi along with sodium during active absorption (Figure 6-14).[11] The energy used in the process is actually needed to pump the sodium ion back out of the absorptive cell. Once glucose, galactose, and fructose enter the villi, they are transported via the portal vein to the liver for glycogen production, fat production, energy use, or direct release into the blood.[13]

ABSORPTION IS COMPLETED IN THE LARGE INTESTINE

The small intestine is responsible for 85% to 90% of the water absorbed from the GI tract. This absorption reduces the 9 L the GI tract receives (2 L of dietary fluid plus 7 L of GI tract secretions) to about 1.5 L. The remnants of digestion that enter the large intestine are the remaining water, some minerals, and undigested food fibers and starches. Only a minor amount (5%) of carbohydrate, protein, and fat escapes absorption in the small intestine (Figure 6-15).[15]

The large intestine absorbs primarily sodium and potassium, along with some water, leaving only about 200 ml of water unabsorbed. This occurs mostly in the first half of the large intestine. Short-chain fatty acids made from both the metabolism of some plant fibers and undigested starches are also absorbed in the

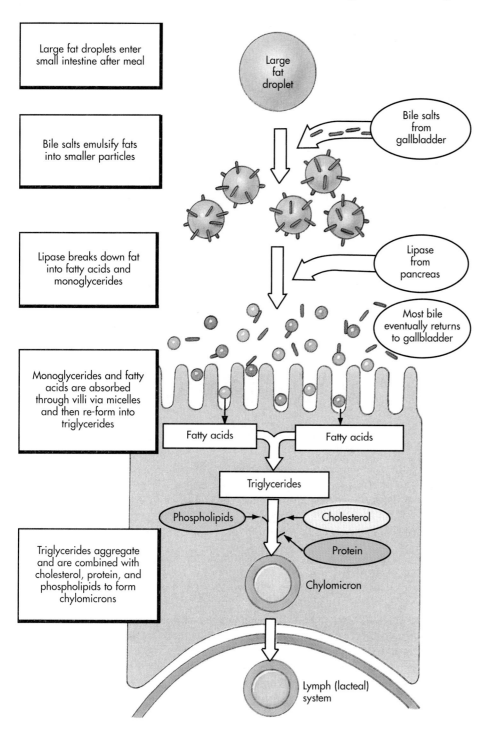

Large fat droplets enter small intestine after meal

Bile salts emulsify fats into smaller particles

Lipase breaks down fat into fatty acids and monoglycerides

Monoglycerides and fatty acids are absorbed through villi via micelles and then re-form into triglycerides

Triglycerides aggregate and are combined with cholesterol, protein, and phospholipids to form chylomicrons

Large fat droplet

Bile salts from gallbladder

Lipase from pancreas

Most bile eventually returns to gallbladder

Fatty acids

Fatty acids

Triglycerides

Phospholipids

Cholesterol

Protein

Chylomicron

Lymph (lacteal) system

Figure 6-13 A simplified look at fat absorption. Triglycerides made up of long-chain fatty acids primarily form monoglycerides and free fatty acids. These are absorbed using bile and then re-formed into triglycerides in the absorptive cells. The triglycerides are then formed into chylomicrons and enter the lymphatic system. Note that short- and medium-chain fatty acids pass directly into the portal circulation.

large intestine, along with some vitamins synthesized by bacteria, such as vitamin K and biotin.[3,15] By the time the contents of the large intestine pass through the first two thirds of its length, a semisolid mass is formed. This remains in the large intestine until peristaltic waves and mass movements push it into the rectum for elimination.

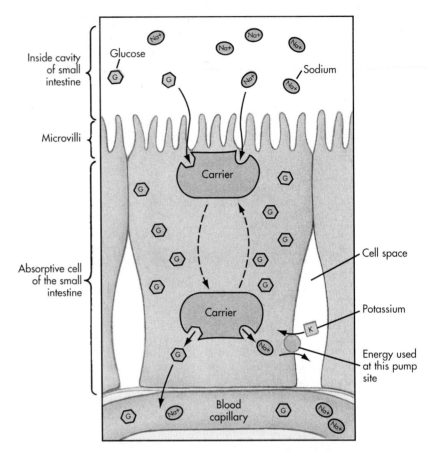

Figure 6-14 Active absorption of glucose. Glucose and sodium pass across the cell membrane of the intestinal absorptive cell in a carrier-dependent, energy-requiring process. The energy is used for maintaining a low concentration of sodium in the cell. Once inside the absorptive cell, glucose can exit by facilitated diffusion down its concentration gradient and enter the bloodstream.

The presence of feces in the rectum powerfully stimulates defecation. This process involves muscular reflexes in the sigmoid colon and rectum, as well as relaxation of the anal sphincters. The feces primarily consist of indigestible plant fibers, tough connective tissue from animal foods, and bacteria from the large intestine (Figure 6-16).[6]

FRANK & ERNEST® by Bob Thaves

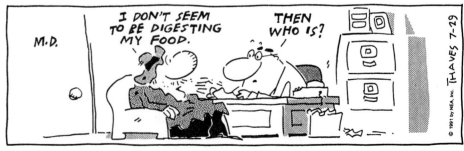

Figure 6-15 Frank & Ernest.
Reprinted by permission of NEA, Inc.

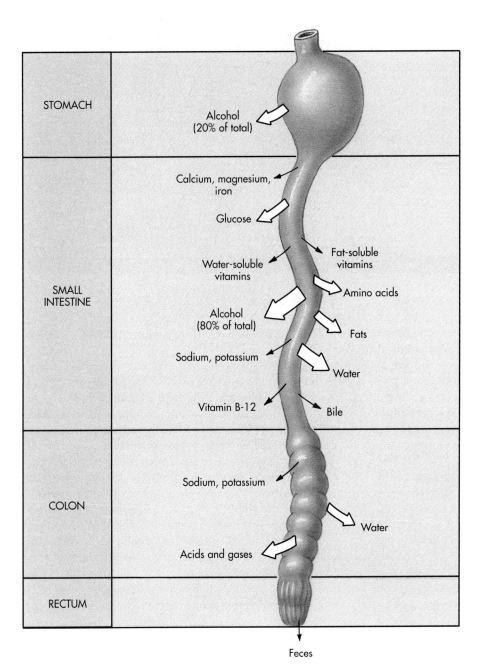

Figure 6-16 Major sites of absorption along the GI tract. The size of the arrow indicates the relative amount of absorption at that site.

CONCEPT CHECK

The breakdown products of protein digestion—namely, peptides and amino acids—are actively absorbed into the absorptive cells, and peptides are broken down into amino acids. These enter the portal vein for delivery to the liver. The breakdown products of fat digestion, mostly monoglycerides and free fatty acids, are passively absorbed into the absorptive cells from micelles. These products are mostly synthesized back into triglycerides and combined with cholesterol, protein, phospholipid, and other substances to yield chylomicrons. Chylomicrons enter the lymphatic system and eventually the bloodstream. The single sugars glucose and galactose, which arise from carbohydrate absorption, are actively absorbed into the absorptive cells; however, fructose follows facilitated absorption, in which a carrier is used but no energy is expended. These single sugars then travel via the portal vein to the liver. Some water and mineral absorption occurs in the large intestine. The remaining contents form the feces, which consist primarily of indigestible plant fibers, tough connective tissue from animal foods, and bacteria.

Summary

1. The gastrointestinal (GI) tract consists of the mouth, esophagus, stomach, small intestine, large intestine (colon), rectum, and anus. Most absorption of nutrients occurs in the small intestine.

2. The salivary glands, liver, gallbladder, and pancreas participate in digestion and absorption. Products from the last three organs enter the small intestine, where enzymes and bile play important roles in digesting protein, fat, and carbohydrates.

3. The GI tract contains valves (sphincters) that control the flow of food. Muscular contractions, called *peristalsis,* propel the food down the GI tract. Segmentation contractions mechanically break down and mix the intestinal contents. Nerves, hormones, and hormonelike compounds control the activity of sphincters and peristaltic and segmentation processes.

4. The mouth chews food to break it into smaller parts, increasing its surface area, which enhances enzyme activity. Some starch digestion occurs in the mouth. Much protein digestion occurs in the stomach. Carbohydrate and protein digestion are finished in the small intestine, where fat digestion begins in earnest and is completed. Some plant fibers are digested by the bacteria present in the large intestine; undigested plant fibers exit the body in the feces.

5. Digestive enzymes are secreted by the mouth, stomach, pancreas, and cells forming the wall of the small intestine. Pancreatic enzyme release is controlled by the hormone cholecystokinin (CCK) and stimulated by fat and protein entering the small intestine. Bile needed for fat digestion is synthesized by the liver, stored in the gallbladder, and released in digestion due to the action of CCK.

6. The major absorptive sites are fingerlike projections in the small intestine called *villi.* The absorptive cells that cover the villi have a life span of 2 to 5 days. Thus the intestinal lining continually renews itself. Absorptive cells can perform passive, facilitated, and active absorption, as well as endocytosis (phagocytosis/pinocytosis, specific types of active absorption.)

7. The products of protein digestion—namely, amino acids and peptides—are actively absorbed into the absorptive cells of the villi. Most of the end products of fat digestion are passively absorbed and rebuilt into triglycerides. The single sugars glucose and galactose, from carbohydrate digestion, are actively absorbed; fructose undergoes facilitated absorption.

8. Water-soluble compounds in the absorptive cells, such as glucose and amino acids, enter the portal vein and travel to the liver. Fat-soluble compounds, such as triglycerides, are incorporated into chylomicrons and enter the lymphatic system, which eventually connects to the bloodstream. Some substances used in digestion, such as bile, are absorbed by the small intestine, sent back to the liver, and sent to the small intestine again to act in further digestion of food. This recycling is called enterohepatic circulation.

9. Final water and mineral absorption takes place in the large intestine, as well as absorption of products from bacterial metabolism of some plant fibers. Once the feces enter the rectum, the impetus for elimination is strong.

Study Questions

1. Describe the nerve and hormone interactions involved in "priming" the digestive tract.
2. Depict the physiological mechanisms by which the health and absorptive abilities of the cells of the small intestine are protected.
3. Outline the possible results of a highly diseased pancreas throughout the digestive process.
4. Describe why the small intestine is better suited than the other GI tract organs to carry out the absorptive process.
5. Explain how each of the following nutrients is absorbed:
   a. The three main monosaccharides
   b. Long- and short-chain fatty acids
   c. Amino acids
   d. Water
6. Where is hydrochloric acid secreted, and how is its production regulated? What are its roles in digestion?
7. Describe the actions of the digestive hormones and explain how their production is "turned on."
8. Describe the actions of the digestive enzymes and explain how those that exist as zymogens can be "turned on."
9. How is blood routed through the digestive system? Which nutrients enter the bloodstream directly? Which nutrients are first absorbed into the lymph?

REFERENCES

1. Caspray WF: Physiology and pathophysiology of intestinal absorption, *American Journal of Clinical Nutrition* 55:299S, 1992.
2. Cramer T: When do you need an antacid? *FDA Consumer*, p 19, Jan/Feb 1992.
3. Cummings JH, Euglyst HN: Gastrointestinal effects of food carbohydrates, *American Journal of Clinical Nutrition* 61:938S, 1995.
4. Donowitz M and others: Evaluation of patients with chronic diarrhea, *New England Journal of Medicine* 332:725, 1995.
5. Evans MA, Shrouts EP: Intestinal fuels: glutamine, short-chain fatty acids, and dietary fiber, *Journal of the American Dietetic Association* 92:1239, 1992.
6. Ganong WF: *Review of medical physiology*, ed 15, Norwalk, Conn, 1995, Appleton & Lange.
7. Lentze MJ: Molecular and cellular aspects of hydrolysis and absorption, *American Journal of Clinical Nutrition* 61:946S, 1995.
8. Levin RJ: Digestion and absorption of carbohydrates—from molecules and membranes to humans, *American Journal of Clinical Nutrition* 59:690S, 1994.

9. Lewis R: Surprise cause of gastritis revolutionizes ulcer treatment, *FDA Consumer*, p 5, December 1994.
10. Lynn RB, Friedman LS: Irritable bowel syndrome, *New England Journal of Medicine* 329:1940, 1993.
11. Marshall JB: Severe gastroesophageal reflux disease, *Postgraduate Medicine* 97(5):98, 1995.
12. Mattes RD, Cowart BJ: Dietary assessment of patients with chemosensory disorders, *Journal of the American Dietetic Association* 94:50, 1994.
13. Mayes PA: Nutrition, digestion, and absorption. In Murray RK and others, editors: *Harper's biochemistry*, Norwalk, Conn, 1993, Appleton & Lange.
14. NIH Consensus Development Panel: *Helicobacter pylori* in peptic ulcer disease, *Journal of the American Medical Association* 272:65, 1994.
15. Nordgaard I, Mortensen PB: Digestive processes in the colon, *Nutrition* 11:37, 1995.
16. Pope CE: Acid-reflux disorders, *New England Journal of Medicine* 331:656, 1994.

17. Raymond KF: Gastroenterology and hepatology, *Journal of the American Medical Association* 273:1679, 1995.
18. Riby JE and others: Fructose absorption, *American Journal of Clinical Nutrition* 58:748S, 1993.
19. Saltzam JR, Clifford BD: Identification of the trigger of celiac sprue, *Nutrition Reviews* 52:317, 1994.
20. Schiffman SJ, Gatlin CA: Clinical physiology of taste and smell, *Annual Review of Nutrition* 13:405, 1993.
21. Schneeman B: Nutrition and gastrointestinal function, *Nutrition Today* p 20, Jan/Feb 1993.
22. Stehlin D: No strain, no pain: the bottom line in treating hemorrhoids, *FDA Consumer*, p 31, March 1992.
23. Wilson JD and others: *Harrison's principles of internal medicine*, ed 13, New York, 1994, McGraw-Hill.
24. Zeman FJ: *Clinical nutrition and dietetics*, ed 2, New York, 1991, Macmillan.

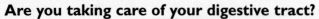

TAKE ACTION

Are you taking care of your digestive tract?

People need to think about the health of their digestive tracts. There are symptoms we need to notice as well as habits we need to practice in order to protect it. The following assessment is designed to help you examine your habits and symptoms associated with the health of your digestive tract. The Nutrition Perspective explains why these habits are important to examine. Put a Y in the blank to the left of the question to indicate yes and an N to indicate no.

—— 1. Are you currently experiencing greater-than-normal stress and tension?

—— 2. Do you have a family history of digestive tract problems (ulcers, hemorrhoids, diverticulosis, constipation, lactose intolerance)?

—— 3. Do you experience pain in your stomach region about 2 hours after you eat?

—— 4. Do you smoke cigarettes?

—— 5. Do you take aspirin frequently?

—— 6. Do you have heartburn at least once per week?

—— 7. Do you commonly lie down after eating a large meal?

—— 8. Do you drink alcoholic beverages more than two or three times per day?

—— 9. Do you experience abdominal pain, bloating, and gas about 30 minutes to 2 hours after consuming milk products?

—— 10. Do you often have to strain while having a bowel movement?

—— 11. Do you consume less than 6 to 8 cups of a combination of water and other fluid per day?

—— 12. Do you perform physical activity (e.g., jog, swim, walk briskly, row, stair climb) less than 20 to 30 minutes three times per week?

—— 13. Do you eat a diet relatively low in dietary fiber (recall that significant dietary fiber is found in whole fruits, vegetables, legumes, nuts and seeds, whole-grain breads, and whole-grain cereals)?

—— 14. Do you frequently have diarrhea?

—— 15. Do you frequently use laxatives or antacids?

Interpretation

Add up the number of "yes" answers you gave and record the total in the blank to the right. ————————

If your score is from 8 to 15, your habits and symptoms put you at risk for experiencing future digestive tract problems. Take particular note of the habits to which you answered yes. Consider trying to cooperate more with your digestive tract.

NUTRITION PERSPECTIVE

When the Digestive Processes Go Awry

T he GI tract can develop problems; knowing about these problems can help you avoid them.

Ulcers

Many adults develop ulcers each year. For some people, stress and tension greatly excite the nerves that control the stomach, which increases acid secretion by the stomach's parietal cells.[23] Eventually the acid erodes through the mucus layer in the stomach and into the stomach tissue, which results in a gastric ulcer. Acid can also erode the tissue lining the duodenum, which results in a duodenal ulcer. A *peptic ulcer* is the general term for either of these.

Some people are more susceptible to ulcers than others because of decreased ability of their stomach and intestinal cells to protect themselves from acid. In addition, recent research suggests that an infection by bacteria (specifically *Helicobacter pylori*) is the cause of most ulcers.[14] Antibiotic and bismuth therapy directed at this bacterium is currently being evaluated as part of treatment in ulcer patients who show evidence of a *Helicobacter pylori* infection.[9,17]

Most ulcers in young people occur in the duodenum; in older people they occur mostly in the stomach. The typical symptom of an ulcer is pain about 2 hours after eating, when digestive acids irritate the ulcer after most of the meal has moved to the jejunum area of the small intestine.[23]

The primary risk of an ulcer is the possibility of its eating entirely through (perforating) the stomach or intestinal wall. The GI contents could then spill into the adjacent body cavity, causing a massive infection called *peritonitis*. In addition, an ulcer may erode a blood vessel, leading to massive blood loss (hemorrhage). For these reasons early warning signs of ulcer development should not be ignored.[23]

In the past, milk and cream therapy—the Sippy diet—was used to help cure ulcers. Today we know that milk and cream are two of the worst foods for an ulcer. The calcium in these foods stimulates gastrin, the hormone that increases stomach acid secretion. Thus this therapy actually inhibits ulcer healing.[24]

Today, antacid medications are a first line of treatment for ulcers. Added to these is a class of medicines called **H₂ blockers.** These include cimetidine (Tagamet), ranitidine (Zantac), and famotidine (Pepcid). They prevent histamine-related acid secretion in the stomach and gastrin release (see Figure 6-9). The stomach cells produce histamine, and the diet supplies histamine from the breakdown of the amino acid histidine. By preventing histamine from increasing acid secretion, the H₂ blockers greatly accelerate ulcer healing and have reduced the need for surgical treatment. Agents that coat the ulcer, such as sucralfate (Carafate), are also commonly used today. Finally, an agent to reduce acid release from the parietal cells (omeprazole [Prilosec]) is used in cases resistant to the other therapies.[23]

People with an ulcer should stop smoking, if they smoke, and minimize the use of aspirin and aspirinlike compounds. Smoking and aspirin use reduce the amount of mucus secreted by the stomach. This combination of therapies has so revolutionized ulcer therapy that dietary changes are of minor importance today (Table 6-4). Current diet-therapy approaches recommend simply avoiding foods that increase ulcer symptoms.[24]

Stomach acid is not a problem for those not prone to ulcers. The acid in the stomach enhances absorption of iron, calcium, and vitamin B-12. Acid also minimizes bacterial growth in the stomach; the stomach is essentially bacteria free because of its high acid content. Bacteria in food are quickly destroyed, which reduces the risk of these bacteria forming cancer-causing agents or leading to food-borne illness (see Chapter 19). Thus acid production by the stomach is an important part of the physiology of digestion and absorption.[13] This means that despite their usual presence alongside the breath mints in a convenience store, antacids should not be used excessively.[2]

H₂ blockers Medications, such as cimetidine (Tagamet), that block the increase of stomach acid production caused by histamine.

TABLE 6-4

Recommendations to prevent ulcers and heartburn from occurring or recurring[23]

Ulcers

1. *Stop smoking, if you are now a smoker.*
2. Avoid aspirin, ibuprofen, and other aspirinlike compounds unless a physican advises otherwise.
3. Limit coffee, tea, and alcohol (especially wine).
4. Limit pepper, chili powder, and other strong spices, if this helps.
5. Eat nutritious meals on a regular schedule.
6. Chew foods well.
7. Lose weight if now overweight.

Heartburn

1. Wait about 3 hours after a meal before lying down.
2. Don't overeat at mealtime. Smaller meals low in fat are advised.
3. Observe the recommendations for ulcer prevention.

CRITICAL THINKING

Mrs. Obonue is obese. She has difficulty breathing and is always tired. She also complains of a burning sensation in her chest that frequently occurs after meals. Her doctor recommends that she lose weight. He believes that if she loses weight her heartburn condition will improve or perhaps even go away. How can you explain the reason for this to Mrs. Obonue?

Heartburn

Many adults regularly have heartburn. This gnawing pain in the upper chest is caused by the reflux of acid from the stomach into the esophagus.[16] Unlike the stomach, the esophagus has no mucous lining to protect it, so acid quickly erodes the lining of the esophagus, causing pain.

An important dietary measure for avoiding heartburn is to eat smaller meals, and especially meals that are low in fat (see Table 6-4). Fatty meals remain in the stomach longer than low-fat meals. The large volume of food and secretions that remains in the stomach creates pressure that can force the stomach contents up into the esophagus.[11]

Several other steps may be taken to prevent heartburn. Cigarette smokers should quit smoking. In addition, it is best not to lie down after eating and to avoid foods and other substances that can specifically contribute to heartburn, such as chili powder, onions, garlic, peppermint, caffeine, alcohol, and chocolate. Each person must discover what bothers him or her and tailor the diet accordingly.[24]

Certain physical conditions can lead to heartburn. For example, both pregnancy and obesity result in increased production of estrogen and progesterone. These hormones relax the lower esophageal (cardiac) sphincter, making heartburn more likely.[23] A pregnant woman may find it helpful to eat more frequent but smaller meals. An obese person should slim down to a more healthy weight so that blood concentrations of these hormones decrease. Adipose (fat) tissue turns circulating hormones into estrogen; thus, the more adipose tissue, the more estrogen is produced.

Heartburn that recurs several times a week for at least a month should be investigated by a physician. Long-standing heartburn may require aggressive medical therapy because it can lead to alteration in the cells of the esophagus, which increases the risk of a rare form of cancer.[23]

Constipation and Laxatives

Constipation, which is difficult or infrequent evacuation of the bowels, is commonly reported by adults. Constipation is caused by slow movement of fecal material through the large intestine. As fluids are increasingly absorbed during the extended time the feces stay in the large intestine, they become dry and hard.

Constipation can result when people regularly inhibit their normal bowel reflexes for long periods.[23] People tend to ignore normal urges when it is inconvenient to interrupt occupational or social activities. Muscle spasms of an irritated large intestine can also slow the movement of feces and contribute to constipation. Medications, such as antacids, can also cause constipation.

Constipation is difficult to diagnose. The normal frequency of bowel movements is 3 to 12 times per week, varying from person to person. The best indication of constipation is unusually hard, dry feces at infrequent intervals, rather than failure to meet a general prescription of "once a day." Sudden, prolonged changes in frequency of bowel movements should be evaluated by a physician. This may be a warning that a more serious intestinal disorder is developing.[23]

Eating foods with plenty of dietary fiber, such as whole-grain breads and cereals, is the best alternative for treating typical cases of constipation. Dietary fibers stimulate peristalsis by drawing water into the large intestine and helping form a bulky, soft fecal output. A person with constipation should also drink more fluids. Eating dried fruits can help stimulate the bowel.[24] In addition, the person may need to develop more regular bowel habits; allowing the same time each day for a bowel movement can help train the large intestine to respond routinely. Finally, relaxation facilitates regular bowel movements, as does regular exercise.

Laxatives can also lessen constipation. They work by irritating the intestinal nerve junctions to stimulate the peristaltic muscles or by drawing water into the intestine to enlarge fecal output. The larger output stretches the peristaltic muscles, making them rebound and then constrict. Regular use of laxatives, especially of irritating ones, can decrease muscle action in the large intestine, causing more constipation. The GI tract in time can actually become dependent on laxatives. Thus it is unwise to use laxatives routinely, although people in certain circumstances—those who are bedridden or quite elderly—may need periodic help from laxatives to relieve constipation.[23]

Perhaps you have heard that taking laxatives after overeating prevents deposition of body fat from the excess energy intake. This erroneous and dangerous premise has gained popularity among followers of numerous fad diets. You may temporarily feel less full after using a laxative because laxatives hasten emptying of the large intestine and increase fluid loss. Most laxatives, however, do not speed the passage of food through the small intestine, where digestion and most nutrient absorption take place.[13] As a result, laxatives do not prevent fat gain from excess energy intake.

Hemorrhoids

Hemorrhoids, also called *piles,* are swollen veins of the rectum and anus. The blood vessels in this area are subject to intense pressure, especially during bowel movements. Added stress to the vessels from pregnancy, obesity, prolonged sitting, violent coughing or sneezing, or straining during bowel movements can lead to a hemorrhoid.[22] Hemorrhoids can develop unnoticed until a strained bowel movement precipitates symptoms, which may include pain, itching, and bleeding.

Itching, caused by moisture in the anal canal, swelling, or other irritation, is perhaps the most common symptom. Pain, if present, is usually aching and steady. Bleeding may result from a hemorrhoid and may appear in the toilet as a bright red streak in the feces. The sensation of a mass in the anal canal after a bowel movement is symptomatic of an internal hemorrhoid that protrudes through the anus.[23]

Anyone can develop a hemorrhoid, and about half of adults over age 50 do. Pressure from prolonged sitting or exertion is often enough to bring on symptoms, although diet, lifestyle, and possibly heredity play a role. If you think you have a hemorrhoid, you should consult your physician. Rectal bleeding, although usually caused by hemorrhoids, may also indicate other problems, such as cancer.

A physician may suggest a variety of self-care measures for hemorrhoids. Pain can be lessened by applying warm, soft compresses or by sitting in a tub of warm water for 15 to 20 minutes.[23] Dietary recommendations are the same as those for treating constipation, especially a focus on consuming enough dietary fiber. Over-the-counter remedies also can offer relief of symptoms.

Irritable Bowel Syndrome

Many adults have irritable bowel syndrome, a combination of cramps, gassiness, bloating, and irregular bowel function (diarrhea, constipation, or alternating episodes of both).[4] It is more common in women than in men. A hallmark of the disease is pain relief after a bowel movement. The cause is thought to be altered intestinal motility, coupled with a decreased pain threshold for abdominal distention. In other words, a minor amount of abdominal bloating causes pain that the average person would not sense.[10]

Therapy is individualized and can include a trial of high-fiber foods (especially foods rich in wheat bran); elimination diets that focus on avoiding dairy products and gas-forming foods, such as legumes and certain other vegetables; medications to treat the diarrhea or constipation; stress-reduction strategies; and psychological counseling. Low-fat meals and smaller, more frequent meals may also help, as large meals can trigger large intestine contractions.[24] Currently, reassurance is the most a physician can offer. Although irritable bowel syndrome can be uncomfortable and upsetting, it is harmless; it carries no risk for cancer or other serious digestive problems.

CHAPTER **S EVEN**

Metabolism

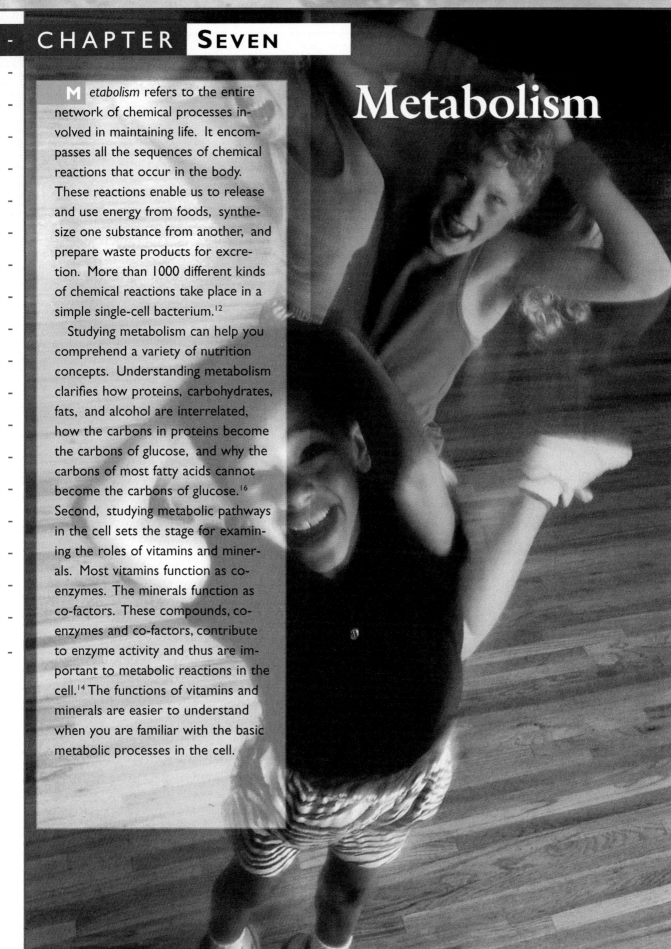

M *etabolism* refers to the entire network of chemical processes involved in maintaining life. It encompasses all the sequences of chemical reactions that occur in the body. These reactions enable us to release and use energy from foods, synthesize one substance from another, and prepare waste products for excretion. More than 1000 different kinds of chemical reactions take place in a simple single-cell bacterium.[12]

Studying metabolism can help you comprehend a variety of nutrition concepts. Understanding metabolism clarifies how proteins, carbohydrates, fats, and alcohol are interrelated, how the carbons in proteins become the carbons of glucose, and why the carbons of most fatty acids cannot become the carbons of glucose.[16] Second, studying metabolic pathways in the cell sets the stage for examining the roles of vitamins and minerals. Most vitamins function as co-enzymes. The minerals function as co-factors. These compounds, co-enzymes and co-factors, contribute to enzyme activity and thus are important to metabolic reactions in the cell.[14] The functions of vitamins and minerals are easier to understand when you are familiar with the basic metabolic processes in the cell.

NUTRITION AWARENESS INVENTORY

Answer these 15 statements about metabolism to test your current knowledge. If you think the statement is true or mostly true, circle T. If you think the statement is false or mostly false, circle F. Use the scoring key at the end of the book to compute your total score. Repeat this test after you have read the chapter, and compare your results.

1. **T F** Carbohydrates can be used for energy needs or stored as glycogen.
2. **T F** Fats can be used for energy needs or stored as fat.
3. **T F** Eating protein can't lead to fat formation.
4. **T F** The brain obtains most of the energy it needs in the form of glucose.
5. **T F** Fasting increases blood ketone concentrations.
6. **T F** Alcohol never turns to fat, no matter how much is consumed.
7. **T F** The B vitamins thiamin, niacin, and riboflavin participate in energy metabolism.
8. **T F** Protein metabolism requires vitamin B-6.
9. **T F** Iron and copper play key roles in energy metabolism.
10. **T F** Carnitine is used in carbohydrate metabolism.
11. **T F** Ketones are formed primarily from glycerol.
12. **T F** Mitochondria supply most of the energy for cell use.
13. **T F** Acetyl-CoA plays a central role in energy metabolism.
14. **T F** Plants obtain energy from photosynthesis.
15. **T F** When fasting, humans use proteins to synthesize glucose via a process called *gluconeogenesis*.

Metabolism

A s noted in the chapter overview, *metabolism* refers to the entire network of chemical processes involved in maintaining life and encompasses all of the sequences of chemical reactions that occur in the body. These reactions enable us to release and use energy from foods, convert one substance into another, and prepare waste products for excretion.[16] Examining cell metabolism is important at this stage in your study of nutrition because it helps clarify how proteins, carbohydrates, fats, and alcohol are interrelated and how vitamins and minerals contribute to these relationships.

A progression of metabolic chemical reactions from beginning to end is called a *pathway*. Compounds formed as the pathway proceeds are called **intermediates. Anabolic** pathways build compounds. Energy must be expended for these processes to take place. The chemical elements and compounds used to form the new substances often are called *building blocks*. Conversely, **catabolic** pathways break down compounds into small units. For example, complete catabolism of glucose results in the release of carbon dioxide (CO_2) and water (H_2O). Energy is released in the process; some is trapped for cell use, and the rest is lost as heat. Virtually every step in any pathway depends on an enzyme to initiate the necessary chemical reaction.[12]

The production of energy for cell use occurs in three separate stages. In the first stage, large food molecules, such as proteins, starches, and triglycerides, are broken down during digestion and absorption into smaller units, such as amino acids, monosaccharides, and free fatty acids. In the second stage, most of these smaller compounds are further degraded to the two-carbon intermediate

compound acetic acid ($CH_3\overset{\overset{O}{\|}}{C}-OH$), the acid found in vinegar. In the third stage, acetic acid (acetate for short) is degraded to carbon dioxide and water. The electrons and hydrogen ions released during this process are donated to oxygen atoms to form water. Some of the energy released in this catabolic process drives the synthesis of **adenosine triphosphate (ATP)**.[12] ATP is energy in a form that cells can

intermediate A chemical compound formed in one of many steps in a metabolic pathway. For example, pyruvate is an intermediate in the glycolysis pathway.

anabolic Describes the building of compounds.

catabolic Describes the breaking down of compounds.

Acids commonly lose a hydrogen ion at the pH found in human cells (pH 7.4). When that ion is lost, the name of the acid is changed by dropping the reference to acid and adding an *ate* ending. Thus acetic acid becomes acetate.

---

adenosine triphosphate (ATP) The main energy source for cells; ATP energy is used to promote ion pumping, enzyme activity, and muscular contraction.

use. Chapter 6 focused on the first stage, digestion and absorption. Let's now examine the last stage, specifically the metabolism of carbohydrate, fat, protein, and alcohol.

The Cell—Primary Site for Metabolism

The cell is the basic unit of body structure, and it is where most metabolic reactions occur (Figure 7-1). The human body is composed of at least 1×10^{14} cells.[12] A quick review of the basic structure of these cells will aid in understanding metabolism.

The cell is surrounded by a membrane that controls the passage of nutrients and other substances in and out of it. Within the cell is fluid called the *cytosol*. Within the cytosol are organelles, which are small bodies that perform specific metabolic functions. The names and activities of the various cell organelles follow:

Cell membrane. This double-layered structure is composed of lipids and protein. It contains channels to admit specific molecules into the cell; receptors that bind hormones and other compounds that send signals to cell components; and protein markers on the exterior that allow the immune system to recognize it as a human cell, as opposed to an invading bacterium (see Figure 7-1). The double-layered structure allows for membrane flexibility and contributes to the function of embedded receptors. Because of their lipid-rich composition, cell membranes are generally permeable to fat-soluble compounds such as fatty acids and cholesterol, but not water-soluble compounds such as glucose and amino acids.[16] Glucose, amino acids, and other water-soluble compounds primarily use specific pumps and receptors to enter cells, as discussed in Chapter 6.

Nucleus. This spherical structure is bound by its own double membrane. Within the nucleus are chromosomes, long threads of DNA that contain genetic information for directing cell protein synthesis and cell reproduction.[2] Most cells have two sets of DNA; sperm and egg cells have only one set. During cell fertilization the single sets are combined to yield the two sets found in the offspring. Inside the nucleus is a nucleolus, where a type of RNA (ribosomal RNA) is synthesized. Ribosomal RNA eventually helps assemble proteins in the cell. To direct protein synthesis, the genetic code in DNA is transcribed to messenger RNA (mRNA). The mRNA leaves the nucleus and is translated into proteins by the ribosomes that reside in the cytosol as part of the endoplasmic reticulum (see below). Amino acids are added one by one to the growing polypeptide chain based on the directions that ultimately originate from the DNA.[19]

Mitochondria. These have their own outer and inner membranes. The mitochondria are the major sites of cellular ATP production, which is carried on primarily within the highly folded inner membrane. Mitochondria are capable of synthesizing important cell components, such as carbon skeletons for nonessential (dispensable) amino acids.[12]

Endoplasmic reticulum. This network of internal membranes serves as a communication network within the cell. Small granules called *ribosomes* cover parts of the endoplasmic reticulum. These areas, known as the *rough endoplasmic reticulum,* are the sites of protein synthesis in the cell. Fat is synthesized in other areas of the endoplasmic reticulum, namely, the *smooth endoplasmic reticulum.*[16]

The Golgi complex. This consists of stacks of flattened structures that package proteins for export from the cell and help form other cell organelles. Budding off the Golgi complex are Golgi vesicles, which are fluid-filled sacs destined for other parts of the cell or for excretion from the cell.[16]

Lysosomes. These are small bodies that contain **hydrolytic enzymes** that degrade worn-out cell components and other cell debris. Lysosomes cannot digest the entire cell because each lysosome maintains very high acidity, which inhibits the hydrolytic enzyme action. When a lysosome fuses with a particle to be degraded, the acidity in the lysosome falls, promoting hydrolytic enzyme activity.[19]

hydrolysis A chemical reaction in which a compound is broken down by the addition of water. One product receives the hydrogen ion (H^+) while the other product receives the hydroxyl ion (OH^-). Hydrolytic enzymes break down compounds using water in the manner just described.

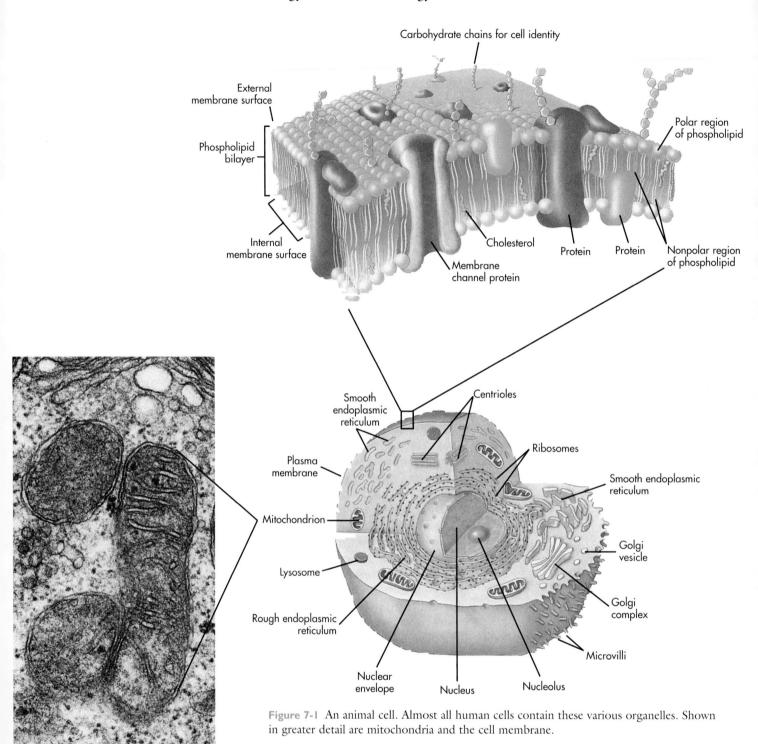

Figure 7-1 An animal cell. Almost all human cells contain these various organelles. Shown in greater detail are mitochondria and the cell membrane.

Cytosol. This is the fluid within the cell, in which the various organelles are suspended. The fluid plus all organelles (except the nucleus) is called the *cytoplasm*.

Storage forms of energy. These exist as glycogen granules and lipid droplets.

Peroxisomes. These contain enzymes, such as catalase, that can break down peroxides and alcohol.

Attachment sites. Cell membranes contain specialized structures used for attachment and communication with adjoining cells. At tight junctions, no space appears between the adjoining cells. Gap junctions provide small reinforced openings between cells, through which electric currents, ions, and small molecules can pass.

Let's now review energy metabolism in general. Later we identify the types of metabolic pathways and where they occur in the cell.

Energy for the Cell

The energy that human cells use comes from chemical bonds found in carbohydrate, fat, protein, and alcohol. This energy is originally produced during photosynthesis, when plants use solar energy to make glucose and other organic (carbon-containing) compounds (Figure 7-2). In doing so, plants trap the sun's energy in the form of chemical bonds. The chemical reactions in photosynthesis form compounds that contain more energy than carbon dioxide and water, the building blocks used. Virtually all organisms use the sun—either directly or indirectly, as we do—as their source of energy.[19]

The body transforms the bond energy trapped in carbohydrate, fat, and protein into other forms of energy[19]:

- chemical energy, which helps build glycogen from many glucoses
- mechanical energy, which propels muscular movements
- electrical energy, which promotes nerve transmissions
- osmotic energy, which maintains ion balance within cells

The by-products of these energy transformations are carbon dioxide, water, and heat. Chemical energy from ingested food that passes through body cells is eventually and irretrievably dissipated to the environment as heat (Figure 7-3).[16]

Thus in human **respiration** the starting materials are energy-yielding compounds such as glucose, which through an elaborate process are converted to end products such as carbon dioxide and water. This process results in the transfer of energy from food to cells, which in turn allows energy-requiring pathways in cells to function.

Many chemical reactions in the body could not occur without the addition of outside energy supplied by food. Outside energy permits compounds such as glucose to be transformed into products such as glycogen, as mentioned earlier. Although glucose molecules themselves contain the energy needed for glycogen synthesis, individual glucose molecules provide neither the right amount of energy for a chemical reaction nor a form of energy that cells can directly use. A glucose molecule contains over 100 times more energy than required to drive an individual chemical reaction in a cell. A triglyceride molecule contains about 500 times more energy than is needed. So a cell must have a means of breaking down the glucose and fatty acid molecules to release and then convert the chemical energy trapped in them into smaller, usable energy forms.[16]

respiration The utilization of oxygen; in the human organism, the inhalation of oxygen and the exhalation of carbon dioxide; in cells, the oxidation (electron removal) of food molecules, particularly in the citric acid cycle, to obtain energy.

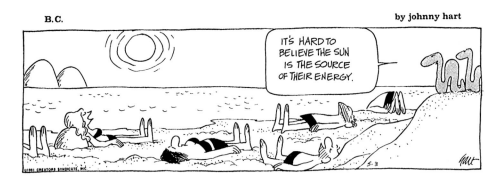

B.C.   **by johnny hart**

IT'S HARD TO BELIEVE THE SUN IS THE SOURCE OF THEIR ENERGY.

Figure 7-2 B.C.

Reprinted by permission of Creators Syndicate, Inc.

EXPERT OPINION

MOLECULAR BIOLOGY IN NUTRITION

DENIS M. MEDEIROS, Ph.D., R.D.

The vast amount of information pertaining to our understanding of how living cells function, remain viable, and propagate has seen tremendous growth in the last several years. Much of this increased knowledge has been made possible by recent advances both in the field of molecular biology and in the tools used to study the fundamental aspect of life.

Molecular biology allows us to understand how cells function at the very basis of life—genetic material or DNA. DNA contains the code on how proteins are assembled. It is important to know how certain genes or segments of DNA are expressed or activated in cells, which other segments are repressed, and the location of these genes in reference to chromosome number, location of the chromosome, and relation to other genes.

All cells that compose an organism have the same copy of DNA, but not all DNA is transcribed to messenger RNA (mRNA). The transcription process is both cell specific and life cycle specific. For instance, during gestation various cell types that compose the fetal heart can make the protein elastin, which is a component of heart vessels and valves. After birth very little, if any, elastin is made by the heart. How these events occur and how they are controlled is part of molecular biology. How does the cell know when to transcribe the genetic code to mRNA and subsequently to the building of a new protein?

More important, some cells, and consequently some individuals, may have a gene or DNA segment that causes the production of a defective protein that leads to a serious disease. Also, missing DNA segments can prevent some individuals from being able to make one or more proteins.

Why should nutritionists be concerned about molecular biology? At one time it was thought that nutrients could not affect the expression of genes. New information tells us differently. Vitamins A and D and the trace element zinc are now known to exert some of their influence at the gene level. For instance, vitamin D is responsible for causing cells in the small intestine to synthesize a calcium-binding protein to aid in the absorption of dietary calcium.

The absorption of dietary zinc and copper by the cells in the small intestine is also regulated at the gene level. It is known that an increase in dietary zinc does not always result in a proportional increase in absorption. Furthermore, excess zinc often results in decreased copper absorption. Since both elements have a 2+ ionic charge, the interpretation to explain these observations was that zinc simply blocked copper absorption by competing for the same absorption-binding site on the cell membrane in the small intestine. It turned out that this interpretation, although simple and logical, was not entirely correct. Subsequent studies revealed that when zinc in the diet increased, the cells in the small intestine increased the synthesis of a small protein, metallothionein. This protein bound to zinc and trapped it in the cell, preventing its transfer to the blood, providing an elegant way of preventing too much zinc from entering the body. When dietary zinc declined, metallothionein declined and zinc absorption and subsequent transfer to the blood increased. In concert, mRNA for metallothionein increased with elevated zinc and dropped when dietary zinc decreased.

Metallothionein, however, can also bind up other elements, copper included. In fact, metallothionein, the concentration of which is regulated by zinc, has a greater binding affinity for copper than zinc. This means that the reason excess dietary zinc can decrease copper absorption is that it causes increased metallothionein synthesis and copper binding, thereby decreasing the absorption of copper as well as zinc.

Molecular biology is useful in clinical medicine, where a related field known as *recombinant DNA technology* has led to the production of insulin and erythropoietin by bacteria. Insulin is the protein hormone produced by cells of the pancreas for glucose utilization. Erythropoietin is a protein hormone produced by cells of the kidneys that stimulates red blood cell production. It is critical in correcting certain types of anemia. Simply stated, scientists insert the human genes that code for either insulin or erythropoietin into bacteria. In turn the bacteria produce these proteins in large quantities, becoming production factories. Insulin and erythropoietin produced in this way are better tolerated by patients than these two proteins taken from other species, such as swine, and given to humans.

Molecular biology tools are also useful in cases of hereditary diseases that may be modulated or controlled by diet. For instance, some people lack low-density lipoprotein (LDL) receptors. Molecular biology tests are available that allow us to determine which individuals have this problem. As these people age, they develop atherosclerosis because of cholesterol build-up in the arteries. Determining which individuals lack the gene or DNA segment responsible for the receptor through a test helps identify candidates for a low-fat diet to minimize cholesterol build-up.

The recent identification of genes that lead to a type of colon cancer and to a type of breast cancer will allow identification of individuals with these genes and perhaps prescription of aggressive dietary modification (low-fat and high-fiber diet) to delay the onset of disease.

An exciting application of molecular biology involves "gene therapy" to compensate for a segment of DNA that is either missing or abnormal. The correct gene then may be inserted into living cells to correct the problem. Clinical trials for treatment of such diseases as muscular dystrophy and cystic fibrosis thus far have yielded promising results.

Forensic science makes extensive use of molecular biology tools in performing genetic analysis or sequencing of nucleic acids (the constituents of DNA) on human specimens obtained from crime scenes. Nucleic acid sequences are almost unique, with a high improbability of two subjects having the same sequence except in the case of identical twins. Such testing has caused the overturning of a number of convictions made prior to the availability of such methods by proving that specimens at the crime scene came from someone other than the alleged perpetrator.

As we look to the future, nutritionists are asking this question: do other diseases with nutrition implications have genetic origins? One nutrition condition that may have a genetic connection is obesity. While environmental factors, such as lifestyle, lack of physical activity, and overeating, play a large role in obesity, much of obesity probably has a genetic basis. Appetite-controlling signals are known to be regulated by the production of certain proteins in various tissues and by feedback to the brain. Either abnormal production or a defect in signaling proteins or brain receptors may have a molecular basis. A gene in mice known as the *ob gene* produces a protein that tells the brain to stop eating. However, in some strains of obese mice the protein does not function correctly or is altered, so the brain doesn't get the signal to stop eating. Humans are thought to have such a gene in addition to others that may influence weight and appetite. There may be a series of several genes that act in concert. Finding the human genes responsible for obesity would be one of the most significant nutrition discoveries in decades! Correcting such a defect might be possible after identification of the gene, perhaps limiting the high incidence of obesity in Western cultures.

Molecular biology aspects of nutrition have also produced a greater understanding of why humans require vitamins and minerals to maintain optimal health. The investment into this area has already paid large dividends to the knowledge base and will continue to do so in the near future.

Dr. Medeiros is a professor of Human Nutrition and Associate Dean of Research for the College of Human Ecology at The Ohio State University. His research interests include the role of trace elements such as copper, zinc, iron, and selenium in heart disease from molecular biology and ultrastructural perspectives.

NUTRITION FOCUS

OXIDATION-REDUCTION REACTIONS—KEY PROCESSES IN METABOLISM

Oxidation-reduction reactions form a vital link between the energy-yielding nutrients and ATP—the form of energy cells use. The formal meaning of oxidation and reduction can be summarized as:

A substance is **oxidized** when it loses one or more electrons.

A substance is **reduced** when it gains one or more electrons.

Electron flow governs oxidation-reduction processes. If one substance loses electrons (is oxidized), another substance must gain electrons (must be reduced). The two processes go together; one cannot proceed without the other.[16]

Consider the oxidation-reduction reaction between zinc and the copper ion Cu^{2+}.

$$Zn + Cu^{2+} \ 0 \ Zn^{2+} + Cu$$

Here Zn has lost two electrons (has been oxidized) ($Zn \ 0 \ Zn^{2+} + 2e^-$). At the same time copper has gained two electrons (has been reduced) ($Cu^{2+} + 2e^- \ 0 \ Cu$). Another example is the iron in hemoglobin, which can be oxidized from Fe^{2+} to Fe^{3+} and reduced from Fe^{3+} to Fe^{2+}. This occurs during the transport of oxygen to body cells.

Oxidation-reduction reactions involving carbon-containing compounds are somewhat more difficult to visualize. A simple rule has been developed to determine oxidation-reduction in these compounds.

If the compound gains oxygen or loses hydrogen it has been oxidized. If it loses oxygen or gains hydrogen the compound has been reduced.

The process below illustrates this definition.

$$CH_3 - CH_3 \xrightarrow[\text{reduction}]{\text{oxidation}} CH_3 - CH_2 - OH$$
ethane   ethanol

pyruvic acid   lactic acid

This method of determining oxidation and reduction—determining oxygen and hydrogen exchange—is extensively used in nutrition. For example, in the above reaction pyruvic acid (made from glucose) is reduced to form lactic acid by gaining two hydrogens. This happens during intense exercise (see Chapter 10). Lactic acid is oxidized back to pyruvic acid by losing two hydrogens.

Scientists generally use the terms *oxidation* and *reduction* as verbs or adjectives. As a verb, pyruvic acid is said to be reduced to lactic acid, and lactic acid is oxidized to pyruvic acid. As an adjective, lactic acid is said to be the reduced form of pyruvic acid, while pyruvic acid is the oxidized form of lactic acid.

Oxidation-reduction reactions in the body are controlled by enzymes. One important class of these enzymes, designated *dehydrogenases*, removes hydrogens from energy-yielding nutrients or their breakdown products and donates the hydrogens to the final acceptor, oxygen, to form water. In the process, large amounts of energy are transferred to ADP plus Pi to make ATP.[16]

Two B vitamins, niacin and riboflavin, assist dehydrogenase enzymes and in turn play a role in transferring the hydrogens from glucose to oxygen in the metabolic pathways of the cell. Niacin functions as the coenzyme niacin adenine dinucleotide (NAD). This is the oxidized form, which can accept one hydrogen ion and two electrons to become NADH. In other words, the oxidized form of niacin, NAD, is reduced to NADH. Note that NAD is actually NAD^+, indicating one less electron than in its complete configuration. By accepting two electrons and one hydrogen ion, NAD^+ becomes NADH, with no net charge. We ignore the charge on NAD to simplify chapter discussions.

Riboflavin plays a similar role. In its oxidized form it is known as flavin adenine dinucleotide (FAD). When it is reduced (gains two hydrogens, equivalent to two hydrogen ions and two electrons), it is known as $FADH_2$.

The reduction of oxygen (O) to form water (H_2O) provides the driving force for life, as it is vital to the way cells synthesize ATP.[16] Thus oxidation-reduction reactions are a key to life.

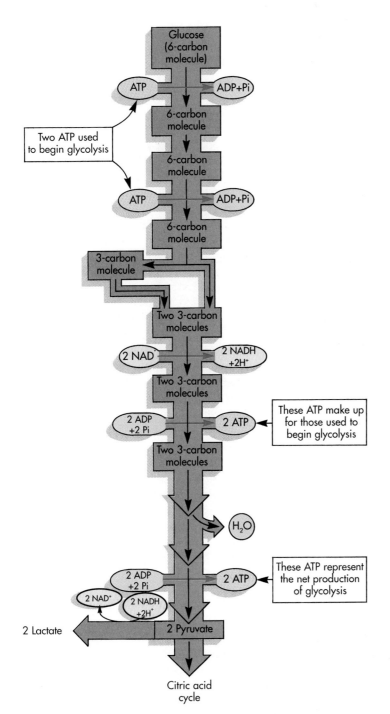

Figure 7-5 Glycolysis simplified. The process begins with one glucose ($C_6H_{12}O_6$) and ends with two pyruvates ($C_3H_4O_3$). Some ATP is produced by the process. The four electrons and two of the hydrogen ions released are captured by two NAD. The other two hydrogen ions float free in the cytosol.

the process four hydrogens (containing a total of four electrons) are removed and four ATP are generated. The electrons and hydrogen ions are picked up by the carrier, called **nicotinamide adenine dinucleotide (NAD).** Each NAD accepts two electrons and one hydrogen ion, yielding the reduced form NADH. Thus an end result of glycolysis is also the synthesis of two NADH, with the release of two hydrogen ions.[12]

Throughout this chapter we simplify many metabolic pathways by including only the most important steps, to give you an overview of metabolism. Other courses will cover the pathways step-by-step, enzyme-by-enzyme. To look at any particular pathway in detail, see Appendix J.

aerobic Requiring oxygen.

anaerobic Not requiring oxygen.

Regenerating NAD by using lactate represents a fermentation reaction. Some yeasts produce alcohol (ethanol) instead of lactate to regenerate NAD in anaerobic conditions. This is also a fermentation reaction.

SO WHERE IS THE ATP?

In glycolysis, the first reaction involves one ATP donating a phosphate group to glucose. In the second step another ATP is used to add a second phosphate group. Thus to begin the pathway, a cell uses two ATP. As the two three-carbon molecules are converted to pyruvate, each one generates two ATP, for a total of four ATP. The net energy produced thus far from glycolysis is two ATP, as two ATP prime the system and four ATP are produced. There are more ATP to come; this represents only about 6% of the ATP possible from one glucose molecule.[12]

Chemical energy stored in the bonds of NADH can eventually be transferred to ATP. Generally each NADH provides enough energy to yield three ATP. Thus NADH is a form of potential energy for the cell; as chemical energy is released from the carbon-hydrogen bonds originally present in glucose, NADH traps some of the energy. A cell eventually uses the energy in NADH to form ATP. Later we will show how this happens.

The other monosaccharides, fructose and galactose, are converted to intermediate compounds of the glycolytic pathway and follow the same sequence of events as glucose. Pyruvate is eventually formed.[16]

LACTATE PRODUCTION IS THE ENDPOINT OF ANAEROBIC GLYCOLYSIS

Some cells lack the oxygen-requiring (**aerobic**) pathway needed for using NADH for ATP synthesis, and in turn also lack the ability to use this process to recycle NADH back to NAD. The red blood cell is an example. Thus as a red blood cell converts glucose to pyruvate, NADH builds up in the cell. Eventually the NAD concentration falls too low to permit glycolysis to continue, since most of the NAD present is in the form NADH.

To compensate, a red blood cell reacts to pyruvate with an NADH and a free hydrogen ion to form lactate (see Figure 7-5). In the process, NADH turns into NAD. This process allows the red blood cell to resupply itself with NAD. Exercising muscles produce lactate for the same reason; they run out of NAD (see Chapter 10). The production of lactate allows **anaerobic** glycolysis to continue, as there remains a steady supply of NAD. Again, this pathway yields only about 6% of the potential ATP per glucose molecule. But for some cells, such as red blood cells, anaerobic glycolysis is the only available method for making ATP. The lactate is released into the bloodstream, picked up primarily by the liver, and synthesized into glucose.[16]

CONCEPT CHECK

Carbohydrate metabolism begins when a cell releases glucose from glycogen or takes glucose from the bloodstream. Glucose is then degraded through a sequence of steps into two pyruvate molecules. This pathway, called *glycolysis*, yields NADH, a potential form of energy, and ATP, an actual energy source for a cell. Both fructose and galactose are also metabolized via glycolysis to pyruvate. Pyruvate is either broken down further or converted to lactate. Red blood cells perform the latter reaction, as part of *anaerobic glycolysis*. The conversion of pyruvate to lactate allows the cell to oxidize NADH into NAD. This provides the NAD needed for glycolysis. NADH can also be oxidized to NAD via oxygen-requiring pathways found in most cells.

The Citric Acid Cycle Completes Glucose Catabolism

The two pyruvate (or lactate) molecules formed at the end of glycolysis still contain much stored energy. Pyruvate passes from the cell cytosol into the mitochondria. A cell then uses pathways found there to extract the remaining energy from pyruvate to form more ATP. One key pathway is called the *citric acid cycle*.

PYRUVATE TO ACETYL-CoA IS AN IRREVERSIBLE STEP

Before the citric acid cycle can begin, pyruvate must lose a carbon dioxide group and eventually form acetyl-CoA. This overall reaction is irreversible, which has important metabolic consequences.[12] As pyruvate is converted to acetyl-CoA, another NADH is formed from NAD, so more potential ATP molecules are produced. The conversion of pyruvate to acetyl-CoA requires the B vitamin thiamin. For this reason dietary carbohydrates increase thiamin needs.

From the point of view of energy metabolism, acetyl-CoA is essentially the two-carbon compound acetate. Attached to the acetate is a large coenzyme A (CoA) molecule. CoA contains the B vitamin pantothenic acid. The CoA molecule activates acetate in the same way a phosphate group activates glucose. Without a CoA molecule attached, acetate does not participate in the first reaction of the citric acid cycle.[12]

THE CITRIC ACID CYCLE

The citric acid cycle is an elegant sequence of chemical reactions used by cells to convert the carbons of acetate to carbon dioxide and to produce energy. Acetyl-CoA enters the cycle, and the reactions eventually yield two molecules of carbon dioxide. In the process the cell produces NADH and other related molecules, which eventually are used to form many ATP.

To begin the citric acid cycle, acetyl-CoA combines with a four-carbon compound, oxaloacetic acid (or oxaloacetate) to form the six-carbon compound citric acid (or citrate) (Figure 7-6). In the process the CoA molecule is released. During

Other names for the citric acid cycle are the tricarboxylic acid cycle (TCA cycle) and the Krebs cycle, named after Sir Hans Krebs, the scientist who first described it.

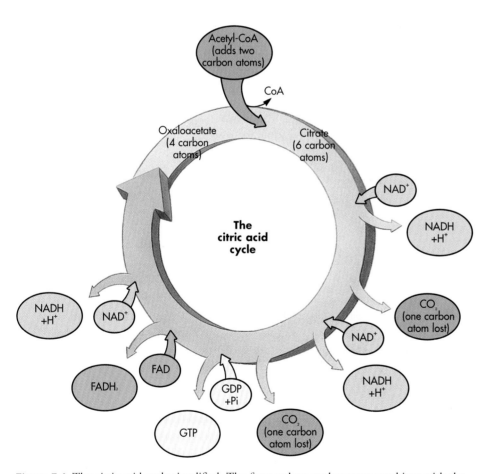

Figure 7-6 The citric acid cycle simplified. The four-carbon oxaloacetate combines with the two-carbon acetyl-CoA to form the six-carbon compound called *citric acid*, or citrate. The citrate is ultimately re-formed into the original four-carbon oxaloacetate, with a net loss of two carbons as carbon dioxide. The pathway thus begins and ends with the same compound, oxaloacetate, which makes it a cycle.

the citric acid cycle the six-carbon citrate molecule is broken down into a four-carbon oxaloacetate molecule and two carbon dioxide molecules. More important, the process produces potential ATP in the form of three more NADH and one $FADH_2$. Each $FADH_2$ provides enough energy to synthesize two ATP, one less than NADH. Finally, guanosine triphosphate (GTP, which is analogous to ATP) is made from GDP and Pi.[16]

To review carbohydrate metabolism so far, we started with a six-carbon glucose and eventually produced six carbon dioxide molecules. Thus all the carbons in glucose end up in the form of carbon dioxide. The carbon dioxide eventually leaves the body by way of the lungs. In the process, ATP is made directly using both the glycolysis and citric acid cycle pathways, and NADH and $FADH_2$ are formed from NAD and FAD. The NADH and $FADH_2$ molecules can be used to drive ATP synthesis in the electron transport chain.[12]

In this way some of the energy in the chemical bonds of glucose is transferred to ATP. So some of the energy in food yields a form of energy that cells can use, rather than just being converted to heat, as would have happened if we had ignited the food with a match. In engineering terms, cells capture about 40% of the chemical energy in glucose and store it in a useful form for later use, namely ATP. The remaining energy (60%) escapes as heat via all the reactions that take place in which ATP, GTP, NADH, or $FADH_2$ is not made. This includes many steps in glycolysis and citric acid cycle pathways. The same 40:60 ratio applies for energy metabolism of fatty acids and amino acids. That's fairly efficient compared with an automobile engine, which captures only about 10% of the chemical energy in gasoline.[19]

The Electron Transport Chain Is the Primary Site for ATP Synthesis

During the metabolism of protein, carbohydrate, fat, and alcohol, cells generate NADH and $FADH_2$. Most cells can use these compounds for ATP synthesis (Figure 7-7). The pathway that performs this exchange is called the **electron transport chain.** The process, which occurs in the inner membrane of mitochondria, is called *oxidative phosphorylation.* The minerals iron and copper are needed for this process.[16]

In the electron transport chain, NADH donates its chemical energy to an FAD-related compound called *flavin mononucleotide (FMN).* As high-energy NADH becomes low-energy NAD, the reaction liberates some energy to form one ATP mol-

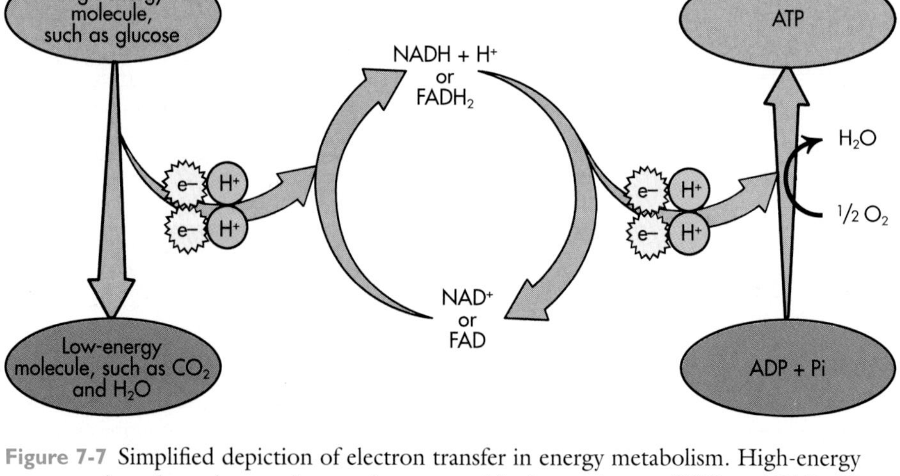

electron transport chain A series of reactions using oxygen to convert NADH and $FADH_2$ molecules to free NAD and FAD molecules by the donation of electrons and hydrogen ions, yielding water and ATP.

Figure 7-7 Simplified depiction of electron transfer in energy metabolism. High-energy compounds such as glucose give up electrons and hydrogen ions to NAD and FAD. The NADH and $FADH_2$ that are formed transfer these electrons and hydrogen ions, using specialized electron carriers, to oxygen to form water (H_2O). The energy yielded by the entire process is used to generate ATP from ADP and Pi.

ecule and to yield $FMNH_2$. The $FMNH_2$, through a series of steps that uses other electron carriers, called **cytochromes,** donates its electrons and hydrogen ions to oxygen. Water and a free FMN are formed, and the energy liberated yields an additional two ATP. Thus the net result of the electron transport chain is the production of ATP and water. Recall also that some metabolic pathways yield $FADH_2$. $FADH_2$ donates its electrons and hydrogen ions directly to the cytochrome chain, bypassing FMN and yielding two ATP (Figure 7-8).[12] Since oxygen is essential to these processes, the electron transport chain represents the aerobic side of metabolism. And although we can describe these processes, there are still questions about how the electron transport chain works.

Although oxygen does not participate directly in the citric acid cycle, it is part of the aerobic side of metabolism, since the cycle operates only under aerobic conditions. NADH and $FADH_2$ produced during the citric acid cycle can be regenerated into NAD and FAD only by the eventual transfer of their electrons and hydrogen ions to oxygen. The citric acid cycle has no way to oxidize NADH and $FADH_2$ back to NAD and FAD analogous to the way that anaerobic glycolysis produces lactate. This is ultimately why oxygen is essential to life; a final acceptor of the electrons and hydrogen ions generated from the breakdown of energy-yielding nutrients is needed. Without oxygen, most of our cells are unable to extract enough energy from fuels to sustain life.[16]

• • •

This entire description of the metabolism of glucose depicts the essence of metabolism. Cells need to release energy stored in food fuels and then trap as much as possible as ATP. The body cannot afford to lose all energy as heat. Some heat is necessary for warmth, but the body also needs mobilizing energy. Glycolysis, the citric acid cycle, and the electron transport chain accomplish many things. Most important, however, they enable cells to capture the chemical energy in food in the form of ATP, which acts as cellular fuel. In effect, ATP allows cells "to get up and do what needs to be done."

cytochromes Electron-transfer compounds that participate in the electron transport chain.

- - - - - - - - - - - - -

An alternative pathway for the metabolism of glucose is the pentose phosphate pathway. This yields ribose for RNA and DNA synthesis, as well as a variation of NAD (NADPH) used in synthetic reactions, such as the synthesis of fatty acids. The pentose phosphate pathway is active in cells that synthesize fatty acids, such as liver cells.

- - - - - - - - - - - - -

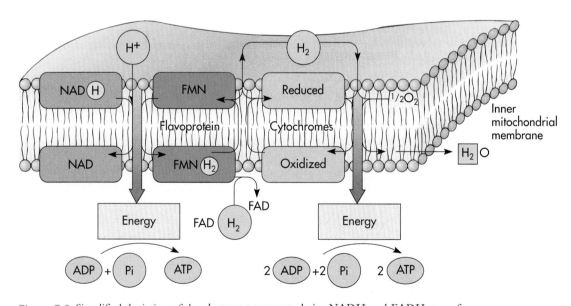

Figure 7-8 Simplified depiction of the electron transport chain. NADH and $FADH_2$ transfer their hydrogen ions and electrons to electron carriers located on the inner mitochondrial membrane. The electrons and hydrogen ions combine with oxygen to form water (H_2O). The energy yielded by the entire process is used to generate ATP. The oxygen atoms attract the electrons down the electron transport chain. Each NADH in the mitochondria releases enough energy to form three ATP, while each $FADH_2$ releases enough energy to form two ATP. Of the 36 to 38 ATP yielded by the complete oxidation of glucose, almost 90% are synthesized in the electron transport chain.

Figure 7-9 A bird's-eye view of cell metabolism. Note that acetyl-CoA forms a crossroads for many pathways and that the citric acid cycle can also be used to help build compounds, such as certain amino acids. Anabolic and catabolic processes may appear to share the same pathways, but generally this is only true for a few steps. Separate enzymes control anabolic and catabolic flow in a pathway. This allows the cell much control over metabolism, since a specific set of enzymes can be activated to promote either anabolism or catabolism. If the chemical reactions in anabolism and catabolism were catalyzed by the same set of enzymes, the direction of flow of compounds through these pathways would be dictated exclusively by the concentration of the starting materials, rather than by the cell's changing needs for energy or synthesis of needed compounds.

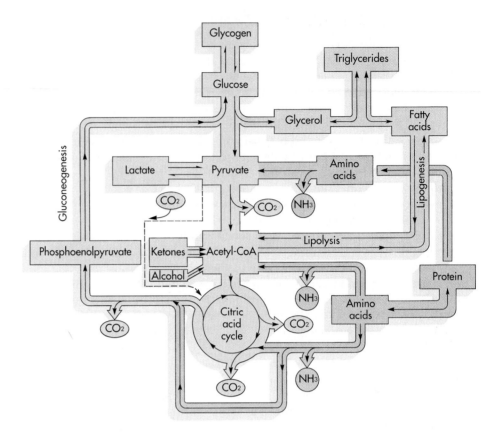

The metabolism of virtually all energy-yielding compounds produces acetyl-CoA at some point. Acetyl-CoA plays a central role in energy metabolism. No matter what type of diet you consume—high carbohydrate, high protein, or high fat—most of the energy-yielding nutrients pass through acetyl-CoA.[12] Acetyl-CoA is the common denominator that links all human diets (see Figure 7-9).

Glycogen Metabolism

Glycogen synthesis uses a form of glucose, adding more glucose molecules to an existing glycogen chain. This provides liver and muscle cells with a short-term storage form of glucose. Later, when glucose is needed, glycogen breakdown yields glucose as a glucose-phosphate compound, which eventually begins glycolysis. An enzyme involved in glycogen breakdown uses vitamin B-6.[16]

CONCEPT CHECK

In the citric acid cycle a two-carbon acetate molecule in the form of acetyl-CoA combines with a four-carbon oxaloacetate molecule to form the six-carbon citrate molecule. Through various chemical reactions, the cycle releases two carbon dioxide molecules and eventually yields another oxaloacetate, the starting material. This new oxaloacetate can combine with another acetyl-CoA molecule to begin the process again. The NADH and $FADH_2$ produced in the citric acid cycle donate their electrons and hydrogens to the electron transport chain, yielding free NAD and FAD, water, and ATP.

Lipolysis: Fat Breakdown

Lipolysis is part of a process of splitting—breaking down—triglycerides into free fatty acids and glycerol. The further breakdown of the fatty acids for energy production is called *fatty acid oxidation,* since the donation of electrons from fatty acids to oxygen is the net reaction in the energy-yielding process. This takes place in the mitochondria and peroxisomes of the cell, but only mitochondria can use the energy released to form ATP.[16]

Fatty acids are liberated from lipid storage in adipose cells by an enzyme called *hormone-sensitive lipase.* The activity of this enzyme is increased by the hormones glucagon, growth hormone, epinephrine, and others.[20] The fatty acids are taken up from the bloodstream by cells and are shuttled from the cell cytosol into the mitochondria using a carrier called **carnitine.** Cells produce the carnitine needed for this process. Healthy adults do not need to consume carnitine supplements, although they are sold in health food stores (see Chapter 13).[16]

Almost all fatty acids in nature are composed of an even number of carbons, ranging from 2 to 26. The first step in transferring the energy in a fatty acid to ATP (fatty acid oxidation) is to cleave the carbons, two at a time, and convert the two-carbon fragments to acetyl-CoA. The process of converting a free fatty acid to multiple acetyl-CoA molecules is more specifically called **beta-oxidation,** since the second carbon on a fatty acid (counting from the methyl [$-CH^3$] end) is called the *beta carbon.*[16] During beta-oxidation, NADH and $FADH_2$ are produced. So, as with glucose, a fatty acid is eventually degraded into the two-carbon compound acetate in the form of acetyl-CoA. Some of the chemical energy is also trapped, in this case as NADH and $FADH_2$.

The acetyl-CoA enters the citric acid cycle and two carbon dioxides are released, just as with the acetyl-CoA produced from glucose. Thus the breakdown product of both glucose and fatty acids, acetyl CoA, uses a common pathway—the citric acid cycle—for energy production. One big difference, however, is that a 16-carbon fatty acid yields 129 ATP, while the 6-carbon glucose yields 36 to 38 ATP. That results in a ratio of about 8 ATP per carbon for fatty acids versus about 6 ATP per carbon for glucose.[12] This difference results from the greater number of C–H bonds per carbon in a fatty acid compared with glucose. It is the oxidation of these chemical bonds that provides the energy to drive ATP synthesis. The carbons in glucose are also bonded to hydroxyl groups (–OH), rather than only to hydrogen atoms, as is primarily the case in a fatty acid. Thus, as a whole, the carbons of glucose exist in a more oxidized state. This is why fats yield more kilocalories per gram than carbohydrates—fats are less oxidized (more reduced) than carbohydrates.

No matter how many carbons a fatty acid contains, it is usually broken down into acetyl-CoA. Occasionally a fatty acid has an odd number of carbons, so the cell forms many acetyl-CoA, plus one three-carbon compound, propionyl-CoA. The propionyl-CoA enters the citric acid cycle directly, bypassing acetyl-CoA.[12] It can then go on to yield carbon dioxide and other products.

CARBOHYDRATE AIDS FAT METABOLISM

In addition to its role in energy production, the citric acid cycle provides compounds that leave the cycle and enter biosynthetic pathways, such as those used to make the red blood cell protein hemoglobin. This means that even though oxaloacetate is reused in the cycle, a minimum amount of it must be maintained because its removal from the citric acid cycle for biosynthetic reactions could prevent completion of the cycle.[12] One potential source of this additional oxaloacetate is pyruvate. So as fatty acids create acetyl-CoA, carbohydrates such as glucose keep the concentration of pyruvate high enough to resupply oxaloacetate to the citric acid cycle.[19] We could say that "fats burn in a fire of carbohydrate," since the entire pathway for fatty acid oxidation works better when carbohydrate is available.

lipolysis The breakdown of triglycerides to glycerol and fatty acids.

carnitine A compound used to shuttle fatty acids from the cytosol of the cell into mitochondria.

beta-oxidation The breakdown of a fatty acid into numerous acetyl-CoA molecules.

Critical Thinking

Sandy bought a large bottle of "carnitine" at her local health food store because the retailer promised her that it would help her lose fat quickly. How would you explain carnitine's role to her? Was her purchase a good choice?

NUTRITION FOCUS

HOMEOSTASIS IS THE OVERRIDING THEME OF BODY METABOLISM

All living things maintain a relatively constant internal environment that is quite different from their surroundings, with more of certain chemical compounds and less of others. **Homeostasis** is the result of the dynamic processes by which an organism maintains this constant internal environment despite changes in the external environment.[14] *Homeo* is Greek for "same" and *stasis* is Greek for "staying." This is a major function of most organs in the human body. Homeostatic effects include regulation of blood pressure, blood glucose concentration, and body temperature. The liver is an especially important organ in nutritional homeostasis because it processes and stores a wide variety of nutrients.

Homeostasis plays a vital role in the body because tissues and organs can function efficiently only within a narrow range of conditions. The range of temperatures in which life is possible is a tiny fraction of those found in nature. Cooler temperatures favor preservation of cellular structure but slow the rates of the chemical reactions carried out by cells. Higher temperatures accelerate chemical reactions but also may disrupt the structures of the proteins and other large molecules within cells. Furthermore, each cell of the body is surrounded by a small amount of fluid, and the normal function of that cell depends on the maintenance of its fluid environment within a narrow range of conditions, including volume, temperature, and chemical content. If the fluid surrounding cells deviates from homeostatic ranges, the cells, and possibly the entire organism, may die.[14]

METHODS OF MAINTAINING HOMEOSTASIS

Methods for maintaining homeostasis include control of intake and output of substances by cells, negative feedback, and hormone and nerve input.

Intake and Output

Homeostasis requires that the intake of some substances, such as water and various ions, equal their elimination. Ingestion of water and various ions adds them to the body; excretion by organs, such as the kidneys and liver, removes them from the body. The regulation of water and ion balance involves the coordinated participation of several organ systems. The kidneys, along with the respiratory, integumentary (skin), and gastrointestinal systems, regulate these parameters. The nervous and endocrine systems coordinate the activities of these systems.[20]

Passive and Active Transport

Much of the exchange between cells and their immediate surroundings occurs by diffusion (see Chapter 6), a process in which individual molecules move if there is a concentration gradient—a difference in the concentration of the substance from one place to another. However, some substances are actively transported across cell membranes.[16] The concentration of substances (e.g., various ions) in the numerous fluid compartments in the body is determined by these transport processes. Virtually all cells contain a high concentration of potassium and low concentrations of sodium, chloride, magnesium, and calcium. Most large molecules (e.g., proteins) that are synthesized within the cell remain within the cell.

Some substances must be exchanged with the environment. In particular, the production of chemical energy in most cell types requires that oxygen and nutrients reach the interior of cells and that carbon dioxide and other chemical end products be transferred to the environment. In the circulatory system, blood is rapidly moved between the respiratory system, where gases are exchanged; the kidney, where nongaseous wastes and excess fluid and solutes are removed; and the digestive system, where nutrients are absorbed.

The body relies on blood flow for rapid transport of the substances within the internal environment to overcome the diffusional limit imposed by the size of human bodies. The volume of fluid outside human cells is about one third the volume of that within cells. The circulatory

Ketogenesis: Producing Ketones from Fatty Acids

ketones (ketone bodies) Products of acetyl-CoA metabolism containing three to four carbons: they are acetoacetic acid, beta-hydroxybutyric acid, and acetone.

Ketones, also called *ketone bodies,* are products of incomplete fatty acid oxidation. Hormonal imbalances, chiefly inadequate insulin production to balance glucagon action in the body, allow some metabolic conditions to develop that lead to significant ketone production, called *ketosis* [16]:

system makes it possible for this relatively small extracellular fluid volume to serve the much larger fluid pool that forms part of every cell.[14]

Negative Feedback

An important homeostatic mechanism used for regulation of most conditions is negative feedback. *Negative* means that any deviation from a normal value is resisted or negated. Negative feedback does not prevent variation, but instead maintains that variation within a normal range.[12] When a certain factor varies from its optimal set point, automatic regulatory mechanisms act to counterbalance the disturbance and reestablish the internal equilibrium. For example, when the body overheats, sweating is stimulated until the temperature returns to normal. Similarly, when the concentration of oxygen in the blood is low, breathing is stimulated; when blood pressure falls, heart rate increases.

Hormone and Nerve Input

The endocrine system is a key component in the adaptation of the human organism to changes in the internal and external environment. Specific endocrine cells, usually grouped in glands, sense a "disturbance" and respond by secreting hormones into the bloodstream. These special molecules are carried by the blood to various tissues, where they act on their target cells. The target cells respond in a manner that opposes the direction of the change that evoked the secretion of the hormone. This helps restore the organism to its original stable state.[20]

For example, when the blood glucose concentration increases, insulin is released by the pancreas. This hormone promotes changes that cause the blood glucose concentration to fall, in part because glucose is taken into adipose and muscle cells and synthesized into glycogen by liver cells. The endocrine system may act independently of, or may be integrated with, the nervous system, which is another major component in the organism's adaptability to internal or external change. When the blood glucose concentration falls, nerve endings and the adrenal glands release the hormones epinephrine and norepinephrine, which cause the liver to release stored glucose, while also directing other tissues to reduce glucose utilization. In addition, neurons in the hypothalamus sense low blood glucose and stimulate the adrenal cortex to secrete the hormone cortisol. This hormone augments synthesis of glucose in the liver to help maintain the supply in case initial stores become depleted. Together these endocrine and neural responses to hypoglycemia raise blood glucose back to normal (see Figure 3-4).[20]

HOMEOSTATIC VERSUS CHEMICAL INDIVIDUALITY

There is much variation in the whole body and tissue content of chemical compounds, from proteins to sugars to trace minerals. But this variability in biochemical and chemical constitution is largely confined to substances within cells.[14] In contrast, the body maintains a constancy in the fluid environment outside cells. It is here that the term *homeostasis* most aptly applies. This fluid composes nearly 20% of the total body weight and includes the blood. Accordingly, most compounds in the blood are maintained within a fairly narrow range. Sodium and potassium concentrations typically vary to only a small degree; the range for glucose and protein is a bit wider but still shows considerable regulation. Overall, homeostasis is an overriding characteristic of the human body, with fine tuning available to respond to various body stresses.[14]

1. Fatty acids stored in adipose cells flood into the bloodstream. The bulk of these fatty acids are taken up by the liver.
2. Fatty acid oxidation to acetyl-CoA predominates over fatty acid synthesis in the liver.
3. As the liver takes up the fatty acids and degrades them to acetyl-CoA, the capacity of the citric acid cycle to process the resulting acetyl-CoA molecules de-

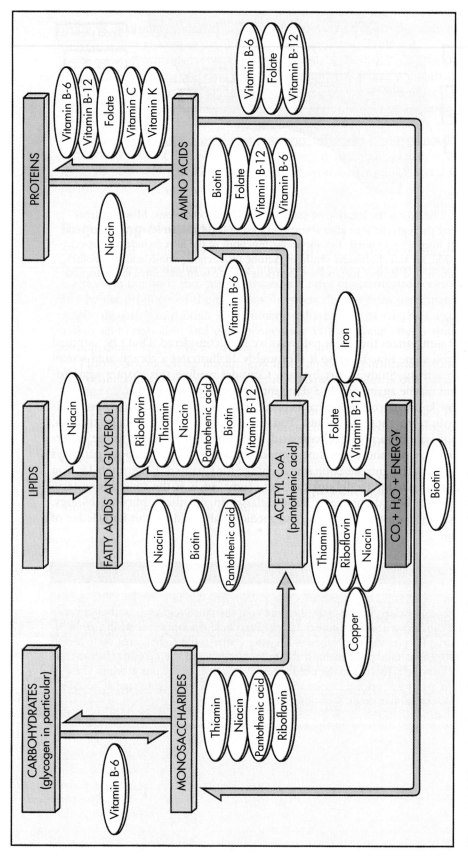

Figure 7-13 Many vitamins and minerals participate in the metabolic pathways. Most notable are the B vitamins thiamin, riboflavin, niacin, pantothenic acid, biotin, vitamin B-6, folate, and vitamin B-12, as well as the minerals iron and copper. Many systemic health problems can develop from nutrient deficiencies, since so many key pathways depend on nutrient input.

Summary

1. A cell is the basic unit of structure in the body. Within the cell is a nucleus containing DNA to direct protein synthesis and cell division. Mitochondria produce a usable form of energy. Golgi bodies package cell products. Endoplasmic reticula are separate structures involved in protein and fat synthesis. Storage granules of glycogen and droplets of fat are present in some cells.

2. ATP is the major form of energy used for cellular metabolism. As ATP breaks down to ADP plus Pi, energy is released from the broken bond. This energy is used to pump ions, promote enzyme activity, and contract muscles. All energy available to humans ultimately comes from the sun as solar energy. Plants capture solar energy by way of photosynthesis. In humans, metabolic pathways make it possible to extract energy from food and transform it to ATP; in the process some energy is lost as heat.

3. In glycolysis, glucose is degraded into two pyruvate molecules, yielding NADH (a form of potential energy) and ATP. Pyruvate can proceed through other aerobic pathways to form carbon dioxide and water. Pyruvate also can react with NADH in an anaerobic pathway to form lactate. Both pathways allow NADH to eventually be re-formed into NAD, which is needed for glycolysis to continue.

4. In the citric acid cycle, acetyl-CoA is formed as a carbon dioxide is lost from pyruvate. Acetyl-CoA then undergoes many metabolic conversions, eventually yielding two more carbon dioxide molecules. In this way the citric acid cycle accepts two carbons from acetyl-CoA and yields two carbons as carbon dioxide. In the process, NADH, $FADH_2$, and a form of energy that can yield ATP directly (GTP) are formed. The NADH and $FADH_2$ then enter the electron transport chain to yield numerous ATP molecules. Water forms as oxygen combines with the electrons and hydrogen ions are released from NADH and $FADH_2$ in the electron transport chain.

5. In fatty acid oxidation, two-carbon fragments are cleaved from a fatty acid, producing multiple acetyl-CoA molecules. These enter the citric acid cycle and electron transport chain to yield ATP, carbon dioxide, and water. In fat synthesis, acetate molecules in effect are combined to yield a fatty acid, primarily the 16-carbon palmitic acid. These fatty acids can then react with a form of glycerol to produce a triglyceride.

6. During starvation and uncontrolled diabetes, more acetyl-CoA is produced in the liver than can be metabolized to carbon dioxide and water. This excess acetyl-CoA is synthesized into ketones, which flood into the bloodstream and are metabolized by other tissues, such as nerve tissue.

7. Amino acids lose their amino group and become carbon skeletons. These can be metabolized to other compounds that enter the citric acid cycle, eventually yielding energy for ATP synthesis. Some carbon skeletons can be formed into oxaloacetate, an intermediate found in the citric acid cycle, which in turn can be converted to glucose. Converting the carbon skeletons of amino acids to glucose is part of a process known as gluconeogenesis. Acetyl-CoA molecules, and thus fatty acids in general, cannot participate in gluconeogenesis.

8. Glycolysis occurs in the cytosol of a cell, while the citric acid cycle and the electron transport chain occur in the mitochondria. Fatty acid oxidation occurs in the mitochondria, and fatty acids for the most part are synthesized in the cytosol. The synthesis of urea and the pathway for gluconeogenesis both take place partly in the cytosol and partly in the mitochondria.

9. Acetyl-CoA is pivotal in cell metabolism because carbohydrates, proteins, amino acids, and fatty acids all can yield acetyl-CoA during their metabolism. The coordination of various metabolic pathways for food fuels allows the carbons of glucose to become the carbons of fatty acids and the carbons of some amino acids to become the carbons of glucose.

10. The vitamins thiamin, niacin, riboflavin, biotin, pantothenic acid, and vitamin B-6 and the minerals magnesium, iron, and copper play important roles in the metabolic pathways.

Study Questions

1. Many vitamins and minerals are used in energy metabolism. Identify three vitamins and/or minerals and describe their roles in ATP synthesis.

2. Why do cells need ATP energy?

3. Explain how the ATP concentration is maintained in a cell. What is the key stimulus to ATP production?

4. What is the "common denominator" compound of the many pathways of energy metabolism (citric acid cycle, glycolysis, beta-oxidation, etc.)? Why is it considered important in the body's chemical processes?

5. Identify the three stages of cellular metabolism. Which energy nutrients are processed in each stage?

6. What is lactate and how and where is it formed in the cell? Which tissues produce the most lactate? Why?

7. How is energy stored in the body? What factors regulate how much energy is stored at any one time?

8. Trace the steps in gluconeogenesis from body protein to the formation of glucose.

9. What is the meaning of the phrase "fats burn in a fire of carbohydrate"?

REFERENCES

1. Achord JL: Alcohol and the liver, *Scientific American Science & Medicine* March/April 1995, p 16.

2. Bowers DF, Allred JB: Advances in molecular biology: implications for the future of clinical nutrition practice, *Journal of the American Dietetic Association* 95:53, 1995.

3. Fuchs CS and others: Alcohol consumption and mortality in women, *New England Journal of Medicine* 332:1245, 1995.

4. Gaziano JM and others: Moderate alcohol intake, increased levels of high-density lipoprotein and its subfractions, and decreased risk of myocardial infarction, *New England Journal of Medicine* 329:1829, 1993.

5. Gordis E: Unraveling the brain chemistry behind alcohol abuse, *Journal of the American Medical Association* 72:1733, 1994.

6. Hendriks HFJ and others: Effect of moderate dose of alcohol with evening meal on fibrinolytic factors, *British Medical Journal* 308:1003, 1994.

7. Isselbacker KJ and others, editors: *Harrison's principles of internal medicine,* ed 13, New York, 1994, McGraw-Hill.

8. Kitchens JM: Does this patient have an alcohol problem? *Journal of the American Medical Association* 272:1782, 1994.

9. Klatsky AL, Armstrong MA: Alcoholic beverage choice and risk of coronary artery disease mortality: do red wine drinkers fare best? *American Journal of Cardiology* 71:467, 1993.

10. Klesges RC and others: Effects of alcohol intake on resting energy expenditure in young women social drinkers, *American Journal of Clinical Nutrition* 59:805, 1994.

11. Lecomte E and others: Effect of alcohol consumption on blood antioxidant nutrients and oxidative stress indicators, *American Journal of Clinical Nutrition* 60:255, 1994.

12. Lenninger AL and others: *Principles of biochemistry,* ed 4, New York, 1993, Worth Publishing.

13. Lieber CS: Alcohol and the liver: 1994 update, *Gastroenterology* 106:1085, 1994.

14. Linder MC: *Nutritional biochemistry and metabolism,* New York, 1991, Elsevier Science Publishing.

15. Maclure M: Demonstration of deductive meta-analysis: ethanol intake and risk of myocardial infarction, *Epidemiology Reviews* 15:328, 1993.

16. Murray RK and others: *Harper's biochemistry,* Norwalk, Conn, 1993, Appleton & Lange.

17. Ridker PM and others: Association of moderate alcohol consumption and plasma concentration of endogenous tissue-type plasminogen activator, *Journal of the American Medical Association* 272:929, 1994.

18. Rosenthal N: DNA and the genetic code, *New England Journal of Medicine* 331:39, 1994.

19. Stryer L: *Biochemistry,* ed 4, New York, 1995, WH Freeman.

20. Wilson JD, Foster DW, editors: *Williams textbook of endocrinology,* Philadelphia, 1992, WB Saunders.

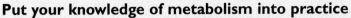

TAKE ACTION

Put your knowledge of metabolism into practice

A friend is very overweight and describes to you his method of weight loss. He fasted completely for 1 week and then initiated a strict diet of 400 to 600 kcal/day under a physician's supervision. The food energy comes from a liquid formula that he drinks for breakfast. He skips lunch and eats a small dinner of 3 ounces of protein, ½ cup of vegetables, 1 cup of fruit, and two starch items (a small potato, a piece of bread, etc.). He has lost approximately 25 pounds in 12 weeks.

- -

Based on your knowledge of energy metabolism, answer the following questions he poses:
1. During the fasting stage, what were the likely sources of energy for the body's cells? What metabolic processes occurred to provide glucose for red blood cells? brain? kidneys?
2. During the low-kilocalorie phase, how did the metabolic processes in the body most likely change from the fasting state?

POSSIBLE ANSWERS
1. While fasting, gluconeogenesis initially supplied the glucose needed for the brain, red blood cells, and kidneys. The carbons used came mostly from body protein, leading to a decrease in lean body mass. Eventually ketone production from fatty acid breakdown increased, leading to elevated ketones in the blood and greater ketone use by many types of body cells. Insulin output fell, leading to glycogen depletion in the liver. Fatty acids from fat stores were "dumped" into the bloodstream. Thus fatty acids became the major energy-yielding fuel for the body.
2. During the low-kilocalorie phase, insulin output in the body rose as carbohydrate intake increased. This led to a reduction in ketone production and spared some body protein from being used as a source of carbons for glucose synthesis. The body switched from using primarily fat as fuel to using more of a mixture of fat and carbohydrate.

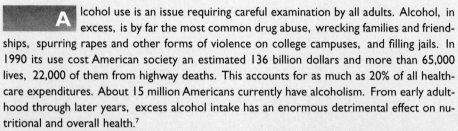
Alcohol—Metabolic, Nutritional, and Social Implications

Alcohol use is an issue requiring careful examination by all adults. Alcohol, in excess, is by far the most common drug abuse, wrecking families and friendships, spurring rapes and other forms of violence on college campuses, and filling jails. In 1990 its use cost American society an estimated 136 billion dollars and more than 65,000 lives, 22,000 of them from highway deaths. This accounts for as much as 20% of all healthcare expenditures. About 15 million Americans currently have alcoholism. From early adulthood through later years, excess alcohol intake has an enormous detrimental effect on nutritional and overall health.[7]

The American Medical Association defines alcoholism as an illness characterized by significant impairment directly related to persistent, excessive use of alcohol. Impairment can involve physiological, psychological, and social dysfunction. Causes of alcoholism include genetic, psychosocial, and environmental factors.[5]

Some studies suggest that as much as 50% of a person's risk for alcoholism comes from genetic factors. Children of people with alcoholism have a four-fold increased risk of alcoholism, even when adopted by people with no history of alcoholism.

Other studies question how strong the genetic component is. Children of people with alcoholism account for only a fraction of the alcohol abusers in the United States. Any one of us can become addicted if we drink long enough and hard enough.[8]

After a person drinks an alcoholic beverage, his or her blood concentration of alcohol rises rapidly. Alcohol, technically known as *ethanol,* is readily absorbed into the blood from all parts of the gastrointestinal tract. You've probably been warned, with good reason, not to drink on an empty stomach. Alcohol absorption depends partly on the rate of stomach emptying. Food slows the stomach's emptying rate and stimulates secretions, such as gastric acid, which dilute the alcohol and slow its absorption into the bloodstream.

Some alcohol is metabolized in the cells lining the stomach, more so in men than women. Most of the remaining alcohol is metabolized in the liver.[13] About 10% of the ethanol in the body is directly eliminated by diffusion through the kidneys or lungs. A social drinker who weighs 150 pounds and has normal liver function metabolizes about 7 to 14 g of alcohol per hour (100 to 200 mg/kg of body weight per hour). This is about 8 to 12 ounces of beer or half an ordinary-sized drink. When the rate of alcohol consumption exceeds the liver's metabolic capacity, blood alcohol rises and symptoms of intoxication appear (Table 7-2).

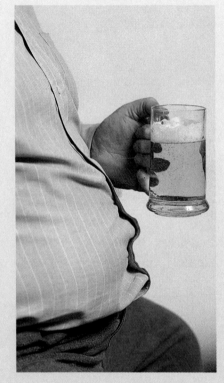

Alcohol intake encourages fat deposition, especially in the abdominal region.

alcohol dehydrogenase An enzyme used in alcohol (ethanol) breakdown; the major enzyme used in the liver when alcohol is in low concentration.

microsomal ethanol oxidizing system An alternative pathway for alcohol metabolism when alcohol is in high concentration in the liver; uses rather than yields energy for the body, in contrast to alcohol dehydrogenase activity.

Metabolic Pathways for Alcohol Metabolism

Alcohol at low doses first reacts with NAD to form the compound acetaldehyde and NADH. The enzyme used is **alcohol dehydrogenase** (Figure 7-14).[16] Distinctly different forms of alcohol dehydrogenase are found in the liver and the stomach. Each varies in its rate of alcohol metabolism. This enzyme requires the mineral zinc for activity.

The acetaldehyde formed is then converted into acetyl-CoA, again yielding NADH. The acetyl-CoA enters the citric acid cycle, and the NADH, $FADH_2$, and GTP molecules produced in the citric acid cycle can then be used to synthesize ATP.[16]

Structurally, ethanol with its hydroxyl group (–OH) resembles a carbohydrate. But since it is converted directly into acetyl-CoA, alcohol carbons cannot support glucose production. Thus alcohol is metabolized more like a fat than a carbohydrate and is considered a fat in metabolic terms.

When a person drinks lots of alcohol, the enzyme alcohol dehydrogenase cannot keep up with the demand to metabolize all of the alcohol into acetaldehyde. For this and other reasons, another enzyme system exists to metabolize alcohol. This system is called the **microsomal ethanol oxidizing system (MEOS).**[13]

The MEOS is normally used by the liver to metabolize drugs and other "foreign" substances. When the liver registers excessive alcohol as a foreign substance, the MEOS kicks

TABLE 7-2

Blood alcohol concentration and symptoms

Concentration (mg/dl)	Sporadic drinker	Chronic drinker	Hours for alcohol to be metabolized
50 (party high)	Congenial euphoria; decreased tension	No observable effect	2-3
75	Gregarious	Often no effect	
100 (0.1%)	Uncoordinated; legally drunk (as in drunk driving) in most states; a level of 0.08% is legal drunkenness in a growing number of areas in the United States.	Minimal signs	4-6
125-150	Unrestrained behavior; episodic uncontrolled behavior; legally drunk at 0.15% in all states.	Pleasurable euphoria or beginning of uncoordination	6-10
200-250	Alertness lost; lethargic	Effort required to maintain emotional and motor control	10-24
300-350	Stupor to coma	Drowsy and slow	
>500	Some will die	Coma	>24

Modified from Wyngaarder JB, Smith LH: *Cecil textbook of medicine,* Philadelphia, 1988, WB Saunders.

in. Once the MEOS is active, alcohol tolerance increases because the rate of alcohol metabolism increases.

There are two interesting aspects to the body's reliance on MEOS. First, rather than forming NADH with use of alcohol dehydrogenase, the MEOS uses NADPH, a compound analogous to NADH. Now, instead of yielding "potential" ATP molecules from the first step in alcohol metabolism via formation of NADH, the MEOS uses "potential" ATP energy in the form of NADPH, as NADPH converts to NADP. This helps explain why people with alcoholism do not gain as much weight as might be expected from the amount of alcohol-derived energy they consume. High doses of alcohol are inefficiently used by the liver because they require energy for the first metabolic step. A person with alcoholism wastes some energy by inducing this alternate metabolic pathway. Liver damage from alcohol, such that other metabolic pathways are hampered, also is implicated in the reduced energy yield associated with high alcohol use.[13] In addition, a recent study suggests that alcohol increases metabolic rate.[10]

Use of the MEOS also increases the potential for a drug overdose. While the MEOS is metabolizing alcohol, its capacity for metabolizing drugs, such as many sedatives, is reduced. If large amounts of both alcohol and sedatives are consumed, the user may lapse into coma and die, because the liver is not able to metabolize the sedatives in the body fast enough. Alcohol itself is toxic in high quantities. Mixed with sedatives it creates an extremely toxic combination.

Alcohol affects the brain more than any other organ. Acting as a sedative, alcohol tends to relieve the drinker's anxiety, cause slurred speech, reduce coordination in walking, im-

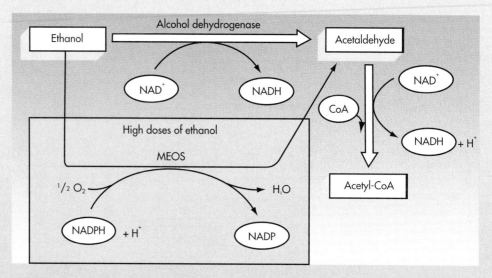

Figure 7-14 Alcohol metabolism. At low alcohol intake, the alcohol dehydrogenase pathway is used. At high alcohol intake, the microsomal ethanol oxidizing system (MEOS) also is used. The MEOS uses rather than yields energy; use of the pathway reduces the body's ability to detoxify drugs, increasing the risk of a drug overdose if large amounts of alcohol are consumed at the same time.

pair judgment, and encourage uninhibited behavior. The mechanism for these effects is thought to be linked to changes in neurotransmitter synthesis and altered cell membrane fluidity in the brain. Because alcohol lowers inhibitions, it appears to act as a stimulant, but in fact it is a powerful depressant. As William Shakespeare wrote, "It stirs up desire, but takes away the performance." Because it reduces secretion of the body's antidiuretic hormone, alcohol increases urination.[16] It also causes the blood vessels to dilate, releasing body heat.

When a man and woman of similar size drink the same amount of alcohol, the woman retains more alcohol in her bloodstream; women have lower amounts of the key alcohol-metabolizing enzyme, alcohol dehydrogenase. And we already noted that a woman also does not metabolize as much alcohol in her stomach as a man does. In addition, women more quickly develop alcohol-related ailments, such as cirrhosis of the liver, than do men with the same drinking history.[7]

Alcohol and Overall Health

About 32% of all Americans have three drinks or less each week, while 22% have two drinks or less a day. Only 11% have more than two drinks a day. Although the public health impact of alcohol abuse is still being calculated, misuse of alcohol is one of the most preventable health problems in the United States. Drinking alcohol excessively contributes significantly to 5 of the 10 leading causes of death in the United States—certain forms of cancer, cirrhosis of the liver, motor vehicle and other accidents, suicides, and homicides. Tobacco reacts with alcohol in a way that reinforces alcohol's effects in causing esophageal and oral cancer. In addition, excessive alcohol intake increases the risk of some types of heart disease (specifically, cardiomyopathy), high blood pressure (especially among African-Americans), nerve diseases, nutritional deficiencies, damage to a fetus, and many other disorders. As we cover in Chapter 16, a major cause of lasting mental retardation that is first seen in infancy results from fetal exposure to alcohol.

Social consequences of dependence on alcohol include violent episodes, incarceration, divorce, unemployment, and poverty. An estimated 27 million American children are more likely to develop abnormally in psychosocial skills and relationships because their parents abuse alcohol.

All this must tell us—use alcohol cautiously and in moderation, if at all. Drinking even small amounts of alcohol can lead to dependence.

People aged 20 to 40 drink the most alcohol. Excessive drinking often begins earlier; many high school seniors report having consumed alcohol in the past month; about 5% described themselves as daily drinkers.

CIRRHOSIS

Long-term alcohol use causes fatty liver, alcoholic hepatitis, and cirrhosis. Cirrhosis is a chronic and usually relentlessly progressive disease characterized by fatty infiltration of the liver. Eventually the fat chokes off the blood supply, depriving the liver cells of oxygen and nutrients (Figure 7-15).[1] Liver cells die and are replaced by connective (scar) tissue. This scarring process is called *cirrhosis*. Most cases of cirrhosis in the United States are caused by alcohol consumption. Cirrhosis develops in 12% to 31% of cases of alcoholism. In addition to the amount and duration of alcohol consumption, genetic factors and individual differences determine a person's risk for cirrhosis. Once a person has cirrhosis there is a 50% chance of death within 4 years, which is a worse prognosis than in many forms of cancer. Most of the deaths from alcoholic cirrhosis occur in people ages 40 to 65.

There are a number of possible mechanisms that underlie the liver damage from alcohol abuse, such as production of free radicals that damage liver cells. Acetaldehyde, a major metabolite of alcohol, may also contribute to liver destruction.[1,13]

No specific amount of alcohol consumption guarantees cirrhosis. One observable pattern is that cirrhosis commonly results from a 15-year consumption of approximately 80 g of alcohol per day. This is equivalent to 7 beers per day (Table 7-3). Some evidence suggests that damage is caused by a dose as low as 40 g/day for men and 20 g/day for women. Early stages of alcoholic liver injury are reversible, while advanced stages usually are not.[13]

A nutritious diet helps prevent some complications associated with alcoholism, but usually alcoholism wreaks serious destruction on the body in spite of an adequate diet. Laboratory animal studies show clearly that even when a nutritious diet is consumed, alcoholism can lead to cirrhosis. Still, deficient nutritional status compounds the problem of cirrhosis as it makes the liver more vulnerable to toxic substances by depleting supplies of antioxidants, such as vitamin E and vitamin C, which can reduce free radical damage to the liver if present in adequate amounts.[13]

ALCOHOL AND NUTRITION

Nutritional problems in a person with alcoholism result from deficiencies of a variety of nutrients:[7,11,13]

Vitamin A deficiency may be caused by a deficient diet, or inability of the liver to produce retinol-binding protein. In addition, the chemical-detoxifying systems in the liver induced by chronic alcohol consumption may hasten the degradation of vitamin A in the liver.

Thiamin deficiency can be caused by decreased thiamin absorption or decreased liver synthesis of the active thiamin coenzyme. People with alcoholism often exhibit nervous system problems similar to those seen in a thiamin deficiency called Wernicke's syndrome (see Chapter 13).

Niacin deficiency and resulting pellagra can be caused by a deficient diet.

Vitamin B-6 deficiency probably stems from a deficient intake of the vitamin and possibly increased breakdown of the vitamin B-6 coenzyme.

Folate deficiency can be caused by a deficient diet and reduced nutrient absorption.

Vitamin D deficiency is usually due to the liver's decreased capacity to convert vitamin D into the final hormonal form, called *calcitriol*. Alcohol may cause bone cell dysfunction that diminishes bone formation and reduces bone mineralization. This can lead to osteoporosis.

Vitamin C deficiency may result primarily from a decrease in dietary intake or altered liver metabolism, or both.

Vitamin K deficiency probably occurs because less is synthesized by intestinal bacteria, less is consumed, and less is absorbed.

CRITICAL THINKING

As a nutrition student, you have become aware of the potential effects of alcohol consumption. You also know that one of the main health problems facing women today is osteoporosis, the decalcification of bone. Explain how alcohol can contribute to the development of this condition.

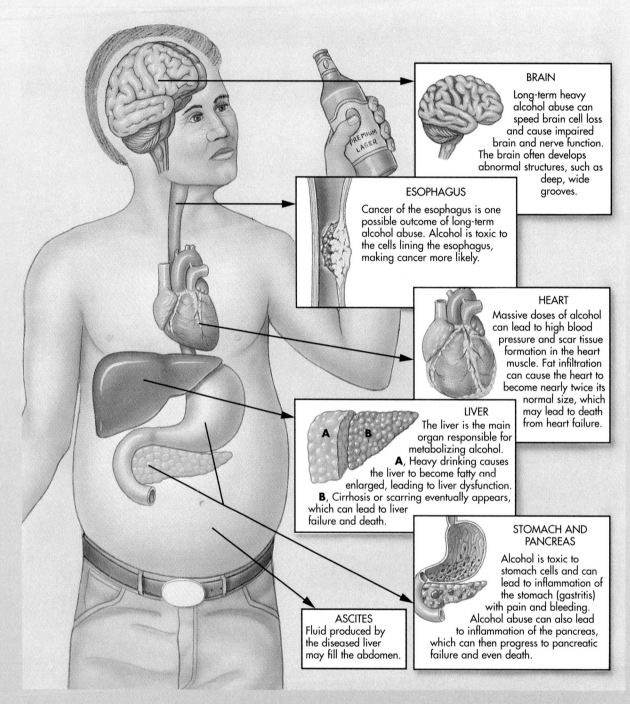

BRAIN
Long-term heavy alcohol abuse can speed brain cell loss and cause impaired brain and nerve function. The brain often develops abnormal structures, such as deep, wide grooves.

ESOPHAGUS
Cancer of the esophagus is one possible outcome of long-term alcohol abuse. Alcohol is toxic to the cells lining the esophagus, making cancer more likely.

HEART
Massive doses of alcohol can lead to high blood pressure and scar tissue formation in the heart muscle. Fat infiltration can cause the heart to become nearly twice its normal size, which may lead to death from heart failure.

LIVER
The liver is the main organ responsible for metabolizing alcohol. **A**, Heavy drinking causes the liver to become fatty and enlarged, leading to liver dysfunction. **B**, Cirrhosis or scarring eventually appears, which can lead to liver failure and death.

STOMACH AND PANCREAS
Alcohol is toxic to stomach cells and can lead to inflammation of the stomach (gastritis) with pain and bleeding. Alcohol abuse can also lead to inflammation of the pancreas, which can then progress to pancreatic failure and even death.

ASCITES
Fluid produced by the diseased liver may fill the abdomen.

Figure 7-15 Effects of alcohol abuse on the body. The mind-altering effects of alcohol begin soon after it enters the bloodstream. Within minutes alcohol numbs nerve cells in the brain. Heart muscle strains to cope with alcohol's depressive action. If drinking continues, rising blood alcohol causes impaired speech, vision, balance, and judgment. With extremely high blood alcohol, respiratory failure is possible. Over time, alcohol abuse increases the risk of certain forms of heart disease and cancer, and liver and pancreas failure.

TABLE 7-3

Caloric, carbohydrate, and alcohol content of alcoholic beverages

Beverage	Amount (ounce)	Alcohol (grams)	Carbohydrates (grams)	Energy (kilocalories)
Beer				
Regular	12	12	13	140
Light	12	10	4	90
Distilled				
Gin, rum, vodka, whiskey, tequila	1.5	15	—	105
Brandy, cognac	1.0	9	—	65
Wine				
Red	4	11	2	80
Dry white	4	10	1	75
Sweet	4	12	5	105
Sherry	2	9	2	75
Rosé	4	11	2	80
Vermouth, sweet	3	12	14	140
Vermouth, dry	3	13	4	105
Manhattan	3	21	2	165
Martini	3	19	1	180
Bourbon & soda	4	15	0	102
Whiskey sour	3	15	5	122
Margarita cocktail	4	18	11	168

Source: Nutritionist IV, N² computing.

General Guidelines for Alcohol Use

Neither the Surgeon General's office, the National Academy of Science, nor the USDA/DHHS recommends drinking alcohol. All groups caution that if adults do consume alcohol, they should (1) drink alcohol only in moderation (no more than two drinks a day for men and one for women); (2) avoid drinking any alcohol before or while driving, operating machinery, taking medications, or engaging in any other activity requiring sound judgment; and (3) avoid drinking alcohol while pregnant. Although this obviously isn't a plea for teetotalers to start drinking, people who have a drink or so a day and are not prone to abuse should know that there's nothing wrong with moderate drinking. In fact there are some benefits to moderate alcohol intake, such as a reduction in the risk of coronary heart disease.[3] The effective dose of alcohol is between one half and three drinks a day. No further benefit can be seen for consumption beyond that amount. The reason for this reduction in coronary heart disease risk is still debatable but likely involves an increase in HDL concentrations[4] and a reduction in blood clotting.[6,17] Phenol compounds in red wine may also act as antioxidants and thus may make this source of alcohol more potent in reducing coronary heart disease risk than others.[9]

Unfortunately, however, when some of us open the door to alcohol we end up walking into a part of life we wish we had never entered. And for people who regularly take certain

---

CAGE Questionnaire to Screen for Alcohol Abuse

C: "Have you ever felt you ought to *Cut* down on drinking?"

A: "Have people *Annoyed* you by criticizing your drinking?"

G: "Have you ever felt bad or *Guilty* about your drinking?"

E: "Have you ever had a drink first thing in the morning to steady your nerves or get rid of a hangover (*Eye-opener*)?"

medications (such as aspirin or anticonvulsants) or who have diabetes or ulcers, consulting a physician about whether to use alcohol is important.

DO YOU HAVE A PROBLEM WITH ALCOHOL?

Asking a person about the quantity and frequency of alcohol consumption is an important means of detecting abuse and dependence. The CAGE instrument is popular for use in routine screening.[8] More than one positive response to the CAGE questionnaire suggests an alcohol problem. Another key point to probe is tolerance. Does it take more to make you inebriated than it did in the past?

The medication disulfiram (Antabuse) can help the person with alcoholism to make the essential decision to stop drinking. An early step in alcohol metabolism is blocked by the action of this drug. As a result, a highly toxic alcohol by-product accumulates in the blood, producing nausea, vomiting, diffuse flushing, and a shocklike reaction. FDA recently approved naltrexone (Revia) as another agent to aid in the treatment of alcohol dependence. This agent reduces the craving for alcohol and blunts the associated inebriation ("high") from alcohol intake. However, neither medication substitutes for a comprehensive treatment plan, such as Alcoholics Anonymous.

Treatment for Alcoholism

Once a diagnosis of alcohol abuse or dependence is established, a physician should arrange appropriate treatment and counseling for the patient and family. The drinker must confront the immediate problem of how to stop drinking. Total abstinence is currently the primary goal. For people with alcoholism, there generally is no such thing as "controlled drinking." A problem drinker cannot return safely to social drinking. The drinker should enter an Alcoholics Anonymous (AA) or similar program, and the spouse enter Al-Anon. Success is usually proportionate to participation in AA, other social agencies, religious counseling, and other resources. About 2 years of treatment should be expected.[7]

Current research does not support the generally negative public opinion about the prognosis for alcoholism. In most job-related alcoholism treatment programs, where workers are socially stable and—because of the risk to jobs and pensions—well-motivated, recovery rates reach 60% or more. This remarkably high cure rate is probably accounted for by early detection. Once a person moves from problem drinking to an advanced stage of alcoholism, success rates seldom exceed 40% to 50%. Early identification and intervention remain the most important steps in the treatment of alcoholism.[7]

CHAPTER EIGHT

Energy Balance

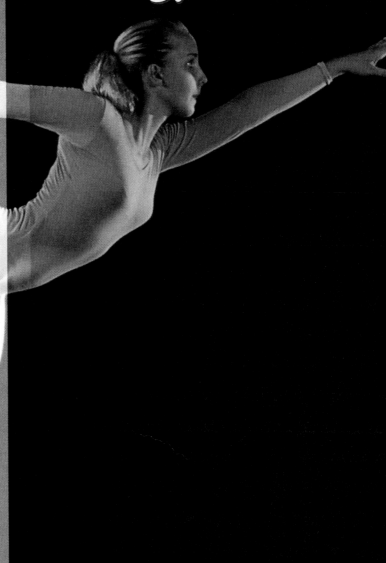

M aintaining energy balance—regulating energy intake so that it matches energy output—contributes to health. Many adults in America maintain a desirable (healthy) body weight; however, adulthood can also be a time of creeping weight gain that eventually turns into obesity. Currently about 33% of adult Americans are obese. The highest proportion of obesity, 42% of men and 52% of women, occurs in those age 50 to 59.[14] This disorder increases the likelihood of many health problems, such as heart disease, cancer, hypertension, bone and joint disorders, and the major form of diabetes.[15]

In this chapter we discuss health problems related to obesity, review the major concepts underlying the components of energy balance, and define the various subtypes of obesity. Since obesity is a major health problem in America, it is important for all of us to understand more about its causes. Prevention of this problem is an important goal. High-fat diets and too little physical activity are two key causes, but others need to be considered.[9,15]

NUTRITION AWARENESS INVENTORY

1. **T F**   Hunger sensations are partially regulated by the liver.
2. **T F**   The desire for specific foods often changes during a meal.
3. **T F**   Adipose cell size regulates eating on an hour-to-hour and day-to-day basis.
4. **T F**   Total energy needs can be accurately estimated using the RDA.
5. **T F**   The energy required to keep the resting body alive represents basal metabolism.
6. **T F**   Brown adipose tissue is more active in adults than in infants.
7. **T F**   Some obese people live at least 80 years, suggesting that obesity doesn't actually affect longevity.
8. **T F**   Excess body fat is a more accurate indicator of risk of poor health than is excess body weight.
9. **T F**   Men and women tend to store most excess fat in the abdomen.
10. **T F**   Health problems related to obesity begin when a person's body mass index (BMI) exceeds 25.
11. **T F**   The more muscle tissue in a body, the higher its resting metabolism.
12. **T F**   Obese people expend more energy during physical activity than lean people do.
13. **T F**   Adult obesity in men is usually tied to childhood obesity.
14. **T F**   The major cause of obesity in America is low thyroid gland activity.
15. **T F**   Most obesity is due to constant overeating throughout life.

energy balance State in which energy intake, in the form of food and/or alcohol, matches the energy expended, primarily through basal metabolism and physical activity.

positive energy balance State in which energy intake is greater than energy expended, generally resulting in weight gain.

negative energy balance State in which energy intake is less than energy expended, resulting in weight loss.

Energy Balance

Energy balance depends on energy input and energy output. This balance influences energy stores, primarily in adipose tissue (Figure 8-1). Energy balance can be thought of as an equation: energy consumed minus energy expended.[1] A person is in positive energy balance when energy consumed is greater than energy expended. The result of positive energy balance is storage of the excess energy, mostly in the form of triglycerides in adipose tissue.[10]

Positive energy balance is necessary during pregnancy, as the surplus of energy supports the developing fetus. Infants and children also need to be in positive energy balance in order to grow. In adults, however, positive energy balance causes creeping weight gain.[10]

Negative energy balance results from an energy deficit. Energy consumed is less than energy expended. Weight loss occurs when a person is in a state of negative energy balance. In adulthood, however, unlike positive energy balance, in which adipose tissue is primarily affected, the weight that is lost consists of a combination of lean and adipose tissue.[15]

As noted in the overview, maintenance of energy balance—energy intake matches energy output—substantially contributes to health and well-being in adults. Maintenance of energy balance is an important goal for everyone who is interested in a long, healthy life. Adulthood can be a time of creeping weight gain that eventually turns into obesity if not checked. However, increasing age is not the primary reason for this weight gain; it is caused primarily by the pattern of food intake and physical activity.[15] Let's look in detail at the factors that affect the relationship between positive and negative energy balance.

Energy Intake: The First Half of Energy Balance

Energy needs are met by food intake. Determining the appropriate amount and type of food to eat is a challenge for many of us. Our ability to consume food and use it

CRITICAL THINKING

A 26-year-old classmate of yours has been thinking about the process of aging. One of the things she fears most as she gets older is gaining weight. How would you explain energy balance to her?

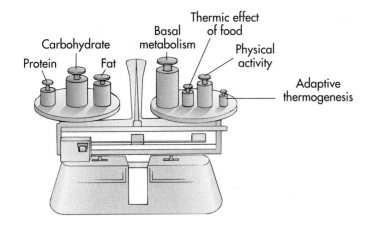

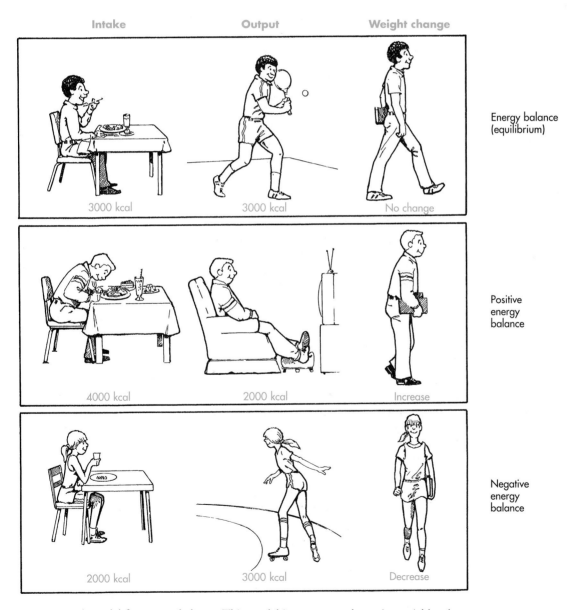

Figure 8-1 A model for energy balance. This model incorporates the major variables that influence energy balance. Note that alcohol is an additional source of energy for some of us.

efficiently is an evolutionary survival mechanism. However, given modern American food supplies, many of us are now too successful in attaining food energy. About one in three adult Americans is obese.[14]

DETERMINING THE ENERGY CONTENT OF FOODS

How much food energy is contained in a meal? A bomb calorimeter is used to determine the amount of energy in a food (Figure 8-2). The process involves burning a portion of food inside a chamber of the calorimeter that is surrounded by water. As the food burns it gives off heat, which raises the temperature of the water surrounding the chamber. The increase in water temperature measured after the food has burned indicates the amount of energy in the food. One kilocalorie is the amount of energy required to increase the temperature of 1 kg of water 1° Celsius. Any food can be burned in the calorimeter to determine energy content, although some foods must be dried first.

The bomb calorimeter provides values for the amount of energy that can be derived from carbohydrate, fat, protein, and alcohol. Carbohydrates yield 4 kcal/g, proteins yield 4 kcal/g, fats yield 9 kcal/g, and alcohol yields 7 kcal/g. These energy figures have been adjusted for (1) digestibility and (2) substances in food, such as waxes and fibrous plant parts, that burn in the bomb calorimeter but are unusable by the human body for energy needs. The figures are then rounded to whole numbers.

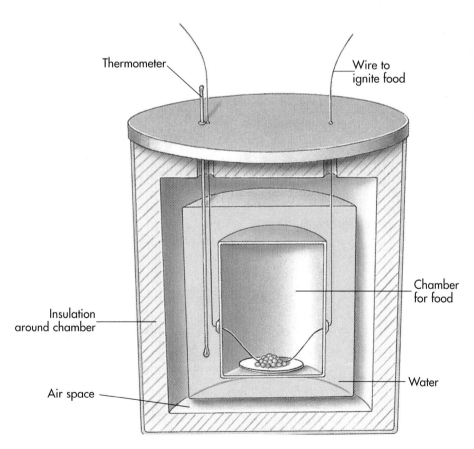

Thermometer

Wire to ignite food

Chamber for food

Insulation around chamber

Water

Air space

Figure 8-2 Cross-section of a bomb calorimeter. To determine energy content, a dried portion of food is burned inside a chamber charged with oxygen and surrounded by water. As the food is burned, it gives off heat, which raises the temperature of the water surrounding the chamber. The amount of increase in water temperature indicates the number of kilocalories contained in the food. Recall that 1 kcal equals the amount of heat needed to raise the temperature of 1 kg of water 1° C.

Once you know the gram quantities of the energy-yielding substances in a food, you can estimate the total energy content in that food using the energy values (Figure 8-3). For example, if a banana milk shake contains 45 g of carbohydrate, 7 g of protein, and 10 g of fat, it contains 298 kcal ([45 × 4] + [7 × 4] + [10 × 9] = 298). If a banana-flavored rum drink has 10 g of carbohydrate, 1 g of protein, 1 g of fat, and 15 g of alcohol, it contains 158 kcal ([10 × 4] + [1 × 4] + [1 × 9] + [15 × 7] = 158).

BOMB CALORIMETER VALUES TELL ONLY PART OF THE STORY

In bomb calorimeter studies, fats produce close to 9 kcal/g. This value alone should warn us about over-consumption of fat. However, absorbed fats are not immediately burned to a great extent in the body for energy needs. Instead, much fat goes directly into storage in adipose tissue. We have an essentially unlimited ability to do this.

In contrast, we have a limited ability to store carbohydrate as glycogen, and essentially no ability to store the excess amino acids yielded from protein intake. As well, most carbohydrate is used at the time of consumption for energy needs or glycogen synthesis; little is converted to fat for storage in the body.[10] Protein is used for tissue synthesis, but adults generally eat more than enough protein for this. Beyond body needs and storage capabilities, excess amounts of amino acids are generally metabolized for energy; only some are metabolized to fat. Carbohydrate and protein intake also stimulate body use of these fuels. This is not true for fat. Finally, excess amounts of carbohydrate or protein are only inefficiently turned into fat and stored as such, if at all.[10]

As we noted in Chapter 4, it is also easier to overeat high-fat foods because they are energy dense and highly palatable. We can more easily eat a few extra cookies than a few extra apples, even though both may contain about the same amount of food energy. High-carbohydrate foods are often too bulky to easily overeat. Laboratory animals become more obese when provided with high-fat foods than with their typical leaner fare.[15] All these findings suggest that to reduce or control body fatness, focus first on controlling fat intake, substituting instead moderate amounts of foods rich in complex carbohydrates and dietary fiber.[3,10,27]

Why Am I Hungry?

Many forces influence when and what we eat. Organs, such as the liver and brain, interact with hormones, hormonelike (**neuroendocrine**) factors, the nervous system, and other aspects of body physiology to influence feeding behavior.[2] Social

neuroendocrine Substances or functions linked to combined action of both endocrine glands and the nervous system. Examples include substances released from glands in response to nerve stimulation.

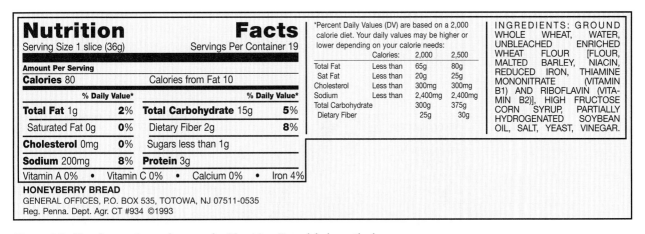

Figure 8-3 Use the nutrient values on the Nutrition Facts label to calculate energy content of a food. A serving of this food contains 81 kcal ([15 × 4] + [3 × 4] + [1 × 9] = 81). The label lists 80, suggesting that the energy value was rounded down.

forces—culture, work schedule, and income to name a few—act in both separate and interrelated fashion with physiological influences to also affect feeding behavior.[6] An interrelationship between social and physiological factors is seen with mood. When depressed, some people eat, while others avoid food. Either of these choices influences hormonal balance in the body, which can affect when and what is eaten later. Overall, a variety of forces—many of which are intertwined and work in concert—influence eating.[5]

The redundancy of forces influencing feeding behavior is important for survival. Because nutrients are vital to the body, it is critical that many factors encourage eating. The system is not perfect; body weight can fluctuate. But some powerful "built-in" and more "social" stimuli greatly affect food intake (Figure 8-4).[16]

WHAT ACTUALLY IS HUNGER?

The influences on feeding behavior can be categorized as either primarily internal or external. The physiological influences of the liver, adipose tissue, gastrointestinal tract, and subconscious brain are part of the internal network, while eating a piece of cake because of a birthday celebration is part of the external forces—the social setting rather than a physiological need.[6]

Internal forces are linked to what is called **hunger.** For our purposes, then, let's define hunger as the physiological forces that encourage us to find and eat food. The associated nagging and irritating feelings prompt the question "When can I eat?"[6] This state is mostly produced by "negative" internal factors, such as low blood concentrations of nutrients. External factors like mental stress and environmental temperature also have a role in hunger. Eating, thereby extinguishing the negative stimuli, should lead to **satiety,** meaning that the desire to eat ceases, at least for a short time.[29]

Satiety is maintained first by the sensory stimulation that food elicits and knowledge that a meal was eaten. Second, the effects of nutrient digestion, absorption, and metabolism are felt.[3] After a time, lack of food intake leads to lack of satiety, and the eating cycle begins again. Together these states, hunger and satiety, and the forces that regulate them greatly influence body weight.

At times when internal forces are not driving us to eat, as when we have just eaten a large meal, external forces may influence us to eat, as in another serving of pie. The question becomes "What do I want to eat?"[6] We use the term **appetite** to describe the motive behind this action. In essence, *appetite* refers to signals that guide dietary selection. You want a piece of pie; you don't want an onion. That drive is very different from the gnawing in the stomach after hours of not eating, or the feelings of faintness or light-headedness (i.e., hunger signals).

Appetite comes mostly from psychological state, but can have some physiological dimensions, such as a desire for salty foods (see Figure 8-5). Furthermore, these forces mostly are "positive" signals that arise to stimulate eating, such as the memory of how good mocha cheesecake tasted the last time you had it.[6]

hunger The primarily physiological drive to find and eat food, mostly regulated by internal cues to eating.

satiety State in which there is no longer a desire to eat.

appetite The external (psychological) influences that encourage us to find and eat food, often in the absence of obvious hunger.

- - - - - - - - - - - - -

Satiety cascade

early   taste of food

knowing a meal was just eaten

influence of stomach distention and receptors in the intestinal tract

late   influence of nutrient metabolism in liver and resulting communication with the brain

- - - - - - - - - - - - -

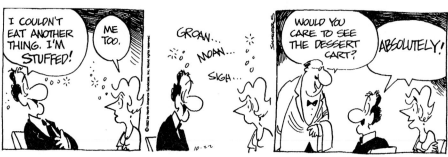

Figure 8-4   The Middletons.

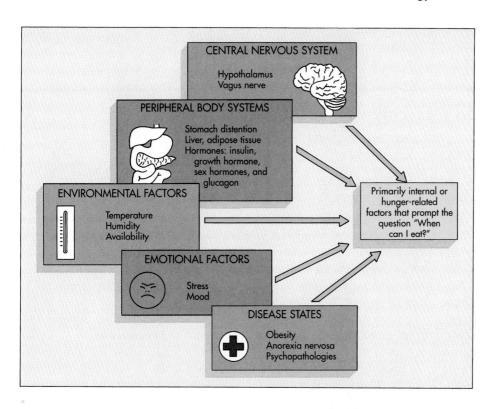

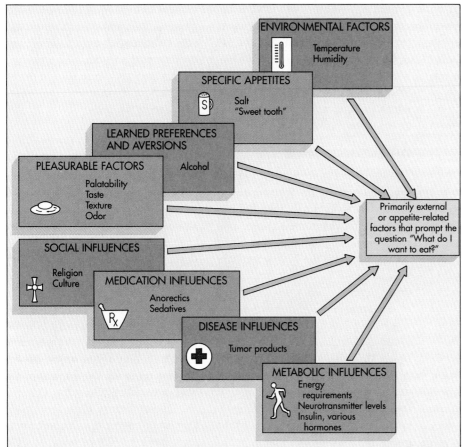

Figure 8-5 A model incorporating many factors that influence satiety. Note that there is some overlap between influences on hunger and appetite. Feeding is regulated by a group of complex and interrelated processes.

EXPERT OPINION

DO CARBOHYDRATES TURN INTO FAT?

MARC HELLERSTEIN, M.D., Ph.D.

At first glance, the answer to the title question seems an obvious "yes." How could it not be so? The scientific evidence reveals a very different, and a more interesting, story, however.

BIOCHEMISTRY OF FAT SYNTHESIS

The ability to convert carbohydrate into fat, also called *de novo lipogenesis (DNL)*, exists in bacteria, plants, and animals. In rats, the liver and adipose cells contribute about equally. In humans, the liver is believed to be the site of most, if not all, DNL.

Fatty acids in the body that do not come from DNL must come from the diet. The research question concerning conversion of carbohydrate into fat can therefore be restated as follows: "What portion of our body's fat comes from diet (exogenous) and what portion is from synthesis (endogenous)?"

INDIRECT EVIDENCE

Thirty years ago, Dr. Jules Hirsch and his colleagues addressed this question indirectly. They analyzed samples of adipose tissue from humans and found that the composition of the fatty acids closely reflected that of the subjects' diet. Moreover, when they put these subjects on controlled diets of different fatty acid composition for 6 months, adipose fatty acids slowly changed to reflect the new dietary fatty acid composition. If endogenous synthesis of fatty acids was important, it would have altered the composition of body fat in a more saturated fat direction, but this was not observed. The conclusion from these studies was that "we are what we eat" with regard to body fat, and that endogenous fat synthesis is not quantitatively important.

Another research tool that has been used to estimate lipogenesis is indirect calorimetry. This technique consists of measuring a person's rates of oxygen consumption and carbon dioxide release. Analyzing their ratio (the respiratory quotient) shows how much carbohydrate and fat are being burned by the body and whether the net rate of fat synthesis exceeds the rate of fat use. An important limitation of this technique, however, is that it measures whether net DNL is occurring in the whole body, but cannot exclude concurrent synthesis *and* use of fat for fuel. By this technique, numerous studies have shown that *net* DNL is absent or very low in humans under most dietary conditions, even after a large meal.

DIRECT EVIDENCE

These indirect approaches suggested that fat synthesis is a minor pathway in normal humans, but they did not prove it. As mentioned above, indirect calorimetry could fail to show *net* lipogenesis if the liver were making a substantial amount of fat but another tissue was using this fat for fuel at the same time. Concurrent synthesis and burning of fatty acids, called *futile cycling*, is very energy costly (this cycle wastes about 25% of the energy in the carbohydrate eaten) and would be important to identify if it were present. Until recently, however, technical problems prevented the direct measurement of DNL in people. The development of new stable isotopic methods for measuring the synthesis of fatty acids has helped to answer the question directly. This technique also has shown that in normal (nonobese, nondiabetic, nonoverfed) men, fat synthesis is minimal, representing < 1 g of satured fat per day, whether the subjects are given large meals, intravenous glucose, or a liquid diet.

But are there any circumstances in which DNL is stimulated? Dr. Jean-Marc Schwarz gave fructose and glucose orally to lean and obese subjects. The dietary fructose increased DNL by about tenfold to twentyfold compared with equal calorie loads of glucose. Nevertheless, fat synthesis still represented only a small percentage of the fructose load given.

My laboratory also studied the effect of 5 to 7 days of carbohydrate overfeeding or underfeeding in normal men. Hepatic synthesis of fat reflected very sensitively the degree of dietary carbohydrate excess. In fact, we were able to determine exactly what diet a person was on by measuring DNL. Even so, the absolute amount of fat synthesis remained low, even on massively excessive carbohydrate intakes, and represented < 20 g fat synthesized per day. Compare that with dietary fat intakes of 100 to 200 g per day. We concluded that lipogenesis might represent a sensitive *signal* of excess carbohydrate in the diet, but is not a quantitatively important route for the disposal of excess ingested carbohydrate.

Similar findings have been made in several other conditions. Very-low-fat diets (10% of energy as fat; 70% as carbohydrate) stimulate lipogenesis, but, again, not a large amount. Young women in the follicular phase of the menstrual cycle synthesize more fat than when in the luteal phase, but the amount is small, representing only 1 to 2 pounds of extra fat per year.

From the point of view of energetics, carbohydrate is therefore not interconvertible with fat. Fat cannot be converted into carbohydrate in animals, including humans, because of the absence of the enzymes composing the glyoxylate pathway. Thus the two major sources of energy in the diet are not interconvertible in the human body—in one direction because of a lack of enzymes and in the other direction because of an unexplained functional block.

ARE CARBOHYDRATE CALORIES THEREFORE "FREE"?

It would be wrong to conclude that the body's apparent resistance to storing excess carbohydrate as fat protects us from becoming fatter if we overeat carbohydrates. Although carbohydrate may be a separate and distinct form of energy, it is a form of energy nevertheless; the laws of thermodynamics are not suspended. A 50% excess of dietary carbohydrate energy did not cause net lipogenesis to occur in one study, but it did markedly reduce the use of fat for fuel by the body. As a consequence of this fat-sparing action, excess dietary carbohydrate *does* cause accumulation of body fat, despite not itself being converted to fat. Therefore dietary carbohydrate is not "free" when the diet also contains fat, because the carbohydrate spares fat use.

WHAT, THEN, ARE THE FUNCTIONS OF LIPOGENESIS?

Why do humans possess this elaborate enzymatic pathway for synthesizing fatty acids if it is not quantitatively important in the body? There are several possibilities (none of which have been proved, however):

- Lipogenesis in fact has no function in humans, but is a vestigial pathway.
- Lipogenesis is mainly an embryonic pathway with less utility in *adult* humans. By this hypothesis, fat synthesis is important in utero but is suppressed by intake of dietary fat, such as in human milk, after birth.
- Lipogenesis is a signal for other processes in the body. It is known that the synthesis of fat inhibits the use of fat for fuel in liver and muscle, that fatty acids signal the pancreas to secrete insulin, and that lipogenic products may have other regulatory functions. DNL may therefore signal carbohydrate availability in tissues.
- Humans in the Western world eat an unnaturally high-fat diet, which suppresses fat synthesis. Under preindustrial conditions, diets were low in fat and lipogenesis might have been an important pathway in adult humans for storing of transient energy surpluses.

WHAT ARE THE HEALTH CONSEQUENCES OF HIGH-CARBOHYDRATE DIETS?

Although high-carbohydrate diets may not be converted into fat, they do have other metabolic consequences. Many individuals exhibit worsening of serum glucose, triglyceride, and cholesterol patterns on 60% to 70% carbohydrate diets.

On the other hand, some investigators have proposed that high-carbohydrate, low-fat diets are more effective at controlling appetite than are high-fat diets because carbohydrate stores in the body may be a satiety signal. If this theory is true, then the apparent functional block in DNL would be essential to the operation of the food-regulatory system, since conversion of carbohydrate to fat would dissipate the signal for satiety and result in increased food intake and accumulation of body fat. Consistent with this hypothesis, a number of studies have found that high-carbohydrate, low-fat diets tend to result in weight loss.

SUMMARY

It is surprising but true that human beings do not convert carbohydrates into fat in significant quantities. The body appears to draw a line between carbohydrates and fats in both directions, at least under typical high-fat Western diets. The reasons for this functional block are unknown but may relate to the appetite-controlling system. Carbohydrate calories are not "free," however, since they spare fat from being used for fuel. Whatever else can be said, it is clear that many questions remain unanswered in this intriguing area and that we can expect more surprises!

Dr. Hellerstein is Associate Professor of Medicine at the University of California, San Francisco, and Associate Professor of Nutritional Sciences at the University of California at Berkeley.

A Closer Look at Internal Forces That Regulate Satiety

Internal (e.g., physiological) forces, such as the concentrations of nutrients in the blood, neurotransmitter production, circulating hormones and medications, gastrointestinal distention, nutrient receptors in the small intestine, adipose cell size, and degree of physical activity, can affect hunger and satiety (see Figure 8-5).[5] Let's look at these forces.

GASTROINTESTINAL EFFECTS ON HUNGER AND SATIETY

Pressure from food and drink in the stomach and intestines and the resulting hormonal and neuroendocrine responses increase satiety for a short period of time.[29] This is especially obvious after eating a large meal. In experiments with animals, the hormone cholecystokinin, which increases in the blood and brain after eating, and **gastrointestinal distention** appear to work together to register satiety (see Chapter 6 for a review of CCK and other gastrointestinal hormones).[2]

Following the influence of stomach distention, **nutrient receptors** in the small intestine are believed to take over in promoting satiety after a meal.[25,26] This concept is supported by experiments in which a subject feels satiated when fats or carbohydrates are infused into his or her small intestine. This effect is not reported, however, when the same fats or carbohydrates are infused directly into the subject's blood.[28]

Applying this information to the control of food intake when dieting, researchers are experimenting with the soluble fiber guar gum. This agent delays gastric emptying and slows nutrient absorption. Therefore, the feeling of fullness brought about by gastrointestinal distention and contact of nutrients with the intestinal receptors may last longer, delaying the desire to eat again.[11]

THE HYPOTHALAMUS CONTRIBUTES TO SATIETY REGULATION

The hypothalamus, a part of the brain, plays a key role in feeding behavior because it helps regulate satiety. Destruction of certain nerve tracts from the hypothalamus to specific target areas in the brain called *nuclei* (paraventricular nuclei and nigrostriatal tract) alters feeding behavior. The responses of these target cells stem in part from the changes in both neurotransmitter synthesis in the brain and **sympathetic nervous system** activity. Overall, as sympathetic nervous system activity declines, food intake increases. The opposite is also true.[5]

Various nuclei in the hypothalamus can be destroyed by specific chemicals, surgery, and certain forms of cancer. When these cells are destroyed, laboratory animals (and humans) continue to eat until they become quite obese. When other cells are destroyed, animals lose the desire to eat and eventually lose weight. Either response is actually quite complex because many nuclei in the vicinity of the destroyed region influence these hypothalamic responses.[2,5]

NUTRIENTS IN THE BLOOD

Accumulating evidence from both human and animal studies on the regulation of hunger suggests that an underlying hunger for food is never actually absent. After a meal, the blood concentrations of glucose, fatty acids, amino acids, and other energy-yielding nutrients increase. At this point, and especially as monosaccharides and amino acids are metabolized by the liver, the brain registers satiety, and hunger is temporarily relieved.[29] Recent studies suggest that an apolipoprotein on the chylomicrons (apolipoprotein A-IV) also signals satiety to the brain as these appear in the blood after a meal.[21]

Several hours after eating, when concentrations of nutrients in the blood begin to fall, the body must begin to utilize fuel from body stores; hunger then returns. This is because satiety is no longer registered by the metabolism of ingested energy-yielding compounds. In other words, feeding signals begin to dominate again. The liver plays a key role in this latter process.[29]

Hunger signals change even while we eat. At the beginning of a meal, we typically consume a variety of foods. By the end of a meal, food choices usually nar-

gastrointestinal distention Expansion of the walls of the stomach or intestines due to pressure caused by the presence of gases, food, drink, or other factors.

nutrient receptor Site in the small intestine that is a proposed mechanism in eliciting a feeling of satiety by communicating with the brain via nerves about the presence of nutrients in the small intestine.

CRITICAL THINKING

A question on your nutrition test asks, "Could adding soluble fiber to foods help control weight?" Using what you know about fiber, how could a positive answer to this question be supported?

sympathetic nervous system Part of the nervous system that regulates involuntary vital functions, including the activity of the heart muscle, smooth muscle, and adrenal glands.

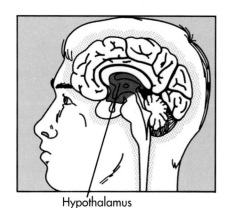

Hypothalamus

row. Consider the last time you went to a buffet. The first trip to the food table you may have chosen meat, pasta, salad, and something to drink. When you returned for a second or third time you probably steered toward the cake, pie, and ice cream. Although this may be partly influenced by social custom, and thus by mostly appetite-related cues, research with laboratory animals suggests that this action is also partly physiological. As nutrients are absorbed, the liver and surrounding organs communicate with the brain through the **vagus nerve.** This changes subsequent food choices by sending information about the rate of digestion and energy metabolism from the gastrointestinal tract and the liver to the brain.[2]

NEUROLOGICAL COMPONENTS

Studies with rats have shown that energy and protein deprivation affect neurotransmitter production. Rats experiencing a long-term protein-energy deficit show a significant decrease in food intake. It is thought that this is caused by an increase in the production of the neurotransmitter **histamine** in the brain. Other chemicals in the brain that have been associated with increased feeding are neuropeptide Y and galanin. Neuropeptide Y is linked to carbohydrate cravings, while a yearning for fat is noticed when blood concentrations of galanin increase.[7,24]

Increased production of **serotonin,** another brain neurotransmitter, has also been linked to intake of various nutrients, especially carbohydrate. High serotonin concentrations in the brain can be calming, induce sleepiness, and reduce food intake.[2]

Overall, certain dietary components can affect hunger and satiety partly through the effect on neuroendocrine compounds. There are possibly 25 of these types of compounds involved in feeding behavior (Table 8-1). Nutrients or their lack in the blood, as well as variation in neurotransmitter production, is involved in short-term satiety regulation—hour-to-hour and day-to-day.[2]

HORMONAL INFLUENCES ON FEEDING

Many hormones and drugs affect feeding behavior and satiety (see Table 8-1). After a meal, blood concentrations of cholecystokinin, secretin, gastrin, and other gastrointestinal hormones increase. These hormones increase satiety.[5]

On the other hand, **endorphins,** the body's natural pain killers, and the hormones cortisol and insulin all lead to increased feeding. The presence of cortisol is especially significant if animals are genetically prone to developing obesity. Insulin actually affects both hunger and satiety. Insulin increases liver metabolism of energy-yielding compounds and interacts with a receptor in the hypothalamus, promoting satiety. However, after insulin has done its job throughout the body, blood concentrations of energy-yielding compounds and insulin itself are low, which causes hunger to return.[29] In general, then, the body's hormonal balance influences the tendency to feel hungry or satiated. In a related fashion, menstrual status in women also influences energy intake and fat intake, which tend to be higher after ovulation than before ovulation.[19] Also notice in Table 8-1 that medications like some tranquilizers and antidepressants can increase hunger.

CONTROL OF FEEDING THROUGH BODY COMPOSITION

One recent theory is that feeding behavior changes in response to body fat content. When body fat is surgically removed from animals, their food consumption increases.[31] Based on work with genetic forms of obesity in animals, there is a substance or group of substances that circulates in the blood and communicates the degree of body fatness to the central nervous system. The gene for one such substance in mice and humans has been isolated.[17] The gene product has been named *leptin.* Reduced production of this protein is likely related to some human forms of obesity. Theoretically, when adipose tissue stores are increasing, leptin (or related substances) causes satiety. Conversely, when adipose tissue stores are decreasing, leptin (or related substances) is not released into the bloodstream and the desire to eat is enhanced. Research on this topic is continuing. Human tests with leptin are slated to begin in 1996. Widespread use will likely follow in 5 to 7 years if it is found to be safe and effective

vagus nerves Nerves arising from the brain that branch off to other organs that are essential for control of speech, swallowing, and gastrointestinal function.

histamine A neurotransmitter synthesized from the amino acid histidine that appears to decrease hunger and food intake.

serotonin A neurotransmitter synthesized from the amino acid tryptophan that appears to decrease the desire to eat carbohydrates and to induce sleep.

endorphins Natural body tranquilizers that may be involved in the feeding response.

- - - - - - - - - - - - - -

While a person is resting, the percentage of total energy use by various organs is about as follows:

Liver	29%
Muscle	18%
Brain	19%
Heart	10%
Kidney	7%
Other	17%

- - - - - - - - - - - - - -

- - - - - - - - - - - - - -

It was once thought that weight cycling—weight loss followed by regain—contributed to a decrease in basal metabolism. However, many current studies have not been able to demonstrate this effect.

- - - - - - - - - - - - - -

Energy Use: The Other Side of Energy Balance

We have examined some stimuli for consuming energy. Now let's look at the other side of the relationship, energy output.

Energy Use by the Body

The body uses energy for four general purposes: (1) **basal metabolism,** (2) **thermic effect of food,** and (3) physical activity are the most important. A fourth use, **adaptive thermogenesis,** is heat production during long-term excess energy intake or exposure to cold temperatures (see Figure 8-1).[32]

BASAL METABOLISM

Basal metabolism represents the minimum energy it takes to keep the resting, awake body alive. This includes maintaining a heart beat, respiration, correct body temperature, and other functions.[32] It does not include energy needs for physical activity or digesting food. Basal metabolism amounts to about 1 kcal/kg of body weight per hour in men and 0.9 kcal/kg of body weight per hour in women (or roughly 1 kcal per minute). Sleep reduces basal metabolism by about 10%.

To determine basal metabolic rate (BMR), the subject must have just awakened, be in a warm room, remain as relaxed as possible, and not have eaten for at least 12 hours. Oxygen consumption (and usually carbon dioxide output) is measured for approximately 20 to 30 minutes. These gas measurements are then used to calculate energy use (see the section on indirect calorimetry).[32] A less accurate value, the **resting metabolic rate (RMR),** is derived when measuring energy use under less stringent conditions. The subject must not have eaten for at least a few hours and be at rest. RMR is often slightly higher than BMR; however, they often differ by less than 3%. Thus the terms *BMR* and *RMR* often are used interchangeably.

Within the general population there is a variation in BMR of about 25% to 30%. This variation influences the risk for developing obesity. BMR usually accounts for about 60% to 70% of daily energy expenditure in people of average physical activity.[9]

About 70% to 80% of basal metabolism depends on the amount of **lean body mass** (Table 8-2).[5] The tissues involved, especially heart, liver, brain, and kidney—show high metabolic activity at rest and thus greatly influence energy needs. Other influences that determine basal metabolism are as follows:

- Body surface area (the greater the area, the greater the heat loss)
- Gender (males average higher energy use because of greater lean body mass)
- Body temperature (fever increases metabolic rate)
- Thyroid hormone (higher concentrations increase metabolic rate)
- Aspects of hormone system activity, such as for the sympathetic nervous system
- Age (metabolic rate decreases with advancing age through adulthood)
- Nutritional state (eating less slows metabolic rate in the short term)
- Pregnancy (increases metabolic rate)
- Caffeine and tobacco use (increase metabolic rate)

Low energy intake decreases BMR about 10% to 20% (about 150 to 300 kcal/day). This reduction makes continued dieting success difficult (see Chapter 9).[16] However, this is a survival mechanism for people who are unable to meet their energy needs during a famine. In addition, it is hard to maintain a desirable body weight as we age because BMR declines approximately 2% every 10 years after age 30. This is caused by a slow and steady decrease in actively metabolizing cells, which is linked to aging (see Chapter 18). However, people who remain active into their elderly years do not show such a great decline in basal metabolism, in part because lean body mass is better maintained.

TABLE 8-2

Factors that increase or decrease basal metabolism

Increase	Decrease
Muscle mass (fat-free mass)	Age (primarily if lean body mass decreases during adulthood)
Fever	Reduction in energy intake, undernutrition
Recent food intake	Genetics
Ovulation	
Surface area	
Recent exercise (effect has limited duration)	
Thyroid hormone	
Trauma	
Epinephrine	
Male gender (greater lean body mass)	
Growth, such as childhood and pregnancy	
Genetics	
Nicotine	
Caffeine	

THERMIC EFFECT OF FOOD

Thermic effect of food (TEF) represents the amount of extra energy used by the body during digestion, absorption, metabolism, and storage of energy-yielding nutrients.[32] This elevates body temperature for several hours after eating. The energy expended is equivalent to about 10% of total energy absorbed, which in turn is essentially 10% of total energy consumed.[9] To supply the body with 100 kcal, a person must eat about 110 kcal to account for the 10 kcal lost to TEF. The processes of digestion, absorption, and metabolism use the extra energy to modify the nutrients so that they are available for use. Given a daily energy intake of 3000 kcal, TEF would use about 300 kcal. The TEF value for a carbohydrate-rich or a protein-rich meal is higher than for a fat-rich meal.[26] This is because it takes less energy to transfer absorbed fat into adipose stores than to convert glucose into glycogen or metabolize excess amino acids into fat.

Large meals show higher values for TEF than the same amount of food eaten over many hours. Some possible mechanisms for this phenomenon include changes in central nervous system activity, greater production and release of hormones (such as insulin) and enzymes, and the rate of absorption and storage of macronutrients.

Other names for the thermic effect of food include *specific dynamic action* and *diet-induced thermogenesis.*

PHYSICAL ACTIVITY

Body energy fuels physical activity. Physical activity is the aspect of energy expenditure over which we have the most control. The biggest difference in energy use among people results from different expenditures for physical activity. Some people are very active and others are very sedentary. Together, basal metabolism and the thermic effect of food represent about 70% to 80% of total energy use, while physical activity accounts for roughly 15% to 30% of energy use in sedentary people.[9]

Physical activity includes sports, such as handball and bicycling, as well as everyday activities. Climbing stairs rather than using the elevator and walking rather than driving increase physical activity and hence energy use. Rates of obesity in America are alarming. We do not consume much more energy than people did at the turn of this century, but as a group we are considerably less active. This inactivity contributes to the increase in obesity.[9,15] For many adults, physical activity consists of little more than walking to and from their automobiles.

Because most of the energy for physical activity is converted to heat, this contributor to energy expenditure is sometimes called the *thermic effect of exercise.*

ADAPTIVE THERMOGENESIS

Adaptive thermogenesis is energy expended via heat production linked to exposure to stimuli such as cold environmental conditions and overfeeding. Heat is produced without work being done.[32] This subject has produced much controversy and interest. Much of the work on this topic deals with the fact that when people are overfed, they do not gain the amount of weight that is expected based on energy intake.

In many animals, including humans to a yet undetermined extent, adaptive thermogenesis is linked to the presence of **brown adipose tissue.** Most fat is stored in white adipose tissue. Brown adipose tissue is less than 1% of body weight in humans. This tissue is a specialized form of fat storage found primarily in the shoulder area. For hibernating animals it is a main source of heat during their long winter sleep. The brown tint derives from (1) the ample supply of arteries and veins that provide the tissues with blood, (2) the numerous mitochondria present that allow greater energy metabolism, and (3) myoglobin that is part of the structural material and is needed for oxygen utilization.

Brown adipose tissue yields heat by failing to form much ATP during the metabolism of energy-yielding nutrients. Most energy is simply lost as heat. Thus these cells provide a lot of heat and, in turn, warm the body.

Decreased activity of brown adipose tissue during overfeeding and cold adaptation is associated with obesity in rats. Researchers are not in agreement, but there is some evidence that impaired adaptive thermogenesis due to abnormalities in the functioning of brown adipose tissue may be a factor in human obesity. Activation of the sympathetic nervous system in response to overfeeding and cold may be the link between these stimuli and activity of brown adipose tissue. Substances such as ephedrine, caffeine, and nicotine increase energy expenditure partially by increasing the activity of the sympathetic nervous system.[1] They appear to increase adaptive thermogenesis and reduce hunger.

The extent to which brown adipose tissue is present and operative in humans has not been clearly determined. If you touch an infant's back, you can feel the heat produced by brown adipose tissue. Sensitive instruments can demonstrate hotter spots around the shoulder area of adults, as well. However, it is difficult to determine how much energy use this represents in adults. Although it seems unlikely that brown adipose tissue serves a pivotal role in weight reduction in adults, information is too sketchy to permit any definite conclusions. Still, some drug manufacturers are trying to find agents that can increase activity of these cells. Overall, it is estimated that adaptive thermogenesis represents up to about 7% of energy use.[9]

brown adipose tissue A specialized form of adipose tissue that produces large amounts of heat by metabolizing energy-yielding nutrients without synthesizing much ATP. The energy is released as heat.

Concept Check

Four factors contribute to energy expenditure: (1) Basal metabolism is the minimum amount of energy needed to maintain a body in an awake, resting state. A person's basal metabolism to a large extent depends on his or her lean body mass, surface area, and thyroid hormone status. (2) The thermic effect of food is the additional energy needed to digest, absorb, and process nutrients. This corresponds to about 10% of total energy intake. (3) Physical activity represents energy use above what is needed for basal metabolism and the thermic effect of food. (4) Adaptive thermogenesis is heat production in response to cold or overfeeding. This phenomenon may be linked to the presence of brown adipose tissue. In a sedentary person, about 70% to 80% of energy is used for basal metabolism and the thermic effect of food; the remainder is used for physical activity and adaptive thermogenesis.

Measuring Energy Use by the Body

Scientists use several methods to quantify energy usage in humans. Some are convenient but not very accurate, while others are very accurate but more cumbersome. While learning about these methods, consider which you would prefer be used if you were the research subject.

DIRECT AND INDIRECT CALORIMETRY

There are two primary ways to *measure* the amount of energy the body uses: **direct calorimetry** and **indirect calorimetry.** When using direct calorimetry, a person is placed in an insulated chamber and the amount of heat he or she releases is calculated by measuring the increase in the temperature of the water surrounding the chamber. Recall that a kilocalorie is defined as the amount of heat it takes to raise the temperature of 1 L of water 1° C. By measuring the temperature of the water surrounding the calorimeter before and after the study, the number of kilocalories expended can be determined. This method resembles that of using a bomb calorimeter to measure the energy content of a food. Direct calorimetry works because almost all the energy used by the body eventually exits as heat (see Chapter 7).

Older direct calorimeters were quite large, about the size of a small room. Newer calorimeters can be the size of a phone booth or even smaller, about the size of a space suit. Nevertheless, few investigators use direct calorimetry, mostly because of its expense and complexity.[32]

In using indirect calorimetry, instead of measuring heat, a technician measures something associated with body metabolism, such as oxygen uptake or oxygen uptake plus the carbon dioxide output (Figure 8-6).[32] There is a predictable relationship between the body's use of energy and its use of oxygen or output of carbon dioxide. For example, when metabolizing a typical mixed diet containing carbohydrate, fat, and protein, the body uses 1 L of oxygen to expend about 4.85 kcal.

Instruments used to measure oxygen consumption (and often carbon dioxide output as well) for indirect calorimetry are widely available. They can be attached to a small room, mounted on carts and rolled up to a hospital bed, or carried in backpacks while a person plays tennis or jogs. The latter method enables scientists to determine the amount of energy used when performing various activities, while using these instruments at a hospital bedside allows medical personnel to determine how much energy a patient is using and therefore how much to feed him or her. Tables showing the amount of energy used to perform various exercises rely on indirect calorimetry to determine the values (see Appendix K).

The newest approach to indirect calorimetry uses **stable isotopes** of oxygen and hydrogen. In this method a person consumes isotopically labeled water ($^2H_2^{18}O$). A technician measures the ^2H_2O and the $H_2^{18}O$ later found in body fluids, such as urine. Using these values and some mathematical formulas, total carbon dioxide (CO_2) output per day can be estimated. This estimate of CO_2 output is used to calculate energy use, just as is done with oxygen use in indirect calorimetry.[32] ^2H and ^{18}O are stable isotopes of hydrogen and oxygen (therefore they are nonradioactive); special equipment can measure them in body fluids.

This stable isotope method is quite accurate but also very expensive. With wider use, it is expected to extend our knowledge of variation in energy use by people over entire days. This information may further reveal why some people can regulate their body weight more easily than others, and it has demonstrated that people often underreport their food intake when interviewed.

Estimating Energy Needs

A variety of methods can be used to *estimate* the body's energy needs.

HARRIS-BENEDICT EQUATION

A method of estimating resting energy needs that is widely used by registered dietitians for hospitalized patients is the **Harris-Benedict equation.** This equation

direct calorimetry A method of determining a body's energy use by measuring heat that emanates from the body, usually using an insulated chamber.

indirect calorimetry A method of measuring a body's energy use by measuring its oxygen uptake (and often carbon dioxide output as well) and then using formulas to convert that gas exchange into energy use.

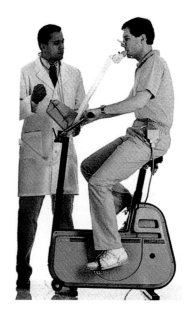

Figure 8-6 Indirect calorimetry. This method can be used to measure energy output during daily activities by monitoring oxygen uptake and carbon dioxide output.

stable isotope An isotope is a specific form of a chemical element. It differs from atoms of other forms (isotopes) of the same element in the number of neutrons in its nucleus. "Stable" means that the isotope is not radioactive, in contrast to some other types of isotopes.

Harris-Benedict equation An equation that predicts resting metabolic rate based on a person's weight, height, and age.

considers weight, height, and age.[31] The Nutrition Focus on the next page illustrates how to use the Harris-Benedict equation. The value for resting energy needs is then multiplied by predetermined factors to reflect a patient's degree of physical activity and illness, both of which raise energy needs above resting needs. The final value calculated gives total energy needs.

A rough estimate for total energy needs uses a person's weight and degree of physical activity. Sedentary energy needs are set at 9 to 10 kcal/pound. The value is then decreased by 100 kcal for every 10 years of age over age 30. Light activity starts with 12 to 13 kcal/pound; heavy activity starts at 20 kcal/pound; values are then adjusted for age. For example, a sedentary 40-year-old who weighs 160 pounds needs about 1500 kcal to meet energy needs: ([160 × 10] − 100 = 1500).

Finally, some rough guidelines for energy needs found in the Food Guide Pyramid publication are:

- Sedentary women and some older adults   1600 kcal
- Children, teenage girls, active women, most men   2200 kcal
- Teenage boys, active men, very active women   2800 kcal
- Young children, pregnant and breast-feeding   Check with a registered
  women   dietitian

These values then need to be fine-tuned based on personal characteristics and experiences, such as amount of physical activity performed.

A simple method of tracking your energy expenditure, and thus your energy needs, is to use the forms in Appendix G. Appendix K lists the energy costs of various activities. The values account for energy use for basal metabolism, the thermic effect of food, and physical activity. Begin by taking an entire 24-hour period and list all activities performed, including sleep. Record the number of minutes spent in each activity; the total should equal 1440 minutes (24 hours). Next record the energy cost for each activity in kilocalories per minute, based on your weight in kilograms (pounds ÷ 2.2). Multiply the energy cost by the minutes. This gives the energy expended for each activity. Total all the kilocalorie values. This gives your estimated energy expenditure for the day.

CONCEPT CHECK

Energy use by the body can be measured by direct calorimetry, as heat given off, and by indirect calorimetry, as oxygen uptake (with or without carbon dioxide output). Energy needs, both resting and total, can be estimated using formulas based on factors such as weight, height, and age, or simply on weight. In addition, the RDA and Food Guide Pyramid publications both provide guidelines for energy intake.

Estimating a Desirable (Healthy) Weight

There are numerous methods used to define a desirable (some scientists prefer the term *healthy*) weight. Several tables exist, based on weight and one or more factors, including height, age, and body frame size. These tables arise from studies of large population groups. When applied to a population, they provide good estimates of weight associated with good health and longevity. These tables, however, do not necessarily refer directly to an individual's weight and health status.

Ideally, family history of obesity-related disease and current health parameters should be considered when establishing a desirable weight for an individual, in addition to weight-for-height. Evidence of the following obesity-related conditions is important[15]:

- Hypertension
- Elevated serum LDL
- Family history of obesity, heart disease, or cancer
- Pattern of fat distribution in the body
- Elevated blood glucose

Recall from Chapter 2 that the RDA publication also lists recommendations for energy intake for lightly to moderately active persons (see the inside cover of this textbook).

Men ages 19 to 50: 2900 kcal

Women ages 19 to 50: 2200 kcal

Medical literature currently uses the terms *desirable* or *healthy*, rather than *ideal*, when referring to body weight. The term *desirable body weight* was first used in 1959 by the Metropolitan Life Insurance Company to replace the term *ideal body weight*. The 1983 tables used neither term.

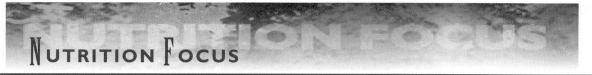

Nutrition Focus

CALCULATING ENERGY USE

The following examples illustrate how to estimate energy expenditure. Adaptive thermogenesis is not included because of limited knowledge regarding its contribution.

Bill weighs 154 pounds (70 kg), is 5 feet 9 inches tall (175 cm), is 35 years old, and is involved in moderate muscular activity each day.

BASAL METABOLISM

Use the value 1 kcal/kg body weight/hour for **MEN.**
  0.9 kcal/kg body weight/hour for **WOMEN.**
For Bill:

1. Multiply his weight in kilograms by the appropriate value for men.

$$70 \text{ kg} \times 1 \text{ kcal/kg/hour} = 70 \text{ kcal/hr.}$$

2. Multiply kilocalories used in an hour by hours in a day.

$$70 \text{ kcal/hr} \times 24 \text{ hr/day} = 1680 \text{ kcal/day.}$$

Basal metabolism = 1680 kcal/day.

PHYSICAL ACTIVITY

Select one of the following categories based on the amount of muscular activity performed in a day:

  Sedentary activity (mostly sitting): add 20% to 40% of BMR.

  Light activity (a clerk involved in a daily walking program): add 55% to 65% of BMR.

  Moderate activity (a teacher involved in daily vigorous exercise): add 70% to 75% of BMR.

  Heavy activity (a mail carrier who walks the route or an adult involved in a daily exercise program): add 80% to 100% or more of BMR.

If Bill performs moderate activity:

1. Take 70% of his basal metabolism.

$$1680 \text{ kcal/day} \times 0.70 = 1176 \text{ kcal/day.}$$

Physical activity = 1176 kcal/day.

THERMIC EFFECT OF FOOD

A quick way to approximate this value is to take 10% of the sum of the BMR and physical activity kilocalories. For Bill:

1. $1680 \text{ kcal/day} + 1176 \text{ kcal/day} = 2856 \text{ kcal/day.}$

2. $2856 \text{ kcal/day} \times 0.10 = 286 \text{ kcal/day.}$

Thermic effect of food = 286 kcal/day.

TOTAL ENERGY USE

Sum of the energy contributions from each factor. For Bill:

$$1680 \text{ kcal/day} + 1176 \text{ kcal/day} + 286 \text{ kcal/day} = 3142 \text{ kcal/day.}$$

Total energy use = 3142 kcal/day.

CALCULATING RESTING ENERGY USE USING HARRIS-BENEDICT EQUATIONS

We have estimated Bill's total energy use. Let's calculate Bill's resting energy expenditure using the appropriate Harris-Benedict equation and compare it with the basal metabolism we determined for him.

Harris-Benedict equation:

$$66.5 + 13.8 \text{ (weight in kg)} + 5 \text{ (height in cm)} - 6.8 \text{ (age in years)}$$

Bill weighs 70 kg, is 175 cm tall, and is 35 years old. Therefore Bill's resting energy expenditure is as follows:

$$66.5 + 13.8 \text{ (70 kg)} + 5 \text{ (175 cm)} - 6.8 \text{ (35)} = 1671 \text{ kcal/day.}$$

Resting energy use = 1671 kcal/day
Compare this with the estimate of basal metabolism of 1680 kcal/day we determined previously. The values are not very different. Note also that the Harris-Benedict equation for women is 66.5 + 9.6 (weight in kg) + 1.8 (height in cm) − 4.7 (age in years).

One way to view a height-weight table is to consider the values a "statistical" estimate of desirable weight. If you weigh somewhat more or less than the tables suggest for your height, this does not necessarily imply adverse health consequences. However, extra body fat can set the stage for future disease,[33] although even that is not guaranteed for a specific person. The individual, under a physician's guidance, should establish a "personal" desirable weight (or need for weight reduction), based on weight history, fat distribution patterns, family history of obesity-related disease, and current health status. Current height/weight standards are only a rough guide.

Striving for body weights and shapes presented in the media is not the way to establish desirable weight. For example, consider a woman who is 5 feet 2 inches tall and has weighed 250 pounds for 25 years. Theoretically she should weigh around 120 pounds according to height and weight tables, but this is not necessarily a realistic weight goal for her. Attempting massive weight loss almost invariably results in rapid weight regain. The most important factor in determining desirable weight for this person is the amount of weight loss that results in a final body weight that is not an impediment to health, employment, or life's normal activities.

Furthermore, a healthy lifestyle may make a more important contribution to a person's health status than the number on the scale. We discuss this at greater length in Chapter 9 with regard to appropriateness of weight loss. Overall, height-weight tables provide a guide for desirable weight, but some fine-tuning is often necessary.

USING BODY MASS INDEX (BMI) TO SET DESIRABLE WEIGHT

Body mass index (BMI) is currently the preferred weight-for-height standard used to define desirable weight. This is calculated as:

$$\frac{\text{body weight (in kilograms)}}{\text{height}^2 \text{ (in meters)}}$$

Table 8-3 lists BMI for various heights and weights. Figure 8-7 shows that health risks from excess weight begin when the body mass index exceeds 25. A desirable weight for height is a BMI of 20 to 25. What is your BMI? How much would your weight need to change to yield a BMI of 27? 30? These are general cut-off values for the presence of obesity (see later section).[15]

The graph in Figure 8-7 is curvilinear rather than linear, so as body mass index increases, health risk increases to a greater degree than body mass index. Also, at lower body mass index values health problems increase. This primarily reflects the lower weight and poorer health of people who smoke. We discuss other links between low body weight and poor health in Chapters 9 and 11.

The concept of body mass index is convenient to use because the values apply to both men and women. However, any body weight-for-height standard is actually a crude measure because we are concerned about overfat, not simply overweight, individuals when setting guidelines for desirable weight. The husky athlete is a notable exception; he or she may be overweight but not overfat. Still, overfat and overweight conditions almost always appear together. We focus on body weight-for-height standards in clinical settings mainly because these are easier to measure than total body fat.

USING THE METROPOLITAN LIFE INSURANCE TABLE TO ESTIMATE DESIRABLE WEIGHT

The Metropolitan Life Insurance Table (see inside cover) provides another common standard for estimating desirable weight. The table lists for any height the weight that is associated with a maximum lifespan. The table does not tell the healthiest weight for a living person; it simply lists the weight associated with longevity.

There are many criticisms of this method. One is that the table's data are derived only from purchasers of life insurance, so the results under-represent poor people and many minorities. Smokers are included in the table, and they often have both lower body weights and earlier ages of death because of their increased risk for lung cancer and heart disease. This distortion may mean that the table overestimates the best weight for maximum longevity. Another problem, body weight, is determined only at the time the insurance policy is purchased; no follow-up weights are recorded.

- - - - - - - - - - - - -

BMI is not a standard for everyone. BMI should not be applied to children, adolescents who are still growing, adults over 65, pregnant and lactating women, or highly muscular individuals.

- - - - - - - - - - - - -

TABLE 8-3

Body weight in pounds according to height and body mass index (BMI)

	BMI (kg/m²)													
	19	20	21	22	23	24	25	26	27	28	29	30	35	40
Height (inches)	**Body weight (pounds)**													
58	91	96	100	105	110	115	119	124	129	134	138	143	167	191
59	94	99	104	109	114	119	124	128	133	138	143	148	173	198
60	97	102	107	112	118	123	128	133	138	143	148	153	179	204
61	100	106	111	116	122	127	132	137	143	148	153	158	185	211
62	104	109	115	120	126	131	136	142	147	153	158	164	191	218
63	107	113	118	124	130	135	141	146	152	158	163	169	197	225
64	110	116	122	128	134	140	145	151	157	163	169	174	204	232
65	114	120	126	132	138	144	150	156	162	168	174	180	210	240
66	118	124	130	136	142	148	155	161	167	173	179	186	216	247
67	121	127	134	140	146	153	159	166	172	178	185	191	223	255
68	125	131	138	144	151	158	164	171	177	184	190	197	230	262
69	128	135	142	149	155	162	169	176	182	189	196	203	236	270
70	132	139	146	153	160	167	174	181	188	195	202	207	243	278
71	136	143	150	157	165	172	179	186	193	200	208	215	250	286
72	140	147	154	162	169	177	184	191	199	206	213	221	258	294
73	144	151	159	166	174	182	189	197	204	212	219	227	265	302
74	148	155	163	171	179	186	194	202	210	218	225	233	272	311
75	152	160	168	176	184	192	200	208	216	224	232	240	279	319
76	156	164	172	180	189	197	205	213	221	230	238	246	287	328

From Bray GA, Gray DS: *Western Journal of Medicine* 149:429, 1988.
Each entry gives the body weight for a person of a given height and BMI. Pounds have been rounded off. To use the table, find the approximate height in the far left column. Move across the row to a given weight. The number at the top of the column is the BMI for that height and weight.

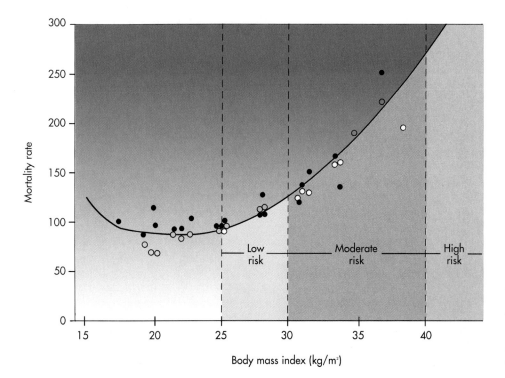

Figure 8-7 The relationship between body mass index and death rate (100 equals normal death rate). Solid circles show men and open circles show women. One estimate of desirable (healthy) body weight is a BMI of 20 to 25, but other health factors need to be considered as well.

The weight and height values in the Metropolitan Life Insurance Table assume the subject is wearing clothes and shoes. The table also refers only to people under 60 years old. An overweight elderly person may have already avoided the typical causes of death, such as stroke, heart disease, and cancer, to which obesity contributes. The fact that they have survived into their 70s and 80s suggests that they are somewhat resistant to the effects of obesity.

The Metropolitan Life Insurance Table adjusts for small, medium, and large frames. Methods for estimating frame size use measurements of wrist width or elbow breadth (see Appendix L). Overall, obviously small and thin people have a small frame, obviously big and bulky people who have large bones have a large frame, and everyone else has a medium frame.

Weighing slightly more or less than the range listed in the table is not necessarily cause for alarm. In addition, the weight ranges listed do not guarantee health when alive. They simply attempt to maximize the chances of a long life.

ADDITIONAL METHODS OF SETTING DESIRABLE WEIGHT

Another height-weight table that is currently in use is the USDA/DHHS table (Table 8-4). This method considers age but not gender or frame size. The range of suggested weight for height is very large, since both males and females and small, medium, and large frames are included. The greatest criticism of this table is that it allows weight gain with age. Some researchers believe that a small amount of fat gain is to be expected with aging, about 2 pounds per decade after age 30, as long as the person does not become overweight. Other researchers believe that no weight gain after age 25 should be the goal.[33] They note that simply the fact that there seems to be a tendency to gain weight with age does not indicate that this is healthy. Overall, maintaining a stable weight (or close to it) in adulthood is an important goal for health.

Still another method of estimating desirable body weight is the pounds per inch of height method. For women, allow 100 pounds for the first 5 feet, then add 5 pounds for every inch thereafter. To estimate a man's desirable body weight, allow 106 pounds for the first 5 feet and then add 6 pounds for each inch thereafter. Based on this system, a 6-foot-tall man should weigh about 178 pounds ($106 + [12 \times 6]$).

PUTTING DESIRABLE WEIGHT INTO PERSPECTIVE

One current school of thought is to let nature takes its course with regard to body weight. According to this proposal, by trying to lose weight in order to fall within a specific height-weight range, people often regain their original weight plus more. In contrast, listening to the body for hunger cues, eating a healthy diet, and remaining physically active eventually maintains an appropriate height-weight value.

Overall, the clearest idea regarding a desirable (healthy) weight is that it is a personal matter. Weight has to be considered in terms of health, not simply fashion. For now a BMI of 20 to 25 is a reasonable goal, but does not represent rigid cut-off values for a person's desirable weight.[15]

CONCEPT CHECK

Desirable (healthy) body weight is generally determined in a clinical setting using a body mass index or some other weight-for-height standard. The presence of existing weight-related disease should be considered in determining desirable body weight. Overall health and a healthy lifestyle, not simply fashion, should be the major considerations when determining desirable weight.

TABLE 8-4

Age-related weight-for-height standards. (The research community is not in agreement that weight gain in adulthood is desirable.)

A. Suggested desirable weights for adults (men and women)

Height*	Weight in pounds†	
	19 to 34 years	35 years and over
5'0"	97-128‡	108-138‡
5'1"	101-132	111-143
5'2"	104-137	115-148
5'3"	107-141	119-152
5'4"	111-146	122-157
5'5"	114-150	126-162
5'6"	118-155	130-167
5'7"	121-160	134-172
5'8"	125-164	138-178
5'9"	129-169	142-183
5'10"	132-174	146-188
5'11"	136-179	151-194
6'0"	140-184	155-199
6'1"	144-189	159-205
6'2"	148-195	164-210
6'3"	152-200	168-216
6'4"	156-205	173-222
6'5"	160-211	177-228
6'6"	164-216	182-234

From USDA/DHHS: *Dietary guidelines for Americans,* 1990.
*Without shoes.
†Without clothes.
‡The higher weights in the ranges generally apply to men, who tend to have more muscle and bone; the lower weights more often apply to women, who have less muscle and bone.

B. Desirable body mass index in relation to age

Age (yr)	Body mass index (kg/m²)
19-24	19-24
25-34	20-25
35-44	21-26
45-54	22-27
55-64	23-28
>65	24-29

From *Diet and health: implications for reducing chronic disease risk,* Washington, DC, 1989, National Academy Press.

Energy Imbalance

If energy intake exceeds expenditure over time, **obesity** is likely to result. Health problems often soon follow. In this context, medical experts believe that a cut-off for obesity for an individual person should not be based primarily on body weight, but rather on the total amount of fat in the body, the location of body fat, and the presence or absence of weight-related medical problems.

Typical health problems associated with obesity include[15]:

• Increased risk in surgery
• Non–insulin-dependent (adult-onset) diabetes
• Hypertension

obesity A condition characterized by excess body fat. In clinical settings it is often defined in one of two ways: (1) a body mass index above 27 to 30; or (2) weighing 20% above desirable weight, based on height-weight tables.

Figure 8-9 Underwater weighing. To get an accurate estimate of body fat, the subject exhales as much air as possible and then holds his breath and bends over at the waist. Once he is totally submerged, the underwater weight is recorded.

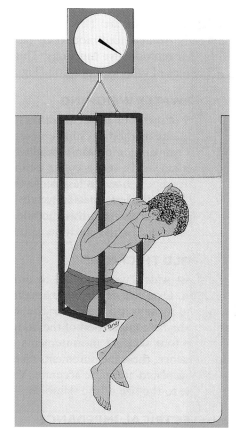

Figure 8-10 Skinfold measurements. Using proper technique, calibrated equipment, and standards, skinfold measurements can be used to accurately estimate total body fat content in about 20 minutes. Commonly measured skinfolds are **A,** subscapular, **B,** thigh, **C,** suprailiac, and **D,** triceps.

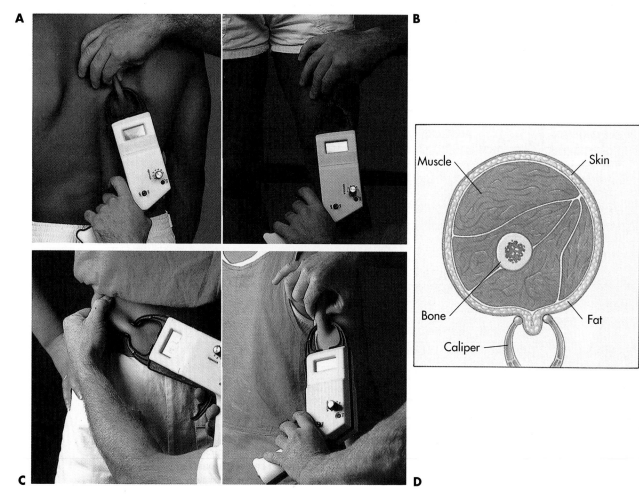

TABLE 8-4

Age-related weight-for-height standards. (The research community is not in agreement that weight gain in adulthood is desirable.)

A. Suggested desirable weights for adults (men and women)

Height*	Weight in pounds†	
	19 to 34 years	35 years and over
5'0"	97-128‡	108-138‡
5'1"	101-132	111-143
5'2"	104-137	115-148
5'3"	107-141	119-152
5'4"	111-146	122-157
5'5"	114-150	126-162
5'6"	118-155	130-167
5'7"	121-160	134-172
5'8"	125-164	138-178
5'9"	129-169	142-183
5'10"	132-174	146-188
5'11"	136-179	151-194
6'0"	140-184	155-199
6'1"	144-189	159-205
6'2"	148-195	164-210
6'3"	152-200	168-216
6'4"	156-205	173-222
6'5"	160-211	177-228
6'6"	164-216	182-234

From USDA/DHHS: *Dietary guidelines for Americans,* 1990.
*Without shoes.
†Without clothes.
‡The higher weights in the ranges generally apply to men, who tend to have more muscle and bone; the lower weights more often apply to women, who have less muscle and bone.

B. Desirable body mass index in relation to age

Age (yr)	Body mass index (kg/m²)
19-24	19-24
25-34	20-25
35-44	21-26
45-54	22-27
55-64	23-28
>65	24-29

From *Diet and health: implications for reducing chronic disease risk,* Washington, DC, 1989, National Academy Press.

Energy Imbalance

If energy intake exceeds expenditure over time, **obesity** is likely to result. Health problems often soon follow. In this context, medical experts believe that a cut-off for obesity for an individual person should not be based primarily on body weight, but rather on the total amount of fat in the body, the location of body fat, and the presence or absence of weight-related medical problems.

Typical health problems associated with obesity include[15]:
- Increased risk in surgery
- Non–insulin-dependent (adult-onset) diabetes
- Hypertension

obesity A condition characterized by excess body fat. In clinical settings it is often defined in one of two ways: (1) a body mass index above 27 to 30; or (2) weighing 20% above desirable weight, based on height-weight tables.

- Heart disease
- Arthritis
- Gallstones
- Pregnancy risks
- Premature death
- Various forms of cancer, such as colon, rectal, and prostate cancer in men and breast (especially after menopause), uterine, and ovarian cancer in women.
- Sleep disorders

Possible explanations of why obesity is associated with these disorders are listed in Table 8-5.

Furthermore, discrimination against obese people is very common. Overweight women have household incomes that average $6,700 less and are 10% more likely to be poor than women who are not obese. Other examples of discrimination include decreased chance of marriage, fewer choices in clothing, and rude remarks.

Overweight versus Overfat

Health risks of being obese actually apply only to people who are overfat. Body fat can range from 2% to upwards of 70% of body weight. In this regard, men with over 25% body fat and women with over 30% to 35% body fat are considered obese.[15]

TABLE 8-5

Health problems associated with excess body fat	
Health problem	**Partially attributable to:**
Surgical risk	Increased anesthesia needs and greater risk of wound infections
Pulmonary disease and sleep disorders	Excess weight over lungs and pharynx
Adult-onset diabetes (non–insulin-dependent diabetes mellitus)	Enlarged fat cells, which poorly bind insulin and also poorly respond to the message insulin sends to the cell
Hypertension and stroke	Increased miles of blood vessels found in the fat tissue; increased blood volume; increased resistance to blood flow
Coronary heart disease	Increases in blood cholesterol (LDL) and triglyceride values, low HDL values, decreased physical activity
Bone and joint disorders	Excess pressure put on knee, ankle, and hip joints
Gallbladder stones	Increased cholesterol content of bile
Skin disorders	Trapping of moisture and microbes in fat folds
Various cancers	Estrogen production by adipose cells; animal studies suggest excess energy intake encourages tumor development
Shorter stature (in some forms of obesity)	Earlier onset of puberty
Pregnancy risks	More difficult delivery and increased needs for anesthesia (if the latter is needed)
Reduced physical agility and increased risk of accidents and falls	Excess weight impairs movement
Premature death	A variety of risk factors for disease, listed above

The greater the degree of obesity, the more likely and the more serious these health problems generally become. They are much more likely to appear in people who show an android fat distribution pattern and/or greater than twice desirable body weight (see later chapter discussions).

Desirable amounts are 12% to 18% body fat for men and 20% to 25% fat for women.[32] Women need more body fat because some "sex-specific" fat is associated with their reproductive functions. This fat is normal and therefore is factored into calculations of body composition (Figure 8-8).

UNDERWATER WEIGHING

A variety of methods can be used to estimate how much body fat a person has. The most accurate method of estimating total body fat is **underwater weighing** (Figure 8-9).[32] Comparing a person's weight on a standard scale to his or her weight underwater can yield a very accurate estimate of total body fat. This works on the principle that adipose tissue is less dense than lean tissue, and so the more adipose tissue in a body, the less a person weighs when submerged (the more he or she tends to float). Unfortunately, this method requires expensive equipment that is not widely available.

SKINFOLD THICKNESS

The most widely used method to estimate total body fat is to measure skinfold thickness. Over half of the body lies directly under the skin. Clinicians use a special caliper to measure this fat layer. The amount of fat under the skin (subcutaneous) reflects the fat composition of the body.[32] More accurate results are obtained using three or four skinfold measurements taken throughout the body (Figure 8-10). With practice, these measurements take less than 10 minutes, and the total body fat values calculated are quite accurate. Very obese people are hard to measure, however, due to the size of the skinfolds.

BIOELECTRICAL IMPEDANCE

Clinicians can also estimate total body fat using **bioelectrical impedance,** a technique that uses a low-energy electrical current (Figure 8-11).[13] Researchers surmise that fat resists the flow of electricity because it contains little water and few electrolytes, such as potassium. Lean tissue, in comparison, is about 73% water and is rich in electrolytes. Thus the more fat a person has per inch of height, the more re-

underwater weighing A method of estimating total body fat by weighing the individual on a standard scale and then weighing him or her again submerged in water. The difference between the two weights is used to estimate total body fat.

bioelectrical impedance A method used to estimate total body fat by measuring the impedance (resistance) in a low-energy electrical current passed through the body; the more fat storage a person has, the more impedance to electrical flow is exhibited.

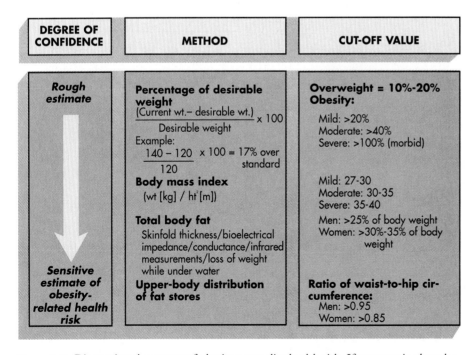

Figure 8-8 Diagnosing the extent of obesity to predict health risk. If a person is obese by any of these measures and has android distribution of fat stores, the risk of complications is greater than if the fat distribution were gynecoid.

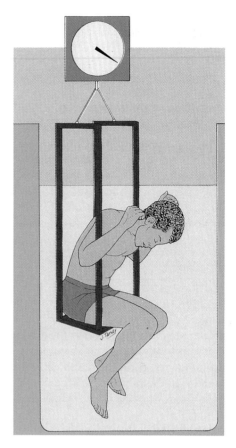

Figure 8-9 Underwater weighing. To get an accurate estimate of body fat, the subject exhales as much air as possible and then holds his breath and bends over at the waist. Once he is totally submerged, the underwater weight is recorded.

Figure 8-10 Skinfold measurements. Using proper technique, calibrated equipment, and standards, skinfold measurements can be used to accurately estimate total body fat content in about 20 minutes. Commonly measured skinfolds are **A,** subscapular, **B,** thigh, **C,** suprailiac, and **D,** triceps.

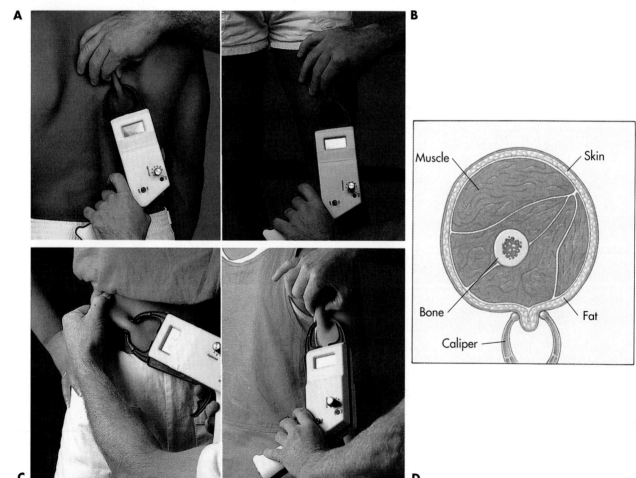

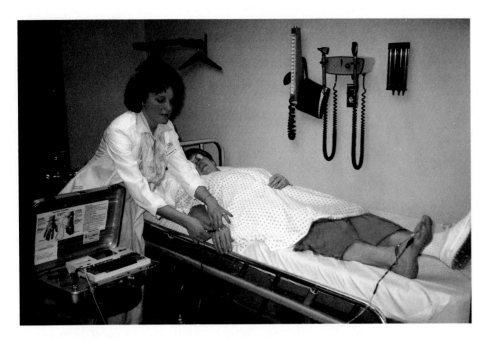

Figure 8-11 Bioelectrical impedance. This method can estimate total body fat in less than 5 minutes and is based on the principle that fat in the body resists the flow of applied low-energy electricity. The degree of resistance to the flow of electricity per increment of body height is used to estimate body fatness.

sistance. So although it is still unclear what aspect of body physiology bioelectrical impedance analyzers are actually measuring, they do provide a rapid and fairly accurate estimate of the percentage of the body that is fat.

TOTAL BODY ELECTRICAL CONDUCTIVITY (TOBEC)

The fat-rich and more lean components of the body also have different electrical properties. The TOBEC method uses this principle to estimate body composition and is based on the change measured in electrical conductivity when a person is placed in an electromagnetic field. Subjects lie face up on a platform, which is slowly rolled into the TOBEC instrument. The instrument then induces an electrical current in the person, and resulting changes in electrical conductivity are measured. The actual changes arise from differences in electrolyte concentration in lean versus fat tissue. While the TOBEC procedure is fast and safe, the equipment is very expensive. In addition, there is currently rather limited information regarding the use of this instrument in various population groups.

INFRARED REACTANCE

Still another method for estimating total body fat uses infrared light interactions with the fat and protein in arm muscle. A device the size of a flashlight is held on the biceps muscle. Total body fat is then estimated after a few seconds of infrared exposure.

DUAL-ENERGY X-RAY ABSORPTIOMETRY

For dual-energy x-ray absorptiometry the subject lies on a table while two different x-ray energies are passed above the body by a scanning arm. The pattern produced as these x-rays pass through the body indicates which parts of the body are fat, bone, or lean. Then two mathematical equations are used to calculate tissue mass and bone mass.[22] Tissue mass is further divided into fat mass and nonfat mass. This method is easier on the subject than underwater weighing, but it has disadvantages, including the size of the scanning table, which may exclude people who are very tall. In addition, substantial body thickness may affect the precision of the measurement.

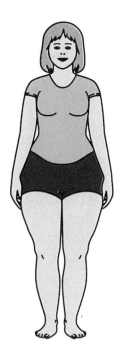

Lower-body obesity
(gynecoid obesity)

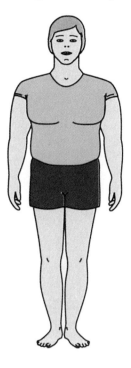

Upper-body obesity
(android obesity)

Figure 8-12 Body fat distribution, showing gynecoid and android obesity. The android form brings higher risks for ill health associated with obesity.

BODY FAT DISTRIBUTION ALSO DESERVES CONSIDERATION

Calculating distribution of fat stores, in addition to the amount of fat, is also instrumental in predicting health risks from obesity (see Figure 8-8). Obese people can be categorized as **android** or **gynecoid** (sometimes called *gynoid*) (Figure 8-12). Android obesity is the characteristic male obesity, with a large abdomen (pot belly) and small buttocks and thighs ("apple" appearance).[15] High blood testosterone and cortisol concentrations, as well as increased sympathetic nervous system activity and alcohol intake, are thought to encourage central body fat deposition.

Gynecoid obesity is the typical female obesity pattern, showing a moderate abdomen and much larger buttocks and thighs ("pear" appearance). Low blood cortisol and high estrogen concentrations relative to testosterone encourage this type of development. After menopause blood estrogen falls and android fat distribution is favored.

The cells in the gynecoid area contain more lipoprotein lipase, the enzyme that enables fat from the bloodstream to enter adipose cells. Furthermore, progesterone, a female hormone, increases the action of lipoprotein lipase in the lower torso region. Overall, there are biological reasons why men tend toward android fat distribution and women tend toward gynecoid fat distribution.

A ratio of waist circumference (at the level of the umbilicus with stomach relaxed) to maximum hip circumference greater than 0.95 in men and 0.85 in women indicates an android shape. The cut-off values are based on studies of Caucasians. Researchers note that more study of minorities is needed to verify use in those populations.[8] Android obesity is associated with more heart disease, hypertension, and diabetes than in the gynecoid form.[15] This may be because adipose tissue in the abdominal area is more likely to resist the action of insulin, increasing the risk of diabetes. The development of diabetes leads to an increased risk for heart disease and hypertension. In addition, fats released from the abdomen appear rapidly in the liver, interfering with the liver's ability to clear fat from the bloodstream. This can lead to further insulin resistance.

Overall, researchers suggest that women with gynecoid fat distribution must be about 20 pounds more obese than men with an android shape to show the same health risks. Only a small percentage of women have android obesity.

Using Height-Weight Tables to Define Obesity

BMI is the simplest height-weight method to define obesity. Figure 8-7 shows that health risks from obesity begin when body mass index exceeds 25.[15] A body mass index above 30 poses an even greater risk for health problems. Thus a value of 27 to 30 is often used as the cut-off for obesity. A body mass index above 40 represents quite a high risk for health problems.

A practical approach to using BMI is to consider a value between 25 and 30 of minor concern if health problems are not present and fat distribution is not in an android pattern. A value greater than 30 is cause for concern, and further medical evaluation should be sought.

Obesity is more crudely defined as body weight 20% higher than desirable body weight based on height-weight tables, such as the Metropolitan Life Insurance Table. Overweight is body weight between 10% and 20% more than the standard. To further define obesity, body weight 20% to 40% more than desirable body weight represents mild obesity, body weight 41% to 99% more than desirable body weight represents moderate obesity, and body weight more than twice desirable body weight represents severe (morbid) obesity. In the United States, about 90% of obese people are mildly obese. This condition carries little health risk. About 0.2% of cases are severe, which carries a twelvefold increase in health risk.

TABLE 8-6

Types of obesity	
Juvenile-onset:	Hyperplastic—increased fat cell number
	Hypertrophic—larger fat cells
Adult-onset:	Mainly hypertrophic
	About 80% to 90% of obesity is adult-onset
Endocrine-related:	Hypothyroidism, hypercorticoidism, brain tumors, Prader-Willi syndrome, Turner's syndrome, and other

Using Age of Onset in the Diagnosis of Obesity

Obesity can be classified as juvenile-onset, adult-onset, or endocrine-onset (Table 8-6). The latter includes obesity caused by relatively rare hormonal abnormalities and even rarer genetic disorders.

When obesity develops in infancy or childhood (especially during puberty), more adipose cells are developed, and each adipose cell grows to a large size. When obesity develops in adulthood, a normal number of adipose cells are usually present, but each cell contains a large amount of fat. Adipose tissue consisting of a large number of cells shows **hyperplasia.** Adipose tissue consisting of large cells shows **hypertrophy.** Juvenile-onset obesity tends to be both hyperplastic and hypertrophic. Adult-onset obesity is mainly hypertrophic, but in cases of extreme obesity it can be both hyperplastic and hypertrophic.

There is concern that in cases of juvenile-onset obesity it is more difficult to lose weight and keep it off than in adult-onset obesity. It is thought that the increased number of fat cells accompanying juvenile-onset obesity may increase the body's resistance to reducing fat stores. It is clear that the more longstanding the obesity, the more difficult it is to correct the problem.

hyperplasia An increase in cell number.

hypertrophy An increase in cell size.

The Individual Path to Obesity

Many paths lead to obesity, and each obese person has unique characteristics and problems. The clinician must tailor a treatment plan to deal with these different problems. Some characteristics of obese people that help clinicians understand more about a particular client, other than body fat content, body weight-for-height measures, body fat distribution, and age of onset include:

- Family history of obesity
- Current energy expenditure
- Blood glucose concentration
- Erroneous nutrition beliefs

The variety in this list illustrates the many possible factors associated with an individual case of obesity.[15]

Obesity is a very personal disorder. From our previous discussion, you can imagine that dysfunctions of the hunger-related (internal) or appetite-related (external) forces that affect satiety may promote overeating. Lower-than-normal energy expenditure can result from impairment of one or a combination of the four contributors to energy use. Therefore the reasons for obesity in an individual can be complex. Multiple causes make obesity a very heterogeneous disorder. As we discuss in Chapter 9, that is why individualized treatment is necessary.

CONCEPT CHECK

Obesity refers to excessive body fat storage. Obesity is defined as a body fat percentage greater than 25% in men and 30% to 35% in women. Fat storage distribution further defines an obese state as android or gynecoid. The actual amount of body fat storage can be estimated using techniques including skinfold thickness or bioelectric impedance. In a clinical setting obesity usually corresponds to a body mass index over 27 to 30 (calculated as weight in kilograms divided by height in meters squared) or body weight 20% over desirable body weight as listed in the current Metropolitan Life Insurance Table. However, if a healthy lifestyle is being followed and there are no current health problems, strict interpretation of these guidelines needs to be reevaluated. Obesity is associated with an increased risk for heart disease, some types of cancer, hypertension, adult-onset diabetes, bone and joint disorders, gallbladder stones, and some sleep disorders. The risks for some of these diseases are especially high if the fat storage is in an android distribution.

Energy Use in Obesity

Does energy use differ in obese and desirable weight individuals? Is there something inherent in an obese person that causes more efficient energy use than in a leaner person? For some obese people these answers are probably "yes." Some laboratory and farm animals more efficiently turn food energy into fat storage. Farmers once selected cows and hogs based on their abilities to acquire fat. Today we know that eating too much animal fat increases the risk for heart disease in some people, so farmers now select animals that produce more lean and less fat tissue (see Chapter 4).

We humans are not so fortunate. Our parents did not choose each other based on genetic counseling. Some of us probably inherited a tendency for leanness, while others inherited a tendency for obesity. There is no way to determine which tendency you inherited without extensive testing of your resting and total energy needs. However, a person who is constantly struggling to maintain body weight probably has some genetic component to the weight problem.[4]

Some families tend toward low basal metabolic rates, when expressed on a body weight basis. The families with lower basal metabolic rates also show higher rates for obesity. Even after adjusting for the amount of fat a person has, research shows that basal metabolic rate can vary as much as 30% between leaner and more obese families.

Unfortunately, at this time nothing can be done to change this genetic background. Nevertheless, we should all keep in mind that genetic differences do exist, which can create a greater struggle for body weight regulation for some people than for others.

DIFFERENCES IN BASAL METABOLISM

Basal metabolism tends to be higher in obese people when based on energy expended per day because their extra fat stores require the addition of extra lean tissue, such as connective tissue, for support. The more lean tissue present, the higher the total basal metabolism. Basal metabolism of an obese person appears to be lower if expressed as energy expenditure per unit of body weight, because adipose tissue shows low metabolic activity. However, when comparing two people, the obese person has a higher total basal metabolism.[32] Still, it doesn't take much more energy to maintain an obese state, just as energy intake per day does not need to be very excessive to cause obesity (as we discuss in the Nutrition Perspective).

THERMIC EFFECT OF FOOD IN OBESITY

Thermic effect of food (seen in response to a meal) is lower in some obese people than in those at leaner weights.[12] This is partially caused by insulin resistance of adipose cells, a characteristic often present with obesity.[30] Thus the thermic effect of eating carbohydrate is decreased in some obese people because insulin action is insufficient to promote normal carbohydrate metabolism.

ENERGY USED IN PHYSICAL ACTIVITY

Obese people use more energy when performing physical activity than do lean people because their extra body weight requires more energy to perform muscular activity. Nevertheless, many obese people expend less total energy in physical activity because they are less active. Obese teenagers in studies avoid vigorous activity when they play tennis. Obese adults in studies perform weight-bearing exercises, such as walking, less vigorously. Recent studies show an association between hours of television watching and obesity in children, adolescents, and adults. Long hours of watching television promote a very sedentary lifestyle. A key component in treating or preventing obesity is performing regular physical activity.[9]

DEFICITS IN ADAPTIVE THERMOGENESIS

Some obese adults may have deficits in heat production in response to stimuli such as overfeeding.[12] This could be caused by less sympathetic nervous system activity or deficiencies in brown adipose tissue metabolism.[5] Several medications are being examined with the intent of increasing adaptive thermogenesis in obese people.

Why Obesity Develops—Nature versus Nurture

In the broadest sense, obesity is a disorder of energy balance. Both genetic traits and psychological influences affect this balance and thus increase the risk for obesity. These two very different types of influences give rise to a "nature versus nurture" question concerning causes of obesity. To date, we simply do not know why one third of the public is susceptible to an abundance of delicious foods and the opportunity to be sedentary, with the result that they eventually become obese.

HOW INFLUENTIAL IS NATURE IN CONTRIBUTING TO OBESITY?

Identical twins raised apart tend to have similar weight gain patterns and deposit fat in the same body pattern (android versus gynecoid). If one twin is obese, the other is usually obese. This research suggests that as much as 80% of obesity is linked to genetics.[4] Being raised apart reduces the effect of nurture, what a person learns about eating habits and nutrition.

It is reasonable to assume that some people inherit a **"thrifty" metabolism.** This is not likely due to a single gene, but to the influences of multiple genes. Genetically obese mice and rats are good examples of animal species destined to become obese (Figure 8-13). Both species overeat and are much more efficient than the normal animal at turning energy intake into fat storage. As we mentioned earlier, one gene likely to promote the overeating has recently been isolated from mice. It is thought that the gene product leptin travels from the adipose tissue to the brain to signal less feeding when adipose tissue stores are ample. However, obese mice have a defective copy of this gene and thus produce a gene product that does not reduce feeding when adipose tissue stores are ample.[17] We also mentioned that there is interest in using leptin as an antiobesity medicine in humans, but it will take many more years of research to determine whether it is safe and effective for human use.

Genetically obese rats and mice even make fat at the expense of synthesizing muscle tissue when food intake is restricted, which indicates how genetically prone they are to fat deposition and eventual obesity. Part of this tendency is reversible if blood cortisol concentration is reduced by removal of the adrenal glands, indicating a hormonal link to this obesity as well, as we mentioned earlier.[5] Certain tribes of Native Americans also show a greater tendency to develop obesity. Researchers surmise that many of these individuals exhibit limited ability to use fat for energy needs, partly linked to altered hormone receptors on adipose cells. Fat intake is mostly stored in adipose tissue instead of being used.

"thrifty" metabolism A metabolism that characteristically conserves more energy than normal, enhancing the risk of weight gain and obesity.

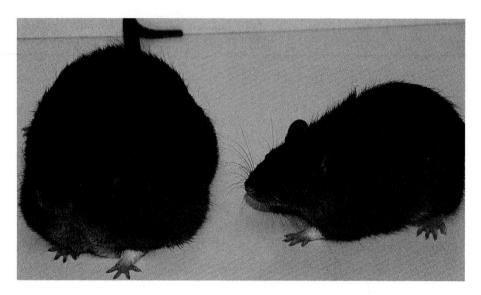

Figure 8-13 A rat with genetic obesity. No matter what type of diet the animal on the left eats, it makes more fat than the normal rat on the right. Genetics can have a powerful effect on the body composition of animals.

A very thrifty metabolism requires less energy for body maintenance and physical activity. In earlier times, when food supplies were scarce, a thrifty metabolism was a great advantage. Today, with a wide variety of energy-dense food so readily available, a thrify metabolism requires high physical activity and wise food choices to balance energy intake with output.[9]

If you feel you have a thrifty metabolism, chances are that you inherited aspects of that characteristic. A child with no obese parent has only a 10% chance of becoming obese. With one obese parent, the child has about a 40% chance of becoming obese. A child who has two obese parents has about an 80% chance of becoming obese.

It can be argued that these probabilities are due to the way a child is raised. Fraternal twins show less variation in weight than two unrelated people. This supports the theory promoting the effects of environment, while the close association of body weights between identical twins supports the theory promoting a genetic explanation. Overall, it is complicated to separate nature influences from nurture influences when searching for the causes of obesity.

DOES NURTURE HAVE A ROLE?

As we just discussed, nurture, how a person is raised, can also strongly influence obesity. Family members often have similar eating habits, make similar food choices, and have similar degrees of fatness. They may find solace in being part of a "clan." This is true even for husbands and wives, two people who have no genetic commonality. So the environment in which a person is raised or currently lives can influence food habits and fatness.

Obesity is related to socioeconomic status in America. Men and women in lower socioeconomic groups are more likely to be obese than people in upper socioeconomic groups. Much of this has to do with the expectations people have of each other within a social class. Race similarly follows this pattern, as obesity is more common in African-Americans than Caucasians, in part linked to cultural expectations. Both patterns are especially true for women. Obesity is also more common in the Midwest than in the Northeast or West Coast states. Individuals in sedentary occupations also exhibit more obesity than those in more physically demanding occupations.

Gender also influences obesity risk. Adult obesity in women can often be tied to childhood obesity, but the same does not hold true for men. Men tend to become obese after age 30, probably as they become more financially successful and therefore more sedentary. This is probably the best evidence for a critical role of nurture in male obesity. If nature is an important reason for obesity in men, obesity should be present much earlier in life.

Early research suggested that infant feeding practices may influence a child's chance to become obese in later life. Specifically, it was thought that bottle feeding, as well as an early introduction of solid foods (before the age of 6 months), encouraged the infant to gain too much weight. This then increased the chance of becoming obese. However, many recent studies reexamining this issue show that very little relationship exists between feeding practices, or even obesity in infancy, and obesity in childhood. The exception could be the infant who gains weight very rapidly in the first 6 weeks of life. Most overweight or obese infants are of normal weight by the time they enter school. However, if a child remains obese at 5 years old or has become obese by this age, immediate attention is necessary. Obesity in childhood is highly related to obesity in adulthood, especially in females. We discuss this further in Chapter 17.

NATURE AND NURTURE TOGETHER

In summary, both nature and nurture influence the tendency for obesity (Table 8-7).[15] We can view the development of obesity as nurture allowing nature to be expressed. Some people may begin with a lower rate of energy metabolism. When these people are put into an inactive environment that is full of both energy-dense foods and social reinforcement, they are nurtured into expressing their natural ten-

CRITICAL THINKING

Sandy noticed at her 4-year-old's party that the children were all eating cookies and ice cream and barely touching the vegetables also available. Why do you think the children preferred the fatty foods?

- - - - - - - - - - -

One eminent obesity researcher has proposed that foods with a high-fat and low-nutritional-value profile be taxed to discourage consumption and thus help prevent or limit development of obesity in our population. Banning advertising of these foods directed at children was also suggested, as is currently done for alcohol and tobacco products.

- - - - - - - - - - -

TABLE 8-7

What encourages excess body fat stores?	
Factor	**How fat storage is affected**
Age	Excess body fat is more common in adults and middle-aged individuals.
Menopause	Increase in abdominal fat deposition is favored.
Gender	Females have more fat.
Insulin resistance	Often develops as obesity develops.
Positive energy balance	Especially important if over a relatively long period.
Composition of diet	High fat intake and preference for sugary, fat-rich foods are likely to contribute to obesity.
Physical activity level	Low or decreasing amount of physical activity affects energy balance and body fat stores.
Resting metabolic rate	A low value with respect to lean body mass is linked to weight gain.
Sympathetic nervous system	Low activity favors weight gain.
Thermic effect of food	Low for some obesity cases.
Use of fat for energy	Poor fat clearance from the bloodstream.
Ratio of fat to lean tissue	A high ratio of fat mass to lean body mass is correlated with weight gain.
Adipose tissue lipoprotein lipase activity	High in some obese individuals and remains high (perhaps even increases) with weight loss.
Blood cortisol value	Elevated values promote weight and fat gain.
Variety of social and behavioral factors	Obesity is associated with socioeconomic status, familial conditions, network of friends, busy lifestyles that discourage balanced meals, easy availability of inexpensive, high-fat food, such as in quick-service restaurants, pattern of leisure activities, television time, smoking habits, alcohol intake, and number of meals eaten away from home.

Continued.

TABLE 8-7—cont'd

What encourages excess body fat stores?

Factor	How fat storage is affected
Undetermined genetic characteristics	These affect energy balance, particularly via the energy expenditure components, the deposition of the energy surplus as fat or as lean tissue, and the relative proportion of fat and carbohydrate use by the body.
Race	In some races higher body weight may be more socially acceptable.
Certain medications	Food intake increases.
Childbearing	Women may not lose all weight gained in pregnancy, leading to creeping weight gain.
National region	Regional differences, such as high-fat diets and sedentary lifestyles in the Midwest, cause different rates of obesity in different places.

Modified from Bouchard C: Current understanding of the etiology of obesity: genetic and nongenetic factors, *American Journal of Clinical Nutrition* 53:1561S, 1991.

dency for obesity (Figure 8-14). This is speculation on our part, but it seems a reasonable assertion.

We feel it is important for everyone to try to determine his or her own risk for obesity and to discover what specific lifestyle factors contribute to this risk. Only then can a person make an individual plan to reduce the risk. We talk more about that plan in Chapter 9.

Keep in mind also that, although you may be fatter than you would like to be, a small amount of extra fat may pose no significant health risk, especially if in a gynecoid distribution.[15] We discussed this idea earlier. Such information may help you

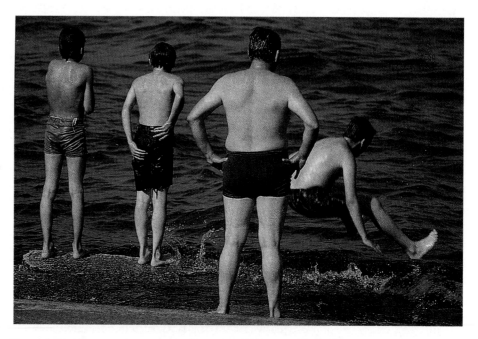

Figure 8-14 Nature versus nurture. Does the difference in body fat between the father and his three sons arise from nature, nurture, or both?

put weight loss into perspective. Knowing that weight loss is difficult and that current body weight poses no serious health threat, some people decide to just stay at their current weight and simply work to not gain any more. That alone is a positive step for some people, as the odds of a young adult (i.e., college student) gaining about 10 to 15 pounds of body fat by age 35 to 40 are high.

CONCEPT CHECK

Genetic background plays a role in the cause of obesity. Body fat distribution and degree of basal metabolism are partially inherited. Nurture is also important. Family members often have similar eating habits, similar activity habits, and similar degrees of fatness. In addition, men tend to develop obesity after age 30, and women tend to develop it throughout their childhood and adult years. Putting both factors together, we can speculate that a proper nurturing state may allow a genetic tendency for obesity to be either expressed or overcome.

Summary

1. Energy balance is energy intake minus energy output. Negative energy balance occurs when energy output is greater than energy intake, resulting in weight loss. Positive energy balance occurs when energy intake is greater than energy output. The result is weight gain.

2. Groups of cells in the hypothalamus and other regions in the brain affect hunger, the primarily physiological desire to find and eat food. These cells may monitor nutrients and other substances in the blood and read low amounts as a signal to promote feeding.

3. A variety of internal (hunger-related) and external (appetite-related) forces affect satiety. Hunger cues combine with appetite cues, such as easy availability of food, to promote feeding.

4. In America, the major determinants of food intake likely are appetite-driven forces because food is so readily available. The physiological influences affecting food consumption are often suppressed or ignored.

5. Total energy use by the body is accounted for by basal metabolism, the thermic effect of food, physical activity, and adaptive thermogenesis. Basal metabolism represents the minimum energy expenditure needed to keep the resting, awake body alive. It is primarily affected by lean body mass, surface area, and thyroid hormone concentrations. The thermic effect of food represents the increase in metabolism to facilitate the digesting, absorbing, and processing of nutrients recently consumed. Physical activity represents energy use that is not related to the other two categories. Adaptive thermogenesis is heat production caused by overfeeding or a cold environment. Brown adipose tissue may be the active heat-producing tissue in adaptive thermogenesis. About 70% to 80% of energy use is accounted

for by basal metabolism and the thermic effect of food in a primarily sedentary person.

6. Energy use by the body can be measured directly from heat output or indirectly by measuring oxygen uptake and/or carbon dioxide output. Energy use by the body can be estimated using formulas based on various combinations of body weight with height, lean body mass, age, and frame size.

7. A person of desirable weight shows good health and performs daily activities without weight-related problems. A body mass index (weight [in kg] ÷ height^2 [in m]) of 20 to 25 is one measure of desirable weight, although weight in excess of this value may not lead to ill health. This suggests that desirable weight is best set in conjunction with a thorough health evaluation by a physician.

8. Obesity is usually defined as total body fat percentage over 25% in men and 30% to 35% in women. A body mass index over 27 to 30 also represents obesity. Being 20% over desirable body weight based on one of many height-weight tables is another measure of obesity.

9. Fat distribution partially determines health risks from obesity. Android fat storage distribution (waist-to-hip circumference ratio greater than 0.95 in men or greater than 0.85 in women) suggests higher risks of hypertension, heart disease, and diabetes associated with obesity than does gynecoid fat distribution.

10. Genetic factors influence the tendency to obesity. Basal metabolism and body fat distribution both have genetic links. How a person is raised (or nurtured) also influences the tendency for obesity, since family members often develop similar eating habits and activity patterns. Obesity can be viewed as nurture allowing nature to be expressed.

Study Questions

1. After reexamining the internal and external forces associated with hunger, satiety, and food intake, propose three hypotheses for the development of obesity.
2. What are two forces that affect appetite?
3. Knowing the four contributors to human energy expenditure, propose four hypotheses for the development of obesity, based on the classes of energy expenditure.
4. Discuss one advantage and one problem associated with using the 1983 Metropolitan Life Insurance Table to assess weight status.
5. Describe the way to define a desirable (healthy) weight that makes the most sense to you.
6. Describe a practical method of defining obesity in a clinical setting.
7. Describe four methods for determining body fatness. List one advantage and drawback for each.
8. What are the two most convincing pieces of evidence that both genetic and environmental factors play significant roles in the development of obesity?
9. What three health problems do obese people typically face? Describe a possible reason that each problem arises.
10. Obesity is not simply caused by lack of will-power. Justify this statement.

REFERENCES

1. Acheson KJ: Influence of autonomic nervous system on nutrient-induced thermogenesis in humans, *Nutrition* 9:373, 1993.
2. Anderson GH: Regulation of food intake. In Shils ME and others, editors: *Modern nutrition in health and disease,* Philadelphia, 1994, Lea & Febiger.
3. Blundell JE and others: Carbohydrates and human appetite, *American Journal of Clinical Nutrition* 59:728S, 1994.
4. Bourchard C, Perusse L: Genetics of obesity, *Annual Review of Nutrition* 13:337, 1993.
5. Bray GA: Appetite control in adults. In Fernstram JD, Miller GP, editors: *Appetite and body weight regulation,* Boca Raton, Fla, 1994, CRC Press.
6. Castonguay TW, Stern JS: Hunger and appetite. In Brown ML, editor: *Present knowledge in nutrition,* Washington, DC, 1990, International Life Sciences Institute.
7. Chance WT, Fischer JE: Neurotransmitters and food intake, *Nutrition* 9:470, 1993.
8. Croft JB and others: Waist-to-hip ratio in a biracial population: measurement, implications, and cautions for using guidelines to define high risk for cardiovascular disease, *Journal of the American Dietetic Association* 95:60, 1995.
9. de Groot LCPGM, van Staveren WA: Reduced physical activity and its association with obesity, *Nutrition Reviews* 53:11, 1995.
10. Flatt JP: Use and storage of carbohydrate and fat, *American Journal of Clinical Nutrition* 61:952S, 1995.
11. French SJ, Read NW: Effect of guar gum on hunger and satiety after meals of differing fat content: relationship with gastric emptying, *American Journal of Clinical Nutrition* 59:87, 1994.

12. Garrel DR, de Jonge L: Intragastric vs oral feeding: effect on the thermogenic response to feeding in lean and obese subjects, *American Journal of Clinical Nutrition* 59:971, 1994.
13. Holt TL: Clinical applicability of bioelectric impedance to measure body composition in health and disease, *Nutrition* 10:221, 1994.
14. Kuczmarski RJ and others: Increasing prevalence of overweight among US adults, *Journal of the American Medical Association* 272:205, 1994.
15. Lachance PA: Scientific status summary—human obesity, *Food Technology,* p 127, Feb 1994.
16. Leibel RL and others: Changes in energy expenditure resulting from altered body weight, *New England Journal of Medicine* 332:621, 1995.
17. Lindpainter K: Finding an obesity gene in a tale of mice and man, *New England Journal of Medicine* 332:679, 1995.
18. Manson JE and others: Parity, ponderosity, and the paradox of a weight-preoccupied society, *Journal of the American Medical Association* 271:1788, 1994.
19. Martini MC and others: Effect of the menstrual cycle on energy and nutrient intake, *American Journal of Clinical Nutrition* 60:895, 1994.
20. Mercer LP and others: Histidine, histamine and the neuroregulation of food intake, *Nutrition* 6:273, 1990.
21. Merrill AH: Apo A-IV: a new satiety signal, *Nutrition Reviews* 51:273, 1993.
22. Ogle GD and others: Body-composition assessment by dual-energy x-ray absorptiometry in subjects aged 4-26y, *American Journal of Clinical Nutrition* 61:746, 1995.

23. Owen OE: Regulation of energy and metabolism. In Kinney JM and others, editors: *Nutrition and metabolism in patient care,* Philadelphia, 1988, WB Saunders.
24. Pennisi E: Food cravings tied to brain chemicals, *Science News* 144:310, 1994.
25. Pennisi E: Gut counts calories even when we do not, *Science News* 146:359, 1994.
26. Read N and others: The role of the gut in regulating food intake in man, *Nutrition Reviews* 52:10, 1994.
27. Rolls BJ: Carbohydrates, fats, and satiety, *American Journal of Clinical Nutrition* 61:960S, 1995.
28. Shide DJ and others: Accurate energy compensation for intragastric and oral nutrients in lean males, *American Journal of Clinical Nutrition* 61:754, 1995.
29. Stricker EM, Verbalis JG: Control of appetite and satiety: insights from biologic and behavioral studies, *Nutrition Reviews* 48:49, 1990.
30. Tataranni PA and others: Thermic effect of food in humans: methods and results from use of a respiratory chamber, *American Journal of Clinical Nutrition* 61:1013, 1995.
31. Weigle DS: Appetite and the regulation of body composition, *FASEB Journal* 8:302, 1994.
32. Westerterp KR: Energy expenditure and body composition. In Westerterp-Plantenza MS and others, editors: *Food intake and energy expenditure,* Boca Raton, Fla, 1994, CRC Press.
33. Willett WC and others: Weight, weight change, and coronary heart disease in women: risk within the "normal" weight range, *Journal of the American Medical Association* 273:461, 1995.

TAKE ACTION

> ## Am I a candidate for weight loss?
> *Determine the following two indices of your body status: body mass index and waist-to-hip ratio.*

- -

BODY MASS INDEX (BMI)

Record your weight in pounds: _____ lbs.

Divide your weight in pounds by 2.2 to determine your weight in kilograms: _____ kg.

Record your height in inches: _____ in.

Divide your height in inches by 39.3 to determine your height in meters: _____ m.
Calculate your BMI using the following formula:
  $BMI = Weight (kg)/height(m)^2$

  BMI = _____ kg/ _____ m² = _____

WAIST-TO-HIP RATIO

Use a tape measure to measure the circumference of your waist (at the umbilicus with stomach muscles relaxed) and hips (widest point).

  Circumference of waist (umbilicus) = _____ in.

  Circumference of hips = _____ in.
Calculate your waist-to-hip ratio using the following formula:
  Circumference of waist/circumference of hips

  Waist to hip ratio = _____ in/ _____ in = _____

INTERPRETATION

1. When BMI is greater than 25, health risks from obesity begin. It is especially advisable to attempt weight loss if your BMI exceeds 30. Does yours exceed 25?

   Yes _____ No _____
2. When a person is greater than 20% above desirable weight, a waist-to-hip ratio exceeding 0.95 in men and 0.85 in women suggests android obesity. This is associated with an increased risk of heart disease, hypertension, and diabetes.
     If appropriate, does your ratio exceed the standard for your gender?

   Yes _____ No _____
3. Do you feel you need to pursue a program of weight loss?

   Yes _____ No _____

APPLICATION

From what you've learned in this chapter, what habits could you change in patterns of eating and physical activity to lose weight and help ensure maintenance of loss?

_____

_____

_____

Do You Have a Set Point for Body Weight?

William Bennett and Joel Gurin popularized the "set-point theory of weight maintenance" in 1982 in their book, *The Dieter's Dilemma.* This theory espouses the notion that weight is closely regulated by the body. It proposes that humans have a genetically predetermined body weight or body fat content that the body attempts to defend. Some research suggests that the hypothalamus monitors the amount of body fat in humans and tries to keep that amount constant over time.[17] This regulation of body fat content is referred to as a "set point." We have already seen in this chapter that in laboratory animals the protein called leptin may form one communication link between adipose cells and the brain that allows for some weight regulation.[17]

Analogies to the tight regulation of blood pressure and body temperature are used to support this concept. You could view the set point as a coiled spring: the further you stray from your usual weight, the harder the force acts to pull you back to that weight.

In the major studies in humans cited to support the set-point theory, volunteers who lost weight through starvation later ate in a way to gain weight back to their original state or a little higher. In addition, studies in the 1960s using prisoners with no history of obesity found it was hard for the men to gain weight, and after gaining weight, they quickly returned to their previous weight when returning to their previous habits. Also, after an illness is resolved, a person generally gains lost weight.

There also is sound physiological evidence that body weight tends to be regulated.[16] If energy intake is reduced, the blood concentration of a thyroid hormone (T_3) falls, and the metabolic rate slows. In addition, lower body weight decreases the energy cost of each future weight-bearing activity, and the total energy used by lean tissues falls because some of these tissues are also lost. Furthermore, the enzyme used by adipose and muscle cells to take up fat from the bloodstream (lipoprotein lipase) often increases its activity. Through these changes the body resists further weight loss.

If a person overeats, in the short run the metabolic rate tends to increase.[16] This causes some resistance to further weight gain. People often recognize the body's resistance to weight loss when dieting but do not think much about the resistance to weight gain after eating a big holiday meal. However, in the long run resistance to weight gain is much less than resistance to weight loss. When a person gains weight and stays at that weight for a while, the body tends to defend the new weight.

Let's explore set-point regulation of weight in concrete terms. The amount we eat varies from day to day. Daily energy intake varies from about 20% (about 400 kcal) below to 20% above a person's 28-day average energy intake. In comparison, even as little as a 2% (40 kcal) over-consumption of energy per day, if continued for 20 years, could result in an over 100-pound gain in fat stores. This significant effect from such a small variation points out how easy it is to follow the road to obesity. However, the average weight gain between the ages of 18 and 54 is only 15 to 20 pounds. It appears that some powerful forces encourage a balance of overeating with undereating.[16] Thus, over time, daily energy imbalances cancel each other, with high energy intake days balancing low energy intake days. Considering that over a 35-year period an adult eats about 35 tons of food (yielding 30 million kcal), the ability to regulate weight, though imperfect, is still quite impressive.[32]

Arguments against the set-point theory cite the fact that during pregnancy women slowly increase body weight and fat with little fight to maintain this trend. Also, an average person's weight does not remain constant throughout adulthood; it usually increases slowly, at least until old age. This means that a person must be able to shift his or her set point. It is also argued that if an individual is placed in a different social, emotional, or physical environment, weight can become markedly higher or lower and is maintained. These arguments suggest that humans, rather than having a set point determined by genetics or number of adipose cells, actually settle into a particular stable weight based on an interaction between nature and nurture influences.

Other researchers argue that the concept of a set point can actually undermine therapy for those who are obese. The idea that the body strongly resists the maintenance of weight

A pound of adipose tissue gained or lost represents about 2700 kcal. The fat itself in the adipose tissue represents 3500 kcal per pound. But as fat storage is lost or gained, so is lean support tissue. This lean tissue has a much lower energy value, and thus the net energy transfer for a pound of fat tissue is closer to 2700 kcal.[23] Use this 2700 figure to calculate the various numbers listed in this section relating energy intake to fat gain or loss.

loss can be discouraging and depressing. Obese individuals may fall victim to a self-fulfilling prophecy. A person may believe that maintenance will be so difficult or impossible that he or she may give up at the slightest lapse or weight gain.

In the final analysis, we must bear much of the responsibility for weight maintenance ourselves. The odds are against the likelihood that, even with a set point helping us, we can avoid creeping weight gain in adulthood without great attention to this tendency. Ideally this includes following a diet both moderate in fat and ample in complex carbohydrates and dietary fiber and a lifestyle rich in opportunities for physical activity.

CHAPTER NINE

Weight Control

D ieting is an American pastime. At any given time, about 25% of men and 50% of women are trying to lose weight—not to mention up to 70% of teenage girls. Still, the number of obese people in America remains disturbing.[13] Each new diet is promoted as the "diet of the century" or the "diet to end all diets." However, most diets fizzle; they are usually ineffective and monotonous and, worse, can be dangerous if followed for a long period or by the wrong people—especially by pregnant women, young children, and teenagers.

Fad diet books use come-ons like "easy to follow, fast, and effective" and perhaps even describe the diet as "a scientific breakthrough previously available only in Europe." The descriptions sound terrific, almost too good to be true, which for the most part they are. The word *fad* is a shortened version of *fiddle-faddle,* which means "to play with and then cast aside."

This chapter leads you through the issue of weight control. After reading it, you will know when diet books are truthful and when they are deceptive. And if these diets do not promote lifestyle overhaul—moderating fat intake, maximizing intake of nutrient-dense foods, and performing regular physical activity—deception is a distinct possibility.[2]

NUTRITION AWARENESS INVENTORY

1. **T F** Increasing physical activity is more important than eating less in losing weight.
2. **T F** Scientists understand little about the psychology of weight regain after weight loss.
3. **T F** Weight-loss diets should contain at least 1000 kcal/day.
4. **T F** Success rates of weight-loss programs are reasonably good.
5. **T F** Rapid weight loss likely means loss of considerable muscle tissue.
6. **T F** A weight-loss program should include close examination of current eating behavior.
7. **T F** A weight-loss program should discourage the consumption of meat right after consumption of milk products.
8. **T F** The best foods to emphasize for weight loss are high-carbohydrate foods.
9. **T F** Eating a low-fat diet for weight control is impractical.
10. **T F** Changing habits is the single most important factor in maintaining weight loss.
11. **T F** *Stimulus control* refers to controlling factors that encourage eating.
12. **T F** You can lose 1 pound of stored fat each week by expending at least 200 kcal/day beyond your normal energy output.
13. **T F** Most weight-loss attempts are followed by equivalent weight regain within a few years.
14. **T F** A 25-minute brisk walk uses about 100 kcal.
15. **T F** Severe (morbid) obesity is defined as 100 pounds over desirable weight.

Treatment of Obesity

Obesity, storage of excess body fat, should be considered similarly to any chronic disease. Treatment of this disease requires long-term lifestyle changes, rather than simply taking medicine for 2 weeks, as for a sore throat, or following some quick fix promoted by a fad diet book.[7] Chronic diseases such as high blood pressure and diabetes require lifelong dietary management and ample physical activity in addition to medical care. Let's explore why obesity must be regarded and treated in the same way.

NATIONAL GOALS FOR TREATMENT OF OBESITY

Health Objectives for the year 2000, issued by the U.S. Public Health Service, include some directed at obesity. Three specific actions are indicated:
1. Teach 90% of all adults that increasing physical activity while decreasing energy intake is the best way to lose weight.
2. Have 90% of the adults already at desirable body weight remain that way.
3. Motivate 90% of overweight Americans to adopt a plan to reduce energy intake and increase physical activity, ultimately attaining and then maintaining desirable weight.

Improving the health of Americans, and others in most of the Western World, hinges on both reducing the **prevalence** of obesity and encouraging healthy weight-loss programs. Even a small amount of weight loss often can improve health status, even though the obesity itself is not corrected. This would provide a healthier life for many people.[13]

prevalence The number of people at any one time who have a specific disease, such as obesity or cancer.

SOME BASIC PREMISES

As we begin our look at current treatment options for obesity, we first must focus on five important principles concerning weight loss in general for adults (see Chapter 17 for weight-loss suggestions for children).

Much of the Current Mania Surrounding Dieting Is Misdirected

People on diets often fall within a BMI of 20 to 25, the height-weight standard experts term a desirable (healthy) body weight. These individuals should instead be focusing on a healthy lifestyle that allows for weight maintenance, and not primarily on weight loss. Lifestyle change rather than dieting is the recommendation; we discussed one such approach in the Nutrition Focus in Chapter 2. Issues such as food choice, physical activity, and various psychological and social problems germane to weight control will be reviewed in this chapter.

Actually this dieting mania can be viewed as mostly a societal problem, stemming from unrealistic weight expectations (especially for women), lack of appreciation for the natural variety in body shape and weight, ready availability of energy-dense foods, and encouragement of a spectator mentality. Not every woman can be size 10, nor can every man look like a Greek god, but all of us can strive for good health and, if physically possible, an active lifestyle.

The Body Defends Itself against Weight Loss

Thyroid hormone concentrations, and consequently basal metabolism, drop during weight loss.[14] This fall in metabolic rate is also a consequence of weight loss, caused by loss of metabolizing tissue. Declines in basal metabolism average 8% to 22% in some studies.[16] This drop makes it difficult to lose weight. Table 9-1 gives some ideas to help reduce the decline.

In addition, the activity of the enzyme lipoprotein lipase increases after weight loss.[5] This enzyme is responsible for breaking down triglyceride from lipoproteins into free fatty acids and glycerol so the lipid can enter cells (see Chapter 4). So after dieting, the body more efficiently takes up fat from the bloodstream for storage. Often fat use for energy needs also remains depressed in people who have recently lost weight.[8] This is a good reason to stay on a low-fat diet for weight maintenance. Insulin action on fat cells also improves with weight loss, which reduces fat release by adipose cells.

Weight Cycling Is a Common Phenomenon

Only about 5% of people who follow commercial diet programs actually lose weight and then remain close to that weight. Typically, one third of the weight lost during dieting is regained within 1 year of the end of dietary restriction, and almost all weight lost is regained within 3 to 5 years. Some programs have slightly higher success rates than 5%, as do some people who simply lose weight on their own without

CRITICAL THINKING

Hal has been dieting to lose weight for 2½ months. However, like many dieters, he has reached a plateau. Although he continues to restrict his kilocalorie intake, he's no longer losing weight. How would you explain to Hal the physical factors that fight weight loss?

TABLE 9-1

Practices that can stimulate metabolism

- Perform physical activity regularly throughout the day. Find opportunities for increasing activity, such as quick walks, stair climbing, or calisthenics (sit-ups, push-ups, etc.).
- Fidget when sitting and standing.
- Eat breakfast, so food intake is spread throughout the day. Each time food is consumed metabolism increases.
- Follow a carbohydrate-rich diet; much of this is further processed by the liver, which uses energy.
- Avoid "crash" dieting. Slow weight loss is a better idea because it leads to a smaller decline in metabolism during a diet.

enrolling in any supervised plan. But overall the statistics are grim. Dieting often results in eventual weight regain.[21] The weight gained includes not only the weight that was lost, but often additional weight as well, causing a person to be worse off than prior to the diet.

Furthermore, the weight gained may consist primarily of adipose tissue, while the weight that was lost consisted more of a mix of adipose and lean tissue. Therefore, the long-term effect is not only an increase in total weight, but also an increase in percentage of body fat.

This gain and lose predicament is referred to as *weight cycling* or yo-yo dieting. There are additional negative health consequences associated with weight cycling, such as an increased risk for abdominal fat deposition and profound discouragement and erosion of self-esteem. Nevertheless, experts still encourage obese people to attempt weight loss, with a strong focus on maintaining that lower weight. It is important to avoid the trap of today's crash diet leading to next month's weight gain.[21] A weight-loss program should be considered successful only when its subjects remain at or close to their lower weights.[13]

Overall, current treatments for obesity are deceptively simple, but usually unsuccessful in the long term. We are groping in the dark with regard to obesity treatment.[12] Keep in mind that (1) no single approach to weight loss is suitable for everyone; (2) the more knowledge a person has about weight loss interventions the better; and (3) we are still a long way from knowing which individuals benefit most from specific approaches.

Weight Gain in Adulthood Is All Too Common

From ages 25 to 44, danger of weight gain exists, especially for women.[13] Particular prudence should be practiced in these decades, although childhood and adolescent years also deserve attention. Rapid weight gainers should closely monitor food intake and activity level in an attempt to discover the causes, and in turn moderate the increases or reverse the trend in appropriate ways. Later we show how to do this.

Changes in Body Composition Deserve a Primary Focus in Weight Loss

Weight should be lost mostly from fat stores, not from muscle and other lean tissues. Rapid weight loss at the start of a diet program often represents fluid lost due to decreased salt intake, and loss of glycogen from the liver and muscles. Much muscle tissue may be lost as well, and this is mostly (about 73%) water. People are fooled when they weigh themselves after starting a fad diet. They lose weight, but very little of it represents fat loss. Any loss of lean tissue means a decrease in basal metabolism and thus a decrease in overall energy expenditure.[16]

All this makes clear that preventing obesity should be emphasized, as curing the disorder is very difficult.[2] Only the very motivated should try to lose weight, and ideally this attempt should be preceded by a period of weight maintenance in order to begin the process of balancing energy intake with a degree of energy output that can be maintained. Nutrition experts strongly endorse this point and note, as we said at the outset, that many people would be healthier if they simply focused on improving food habits, minimizing signs and symptoms of any weight-related chronic disease present (such as high blood pressure), and increasing physical activity, rather than remaining focused on a particular body weight and shape. This is partly because obtaining and maintaining a substantially lower body weight is so difficult.

Weight loss and subsequent maintenance of a lower weight are possible. Many of us know people who have done so, but it takes great motivation. This chapter provides the tools for weight maintenance and loss. The missing ingredient is the motivation and the supportive environment needed to put these tools to use for a lifetime. Knowledge alone is not enough, since some nutrition professionals are themselves obese. This brings us back to an earlier concept that is worth repeating—prevention of obesity is the most reliable therapy.[13]

WISHFUL SHRINKING—WHY QUICK WEIGHT LOSS CAN'T BE MOSTLY FAT

We know that rapid weight loss cannot consist mostly of fat loss because of the high energy deficit needed to lose a large amount of fat tissue. Body fat contains about 3500 kcal/pound. Fat storage, body fat tissue plus supporting tissues, contains approximately 2700 kcal/pound.[22] To lose 1 pound of fat stores per week, energy intake must be decreased by approximately 400 kcal/day (2700/7 = 386). Diets that promise 10 to 15 pounds weight loss per week cannot ensure that the weight loss is from fat stores alone. Producing an energy deficit sufficient to lose that amount of fat storage is simply not practical. What is lost rapidly is not mostly fat, but rather much lean tissue.

WHAT TO LOOK FOR IN A SOUND WEIGHT-LOSS DIET

A dieter can try to devise a plan of action or seek advice of professionals or current books. Either way, a sound weight-loss program should include three components: control of energy intake, especially fat intake; increased energy expenditure through physical activity; and acknowledgement that life-long change in habits is required, not simply a short-term weight-loss period.[13,23] Focusing on just eating less energy represents a difficult path to success, as we will show. Adding regular physical activity and an appropriate psychological component contributes to success and later maintenance of the weight loss.[23]

Specifically, any weight-loss plan should include the following characteristics:

1. The plan should meet nutritional needs, except for energy. To do that, it should follow the Food Guide Pyramid, emphasizing low-fat choices. Overall, eating should remain a satisfying and pleasurable experience.

2. Slow and steady weight loss, rather than rapid weight loss, should be stressed. A loss of 1 to 2 pounds of fat storage per week is desirable. Once about 10% of excess weight is lost, maintenance of that loss for 6 months or so is desirable before more weight loss is attempted. That may seem like a disappointing prescription, but a more radical approach to weight loss is likely to produce a yo-yo episode. Then careful evaluation should be made as to whether further weight loss is needed, based on current health state.

3. The plan should allow adaptations to individual habits and tastes. The same plan does not work for everyone.

4. The plan should minimize hunger and fatigue. To do this, it should contain at least 1200 to 1500 kcal/day. Otherwise, consuming sufficient vitamins and minerals, especially enough iron for young women, is difficult. In reality, however, 1000 kcal/day is generally regarded as the minimum energy intake since many dieters perform so little physical activity and so need very restricted energy allowances. If the eating plan calls for an energy intake below 1200 to 1500 kcal/day, it should recommend use of either fortified foods (breakfast cereals, for example) or a balanced vitamin and mineral supplement (see Chapter 12 for advice on supplements).[4]

5. The plan should contain common foods. There is no magical food that can speed weight loss. If a diet suggests that there is, whether ginseng, tofu, or garlic, advice should be sought elsewhere. Furthermore, if special foods were required, it would be difficult to maintain this practice indefinitely.

6. The plan should fit into any social situation. The healthier lifestyle should allow attendance at parties, eating at restaurants, and participation in normal daily activities.

7. The plan should help change problem eating habits. It should promote reshaping food habits and lifestyle to make weight loss, and then weight maintenance, possible, and so thwart weight regain. Maintenance should be a key concern of any plan—the plan must have a lifetime focus.[7] For example, a 150-pound person should reduce energy intake, increase physical activity, and start eating like a 130-pound person to become a 130-pound person. But once the weight is lost, the person can't go back to the habits of his or her 150-pound self. The program

CRITICAL THINKING

Jenny's been invited to be a guest speaker at a very important social at her job. Looking at her wardrobe, she realizes that she's gained 10 pounds since she wore her special black dress. Since she only has 1 week to lose the excess weight, she's going to resort to a low-carbohydrate diet. What could the consequences be if Jenny goes on this diet?

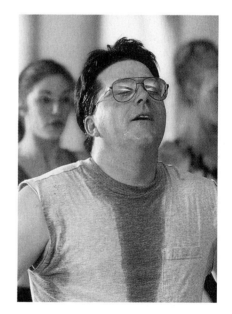

Regular physical activity is one component of a healthy weight-loss plan.

should also focus on changing obesity-promoting beliefs and rallying healthy social support.

8. The plan should improve overall health. It should emphasize proper rest, stress reduction, and other healthy changes in lifestyle. All too often people know how to diet, but they don't know how to live. They find it easier to count kilocalories and follow a plan than to deal with underlying issues that encourage eating, such as stress.[29]

9. The plan should insist that the person see a physician before starting if he or she:
   - Has existing health problems
   - Plans to lose weight as quickly as possible
   - Is over 35 years of age and plans to perform substantially increased physical activity.

Controlling Energy Intake

A goal of losing 1 to 2 pounds of stored fat per week often requires limiting energy intake to 1000 to 1600 kcal/day for women and 1600 to 2000 kcal for men, with less than 30% of energy intake coming from fat. The range for each gender arises because of the range of physical activity that may be performed. Another approach to setting energy needs is to allow 10 kcal/pound of desirable weight for sedentary people and 13 kcal/pound for active people. Then subtract 400 kcal for each pound per week of fat tissue loss desired. For example, an active 160-pound woman who should weigh 140 pounds and wants to lose 1 pound per week could start with 1820 kcal (13 × 140) and then subtract 400 kcal, which allows about 1400 kcal for her diet.

Traditionally dieters have counted kilocalories. There is a growing call to count fat grams mostly, assuming kilocalorie control follows. This makes sense as it is almost impossible to restrict energy intake forever, whereas it is easier to follow a low-fat diet indefinitely if it allows consumption of enough food to satisfy hunger. The new food labels ease the task of counting fat grams. However, as we noted in Chapter 4, many of the fat-reduced products flooding the market substitute sugar for fat in order to maintain flavor and in turn end up not much lower in kilocalories. This makes it easy to gain weight even on a low-fat diet without careful portion control of fat-reduced foods.

A better low-fat diet focuses primarily on foods that are naturally low in fat—such as fruits, vegetables, plain breads and cereals, lean cuts of meats, and nonfat dairy products—rather than foods that have been "tweaked" a bit to reduce fat content enough to satisfy food labeling regulations. This low-fat approach helps train the palate to enjoy a leaner diet and generally increases vitamin and mineral content of the diet, while reducing saturated fat and total fat intake. Some experts think that certain fat-reduced foods, like nonfat sour cream, in effect are a reminder of what is missing from the diet, driving the dieter back to the high-fat food choice. These experts believe it is better to simply not use a high-fat food product or its fat-reduced look-alike when possible, replacing it with a food choice naturally low in fat, such as nonfat yogurt for sour cream or a plain warm bagel for a doughnut.

In any case, a dieter should consume at least 1000 kcal daily; fewer than that causes so much hunger that he or she will probably not be able to stick to the plan. A better idea is to first increase physical activity, allowing at least 1000 kcal (ideally closer to 1500 kcal) to be eaten each day.

Two ways for a dieter to monitor energy intake are the exchange system and label reading (Figure 9-1). See the menu patterns listed in Table 2-9 for some possible exchange system approaches. Another method is to write down food intake throughout the day and then calculate energy intake from food tables in Appendix A in the evening, adjusting future food choices as needed.

It is common for people to inaccurately estimate portion sizes. During the first week of a weight loss program, it is best to measure food as precisely as possible. Including estimated amounts of toppings, gravies, and garnishes is important. If an

---

How many fat grams can I consume?

Energy intake	30% of energy	20% of energy
1000	33 g	22 g
1200	40 g	27 g
1500	50 g	33 g
1800	60 g	40 g
2100	70 g	47 g
2400	80 g	53 g
2700	90 g	60 g
3000	100 g	67 g
3600	120 g	80 g
3900	130 g	87 g

When following an exchange plan it is very important to consume an accurate serving. Measuring cups and a small kitchen scale are extremely useful tools in portion control.

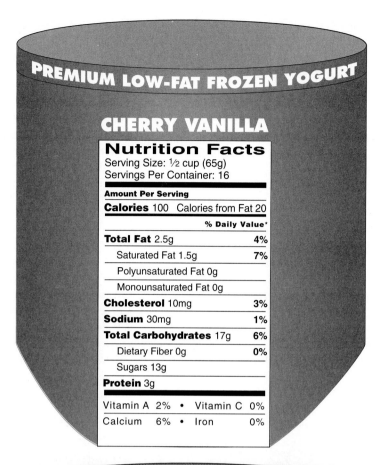

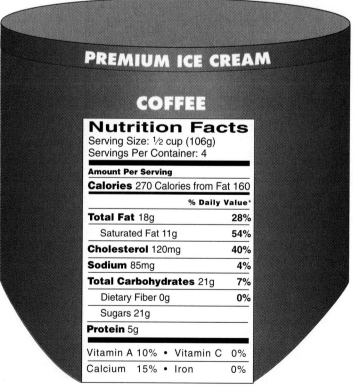

Figure 9-1 Reading labels helps you choose foods with less fat and energy. Which frozen dessert is the best choice for a person on a weight-loss diet? The % Daily Values are based on a 2000 kcal diet.

eating plan allows only 3 ounces of skinless chicken breast, it is necessary to know that a 3-ounce portion on a plate is not much bigger than a pack of playing cards or the palm of your hand. A kitchen scale may serve as well as the bathroom scale.

Minimizing fat intake is a very important goal when trying to lose body fat. Diets containing as little as 20% of energy from fat are well tolerated, especially when high in complex carbohydrates and dietary fiber. Complex carbohydrates and dietary fiber in a diet help ensure adequate satiety when less total energy intake comes from fat.[27] One study showed that when diets were reduced from energy intake from fat of 40% to 30% and then to 20%, subjects ate slightly more food on the lower-fat diet. However, the end result was that the lower-fat diet provided far less energy, allowing more weight loss even though more food was consumed.

An eating plan that contains 20% to 30% of energy as fat permits incorporation of most commonly eaten foods. The lower fat allowance, however, requires much attention to food choice at the outset. A registered dietitian can help with the early stages of implementation if needed. Still, subtle changes in food habits can aid desired weight loss (Figure 9-2). For example, simply substituting pretzels for potato chips saves 9 g of fat and 40 kcal/ounce. If 2 ounces of such snack foods are eaten every day, that one diet change saves 800 kcal and 180 g of fat every 10 days. For another example, rather than grabbing two cookies a person could choose two apples. Besides the obvious nutritional benefit of added vitamins, minerals, dietary

Keeping low-fat snack foods close at hand, especially during peak snacking periods, is a good idea. Fruit nearby may prevent snacking on fat-laden foods. Although it is desirable to have the willpower to refuse high-fat foods, most people find it is best simply to avoid the temptation.

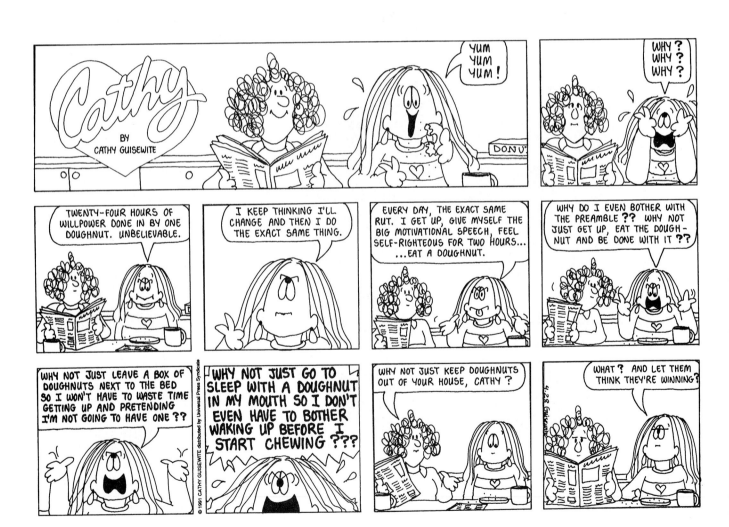

Figure 9-2 Cathy.

fiber, and 7 fewer grams of fat, the apples are more satiating and take longer to eat. It is also harder to overeat fruit than cookies. Table 9-2 offers more examples of healthy food substitutes. Recall that carbohydrates provide less than half as many kilocalories per gram as fat.

A weight-loss diet should include at least 150 g (600 kcal) of carbohydrate daily. This prevents ketosis and reduces the risk of bingeing on large amounts of food, particularly sweets, because of intense hunger.

WHAT SHOULD BE EATEN?

The easiest way to eat in a healthy manner, thereby obtaining enough nutrients, is to begin with the Food Guide Pyramid, spreading out the food choices into a regular meal pattern (3 or more meals).[26] As a review, this consists of 6 servings (½ cup, 1 ounce, or 1 slice) of breads, cereals, rice, and pasta. It is important to emphasize whole grains, with limited amounts of sugar and fat.[18] Two to 4 servings

One of the biggest obstacles to staying on a reduced-fat diet is lack of taste. One way to overcome this is to savor foods:
- **Choose foods with eye appeal.** They will stimulate saliva.
- **Serve foods hot or warm to increase their aroma.**
- **Take time to smell the food.**
- **Enjoy the flavor by holding the food in your mouth before swallowing.**
- **Chew foods thoroughly to release their flavor.**
- **Eat several foods at each meal, and alternate foods as you eat to reduce taste bud fatigue.**

TABLE 9-2

Choosing "thin" foods

The chart below can help you plan your meals while following the simple guidelines for healthful eating. When you select a variety of foods from those listed in the far left column, you'll be eating foods that are low in fat and/or high in dietary fiber.

Types of food	Select most often	Select moderately often	Select least often
Animal protein	Lean cuts of beef/pork Salmon, halibut (broiled) Canned tuna in water Poultry (without skin) Egg Crab	Untrimmed beef and pork Canned tuna in oil Poultry (with skin) Lobster, shrimp Canadian bacon	Fatty beef, lamb, pork Luncheon meats/hot dogs Fried chicken Fried fish Liver, kidneys Bacon
Dairy	Nonfat yogurt Nonfat milk (or ½%) Nonfat dry milk Nonfat frozen yogurt	Reduced-fat and part-skim cheeses Low-fat cottage cheese Low-fat milk Low-fat yogurt 95% fat-free frozen yogurt	Whole-milk cheese (cheddar, muenster) Whole-milk Sour cream, ice cream Cream, half-and-half
Vegetable protein	Dried beans and peas (kidney, lima, and soy beans; lentils; split peas) Tofu (bean curd)	Raw or dry-roasted nuts and seeds Peanut and other nut butters (moderate amounts)	Oil-processed nuts and seeds
Vegetables	Raw, fresh vegetables Fresh or frozen, slightly cooked vegetables	Canned vegetables Canned tomato or vegetable juice	Vegetables in cream or butter sauces Fried vegetables
Fruits	Fresh, raw fruit Dried fruit Frozen and fresh fruit juices	Canned fruit packed in juice Canned fruit juices Frozen fruit	Fruit-flavored beverages Canned fruit packed in syrup Avocados Olives
Grain products	Shredded wheat, oats Whole-grain cereals Whole-grain breads Brown rice Wheat bran, oat bran Bagels Fig bars	Refined cereals Enriched white breads Refined pasta White rice Granola Toast with margarine Plain cookies	Cookies, cakes, pies Sweetened cereals Tortilla chips Oil-processed crackers Cream-filled cookies Croissants, doughnuts Fat-rich salad dressings
Other (limit quantity)	Popcorn (air popped)	Low-fat salad dressing Low-fat mayonnaise Pretzels	Mayonnaise Gravies, cream sauce Potato chips

TABLE 9-3

Saving kilocalories: ideas to help get started

Check out the following kilocalorie-saving ideas. Then think of other changes to help cut kilocalories.

Instead of:	Try:	Kilocalories saved:
3 ounces well-marbled meat (prime rib)	3 ounces lean meat (eye of round)	140
½ chicken breast, batter-fried	½ chicken breast, broiled with lemon	175
½ cup beef stroganoff	3 ounces lean roast beef	210
½ cup home-fried potatoes	1 medium baked potato	65
½ cup green bean-mushroom casserole	½ cup cooked green beans	50
½ cup potato salad	1 cup raw vegetable salad	140
½ cup pineapple chunks in heavy syrup	½ cup pineapple chunks canned in juice	25
2 tablespoons bottled French dressing	2 tablespoons low-calorie French dressing	150
⅐ 9-inch apple pie	1 baked apple	185
3 oatmeal-raisin cookies	1 oatmeal-raisin cookie	125
½ cup ice cream	½ cup ice milk	45
A danish pastry	Half an English muffin	150
1 cup sugar-coated corn flakes	1 cup plain corn flakes	60
1 cup whole milk	1 cup 1% low-fat milk	45
7-fluid-ounce gin and tonic	6-fluid ounce wine cooler made with sparkling water	150
1-ounce bag potato chips	1 cup plain popcorn	120
1/12 8-inch white layer cake with chocolate frosting	1/12 angel food cake, 10-inch tube	185
Regular beer	Light beer	40

(one medium or ½ cup) of fruit and 3 to 5 servings of vegetables are then added. To finish, add 2 to 3 servings of nonfat or low-fat milk/dairy products (1 cup) and 4 to 6 ounces of lean meat or alternatives each day. Sweets and fats should be kept to minimal amounts. Remember that potato chips and cheese are rich in fat, and fruit punches are considered a sweet. Table 9-3 shows how to start reducing energy intake.

As you should realize by now, it is best to consider healthy eating a lifestyle change rather than simply a weight-loss plan.[7] You should make reasonable choices, consume adequate portions, and not expect a miracle overnight. Starting out with limited food selections and rapid weight loss can sabotage efforts to maintain healthy eating by encouraging bingeing and feelings of failure that often accompany those types of dieting experiences (Figure 9-3).[26]

One suggested reason for failure of restrictive diets is the sense of **restraint** people feel from limitations in the amount and types of food they can eat. Often a trade-off is constructed, classifying some foods as "good" and others as "bad." One violation of the diet is considered a failure, which exerts considerable pressure on the dieter. One small emotionally disturbing event or environmental change now may "release" the dieter, who eats a little forbidden food, feels a sense of relief from restraint, and has a binge. This leads them to classify themselves as failures and to abandon the weight-loss attempt.[29] Later we address behavioral methods to avoid this trap.

restraint A feeling of constraint caused by restricted food intake, often associated with the belief that there are good and bad foods.

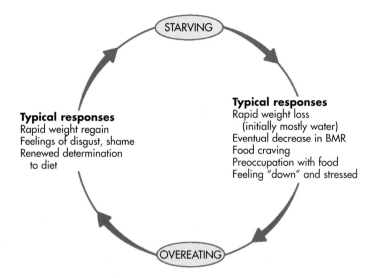

Figure 9-3 A poor start often leads to a poor finish. When dieting to lose weight, changing habits is often the key.

CONCEPT CHECK

Obesity is a chronic disease that necessitates lifelong treatment. Key points to consider when attempting to treat obesity include: (1) the primary focus should be on a healthy lifestyle that can be maintained; (2) the body resists weight loss; (3) typical weight-loss attempts often are followed by weight regain; (4) emphasis should be placed on preventing obesity, since curing this disorder is very difficult; (5) weight should be lost from fat stores, not mostly from lean tissues. Appropriate weight-loss programs have the following characteristics in common: (1) they meet nutritional needs—this can be evaluated by checking for mostly low-fat and non-fat choices from the Food Guide Pyramid; (2) they can adjust to accommodate habits and tastes; (3) they emphasize readily obtainable foods; (4) they promote changing habits that lead to overeating; (5) they encourage regular physical activity; and (6) they help change obesity-promoting beliefs and rally healthy social support.

Regular Physical Activity—A Second Key to Weight Loss

Regular physical activity is very important for everyone, especially those who are trying to lose weight or maintain a lower body weight.[7,25] Many of us rarely do more than sit, stand, and sleep. Obviously, much more energy is used during physical activity than at rest. In addition, expending only 200 to 300 extra kcal/day above and beyond normal activity level, while maintaining energy intake, can eliminate about a half pound of fat stores per week; about 25 pounds of fat loss in a year. Physical activity also increases fat use by the body and often boosts overall self-esteem.

Adding any of the activities in Figure 9-4 to the lifestyle leads to expenditure of an extra 200 kcal; note that sitting is not a recommended "activity." Duration and regular performance, rather than intensity, are the keys to success with this approach to weight loss. Walking vigorously 2 miles per day can be as helpful as sophisticated aerobic dancing or jogging. Moreover, walking is less likely to lead to injuries.

The easiest way to increase physical activity is to make it part of a daily routine. As a start the person could consider walking every day and then try to incorporate some stair climbing every day. A simple trick is to park your car farther from school or the shopping mall so you must walk farther.

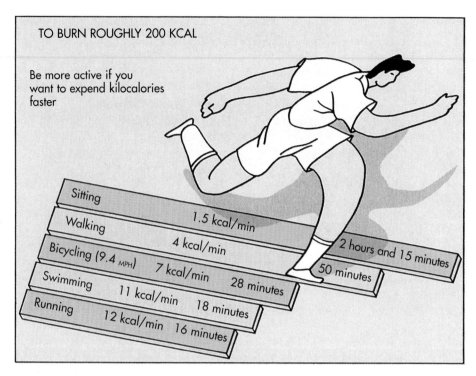

TO BURN ROUGHLY 200 KCAL

Be more active if you want to expend kilocalories faster

Sitting

Walking   1.5 kcal/min

Bicycling (9.4 MPH)   4 kcal/min   2 hours and 15 minutes

Swimming   7 kcal/min   28 minutes   50 minutes

Running   11 kcal/min   18 minutes

12 kcal/min   16 minutes

Figure 9-4 Physical activity improves any diet. Weight loss is enhanced because much more energy is used in physical activity than at rest. In addition, physical activity facilitates fat loss while preserving most lean body mass. Each of these activities uses approximately 200 kcal.

Spot-reducing using diet and physical activity is not possible. Physical activity may firm the tissue by tightening the muscles present, but the fat decreases only as other fat stores in the body generally decrease. "Problem" local fat deposits can be reduced in size, however, using suction lipectomy. Lipectomy simply means surgical removal of fat. A pencil-thin tube is inserted into an incision in the skin, and the fat tissue, such as that in the buttocks and thigh area, is suctioned off. This procedure, developed in the early 1980s, carries risks such as infection, lasting depressions in the skin, and blood clots that can lead to kidney failure. Also, it is often quite painful. It is not designed to help a person lose 30 to 40 pounds, but rather about 4 pounds per treatment. It can be used as part of cosmetic surgery by an experienced physician to help reduce localized fat deposits that are very diet-resistant, such as those in the outer and inner thighs and stomach. Over 100,000 procedures were performed in 1990, with women receiving 85% of them. Cost is about $1500 per site. People who are able to maintain the loss of fat are generally those who make substantial changes in eating habits and physical activity.

Besides using energy, increased physical activity has the advantage of reducing the stress and boredom of a diet and increasing the likelihood of later weight maintenance. In essence, eating less and performing more physical activity go hand-in-hand in a weight-loss plan. Physical activity can also take the dieter out of the house and away from snacks.

Eventually, increased physical activity can lead to modest increases in muscle mass as well. More lean tissue raises basal metabolism so that, even while sitting quietly, more energy is used than when the same body contains a higher proportion of adipose tissue. The extra energy used in physical activity, coupled with any increase in muscle mass, can pay dividends. Performing physical activity can also help maintain lean body tissue when on a weight-loss diet; therefore more of the weight lost is fat.

Whatever means of increasing physical activity is chosen, the activities should be enjoyable so that they are practiced regularly (Figure 9-5). They should also be convenient, should be within the budget, and should provide options for bad weather. One suggestion is to find several different activities and vary them to prevent boredom.

Once a regular program of physical activity is established, the rate of weight loss often begins to diminish. In other words, after 4 or 5 weeks of the same energy intake and the same activity level, weight is not lost as fast as during the first month. One cause of this slower weight loss is the lowered body weight, which reduces the energy cost of each activity.[16] Also, if lean tissue is partially replacing fat tissue, the health advantage of physical activity may not be apparent on the scale. At this point the activity level should be increased. For example, walking 15 minutes more or doing more stair climbing each day is needed to obtain the same amount of energy output.

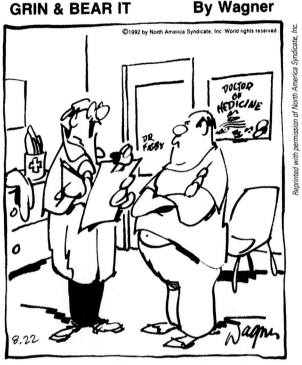

GRIN & BEAR IT   By Wagner

©1992 by North America Syndicate, Inc. World rights reserved.

"Opening the refrigerator is *not* exercise!"

Figure 9-5 Grin & Bear It

Behavior Modification—Changing Problem Habits Adds a Third Key Element

Behavior modification helps control energy intake in a weight-loss program.[7] Table 9-4 lists behavior modification principles for weight loss. Each person must decide which behavior contributes to obesity and then find ways to modify that behavior. Food often is used to cope with depression, stress, unsatisfying relationships, and childhood psychological wounds. If these stressors are not addressed, any pounds that are shed are likely to creep back.[29] Professional help is available to help dieters confront and resolve these problems.

One aim of counselors is to get people to listen to their bodies—to eat when they are hungry and stop when they are full. In essence, lifestyle and environment should be reshaped so that weight maintenance, rather than weight gain, is the overwhelming thrust, and self-control is not constantly tested.[11]

To do this, a person should consider the events that cause him or her to start eating, factors that influence food choices, and factors associated with eating cessation.[28] Psychologists often use terms like **chain-breaking, stimulus control, contingency management,** and **self-monitoring** when discussing behavior modification. This terminology helps place the problem in perspective and organize the entire intervention strategy into manageable steps.

Chain-breaking is separating activities that tend to occur together; for example, snacking on chips and peanuts while watching television. Although these activities do not have to occur together, they often do and need to be clearly separated when striving to eat less energy (Figure 9-6). An easy way to break the chain is to substitute an alternative activity. The earlier the chain is broken, the better, and the easier it is to reduce energy intake. Once the snack touches the taste buds, it's often too late.

chain-breaking Breaking the link between two or more activities that encourage overeating, such as snacking while watching television.

stimulus control Altering the environment to minimize the stimuli for eating; for example, removing foods from sight by storing them in kitchen cabinets.

contingency management Forming a plan of action to respond to a situation in which overeating is likely, such as when snacks are within arm's reach at a party.

self-monitoring A process of tracking foods eaten and conditions affecting eating; actions are usually recorded in a diary, along with location, time, and state of mind. This is a tool to help a person understand more about his or her eating habits.

TABLE 9-4

Behavior modification principles for weight loss

Stimulus control
Shopping

1. Shop for food after eating—buy nutritious foods.
2. Shop from a list; do not buy irresistible "problem" foods.
3. Avoid ready-to-eat foods.
4. Put off shopping until absolutely necessary.

Plans

1. Plan to limit food intake as needed.
2. Substitute exercise for snacking.
3. Eat meals and snacks at scheduled times; don't skip meals.

Activities

1. Store food out of sight, preferably in the freezer, to discourage impulsive eating.
2. Eat all food in the same place.
3. Keep serving dishes off the table, especially dishes of sauces and gravies.
4. Use smaller dishes and utensils.

Holidays and parties

1. Drink fewer alcoholic beverages.
2. Plan eating behavior before parties.
3. Eat a low-kilocalorie snack before parties.
4. Practice polite ways to decline food.
5. Don't get discouraged by an occasional setback.

Eating behavior

1. Put fork down between mouthfuls.
2. Chew thoroughly before taking the next bite.
3. Leave some food on the plate.
4. Pause in the middle of the meal.
5. Do nothing else while eating (e.g., reading, watching television).

Reward

1. Solicit help from family and friends and suggest how they can help you.
2. Help family and friends provide this help in the form of praise and material rewards.
3. Use self-monitoring records as basis for rewards.
4. Plan specific rewards for specific behavior (behavioral contracts).

Self-monitoring
Diet Diary

1. Note time and place of eating.
2. List type and amount of food eaten.
3. Record who is present and how you feel.
4. Use diet diary to identify problem areas.

Cognitive restructuring

1. Avoid setting unreasonable goals.
2. Think about progress, not shortcomings.
3. Avoid imperatives like "always" and "never."
4. Counter negative thoughts with positive restatements.

From Frankle RT, Yang M: *Obesity and weight control,* Rockville, Md, 1988, Aspen Publishers.

ALTERNATIVE ACTIVITY SHEET

SUBSTITUTE ACTIVITIES

Pleasant activities
1. *Singing/washing hair*
2. *Reading comics/biking*
3. *Sewing/ calling a girlfriend*

Necessary activities
1. *Ironing*
2. *Vacuuming*
3. *Straightening apartment*

Situations when used
1. *Wanted ice cream – delayed with bath*
2. *Wanted wheat thins – cleaned up apt.*
3. *Wanted snack – went for walk*
4. *Wanted cookies – did dishes first*
5. *Saw leftovers – went for bike ride*
6. *Tempted by cookies – set timer*
7. *Wanted snack – read comics*

BEHAVIOR CHAIN

Identify the links in your eating response chain on the following diagram. Draw a line through the chain where it was interrupted. Add the link you substituted and the new chain of behavior this substitution started.

ALTERNATIVE ACTIVITY SHEET

SUBSTITUTE ACTIVITIES

Pleasant activities
1. _____
2. _____
3. _____

Necessary activities
1. _____
2. _____
3. _____

Situations when used
1. _____
2. _____
3. _____
4. _____
5. _____
6. _____
7. _____

BEHAVIOR CHAIN

Identify the links in your eating response chain on the following diagram. Draw a line through the chain where it was interrupted. Add the link you substituted and the new chain of behavior this substitution started.

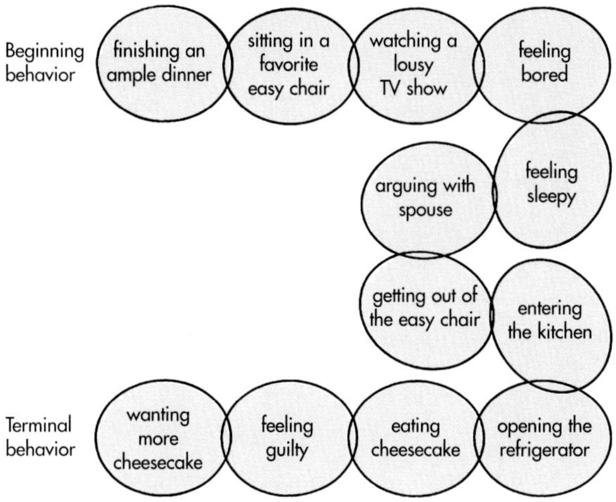

Beginning behavior: finishing an ample dinner → sitting in a favorite easy chair → watching a lousy TV show → feeling bored → feeling sleepy → arguing with spouse → getting out of the easy chair → entering the kitchen → opening the refrigerator → eating cheesecake → feeling guilty → wanting more cheesecake

Terminal behavior: wanting more cheesecake, feeling guilty, eating cheesecake, opening the refrigerator

Beginning behavior (blank circles)

Terminal behavior: feeling guilty, eating

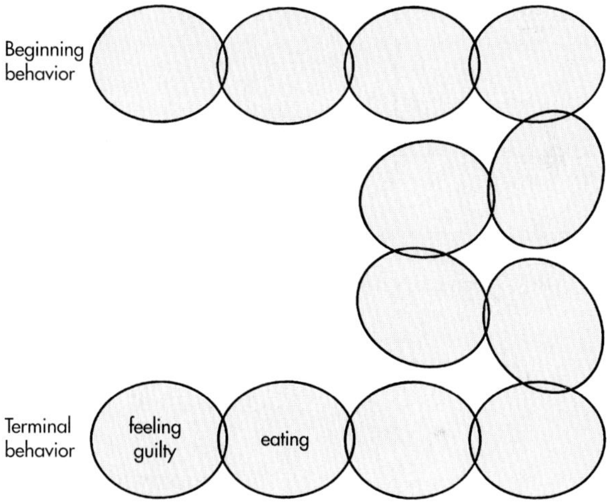

Figure 9-6 Identifying behavior chains is a good tool for understanding more about your habits and pinpointing ways to change unwanted habits.

Four types of behavior can be substituted in an ongoing behavior chain:
1. Fun activities, such as reading a book.
2. Necessary activities, such as cleaning a room.
3. Incompatible activities, such as taking a shower.
4. Urge-delaying activities, such as waiting 20 minutes before eating.

Stimulus control involves controlling factors that encourage eating. That may mean hiding irresistible food in the back of the refrigerator, taking the light bulb out of the refrigerator, moving foods from the counter into cabinets, or avoiding a certain vending machine on the way to class.

Contingency management focuses on planning ahead for responses to possible pitfalls and high-risk situations. One strategy, for example, is to rehearse what to say when people offer food and what to do when irresistible foods are within arm's reach at a party, such as moving to the other side of the room.

Self-monitoring, a key practice in behavior modification, usually begins with keeping a diary of foods eaten and the circumstances that lead to eating. The record can reveal general patterns that provide a better understanding of eating habits (Figure 9-7). (You completed a food record as part of the Take Action activity in Chapter 1.) Self-monitoring is an efficient way to spot problems in eating habits, especially times of overeating.[11]

Time	Minutes spent eating	M or S*	H†	Activity while eating	Place of eating	Food and quantity	Others present	Reason for choice
7:10 a.m.	15	M	2	standing, fixing lunch	kitchen	1 cup orange juice 1 cup raisin bran ½ cup 2% milk 2 tsp sugar Black coffee	—	health habit health taste habit
10:00 a.m.	4	S	1	sitting, taking notes	classroom	12 oz diet cola	class	weight control
12:15 p.m.	40	M	2	sitting, talking	student union	1 chicken sandwich with lettuce and mayonnaise 1 pear 1 cup 2% milk	friends	taste health health
2:30 p.m.	10	S	1	sitting, studying	library	12 oz regular cola	friend	hunger
6:30 p.m.	35	M	3	sitting, talking	kitchen	1 pork chop 1 baked potato 2 tbsp margarine Lettuce and tomato salad 2 tbsp ranch dressing ½ cup peas 1 cup whole milk 1 piece cherry pie	boyfriend	convenience health taste health taste health habit taste
9:10 p.m.	10	S	2	sitting, studying	living room	1 apple 1 glass mineral water	—	weight control weight control

*M or S: Meal or snack
†H: Degree of hunger (0 = none; 3 = maximum).

Figure 9-7 A food record can illuminate eating habits.

Self-monitoring can be a persuasive means of encouraging new habits to counteract unwanted behavior. These new habits include limiting eating to only one place in the house, which could reduce snacking in front of the television, as well as in the kitchen while preparing meals. People who eat very rapidly should put down their utensils while chewing. This practice slows the rate of eating and helps the hormone cholecystokinin (CCK) signal a natural satiety response. It also gives the stretch receptors in the stomach and the nutrient receptors in the intestines time to signal fullness. Both of these actions naturally encourage cessation of eating. People who tend to eat anything available should not purchase foods they cannot resist.

Current discussions of behavior modification for obesity also include **cognitive restructuring,** social support, providing rewards, and relapse prevention as other helpful strategies. Cognitive restructuring is a strategy for helping people change negative, self-defeating, or pessimistic thoughts. Thinking "I want that cheesecake but I can't have it because I'm on a diet and don't want to be bad," will cause a diet to fail because people don't do well in an atmosphere of deprivation. Instead thinking "I want it but it's not healthful, so I choose not to work it in today," gives a better feeling about a diet and, therefore, a better chance of success.

Self-talk is another factor to aid behavior modification. People carry on an internal dialogue—self-talk—to sort out their own truths, beliefs and attitudes, and responses to events around them. Positive self-talk leads us kindly through changes, like choosing to lose weight.[6] We praise ourselves for success. Negative self-talk is different. Praise is replaced with self-deprecating remarks, self-blame,

cognitive restructuring Changing negative, self-defeating, or pessimistic thoughts that undermine weight-control efforts to ones that are positive, optimistic, and supportive of weight control.

self-talk The internal dialogue everyone carries on in their heads to sort out beliefs, feelings, attitudes, and events happening in their lives.

and angry, guilt-producing put-downs. Negative self-talk undermines efforts at self-control, particularly when trying to lose weight, and leads to anxiety and depression. Beliefs and self-talk influence how we interpret events of today and expectations of the future, as well as how we feel and react. Positive self-talk and problem-solving efforts and realistic beliefs and goals lead to a healthful, self-caring lifestyle.[6]

A key way that self-talk fits into behavior modification is through the concept of cognitive restructuring just mentioned. People are trained to change thoughts that promote being obese. Thoughts like "I hate exercise and can never enjoy it," or "I can't have any fun if I don't eat a luscious dessert when I go out with my friends," can undermine a weight-control program. By challenging and stopping these thoughts, as well as substituting more appropriate thoughts, adhering to a weight-control program becomes easier. Self-talk that reminds us of our achievements, with weight loss and with other activities in life, helps increase our self-esteem and likelihood of success.[6]

RELAPSE PREVENTION ALSO DESERVES ATTENTION

Relapse prevention is a series of strategies to help people on diets and weight-maintenance programs anticipate and cope with problems. Advance planning attempts to prevent slips, called *lapses,* and deal with them when they occur. A lapse is one mistake, but a relapse is total abandonment of the weight-control program. A person who is unprepared for a lapse may interpret it as failure and abandon weight-control efforts.

Relapse often starts with a high-risk situation, like going on vacation. Most people don't recognize when they are at high risk for relapse, and just one slip becomes a series of lapses that leads to complete relapse into old behavior. The first lapse should be a signal to the person that he or she is stressed, having interpersonal conflicts, and not coping adequately with everyday events. This is a high-risk situation. One or two slips is not fatal. Healthful behavior can be recovered if the potential for relapse is planned in advance and even expected.[6]

The following are some helpful strategies for relapse prevention:
1. Identify high-risk situations—if and when backsliding occurs, question whether it is linked to a high-risk situation. This should help put the focus on the event, rather than on feeling guilty about backsliding.
2. Mentally rehearse a response to backsliding behavior—imagine both backsliding and then taking positive action to recover. Rehearsing responses to as many potential lapses as possible is important.
3. Remember goals set—keep in mind the reasons for making the commitment to change behavior and the hard work that has gone into achieving progress.
4. Stay calm when errors are made—take charge immediately. Ask for help if needed.

It is important for a person to analyze his or her particular behavior shortcomings and then be sensitized to facets of lifestyle that make healthy living difficult. Is snacking, compulsive eating, or overeating at each meal a constant problem? Specific problems must be addressed.[7] There are many options for changing shopping and eating behavior (see Tables 9-3 and 9-4). It is best to integrate many strategies and tactics into a behavior plan. Overall, maintenance of weight loss is fostered by the "3 M's": motivation, movement, and monitoring.

relapse prevention A series of strategies used to help prevent and cope with weight-control lapses, such as recognizing high-risk situations and deciding beforehand on appropriate responses.

SOCIAL SUPPORT AIDS BEHAVIOR CHANGE

Healthy social support is helpful in weight control. Helping others understand how they can be supportive can make weight control easier.[6] Family and friends can provide praise and encouragement. A weight-control professional can keep the dieter accountable and help him or her learn from difficult situations. Long-term contact with a professional can be quite helpful for later weight maintenance. Groups of individuals attempting to lose weight or maintain losses can provide empathetic support.

CONCEPT CHECK

Increasing physical activity as part of daily life should be part of any weight-loss plan. A goal of 200 to 300 kcal spent in daily activity such as walking and stair climbing is recommended. Behavior can be modified to improve conditions for losing weight. One behavior area that requires change is habit chains that encourage overeating, such as snacking while watching television. Another tactic is to modify the environment to reduce temptation; for example, putting foods into cupboards to keep them out of sight. In addition, rethinking attitudes about eating—for example, substituting pleasures other than food as a reward for coping with a stressful day—can be important for altering undesirable eating behavior. Advance planning to prevent and deal with lapses is vital, as is rallying healthy social support. Finally, careful observation and recording of eating habits in a diary can reveal subtle behavior that leads to overeating.

The Behavior Change Process

Integration of the previously mentioned techniques into the lifestyle is very complex. Remember, a complete lifestyle change is being made. First, the person attempting weight loss should learn more about the problem. This interest in learning is referred to as a **receptive framework.** Personal responsibility for lifestyle change must be accepted by the individual.

receptive framework An attitude of openness to learning and responding to a problem; usually involves seeking more information about the issue from books and people.

GATHERING BASELINE DATA

Next, the person should gather baseline data about present eating and activity patterns. By looking at current behavior, specific areas where changes are needed are revealed. For example, if after coming home from work at 4:30 pm, the person tends to turn on the television and grab a bag of chips until dinner-time, that is the time of day at which a brisk walk could be substituted for the television and chips.

CHARTING THE PLAN FOR CHANGE

Learning more about present behavior is the first step of charting the plan for change. The next step is to set attainable goals. An example of an attainable goal from the discussion above is walking for 30 minutes every day after work instead of eating potato chips and watching television. The goal should be realistic and measurable. Another part of developing a plan may consist of finding a good weight-loss program and joining.

MAKING IT OFFICIAL

People often find it helpful to develop a behavior contract to encourage follow-through. The contract can list goal behavior and objectives, mileposts for measuring progress, and regular rewards for meeting the terms of the contract. The main criteria for effective rewards or outlets for stress are that they be of value and can be frequently given. Music tapes or compact discs, clothing, and tickets to sporting events or concerts can serve as effective rewards, based on the preferences of the in-

numb
the ch
eas of
ments
ing si
and h
by me

Ra
chang
record
serum
weigh

REEV

After
sues.
be cha
dresse

A Re

When
tors th
should
1. M
 to
2. Ti
3. A
4. Ta
5. Fo
6. Po
7. So
 ho
8. Su
 mu
9. Re
10. Ke
 cha
Failure
1. Neg
2. Out
 leng
 or i
3. Rev
 A di
regaine
less hea
formati
not be
needed
propriat
goals th
Wou
them. T
modifica
tools ar
lifestyle

Name _Chris Willer_

Goal

I agree to _spend at least 20 minutes eating._
(specify behavior)

under the following circumstances: _in my home, during dinner_
(specify where, when, how much, etc.)
5 times per week.

Substitute behavior and/or reinforcement schedule _I will reward myself at the end of week if I fulfill my goal._

Environmental planning

In order to help me do this, I am going to (1) arrange my physical and social environment by _eat more dinners at home, place a timer set for 20 minutes on the dinner table._

and (2) control my internal environment (thoughts, images) by _put a note on the refrigerator reminding me._

Reinforcements

Reinforcements provided by me daily or weekly (if contract is kept): _rent one of my favorite VCR movies at the end of the week._

Reinforcements provided by others daily or weekly (if contract is kept): _will ask me at the end of the week if I achieved my goal and if so will complement me._

Social support

Behavior change is more likely to take place when other people support you. During the quarter/semester, please meet with the other person at least three times to discuss your progress.

The name of my "significant helper" is: _Shawn Jones_

This contract should include:
1. Baseline data (one week)
2. Well-defined goal
3. Simple method for charting progress (diary, counters, charts, etc.)
4. Reinforcements (immediate and long term)
5. Evaluation method (summary of experiences, success, and/or new learning about self).

Figure 9-8 Behavior contracts aid behavior change.

dividual. A system of rewards can increase the likelihood of appropriate weight-control behavior in the future.

Positive reinforcement contributes more to successful behavior change than negative reinforcement. Initially, the focus should be on positive behavior rather than on positive results.[6] Positive behavior, such as regular physical activity, eventually leads to positive outcomes, although it may take months to see the effects. A behavior contract for weight loss is shown in Figure 9-8. When finished, the contract should be signed in the presence of friends to publicly affirm it. Contracts can help promote adherence to the program.

FOLLOWING THE PLAN

Once the best weight-control plan is determined and perhaps a contract written, it is time to implement the plan. To begin, it is best to plan a trial of at least 6 to 8 weeks. Thinking of a lifetime commitment can be overwhelming. Remember that games are won one point at a time. Then, if successful, aim for a total of 6 months of new activities to provide a reasonable test. It is difficult to overcome the inertia

best chance of losing weight and maintaining the loss, the person must explore his or her own strengths and weaknesses.

If this lifelong commitment is a struggle for you, make dieting choices wisely so that each pound is lost forever. If you have a healthy, acceptable body weight, simple weight maintenance is a positive step. Otherwise healthy people who do not exceed a BMI of 25 to 27 do not necessarily need weight loss for health's sake. These people would be better served if our culture simply rethought its obsession with slimness.[1] For people who have heart disease, hypertension, diabetes, arthritis, or another disorder that is often worsened by obesity, weight loss is recommended. Overall, in terms of both health and self-esteem, a plan must strive to make sure the life of the dieter improves as weight is lost.

Concept Check

Once a person decides to lose weight a series of steps is necessary for effective behavior change. The behavior change process involves (1) charting a plan based on an assessment of current habits; (2) setting attainable goals; (3) working out the details of the plan; (4) making it official by drawing up a contract; (5) measuring progress; (6) being assertive with others while following the plan; and (7) reevaluating the plan. This process increases the chances of losing weight and keeping it off in the future. Permanent weight loss is difficult to attain; a serious plan of action is needed when weight loss is attempted.

Professional Help for Weight Loss

The first professional to see for advice about a weight-loss program is the family physician. Doctors are best equipped to assess overall health and the appropriateness of weight loss. The physician may refer the person to a registered dietitian for a specific weight-loss plan and for answers to diet-related questions. Registered dietitians are uniquely qualified to help design a weight-loss plan because they understand both food composition and what food means to people. Exercise physiologists can provide advice on a program to increase physical activity.

Many communities have a variety of weight-loss organizations. These may include self-help groups, such as Take Off Pounds Sensibly and Weight Watchers. Other programs, such as Jenny Craig and Physicians' Weight Loss Center, are less desirable for the average dieter. These programs are generally expensive because of their requirements for intense counseling and/or mandatory diet foods and supplements. In addition, the Federal Trade Commission has charged these and other commercial diet program companies with misleading consumers with unsubstantiated weight-loss claims and deceptive testimonials.

TREATING SEVERE (MORBID) OBESITY

Severe (morbid) obesity refers to the status of a body at least 100 pounds over desirable body weight, body mass index greater than 39, or twice desirable body weight. Currently about 1.5 million people in the United States have severe obesity. Severe obesity causes the worst obesity-related health problems. More drastic treatment may be used in these cases if conservative plans have failed.

Gastroplasty

gastroplasty Surgery on the stomach to limit its volume to approximately 50 ml, the size of a shot glass.

The most common surgical procedure for treating severe obesity today involves modifying the stomach by **gastroplasty,** also known as *stomach stapling.* One of two specific surgical procedures is commonly used, either a vertical-banded gastroplasty or a roux-en-Y gastric bypass.[9] The latter surgical procedure is more effective, but more technically difficult. The goal is to reduce the volume of the stomach to ap-

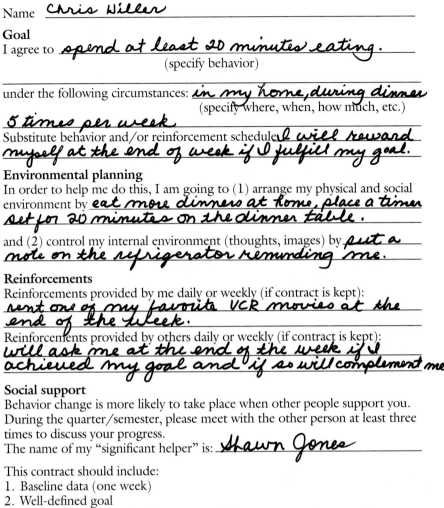

Name *Chris Willer*

Goal
I agree to *spend at least 20 minutes eating.*
 (specify behavior)

under the following circumstances: *in my home, during dinner*
 (specify where, when, how much, etc.)
5 times per week
Substitute behavior and/or reinforcement schedule *I will reward myself at the end of week if I fulfill my goal.*

Environmental planning
In order to help me do this, I am going to (1) arrange my physical and social environment by *eat more dinners at home, place a timer set for 20 minutes on the dinner table.*

and (2) control my internal environment (thoughts, images) by *put a note on the refrigerator reminding me.*

Reinforcements
Reinforcements provided by me daily or weekly (if contract is kept):
rent one of my favorite VCR movies at the end of the week.
Reinforcements provided by others daily or weekly (if contract is kept):
will ask me at the end of the week if I achieved my goal and if so will complement me.

Social support
Behavior change is more likely to take place when other people support you. During the quarter/semester, please meet with the other person at least three times to discuss your progress.
The name of my "significant helper" is: *Shawn Jones*

This contract should include:
1. Baseline data (one week)
2. Well-defined goal
3. Simple method for charting progress (diary, counters, charts, etc.)
4. Reinforcements (immediate and long term)
5. Evaluation method (summary of experiences, success, and/or new learning about self).

Figure 9-8 Behavior contracts aid behavior change.

dividual. A system of rewards can increase the likelihood of appropriate weight-control behavior in the future.

Positive reinforcement contributes more to successful behavior change than negative reinforcement. Initially, the focus should be on positive behavior rather than on positive results.[6] Positive behavior, such as regular physical activity, eventually leads to positive outcomes, although it may take months to see the effects. A behavior contract for weight loss is shown in Figure 9-8. When finished, the contract should be signed in the presence of friends to publicly affirm it. Contracts can help promote adherence to the program.

FOLLOWING THE PLAN

Once the best weight-control plan is determined and perhaps a contract written, it is time to implement the plan. To begin, it is best to plan a trial of at least 6 to 8 weeks. Thinking of a lifetime commitment can be overwhelming. Remember that games are won one point at a time. Then, if successful, aim for a total of 6 months of new activities to provide a reasonable test. It is difficult to overcome the inertia of 20, 30, or 40 or more years. The value of continuing the behavior-change program may have to be recalled more than once. Backsliding may occur. Backsliding is not totally disastrous if the focus is kept on reducing, but not necessarily extinguishing, undesirable behavior. It is usually unrealistic to say "I will never eat chocolate ice cream again." Better to say "I will not eat chocolate ice cream as often as before."

Being assertive with others is important when pursuing goals. A person wishing to change is likely to get feedback from people who support the planned changes, but also from some who prefer to keep things the way they are and may try to stand in the way of a plan. Even dieters may have days or moments when they try to talk themselves out of the plan. We all respond to others' opinions, especially about ourselves. We like approval, generally, and are influenced by others to behave in certain ways. One problem in undertaking behavior change is to be strong enough to behave in a chosen manner when others encourage, consciously or not, behavior inappropriate to the desired goal.

A certain amount of "psyching up" is sometimes necessary to pursue goals in spite of others' expectations. Almost everyone benefits from some assertiveness training when it comes to changing behavior. Here are a few suggestions:

- No feelings should be hurt if you say, "No, thank you," firmly and repeatedly, when others try to dissuade you from a plan. Rather, ask them, and yourself, why they want you to eat their way. Your needs are as important as theirs.
- It's not necessary to order "big" to accommodate anyone—mother, business clients, or the chef. Ordering "big" just because someone else is paying for the meal is a trap.
- Lighter, more healthful low-fat meals can be served when entertaining. Some new recipes may have to be tried, but that will be a useful step en route to changing the overall approach to cooking.
- Dealing with parties and social occasions built around food is possible but difficult. Friends can plan celebrations around a hike or a tennis court, rather than around cake and ice cream. At parties where food is everywhere, eat before going, take low-kilocalorie foods along, and converse far from the food table.
- Learn ways to handle "put-downs"—inadvertent or conscious. The most effective response may be to communicate feelings honestly, without hostility. A person can tell critics that they have hurt his or her feelings, that habits are being changed and what is really needed is understanding and support.

Fostering feelings of self-worth facilitates behavior changes. Getting rid of the habit of self-criticism requires strong self-retraining. Creating and memorizing lists of strengths, giving credit where deserved, is important. Practicing forgiveness is helpful, as is lowering unrealistic expectations.[6] Stopping negative thoughts and purposely switching to positive thoughts should be a goal.

In all, a long-term vision for a nutrition and health plan should be cultivated and occasional indiscretions forgiven. The focus should be on behavior that has been established and performed day after day. An occasional lapse does not justify a relapse and certainly not a collapse. Especially watch for **rationalization,** an attempt at self-deception—distorting information and denying facts to support wishful thinking are ways of rationalizing. Trying to justify backsliding by saying "I can't do it" when one has done it for 4 months already is rationalizing.

rationalization The process of distorting information and denying facts in an attempt to hold on to a certain opinion.

MEASURING PROGRESS

There are a few good ways to measure progress in a weight-loss program. The first is to track weekly whether the two or three behavioral goals were accomplished and to what degree.

People attempting to lose weight like to see changes in their body composition. Simple daily or weekly weighing is not recommended because weight can vary for a number of reasons besides the amount of fat gained or lost, as we noted earlier in the chapter. A better way to track progress is to use a tape measure to monitor areas of the body like the neck, waist, upper thigh, and upper arm. These measurements are closely related to body fat changes. Monitoring changes in waist or clothing size is an additional way to track long-term progress. Changes in fitness level and health are good indicators of progress, as is percentage of body fat, determined by measuring skinfold thickness.

Rather than just setting a goal weight, it is better for an individual to primarily change his or her lifestyle and then see ultimately where weight settles.[1] Keeping records of diet, physical activity, changes in body fat or weight, blood pressure, serum cholesterol values, and clothing size over time can help track progress in a weight-loss program. Seeing progress over time is good reinforcement.

REEVALUATING THE PLAN

After practicing a program for several months, reevaluating it may clarify some issues. Are goals being accomplished and progress made? If not, how must the plan be changed? Is there other behavior that needs to be changed that hasn't been addressed? These are all pertinent questions. The plan should be modified as needed.

A Recap

When weight-loss experts pool their collective experience, they identify certain factors that characterize success and failure in weight loss. Based on this chapter, it should be clear that success is encouraged by[6]:

1. Moderation in fat/energy intake. A first step should be use of this intervention to establish weight maintenance behavior before attempting to lose weight.
2. Time and inclination to perform regular physical activity.
3. A sense of control of personal destiny and likelihood of success.
4. Taking charge of the plan with a strong motivation to succeed.
5. Focusing on improved health status to spur success.
6. Positive self-talk.
7. Social support via family/friends, in turn balancing life with friendships, work, hobbies, and other interests.
8. Sustained vigilance in pursuit of goals—realizing it is a lifetime pursuit that must be suited to one's specific needs.
9. Realistic goals that promote gradual change.
10. Keeping track of body weight and body measurements and quickly making changes in a plan if relapse is noticed.

Failure is encouraged by[6]:

1. Negative feelings.
2. Out-of-control situations, such as family life or lifestyle that constantly challenges the will to succeed; prior or current practices of bingeing, laxative abuse, or induced vomiting. In these cases professional help should be sought.
3. Reverting to old habits.

A disturbing fact about dieting for weight loss is that often the weight is quickly regained.[21] Dieters may then end up with a greater percentage of body fat and be less healthy after their diet-and-regain cycle than when they began. Based on this information, it appears that dieting itself can promote obesity. Thus dieting should not be undertaken lightly. If a person is not highly motivated and does not have the needed social support, dieting for weight loss should be delayed until a more appropriate time.[6] In the meantime, the person can strive to give up unrealistic weight goals that he or she may have harbored for a lifetime.

Would-be dieters should choose and follow diet plans that are appropriate for them. There is a smorgasbord of options: lowered energy and fat intakes, behavior modification, increased physical activity, and group or individual counseling. Many tools are effective, but some are more useful than others, depending on the dieter's lifestyle, personality, and motivation. To discover which techniques promote the best chance of losing weight and maintaining the loss, the person must explore his or her own strengths and weaknesses.

If this lifelong commitment is a struggle for you, make dieting choices wisely so that each pound is lost forever. If you have a healthy, acceptable body weight, simple weight maintenance is a positive step. Otherwise healthy people who do not exceed a BMI of 25 to 27 do not necessarily need weight loss for health's sake. These people would be better served if our culture simply rethought its obsession with slimness.[1] For people who have heart disease, hypertension, diabetes, arthritis, or another disorder that is often worsened by obesity, weight loss is recommended. Overall, in terms of both health and self-esteem, a plan must strive to make sure the life of the dieter improves as weight is lost.

CONCEPT CHECK

Once a person decides to lose weight a series of steps is necessary for effective behavior change. The behavior change process involves (1) charting a plan based on an assessment of current habits; (2) setting attainable goals; (3) working out the details of the plan; (4) making it official by drawing up a contract; (5) measuring progress; (6) being assertive with others while following the plan; and (7) reevaluating the plan. This process increases the chances of losing weight and keeping it off in the future. Permanent weight loss is difficult to attain; a serious plan of action is needed when weight loss is attempted.

Professional Help for Weight Loss

The first professional to see for advice about a weight-loss program is the family physician. Doctors are best equipped to assess overall health and the appropriateness of weight loss. The physician may refer the person to a registered dietitian for a specific weight-loss plan and for answers to diet-related questions. Registered dietitians are uniquely qualified to help design a weight-loss plan because they understand both food composition and what food means to people. Exercise physiologists can provide advice on a program to increase physical activity.

Many communities have a variety of weight-loss organizations. These may include self-help groups, such as Take Off Pounds Sensibly and Weight Watchers. Other programs, such as Jenny Craig and Physicians' Weight Loss Center, are less desirable for the average dieter. These programs are generally expensive because of their requirements for intense counseling and/or mandatory diet foods and supplements. In addition, the Federal Trade Commission has charged these and other commercial diet program companies with misleading consumers with unsubstantiated weight-loss claims and deceptive testimonials.

TREATING SEVERE (MORBID) OBESITY

Severe (morbid) obesity refers to the status of a body at least 100 pounds over desirable body weight, body mass index greater than 39, or twice desirable body weight. Currently about 1.5 million people in the United States have severe obesity. Severe obesity causes the worst obesity-related health problems. More drastic treatment may be used in these cases if conservative plans have failed.

Gastroplasty

The most common surgical procedure for treating severe obesity today involves modifying the stomach by **gastroplasty,** also known as *stomach stapling*. One of two specific surgical procedures is commonly used, either a vertical-banded gastroplasty or a roux-en-Y gastric bypass.[9] The latter surgical procedure is more effective, but more technically difficult. The goal is to reduce the volume of the stomach to ap-

gastroplasty Surgery on the stomach to limit its volume to approximately 50 ml, the size of a shot glass.

NUTRITION FOCUS

MEDICATIONS TO AID WEIGHT LOSS

Over-the-counter medications that claim to facilitate weight loss sell briskly. Some can be effective, but so far none can substitute for the basic approach outlined in this chapter to promote weight loss. Diet aids include fiber pills, **phenylpropanolamine,** and benzocaine. Phenyl-propanolamine is an epinephrine-like drug that can cause a slight decrease in food intake.[3] At a typical dose of 75 mg/day, the degree of appetite suppression varies among people. FDA recommends that phenylpropanolamine be used with caution in people with hyperthyroidism, cardiovascular disorders (including hypertension), and diabetes. Adverse reactions may also occur in people taking various other medications or consuming caffeine at the same time. Benzocaine numbs the tongue, so a person tends to eat less.

Fiber pills can increase bulk in the stomach and ideally lead to satiety. Only soluble fiber, the type found in beans, oats, and guar gum, is effective in decreasing food intake. Bran fiber, such as that found in fiber pills, is not effective. However, when people consume enough soluble fiber (23 g) incorporated into crackers to decrease food intake, they also experience significant intestinal gas.

Physicians sometimes prescribe amphetamines for weight loss. Amphetamines cause a person to eat less, but they can also be addictive. In addition, amphetamines can increase heart rate and nervousness and lead to insomnia. Work on related medications continues. Thyroid hormone preparations were once popular, but these caused significant loss of lean tissue.

Fenfluramine (Pondimin) and related medications are prescribed by physicians to promote weight loss. These drugs increase the action of serotonin in the brain, which may lead to less food craving, especially for high-carbohydrate foods (see Chapter 8).[3] Rapid weight gain after dis-

continuing the drug is a problem. Addition of behavior therapy to this approach may improve weight maintenance. Some medication regimens add a form of amphetamine-like medications (phentermine) as well to increase efficacy. These therapies are effective for some people in the short run, but it remains to be seen if they are safe and effective in the long run.[10] Studies are ongoing. Most state medical boards currently limit use to 12 weeks unless the person is participating in a medical study using the product.

Studies are being done on a medication that inhibits lipase activity in the small intestine (Orlistat). With less lipase activity, fewer triglycerides are broken down into free fatty acids and monoglycerides, which reduces absorption of dietary fat. The drawback of this drug is that it is only 30% effective, no matter what the dose is, so a reduced energy diet is also needed for this approach to be efficacious. Therefore, this product has the potential to give only a slight boost to someone already following a healthy lifestyle for weight loss. A common side effect of this drug is diarrhea; a low-fat diet reduces this problem.

A medication that is used for treatment of ulcers, cimetidine, is being tested as a hunger-suppressing agent. Cimetidine is an H_2 blocker that reduces acid output by the parietal cells in the stomach, as described in Chapter 6. The theory is that if there is reduced acid in the stomach, there will be a diminished sensation of hunger. Further studies are needed with this drug before the overall efficacy is known, but results are promising to date.

Overall, in skilled hands, prescription medications can aid weight loss.[10] However, they do not supplant the need for reducing energy and fat intake, modifying problem behavior, and increasing physical activity.

proximately 50 ml, the size of a shot glass, which prevents overeating, except of liquids. Overeating solid foods rapidly results in vomiting. The gastric bypass approach also reduces absorption of consumed food. About 75% of people with severe obesity eventually lose about 50% of body weight after gastroplasty, and they can maintain much of that weight loss over time.[24] This dramatic loss occurs because only small amounts of food can be eaten throughout the day. So people who have had gastroplasty are forced to do what was difficult to do before—eat less.

EXPERT OPINION

VERY-LOW-CALORIE DIETS IN THE TREATMENT OF OBESITY

JUDY LOPER, Ph.D., R.D., L.D.

In the early 1970s, research in Boston and Cleveland examined the use of supplemental fasting for the treatment of severe (morbid) obesity. Since that time the popularity, composition of the regimens, and public perception of this method of weight control have varied. Many diet plans have evolved.

In the late 1970s, there were 58 deaths reported among obese adults using "liquid protein" diets. These diets provided 300 to 500 kcal/day and contained protein of low biological value (collagen or gelatin). No medical supervision accompanied these very-low-calorie diets, as they were self-prescribed. These deaths were thought to be linked to the inadequate amino acid composition and low amounts of potassium and other minerals, which contributed to considerable loss of muscle mass, including heart muscle.

TODAY'S MEDICALLY SUPERVISED VERY-LOW-CALORIE DIETS

Very-low-calorie diets (VLCDs) today supply 400 to 800 kcal/day. They are designed to promote considerable weight loss while preserving lean body mass. To do this, these diets provide 70 to 100 g/day of high-quality protein (egg or milk) either (1) in a powdered formulation that must be mixed with water or a low-calorie fluid or (2) in the form of lean meat, fish, or fowl. The liquid forms of the diet often contain 30 to 120 g of carbohydrate and supplemental vitamins and minerals, including potassium. These are added to promote retention of lean body mass and to minimize some medical complications.

The VLCD using lean meat generally contains 1.2 g of protein per kg of desirable body weight and very little carbohydrate. Extra vitamins and minerals are given along with this diet. These VLCDs promote weekly weight losses of about 3 pounds in women and 4 pounds in men.

INDICATIONS FOR THE VLCD

There are a limited number of therapeutic alternatives in the treatment of the severely obese person. Most programs that use the VLCD limit the use of it to persons who are 30% or greater above desirable body weight. Many of these people have concurrent health problems (i.e., hypertension, diabetes, hyperlipidemia, arthritis, sleep apnea, and coronary heart disease). Even with a modest weight loss on a VLCD, many of these medical problems can be minimized or reduced.

CONTRAINDICATIONS

Contraindications for the VLCD are pregnancy or lactation, ongoing substance abuse, recent myocardial infarction (within 3 months), kidney or liver failure, cerebrovascular disease (stroke), transient ischemic heart disease, and only mild overweight status. Mildly overweight individuals have less fat stores and may tend to lose more lean body mass than the more obese person who follows a VLCD. Less drastic weight loss methods are generally more appropriate for this population group.

MEDICAL MONITORING

Medical monitoring by experienced physicians includes initial screening,

laboratory work, an electrocardiogram, physical examination, and body composition analysis. Safe use of these diets includes medical monitoring through refeeding and weight maintenance.

The length of time a person should diet depends on the person's initial weight, medical history, and the rate of weight loss. Twelve to 16 weeks of a VLCD has been shown to be safe; some studies have reported safe use for longer than that.

Unsupervised use of VLCDs is dangerous. This includes the use of powdered diets that can be purchased at health food stores and in the supermarket and are self-administered. Careful physician scrutiny must be part of the process.

THE PROGRAM

A comprehensive VLCD program includes behavior modification, nutrition education, plus some cognitive therapy (see Chapter 11 for examples) and exercise instruction. Reports of the effectiveness of the VLCD without behavior modification and nutrition education are dismal. Preparation for refeeding and maintenance needs to be made early. Some programs use the "open-group" approach, in which a person stays on the VLCD until he or she reaches goal weight. Then the person refeeds gradually back to a regular food diet. Other programs use the "closed-group" approach, in which a group of people start the program together, and they stay on the same time sequence for weight loss, refeeding, and maintenance. In this program the VLCD may be limited to 12 weeks. Some physicians may provide the medical monitoring out of their offices without the help of ancillary personnel, such as the registered dietitian, exercise physiologist, and psychologist. This is not thought to be as effective as multidisciplinary care.

VLCDs can have some temporary side effects, such as dizziness, muscle cramping, headaches, cold intolerance, and constipation or diarrhea. When quickly identified and medically managed, these problems can be easily corrected or minimized.

RISKS OF VLCD THERAPY

Studies now under way are exploring the risk of gallstones and VLCD-linked weight loss. People are at risk for gallstones just by being obese (1% risk). Results of some of the studies show up to a 4% risk of developing symptomatic gallstones from various VLCDs. This again points to the necessity of medical monitoring when on the VLCD.

Those people who diet without medical monitoring risk having short-term complications turn into more serious ones, like heart dysfunction and potassium depletion. Currently there are formulas being promoted by the media that are to be used as replacements for not more than two meals per day. Misuse of these can have dangerous consequences. Their unsupervised nature opens the door to abuse, such as skipping the balanced meals that are supposed to accompany the diet plan.

OVERALL WEIGHT LOSS

Overall weight loss with VLCDs has been substantial. In one study with a period of 13 to 14 weeks, 66% of males and 49% of females lost 40 pounds (18 g) or more. In comparison to behavior therapy alone, the weight loss on a VLCD was nearly double.

MAINTENANCE OF WEIGHT LOSS

The biggest criticism of weight-loss programs in general is the dismal experience of people unable to maintain their weight loss. Very little data exist in the literature on this for VLCDs, whether commercial programs or programs administered by health professionals.

Large clinical trials have shown some results of VLCDs. In one study, of the people who completed treatment, successful weight maintenance (defined as maintaining 60% or more of the lost excess weight at 18 months) was achieved in 46%. A five-year follow up study revealed results of post-VLCDs at 33 diverse sites across the country. One fourth of the patients showed a 20% decrease of initial body weight from treatment entry after 5 years. These patients maintained significant improvement in health risk factors. Another fourth showed a 7% decrease of initial body weight from entry, and a third group was 2% above entry.

There still is no clear standard in the scientific community for defining success of obesity treatment. Success could be defined as risk-factor reduction, such as the lowering of blood pressure levels. It could also be defined as a partial normalization of body weight or prevention of continued weight gain. Another evaluation of success might be psychosocial factors, such as improvement of the quality of life with weight loss.

Some research is now being done examining a combination of approaches to aid in long-term weight maintenance. There has been a reevaluation of the use of anti-obesity drugs either for weight loss or weight maintenance. Initial results are encouraging and have shown a beneficial effect when treatments are combined. Patients lose weight first on a VLCD, and follow-up utilizes anti-obesity medications. Some success has also been shown when patients have continued to use some formula diets and prepackaged foods in maintenance to help control food intake.

Some programs, but not all, offer a maintenance phase and an ongoing maintenance program. Ideally, follow-up should be long-term and should include further reinforcement of eating, exercise, and lifestyle habits conducive to weight maintenance. One thing is clear from evaluating studies dealing with weight maintenance: people who complete the entire treatment have a better chance of maintaining the weight that they have lost. Also, multidisciplinary care appears to improve long-term results.

Dr. Loper practices dietetics in Columbus, Ohio, and has many years of experience working with people following VLCD therapy.

Gastroplasty is costly and often not covered by medical insurance. There is also nothing magical about the surgery. The person does not awaken from anesthesia thin. Instead, torturous months must be endured while weight loss occurs. A side effect of this surgery can be deficiencies of nutrients, such as vitamin B-12, folate, and iron, since it is difficult to ingest and/or absorb sufficient quantities of these nutrients to meet body needs. This side effect can be treated with vitamin and mineral supplementation.[9]

People who have had gastroplasty and lost much weight typically no longer need medication for the **co-morbid** conditions commonly associated with obesity (i.e., diabetes, hypertension, and high blood lipids).

co-morbidity Disease linked to another disease, such as heart disease and certain forms of cancer that are more common in someone who has obesity. *Morbidity* refers to disease.

very-low-calorie diet (VLCD) Also known as a *protein-sparing modified fast (PSMF)*, this diet allows the consumption of 400 to 800 kcal/day, generally in a liquid form. Of this, about 120 to 480 kcal comes from carbohydrate; the rest comes from mostly high–biological value protein.

Very-Low-Calorie Diets

If more traditional diet changes have failed, treating severe obesity with a **very-low-calorie diet (VLCD)** is possible.[20] Commercial programs include Optifast. Some researchers believe people with body weight greater than 30% above desirable weight are also appropriate candidates. The diet allows a person to eat 400 to 800 kcal/day, often in liquid form. (These diets were known earlier as *protein-sparing modified fasts.*) Of this amount, about 30 to 120 g (120 to 480 kcal) is carbohydrate. The rest is high–biological value protein, supplying about 70 to 100 g/day (280 to 400 kcal). This low carbohydrate intake often causes ketosis, which may decrease hunger. However, the main reasons for weight loss are the minimal energy allowed and the absence of food choice. About 3 to 5 pounds can be lost per week: men tend to lose at a higher rate than women. When physical activity and weight training are combined with this diet, a greater loss of adipose tissue occurs.

Weight regain is a nagging problem with this type of therapy to date. If behavior therapy and physical activity are used with a long-term support program, maintenance of the weight loss is more likely.[20] Dr. Judy Loper discusses this therapy approach in her Expert Opinion.

CONCEPT CHECK

When a person is faced with severe obesity and previous failures with conservative weight-loss strategies, other options can be considered. Either surgery to reduce the volume of the stomach to approximately 50 ml or a very-low-calorie diet of 400 to 800 kcal/day may be used.

Fad Diets—Why All the Commotion?

Many overweight people try to help themselves using the latest fad diet book. But as you will see, most of these diets do not help, and some can actually harm those who follow them (Table 9-5).

You may wonder why fad diet books exist at all. Why doesn't the government put a stop to them? Many contain blatant misinformation. However, FDA concerns itself only when products are suspected of doing serious harm, as in the case of earlier forms of liquid protein diets. FDA is too busy to pursue every new fad diet plan. So ancient advice is still valid: "Let the buyer beware." Responsibility rests with the authors and publishers, who want to sell books and earn money, and know there is little risk involved. Making outrageous claims sells more books than writing "eat less fat and walk more." Diet quackery has existed for many years (Figure 9-9). Dr. Stephen Barrett discusses the psychology behind diet quackery in the Nutrition Perspective for this chapter.

- - - - - - - - - - - - - -
It is illegal in the United States to falsely represent worthless or dangerous cures and medical devices. Thus U.S. citizens can use their rights under federal law to have FDA pursue a seller of a dangerous fad diet book in an attempt to have it removed from the market.
- - - - - - - - - - - - - -

HOW TO RECOGNIZE A FAD DIET

We listed criteria earlier in this chapter for evaluating weight-loss programs with regard to their safety and effectiveness. In contrast, fad diets typically share some different common characteristics. We list a few here:

1. They promote quick weight loss. As mentioned before, this loss is primarily due to glycogen, sodium, and lean muscle mass depletion. All lead to a loss of body water.
2. They limit food selections and dictate specific rituals, such as eating only fruit for breakfast.
3. They use testimonials from famous people and tie the diet to well-known cities, such as Beverly Hills and New York.
4. They bill themselves as "cure-alls." Whatever the type of obesity or whatever a person's specific strengths and weaknesses, these diets claim to work for everyone.
5. They often recommend expensive supplements. Some of these supplements can be harmful because of high doses of vitamin A, vitamin D, vitamin C, or vitamin B-6 (pyridoxine).
6. No attempts are made to permanently change eating habits. The dieter follows the diet until the desired weight is reached and then reverts to old eating habits. Eat rice for a month, lose weight, and then return to old habits.
7. They are generally critical of and skeptical about the scientific community. They suggest that physicians and registered dietitians do not really want people to lose weight. They encourage people to look outside the medical establishment for correct advice.

Probably the cruelest characteristic of fad diets is that they essentially guarantee failure for the dieter. These diets are not designed for permanent weight loss. Habits are not changed, and the food selection is so limited that the person cannot follow the diet for more than 1 or 2 weeks. Although dieters assume they have lost fat, they have actually lost mostly muscle and other lean tissue mass. As soon as they begin eating normally again, the lost tissue is replaced. In a matter of weeks, most of the lost weight is back. The dieter appears to have failed, when actually the diet has failed. This whole scenario can add more blame and guilt to the psyche and challenge the self-worth of the dieter—and that is very unfortunate. If someone needs help losing weight, professional help is the answer. Sound nutrition and regular physical activity are the only approaches that come close to offering hope for weight loss and later weight management, and that is something fad diets rarely offer.[13]

TYPES OF FAD DIETS
Low-Carbohydrate Approaches

This is the most common form of fad diet. The low carbohydrate intake forces the liver to perform gluconeogenesis (see Chapters 3 and 7). The source of carbons for gluconeogenesis is mostly protein tissue. Thus a low-carbohydrate diet results in protein tissue loss, as well as urinary loss of essential ions, such as potassium. Since protein tissue is mostly water, the dieter loses weight very rapidly. When a normal diet is resumed, the protein tissue is rebuilt and the weight is regained.

There is nothing special about a low-carbohydrate diet in terms of weight loss. If the diet is also low in energy, then it is likely to result in weight loss. But a low-carbohydrate diet by itself does not result in more weight loss than any other type of diet.

Diet plans that use a low-carbohydrate approach are the Dr. Atkins' Diet Revolution, Dr. Stillman's Calories Don't Count Diet, the Scarsdale Diet, the Drinking Man's Diet, Four Day Wonder diet, and the Air Force Diet. When you see a new fad diet advertisement, look first to see how much carbohydrate it contains. If breads, cereals, fruits, and vegetables are extremely limited, you are probably looking at a **ketogenic** diet.

Low-Fat Approaches

The very-low-fat diet turns out to be a very-high-carbohydrate diet. These diets contain approximately 5% to 10% of energy intake as fat. The most notable is the Pritikin Diet. This approach is not harmful for healthy adults, but it is extremely difficult to follow. People get bored with this type of diet very quickly because many of their favorite foods cannot be eaten. The dieter primarily eats grains, fruits, and

Marie's been reading a lot about new ways to lose weight. She's a typical teenager, obsessed with her weight. You want to prevent the serious health consequences that may occur if she goes on a fad diet. What are the criteria you would advise her to look for to avoid fad diets and instead choose a healthy one?

ketogenic Describes diets that lead to the production of ketones by the liver due to low carbohydrate intake.

TABLE 9-5

Summary of popular diet approaches to weight control

Approach and examples*	Characteristics and possible negative health consequences
Moderate kilocalorie restriction	
The Setpoint Diet	Usually 1000-1800 kcal/day, with moderate fat intake
Slim Chance in a Fat World	Reasonable balance of macronutrients
Weight Watcher's Diet	Encourages exercise
The American Heart Association Diet	May employ behavioral approach
Mary Ellen's Help Yourself Diet Plan	
The Beyond Diet	Acceptable if vitamin and mineral supplement is used and permission of family physician is granted
Nutripoints	
The Good Calorie Diet	
The Callaway Diet	
Fast Food Diet	
50 Ways to Lose Your Blubber	
Macronutrient restriction	
Low carbohydrate	
Dr. Atkins' Diet Revolution	Less than 100 g of carbohydrate per day
Calories Don't Count	
Wild Weekend Diet	Ketosis; poor exercise capacity due to poor glycogen stores in the muscles; excessive animal fat intake
Miracle Diet for Fast Weight Loss	
Drinking Man's Diet	
Woman Doctor's Diet for Women	
The Doctor's Quick Weight Loss Diet	
The Complete Scarsdale Medical Diet	
Four Day Wonder Diet	
Endocrine Control Diet	
Air Force Diet	
Low fat	
The Rice Diet Report	Less than 20% of energy from fat
The Macrobiotic Diet (some versions)	Limited (or elimination of) animal protein sources; also all fats, nuts, seeds
The Pritikin Diet	
The Tokyo Diet	
The Palm Beach Lifelong Diet	Little satiety; flatulence; possibly poor mineral absorption from excess fiber; limited food choices leads to deprivation
The James Coco Diet	
The 35+ Diet	
7-Week Victory Diet	
Fat to Muscle Diet	
T-Factor Diet	
Fit or Fat	
Two Day Diet	
Complete Hip and Thigh Diet	
The Maximum Metabolism Diet	
The Pasta Diet	
The McDougall Plan	
Ultrafit Diet	
Stop the Insanity	
G-Index Diet	
Eat More, Weigh Less	
Outsmarting the Female Fat Cell	
Foods that Cause You to Lose Weight	

*Diets may be listed in more than one category if multiple characteristics apply.

TABLE 9-5—cont'd

Summary of popular diet approaches to weight control

Approach and examples	**Characteristics and possible negative health consequences**
Novelty diets	
Dr. Abravanel's Body Type and Lifetime Nutrition Plan (or his other books) Dr. Berger's Immune Power Diet	Promotes certain nutrients, foods, or combinations of foods as having unique, magical, or previously undiscovered qualities Malnutrition; no change in habits leads to relapse; unrealistic food choices leads to possible bingeing
Fit for Life The Rotation Diet The Hilton Head Metabolism Diet The Junk Food Diet The Beverly Hills Diet Dr. Debetz Champagne Diet Sun Sign Diet F-Plan Diet Fat Attack Plan Popcorn Plus Diet Jean Simpson's Numbers Diet Autohypnosis Diet The Ultrafit Diet The Princeton Plan The Diet Bible Bloomingdale's Diet The Love Diet Eat to Succeed The Underburner's Diet Eat to Win Two Day Diet Paris Diet	
Very-low-calorie diets (VLCDs)	
Optifast Cambridge Diet The Last Chance Diet Genesis Medifast New Direction	Less than 800 kcal/day Also known as protein-sparing modified fasts Must be under close physician scrutiny Organ tissue loss—especially from the heart; low serum potassium leads to heart failure; expense; kidney stones; gout
HMR Ultrafast Thin So Fast	
Formula diets	
U.S.A. (United States of America), Inc. Optifast	 Can help people who find it easier not to eat whole foods while dieting to lose weight
Genesis Cambridge Diet Herbalife The Last Chance Diet	 Based on formulated or packaged products Many are very low-kilocalorie diet regimens (see above); no change in habits leads to increased chance of relapse; expense; constipation
Slimfast	
Premeasured diets	
Jenny Craig	Most food supplied in premeasured servings to take much of the decision making out of the process of eating Expense; may not allow for easy sound eating later

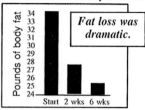

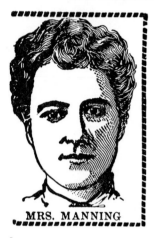

35 Pounds of Fat.

DR. EDISON'S OBESITY PILLS AND REDUCING TAB-LETS CURED MRS. MANNING.

No Other Remedies But Dr. Edison's Reduce Obesity—Take No Others.

SAMPLES FREE—USE COUPON.

Mary Hyde Manning, one of the best known of Troy's, New York, society women, grew too fleshy, and used Dr. Edison's Obesity Remedies. Read the letter telling of her reduction and restoration to health:—"In six weeks I was reduced 35 pounds, from 171 to 136, by Dr. Edison's Obesity Pills and Reducing Tablets. I recommend these remedies to all fat and sick men and women."

The following well-known men and women have been reduced by DR. EDISON'S OBESITY REMEDIES:

Mrs. H. Mershon, 156 South Jackson St., Lima, O., 148 lbs.
Mrs. Josephine McPherson, 7916 Wright St., Chicago, 42 lbs.
Rev. Edward R. Pierce, 410 Alma St., Chicago, 42 lbs.
C. C. Nichols, 145 Clark St., Aurora, Ill., 86 lbs.
Mrs. W. Davlin, Whitemore, O., 149 lbs.
W. H. Webster, 618 2d Ave., Troy, N. Y., 26 lbs.
J. M. McKinney, 4504 State St., Chicago, 30 lbs.
Mrs. J. M. McKinney, 4504 State St., Chicago, 33 lbs.
Mrs. A. Walker, 1104 Milton Place, Chicago, 20 lbs.

MRS. MANNING

A

22% LESS BODY FAT IN SIX WEEKS

University studies have identified CHROMIUM PICOLINATE as a "trigger" for fat loss and lean muscle enhancement. 200 micrograms taken daily caused a 22% fat loss in only 6 weeks.

Fat loss was dramatic.

Men and women of every age are talking about the amazing benefits of this safe, essential nutrient:

WEIGHT LOSS • FAT LOSS
MORE ENDURANCE AND STAMINA
MORE LEAN MUSCLE

BODY GOLD is made to the exact specifications of the capsules used in the studies cited above. Each bottle of 60 capsules is a 2-month supply.

SATISFACTION GUARANTEED
(Check or money order only. Canada: U.S. $ m.o.)

Please rush _____ bottles of BODY GOLD @ $10.95 each + $2.50 total delivery.

Name_____

Address_____

City_____ State_____ Zip_____

BODY GOLD, 5930 La Jolla Hermosa, Dept. NH-123, La Jolla, CA 92037

B

Figure 9-9 Quackery has been with us for ages. **A,** Even at the turn of the century, people wanted to believe that fat could be lost without changing habits or without much effort, and **B,** many still do.

vegetables, and most people cannot do this for very long. Eventually, the person wants some foods higher in fat or protein. Thus the dieter suffers a lapse, then a relapse, and probably a collapse. These diets are just too different from the typical American diet to follow consistently. A popular diet marketed recently, the T-Factor Diet, focuses on restricting fat but is a more moderate approach than the Pritikin diet.

Novelty Diets

A whole variety of diets are built on gimmicks. The Rotation Diet, for example, rotates the amount of energy ingested in an attempt to prevent the usual drop in basal metabolism associated with dieting. A woman is supposed to eat 600 kcal/day for 3 days, then 900 kcal/day for 4 days, and then 1200 kcal/day for 7 days, repeating this cycle over and over again. For men, the levels are 1200, 1500, and 1800 kcal. No scientific data show that this diet works or even how it could work. Thus it must be considered a fad diet.

Other novelty diets emphasize one food or food group and exclude almost all others. A rice diet was designed in the 1940s to lower blood pressure; now it has resurfaced as a weight-loss diet. The first phase consists of eating only rice and fruit until you cannot stand them any longer. Another novelty diet is the egg diet, on which you eat all the eggs you want. On the Beverly Hills Diet, you eat mostly fruit.

The rationale behind these diets is that you can eat only eggs, fruit, or rice for just so long, and that you will soon become bored and, in theory, reduce energy intake. However, chances are that you will abandon the diet entirely before losing much weight.

Since the 1960s grapefruits have been touted for their supposed unique ability to cause weight loss. No studies back up this claim. To add appeal to a grapefruit diet, proponents even suggest adding several "diet aids": lecithin to help release fat from the tissues, vitamin B-6 to act as a diuretic, vinegar to provide potassium, and kelp to stimulate the thyroid gland.

The most bizarre of the novelty diets proposes that "food gets stuck in your body." Fit for Life and the Beverly Hills Diet are examples. The supposition is that food gets stuck in the intestine, putrefies, and creates toxins that invade the blood and cause disease. This is utter nonsense (see Chapter 6). Nevertheless, the same idea has been promoted in health food books since the 1800s. Today, Fit for Life suggests that meat eaten with potatoes is not digested and that fresh fruit only be consumed before noon. These recommendations are absurd. They are gimmicks that appear controversial but are really designed to sell books.

Finally, some commercial schemes are used to sell diet books. Books describing the allergy approach to dieting, for instance, suggest that diseases, including obesity, are due to food allergies. Supposedly, once your food allergies are found and treated, you will no longer have the disease. However, we know of no research that supports the claim that 30% of people have food allergies, as suggested in Dr. Berger's Immune Power Diet Book. In addition, see the Sun Sign Diet if you believe in astrology, the Champagne Diet if you need a drink, or the Body Type and Lifetime Nutrition Diet if you have a "dominant" gland.

QUACKERY IS CHARACTERISTIC OF FAD DIETS

Fad diets fall under the category of quackery, people taking advantage of others. There is usually a product or service involved that costs a considerable amount of money. Often those offering the product or service don't realize that they are promoting quackery, because they were victims themselves. For example, they tried the product and by pure coincidence it worked for them, so they wish to sell it to all their friends and relatives.

Victims of quackery may be desperate people who cannot be helped by conventional methods so they are willing to try anything. However, a victim can be anyone who hears of a "scientific breakthrough" and wishes to give it a try.

Recent examples of quackery in the field of weight loss are thigh-reducing creams, chromium picolinate, and "Quickly." The thigh-reducing creams contain aminophylline, an asthma drug, that is thought to increase fat metabolism. The product was in fact developed by obesity researchers famous in the scientific community. So there is a legitimate science behind the concept. However, the researchers did not intend their work to be on the market yet. Few people using the product have been carefully studied, and there are still many other unanswered questions that have serious implications, such as "Where does the fat go?" Allergic reactions to the product are also possible.

Chromium picolinate, a nutritional supplement, has been touted as an aid for reducing body fat, increasing lean body mass, suppressing hunger, and increasing metabolic rate. However, chromium picolinate has not been approved for weight loss by FDA, nor has the agency seen any data on the claims being made (see the Expert Opinion in Chapter 15 for more details).

"Quickly" is a product that was marketed for weight loss. After about 5000 containers were sold, they were found to contain significant amounts of the prescription drug furosemide, a powerful diuretic. Furosemide is used for people who have congestive heart failure, liver and kidney disease, and hypertension. The unsupervised use of this product could have serious health implications.

Usually, quackery harms only the bank account. However, it can lead to life-threatening results. The rule of thumb upon seeing a new product on the market is that if it sounds too good to be true, it probably is.

Numerous other gimmicks for weight loss have come and gone and are likely to resurface. If in the future an important aid for weight loss is discovered, you can feel confident that major journals, such as the *Journal of the American Dietetic Association*, the *Journal of the American Medical Association*, or the *New England Journal of Medicine*, will report it. You don't need to rely on paperback books or newspaper advertisements for information about weight loss.

CONCEPT CHECK

Fad diets characteristically promote quick weight loss and limited food selections, use testimonials from famous people, bill the plan as a cure-all, include expensive supplements, and show little concern for permanently changing food habits. Typical approaches include low-carbohydrate regimens, low-fat regimens, and novel approaches, which often consist of complex food-combining rules or a focus on one type of food, such as rice or fruit. Quackery is ubiquitous and not always easy to recognize. New products and services are often introduced to the public through the media. Recent examples of quackery are thigh-reducing creams, chromium picolinate, and "Quickly."

Treating Underweight

underweight Body weight for height about 15% to 20% below desirable weight, or a body mass index below about 19. These cut-offs are less precise than for obesity, since this condition has been less studied.

Underweight can be caused by a variety of factors, such as anorexia nervosa, cancer, infectious disease, digestive tract disorders, and excessive physical activity. Genetic background may also lead to a higher resting metabolic rate and/or a slight body frame. As you can see in Figure 8-7, underweight is also associated with increased death rates, especially when combined with cigarette smoking.[15] Most of the time we hear about the risks of obesity, but not underweight. In our society being underweight is much more socially acceptable than being obese.

Sometimes being underweight requires medical intervention. A physician should be consulted first to rule out hormonal imbalances, depression, cancer, infectious disease, digestive tract disorders, excessive physical activity, and other hidden disease, such as anorexia nervosa or bulimia nervosa. Risks associated with being underweight include the loss of menstrual function in women, complications during pregnancy and surgery, and slow recovery after illness. Underweight women may have menstrual irregularities, stop menstruating altogether (which is associated with bone loss—see Chapter 11), risk infertility, and deliver low-birthweight babies.

The causes of underweight are not altogether different from the causes of obesity. Internal and external satiety signal irregularities, rate of metabolism, hereditary tendencies, and psychological traits can all contribute to being underweight.

In growing children, the demand for energy to support physical activity and growth can cause underweight. During growth spurts in adolescence, an active child may not take the time to consume enough energy to support his or her energy needs. And gaining weight can be a formidable task for an underweight person. More than 500 extra kilocalories per day may be required to gain weight, even at a slow pace, due in part to the expenditure of energy in adaptive thermogenesis. In contrast to the weight loser, the weight gainer may need to increase portion sizes and learn to like new energy-dense foods.

When underweight requires intervention, one approach for treating adults is to gradually increase their consumption of energy-dense foods (foods that provide much energy in a small volume), especially those high in vegetable fat. Italian cheeses, nuts, and granola are good energy sources with low saturated fat content. Dried fruit and bananas are energy-dense fruit choices. If eaten at the end of a meal, they don't cause early satiety. Underweight people should replace such foods as diet soft drinks with good energy sources like fruit juices.

Keeping a daily food record for weekly review can help point toward wise high-energy food choices (the right side of Table 9-2 lists some possible choices). In addition, encouraging a regular meal and snack schedule aids in weight gain and maintenance. Sometimes people who are underweight have experienced stress at work or have been too busy to eat. Making regular meals a priority can not only aid with attaining an appropriate weight, but can also help with digestive disorders, such as constipation, which are sometimes associated with irregular eating times.

A physically active person can reduce activity. If weight still stays low, a weight-lifting program could be used to add muscle mass, but energy intake must be increased to support that physical activity. Otherwise, weight gain will be hindered.

If these efforts fail to achieve the desired weight, they should at least prevent health problems associated with being underweight. After achieving that, the person may have to accept his or her very lean frame.

Summary

1. When considering a treatment for obesity, five points should be remembered: (1) a focus on healthy lifestyle rather than weight loss per se would be more appropriate for many potential and current dieters; (2) the body resists weight loss; (3) the emphasis should be on preventing obesity, since curing the disorder is very difficult; (4) weight loss on a diet should represent mostly a loss of fat storage and not primarily the loss of muscle and other lean tissues; and (5) rapid weight loss and quick regain can be harmful to physical and emotional health both short and long term.

2. A sound weight-loss diet meets the dieter's nutritional needs by emphasizing low-fat and nonfat food choices from the Food Guide Pyramid; it adapts to the dieter's habits, consists of readily obtainable foods, strives to change poor eating habits, recommends regular physical activity, and insists the person see a physician if weight is to be lost rapidly or if the person is over 35 years of age and plans to perform substantially greater physical activity than usual.

3. A pound of adipose tissue lost or gained represents approximately 2700 kcal. Thus if energy output exceeds energy intake by about 400 kcal/day, a pound of fat storage can be lost per week. Decreasing the intake of high-fat foods is probably the best way to obtain this energy deficit, along with increasing physical activity.

4. Physical activity as part of a weight-loss program should be focused on duration rather than intensity. Ideally, approximately 200 to 300 kcal should be expended in vigorous activity each day.

5. Behavior modification is a vital part of a weight-loss program because the dieter may have many habits that encourage overeating and thus discourage weight maintenance. Specific behavior-modification techniques, such as stimulus control and self-monitoring, can be used to help change problem behavior.

6. It is important to have a personal behavior-change plan to lose weight and keep it off. Assessing commitment and current behavior is an important first step. After that, goals should be established with appropriate rewards. These goals should be written in a contract and witnessed by significant others.

7. Treatment of severe obesity includes surgery to reduce stomach volume to approximately 50 ml or very-low-calorie diets containing 400 to 800 kcal/day. Both these procedures should be reserved for people who have failed at more conservative approaches to weight loss. They require medical supervision.

8. Medications to aid weight loss that are available over-the-counter in drug stores include phenylpropanolamine, benzocaine, and fiber pills. None of these, however, can substitute entirely for a good diet, behavior, and physical activity plan.

9. Fad diets are easy to recognize. They often promote rapid weight loss, have limited food selections, offer testimonials from famous people, are billed as "cure-alls," include expensive supplements, and make little or no attempt to permanently alter food habits. General criticism of and skepticism about the scientific community is also common.

10. Fad diets can be classified as low-carbohydrate approaches, low-fat approaches, and novel approaches. The latter category includes diets with complex food-combining rituals and those that focus on one type of food to the exclusion of most others. A fad diet is a form of quackery.

Study Questions

1. What are the major psychological and physiological problems associated with rapid weight loss?

2. When searching for a sound weight-loss program, what key characteristics would you look for?

3. You are following a nutritional plan for weight loss. What are five specific ways you could reduce energy intake?

4. Describe the term *behavior modification*. Relate it to the terms *stimulus control, self-monitoring, chain breaking, relapse prevention,* and *cognitive restructuring*. Give examples of each of the latter.

5. Describe the type of physical activity you would suggest for someone who is obese.

6. Why should the treatment of obesity be viewed as a lifelong commitment, rather than just a short episode of weight loss?

7. What are some current examples of quackery related to weight loss?

8. In a weight-loss program for someone who is obese, how would you approach the problem of later weight maintenance?

9. Since there are many co-morbid conditions associated with being overweight, is it healthier to weigh significantly less than one's desirable body weight? Why or why not?

10. If a friend or relative told you they found a great new vitamin and mineral supplement that will allow them to lose 12 pounds in 2 weeks, how would you respond?

REFERENCES

1. Abernathy RP, Black DR: Is adipose tissue oversold as a health risk? *Journal of the American Dietetic Association* 94:641, 1994.

2. ADA Reports: Position of the American Dietetic Association and the Canadian Dietetic Association: women's health and nutrition, *Journal of the American Dietetic Association* 95:362, 1995.

3. Atkinson RL, Hubbard VS: Report on the NIH workshop on pharmacologic treatment of obesity, *American Journal of Clinical Nutrition* 60:153, 1994.

4. Committee to Develop Criteria for Evaluating the Outcomes of Approaches to Prevent and Treat Obesity, Food and Nutrition Board, Institute of Medicine, National Academy of Sciences: Summary: weighing the options—criteria for evaluating weight-management programs, *Journal of the American Dietetic Association* 95:96, 1995.

5. Eckel RH, Yost TJ: Weight reduction increases adipose tissue lipoprotein lipase responsiveness in obese women, *Journal of Clinical Investigation* 80:992, 1987.

6. Fletcher AM: *Thin for life: 10 keys to success from people who have lost weight and kept it off,* Shelburne, VT, 1994, Chapters Publishing.

7. Foreyt JP, Goodrick GK: Weight management without dieting, *Nutrition Today,* p 4, March/April 1993.

8. Froidevaux F and others: Energy expenditure in obese women before and during weight loss, after refeeding, and in the weight-relapse period, *American Journal of Clinical Nutrition* 57:35, 1993.

9. Gastrointestinal surgery for severe obesity: National Institutes of Health Consensus Development Conference Statement, *American Journal of Clinical Nutrition* 55:615S, 1992.

10. Goldstein DJ, and Potvin JH: Long-term weight loss: the effect of pharmacologic agents, *American Journal of Clinical Nutrition* 60:647, 1994.

11. Haus G and others: Key modifiable factors in weight maintenance: fat intake, physical activity, and weight cycling, *Journal of the American Dietetic Association* 94:409, 1994.

12. Hirsh J: Herman Award Lecture, 1994: Establishing the biological basis for obesity, *American Journal of Clinical Nutrition* 60:613, 1994.

13. Institute of Food Technologists' Expert Panel on Food Safety and Nutrition: Human obesity, *Food Technology,* p 127, Feb 1994.

14. Karklin A and others: Restricted energy intake affects nocturnal body temperature and sleep patterns, *American Journal of Clinical Nutrition* 59:346, 1994.

15. Kushner RF: Body weight and mortality, *Nutrition Reviews* 51:127, 1993.

16. Leibel RL and others: Changes in expenditure resulting from altered body weight, *New England Journal of Medicine* 332:621, 1995.

17. Lewitsky DA: Imprecise control of food intake on low-fat diets. In Kotsonis FN, Mackey MA, editors: *Nutrition in the 90's,* New York, 1994, Mercel Dekker.

18. Miller WC and others: Dietary fat, sugar, and fiber predict body fat content, *Journal of the American Dietetic Association* 94:612, 1994.

19. Mortenson GM and others: Predictors of body satisfaction in college women, *Journal of the American Dietetic Association* 93:1037, 1993.

20. National Task Force on the Prevention and Treatment of Obesity: Very low-calorie diets, *Journal of the American Medical Association* 270:967, 1993.

21. NIH Task Force on the Prevention and Treatment of Obesity: Weight cycling, *Journal of the American Medical Association* 273:999, 1995.

22. Owen OE: Regulation of energy metabolism. In Kinney JM and others, editors: *Nutrition and metabolism in patient care,* Philadelphia, 1988, WB Saunders.

23. Racette SB and others: Effects of aerobic exercise and dietary carbohydrate on energy expenditure and body composition during weight reduction in obese women, *American Journal of Clinical Nutrition* 61:486, 1995.

24. Reinhold RB: Late results of gastric bypass surgery for morbid obesity, *Journal of the American College of Nutrition* 13:326, 1994.

25. Rising R and others: Determinants of total daily energy expenditure: variability in physical activity, *American Journal of Clinical Nutrition* 59:800, 1994.

26. Robinson JI and others: Redefining success in obesity intervention: the new paradigm, *Journal of the American Dietetic Association* 95:422, 1995.

27. Shah M and others: Comparison of a low-fat, ad libitum complex-carbohydrate diet with a low-energy diet in moderately obese women, *American Journal of Clinical Nutrition* 59:980, 1994.

28. Wing R: Behavioral treatment of severe obesity, *American Journal of Clinical Nutrition* 55:545S, 1992.

29. Wooley SC, Garner DM: Obesity treatment: the high cost of false hope, *Journal of the American Dietetic Association* 91:1248, 1991.

TAKE ACTION

➤ Is the Lipoloss Weight-Loss Plan for you?

Read the following discussion of the Lipoloss Weight-Loss Plan. See if it is one you would want to follow.

- -

Do you want to turn your body into a high-powered fat burner? Try the Lipoloss Weight-Loss Plan, scientifically proven to be the quickest and most permanent fat-loss miracle in America. The nutritional part of the Lipoloss Plan consists of eating 800 kcal of delicious tuna, turkey, fruits, and vegetables. Combine the fruits with the turkey and the vegetables with the tuna to achieve the greatest lipoloss effect (remember, *lipo* means "fat").

We encourage at least 30 minutes of aerobic physical activity—brisk walking, jogging, swimming, or biking—daily. And we haven't forgotten those diet-wrecking urges and cravings. Fight them with our high-fiber Urgesmasher Wafers. These wafers fill you up, fighting the gnaw of hunger.

If you have any health problems, see your physician for approval and clearance for regular physical activity.

Overall, with the Lipoloss Plan you can lose 3 to 5 pounds each week and enjoy a variety of tasty foods.

- -

Now rate this diet based on the following questions: a perfect score of 100 points indicates a good weight-loss plan. For every "no" answer to the questions below, subtract 10 points.

1. Will the diet meet all nutritional needs with a wide variety of foods? IF NOT, SUBTRACT 10 POINTS.
2. Does the program stress slow and steady weight loss of about 1 to 2 pounds per week, rather than rapid loss? IF NOT, SUBTRACT 10 POINTS.
3. Is the diet tailored to individual habits and tastes, diminishing feelings of deprivation? IF NOT, SUBTRACT 10 POINTS.
4. Does the plan avoid rigid rituals, such as eating fruits only in the morning or not eating meat after milk products? IF NOT, SUBTRACT 10 POINTS.
5. Does the diet minimize hunger and fatigue by containing at least 1000 kcal/day? IF NOT, SUBTRACT 10 POINTS.
6. Does the diet include readily obtainable foods, with no special products to buy to speed weight loss? IF NOT, SUBTRACT 10 POINTS.
7. Is the diet socially acceptable, allowing the dieter to attend parties, eat at restaurants, and participate in normal daily activities? IF NOT, SUBTRACT 10 POINTS.
8. Does the plan promote changes in eating habits and lifestyle so that weight maintenance will be possible? IF NOT, SUBTRACT 10 POINTS.
9. Does the plan emphasize regular physical activity? IF NOT, SUBTRACT 10 POINTS.
10. Does the plan encourage the dieter to see a physician before starting if the person has existing health problems, wants quick weight loss, is over 35 years of age, or plans to perform vigorous physical activity? IF NOT, SUBTRACT 10 POINTS.

Having assessed the Lipoloss Weight-Loss Plan, how many points would you give it? _____ SCORE

Would you choose this weight-loss plan if you were attempting to lose fat and keep it off? _____ Yes _____ No

Ten Common Misconceptions about Quackery

STEPHEN BARRETT, M.D.

Misconception 1: Quackery Is Easy to Spot

Quackery is far more difficult to spot than most people realize. Modern promoters use scientific jargon, which can fool people unfamiliar with the concepts being discussed. Even health professionals can have difficulty separating fact from fiction in fields unrelated to their expertise.

Misconception 2: Personal Experience Is the Best Way to Tell Whether Something Works

When you feel better after having used a product or procedure, it is natural to give credit to whatever you have done. This effect can be misleading, however, because most ailments resolve by themselves, and those that don't can have variable symptoms. Even serious conditions can have sufficient day-to-day variation to enable quack methods to gain large followings. In addition, taking action often produces temporary relief of symptoms (a placebo effect). For these reasons, scientific experimentation is usually necessary to establish whether health methods actually work.

Misconception 3: Most Victims of Quackery Are Gullible

Individuals who buy one diet book or "magic" diet pill after another are indeed gullible. And so are many people who follow whatever health fads are in vogue. But the majority of quackery's victims are merely unsuspecting. People tend to believe what they hear the most. And quack ideas, particularly regarding nutrition, are everywhere. Another large group of quackery's victims is composed of individuals who have serious or chronic disease that makes them feel desperate enough to try anything that offers hope.

Alienated people, many of whom are paranoid, form another victim group. These people tend to believe that our food supply is unsafe, that drugs do more harm than good, and that doctors, drug companies, large food companies, and government agencies are not interested in protecting the public.

Misconception 4: Victims of Quackery Deserve What They Get

This misconception is based on the feeling that people who are gullible should "know better" and therefore deserve whatever they get. This feeling is a major reason why journalists, law enforcement officials, judges, and legislators seldom give priority to combating quackery. As noted earlier, however, most victims are not gullible. Nor do people deserve to suffer or die because of ignorance or desperation.

Misconception 5: Quacks Are Frauds and Crooks

Quackery is often discussed as though all its promoters were engaged in deliberate deception. This is untrue. Promoters of mail-order quackery are almost always hit-and-run artists who know their products are fakes but hope to profit before the Postal Service shuts them down. But most promoters of quackery sincerely believe in what they do.

Most people think of quackery as being promoted by quacks, charlatans, or others who are deliberately taking advantage of others. Actually, most of it is promoted by victims of quackery who share their misinformation and personal experiences with others. Quackery is also involved in misleading advertising of nonprescription drugs.

Misconception 6: Most Quackery Isn't Dangerous

Quackery can seriously harm or kill people by inducing them to abandon or delay effective treatment for serious conditions. Although the number of people harmed in this manner cannot be determined, it is not large enough or obvious enough to arouse a general public outcry. Most victims of quackery are harmed economically rather than physically. Moreover, many people believe that an unscientific method has helped them. In most cases, they have confused cause-and-effect and coincidence.

Misconception 7: "Minor" Forms of Quackery Are Harmless

Quackery involving small sums of money and no physical harm is often viewed as harmless. Examples are "nutrition insurance" with vitamin pills and wearing a copper bracelet for arthritis. But their use indicates confusion on the part of the user and vulnerability to more serious forms of quackery. There is also harm to society. Money wasted on quackery would be better spent for research, but much of it goes into the pockets of people who are spreading misinformation and trying to weaken consumer protection laws.

The Feingold diet—based on the notion that food additives cause children to be hyperactive—is an example of quackery whose potential harm is underestimated. Although the diet itself is harmless, it is probably harmful to teach children that the way they behave depends on what they eat rather than on what they feel. Also, social development can be jeopardized if eating habits subject children to ridicule or lead them to avoid group activities where forbidden foods are served.

Misconception 8: The Media Are Reliable

Most people believe that statements about health issues "wouldn't be allowed" if they weren't true. Some media outlets do achieve great accuracy. But most are willing to publish sensational viewpoints that they believe are newsworthy and will increase their audience. Radio and television talk shows abound with promoters of quackery. Even exposés on questionable methods are often "balanced" by including testimonials from satisfied customers.

There is a widespread public belief that if something isn't legitimate, publications and broadcast outlets would not allow it to be advertised. Although most outlets have some limitations, few screen out misleading advertisements for health products.

Misconception 9: Government Protects Us

Although various government agencies are involved in fighting quackery, most don't give it sufficient priority to be effective.

Misconception 10: Quackery's Success Represents Medicine's Failure

It is often suggested that people turn to quacks when doctors are brusque with them and that if doctors were more attentive, their patients would not turn to quacks. It is true that this sometimes happens, but most quackery does not involve medical care. Blaming medicine for quackery is like considering the success of astrology the fault of astronomy.

Dr. Barrett, a retired psychiatrist and consumer advocate, is coauthor/editor of 37 books, including The Health Robbers: A Close Look at Quackery in America *(Prometheus Books, 1993) and* The Vitamin Pushers *(Prometheus Books, 1994).*

CHAPTER TEN

Nutrition for Fitness

Athletes invest a lot of time and effort in training. Because they are often seeking ways to modify their diets to improve their performances, athletes make easy targets for purveyors of nutrition misinformation. Still, most athletes don't want to miss out on any advantage, whether real or perceived, that might give them the winning edge.[27]

Although good eating habits can't substitute for physical training and genetic endowment, proper diet choices are crucial to top-notch performance, contributing to endurance and helping speed repair of injured tissues. Thus nutrition knowledge helps open the door to victory. Especially for athletes who expend 2000 or more kcal/day in physical activity, diet choices can really make a difference in performance.[23]

In this chapter you will also discover how physical fitness benefits the entire body: it is essential to achieving maximum health.[2] Being physically fit, of course, is also fun, feels good, and even lessens the strain of daily activities around the house and yard. Let's now look at these concepts further.

NUTRITION AWARENESS INVENTORY

Answer these 15 statements about nutrition and fitness to test your current knowledge. If you think the statement is true or mostly true, circle T. If you think the statement is false or mostly false, circle F. Use the scoring key at the end of the book to compute your total score. Repeat this test after you have read the chapter, and compare your results.

1. **T F** A cell can use the energy stored in carbohydrate to fuel a muscle's energy demands without further modification.
2. **T F** Carbohydrates can be used to meet energy needs, but fat cannot.
3. **T F** Complete metabolism of carbohydrate does not require oxygen.
4. **T F** Carbon dioxide is a by-product of energy metabolism.
5. **T F** Even when athletes are getting RDA quantities of vitamins and minerals in their diet, consumption of certain vitamin and mineral supplements will increase their athletic performance.
6. **T F** There are no disadvantages for an athlete who attempts to lose weight during the competitive season.
7. **T F** It is particularly important for athletes to consume protein and amino acid supplements because it is hard for them to get enough through their diets.
8. **T F** A large amount of carbohydrate foods such as starches and fruits should be consumed within 2 hours after an exercise to maximize glycogen synthesis, because this is when glycogen synthesis is the greatest.
9. **T F** Sports-type drinks like PowerAde and Gatorade are not significantly better beverages for fluid replacement than water for the everyday athlete. However, for endurance athletes they may be advantageous.
10. **T F** Caffeine use has improved athletic performance in some cases.
11. **T F** A target heart rate for cardiovascular fitness is 80% to 95% of maximum heart rate.
12. **T F** Cool-down exercises are not as important as a good warm-up.
13. **T F** Thirst is a good guide for fluid replacement after hard physical activity.
14. **T F** Eating lots of carbohydrate before a 100-meter dash is important for peak performance.
15. **T F** Anabolic steroids are illegal ergogenic aids used by some athletes.

Relationship between Nutrition and Fitness

The ability to engage routinely in vigorous physical activity requires good health. The ability to perform also depends on a nutritious diet that supplies all the needed nutrients. Adequate carbohydrate intakes are especially important for enhancing the endurance of athletes and nonathletes who expend more than 2000 kcal daily.[17]

Once muscles have nutrients available to them, what determines the type of fuel muscles will use? The athlete does, to an extent, depending on how physically fit he or she is and how hard one performs. This physical fitness—defined as the ability to do moderate to vigorous activity without undue fatigue—affects fat use by the body. The greater one's fitness, the more fat used to supply energy needed for activity, especially if the activity lasts for 20 minutes or more.

Beyond affecting fuel use, the benefits of regular physical activity include improvement in several aspects of heart function, less injury, better sleep habits, and improvement in body composition (less body fat, more muscle mass).[2] Physical activity also can reduce stress and positively affect blood pressure and blood glucose regulation. In addition, it aids in weight control, both by raising resting energy expenditure and by increasing overall energy expenditure.[1]

Overall, nutrition influences physical activity, while physical activity influences nutrient use and general health.[1] Unfortunately, sedentariness is a way of life for many adult Americans. We hope you will be more than simply a spectator throughout your life (Figure 10-1).

Energy Sources for Muscle Use

As you learned in Chapter 7, cells can't directly use the energy released from breaking down glucose or triglycerides. Rather, to utilize the chemical energy in foods, body cells must first convert the energy to a specific form, called adenosine triphosphate (ATP).

ADENOSINE TRIPHOSPHATE (ATP): IMMEDIATELY USABLE ENERGY

The partial breakdown of ATP by cells to yield ADP and Pi releases usable energy for cell functions, including the muscle contractions required for locomotion. A resting muscle cell, however, contains just a small amount of stored ATP, enough to keep the muscle working maximally for about 2 to 4 seconds. To produce more ATP for muscle contraction over extended periods, the body uses **phosphocreatine (PCr),** which is formed and stored in the muscle cells. Dietary carbohydrates, fats, and proteins are also used as energy sources. Breakdown of all of these compounds releases enough energy to make more ATP. Cells must constantly use and then regenerate ATP over and over again. Depending on the type and extent of exercise, muscle cells draw on several different energy systems (Table 10-1).[15]

phosphocreatine (PCr) A high-energy compound that can be used to re-form ATP from ADP.

PHOSPHOCREATINE: INITIAL RESUPPLY OF MUSCLE ATP

During periods of relaxation, muscles synthesize PCr, a high-energy compound, from ATP and certain amino acids and then store this in small amounts. As soon as ADP from the breakdown of ATP begins to accumulate in a contracting muscle, an enzyme is activated that can transfer a high-energy Pi from PCr to ADP, thus re-forming ATP (Figure 10-2):

$$PCr + ADP\ 0\ \ Cr + ATP$$

If no other system for resupplying ATP were available, PCr could probably maintain maximal muscle contractions for about 10 seconds. But since metabolism of glucose and fatty acids begins to contribute ATP, PCr functions as the major source of energy for all events lasting up to about 1 minute (Table 10-1).[15]

The main advantage of PCr is that it can be activated instantly and can replenish ATP at rates fast enough to meet the energy demands of the fastest and most powerful sports events, including jumping, lifting, throwing, and sprinting actions. The disadvantage of PCr is that not enough is made and stored in the muscles to sustain a high rate of ATP resupply for more than a few minutes.[15]

FRANK & ERNEST® by Bob Thaves

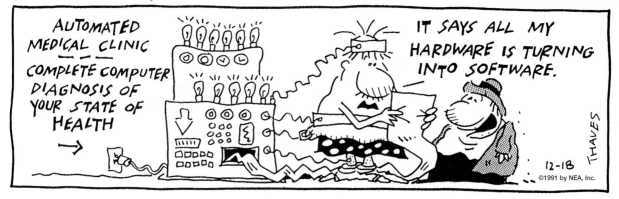

Figure 10-1 Frank & Ernest.

TABLE 10-1

Energy sources used by resting and working muscle cells

Source/system*	When in use	Examples of an exercise
ATP	At all times	All types
Phosphocreatine (PCr)	All exercise initially; extreme exercise thereafter	Shotput, jumping
Carbohydrate (anaerobic)	High-intensity exercise, especially lasting 30 seconds to 2 minutes	200-yard (200-meter) sprint
Carbohydrate (aerobic)	Exercise lasting 2 minutes to 4 to 5 hours; the higher the intensity (e.g., running a 6-minute mile), the greater the use	Basketball, swimming, jogging
Fat (aerobic)	Exercise lasting more than a few minutes; greater amounts are used at lower exercise intensities	Long-distance running, long distance cycling; 70%-90% of fuel used in a brisk walk is fat
Protein (aerobic)	Low quantity during all exercise; moderate quantity in endurance exercise, especially when carbohydrate fuel is lacking	Long-distance running

*Note that at any given time more than one system is operating.

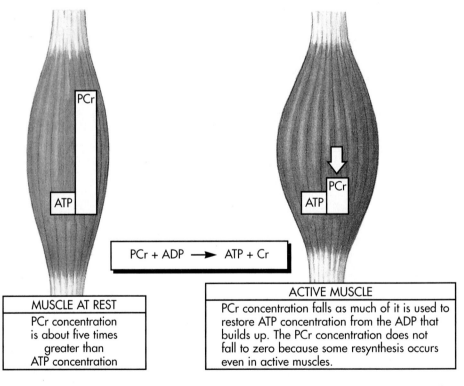

PCr + ADP ⟶ ATP + Cr

MUSCLE AT REST
PCr concentration is about five times greater than ATP concentration

ACTIVE MUSCLE
PCr concentration falls as much of it is used to restore ATP concentration from the ADP that builds up. The PCr concentration does not fall to zero because some resynthesis occurs even in active muscles.

Figure 10-2 Quick energy for muscle use includes a supply of phosphocreatine (PCr). This can rapidly replenish ATP stores as activity begins. Phosphocreatine can be almost depleted in maximally contracting human forearm muscles in less than 60 seconds. It takes 4 minutes of rest to replenish half the PCr and 7 minutes to replenish 95% of the PCr. Similarly, it takes about 7 minutes of rest to replenish 95% of the PCr depleted with repeated knee extensions against resistance.

GLUCOSE: MAJOR FUEL FOR SHORT-TERM HIGH-INTENSITY AND MEDIUM-TERM EXERCISE

Recall from Chapter 7 that glucose breaks down during **glycolysis,** yielding the three-carbon compound called pyruvate. Glycolysis does not require oxygen and yields a small amount of ATP. If oxygen is present, the pyruvate is metabolized further, yielding additional ATP.

Anaerobic Pathway

When the oxygen supply in muscle is limited (**anaerobic** state) or when the physical activity is intense (e.g., running 400 meters or swimming 100 meters), pyruvate resulting from glycolysis accumulates in the muscle and is converted to **lactate.**[17] Since the breakdown of 1 glucose to 2 pyruvates yields 2 ATP, glycolysis can resupply some ATP depleted in muscle activity. Carbohydrate is the only fuel that can be used for this process. The advantage of the anaerobic pathway is that, other than PCr breakdown, it is the fastest way to resupply ATP in muscle.

Glycolysis provides most of the energy for physical activity from about 30 seconds to 2 minutes after it has started. As we'll see shortly, fat utilization simply can't occur fast enough to meet the ATP demands of short-duration, high-intensity physical activity.[5] If fat were the only available fuel, we would be unable to carry out physical activity more intense than a fast walk or jog. High-caliber sports events would be out of the question.

The anaerobic pathway has three major disadvantages: (1) it can't sustain ATP production for long; (2) only about 5% of the energy available from glucose is released during glycolysis; and (3) the rapid accumulation of lactate greatly increases the acidity of muscle cells. Because high acidity inhibits the activity of key enzymes in glycolysis, anaerobic ATP production soon slows and fatigue sets in.[15]

Most of the lactate that accumulates in active muscle cells is eventually released into the bloodstream. The liver picks up the lactate from the blood and resynthesizes it into glucose. This glucose then can reenter the bloodstream, where it is available for cell uptake and breakdown. The heart can also use lactate directly for its energy needs, as can less active muscle cells situated near active ones.

Aerobic Pathway

If there is plenty of oxygen available in muscle (**aerobic** state) and the physical activity is of moderate to low intensity (e.g., jogging or distance swimming), the bulk of the pyruvate produced in glycolysis can be shuttled to the **mitochondria** of muscle cells. There it is further metabolized into carbon dioxide and water in a series of reactions, some of which require oxygen. About 95% of the ATP yielded from the complete metabolism of glucose is formed "aerobically" in mitochondria (Figure 10-3).[15]

Although the aerobic pathway supplies ATP more slowly than does the anaerobic pathway, it releases more energy. Furthermore, ATP production via the aerobic pathway can be sustained for hours. Accordingly, this pathway of glucose metabolism makes an important energy contribution to sports events lasting anywhere from about 2 minutes to 4 or 5 hours (Figure 10-4).[17]

GLYCOGEN VERSUS BLOOD GLUCOSE AS MUSCLE FUEL

Glycogen is the temporary storage form of glucose in the liver (about 100 g) and muscles (about 300 g in sedentary people). It is broken down to a form of glucose, which in turn can be metabolized by both the anaerobic and aerobic pathways just described. Glycogen is, in fact, the primary source of glucose for ATP production in muscle cells during fairly intense activities that last for less than about 2 hours. In such activities, the depletion of glycogen in the liver leads to a fall in blood glucose, while depletion of glycogen in the muscles contributes to fatigue.[5] Once these glycogen stores are exhausted, an athlete can only continue working at about 50% of maximal capacity. Diets high in carbohydrate can be used to build up muscle glycogen stores—up to double the typical amounts—in advance of competition,

Recall from Chapter 7 that when acids lose a hydrogen ion, as typically happens at the pH of the body, they are given the ending "-ate." So pyruvic acid is called *pyruvate* when in the context of body metabolism.

anaerobic Not using oxygen. Anaerobic activities use muscle groups at high intensities that exceed the body's capacity to supply energy using only oxygen-requiring pathways.

lactic acid (lactate) A three-carbon acid formed during anaerobic cell metabolism; a partial breakdown product of glucose.

aerobic Using oxygen. Aerobic activities use large muscle groups at moderate intensities that permit the body to use oxygen-requiring pathways to supply energy at a steady rate for more than a few minutes.

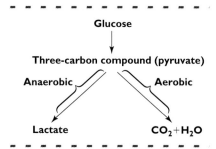

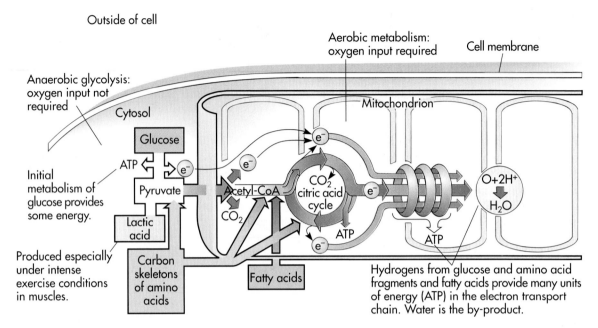

Outside of cell

Anaerobic glycolysis:
oxygen input not
required

Aerobic metabolism:
oxygen input required

Cell membrane

Cytosol

Mitochondrion

Glucose

ATP

Initial
metabolism of
glucose provides
some energy.

Pyruvate

Acetyl-CoA

CO_2

CO_2
citric acid
cycle

ATP

ATP

$O+2H^+$

H_2O

Lactic
acid

Produced especially
under intense
exercise conditions
in muscles.

Carbon
skeletons
of amino
acids

Fatty acids

Hydrogens from glucose and amino acid
fragments and fatty acids provide many units
of energy (ATP) in the electron transport
chain. Water is the by-product.

Figure 10-3 Metabolism of carbohydrate, fat, and protein supports ATP synthesis in a muscle cell. Carbohydrate metabolism occurs via both aerobic and anaerobic pathways, whereas fat and protein are metabolized for the most part via the aerobic pathway. Most of the ATP is produced as the hydrogen released from carbohydrate, fat, and protein metabolism combines with oxygen in the electron transport system to yield water.

thereby forestalling fatigue and improving endurance.[17] The Nutrition Perspective discusses how to do this.

As exercise duration increases beyond about 20 to 30 minutes, blood glucose becomes increasingly important as a fuel for ATP production in muscle cells. This use of glucose from the bloodstream can spare muscle glycogen, saving it in the muscle for sudden bursts of effort that may be required, such as a sprint to the finish in a marathon race. Because it is important to maintain a normal concentration of glucose in the bloodstream during prolonged exercise, many researchers have studied various types of carbohydrate feedings before and during exercise to maximize glucose supply to muscles. Overall, they have found that carbohydrate intake of about 30 to 80 g/hour during strenuous endurance exercise like cycling can help maintain adequate blood glucose concentrations, resulting in a delay of fatigue by 30 to 60 minutes.[19] This delay in the onset of fatigue occurs primarily because glucose intake reduces the use of liver glycogen and some muscle glycogen for fuel.[5] We discuss this issue further in a later section as well.

CONCEPT CHECK

ATP is the main form of energy that cells use. Metabolic pathways transform food energy to ATP energy. Carbohydrate metabolism to form ATP begins as glucose becomes available from the bloodstream or from glycogen breakdown. In a muscle cell, each glucose is broken down through a series of steps to yield either lactate or carbon dioxide (CO_2) plus water (H_2O). The breakdown of glucose to carbon dioxide and water is called the aerobic pathway because it requires oxygen. The conversion of glucose to lactate is called the anaerobic pathway because no oxygen is used. This latter process allows the cell to quickly re-form ATP and supports the demand for energy during intense physical activity, as does phosphocreatine (PCr).

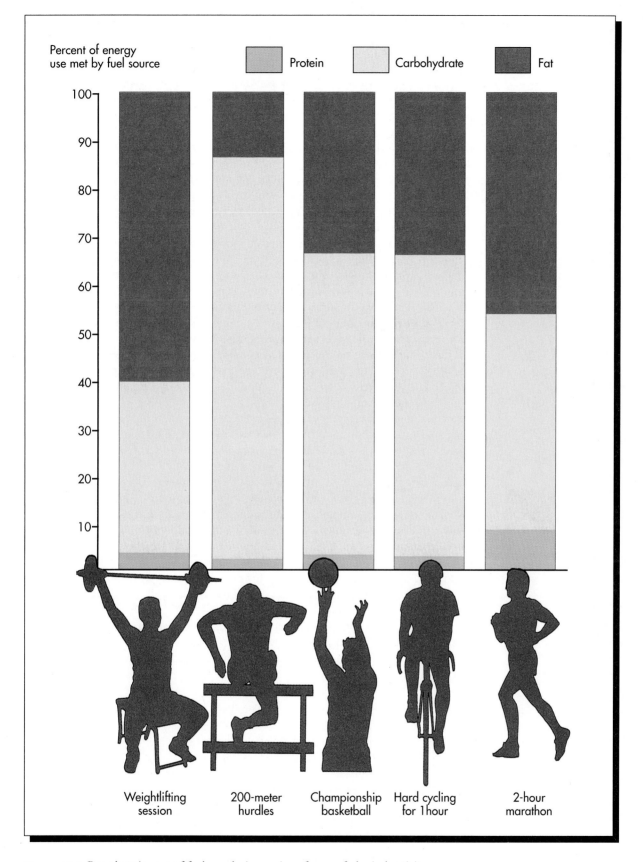

Figure 10-4 Rough estimates of fuel use during various forms of physical activity.

FAT: THE MAIN FUEL FOR PROLONGED LOW-INTENSITY EXERCISE

The majority of the stored energy in the body is found in the fatty acids of stored triglycerides. When fat stores in various adipose tissue depots are broken down for energy, 1 triglyceride molecule first yields 3 fatty acids and 1 glycerol. The free fatty acids are then released into the bloodstream and travel to the muscles, where they are taken into each cell's cytosol. The fatty acids can come from all over the body, not necessarily from depots near the active muscles.[15] This is why spot reducing does not work. Exercise can tone the muscles underlying adipose tissue, but does not preferentially use those stores. If this was not the case, we would all have lean cheeks and necks, as muscles in that vicinity are regularly used! Once fatty acids enter muscle cells, they move into the mitochondria, using a shuttle system that employs carnitine.[18] Then they are broken down into carbon dioxide and water using in part an oxygen-requiring pathway that yields much ATP. The rate at which muscles use fatty acids depends on a number of factors:

- *The more trained a muscle, the greater the ability to use fat as a fuel.* After a period of aerobic training, muscle cells contain more and larger mitochondria. These changes enable muscle cells to produce more ATP via oxygen-requiring pathways, including the pathway used to burn fat for fuel.[15]
- *The greater the concentration of fatty acids in the bloodstream, the greater the use of fat by muscle.* In other words, the more fatty acids that are released from adipose tissue stores into the bloodstream, the more fat will be used by the muscles. Recently some athletes have attempted to raise their blood concentrations of fatty acids by consuming caffeinated beverages. Because this practice actually can increase fatty acid release from the adipose tissue, it may be helpful to some athletes (see the Nutrition Perspective).[27]
- *As exercise becomes increasingly prolonged, fat use predominates,* especially when exercise remains at a low or moderate (aerobic) rate. Fat is not a very useful fuel for intense, brief physical activity, but it becomes progressively more important as an energy source as duration increases (Figure 10-4).[24]

The advantage of fat over other sources of energy is that it provides more "bang for the buck." That is, for a given weight of fuel, fat supplies more than twice as much energy as carbohydrate. On the basis of ATP produced per carbon, fat also comes out ahead of carbohydrate. The aerobic breakdown of a six-carbon glucose molecule yields 36 to 38 ATP (ratio of about 6 ATP to 1 carbon), whereas an 18-carbon fatty acid molecule produces 147 ATP (ratio of about 8.2 ATP to 1 carbon). In addition, when energy is needed for long-duration exercise or physical labor, the body's reserves of carbohydrate are too small to sustain work, but there is almost always plenty of fat that can be called on.

However, carbohydrate is more efficient than fat in one very important way: the amount of ATP produced per unit of oxygen consumed. It takes six O_2 molecules to produce 36 to 38 ATP molecules during the aerobic breakdown of a molecule of glucose (ratio of about 6 ATP to 1 O_2), whereas 26 O_2 molecules are needed to produce 147 ATP molecules from an 18-carbon fatty acid (ratio of about 5.7 ATP to 1 O_2). Thus in situations when an athlete's maximal performance would be limited by the activity of oxygen-requiring pathways (as in competitive endurance exercise), it is important that muscle cells also use carbohydrate as long as the carbohydrate supply, especially muscle glycogen, lasts.[5]

During very lengthy activities, such as a triathalon, ultramarathon, manual labor in a foundry, or even sitting at a desk for 8 hours a day, fat supplies about 70% to 90% of the energy required. Overall, keep in mind that the only fuel we eat that can support "fast-paced" (anaerobic) activity is carbohydrate; slow and steady (aerobic) activity uses all three energy sources: carbohydrate, fat, and protein.[15]

PROTEIN: A MINOR FUEL SOURCE, PRIMARILY FOR ENDURANCE EXERCISE

Although amino acids derived from protein are used to fuel muscles, their contribution is relatively small compared with that of carbohydrate (glucose) and fat (fatty acids). Only about 2% to 5% of the body's general energy needs, as well as the typical energy needs of exercising muscles, is supplied by metabolism of proteins.

However, proteins can contribute significantly to energy needs in endurance exercise, perhaps as much as 10%, especially as glycogen stores in the muscle are exhausted. Most of the energy supplied from protein comes from metabolism of the branched-chain amino acids—leucine, isoleucine, and valine.[12] Because a normal diet provides enough protein to supply this amount of fuel, protein supplements or amino acid supplements are not needed.[20] Contrary to what many athletes believe, protein is used less for fuel in resistance types of exercise (e.g., weight lifting) than for endurance exercise (e.g., running) (Figure 10-4). The primary fuels for weight lifting are phosphocreatine (PCr) and carbohydrate.[15] Recent research also shows that consuming high-carbohydrate, moderate-protein foods immediately after a weight-training workout enhances the anabolic effect of the activity, most likely by increasing the concentrations of insulin and growth hormone in the blood.[8]

CONCEPT CHECK

Fat is a key aerobic fuel for muscle cells, especially at low to moderate exercise intensities. At rest, muscles burn primarily fat for energy needs. On the other hand, little protein is used to fuel muscles. It supplies about 2% to 5% of energy needs and perhaps 10% of energy needs during endurance exercise.

The Body's Response to Physical Activity

We have discussed how muscle cells obtain the ATP energy needed to do work. Let's now focus on how muscles and related organs adapt to an increased work load.

SPECIALIZED FUNCTIONS OF SKELETAL MUSCLE FIBER TYPES

The body actually contains three types of muscle tissue: skeletal muscle, the type involved in locomotion; smooth muscle, the type found in internal organs except the heart; and cardiac (heart) muscle. Skeletal muscle, our primary focus, is composed of three types of muscle fiber, which exhibit distinct functional characteristics[1]:

- Type I (slow twitch—oxidative): Aerobic metabolism of fat primarily fuels type I fibers. These are also called red fibers because of their high myoglobin content.
- Type IIA (fast twitch—oxidative, glycolytic): Glycolysis using glucose (anaerobic) plus aerobic metabolism of both fat and glucose fuels type IIA fibers.
- Type IIB (fast twitch—glycolytic): Glycolysis using glucose (anaerobic) is the primary energy system for type IIB fibers. These are also called white fibers.

Prolonged low-intensity exercise, such as a slow jog, mainly involves use of type I muscle fibers, so the predominant fuel is fat. As exercise intensity increases, type IIA and type IIB fibers are gradually recruited; in turn the contribution of glucose as a fuel increases. Type IIA and type IIB fibers also are important for rapid movements, such as a jump shot in basketball.[1]

The relative proportions of the three fiber types throughout the muscles of the body vary from person to person and are constant throughout each person's life. The individual differences in fiber-type distribution are partially responsible for producing elite marathon runners who could never compete at the same level as sprinters, or elite gymnasts who could never be competitive as long-distance swimmers. Although the proportion of muscle fiber types is largely determined by genetics, appropriate training can develop muscles within limits. For example, aerobic training enhances the capacity of type IIA muscle fibers to produce ATP and may bring about a relative change in size. Overall, great athletes are born, but their genetic potential then must be exploited by training.[1]

EXPERT OPINION

WHAT CAN A PHYSICALLY ACTIVE LIFESTYLE PROMISE?

J. MARK DAVIS, Ph.D.

Concerned about widespread heart disease, diabetes, obesity, and osteoporosis, many Americans have become interested in the potential health benefits of regular physical activity. Increasing evidence suggests that physical activity may delay the onset and/or help treat these diseases. Although increased physical activity is hardly a magic bullet, many people change their habits in hopes that moderate physical activity will improve their chances of living healthier and longer. This hope is not without scientific support.

OVERALL PHYSICAL FITNESS

Physical fitness can be divided into two components: skill-related fitness and health-related fitness. The elements composing skill-related fitness include agility, balance, coordination, speed, power, and reaction time. This component is relatively more important for athletic competition. Health-related fitness is usually emphasized more for the general population and includes the elements of cardiorespiratory endurance, body composition, and musculoskeletal fitness. Musculoskeletal fitness includes flexibility, muscular strength, and muscular endurance.

In general, a program of regular physical activity (aerobic training) will produce beneficial cardiorespiratory changes, including increases in heart size and strength, stroke volume, and blood volume. Muscle strength and flexibility should also improve. In all, these attributes allow a person to do everyday tasks such as climbing stairs and carrying books or groceries with ease, enhance the enjoyment of recreational sports by making it possible to achieve high degrees of performance, provide protection against injury, and improve body composition by increasing lean body mass and decreasing fat mass. All of this promotes a more positive self-image.

HEART DISEASE

How can an active lifestyle reduce the risk of heart disease? Regular physical activity can produce changes in the cardiovascular system that decrease the risk of heart attack, including larger coronary arteries and increased heart size and pumping capacity. It also has a favorable effect on many risk factors for cardiovascular disease, including hypertension, serum lipids, obesity, diabetes, and stress, and even helps to control smoking.

OBESITY

Although obesity is most commonly treated with energy restriction (i.e., dieting), a combination of dieting and physical activity is much preferred to dieting alone. Losing weight by dieting alone usually entails losing lean tissue as well as body fat. Performing regular physical activity along with dieting usually spares some of this lean tissue loss, while promoting the loss of fat tissue.

Physical activity stimulates fat mobilization and the preferential use of fat for energy, assists in better control of appetite, increases energy expenditure during and after exercise, and helps the body more precisely balance energy intake and expenditure after a meal. This all helps to maintain a more optimal body com-position. In addition, physical activity can also help prevent or reverse development of other diseases associated with obesity, including diabetes, hypertension, and heart disease.

DIABETES

Physical activity contributes to weight loss in obesity, which in turn enhances the action of the hormone insulin. Blunted insulin action is characteristic of adult-onset diabetes (NIDDM), the predominant form of diabetes in the United States. Enhancing insulin sensitivity also potentially allows the insulin dosage to be reduced for those with NIDDM who use it.

A person with diabetes must work with a physician to make the correct alterations in diet and medications to perform exercise safely. This is because physical activity can adversely affect some people by inducing low blood glucose. The benefits on insulin action are also short-lived, so regular moderate physical activity is encouraged.

OSTEOPOROSIS

Osteoporosis is a disease that leads to a high risk for bone fracture caused by bone loss. Both genetic and environmental factors are implicated as causes. The decline in estrogen synthesis at menopause is a major factor; prolonged intake of calcium is another contributor.

Physical activity, particularly moderate weight-bearing exercise, can help to prevent osteoporosis. An extremely sedentary lifestyle causes bone loss. Bone loss also occurs under extreme conditions of prolonged bed rest or weightlessness, as astronauts experience in space. Experts agree that regular moderate physical activity is important for bone health, especially among elderly persons, who in general are at great risk of osteoporosis. The agility and strength developed from regular physical activity can reduce both the likelihood of falls and injuries caused by falls.

IMMUNE SYSTEM

Interest in the area of exercise immunology probably began from the common belief that physically fit individuals typically have fewer and less severe colds and flus than unfit people. Alternatively, some people believe that very strenuous physical activity or heavy training can increase the chances of getting sick. Interestingly, scientific evidence is now beginning to emerge in support of both these common beliefs, and a new theory—dubbed the inverted-U theory—has been developed to explain it.

The inverted-U theory suggests that moderate (healthy) physical activity enhances the body's immune system and therefore decreases the risk of infections, whereas strenuous (stressful) physical activity suppresses the immune system and increases the risk of illness. The positive and negative effects of physical activity likely depend, at least in part, on whether the individual perceives an activity as having a stressful or calming effect. While regular, moderate activities such as walking and jogging may be beneficial, acute bouts such as a marathon run and prolonged periods of intense training by athletes preparing for intense competition present highly stressful situations for the body to cope with.

To date many studies have supported this inverted-U theory as it relates to both viral infections and cancer. For example, it is now well established that physical activity can alter the number and functions of various viruses and cancer-fighting immune cells, including lymphocytes, natural killer cells, monocytes and macrophages. There is also good data that an individual's susceptibility to infection and cancer can be altered by physical activity.

PSYCHOLOGICAL HEALTH

One of the most important habits that anyone can develop to improve mood state and manage stress is regular physical activity. There is now good scientific evidence to support the anecdotal reports and the common belief that regular physical activity can reduce depression, anxiety, and mental stress, while increasing psychological well-being and mental cognition. Good evidence is beginning to emerge that physical activity may increase the concentrations and/or activity of dopamine, norepinephrine, serotonin, and other neurotransmitters in the brain. Physical activity also may influence mood by stimulating the release of various endogenous opioid substances that have properties similar to morphine in relieving pain and inducing euphoria.

RECOMMENDED ACTIVITY LEVELS FOR GENERAL HEALTH

In 1990 the American College of Sports Medicine (ACSM) recommended the following standard for development of cardiorespiratory endurance: exercise at an intensity between 60% and 90% of maximum heart rate (50% to 85% VO_2max) for 20 to 60 minutes, 3 to 5 days per week.

For purposes of general health benefits, the ACSM and Centers for Disease Control urge instead that American adults accumulate at least 30 minutes of mild- to moderate-intensity physical activity over the course of most days of the week. Interestingly, it doesn't seem like the activity has to be all at once. It is my opinion that the optimal program for most people lies between these two approaches, depending on the individual and the specific situation.

It is very important to realize that harmful side effects may accompany excessive physical activity. The growing list of complications includes an increased risk of musculoskeletal injuries, heat illness, sudden death from heart attack, upper respiratory infection, bronchospasm, gastrointestinal problems, and disturbances in mood, sleeping habits, and appetite, not to mention impaired performance. The benefits of regular participation in physical activity must be balanced against these risks, which rise exponentially with excessive amounts. In general, activities such as brisk walking are highly recommended, producing many benefits with few risks.

Dr. Davis is a professor in the Department of Exercise Science at the University of South Carolina. His research interests include the area of sports nutrition.

ADAPTATION OF MUSCLES AND BODY PHYSIOLOGY TO EXERCISE

With training, muscle strength also becomes matched to the muscles' greater and lesser work demands. Muscles enlarge after being made to work repeatedly, a response called **hypertrophy.**[15] Certain cells in the muscles gain bulk and improve their ability to work. Conversely, after several days without activity, muscles diminish in size and lose strength, a response called **atrophy.** Both hypertrophy and atrophy are forms of adaptation to the load applied. Thus marathon runners often have well-developed leg muscles but little arm or chest muscle development.[1]

Beyond the effects on individual muscles, repeated aerobic exercise also produces beneficial changes in the heart and blood vessels that are responsible for delivering oxygen to the mitochondria of the muscles. Because the body needs more oxygen during exercise, it responds to training by producing more red blood cells and expanding total blood volume. Training also leads to an increase in the number of very small blood vessels (capillaries) in muscle tissue; as a result, oxygen can be delivered more easily to muscles. Finally, training causes the heart, a muscle itself, to enlarge and strengthen. Then each contraction empties the heart's chamber more efficiently, so more blood is pumped with each beat. As exercise increases the efficiency of the heart, its rate of beating at rest and during submaximal exercise decreases. This effect can be used as an index of fitness: as fitness increases, the resting heart rate decreases.[15]

After a period of aerobic training, muscle cells contain more and larger mitochondria, as we've mentioned. The muscles can then more efficiently fuel themselves from fat stores. These changes in mitochondrial function allow for greater intensity during aerobic exercise. An athlete can then train harder and longer at an "aerobic" pace. Furthermore, training leads to a 20% to 50% increase in muscle glycogen stores, thus making more carbohydrate available as fuel for muscular work.[17]

MEASURING EXERCISE CAPACITY

There is more oxygen in the air we inhale than in the air we exhale. Oxygen taken up by cells and shuttled to mitochondria for use in ATP production accounts for this difference. The amount of oxygen consumed by the mitochondria of the body tissues is directly related to ATP needs during exercise. Every atom of oxygen used in the mitochondrial energy-yielding pathways results in production of 2 to 3 ATP molecules. Thus oxygen consumption indicates how hard a person is exercising. The harder the muscles work, the more oxygen they demand.

The more physically fit a person is, the more work the muscles and body can do, and the more oxygen the person can consume. A treadmill test commonly is used to determine a person's **Vo₂max,** the maximum amount of oxygen that can be consumed in a unit of time. In this test, oxygen consumption is measured as the treadmill speed and/or grade is gradually increased until the subject becomes profoundly fatigued. The oxygen consumption measured right before total exhaustion is assigned the value Vo_2max. Although Vo_2max varies among individuals, most people can improve their Vo_2max by 15% to 20% or more with exercise training.[15]

Because of individual differences in Vo_2max, it is generally best to express exercise intensity as a percentage of Vo_2max. The percentage of Vo_2max required for exercise of various intensity is as follows:

- Low intensity (e.g., fast walk)—30% to 50% of Vo_2max
- Moderate intensity (e.g., fast jog)—50% to 65% of Vo_2max
- High intensity (e.g., 3-hour marathon pace)—70% to 80% of Vo_2max
- Very high intensity (e.g., sprints)—85% to 150% of Vo_2max

In very-high-intensity activities, the ATP equivalent to the "extra" 50% above 100% of Vo_2max is produced anaerobically from PCr and glycolysis, as we discussed already.

FUEL USE IN EXERCISE: A CLOSER LOOK

The fuel used for a specific work load is determined by the intensity (portion of Vo_2max used) and duration of exercise. The availability of certain energy-yielding

---

atrophy A wasting away of tissues, organs, or the entire body.

CRITICAL THINKING

Marty started going to the gym about 8 weeks ago. At first, he noticed that he began "huffing and puffing" about 7 minutes into his aerobic workout. Now, however, he can work out for about 25 minutes without tiring. What is a possible explanation for his ability to work out longer?

Vo₂max Maximum volume of oxygen that can be consumed per unit of time.

pathways in a cell—notably the citric acid cycle and electron transport chain—depends on the work load and how much work has been done already (Table 10-1). Because these pathways were discussed in Chapter 7, we will only summarize them briefly here, focusing mostly on their use in exercise.

Rest and Low-Intensity Workloads

Both resting muscle cells and those engaged in low-intensity exercise such as a brisk walk primarily burn fat, especially beyond 20 minutes of activity. The maximal use of fat to fuel working muscles is delayed because the release of fatty acids from adipose stores into the bloodstream depends on numerous hormonal events. Only after release occurs, which takes some time, can significant amounts of fatty acids be taken up and used for ATP production by working muscle cells.[5]

Fat metabolism supplies about 70% to 90% of the ATP needed to sustain low-intensity work loads (<50% VO_2max). The rest comes mostly from carbohydrate metabolism. And while a muscle cell is busy making ATP using fat energy, it cannot easily make ATP using glucose energy, because high concentrations of ATP and other substances produced during fat metabolism inhibit important enzymes used in glycolysis. On the other hand, there is no such inhibition of the enzymes used in the citric acid cycle and electron transport system, the pathways used for fat metabolism. This tips the balance toward using fat to form ATP.[15]

Brief and Maximally Intense Exercise

Intense exercise, such as running 200-meter sprints, requires maximum effort and cannot be sustained. In fact, this exercise is so intense that it may last for no more than 30 seconds. For such work loads ATP is resupplied primarily from PCr, although the anaerobic pathway of glycolysis provides some ATP. During short bursts of maximally intense work (up to about 10 seconds), the supply of PCr in muscle tissue is depleted rapidly as it re-forms ATP. The PCr system is also used as muscle contractions begin to reinitiate activity after a rest.[15] However, in prolonged exercise at moderate intensity, PCr is not as critical as a muscle fuel because other cell pathways are available for ATP replenishment.

Moderately Intense Exercise

When someone exercises hard and sustains it for more than a few minutes—for example, running a 6-minute mile—fatty acid metabolism via the citric acid cycle and electron transport chain cannot keep pace with the cells' ATP demands. Both the anaerobic and aerobic pathways of glycolysis must provide help. This is partly because the electron transport chain in each mitochondrion takes a few minutes to shift into high gear.[5] Moreover, the amount of fatty acids available as fuel is limited, as we just noted. That being the case, the ATP concentration at the start of exercise in muscle cells drops, and the ADP concentration in muscle cells increases. The PCr system contributes energy, but fades fast. Now the low ATP concentration in the muscle cells allows important enzymes in the glycolytic process to speed up. Glycogen in the muscle then breaks down into glucose, which undergoes glycolysis to form pyruvate. At this point carbohydrate is supplying 80% to 90% of the fuel used.[17] Because so little ATP is produced in the anaerobic glycolytic breakdown of glucose to pyruvate, this pathway must proceed very rapidly in muscle cells to be of much value.

Since the aerobic pathway, involving the citric acid cycle and electron transport chain, is not yet fully engaged, much of the pyruvate is converted to lactate. Lactate production is greatest during the first minute of exercise. After that, some of the pyruvate produced in glycolysis enters the aerobic pathway, which then begins to contribute to meeting ATP demands. It has long been assumed—incorrectly—that lactate accumulation in muscle and blood always meant that muscle was anaerobic (deprived of oxygen) during exercise. We now know that lactate is formed and removed continuously, even when muscles are at rest; only the total amount of lactate produced varies.[15]

NUTRITION FOCUS

DESIGNING A FITNESS PROGRAM

A gradual increase in regular physical activity is recommended for all healthy persons. But the American College of Sports Medicine recommends that those who are 35 years or older, have been inactive for many years, or have an existing health problem, talk to a physician before increasing their activity substantially. Health problems that require medical evaluation before beginning an exercise program are obesity, heart disease (or family history of it), high blood pressure, diabetes (or family history), shortness of breath after mild exertion, and arthritis. Although vigorous exercise involves minimal health risks for those in good health, far greater risks exist for those who are inactive.

PHASE I: GETTING STARTED

During the first phase of a fitness program, begin to incorporate short periods of physical activity into your daily routine. This can include brisk walking, stair climbing, house cleaning, gardening, or other activities that cause you to "huff and puff" a bit. The goal is a total of 30 minutes of this moderate type of physical activity each day, expending an average of 200 kcal.[21]

Any physical activity that leads to energy use of more than 300 kcal/hour in a typical woman or 350 kcal/hour in a typical man is especially helpful (see Appendix K). The more vigorous the activities, the more effective they are for maintaining fitness, but only about 1 in 10 adults practices vigorous activities on a daily basis. Thus exercise experts now suggest starting small, with a total of 30 minutes of activity incorporated into each day's tasks.

The easiest way to increase physical activity is to make it part of your daily routine, similar to other regular activities, such as eating. For many people the best time to exercise is when they need an energy pick-me-up or a break from work. Rather than abandoning an exercise program entirely when obstacles impede, strive to use any small periods of available time. As you begin to enjoy exercising and reaping its benefits, you'll tend to spend more time at it.

Clearly, many of the activities recommended for phase I are not very vigorous. Fitness experts have not given up on the value of vigorous physical activity by recommending phase I for those starting an exercise program. They're just bowing to human nature. Although the experts still advise at least 30 minutes of moderate-intensity physical activity 5 days a week, they're now willing also to consider gardening, raking leaves, and climbing stairs as suitable activities.

PHASE II: SEEKING GREATER FITNESS

Once you've gotten started on regular activity of moderate intensity, you can add more intense activities to reap even more health benefits. Suggested activities include jogging, cycling, and swimming. The goal is 30 minutes of such vigorous activity at least 5 days per week. As well, some resistance exercise, (e.g., push-ups, sit-ups, weight training) should be performed at least 2 days per week. It's fine to try pushing a little past fatigue, but when your arms or legs start shaking uncontrollably, it's time to ease up. Note that ignoring pain can almost guarantee an injury.

This basic exercise program should begin with warm-up exercises, primarily to increase blood flow and warm the muscles. This reduces risk of injuries. Then activities to increase muscular strength, endurance, and flexibility are done. Cool-down exercises finish the program.[15] Table 10-2 shows how to design a cardiovascular workout program. Fitness target heart rates for adults are about 60% or more of their predicted maximum heart rate (220 minus current age).

To determine whether you are in the target exercise zone, learn to count your pulse. Placing a hand over your heart is a simple method. However, since clothing may obscure the beat, it is best to lightly put pressure on either large artery at the side of your neck. A full pulse can also be felt at the wrist or inside the bend of the elbow. Count the pulse immediately on stopping exercise because the rate changes very quickly once exercise is slowed or stopped. Find the beat within a second and count for 10 seconds. Multiply this number by six to obtain the count for a minute. Do not count for the whole minute, or even for 15 seconds, because the fall-off after exercise is too fast.

It's important to include several types of enjoyable physical activities in your fitness program; make sure to start off gradually and work up to longer times. Doing too much too fast is a quick way to extinguish enthusiasm and determination. A new trend in exercising is cross-training, in which a variety of exercises are incorporated into a fitness program. For example, instead of jogging for 30 minutes, a person may swim for 15 minutes and then jog for 15 minutes. Adding variety to your program not only keeps you mentally fresh, but also strengthens different

TABLE 10-2

Your exercise prescription

Fitness component	Definition	Activities
Flexibility	The ability to bend without injury; it is dependent on elasticity of muscles, tendons, and ligaments, and condition of joints.	Stretches will enhance flexibility. They should be held for at least 10 seconds. Never use bouncy, choppy, or painful stretches that twist or put pressure on joints.
Strength	The ability to work against resistance.	Using few repetitions (8-12 per set) with weights as heavy as is safely possible will increase strength.
Muscle endurance	The ability of a muscle to sustain effort over a period of time.	Repetitive exercises, such as push-ups, pull-ups, sit-ups.
Cardiovascular endurance	The ability of the cardiovascular system to sustain effort over a period of time; it should involve larger muscle groups and be performed at 60% or more of maximum heart rate.	Activities include fast walking, jogging, swimming, bicycling, and stair climbing. These can provide the needed sustained, submaximal work if the exercise is performed at an appropriate pace.

The plan

WARM-UP: 5-10 minutes of stretching the whole torso. Start with smaller muscle groups (arms) and work toward larger muscle groups (legs and abdomen).

5-10 minutes more of exercises, such as walking, slow jogging, or any slow version of anticipated activity. Low-intensity movement literally warms up muscles so that muscle filaments slide more easily over one another and will gradually bring heart rate up to target level.

WORKOUT: 20 or more minutes of rhythmic continuous activity 5 times a week. Pace should be set so that exercise raises heart rate to within target range. Modify pace or workload as necessary so that the heart rate reaches and does not exceed target range. A good rule of thumb is that you should still be able to converse, in order to minimize lactate production. Popular aerobic conditioning activities include brisk walking, jogging, swimming, cycling, cross-country skiing, and aerobic dance. Activities such as basketball and racquetball provide a good workout, but because the heart rate jumps up high and then drops and then goes up again, they do not

Continued.

NUTRITION FOCUS

TABLE 10-2

Your exercise prescription—cont'd

Fitness component	Definition	Activities
WORKOUT— cont'd	condition the heart as rhythmic continuous activities do. Exercises that develop muscular strength and endurance can follow the aerobic session or alternate with it on different days. Resistance exercises, such as weight training or calisthenics, encourage muscle maintenance and are particularly important in weight-reducing diets in order to maintain muscle mass.	
COOL-DOWN:	Follow a reverse pattern of warm-up: 5-10 minutes of low-intensity activity and 5-10 minutes of stretching. The same exercises performed during warm-up are appropriate. The cool-down is essential to the prevention of injury and soreness.	

muscle groups and reduces risk of injury. Variety also keeps the program interesting. An exercise partner may offer additional motivation.

Search for opportunities that suit you: heel-to-toe brisk walking is recommended for just about everyone. To ease into a regular aerobic exercise routine, start by walking. Begin with 30 to 45 minutes of brisk walking 5 days a week. After a few weeks, if you find yourself feeling more energetic, speed up to a jog or start an aerobic dance program. More than most other forms of exercise, walking lends itself to sharing, socializing, and enjoying nature. And because it's so easy and pleasurable, you're likely to continue including it in your routine long after you've dropped more exotic or strenuous sports. More vigorous exercise for overweight persons should be non–weight-bearing activities such as swimming and bicycling.

If you do jog or run, or do aerobic dance, pace yourself so that you are able to talk comfortably without becoming short of breath. At this point lactate production remains low, so muscle fatigue from that will be minimized. It is best for a beginner to switch from brisk walking to jogging and back again every couple of minutes. Gradually, the amount of walking time can be decreased while jogging time is extended. Because jogging or running may be stressful on the knees, it is very important to select proper shoes and to seek an appropriate running surface, such as a track.

Whatever physical activities are included in a fitness program, they should be enjoyable. This way they can become routine. Keep in mind convenience, cost, and options for bad weather so that when motivation wanes, you are not adding any further obstacles.

If a person starts exercising regularly four or five times a week, he or she will experience a "training effect." At the start the person might be able to exercise for 20 minutes before tiring. Months later exercise can be extended to an hour before the person feels tired. During the months of training, muscle cells have produced more mitochondria and so can burn more fat. As a result, lactate production decreases. Since lactate contributes to muscle fatigue, the less lactate produced, the longer the person will be able to exercise. Part of the training effect derives also from the increased aerobic efficiency of heart and muscle action. However, when you consider only metabolism, a very important result of training is the increased number of mitochondria in the muscle cells, resulting in less dependence on the anaerobic production of ATP via glycolysis.[15]

Endurance Exercise

Endurance exercise, such as brisk walking or cycling, often involves moderate effort sustained over 1 or more hours. For such prolonged moderate work loads, the aerobic metabolism of fatty acids via the citric acid cycle and electron transport chain can supply about 60% to 80% of the needed ATP. The aerobic pathway of glucose metabolism contributes about 15% to 30% of the energy needs, and protein provides up to 10%. In the aerobic pathway, pyruvate produced from glucose is shuttled to the mitochondria and is metabolized via the citric acid cycle and electron transport chain. Less lactate builds up in endurance exercise than during high-intensity activities because of the lesser demand for glycolysis. At this slower rate of glucose utilization, the oxygen-requiring pathways in the mitochondria can handle most of the pyruvate produced in glycolysis, so less is converted to lactate.

As intensity increases, such as in a 3-hour marathon run at 70% of VO_2max, muscles use about a 50:50 ratio of fat to carbohydrate. When carbohydrate fuel (glycogen) in muscles is eventually used up, it is difficult to maintain the high initial work load unless normal blood glucose concentrations are maintained by carbohydrate feedings. Athletes call this point of glycogen depletion "hitting the wall," as further exertion is hampered. So when exertion meets or exceeds 70% of VO_2max for more than an hour, athletes (e.g., long-distance runners or cyclists) should consider increasing the amount of carbohydrate stored in muscles.[17] Again, the Nutrition Perspective discusses how to do this.

Power Food: Dietary Guidelines for Athletes

Athletic training and genetic makeup are two very important determinants of athletic performance. A good diet won't substitute for either factor, but as we have mentioned, diet can further enhance and maximize an athlete's potential. More important, a poor diet can certainly harm performance.[23]

DETERMINING NEEDED FOOD-ENERGY INTAKE

Athletes need varying amounts of food energy, depending on each athlete's body size and current body composition and on the type of training or competition being considered. A small person may need only 1700 kcal daily to sustain normal daily activities without losing body weight; a large muscular man may need 4000 kcal. These rough estimates can be viewed as starting points that need to be individualized by trial and error for each athlete. The energy required for sports training or competition has to be added to the basal energy needed just to carry on normal activities. Energy use averages 5 to 8 kcal/minute for moderate activity; again, this is just an estimate. For example, an hour of bowling requires little energy in addition to that required to sustain normal daily living. At the other extreme, a 12-hour endurance bicycle race over mountains can require an additional 4000 kcal/day.[10] Therefore some athletes may need as much as 7000 kcal daily just to maintain body weight while training, whereas others may need 1700 kcal or less.

How can we know if an athlete is getting enough energy from food? The first step is to estimate the athlete's body fat percentage by measuring skinfold thicknesses, by using bioelectrical impedance, or by using the underwater weighing technique (see Chapter 8). Body fat should be in the desirable range, that is, about 5% to 15% for most male athletes and 10% to 25% for most female athletes.[23] The next step is simply to monitor body weight changes on a daily or weekly basis. If body weight starts to fall, food energy should be increased; if weight rises and it is because of increases in body fat, the athlete should be encouraged to eat less.

If the body composition test shows that an athlete has too much body fat, the athlete should lower food intake by about 200 to 500 kcal/day, while maintaining a regular exercise program, until the desirable fat percentage is achieved. Reducing fat intake is the best nutrient-related approach. On the other hand, if an athlete needs to gain weight, increasing food intake by 500 to 700 kcal/day will eventually

Joe is a wrestler who qualified for the lightweight division in his annual high school competition. After a few matches, Joe began to feel dizzy and faint. He was disqualified because he was unable to continue the match. Later, the coach found out that Joe had spent 2 hours in the sauna before weighing in, which had made him dehydrated. What are the consequences of dehydration? What can you suggest as an alternative way to lose weight?

lead to the needed weight gain. A mix of carbohydrate, fat, and protein is advised, coupled again with exercise to make sure this gain is mostly from lean tissue, and not mostly added fat stores.

RAPID WEIGHT LOSS BY DEHYDRATION

Wrestlers, boxers, judo players, and oarsmen often try to lose weight so that they can be certified to compete in a lower weight class. This helps them gain a mechanical advantage over an opponent of smaller stature. Most of the time, this weight is lost a few hours before stepping on the scale for weight certification. Athletes can lose up to 22 pounds (10 kg) of body water in 1 day by sitting in a sauna, exercising in a plastic sweat suit, and/or taking diuretic drugs that speed water loss from the kidneys. Losing as little as 3% of body weight by dehydration can adversely affect endurance performance.[1] A pattern of repeated weight loss or gain of more than 5% of body weight by dehydration carries some risk of kidney malfunction and heat illness. We discuss this further in a later section.

The practice of losing weight by dehydration is common in sports such as interscholastic and intercollegiate wrestling. Thus most competitors in these sports probably face an opponent who has gone through the same misery to gain an "advantage." If an athlete wishes to compete in a lower body weight class and has enough extra fat stores, that athlete should begin a gradual, sustained reduction in food-energy intake long before the competitive season starts. In so doing, the athlete will attain a presumably healthier body composition (less fat) while avoiding the potentially harmful and certainly misery-creating effects of severe dehydration. Athletes who have no extra body fat should be discouraged from attempting to compete at a lower body weight class. It is important for coaches and trainers to be aware of the decreased performance and serious side effects of severe dehydration.[1]

MEETING CARBOHYDRATE AND PROTEIN NEEDS IN THE TRAINING DIET

Anyone who exercises regularly, including the dieter, needs to consume a diet that includes moderate to high amounts of carbohydrates. The diet should include a variety of foods, adhering to the Food Guide Pyramid. Numerous servings of starches and fruits will provide enough carbohydrate to maintain adequate liver and muscle glycogen stores, especially for replacing glycogen losses from the previous day.[5]

Carbohydrate intake should be at least 5 g/kg body weight. People engaged in aerobic training and endurance athletes (duration >60 minutes per day) may need as much as 8 to10 g/kg body weight.[24] In other words, triathletes and marathoners should consider eating close to 600 g of carbohydrates daily, and even more if necessary, to (1) prevent chronic fatigue and (2) load the muscles and liver with glycogen.[10] This is especially important when performing multiple training bouts in a day, such as swim practices, or heavy training on successive days, as in cross-country running. Table 10-3 shows sample menus, based on the Food Guide Pyramid, for diets providing food energy ranging from 1500 to 5000 kcal/day. Table 10-4 lists the number of grams of carbohydrate in 1 exchange (serving) of the various groups in the Exchange System and some representative foods in each group. As we saw in Chapter 2, the Exchange System is a very useful tool for planning all types of diets, including diets for athletes.

Note that one does not have to give up any specific food when planning a high-carbohydrate diet. The focus just must turn to more of the best—high-carbohydrate foods—and moderate the rest—concentrated fat sources. Sports nutritionists emphasize the difference between a high-carbohydrate meal and a high-carbohydrate/high-fat meal. Before endurance events, such as marathons or triathalons, some athletes seek to increase their carbohydrate reserves by eating potato chips, french fries, banana cream pie, and pastries. Although such foods contain carbohydrate, they also contain a lot of fat. Better high-carbohydrate food choices include pasta, rice, potatoes, bread, and many breakfast cereals (check the label for carbohydrate content). Sports drinks appropriate for carbohydrate loading, such as GatorLode and UltraFuel, can also help. Consuming a moderate amount of dietary

TABLE 10-3

Sample daily menus based on the Food Guide Pyramid that provide various total energy intakes

1500 kcal diet
Breakfast

Skim milk, 1 cup
Cheerios, ½ cup
Bagel, ½
Cherry jam, 2 tsp
Margarine, 1 tsp

Lunch

Chicken breast (roasted), 2 oz
Figs, 1
Skim milk, ½ cup
Banana, 1

Snack

Oatmeal-raisin cookie, 1
Low-fat fruit yogurt, 1 cup

Dinner

Spagetti w/meatballs, 1 cup
Romaine lettuce, 1 cup
Italian dressing, 2 tsp
Green beans, ½ cup
Cranberry juice, 1½ cups
_____
18% protein (68 g)
64% CHO (240 g)
19% fat (32 g)

2000 kcal diet
Breakfast

Skim milk, 1 cup
Cheerios, 1 cup
Bagel, ½
Cherry jam, 1 tbsp
Margarine, 1 tsp

Lunch

Chicken breast (roasted), 2 oz
Wheat bread, 2 slices
Mayonnaise, 1 tsp
Figs, 2
Cranberry juice, 1½ cups
Banana, 1

Snack

Oatmeal-raisin cookies, 3
Low-fat fruit yogurt, 1 cup

Dinner

Broiled beef sirloin, 3 oz
Romaine lettuce, 1 cup
Italian dressing, 2 tsp
Green beans, 1 cup
Skim milk, ½ cup
_____
17% protein (85 g)
63% CHO (315 g)
20% fat (44 g)

2500 kcal diet
Breakfast

Skim milk, 1 cup
Cheerios, 2 cups
Bagel, ½
Cherry jam, 2 tsp
Margarine, 1 tsp
Banana, 1

Lunch

Chicken breast (roasted),
   2 oz
Wheat bread, 2 slices
Mayonnaise, 1 tsp
Figs, 3
Cranberry juice, 1½ cup
Low-fat fruit yogurt, 1 cup

Snack

Oatmeal-raisin cookies, 3

Dinner

Broiled beef sirloin, 3 oz
Spinach pasta noodles,
   1½ cups
Margarine, 1 tsp
Romaine lettuce, 1 cup
Italian dressing, 2 tsp
Garbanzo beans, ¼ cup
Green beans, 1 cup
Skim milk, ½ cup
_____
17% protein (106 g)
63% CHO (394 g)
20% fat (56 g)

3000 kcal diet
Breakfast

Skim milk, 1 cup
Cheerios, 2 cups
Bagel, 1
Cherry jam, 2 tsp
Margarine, 1 tsp
Oat bran muffins, 2

Lunch

Chicken breast (roasted), 2 oz
Wheat bread, 2 slices
Provolone cheese, 1 oz
Mayonnaise, 1 tsp
Figs, 3
Cranberry juice, 1½ cups
Low-fat fruit yogurt, 1 cup

Snack

Banana, 1
Oatmeal-raisin cookies, 3

Dinner

Broiled beef sirloin, 3 oz
Romaine lettuce, 1 cup
Garbanzo beans, 1 cup
Italian dressing, 2 tsp
Spinach pasta noodles,
   1½ cups
Margarine, 1 tsp
Green beans, 1 cup
Skim milk, ½ cup
_____
17% protein (128 g)
62% CHO (465 g)
21% fat (70 g)

3500 kcal diet
Breakfast

2% milk, 1 cup
Cheerios, 2½ cups
Bagel, 1
Margarine, 1 tsp
Cherry jam, 1 tbsp
Low-fat fruit yogurt, 1 cup

Lunch

Chicken breast (roasted), 2 oz
Wheat bread, 2 slices
Mayonnaise, 1 tsp
Cranberry juice, 2 cups
Banana, 1
Figs, 3
Celery, 1 cup

Snack

Oatmeal-raisin cookies, 4
Wheat Thins, 25 crackers

Dinner

Hamburger patty, 1
American cheese, 1 slice
Macaroni and cheese, ½ cup
Romaine lettuce, 1 cup
Italian dressing, 2 tsp
Garbanzo beans, 1 cup
Green beans, 1 cup
2% milk, 1 cup
_____
14% protein (122 g)
62% CHO (542 g)
24% fat (93 g)

Continued.

TABLE 10-3

Sample daily menus based on the Food Guide Pyramid that provide various total energy intakes—cont'd

4000 kcal diet
Breakfast

Orange, 1
Cheerios, 2 cups
Skim milk, 1 cup
Bran muffins, 2

Snack

Chopped dates, ¾ cup

Lunch

Romaine lettuce, 1 cup
Garbanzo beans, 1 cup
Alfalfa sprouts, ½ cup
French dressing, 2 tbsp
Macaroni and cheese, 3 cups
Apple juice, 1 cup

Snack

Wheat bread, 2 slices
Margarine, 1 tsp
Jam, 2 tbsp

Dinner

Skinless turkey breast, 2 oz
Mashed potatoes, 2 cups
Peas and onions, 1 cup
Banana, 1
Skim milk, 1 cup

Snack

Pasta, 1 cup
Margarine, 2 tsp
Parmesan cheese, 2 tbsp
Cranberry juice, 1 cup
_____
14% protein (140 g)
61% CHO (610 g)
26% fat (116 g)

5000 kcal diet
Breakfast

Cheerios, 2 cups
Bran muffins, 2
Orange, 1
2% milk, 1 cup

Snack

Low-fat yogurt, 1 cup
Chopped dates, 1 cup

Lunch

Apple juice, 1 cup
Chicken enchilada, 1
Romaine lettuce, 1 cup
Garbanzo beans, 1 cup
Alfalfa sprouts, ¾ cup
Grated carrots, ½ cup
Seasoned croutons, 1 oz

French dressing, 2 tbsp
Wheat bread, 2 slices
Margarine, 1 tbsp

Snack

Banana, 1
Bagel, 1
Cream cheese, 1 tbsp

Dinner

2% milk, 1 cup
Beef sirloin, 5 oz
Mashed potatoes, 2 cups
Spinach pasta noodles, 1½ cups
Grated parmesan cheese, 2 tbsp
Green beans, 1 cup
Oatmeal-raisin cookies, 3

Snack

Cranberry juice, 2 cups
Air-popped popcorn, 4 cups
Figs, 3
_____
14% protein (175 g)
63% CHO (813 g)
24% fat (136 g)

C RITICAL T HINKING

Some athletes believe that their diets should consist of 25% of kilocalories from protein because they are body building and working out. Your neighbor is a high school baseball player. He has been listening to many professional athletes talk about diet, and he plans to begin consuming 25% of his kilocalories from protein. How would you explain to him that this is too much protein?

fiber during the final day of training is a good precaution to reduce the chances of bloating and intestinal gas during the next day's event.[1]

As a general rule, athletes should obtain about 60% to 70% of their total energy needs from carbohydrate, rather than the 50% typical of most American diets. Endurance athletes should meet the higher value, especially as exercise duration exceeds 2 hours. With carbohydrate intakes in this range, intake of fat should fall, so that fat provides 20% to 30% of total energy needs rather than the typical 34%. Protein then provides the rest of the total energy—about 15% of total needs.[1] This approach yields a training diet that is about two-thirds carbohydrate-rich foods and one-third protein-rich foods, with fat coming in as part of many of the food choices made.

Looking at protein intake more specifically, typical recommendations for athletes range from 1.2 to 1.6 g of protein per kg of body weight, considerably higher than the RDA of 0.8 g/kg body weight.[13] Again, athletes engaged in endurance sports should aim for the higher value, as protein supplies a greater percentage of the energy used (up to 10%) in these sports than in other athletic endeavors. Overall, the vast majority of athletes can meet protein needs without having to exceed twice the RDA (1.6 g of protein per kg of body weight).

For athletes beginning a weight-training program, some experts recommend 2 to 2.5 g of protein per kg of body weight. That is up to approximately three times the RDA for protein.[5] To date, the importance of such an excessive protein intake during the initial phases of weight training has not been supported by sufficient research. Note that energy needs for weight lifting itself are not the reason for the high protein recommendation, as the fuel used in this activity is primarily carbohydrate. The extra protein theoretically is required for the synthesis of new tissue

TABLE 10-4

Grams of carbohydrate per exchange and serving size of typical foods

Starch list—15 g carbohydrate per serving
One serving:

½-¾ cup dry breakfast cereal*
½ cup cooked breakfast cereal
½ cup cooked grits
⅓ cup cooked rice
½ cup cooked pasta
¼ cup baked beans
½ cup cooked corn
½ cup cooked/dry beans

1 small baked potato
½ bagel
½ English muffin
1 slice bread
¾ oz pretzels
6 saltine crackers
2 pancakes, 4 inches in diameter
2 taco shells

Vegetable list—5 g carbohydrate per serving
One serving:

½ cup cooked vegetables
1 cup raw vegetables
½ cup vegetable juice
Examples: carrots, green beans, broccoli, cauliflower, onions, spinach, tomatoes, vegetable juice

Fruit list—15 g carbohydrate per serving
One serving:

½ cup fresh fruit
½ cup fruit juice
¼ cup dried fruit
1 small apple
4 apricots
1 banana (small)

12 cherries or grapes
½ grapefruit
1 nectarine
1 orange
1 peach
1¼ cups watermelon

Milk list—12 g carbohydrate per serving
One serving:

1 cup milk
¾ cup plain low-fat yogurt

Other carbohydrates list—15 g carbohydrate per serving
One serving:

2-inch square typical slice of cake
2 small cookies
3 ginger snaps

½ cup ice cream
½ cup sherbet

*Note that the carbohydrate content of dry cereal varies widely. Check the labels of the ones you choose and adjust serving size accordingly.
Modified from *Exchange Lists for Meal Planning* by the American Diabetes Association and American Dietetic Association, 1995, Chicago, American Dietetic Association.

brought on by the loading effect of weight training, which will be the greatest during the initial phases of weight training. Once the desired muscle mass is achieved, protein intake need not exceed twice the RDA.[13]

Table 10-5 shows the actual amount of protein that people of different body weights need to consume to meet the RDA and twice the RDA. Any athlete can easily have a protein intake twice the RDA simply by eating a variety of foods (see Table 10-3). For example, a 123-pound (53 kg) woman can consume 82 g of her upper range of 85 g of protein (twice the RDA) by eating 4 ounces of chicken (one chicken breast), 3 ounces of beef (a small lean hamburger), and ½ cup of cooked beans, and drinking 2 glasses of milk during a single day. A 180-pound (77 kg) man needs to consume only 6 ounces of chicken (a large chicken breast), ½ cup of cooked beans, a 6-ounce can of tuna, and 2 glasses of milk during a day to consume 122 g of his upper range of 123 g of protein (twice the RDA). And for both ath-

TABLE 10-5

Grams of protein that meet recommendations for individuals of different weights			
Body weight		**Protein allotment (grams)**	
pounds	kilograms	RDA (0.8 g/kg)	2 × RDA (1.6 g/kg)
110	50	40	80
130	60	48	96
155	70	56	112
175	80	64	128
200	90	72	144
220	100	80	160

Compare these quantities with protein intake from the diets listed in Table 10-3. Note that diets supplying enough total energy for athletes yield plenty of protein, even without making any special attempt to consume high-protein foods.

letes this does not even include the protein in the grains or vegetables they will also eat. In meeting their energy needs, many athletes consume even more protein. Thus protein supplements or amino acid supplements are not needed for athletes because their diets can easily meet protein needs.[20]

However, athletes who either feel they must significantly limit their energy intake or are vegetarians should specifically determine how much protein they eat. They should make sure to choose foods that provide at least 1.2 g of protein per kg of body weight. Skimping on protein is not a good idea.

VITAMIN AND MINERAL INTAKES FOR ATHLETES

Vitamin and mineral needs are the same or slightly higher for athletes compared with sedentary adults. Athletes' needs for vitamin E and vitamin C may be somewhat greater because of the antioxidant protection these nutrients provide; this effect could be especially important in the face of high oxygen use by muscles.[6] Still, use of megadoses of vitamin E and vitamin C requires more study and is not currently an accepted part of the dietary guidance for athletes.[14] Riboflavin, vitamin B-6, potassium, magnesium, iron, zinc, copper, and chromium needs also may increase somewhat because of their role in energy metabolism and/or loss in sweat (Table 10-6).[5] Based on current available research, any extra needs can be met by diet.[1, 9, 23] In addition, because athletes usually have high food-energy intakes, they tend to consume plenty of vitamins and minerals.

Athletes who reduce their energy intake to less than 1500 kcal in order to lose weight should pay very close attention to their vitamin and mineral intake. Vegetarian athletes should heed the same warning, as well as athletes undergoing intense training. A good approach for such athletes is to focus on nutrient-dense foods, such as low-fat and nonfat milk, broccoli, tomatoes, oranges, strawberries, whole grains, lean beef, kidney beans, turkey, fish, and chicken. Vitamin- and mineral-fortified foods, including many breakfast cereals, can also be used. Vitamin and mineral intakes from supplements greatly exceeding 150% of the Daily Values listed on the labels are not advised.

Iron

Athletes, especially female and adolescent athletes, should pay special attention to their iron intake.[16] In all athletes, iron stores can be depleted both by the loss of iron in sweat, urine, and gastrointestinal blood and by the increased use of iron required for the elevated production of red blood cells associated with physical fitness. Another, less important, mechanism of iron loss is foot-strike destruction of red blood cells in the blood passing through the feet; this results from the trauma created at

TABLE 10-6

Vitamins and minerals: functions and usage with regard to exercise

Vitamins and minerals	Exercise-related function	Proposed benefit to performance	Effects of supplementation in excess of RDA/ESADDI
Thiamin	Carbohydrate metabolism	Enhances endurance performance	Likely does not enhance performance
Riboflavin	Energy metabolism	Enhances aerobic performance	Does not enhance performance; needs may increase to 1.5 times the RDA at outset of training program.
Niacin	Energy metabolism	Enhances energy metabolism	Does not enhance performance and may even impair performance by reducing fatty acid release.
Vitamin B-6	Formation of hemoglobin	Enhances exercise performance	Does not enhance performance
Pantothenic acid	Energy metabolism	Enhances aerobic performance	Does not enhance performance
Vitamin B-12	Red blood cell development	Enhances endurance performance	Does not enhance performance
Folate	Cell synthesis; red blood cell formation		Does not enhance performance
Biotin	Fat and glycogen synthesis		No studies available
Vitamin C	Antioxidant capability	Prevents tissue damage; speeds repair	Well-controlled studies show no effect on performance, but some researchers think extra amounts may reduce oxidative damage to muscle from exercise. However, diet can easily supply the 150 mg it takes to saturate body tissues.
Vitamin A and beta-carotene	Antioxidant capability	Prevents tissue damage; speeds repair	Enhanced performance unlikely, but some researchers think extra amounts of carotenoids may reduce oxidative damage to muscle from exercise.
Vitamin D	Bone mineral metabolism	Bone formation during muscle repair	Does not affect work performance; may affect muscle building (one study), but needs likely do not exceed the RDA. Note that excess intakes can be toxic.
Vitamin E	Antioxidant capability	Prevents tissue damage; speeds repair	Does not enhance performance; may reduce exercise damage caused by breakdown in fat structure in cell membranes; research is ongoing. Needs may approach 2 times the RDA.
Zinc	Carbohydrate, fat, and protein metabolism; tissue repair	Repair of exercise damage	Does not enhance performance if diet meets the RDA.
Copper	Red blood cell synthesis; energy metabolism	Enhances aerobic performance	No studies available to show enhanced performance, but sweating increases copper losses.
Chromium	Carbohydrate metabolism; increases effects of insulin	Enhances muscle gain	Currently conflicting results in literature. May enhance muscle gain during weight training, but a study of football players did not support this hypothesis.[10] Any use should be considered experimental and should not exceed 200 μg per day.
Selenium	Antioxidant capability	Protects against exercise damage; delays fatigue	No conclusive studies available; note that it has a high potential for toxicity
Iron	Oxygen transport and delivery	Reduces fatigue; enhances endurance	No effect on performance in nonanemic or non–iron-deficient subjects

Primarily from Brouns F: *Nutritional needs of athletes*, Chichester, 1993, John Wiley & Sons.

At one time in his career, long-distance runner Alberto Salazar experienced problems sleeping and performed poorly because of low iron intake and related iron-deficiency anemia. Thus men and women are at risk, and both should regularly monitor iron status.

stress fracture A fracture that occurs from repeated jarring of a bone. Common sites include bones of the foot.

the point of impact when a foot strikes the ground. Young women are at special risk of iron deficiency because of the additional iron loss during menstruation.

If iron stores are not replenished, iron-deficiency anemia and markedly impaired endurance performance can eventually result. Although true anemia (noted as a depressed blood hemoglobin concentration) is quite rare among athletes, it is a good idea, especially for adult women athletes, to have the blood hemoglobin concentration checked about once a year and to monitor dietary iron intake.[3] Vegetarian female athletes should be especially careful to watch iron status. If blood iron is consistently low, the use of iron supplements by an athlete may be advisable. Iron supplements can improve athletic performance if an athlete is truly anemic, but indiscriminate use of iron supplements is not advised because toxic effects are possible (see Chapter 15).[1]

Calcium

Athletes, especially women trying to lose weight by restricting their intake of dairy products, can have marginal or low dietary intakes of calcium. This practice compromises optimal bone health. Of still greater concern are women athletes who have stopped menstruating because their arduous exercise training interferes with the normal secretion of the reproductive hormones. Disturbing reports show that female athletes who do not menstruate regularly have far less dense spinal bones than both nonathletes and female athletes who menstruate regularly.[11] This places them at increased risk for osteoporosis in later life. We discuss this further in Chapter 11, with respect to the female athlete triad, and in Chapter 14, where we review osteoporosis in detail.

For now, note that research has clearly documented the importance of regular menstruation to maintain bone mineral density. Current studies imply that a woman runner who does not menstruate regularly may also have a higher risk for the development of a **stress fracture.** Female athletes whose menstrual cycles become irregular should consult a physician to ascertain the cause. Decreasing the amount of training and/or increasing energy intake and body weight often restores regular menstrual cycles.[11] If irregular menstrual cycles persist, severe bone loss and osteoporosis can result. Extra calcium in the diet does not necessarily compensate for the effects of menstrual loss, but inadequate dietary calcium can make matters worse. Calcium intakes up to 1500 mg/day have been suggested, but the most effective measure is to have menstruation resume.

MEALS BEFORE ENDURANCE EVENTS

A light meal supplying 300 to 1000 kcal should be eaten about 2 to 4 hours before an endurance event to top off muscle and liver glycogen stores, prevent hunger during the event, and provide extra fluid (see next section).[1] The longer the period before an event, the larger the meal can be, as there will be more time available for digestion. A pre-event meal should consist primarily of carbohydrate (about 50 to 150 g), have little fat (<25% of energy intake) or dietary fiber, and include a moderate amount of protein (Table 10-7). A pre-event meal eaten 1 to 2 hours before an event should be blended or liquid to promote rapid stomach emptying.[1]

Good food choices for a pre-event meal include spaghetti, bagels, muffins, bread, and breakfast cereals with low-fat or nonfat milk. Liquid meal replacement formulas, like Carnation Instant Breakfast, also can be used. Foods rich in dietary fiber should be eaten the previous day to help clear the bowels before an event, but they should not be eaten the night before or in the morning before the event. Foods to avoid are those that are fatty or fried, such as sausage, bacon, sauces, and gravies. A meal high in carbohydrate is quickly digested, promotes maintenance of blood glucose, and avoids the need to dip right away into glycogen stores. If an athlete feels a pre-event meal harms performance, eating a high-carbohydrate diet the day and night before can help meet the same goal.

Specific carbohydrate feeding an hour or so before competition was previously thought to adversely affect performance because it increases release of insulin, which

TABLE 10-7

Convenient pre-event meals	
Breakfast (McDonald's)	**Energy content**
Hot cakes with syrup and margarine	900 kcal
Orange juice, 2 servings	67% from carbohydrate
English muffin (whole) with 2 tsp margarine and 2 tsp jam	(150 g)
• • •	
Cheerios, ¾ cup	450 kcal
Low-fat milk, 1 cup	82% from carbohydrate
Blueberry muffin	(92 g)
Orange juice, 1 serving	
Lunch or dinner (Wendy's)	
Chili, 8 oz portion	900 kcal
Baked potato with sour cream and chives	65% from carbohydrate
Chocolate Frosty, 10 oz	(150 g)
• • •	
Grilled chicken sandwich	425 kcal
Cola, 12 oz	65% from carbohydrate
	(70 g)

causes blood glucose to fall. However, we know now that this practice does not cause premature fatigue nor decrease endurance for most people, especially if they have eaten breakfast and perform adequate warm-up exercises. In fact, recent studies show positive benefits from pre-event carbohydrate feeding.[17] However, some athletes are extremely sensitive to an insulin surge. Thus athletes should experiment with pre-event carbohydrate feedings to see if their performance is adversely or positively affected.[1]

MAXIMIZING BODY FLUIDS AND ENERGY STORES DURING EXERCISE

Water (fluid) needs for an average adult are about 1 ml/kcal expended. This is equivalent to about 6 to 8 cups of fluid per day. Athletes need this and generally even more water intake to maintain the body's ability to regulate its internal temperature and to keep itself cool.[21] Most energy released during metabolism appears immediately as heat. Unless this heat is quickly dissipated, heat exhaustion, heat cramps, and deadly heatstroke may ensue (Figure 10-5).

Heat exhaustion occurs when heat stress causes depletion of blood volume from fluid loss by the body.[4] As environmental temperature rises above 95° F (35° C), virtually all body heat is lost through evaporation of sweat from the skin. Sweat rates during prolonged exercise range from 3 to 8 cups (750 to 2000 ml) per hour. However, as the humidity rises, especially when it rises above 75 percent, evaporation slows and sweating becomes inefficient.

Increased body temperature associated with dehydration is most evident when the amount of water loss exceeds 3% of body weight.[4] This dehydration then leads to a fall in endurance, strength, and overall performance. Wearing football equipment in hot weather can lead to a loss of 2% of body weight in 30 minutes. Marathon runners have been shown to lose 6% to 10% of body weight during a race.[1]

Common symptoms of heat exhaustion include profuse sweating, headache, dizziness, nausea, vomiting, muscle weakness, visual disturbances, and flushing of the skin. A person with heat exhaustion should be taken to a cool environment im-

Heat index

Relative humidity (%)	70°	75°	80°	85°	90°	95°	100°	105°	110°
100	72°	80°	91°	108°					
90	71°	79°	88°	102°	122°				
80	71°	78°	86°	97°	113°	136°			
70	70°	77°	85°	93°	106°	124°	144°		
60	70°	76°	82°	90°	100°	114°	132°	149°	
50	69°	75°	81°	88°	96°	107°	120°	135°	150°
40	68°	74°	79°	86°	93°	101°	110°	123°	137°
30	67°	73°	78°	84°	90°	96°	104°	113°	123°
20	66°	72°	77°	82°	87°	93°	99°	105°	112°
10	65°	70°	75°	80°	85°	90°	95°	100°	105°
0	64°	69°	73°	78°	83°	87°	91°	95°	99°

Air temperature (°F)

Heat index	Heat disorders possible with prolonged exposure and/or physical activity
80° to 89°	Fatigue
90° to 104°	Sunstroke, heat cramps, and heat exhaustion
105° to 129°	Sunstroke, heat cramps, or heat exhaustion likely and heatstroke possible
130° or higher	Heatstroke/sunstroke highly likely

NOTE: Direct sunshine increases the heat index by up to 15° F.

Figure 10-5 Heat index chart, showing associated heat disorders.

mediately, and excess clothing should be removed. The body should be sponged with tap water. Fluid replacement, as tolerated, then should suffice.[4]

Heat cramps are a frequent complication of heat exhaustion, but they may appear alone, without other symptoms of dehydration.[4] They usually occur in individuals exercising for several hours in a hot climate who have large sweat losses and have consumed a large volume of unsalted water. It is important not to confuse heat cramps with other forms of muscle cramps, such as those caused by gastrointestinal upset. Heat cramps occur in skeletal muscles, including those of the abdomen and the extremities. They consist of a contraction for 1 to 3 minutes at a time. The cramp moves down the muscle and is associated with excruciating pain. The best way to prevent heat cramps is to exercise moderately at first in the heat, with adequate salt intake, before engaging in long, strenuous exercise.[4]

Heatstroke can occur when internal body temperature reaches 105° F. Exertional heatstroke results from high blood flow to exercising muscles, which overloads the body's cooling capacity. Sweating generally ceases, and the body temperature may become dangerously high. If left untreated, circulatory collapse, central nervous system damage, and death are likely. Death rate is high, approximately 10%.[4]

Many individuals who suffer heatstroke faint, and their skin becomes hot and dry. Ice packs or cold water is the usual recommended immediate treatment until medical help can be summoned. To decrease the risk of developing heatstroke, athletes should replace lost fluids, watch for rapid body-weight changes (≥3% body weight), and avoid exercise under extremely hot, humid conditions.[4]

Since dehydration during exercise leads to body-weight loss and sets the stage for heat exhaustion, heat cramps, and potentially fatal heatstroke, athletes must avoid becoming dehydrated. Fluid intake during exercise, when possible, should be

The symptoms of heatstroke include:
• **Nausea**
• **Confusion**
• **Irritability**
• **Poor coordination**
• **Seizures**
• **Elevated body temperature**
• **Coma (in severe cases)**

adequate to minimize body-weight loss; this practice is a good idea even in the wintertime, when sweating can go unnoticed.

The recommended goal is a loss of no more than 3% of body weight during exercise.[1] Athletes should first calculate 3% of their body weight and then by trial and error determine how much fluid they must take in to avoid losing more than this amount of weight during exercise. This determination will be most accurate if an athlete is weighed before and after a typical workout. For every 1 pound (½ kg) lost, 2 cups (0.5 L) of water should be consumed during exercise or immediately afterward. However, most athletes find it very uncomfortable to replace more than about 75% to 80% of this sweat loss during exercise.[12]

Thirst is not a reliable indicator of an athlete's need to replace fluid during exercise. An athlete who only drinks when thirsty is likely to take 48 hours to replenish fluid loss. After several days of training, an athlete relying on thirst as an indicator can build up a large enough fluid debt to impair performance. The following fluid-replacement approach can meet athletes' fluid needs in most cases.[12,22]

- Freely drink beverages (e.g., water, diluted fruit juice, sports drinks) up to 2 hours before an event, even if not particularly thirsty.
- About 20 to 30 minutes before an event, consume about 1½ to 2 cups (360 to 500 ml) of these fluids. This is called hyperhydration. The extra fluid in the body will be ready to replace sweat losses as needed.
- During events lasting more than 30 minutes, consume about ½ to 1 cup (150 to 250 ml) of fluid every 15 to 20 minutes as possible, totaling up to about 4 cups (1 L) per hour. Consuming more than 1 L per hour can cause discomfort. On hot days, cold drinks are preferable to help cool the body. Again, the athlete should not wait until he or she feels thirsty.

If the weather is hot and/or humid, even more fluids may be required. Note that skipping fluids before or during events will almost certainly cause problems!

SPORTS DRINKS: MOST HELPFUL FOR ENDURANCE ACTIVITIES

A question that often arises is whether to drink water or a sports-type carbohydrate-**electrolyte** drink, e.g., All Sport, Exceed Energy Drink, Gatorade, PowerAde, and Amino Force, during competition (Figure 10-6). For sports that require less than 30 minutes of exertion or when total weight loss is less than 5 to 6 pounds, the primary concern is replacing the water lost in sweat, because losses of body carbohydrate stores and electrolytes (sodium, chloride, potassium, and other minerals) are not usually too great. Although electrolytes are lost in sweat, the quantities lost in exercise of brief to moderate duration can be easily replaced later by consuming normal foods, such as orange juice, potatoes, and tomato juice.[12] Keep in mind that sweat is about 99% water and only 1% electrolytes and other substances.

Water is certainly cheaper than a sports drink. The use of sports drinks is most critical for athletes engaged in sports events lasting longer than 60 to 90 minutes.[12] Beverages for the endurance athlete must provide water for hydration, electrolytes both to enhance water and glucose absorption from the intestine and to help maintain blood volume, and carbohydrate to provide energy. Beyond 2 to 4 hours of exertion, electrolyte and carbohydrate replacement becomes increasingly important, especially in hot weather. Sports-type drinks may also taste better than water, which may help the athlete drink more often—a clear advantage of this form of fluid replenishment. In addition, the carbohydrate in these drinks quickly replaces carbohydrate used during practice or competition.

Prolonged exercise results in large sweat losses, and some of the fluid for sweating comes from the bloodstream. If plain water is used to replace the fluid lost from the blood, the concentration of essential electrolytes in the bloodstream may become too diluted. Thus when sports drinks are used to help maintain blood volume, they must contain small amounts of sodium and potassium to avoid electrolyte imbalance.[5]

electrolytes Compounds that separate into ions in water and, in turn, are able to conduct an electrical current. These include sodium, chloride, and potassium.

- - - - - - - - - - - -

Alcohol and caffeine both have a dehydrating effect on the body, so fluids containing them should not be part of any hydration plan for exercise.

- - - - - - - - - - - -

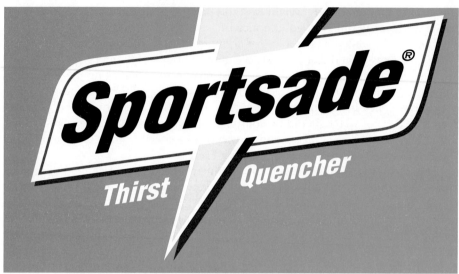

Nutrition Facts
Serving Size 8 fl oz (240ml)
Servings Per Container 4

Amount Per Serving

Calories 50

	% Daily Value*
Total Fat 0g	0%
Sodium 110mg	5%
Potassium 30mg	1%
Total Carbohydrates 14g	5%
Sugars 14g	
Protein 0g	

Not a significant source of Calories From Fat,
Saturated Fat, Cholesterol, Dietary Fiber,
Vitamin A, Vitamin C, Calcium, Iron.

* Percent Daily Values are based on a 2,000
calorie diet.

NO FRUIT JUICE
INGREDIENTS: WATER, SUCROSE SYRUP, GLUCOSE-
FRUCTOSE SYRUP, CITRIC ACID, NATURAL ORANGE
FLAVOR WITH OTHER NATURAL FLAVORS, SALT,
SODIUM CITRATE, MONOPOTASSIUM PHOSPHATE,
YELLOW 6, ESTER GUM, BROMINATED VEGETABLE OIL

Figure 10-6 Sports drinks for fluid and electrolyte replacement typically contain a form of simple carbohydrate plus sodium and potassium. The various sugars in this product total 14 g per 1 cup (240 ml) serving. In percentage terms based on weight, the sugar content is about 6% ([14 g sugar/serving ÷ 240 g/serving] × 100 = 5.8%). Sports drinks typically contain about 6% to 8% sugar. This provides ample glucose and other monosaccharides to aid in fueling working muscles, and it is well tolerated. Drinks with a higher sugar content may cause stomach distress.

Use of sports drinks that contain carbohydrate also has been found to delay fatigue during endurance sports with exercise intensities of a 3-hour marathon pace. The carbohydrate intake improves endurance presumably either by preventing great drops in blood glucose or by providing an outside source of glucose for muscle use. When sports drinks are used as part of fluid replacement, one possible protocol is:

- About 20 to 30 minutes before endurance exercise, consume 1 to 2 cups (250 to 500 ml) of water.[12] Some experts, however, recommend instead consumption of the same amount of a 10% to 20% solution of carbohydrate (25 to 50 g of carbohydrate per 8-ounce cup of fluid). Drinks such as GatorLode, UltraFuel, and CarboForce have carbohydrate concentrations in this latter range.
- Once exercise begins, consume 1 cup (240 ml) of a 6% to 8%, carbohydrate solution (14 to 19 g per cup of fluid) every 15 to 20 minutes, totaling about 45 to 60 g of carbohydrate and up to 4 cups (1 L) per hour.[12] The carbohydrate concentration of many common sports drinks is 6% to 8%, but check the label to be sure (Figure 10-5).

- After 1½ to 2 hours of exertion, switch back to a higher carbohydrate drink (10% to 20% solution) and continue consuming 1 cup every 15 to 20 minutes.[12]

Some sports drinks contain **glucose polymers** (glucoses linked together in short chains). These drinks initially were thought to empty from the stomach faster than drinks containing glucose. We now know that there's little difference in stomach-emptying times between sports drinks containing glucose polymers and those containing simple sugars such as glucose or sucrose. Furthermore, comparisons of drinks containing glucose polymers (more properly known as maltodextrins), glucose, or sucrose show that all of these carbohydrates have similar positive effects on exercise performance and physiological function as long as the carbohydrate concentration is in the 6% to 8% range.[26] Drinks whose only carbohydrate source is fructose are the only exception to this rule. Fructose is absorbed from the intestine more slowly than glucose and often causes bloating or diarrhea.

Overall, then, the decision to use a sports drink hinges primarily on the duration of the activity. As the duration of continuous activity approaches 60 to 90 minutes or longer, the advantages from use of a sports drink over plain water begin to emerge.[12] However, athletes should first experiment with the suggested protocol during practice, instead of trying it for the first time during competition.

CARBOHYDRATE INTAKE DURING RECOVERY FROM EXERCISE

Carbohydrate-rich foods yielding about 50 to 100 g of carbohydrate should be consumed within 2 hours after extended (endurance) exercise, and the sooner the better, because this is when glycogen synthesis is greatest.[24] This process should then be repeated over the next 2-hour interval. Athletes who are training hard can consume a simple sugar candy, sugared soft drink, fruit or fruit juice, or a sports-type carbohydrate supplement right after training as they attempt to reload their muscles with glycogen. At quick-service restaurants, athletes can order thicker crust on pizza and have extra rolls and muffins.

Fluid and electrolyte (i.e., sodium and potassium) intake is also an essential component of an athlete's recovery diet. This helps replenish body fluids as quickly as possible. This is especially important if two workouts a day are followed and if the environment is hot and humid. If food and fluid intake is sufficient to restore weight loss, it generally will also supply enough electrolytes to meet needs during recovery from endurance activities.

It cannot be emphasized enough that any nutrition strategies should be tested out during practice and trial runs before being used in a meet or key event. An athlete should never try a new food or beverage on the day of competition. Some food items or beverages may not be tolerated well, and the day of competition is not the time to find that out.[1]

glucose polymers Carbohydrates used in some sports drinks that consist of a few glucose molecules chemically linked together.

CONCEPT CHECK

All athletes would do well to plan a diet following the Food Guide Pyramid. High-carbohydrate foods should be emphasized, and these should dominate in pre-event meals. Protein intake above twice the RDA is not needed in most cases. If nutrient supplements are used, dosages generally should not exceed 150% of the Daily Value listed on the label. Fluid should be consumed as liberally as possible before, during, and after an event. Carbohydrate and electrolytes in the fluid are helpful when exercise duration exceeds 60 to 90 minutes, to help delay fatigue and maintain electrolyte balance.

Summary

1. Human metabolic pathways extract chemical energy from foodstuffs and transfer it into ATP, the compound that provides energy for body functions.

2. In glycolysis, glucose is broken down (oxidized) into pyruvate, a three-carbon compound, yielding some ATP. The pyruvate is metabolized further via the aerobic pathway to form carbon dioxide (CO_2) and water (H_2O) or via the anaerobic pathway to form lactate.

3. A gradual increase to regular physical activity is recommended for all healthy persons. If one is over age 35, it is recommended that he or she first consult a physician. A minimum plan includes at least a total of 30 minutes of physical activity per day. A more intense program should begin with warm-up exercises, to increase blood flow and warm the muscles, and end with cool-down exercises.

4. Vo_2max is a measure of the maximum volume of oxygen one can consume per unit of time. Oxygen consumption is measured by exercising the subject at an increasing pace and work load until fatigue occurs. The oxygen consumed right before total exhaustion is Vo_2max. The value of Vo_2max varies among individuals, but usually improves with exercise training.

5. At rest, muscle cells mainly use fat for fuel. For intense exercise of short duration, muscles use mostly phosphocreatine (PCr) for energy. During more sustained intense activity, muscle glycogen breaks down into lactate. For endurance exercise, both fat and carbohydrate are used as fuels; carbohydrate is used increasingly as activity intensifies. Little protein is used to fuel muscles.

6. Anyone who exercises regularly should consume a diet that is moderate to high in carbohydrates and that follows the Food Guide Pyramid. Weekend athletes would be well advised to do the same, as the many health benefits experienced add to those from the physical activity.

7. Athletes should consume enough fluid to both minimize loss of body weight and ultimately restore pre-exercise weight. Sports drinks aid fluid, electrolyte, and carbohydrate replacement. Their use should be considered when continuous activity lasts beyond 60 to 90 minutes.

Study Questions

1. How does greater physical fitness contribute to greater aerobic metabolism? Explain the process.

2. The store of ATP in muscle is rapidly depleted once contraction begins. For physical activity to continue, ATP must be resupplied immediately. Describe how this occurs after initiation of exercise and at various times thereafter.

3. What is the difference between anaerobic and aerobic exercise? At what point is the switch made from mostly anaerobic to mostly aerobic fuel metabolism? Explain why aerobic metabolism is increased by a regular exercise routine.

4. What is glycogen? How does the body obtain it? How much can be stored? How long does it last during exercise?

5. Are fat stores used as an energy source during exercise? If so, when?

6. What are some typical measures of fitness? Explain the physiological/biochemical bases for why these are appropriate measures.

7. Physical activity can be classified into four types: low intensity; moderate intensity; prolonged high intensity (endurance); and brief maximal intensity (very high intensity). Compare and contrast the four types of exercise with respect to the percentage of Vo_2max used and the specific fuels employed.

8. List five specific nutrients that athletes need and the ideal food sources from which these nutrients can be obtained.

9. What advice would you give to your neighbor, who is planning to run a 50-kilometer (km) race, concerning fluid intake before and during the event?

10. One of your friends, who is a competitive athlete, asks your opinion about a nutritional supplement sold in a local sporting-goods store. She has read that such supplements, which contain vitamins, minerals, and amino acids, can help improve athletic performance. What would you tell her about the general effectiveness of such products?

REFERENCES

1. Benardot D: *Sports nutrition,* Chicago, 1993, The American Dietetic Association.
2. Blair SN: Diet and activity: the synergistic merger, *Nutrition Today* 30:108, 1995.
3. Brigham DE and others: Changes in iron status during competitive season in female collegiate swimmers, *Nutrition* 9:418, 1993.
4. Bross MH and others: Heat emergencies, *American Family Physician* 50:389, 1994
5. Brouns F: *Nutritional needs of athletes,* Chichester, 1993, John Wiley.
6. Bucci LR: Nutritional ergogenic aids. In Wolinsky I, Hickson JF, editors: *Nutrition in exercise and sport,* ed 2, Boca Raton, Fla, 1994, CRC Press.
7. Burke LM, Read RS: Dietary supplements in sport, *Sports Medicine* 15:43, 1993.
8. Chandler RM and others: Dietary supplements affect the anabolic hormones after weight-training exercise, *Journal of Applied Physiology* 76:839, 1994.
9. Clancy SP and others: Effects of chromium picolinate supplementation on body composition, strength, and urinary chromium loss in football players, *International Journal of Sports Nutrition* 4:142, 1994.
10. Clark N and others: Feeding the ultraendurance athlete: practical tips and a case study, *Journal of the American Dietetic Association* 92:1258, 1992.
11. DiFiori JP: Menstrual dysfunction in athletes, *Postgraduate Medicine* 97:143, 1995.
12. Hawley JA and others: Carbohydrate, fluid, and electrolyte requirements during prolonged exercise. In Kies CV, Driskell JA, editors: *Sports nutrition,* Boca Raton, Fla, 1995, CRC Press.
13. Hickson JF: Research directions in protein nutrition for athletes. In Wolinsky I, Hickson JF, editors: *Nutrition in exercise and sport,* ed 2, Boca Raton, Fla, 1994, CRC Press.
14. Holt WS: Nutrition and athletes, *American Family Physican* 47:1757, 1993.
15. Katch FI, McArdle WD: *Introduction to nutrition, exercise, and health,* ed 4, Philadelpia, 1993, Lea & Febiger.
16. LaManca JJ, Haymes EM: Effects of iron depletion on VO_2max, endurance, and blood lactate in women, *Medical Science Sports Exercise* 12:1386, 1993.
17. Liebman M, Wilkinson JG: Carbohydrate metabolism and exercise. In Wolinsky I, Hickson JF, editors: *Nutrition in exercise and sport,* ed 2, Boca Raton, Fla, 1994, CRC Press.
18. Matson LG, Tran ZV: Effects of sodium bicarbonate ingestion on anaerobic performance: a meta-analytic review, *International Journal of Sports Nutrition* 3:2, 1993.
19. Maughan RJ: Nutritional aspects of endurance exercise in humans, *Proceedings of the Nutrition Society* 53:181, 1994.
20. Millward DJ and others: Physical activity, protein metabolism, and protein requirements, *Proceedings of the Nutrition Society* 52:223, 1994.
21. Pate RR and others: Physical activity and public health—a recommendation from the Centers for Disease Control and Prevention and the American College of Sports Medicine, *Journal of the American Medical Association,* 273:402, 1995.
22. Pivarnik JM, Palmer RA: Water and electrolyte balance during rest and exercise. In Wolinsky I, Hickson JF, editors: *Nutrition in exercise and sport,* ed 2, Boca Raton, Fla, 1994, CRC Press.
23. Position of the American Dietetic Association and the Canadian Dietetic Association: Nutrition for physical fitness and athletic performance for adults, *Journal of the American Dietetic Association* 93:691, 1993.
24. Sherman WM: Metabolism of sugars and physical performance, *American Journal of Clinical Nutrition* 62:228S, 1995.
25. Trappe SW and others: The effects of L-carnitine supplementation on performance during interval swimming, *International Journal of Sports Medicine* 15:181, 1994.
26. Wagaenmakers AJ and others: Oxidation rates of orally ingested carbohydrates during prolonged exercise in men, *Journal of Applied Physiology,* 75:2774, 1993.
27. Williams MH: Ergogenic and ergolytic substances, *Medicine and Science in Sports and Exercise,* 24:S344, 1992.
28. Yesalis CE and others: Anabolic-androgenic steroid use in the United States, *Journal of the American Medical Association,* 270:1217, 1993.

TAKE ACTION

Are you measuring up to the numbers?

In this chapter several key nutrients were highlighted in our discussion of exercise performance. Some of the guidelines are generally useful for maintaining good fitness and apply to athletes and nonathletes alike. These include the following:

- Eat a moderate to high amount of carbohydrates (60% of total energy intake).
- Eat a minimum of 1.2 g of protein (for athletes) or 0.8 g of protein (for nonathletes) per kg body weight.
- Consume the RDA for vitamins and minerals
- Make sure iron and calcium intake meets the RDA, especially in women.

Review the results of the dietary assessment you completed in Chapter 2. Remember that you assessed 1 day's food intake. Now answer the following questions (even if you are not an athlete):

1. What percentage of your energy intake was in the form of carbohydrate? Was 60% or more of your total energy intake supplied by carbohydrate?
2. Was your total protein intake equivalent to at least 0.8 g of protein per kg body weight if you are not an athlete, or at least 1.2 g per kg body weight if you are an athlete?
3. Did you consume at least the RDA for all vitamins and minerals assessed? For which ones were you below the RDA? Pay particular attention to iron and calcium.
4. What can you do to improve your dietary intake to promote general fitness and, if you are an athlete, to promote maximum performance in your chosen event(s)?

Ergogenic Aids: Substances That Can Enhance Athletic Performance

DAVID LAMB, Ph.D.

Diet manipulation to improve athletic performance is not a recent practice. As long as 30 years ago, American football players were encouraged on hot practice days to "toughen up" for competition by liberally consuming salt tablets before and during practice and by not drinking water. Now it is widely recognized that this practice can be fatal. Today's athletes are as likely as their predecessors to experiment: artichoke hearts, bee pollen, dried adrenal glands from cattle, seaweed, freeze-dried liver flakes, gelatin, and ginseng are just some of the worthless substances now used by athletes in hopes of gaining an **ergogenic** (work-producing) edge.

Still, today's athletes can benefit from recently documented scientific evidence that a few dietary substances do have ergogenic properties. These ergogenic aids include sufficient water, lots of carbohydrates, and a balanced and varied diet that adheres to the Food Guide Pyramid. Protein and amino acid supplements are not among these aids, since athletes can easily meet protein needs from foods, as Table 10-4 demonstrates.

Clearly, it is not possible to change average athletes into champions simply by altering their diets. The use of nutrient supplements should be targeted to meet a specific dietary weakness, such as an inadequate iron intake. These and other aids, which often have dubious benefits and may pose health risks, must be given close scrutiny before use. The risk-benefit ratio of these ergogenic aids especially needs to be examined. Athletes must stay on guard against false promises.

CARBOHYDRATE LOADING

For athletes who compete in continuous events lasting 90 to 120 minutes or longer, or in shorter events repeated in a 24-hour period, it is often advantageous to undertake a **carbohydrate-loading** regimen to maximize muscle glycogen stores. One possible regimen includes a gradual reduction or "tapering" of exercise intensity and duration, coupled with a gradual increase in dietary carbohydrate as a percentage of energy intake. The procedure can begin 6 days before competition, with the athlete completing a hard workout lasting about 60 minutes. Workouts for the next 4 days then last about 40, 40, 20, and 20 minutes, respectively, with exercise intensities being progressively reduced each day. On the final day before competition, the athlete rests.

The dietary carbohydrate on the first 3 days of this regimen (about 450 g/day) contributes 45% to 50% of energy intake. This rises to 65% to 75% carbohydrate (about 600 g/day) for the last 3 days before competition. This carbohydrate-loading technique usually increases muscle glycogen stores by 50% to 85% over typical conditions (i.e., when dietary carbohydrate constitutes about 50% of total energy intake). The greater carbohydrate stores then often result in improved athletic endurance. A typical carbohydrate-loading schedule would be:

	Days before competition					
	6	5	4	3	2	1
Exercise time (min)	60	40	40	20	20	REST
Carbohydrate (g)	450	450	450	600	600	600

A potential disadvantage of carbohydrate loading is that some water is stored in the muscles along with the extra glycogen. In some individuals, this additional water weight is sufficient to detract from sport performance. Thus for these athletes, carbohydrate loading is not an ergogenic aid. Athletes considering carbohydrate loading should try it during training (and well before an important competition) to experience its effects on performance. They can then determine if it is worth the effort. Sports activities for which carbohydrate loading is likely to improve performance include marathons, long-distance swimming, cross-country skiing, 30-kilometer runs, tournament play basketball, soccer, triathlons, cycling time trials, and long-distance canoe racing.   Carbohydrate loading is not effective for improving

ergogenic Work-producing. An ergogenic aid is a physical, mechanical, nutritional, psychological, or pharmacological substance or treatment that is intended to directly improve exercise performance.

carbohydrate loading The process of consuming a very-high-carbohydrate diet for about 3 days before an athletic event while tapering exercise duration to try to increase muscle glycogen stores.

performances in American football games, 10-kilometer runs, walking and hiking, most swimming events, single basketball games, most track and field events, and weight lifting.

Carbohydrate loading is safe for adolescents, but the activities this technique is useful for, like marathon runs, may not be. A physician's approval should be sought for the latter.

CARNITINE

The majority of the energy stored in the body for muscle use is found in fat. During physical activity, fatty acids are released from the fat depots into the blood and travel to the muscles, where they are taken into each cell. These fatty acids must enter the cell's mitochondria before they can be broken down to carbon dioxide and water, yielding ATP in the process. Movement of fatty acids from the cytosol of the cell into the mitochondria mostly occurs via a transport system that contains a compound called **carnitine.** Athletes sometimes take a carnitine supplement, hoping it will help them burn fat faster in exercise. But since body cells can make carnitine quite easily, carnitine supplements provide no reliable benefit.[25]

carnitine A compound used to shuttle fatty acids into the mitochondria of a cell, where the fatty acids can be broken down to provide energy.

BICARBONATE LOADING

We saw in this chapter that lactate buildup inhibits the activity of some enzymes involved in anaerobic ATP production by glycolysis, and may lead to early fatigue. Early attempts to counter this lactate accumulation by ingestion of small doses of **sodium bicarbonate** (a base) failed to improve athletic performances. On the other hand, more recent experiments in which large doses of bicarbonate (200 to 300 mg/kg body weight) were consumed with a large volume of water (approximately 1 L) 1 to 2 hours before exercise generally showed improved performance in strenuous activities lasting 2 to 10 minutes. About 20 minutes of warm-up typically preceded the exercise activity in these experiments. Sodium bicarbonate loading apparently speeds removal of lactate from contracting muscle cells and alters the balance of charged particles (e.g., sodium and hydrogen ions) to help reduce acidity.[18] Unfortunate side effects of large doses of sodium bicarbonate are nausea and diarrhea, often at unpredictable times and especially when water intake is insufficient. For this reason, bicarbonate loading has so far not become popular with athletes.

sodium bicarbonate An alkaline substance made basically of sodium and carbon dioxide ($NaHCO_3$).

ALCOHOL

Alcohol has been purported to enhance endurance performance by reducing a person's perception of fatigue and by providing additional energy. Alcohol's ergogenic value is not borne out by research findings, however, and it appears more likely that alcohol impairs rather than enhances physical performance. Alcohol decreases glucose release from the liver, which reduces blood glucose and can lead to hypoglycemia and possible premature fatigue. In cold environments, this hypoglycemia can also contribute to hypothermia.

CAFFEINE

Drinking two to three 5-ounce cups of coffee (equivalent to 3 to 6 mg of caffeine per kg body weight) or using caffeine suppositories about 1 hour before events lasting about 5 minutes or longer than 30 minutes enhances performance in some, but not all, athletes. The effect is sometimes less apparent in those who have ample stores of glycogen, are highly trained, or habitually consume caffeine.

The mechanism of the caffeine effect is not well established. Sparing of muscle glycogen by increasing the use of fatty acids for muscle fuel, psychological effects, or enhancement of glycolysis or the contractile process in muscles all deserve consideration. However, some athletes experience changes in heart rhythm, nausea, or lightheadedness that can actually impair performance. Olympic officials view caffeine as a drug and do not condone its use, but athletes are permitted fairly large amounts of caffeine before competition. Intake of more than about 600 mg (the amount in 4 to 5 cups of coffee) will elicit a urine concentration that would be grounds for disqualification according to standards set by the International Olympic Committee.

ANABOLIC STEROIDS

steroids A group of hormones and related compounds that are derivatives of cholesterol.

Public attention focused on the use of anabolic **steroids** when Ben Johnson, winner of the gold medal for the 100-meter dash in the 1988 Olympic Games, was disqualified. Johnson took anabolic steroids regularly as part of his training regimen. These steroids are used by athletes to enhance performance in a variety of sports, most commonly "strength sports" such as football, power lifting, weight lifting, and certain track-and-field events. Steroids have also been used by some swimmers and cyclists and commonly are used by male and female body builders.[28] Even nonathletic high school students have taken steroids in an attempt to "get big."

Anabolic steroids are synthetic versions of male sex hormones that promote two types of effects: masculinization (**androgenic** effect) and growth promotion (anabolic effect). Athletes have taken these drugs, often in doses 10 to 30 times normal androgen output, to increase muscle size, strength, and performance; note that no reliable cardiovascular benefit has been found.

androgenic A general term for hormones such as testosterone that stimulate development in male sex organs.

Although these steroids often can increase muscle mass and strength, their use in competitive athletics is illegal. In the United States their possession without a prescription is a federal crime. In addition, depending on the dose, steroids have numerous—occasionally devastating—side effects. They can, for example, cause premature closure of growth plates in bones (thus possibly limiting the adult height of a teenage athlete); produce bloody cysts in the liver; increase the risk of heart disease; and lead to high blood pressure, reproductive dysfunction, and many other detrimental physical effects. The psychological consequences of steroid use include increasing aggressiveness, drug dependence (addiction), withdrawal symptoms such as depression and sleep disturbances, mood swings, decreased sex drive, depression, and even "roid-rage" (violence attributed to steroid use).

Athletes often begin to use steroids during high school, some even as early as junior high school. Many serious athletes must make a hard choice: to not use steroids and face a large field of artificially endowed opponents or to use the drugs and risk side effects and legal sanctions.

GROWTH HORMONE

growth hormone A pituitary hormone that stimulates body growth and release of fat from storage, and has other effects.

Growth hormone, which is produced in the pituitary gland, normally promotes synthesis of protein, mobilizes fatty acids from fat stores, and helps control the rate of skeletal growth. Some athletes have used growth hormone injections to increase their muscle mass and strength, but no scientific studies have shown that such injections are effective for this purpose. Furthermore, it is known that the skin, the tongue, and bones of the jaw, fingers, and toes may grow abnormally when stimulated by high-growth hormone. Although treatment with growth hormone at critical ages may increase height, other potential consequences are uncontrolled growth of the heart and other internal organs and even death. All in all, any use of growth hormone is potentially dangerous and requires careful monitoring by a physician.

In addition to growth-hormone injections, supplementation with the amino acids arginine, ornithine, and glycine has been promoted as a way to boost the body's synthesis of growth hormone. Current evidence suggests that any increase in growth hormone after consuming these amino acids in supplement form is rather modest and probably of little physiological consequence.

BLOOD DOPING

blood doping A procedure for increasing an athlete's red blood cell count. Generally, blood is taken from the athlete and the red blood cells are concentrated and frozen; later the red cells are thawed and reinjected into the athlete.

Injection of red blood cells into the bloodstream—known as **blood doping**—is used to try to enhance aerobic capacity. In this procedure, a minimum of 2 pints of blood is drawn from the athlete at least 6 weeks before a competitive event and the red blood cells are isolated and frozen. As is usual following removal of blood, the body over time makes more red blood cells to restore the original number. Then, a day or two before competition, the frozen red blood cells are thawed and reinfused into the donor athlete, thereby elevating the total red blood cell count and hemoglobin concentration above normal. The downside of blood doping is that it thickens the blood, which puts extra strain on the heart.

A simpler, faster, but more dangerous way to "blood dope" is to inject a synthetic form of the hormone called **erythropoietin**. Erythropoietin, which is secreted by the kidney, stimulates red blood cell production by the bone marrow. Erythropoietin can increase the concentration of red blood cells so greatly that blood clots develop in the lungs or brain, leading to strokes that can paralyze or kill. It has been widely speculated in the medical community that misuse of synthetic erythropoietin, after it first became available, was responsible for a sudden dramatic increase in deaths of young competitive cyclists in Europe.

Several studies confirm an aerobic benefit to the athlete as a result of blood doping, but the potential negative health consequences, especially with erythropoietin abuse, are very serious. It is also an illegal practice under Olympic guidelines.

PHOSPHATE LOADING

Contrary to the belief of many athletes and coaches, phosphate pills do not always improve performance or efficiency of heart function during endurance events. Some studies have suggested that loading phosphate for 4 days increases the amount of a metabolically important phosphate compound, **diphosphoglycerate (DPG),** in red blood cells. These studies also showed that increased DPG potentially improves delivery of oxygen to muscles and reduces work by the heart during vigorous exercise. We now know, however, that rigorously trained athletes already have high amounts of DPG in their red blood cells. Thus, although a single dose of phosphate can induce blood-chemistry changes, it does not reliably improve the ability to perform endurance exercise, nor does it necessarily increase the efficiency of aerobic metabolism.

INOSINE

Inosine is a component of DNA and RNA and a breakdown product of ATP metabolism. It has been marketed as a product that could theoretically increase protein synthesis and ATP synthesis, thereby serving both as an anabolic agent to increase muscle mass and as an energy enhancer to improve endurance performance. To date there is no reliable scientific evidence that inosine has any beneficial effect on the performance of exercise, either in laboratory or competitive conditions. Moreover, breakdown of inosine in the liver yields ammonia and uric acid, both potentially toxic compounds.

COENZYME Q-10

Coenzyme Q-10 (CoQ-10), also called ubiquinone, is a component of the electron transport chain in the mitochondria. Because it participates in the metabolism of carbohydrate and fat to produce ATP, CoQ-10 supplements theoretically might enhance the energy-producing capacity of mitochondria during strenuous exercise. The body, however, appears to produce adequate amounts of CoQ-10, and as yet no solid scientific evidence has demonstrated that CoQ-10 aids in athletic performance.

ASPARTATES

Aspartic acid is a nonessential amino acid that may help reduce ammonia accumulation in muscle. Magnesium and/or potassium salts of aspartic acid (i.e., aspartates) have been used as potential aids to endurance performance. However, about the same number of studies have reported inconsequential effects of aspartate supplementation on exercise performance as have reported positive effects. Thus, definitive conclusions about these compounds are premature. There appears to be little or no toxicity with the doses used in the reported studies.

CREATINE

As discussed in this chapter, phosphocreatine (PCr) is a high-energy compound that initially resupplies muscle ATP during brief, intense bursts of activity (e.g., a 100-meter sprint) and during repeated high-power efforts that occur in fast-break basketball, in sprint interval training for track, swimming, and football, and in weight-training sessions. PCr is the phosphorylated form of creatine, which is manufactured in the body from the amino acids glycine and arginine and also is consumed in the diet, especially in red meats.

erythropoietin A hormone that enhances the synthesis and release of red blood cells from bone marrow; it is produced mostly by the kidneys.

diphosphoglycerate (DPG) A compound present in the red blood cells; it is involved in the release of oxygen from hemoglobin.

In the early 1990s a series of studies of the possible ergogenic effects of dietary creatine supplementation was initiated. The results to date indicate that creatine supplementation in a dosage of about 5 g given four times daily for 5 days often improves performance in subjects who undertake repeated bursts of high-power cycling, strength exercises, or sprinting. This creatine loading appears to speed resynthesis of phosphocreatine, so that subsequent exercise bouts can be completed faster and/or more powerfully. Thus creatine loading may be most effective when used during training rather than during competitive events that involve single sprints or lifts.

Creatine loading seems to be effective only in those who begin the dietary treatment with relatively low stores of creatine in their muscles. This finding suggests that muscles can store a certain amount of creatine and no more. Thus creatine supplementation will not increase muscle creatine stores in individuals who have already attained their natural maximal storage level. It remains to be seen if creatine supplementation over many weeks or months has any positive or negative effects on performance. Furthermore, many more studies in sport settings are needed to confirm the findings of ergogenicity that have so far been obtained mostly in laboratory experiments.

• • •

As summarized in Table 10-8, no scientific evidence supports the effectiveness of many substances touted as performance-enhancing aids. Athletes should avoid any substance claimed to boost performance until its ergogenic effects are scientifically verified. Even with substances whose ergogenic effects have been supported by systematic scientific studies, careful attention to how and when they are used is recommended. Finally, rather than waiting for a magic bullet to enhance performance, athletes are well advised to concentrate their efforts on improving their training routines and sport technique, and consuming well-balanced diets as described in this chapter.

TABLE 10-8

Some substances and practices claimed to have ergogenic effects*

Effective in some instances	Ineffective	Effective in some instances but illegal or dangerous
Aspartates	Alcohol	Anabolic steroids
Bicarbonate loading	Carnitine	Blood doping
Caffeine	Coenzyme Q-10	
Carbohydrate loading	Growth hormone	
Creatine	Inosine	
	Phosphate loading	

*The ergogenic effects of substances and practices in the "Effective" column have been supported by scientific evidence for certain activities; use of those in the right-hand column is illegal in competitive sports and may be dangerous. No credible evidence is available to support any ergogenic effect of the substances and practices in the "Ineffective" column.

Dr. Lamb is Professor of Sport and Exercise Science and Professor of Preventive Medicine at The Ohio State University.

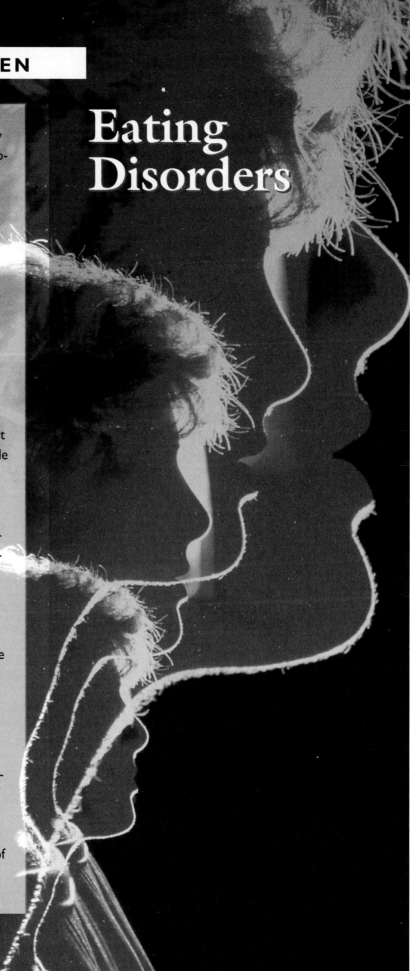

CHAPTER ELEVEN

Eating
Disorders

N ormal eating behavior involves consuming food when we are hungry until satiation (fullness) and then stopping, even if this means leaving some food on our plate. Normal eating also involves consuming a variety of foods, all in moderation, so that we obtain the various nutrients needed to promote health. Depending on individual preferences and health status, consuming three meals a day or small amounts of food more frequently constitutes normal eating behavior. And although we all sometimes overeat and at other times undereat, these occasions generally balance out. Moreover, when we exhibit normal behavior, eating is an enjoyable and important aspect of life, but it is not an obsession that predominates over all else.

In stark contrast, the eating disorders we explore in this chapter represent severe distortions of normal eating behavior.[2] The abnormal behavior associated with true eating disorders is prolonged and significantly affects nutritional status; these disorders can also develop into life-threatening conditions.[6] And what's most alarming about these disorders—anorexia nervosa, bulimia nervosa, binge-eating disorder, and baryophobia—is the increasing number of cases reported each year.[11] Let's examine the causes and treatments of these conditions in detail, since eating disorders touch many of our lives.

NUTRITION AWARENESS INVENTORY

1. **T F** Body images conveyed in American media as desirable can be achieved by most Americans.
2. **T F** Eating disorders are most common among women involved in occupations and sports that place a high value on appearance.
3. **T F** People with anorexia nervosa have an intense fear of losing weight.
4. **T F** Bulimic people often induce vomiting to control their weight.
5. **T F** Girls with anorexia nervosa are often underachievers and are lax in fulfilling responsibilities.
6. **T F** People with anorexia nervosa restrict their food intake to gain a greater sens of control over their lives.
7. **T F** People with bulimia nervosa are aware that their eating patterns are abnormal.
8. **T F** American society favors the lean and angular look.
9. **T F** People with bulimia nervosa tend to come from families that encourage expression of emotions and a balance between dependence and independence
10. **T F** Not having a menstrual period because of food restriction or vigorous exercise poses minimal health risks for a woman.
11. **T F** Restrictive dieting can promote binge eating.
12. **T F** Eating disorders are easier to treat at early stages.
13. **T F** Binge eating and purging are characteristic of bulimia nervosa.
14. **T F** Treatment of bulimia nervosa emphasizes following a strict diet.
15. **T F** Baryophobia is an eating disorder found in children.

From Ordered to Disordered Eating Habits

Eating—a completely instinctive behavior for animals—serves an extraordinary number of psychological, social, and cultural purposes for humans. As we mentioned in Chapter 1, eating practices may take on religious meanings; signify bonds among cultural, ethnic, and family groups; and be a means of expressing hostility and affection, prestige, and class values. Similarly, providing, preparing, and distributing food may be a means of expressing love or hatred, or even power, in family relationships.

In our society we are bombarded daily with images of the "ideal" body. Dieting is promoted to achieve this ideal body—eternally young and acceptable to those around us. Television programs, billboard advertisements, magazine pictures, movies, and newspapers tell us that an ultra-slim body will bring happiness, love, and even success. It is hard not to compare the media images with our own, seemingly less-than-perfect, bodies. People who are overly susceptible to these messages, for both psychological and physical reasons, may be more likely than others to develop eating disorders.[2,17,28]

Given the multiple functions associated with normal eating and the media bombardment about ideal body image, it is not surprising that some people progress from typical responses to hunger and satiety cues, to obsessive weight loss, and then to a full-blown eating disorder, often associated with unusual and strange rituals.[18]

FOOD: MORE THAN JUST A SOURCE OF NUTRIENTS

From birth we link food with personal emotional experiences. As infants we associate milk with security and warmth, so the bottle or breast becomes a source of comfort as well as food. Even when older, some people continue to derive comfort and great pleasure from food. This is both a biological and a psychological phenome-

---

Progression from ordered to disordered eating

Attention to hunger and satiety signals; limitation of energy intake to restore weight to a healthful level

↓

Some "disordered" eating habits begin as weight loss is attempted

↓

Clinically evident eating disorder can be recognized

non. Food can be a symbol of comfort, but eating also can stimulate release of substances called natural opioids, which produce a sense of calm and euphoria in the human body. Thus in times of great stress some people will turn to food for a drug-like calming effect.[12]

Food is also used as a reward or a bribe. Haven't you heard or spoken something like the following comments?

You can't play until you clean up your plate.

I'll eat the broccoli if you let me watch TV.

If you love me, you'll eat what I fixed for dinner.

On the surface, using food as a reward or bribe seems harmless enough. But eventually this practice encourages both caregivers and children to use food to achieve unstated goals. Food then may become much more than a source of nutrients. Regularly using food as a bargaining chip can contribute to abnormal eating patterns. Carried to the extreme, these patterns can lead to disordered eating behavior.[2]

OVERVIEW OF TWO COMMON EATING DISORDERS

The two most common eating disorders—**anorexia nervosa** and **bulimia nervosa**—have been described since the time of the ancient Greeks. Here we briefly describe the characteristics and diagnosis of these disorders. We discuss them in detail and their treatment in the following sections.

Anorexia nervosa is characterized by extreme weight loss, poor and distorted body image, and an irrational, almost morbid fear of obesity and weight gain. People with anorexia nervosa typically see themselves as fat even though they are extremely thin.[2] The term *anorexia* implies a loss of appetite; however, denying one's appetite more accurately describes anorexic behavior. By rough estimate, approximately 1 in 100 girls between the ages of 12 and 18 years suffers from anorexia nervosa. Peak incidence for the disorder occurs among 14- to 19-year-old girls.[14] It occurs less commonly among adult women and rarely in African-American women. Men account for only about 5% to 10% of the cases of anorexia nervosa, partly because the ideal image conveyed for men is big and muscular.[17]

Bulimia nervosa (*bulimia* means "great hunger") is characterized by episodes of binge eating followed by attempts to purge the excess energy taken up by the body, usually by vomiting, strict dieting, taking diuretics, **hypergymnasia,** or using laxatives.[2] People with this disorder may be difficult to identify because they keep their binge-purge behaviors secret and their symptoms are not obvious.[14] Researchers think that approximately 3% to 9% or more of adolescent and college-age women suffer from bulimia nervosa. A growing number of male athletes also report these practices, especially those who participate in sports that require achieving weights to fit weight classes, such as boxers, wrestlers, and jockeys.[17] These athletes will vomit and dehydrate to "make weight." "Get thin and win" is a slogan heard around gyms.

The fourth edition of the *Diagnostic and Statistical Manual of Mental Disorders* (DSM-IV) of the American Psychiatric Association lists specific criteria for diagnosing eating disorders (Table 11-1).[2] People may exhibit some symptoms of an eating disorder but not sufficiently enough to enable a medical worker to diagnose the disease. As is suggested in the diagnostic criteria, some people show characteristics of both anorexia nervosa and bulimia nervosa, since the diseases overlap considerably (Figure 11-1). Studies suggest that about half of the women diagnosed as having anorexia nervosa eventually develop bulimic symptoms.[17] Thus bulimic characteristics are included as part of one type of anorexia nervosa, as shown in Table 11-1. Still, appreciating the differences between the disorders is helpful in terms of understanding various approaches to prevention and treatment.

Anorexia nervosa and bulimia nervosa are both potentially serious diseases that can harm physical and mental health and lead to long-term health problems, especially if medications are used to stimulate vomiting, bowel movements, or urination, since this increases the risk of heart failure.[17]

anorexia nervosa An eating disorder involving a psychological loss or denial of appetite and self-starvation, related in part to a distorted body image and to various social pressures commonly associated with puberty.

bulimia nervosa An eating disorder in which large quantities of food are eaten at one time (binge eating) and then purged from the body by vomiting, use of laxatives, or other means.

- - - - - - - - - - - -

Many people in professions that require ultra-slim bodies have longstanding histories of anorexia nervosa. These include models, actresses, ballet dancers, figure skaters, and gymnasts.

- - - - - - - - - - - -

hypergymnasia Exercising more than is required for good physical fitness or maximal performance in a sport; excessive exercise.

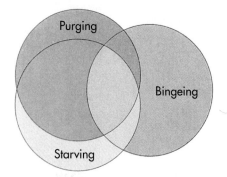

Figure 11-1 The overlap of eating disorders. A combination of binge eating, purging, and/or starving can be found in both anorexia nervosa and bulimia nervosa.

TABLE 11-1

Diagnostic criteria for anorexia nervosa and bulimia nervosa

Anorexia nervosa

A. Refusal to maintain body weight at or above a minimally normal weight for age and height (e.g., weight loss leading to maintenance of body weight less than 85% of that expected; or failure to make expected weight gain during periods of growth, leading to body weight less than 85% of that expected).

B. Intense fear of gaining weight or becoming fat, even though underweight.

C. Disturbance in the way in which one's body weight or shape is experienced, undue influence of body weight or shape on self-evaluation, or denial of the seriousness of the current low body weight.

D. In postmenarcheal females, amenorrhea, i.e., the absence of at least three consecutive menstrual cycles. (A woman is considered to have amenorrhea if her periods occur only following hormone, e.g., estrogen, administration.)

Specify type:

   Restricting type: during the current episode of anorexia nervosa, the person has not regularly engaged in binge-eating or purging behavior (i.e., self-induced vomiting or the misuse of laxatives, diuretics, or enemas)

   Binge-eating/purging type: during the current episode of anorexia nervosa, the person has regularly engaged in binge-eating or purging behavior (i.e., self-induced vomiting or the misuse of laxatives, diuretics, or enemas)

Bulimia nervosa

A. Recurrent episodes of binge eating. An episode of binge eating is characterized by both of the following:
   (1) eating, in a discrete period of time (e.g., within any 2-hour period), an amount of food that is definitely larger than most people would eat during a similar period of time and under similar circumstances
   (2) a sense of lack of control over eating during the episode (e.g., a feeling that one cannot stop eating or control what or how much one is eating)

B. Recurrent inappropriate compensatory behavior in order to prevent weight gain, such as self-induced vomiting; misuse of laxatives, diuretics, enemas, or other medications; fasting; or excessive exercise.

C. The binge eating and inappropriate compensatory behaviors both occur, on average, at least twice a week for 3 months.

D. Self-evaluation is unduly influenced by both body shape and weight.

E. The disturbance does not occur exclusively during episodes of anorexia nervosa.

Specify type:

   Purging type: during the current episode of bulimia nervosa, the person has regularly engaged in self-induced vomiting or the misuse of laxatives, diuretics, or enemas

   Nonpurging type: during the current episode of bulimia nervosa, the person has used other inappropriate compensatory behaviors, such as fasting or excessive exercise, but has not regularly engaged in self-induced vomiting or the misuse of laxatives, diuretics, or enemas

From Diagnostic and Statistical Manual of Mental Disorders (DSM-IV), Washington, DC, 1994, American Psychiatric Association.

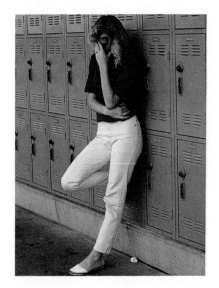

Figure 11-2 The stress of crossing from childhood into adulthood may trigger anorexia nervosa.

Table 11-2 lists some characteristics of people with anorexia nervosa and bulimia nervosa. Do you know someone who is at risk? If so, suggest that the person seek a professional evaluation, because the sooner treatment begins, the better. However, do not try to diagnose eating disorders in your friends or family members. The first step in the evaluation is to rule out other diseases, such as cancer, gastrointestinal disease, cystic fibrosis, allergies, schizophrenia, and depression. Only a professional can exclude such diseases and correctly evaluate the diagnostic criteria required to make a diagnosis of anorexia nervosa or bulimia nervosa.[2] Once an eating disorder is diagnosed, immediate treatment is advisable.[9] As a friend, the best you can do is encourage an affected person to seek professional help. Such help is commonly available at student health centers and student guidance/counseling facilities on college campuses.

There are no simple causes of eating disorders, and there are no simple treatments. The causes are rooted in multiple determinants—biological, psychological, and social. Stress may have an especially strong role in the development of eating disorders.[2] An underlying commonality seems to be the lack of appropriate coping mechanisms as individuals begin to reach adolescence and young adulthood, coupled with dysfunctional family relationships (Figure 11-2).[14]

TABLE 11-2

Typical characteristics of anorexic and bulimic persons

Anorexia nervosa	Bulimia nervosa
• Rigid dieting causing dramatic weight loss	• Secretive binge eating; never overeating in front of others
• False body perception—thinking "I'm too fat," even when emaciated; relentless pursuit of thinness	• Eating when depressed or under stress
• Rituals involving food, excessive exercise, and other aspects of life	• Bingeing followed by fasting, laxative abuse, self-induced vomiting, or excessive exercise
• Maintenance of rigid control in lifestyle; security found in control and order	• Shame, embarrassment, deceit, and depression; low self-esteem and guilt (especially after a binge)
• Feeling of panic after a small weight gain; intense fear of gaining weight	• Fluctuating weight resulting from alternate bingeing and fasting (± 10 lbs or 5 kg)
• Feelings of purity, power, and superiority through maintenance of strict discipline and self-denial	• Loss of control; fear of not being able to stop eating
• Preoccupation with food, its preparation, and observing another person eat	• Perfectionism, "people pleaser"; food is the only comfort/escape in an otherwise carefully controlled and regulated life
• Helplessness in the presence of food	• Erosion of teeth, swollen glands
• Lack of menses after what should be the age of puberty	• Purchase of syrup of ipecac

This listing can be used in a group discussion to help people assess their risk for developing an eating disorder. Those who exhibit only one or a few of these characteristics may be at risk, but probably do not have either disorder. They should, however, reflect on their eating habits and related concerns and take appropriate action.

- - - - - - - - - - - - -
A person with anorexia nervosa may use the disorder to gain attention from the family, sometimes in hopes of holding the family together.
- - - - - - - - - - - - -

In the Nutrition Perspective we review some sociological aspects of these disorders. From this perspective you might see how the disorders develop and why some people are more susceptible than others.

Anorexia Nervosa

Anorexia nervosa evolves from a dangerous mental state to an extremely dangerous physical condition. People suffering from this disorder think they are fat and intensely fear obesity and weight gain. They lose much more weight than is healthful. Still, although food is entwined in this disease, it stems from psychological conflict.[2]

About 3% to 8% of people with anorexia die prematurely—from suicide, heart ailments, and infections. About half of those with anorexia nervosa recover within 6 years; the rest simply exist with the disease. The longer an individual suffers from this eating disorder, the poorer the chances for complete recovery.[6] A young patient with a brief episode and a cooperative family has a better outlook. Prompt and vigorous treatment with close follow-up improves the chances for success.[9]

Anorexia nervosa may begin as a simple attempt to lose weight. A comment from a well-meaning friend, relative, or coach suggesting that the person seems to be gaining weight or is too fat may be all that is needed.[14] The stress of having to maintain a certain weight to look attractive or competent on a job can lead to disordered eating. Physical changes associated with puberty, the stress of leaving childhood, or losing a friend may also trigger extreme dieting (Figure 11-3).[11] Leaving home for boarding school or college or starting a job can reinforce the desire to make oneself more "socially acceptable." Still, looking "good" does not necessarily help a person deal with anger, depression, low self-esteem, or past experiences with sexual abuse. If these issues are pushing the disorder and are not

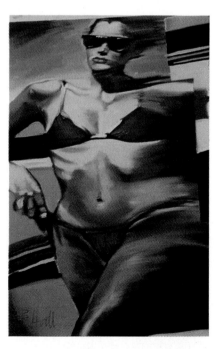

Figure 11-3 Self-image can be ever-changing and deceiving. For people with eating disorders, the difference between the real and the desired body image may be too difficult to accept.

resolved as weight is lost, the individual may intensify efforts to lose weight "to look even better" rather than working through unresolved psychological concerns.

During adolescence, a period of turbulent sexual and social tensions, teenagers seek—and are often expected—to establish separate and independent lives. While declaring independence, they seek acceptance and support from peers and parents, and react intensely to how they think others perceive them. At the same time, their bodies are changing, and much of the change is beyond their control. Adolescents often lack appropriate coping mechanisms for the stresses of the teen years. In the attempt to take charge of their lives, some teenagers try to maintain extreme control over their bodies, promoting anorexia nervosa. Genetic factors also appear to increase the risk for anorexia nervosa: often both identical twins—rather than only one—develop the disorder.[2]

Once dieting begins, a person developing anorexia nervosa does not stop. The result is long periods of rigidly self-enforced semistarvation practiced almost with a vengeance, in a relentless pursuit of thinness. Anorexia nervosa may eventually lead to bingeing on large amounts of food in a short time, then purging. Purging occurs primarily through vomiting, but laxatives, diuretics, and exercise are also used.[2] Thus a person with anorexia nervosa may exist in a state of semistarvation or may alternate periods of starvation with periods of bingeing and purging.

Once a person drops 15% below normal body weight, there is great risk for lifelong suffering from anorexia nervosa. After a person falls 25% below normal body weight, a cure becomes very difficult, hospitalization is almost always necessary, and premature death is more likely.[6,14]

PROFILE OF THE TYPICAL PERSON WITH ANOREXIA NERVOSA

A person with anorexia nervosa refuses to eat enough. This refusal is the hallmark of the disease, whether or not other practices, such as binge-purge cycles, appear. The most typical anorexic person is a Caucasian girl from the middle or upper socioeconomic class. Perhaps her mother also has distorted views of desirable body shape and acceptable food habits. The girl is often described by parents and teachers as "the best little girl in the world."[2]

She is competitive and often obsessive. Her parents set high standards for her. At home, she may not allow clutter in her bedroom. Physicians note that after a physical examination, she may fold her examination gown very carefully and clean up the examination room before leaving. Even though such behavior may be apparent, it takes a skilled professional to tell the difference between anorexia nervosa and other common adolescent complaints, such as delayed puberty, fatigue, and depression.[2]

A common thread underlying many—but not all—cases of anorexia nervosa is conflict within the family structure, especially rooted in an overbearing mother and an emotionally absent father. When family expectations are always too high, resulting frustration leads to fighting. Overinvolvement, rigidity, overprotection, and denial are typical daily transactions of such families.[17]

Often the eating disorder allows an anorexic person to exercise control over an otherwise powerless existence. People with anorexia evaluate their self-worth almost entirely in terms of self-control. Issues of control are central to the development of anorexia nervosa. Some sexually abused children develop anorexia nervosa, believing that if they control their appetite for food, sexual relations, and human contact, they will feel in control and competent and eliminate shameful feelings.[17] Moreover, food restriction, which will arrest development and shut down sexual impulses, may be a strategy to prevent future victimization and guilt feelings in such cases.[2] Often anorexic persons feel hopeless about human relationships and socially isolated because of their dysfunctional families. Thus they substitute the world of food, eating, and weight for the world of human relationships.

In evaluating patients suspected of having an eating disorder, health professionals should compare weight and height to accepted standards. Assessment based merely on appearance is not reliable and may be distorted by the common image of very thin models in advertisements.

Nutrition Focus

ANOREXIA NERVOSA: A CASE STUDY

Jill was 17 years old when she was seen at a sports medicine clinic for stress fractures in her feet and lower left leg. At 5'4" tall and 89 pounds, she was frail and actually seemed more like a little girl than a blossoming adolescent. A gymnast with a promising future, this young woman had experienced a number of muscle and skeletal injuries in the previous 6 months. She had stopped having menstrual cycles at age 15, when she weighed about 100 pounds. When asked why she started eating a modest diet consisting of a frozen yogurt banana shake for breakfast, fruit or salad for lunch, and a baked potato with nonfat cottage cheese for dinner, she replied, "Because my coach said that I could fly through the roof on my routines if I lost some weight." That was back when she was 113 pounds. Jill's coach called the gymnasts with larger bodies "sows."

Her mother reported that Jill was the type of girl who could never sit still. In addition to her daily routine of an hour run, 30 minutes on the exercise bike, and 2 hours of gymnastics practice, she would do deep knee bends while brushing her teeth and bounce on a minitrampoline while watching TV.

Jill's mother and father had been divorced for 2 years. Her father, besides rarely being home because of his sales job, was critical of her behavior when he was home and at times would slap her across the face because of his frustration with her lack of perfection. Jill's mother had multiple sclerosis, and Jill often had to be her mother's caretaker. Despite being popular and well-liked by both teachers and students, Jill felt disconnected from people. Jill stated with great pride, "When I strive for perfection and deprive myself of food, I feel strong, secure, and in control." As she sat in the warm clinic with a bulky sweater and baggy slacks, she proclaimed, "The thinner I get, the greater my chances of competing in the Olympics."

The sports medicine staff who saw Jill immediately referred her to the eating-disorder clinic at the local university medical center. Jill's response was to smile, mumble "okay," and quickly leave. Jill's mother doubted that Jill would be willing to go to the clinic.

EARLY WARNING SIGNS

A person developing anorexia nervosa will exhibit important warning signs. At first, dieting becomes the life focus. The person may feel, "The only thing I am good at is dieting. I can't do anything else." This innocent beginning often leads to very abnormal self-perceptions and eating habits, such as cutting a pea in half before eating it. An anorexic person may cook a large meal and watch others eat it while refusing to eat any.[24]

As the disorder progresses, the range of foods may narrow and be rigidly divided into safe and unsafe ones, with the list of safe foods becoming progressively shorter. For someone developing anorexia nervosa, these practices say "I am in control."[17] The anorexic person may be hungry but denies it, driven by the belief that good things will happen by just becoming thin enough. It becomes a question of willpower.

As we noted at the outset, some Americans feel that a thin body might make life perfect. This ephemeral hope especially appeals to young people (Figure 11-4). Most vulnerable are young women who feel alienated from or suffocated by their parents. For instance, parents may not consider a teenager mature enough to make decisions. She disagrees, and if the situation is very tense, may turn to purging or starving as a way to show her power. "You may try to control my life, but I can do anything I want with my body."

In the words of one young woman: "I couldn't get angry, because it would be like destroying someone else, like my mother. It felt like she would hate me forever. I got angry through anorexia nervosa. It was my last hope. It's my own body and this was my last-ditch effort."

For Better or For Worse   by Lynn Johnston

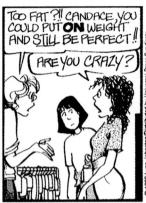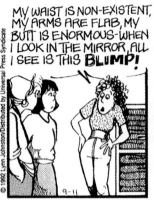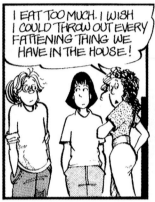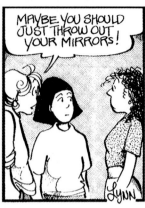

Figure 11-4 For Better or For Worse.

amenorrhea The absence of three or more consecutive menstrual cycles.

CRITICAL THINKING

Jennifer is an attractive 13-year-old. However, she's very compulsive. Everything has to be perfect—her hair, her clothes, even her room. Since her body is beginning to mature, she's quite obsessed with having perfect physical features as well. Her parents are worried about her behavior. The school counselor told them to look for certain signs that could indicate an eating disorder. What are those signs?

Soon the anorexic person becomes irritable and hostile and begins to withdraw from family and friends. School performance generally crumbles.[17] The person refuses to eat out with family and friends, thinking, "I won't be able to have the foods I want to eat," or "I won't be able to throw up afterward." The person also tends to be excessively critical of her- or himself and others. Nothing is good enough. Because it cannot be perfect, life appears meaningless and hopeless. A sense of joylessness colors everything.

As stress increases in the person's life, sleep disturbances and depression are common.[2] Many of the psychological and physical problems associated with anorexia nervosa arise from deficiencies of nutrients, such as thiamin and vitamin B-6, and semistarvation.[19] For a female, these problems—coupled with lower and lower body weight and fat stores—cause menstrual periods to cease, technically called amenorrhea.[6] This may be the first sign of the disease that a mother notices.

Ultimately, an anorexic person eats very little food; 300 to 600 kcal daily is not unusual. In place of food the person may consume up to 20 cans of diet soft drinks and chew many pieces of gum each day.

PHYSICAL EFFECTS OF ANOREXIA NERVOSA

Rooted in the emotional state of the victim, anorexia nervosa produces profound physical effects. The anorexic person often appears to be skin and bones. This state of semistarvation disturbs many body systems as it forces the body to conserve as much energy as possible. Hormonal responses to semistarvation then cause an array of predictable effects[2,6]:

- Lowered body temperature caused by loss of fat insulation.
- Slower basal metabolism caused by decreased synthesis of active thyroid hormone.
- Decreased heart rate as metabolism slows, leading to easy fatigue, fainting, and an overwhelming need for sleep. Other changes in heart function also may occur, including loss of heart tissue itself.
- Iron-deficiency anemia from a deficient nutrient intake, which leads to further weakness.
- Rough, dry, scaly, and cold skin from a deficient nutrient intake and anemia. The skin may also show multiple bruises because of the loss of protection from subcutaneous fat.
- Low white blood cell count caused by a deficient nutrient intake, especially of protein and zinc.[15] This condition increases the risk of infection, one cause of death in people with anorexia.

- Loss of hair caused by a deficient nutrient intake.
- Appearance of lanugo, downy hairs on the body that trap air, reducing heat loss and in turn replacing some insulation lost with the fat layer.
- Constipation from semistarvation and laxative abuse.
- Low blood potassium caused by a deficient nutrient intake and by loss of potassium from vomiting and the use of some types of diuretics. This increases the risk of heart rhythm disturbances, another leading cause of death in anorexic people.
- Loss of menstrual periods because of low body weight, low body fat content, and the stress of the disease. Periods cease when loss of body fat leads to a body weight of around 100 pounds or less in many women. Accompanying hormonal changes cause a loss of bone mass and increase the risk of osteoporosis later in life.
- Eventual loss of teeth caused by frequent vomiting. Loss of teeth and bone mass can be lasting signs of the disease, even if the other physical and mental problems are resolved.[21]
- Muscle tears and stress fractures in athletes because of decreased bone and muscle mass.

A person with anorexia nervosa is psychologically and physically ill and needs help.

CONCEPT CHECK

Anorexia nervosa is an eating disorder characterized by semistarvation. It is found primarily—but not only—in adolescent girls, starting at or around puberty. An anorexic person dwindles essentially to "skin and bones," but often thinks she is fat. Semistarvation produces hormonal and other changes that lower body temperature, slow the heart rate, decrease immune response, stop menstrual periods, and contribute to hair loss. It is a very serious disease that often produces lifelong consequences and may be fatal.

lanugo Downlike hair that appears after a person has lost much body fat through semistarvation. The hair stands erect and traps air, acting as insulation for the body to compensate for the relative lack of body fat, which usually functions as insulation.

CRITICAL THINKING

Jennifer continues her pursuit of the perfect thin body into her late teens. She ignores the advice of her parents and the counselor. As a 19-year-old entering college, she is finally beginning to realize that her anorexic behavior might have serious consequences. She has been fluctuating 15% to 20% below her desirable body weight and has been amenorrheic for a few years. She would like to marry someday and have a family. What might some of the health consequences be for a person like Jennifer with anorexia nervosa?

TREATMENT OF ANOREXIA NERVOSA

Anorexic persons often sink into shells of isolation and fear. They deny that a problem exists. Frequently, friends and family members meet in a group with the person to confront the problem in a loving way. This is called an intervention. They present evidence of the problem and encourage entrance into treatment immediately. Treatment then requires a team of physicians, registered dietitians, psychologists, and other health professionals working together. An ideal setting is an eating disorders clinic in a medical center where the anorexic person can stay as an inpatient. Still, even in the most skilled hands and using the finest facilities, efforts may fail and the person succumbs to the disease. This tells us that prevention of anorexia nervosa is of utmost importance.

Once the medical team has gained the cooperation of the patient, they attempt to work together to restore a sense of balance, purpose, and future. As we said, anorexia nervosa is usually rooted in psychological conflict. However, a person who has been barely existing in a state of semistarvation cannot focus on much besides food. Dreams and even morbid thoughts about food will interfere with therapy until sufficient weight is regained.

Nutrition Therapy

The first goal of therapy, then, is to increase food intake, but the therapist must have the patient's cooperation. Otherwise, no long-term benefit will be realized. Ideally, weight gain must be enough to raise the metabolic rate to normal and to reverse as many physical signs of the disease as possible.[24] Food intake is designed to first minimize or stop any further weight loss. Then the focus shifts to restoring regular food habits. After this is accomplished, the expectation can be switched to slow weight gain, from 1 to 4 pounds (0.5 to 2 kg) each week until weight exceeds 80% to 90% of body weight seen before the disorder began.

Weight stabilization and ultimate gain are achieved by starting the anorexic patient at 1200 to 1500 kcal/day, increasing this to 2500 kcal/day over 1 to 2 weeks as possible, with the ultimate goal being 3000 to 3600 kcal/day while in the hospital. The high energy intake advocated by some clinicians to promote weight gain may seem surprising, but studies have demonstrated that the resting energy expenditure of anorexic persons increases significantly above normal as more energy is consumed, in turn leading to resistance weight gain.[19]

The patient will need considerable reassurance during the refeeding process because of uncomfortable effects such as bloating, increase in body heat, and increase in body fat. These changes can lead to feeling out of control. Weight gain is not the sole goal of treatment, but rather a prelude to fuller engagement in psychological issues. The medical team should assure the patient that she will not be abandoned after gaining weight.

Hyperactivity and hypergymnasia are characteristic of anorexia nervosa. Often patients in treatment insist on exercising, and withdrawal symptoms such as irritability, anxiety, and depression may develop when exercise is limited. Because excessive energy expenditure acts as a barrier to weight gain, professionals must work with anorexic patients to help them moderate their activity. At many treatment centers patients are placed on moderate bed rest in the early stages of their treatment to help promote weight gain.[3]

Experienced, professional help is the key. An anorexic patient may be on the verge of suicide and near starvation. Today suicide is the most common cause of death in people with anorexia nervosa.[2,6,14] In addition, anorexic people are often very clever and resistant. They may try to hide weight loss by wearing many layers of clothes, putting coins in their pockets, and drinking numerous glasses of water.

Psychological Therapy

Once the physical problems of anorexic patients are addressed, the treatment focus shifts to the underlying emotional problems that led to excessive dieting and other symptoms of the disorder. To heal, these patients must reject the sense of accomplishment associated with an emaciated body. If therapists can discover reasons for the disorder, they can develop strategies for restoring normal weight and eating habits by resolving psychological conflicts. Education about the health consequences of semistarvation is also helpful.[14] A key aspect of psychological treatment is showing affected individuals how to regain control of some facets of their lives and how to cope with tough situations. As eating evolves into a normal routine, they then can turn to previously neglected activities.

Therapists may use cognitive therapy, which involves helping the person confront and change irrational beliefs about body image, eating, relationships, and weight.[17] Obviously, issues of sexual abuse need to be addressed as well.

Family therapy is important in treating anorexia nervosa. It focuses on the role of the illness among family members, how individual family members react, and how through their behavior they might unknowingly contribute to the abnormal eating patterns. Therapy involves all family members relevant to the behavior problem. Frequently, a therapist finds family struggles at the heart of the problem. As the disorder resolves, the person has to relate to family members in new ways in order to gain the attention previously tied to the disease. The family needs to help the young person ease into adulthood and to accept its responsibilities as well as its advantages.[9]

Self-help groups for anorexic and bulimic persons, as well as their families and friends, represent nonthreatening first steps into treatment. People can also attend to get a sense of whether they really do have an eating disorder.

With professional help, many people with anorexia nervosa can again lead normal lives. They then do not have to depend on unusual eating habits to cope with daily problems. Although they may not be totally cured, they do recover a sense

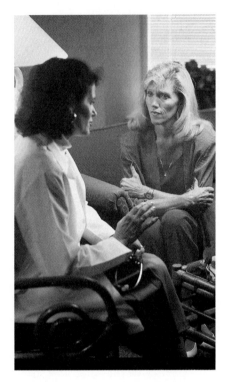

Anorexia nervosa is a potentially fatal disease that requires professional treatment.

A young woman in a self-help group for those with anorexia nervosa explained her feelings to the other group members: "I have lost a specialness that I thought it gave me. I was different from everyone else. Now I know that I'm somebody who's overcome it, which not everybody does."

of normality in their lives. There are no set answers or approaches; each case is different.

There is also no specific pharmacological agent used to treat anorexia nervosa. Increasing intake of food is considered the drug of choice. Medications used typically depend on the physician's preference and the patient's symptoms. Tranylcypromine sulfate (Parnate), imipramine (Tofranil), amitriptyline (Elavil), desipramine (Norpramin), and lithium carbonate (Lithane) are useful mainly when depression accompanies the disorder. Chlorpromazine (Thorazine) has been shown to decrease anxiety about eating. More recently, fluoxetine (Prozac) has proven helpful for alleviating depression and promoting weight gain. It appears to be well tolerated, with few side effects.[17]

Still, establishing a strong relationship with either a therapist or another supportive person is a key to recovery. Once anorexic patients feel understood and accepted by another person, they can begin to build a sense of self and exercise some autonomy. Then they can progress to substituting healthy relationships with others for a relationship with food.

CONCEPT CHECK

To relieve the semistarved condition of most anorexic patients, the initial treatment focuses on weight gain and restoration of normal basal metabolism. Once this is accomplished, psychotherapy can begin to uncover the causes of the disease and to help the person develop skills needed to return to a healthy life. Family therapy is an important tool in treatment.

Bulimia Nervosa

Bulimia nervosa involves episodes of binge eating followed by attempts to purge the food (energy intake). This eating disorder was first classified as a clinical psychiatric disorder by the American Psychiatric Association in 1980.[2] It is found most commonly among young adults of college age, although some high school students also are at risk.[7] Susceptible people often have biological factors and lifestyle patterns that predispose them to becoming overweight, and many try frequent weight-reduction diets as teenagers.[28] Like people with anorexia nervosa, those with bulimia nervosa are usually female and successful. But they are usually at or slightly above a normal weight.[2] Females with bulimia nervosa are also more likely to be sexually active than those with anorexia nervosa.

The person with bulimia nervosa may think of food constantly. In contrast to the anorexic person, who turns away from food when faced with problems, the bulimic person turns toward food in critical situations. Also, unlike those with anorexia nervosa, people with bulimia nervosa recognize their behavior as abnormal. These people often have very low self-esteem and are depressed. Approximately half of people with bulimia nervosa have major depression. Lingering effects of child abuse may be one reason for these feelings. Many bulimic persons report that they have been sexually abused.[27] The world sees their competence, while inside they feel out of control, ashamed, and frustrated.[2]

Bulimic people tend to be impulsive, which may be expressed as stealing, drug and alcohol abuse, self-mutilation, or attempted suicide.[2] It has been suggested that part of the problem may actually arise from an inability to control responses to impulse and desire. Some studies have demonstrated that bulimic people tend to come from disengaged families, ones that are loosely organized. Roles for family members are not clearly defined. Too little protection is given for family members, rules are very loose, and there is a high degree of conflict.[17] This is in contrast to homes of anorexic people, whose families may be so actively engaged that roles may be too well defined.

Among men, athletes who are trying to maintain weight are most likely to suffer from bulimia nervosa.

TYPICAL BULIMIC BEHAVIOR

It is likely that many people with bulimic behavior are not diagnosed. The strict diagnostic criteria specify that to be diagnosed with bulimia nervosa a person must binge at least twice a week for 3 months (Table 11-1).[2] Approximately 2% to 9% of college-age women fit this description. However, people with bulimia nervosa lead secret lives, hiding their abnormal eating habits. Moreover, it is impossible to recognize people with bulimia nervosa simply from their appearance. Since most diagnoses of bulimia nervosa are based on self-reports, estimates of the incidence of this disorder probably are much lower than its true incidence. The disorder, especially in its milder forms, may be much more widespread than commonly thought.

Among sufferers of bulimia nervosa, bingeing often alternates with attempts to rigidly restrict food intake. Elaborate "food rules" are common, such as avoiding all sweets. Thus eating just one cookie or donut may cause bulimic persons to feel they have broken a rule. Then the objectionable food must be eliminated. Usually this leads to further overeating, partly because it is easier to regurgitate a large amount of food than a small amount.

Binge-purge cycles may be practiced daily, weekly, or at longer intervals. A special time is often set aside. Most binge eating occurs at night, when other people are less likely to interrupt, and usually lasts from a half hour to 2 hours. A binge can be triggered by a combination of stress, boredom, loneliness, and depression.[2] It often follows a period of strict dieting and thus can be linked to intense hunger. The binge is not at all like normal eating; once begun, it seems to propel itself. The person not only loses control but generally doesn't even taste or enjoy the food that is eaten during a binge (Figure 11-5).

Most commonly bulimic persons consume cakes, cookies, ice cream, and similar high-carbohydrate convenience foods during binges, because these foods can be purged relatively easily and comfortably by vomiting.[2] In a single binge, foods supplying 10,000 to 15,000 kcal or more may be eaten.[12] Purging follows in hopes that no weight will be gained. But even when vomiting follows the binge very quickly, 20% to 33% of the food energy taken in is still absorbed, in turn encouraging some weight gain. Even more energy is absorbed when laxatives are used for purging. The common belief of bulimic persons that purging soon after bingeing will prevent excessive energy intake and weight gain is clearly a misperception.

Early in the onset of bulimia nervosa, sufferers often induce vomiting by placing their fingers deep into the mouth. They may inadvertently bite down on these fingers if not retracted quickly. Because the resulting bite marks around the knuckles are a characteristic sign of this disorder, physicians should routinely examine the hands of young people suspected of having an eating disorder.[24] Once the disease is established, however, a person can often vomit simply by contracting the abdominal muscles. Vomiting may also occur spontaneously.[2]

Another way bulimic persons attempt to compensate for a binge is by engaging in hypergymnasia—excessive exercise—to expend a large amount of energy. Some bulimic persons try to mentally estimate the amount of energy eaten in a binge and then exercise to counteract this energy intake. This practice, referred to as "debting," represents an effort of bulimic persons to control their weight.[3]

People with bulimia nervosa are not proud of their behavior. After a binge, they usually feel guilty and depressed. Over time they experience low self-esteem and feel hopeless about their situation (Figure 11-6). Compulsive lying and drug abuse can further intensify these feelings.[2] Bulimic persons caught in the act of bingeing by a friend or family member may order the intruder to "get out" and "go away." Sufferers gradually distance themselves from others, spending more and more time preoccupied by and engaging in bingeing and purging.

HEALTH PROBLEMS STEMMING FROM BULIMIA NERVOSA

The induced vomiting that many bulimic sufferers practice is the most physically destructive method of purging. Indeed the majority of health problems associated with bulimia nervosa arise from vomiting.[2,6,17]

Frequent binges can lead to enormous food bills for a bulimic person.

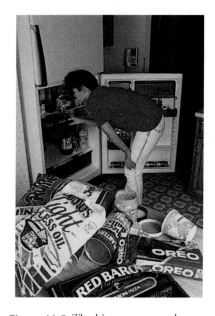

Figure 11-5 The binge-purge cycle can lead to a sense of helplessness.

Nutrition Focus

THOUGHTS OF A BULIMIC WOMAN

I am wide awake and immediately out of bed. I think back to the night before, when I made a new list of what I wanted to get done and how I wanted to be. My husband is not far behind me on his way into the bathroom to get ready for work. Maybe I can sneak onto the scale to see what I weigh this morning before he notices me. I am already in my private world. I feel overjoyed when the scale says that I stayed the same weight as I was the night before, and I can feel that slightly hungry feeling. Maybe it will stop today; maybe today everything will change. What were the projects I was going to get done?

We eat the same breakfast, except that I take no butter on my toast, no cream in my coffee, and never take seconds (until Doug gets out the door). Today I am going to be really good, and that means eating certain predetermined portions of food and not taking one more bite than I think I am allowed. I am very careful to see that I don't take more than Doug. I judge myself by his body. I can feel the tension building. I wish Doug would hurry up and leave so I can get going!

As soon as he shuts the door, I try to get involved with one of the myriad responsibilities on my list. I hate them all! I just want to crawl into a hole. I don't want to do anything. I'd rather eat. I am alone; I am nervous; I am no good; I always do everything wrong anyway; I am not in control; I can't make it through the day, I know it. It has been the same for so long. I remember the starchy cereal I ate for breakfast. I am into the bathroom and onto the scale. It measures the same, but I don't want to stay the same! I want to be thinner! I look in the mirror. I think my thighs are ugly and deformed looking. I see a lumpy, clumsy, pear-shaped wimp. There is always something wrong with what I see. I feel frustrated, trapped in this body, and I don't know what to do about it.

I float to the refrigerator knowing exactly what is there. I begin with last night's brownies. I always begin with the sweets. At first I try to make it look like nothing is missing, but my appetite is huge and I resolve to make another batch of brownies. I know there is half of a bag of cookies in the bathroom, thrown out the night before, and I polish them off immediately. I take some milk so my vomiting will be smoother. I like the full feeling I get after downing a big glass. I get out six pieces of bread and toast one side of each in the broiler, turn them over and load them with pats of butter, and put them under the broiler again until they are bubbling. I take all six pieces on a plate to the television and go back for a bowl of cereal and a banana to have along with them. Before the last piece of toast is finished, I am already preparing the next batch of six more pieces. Maybe another brownie or five, and a couple of large bowls full of ice cream, yogurt, or cottage cheese.

My stomach is stretched into a huge ball below my rib cage. I know I'll have to go into the bathroom soon, but I want to postpone it. I am in never-never land. I am waiting, feeling the pressure, pacing the floor in and out of the rooms. Time is passing. Time is passing. It is getting to be time. I wander aimlessly through each of the rooms again, tidying, making the whole house neat and put back together. I finally make the turn into the bathroom. I brace my feet, pull my hair back and stick my finger down my throat, stroking twice, and get up a huge pile of food. Three times, four times, and another pile of food. I can see everything come back. I am so glad to see those brownies because they are so fattening. The rhythm of the emptying is broken and my head is beginning to hurt. I stand up feeling dizzy, empty, and weak. The whole episode has taken about an hour.

From Hall L, Cohn L: *Bulimia—a guide to recovery,* Carlsbad, Calif, 1992, Gurze Books.

- Repeated exposure of teeth to the acid in vomit causes demineralization, making the teeth painful and sensitive to heat, cold, and acids. Eventually, the teeth may severely decay, erode away from fillings, and finally fall out. Dental professionals are sometimes the first health professionals to notice signs of bulimia nervosa (Figure 11-7).[21]
- Blood potassium can drop significantly with regular vomiting or use of certain diuretics. This can disturb the heart's rhythm and even produce sudden death.

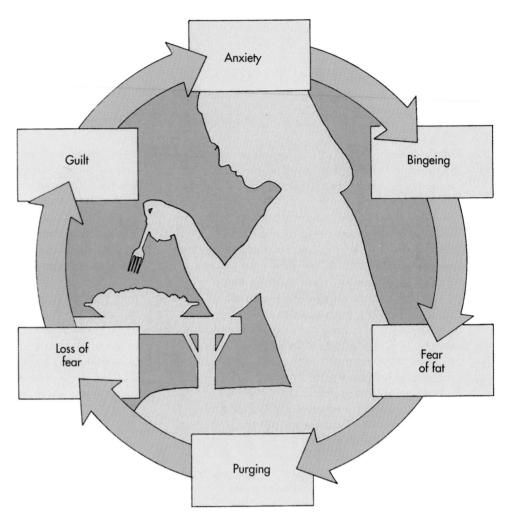

Figure 11-6 Bulimia nervosa's vicious circle of obsession.

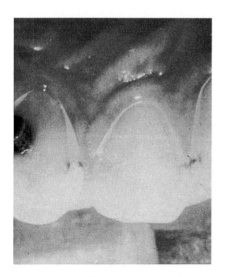

Figure 11-7 Excessive tooth decay is common in bulimic patients.

- Salivary glands may swell due to infection and irritation from the vomit. A link between this swelling and hormonal changes is also suspected.
- Stomach ulcers and bleeding and tears in the esophagus develop in some cases.
- Constipation may result from frequent laxative use.[16]
- Ipecac syrup, also used to induce vomiting, is poisonous to the heart, liver, and kidneys. It has caused accidental poisoning when taken repeatedly.

In all, bulimia nervosa is a potentially debilitating disorder that can lead to death, usually from suicide, low blood potassium, or overwhelming infections.[17]

TREATMENT OF BULIMIA NERVOSA

Therapy for bulimia nervosa, as for anorexia nervosa, requires a team approach. These patients are less likely than those with anorexia to enter treatment in a state of semistarvation. However, if a bulimic patient has lost significant weight, this must be treated before psychological treatment is begun. Although clinicians have yet to agree on the best therapy for bulimia nervosa, they generally agree that treatment should last at least 15 to 20 weeks.

The primary aim of psychotherapy is to improve patients' self-acceptance and help them to be less concerned about body weight. To correct the "all-or-none" thinking typical of bulimic persons—if I eat one cookie, I'm a failure and might as well binge. A patient may be asked to role play a scientist testing assumptions and beliefs about food and weight. Patient and therapist together examine the validity of such beliefs. The premise of this therapy is that if abnormal attitudes and beliefs can be altered, normal eating will follow.[8] In addition, the therapist guides the person to establish food habits that will minimize bingeing: avoiding fasting, eating regular meals, and using alternative methods—other than eating—to cope with stressful situations. Group therapy often is useful.

One goal of therapy is to help bulimic persons accept as normal some depression and self-doubt. Therapists may prescribe antidepressant medications to combat some depression associated with bulimia nervosa.[20] That often also works to reduce binge eating in early phases of treatment. Fluoxetine (Prozac) has been used successfully to decrease binge frequency and treat depression among bulimic patients.[17]

Nutritional counseling is two pronged: correcting misconceptions about food and reestablishing regular eating habits. Patients are given information about bulimia nervosa and its consequences. Avoiding both binge foods and constantly stepping on a scale may be recommended early in treatment. The primary goal, however, is to develop a normal eating pattern.[24] To achieve this goal, some nutrition specialists encourage patients to develop daily meal plans and to keep a food diary in which they record food intake, internal sensations of hunger, environmental factors that precipitate binges, and thoughts and feelings that accompany binge-purge cycles. Keeping a food diary not only is an accurate way to monitor food intake but also may help identify situations that seem to trigger binge episodes. With the help of a therapist, patients then can develop alternative coping strategies.

In general the focus is not on stopping bingeing and purging per se, but on developing regular eating habits. Once this is achieved, the binge-purge cycle should stop by itself. Patients are discouraged from following strict rules about healthy food choices, because this simply mimics the typical obsessive attitudes associated with bulimia nervosa. Rather, encouraging a mature perspective on nutrient intake is a key to helping patients to overcome this disorder, that is, regular consumption of moderate amounts of a variety of foods balanced among the food groups.[1]

Persons with bulimia nervosa must recognize that it is a serious disorder that can have grave medical complications if not treated. Since relapse is likely, therapy should be long term, as mentioned before. Unlike those with anorexia nervosa, most bulimic patients do not require hospitalization. However, those with bulimia nervosa do need professional help because they can be very depressed and are at a high risk for suicide.[2]

Female Athlete Triad

As mentioned previously, women participating in appearance-based and endurance sports are at risk of developing an eating disorder.[4] A recent study of college-age female athletes found that 15% of swimmers, 62% of gymnasts, and 32% of all varsity athletes exhibited disordered eating patterns.[22] A much lower incidence of such disordered eating is typical of college women not involved in competitive sports.

In addition to disordered eating, college women athletes tend to experience amenorrhea more frequently than other college women.[5] Disordered eating, particularly food restriction, can precipitate amenorrhea. Amenorrhea causes women to have less dense and weaker bones than normal because of lower estrogen and higher cortisol concentrations in the blood. Some of these young women have bones equivalent to those of 50- to 60-year-olds, making them overly susceptible to fractures during both sports and general activities. Much of the bone loss is irreversible.

The American College of Sports Medicine (ACSM) has named the syndrome consisting of disordered eating, amenorrhea, and compromised bone density the female athlete triad.[22] The ACSM has issued a call to teachers, coaches, health professionals, and parents to educate female athletes about the triad and its consequences. Those exhibiting the symptoms should get treatment. One treatment plan has the following goals:
- Reduce preoccupation with food, weight, and body fat.
- Gradually increase meals and snacks to an appropriate amount.

EXPERT OPINION

EATING DISORDERS

BRUCE ARNOW, Ph.D.

Three eating disorders are most commonly encountered in clinical practice: bulimia nervosa, binge-eating disorder, and anorexia nervosa. Each has its own distinct set of clinical features and treatment considerations. I will focus on the first two, as their treatments overlap to some extent.

BULIMIA NERVOSA

Bulimia nervosa is characterized by recurrent episodes of binge eating, followed by inappropriate compensatory behavior, that is, behavior intended to prevent weight gain. Such behavior may include self-induced vomiting; abuse of laxatives, diuretics, or enemas; fasting; and excessive exercise.

But what do we mean by binge eating and how does it differ from ordinary overeating? By binge eating, we mean that in a discrete and relatively brief period of time (e.g., within a 2-hour period) an amount of food is consumed that is significantly larger than most people would eat in a similar context, and that the person experiences an inability to stop eating or control what is being eaten. Feelings of guilt, shame, and self-disgust are commonly experienced following the binge. Self-induced purging often brings calm, relief, or relaxation.

People with bulimia nervosa frequently skip meals and often try to adhere to an unrealistic set of self-imposed guidelines regarding what they are permitted to eat and in what amounts. For instance, many try to avoid eating sweets of any kind. Others may avoid all foods that are rich in carbohydrates. Some will purge even following a normal snack or meal, while others will purge only after a binge.

Many of my patients have reported incidents in which they ate very little during the day, perhaps skipping one or two meals, and then found themselves in a situation where they were both hungry and in the presence of "forbidden food," which they found irresistible; this led to bingeing followed by purging to "undo" the effects of the binge. At other times feeling depressed or disappointed, or having a disturbing interaction with another person will undermine their motivation to adhere to their strict diet and precipitate a binge. After bingeing, bulimic persons typically feel "guilty" and purge, resolving the next day to "be perfect," thus re-initiating the cycle.

In the past 15 years, a number of promising approaches to the treatment of bulimia nervosa have been developed and evaluated. One is cognitive-behavioral therapy (CBT); a second is administration of antidepressant medications; and most recently, a specific application of interpersonal therapy (IPT) was shown to be effective.

Cognitive-behavioral therapy for bulimia nervosa involves two major components. The first is to assist the patient in breaking the binge-starve cycle that is thought to maintain the disorder by gradually instituting three meals and one or two snacks daily. Treatment typically begins by having patients self-monitor all episodes of eating and purging; the time of eating; the content and amount of food consumed; the degree of hunger experienced; whether the person considered what was eaten a meal, snack, or binge; whether or not purging took place; and what feelings accompanied the episode. This process helps identify unrealistic dietary guidelines, patterns of eating that are impossible to sustain in the long run, as well as symptom-maintaining assumptions, such as the belief that eating carbohydrate-rich foods or three moderate meals daily will inevitably cause weight gain.

A second focus of treatment is to facilitate the questioning of assumptions about weight and shape and the role that these play in the patient's overall self-esteem. The self-concept of the bulimic patient is overly influenced by weight and shape, even on a short-term basis. Thus patients often report that if they weigh themselves in the morning and their weight is, for example, 120 pounds, they feel satisfied with themselves, but if they weigh themselves at night and the scale indicates 121 or 122 pounds, they "feel crushed" or "like a failure."[11]

Antidepressant medications have also been shown to be helpful in the treatment of bulimia nervosa. A recently published study conducted at Stanford University investigated the efficacy of three treatments: medication with desipramine, a tricyclic antidepressant (given to some patients for 16 weeks and others for 24 weeks), cognitive-behavioral therapy (15 sessions), and a combination of medication and CBT. Patients were followed for 1 year after the conclusion of treatment. The 2-year post-treatment results were as follows: abstinence rates (i.e., complete cessation of binge eating and purging) were 67% for the 24-week medication group, 54% for those receiving CBT, and 78% for the group that received both CBT and 24 weeks of medication. Interestingly, the group receiving medication alone for 16 weeks fared significantly worse (18% abstinent at the 1-year followup), and the combined treatment group in which medication was given for 16 weeks showed a lower abstinence rate (40%) than the combined treatment that included 24 weeks of medication. The study provides some evidence that combining CBT and medication for a sufficient period of time is the most effective treatment available. More recently, clinicians have been prescribing a newer class of antidepressants, including Prozac and Zoloft, and achieving comparable results, in some cases with fewer side effects.

For many years CBT was the only psychosocial treatment for bulimia whose efficacy was supported by research. However, one recent study that compared 18 weeks of interpersonal therapy (IPT) with 18 weeks of CBT found that 1 year following treatment the abstinence rates were roughly equivalent, around 40%. IPT, rather than focusing on the patient's eating habits and assumptions about weight and shape, formulates the problem in terms of the interpersonal context, usually in one or more of four areas: grief, interpersonal problems (e.g., difficulty forming or maintaining close relationships), interpersonal disputes (e.g., unresolved conflict regarding the expectations of significant others in the person's life), or role transitions (e.g., fear of inde-

pendence due to lack of self-confidence). Treatment focuses on assisting the patient to change in one or more of these areas.

BINGE-EATING DISORDER

People with binge-eating disorder differ from bulimia nervosa patients in two important respects. First, those with this problem do not engage in self-induced purging. Second, their weight is less frequently in the normal range. Although binge-eating disorder is encountered in only about 2.5% of the population at large, it is more common among obese people, and even more so among obese people seeking weight-loss treatment. Among those seen in university-based clinics or programs offering very-low-calorie diets (i.e., supplemented fasting programs), the rate of binge-eating disorder is about 30%.

Obese binge eaters have been shown to fare more poorly than obese nonbingers in weight-loss programs, dropping out more frequently and regaining their weight more rapidly. For this reason recent research efforts have attempted to treat the binge-eating disorder before patients enter specific treatment for weight loss. As binge-eating disorder has only recently been recognized and studied, the number of treatment studies is limited. The results so far suggest that both CPT and IPT have promise for treatment of binge-eating disorder.

Although binge eaters may skip meals and adhere to a low-calorie dietary regimen like bulimic patients, their most problematic characteristic is a chaotic eating pattern. They may

have no specific meal routine but simply snack throughout the day. Others report an ad lib pattern regarding choice of foods; for example, they may consume last night's leftovers for breakfast or consume dessert prior to eating a meal. Thus CBT for the obese binge eater focuses on facilitating a healthier pattern of eating, with discrete, moderate meals that are appropriate to the setting and time of day, as well as dealing with any undue restraint. In addition, there is an emphasis on developing alternative coping responses in situations that are associated with emotional eating.

Two studies, both conducted at Stanford, have examined the effectiveness of IPT for binge-eating disorder. In one, those who did not respond to CBT were then given IPT. Results indicated that IPT was of no benefit to the nonresponders. The other study directly compared CBT and IPT administered in a group therapy format and found essentially equivalent results. Further investigations are currently under way to compare these two treatments and to try to ascertain how they work.

Dr. Bruce Arnow is Assistant Professor of Psychiatry and Chief of the Psychology Service at Stanford University Medical Center. He is also Director of the Behavioral Medicine Clinic, in which the Eating Disorders, Obesity, and Anxiety Disorders programs for the Department of Psychiatry are located. He is co-author with Prof. C. Barr Taylor of one book, The Nature and Treatment of Anxiety Disorders, *and has written numerous journal articles on the topic of eating disorders.*

- Rebuild the body to an appropriate weight.
- Establish regular menstrual periods.

The tragic case of Christy Henrich illustrates why anyone at risk for the female athlete triad should seek professional help. As a young teenager Christy weighed 95 pounds and was 4 feet 11 inches tall. She showed promise as a gymnast, but was told by others that she was too fat to excel in gymnastics. Christy continued her training but often starved herself, some days consuming just an apple and then frequently purging by vomiting. Her success in gymnastics continued, but at age 22 her weight had fallen to 52 pounds, and she died in August 1994 of multiple organ system failure.

Other Disordered Eating Patterns

In recent years, two other eating disorders—**binge-eating disorder** and **baryophobia**—have been recognized as requiring professional treatment. Although these disordered eating patterns share some characteristics with anorexia nervosa and bulimia nervosa, they also exhibit distinctive characteristics.

BINGE-EATING DISORDER

binge-eating disorder An eating disorder characterized by recurrent binge eating and feelings of loss of control over eating. Binge episodes can be triggered by frustration, anger, depression, anxiety, permission to eat forbidden foods, or excessive hunger.

With the publication of the DSM-IV in 1994, binge-eating disorder, commonly called compulsive overeating, was formally classified as an eating disorder.[2] The diagnostic criteria for this disorder are listed in Table 11-3. Generally it can be defined as binge-eating episodes not accompanied by purging (as typifies bulimia nervosa) at least two times per week. In the past the catchall term *compulsive overeating* described a range of habitual excessive eating. But now health-care professionals recognize this condition as a separate, unique eating disorder, as complex and serious a problem as anorexia nervosa or bulimia nervosa.

Approximately 30% of subjects in organized weight-control programs have binge-eating disorder, whereas among the general population only 2% to 5% have this disorder.[2] However, many more people in the general population likely have less severe forms of the disorder but do not meet the formal criteria for diagnosis.[23] The incidence of binge-eating disorder is far greater than the incidence of either anorexia nervosa or bulimia nervosa. This disorder is also more common among the severely obese and those with a long history of frequent restrictive dieting.[2]

Development and Characteristics of Binge Eating

Individuals with binge-eating disorder often perceive themselves as hungry more often than normal. They usually started dieting at a young age, began bingeing during adolescence or in their early 20s, and typically are unsuccessful in commercial weight-control programs. Almost half of those with severe binge-eating disorder exhibit clinical depression.[25]

Typical binge eaters isolate themselves with a favorite food and proceed to eat large quantities of it.[2] Stressful events or feelings of depression or anxiety can trigger this behavior. Also, giving themselves permission to eat a forbidden food can precipitate a binge. They sometimes binge on whatever is easy to eat in large amounts—noodles, rice, bread, leftovers. But characteristically binge eaters consume foods that carry the social stigma of "junk" or "bad" foods—ice cream, cookies, sweets, potato chips, and similar snack foods.

In general, people engage in binge eating to induce a sense of well-being and perhaps even numbness, usually in an attempt to avoid feeling and dealing with emotional pain and anxiety. They eat without regard to biological need for nutrients and often in a recurrent, ritualized fashion. Some people with this disorder eat food continually over an extended period, called *grazing;* others cycle episodes of bingeing with normal eating. For example, someone who works at a stressful or frustrating job might come home every night and graze until bedtime. Another person might eat normally most of the time but find comfort in consuming large quantities of food when an emotional setback occurs.[2]

TABLE 11-3

Research criteria for binge-eating disorder

A. Recurrent episodes of binge eating, an episode being characterized by both of the following:
  (1) Eating, in a discrete period of time (e.g., within any 2-hour period), an amount of food that is definitely larger than most people would eat during a similar period of time in similar circumstances.
  (2) A sense of lack of control during the episodes (e.g., a feeling that one can't stop eating or control what or how much one is eating).
B. During most binge episodes, at least three of the following:
  (1) Eating much more rapidly than usual.
  (2) Eating until feeling uncomfortably full.
  (3) Eating large amounts of food when not feeling physically hungry.
  (4) Eating alone because of being embarrassed by how much one is eating.
  (5) Feeling disgusted with oneself, depressed, or very guilty after overeating.
C. Marked distress regarding binge eating.
D. The binge eating occurs, on average, at least two days a week for 6 months.
E. Does not occur only during the course of bulimia nervosa or anorexia nervosa.

From *Diagnostic and statistical manual of mental disorders* (DSM-IV), Washington, DC, 1994, American Psychiatric Association.

Although persons with anorexia nervosa and bulimia nervosa exhibit persistent preoccupation with body shape, weight, and thinness, binge eaters do not necessarily share these concerns. Thus neither purging nor prolonged food restriction is characteristic of binge-eating disorder. Some physicians classify binge-eating disorder as an addiction to food involving psychological dependence. The person becomes attached to the behavior itself and has a drive to continue it, senses only limited control over it, and needs to persist at it despite negative consequences. Food is the means used to reduce stress, produce feelings of power and well-being, avoid feelings of intimacy with others, and avoid life problems.[2] Note that obesity and binge eating are not necessarily linked. Not all obese people are binge eaters, and although obesity may result from trying to numb emotional pain with food, it is not necessarily an outcome.

Binge-eating disorder is most likely to develop in people who never learned to appropriately express and deal with their feelings. Rather than face their problems, they turn to food instead. They continue to do the things that perpetuate the experiences of frustration, anger, and pain. A person, for example, who regularly becomes frustrated because he doesn't assert himself when he needs to may eat to forget his frustration rather than learn to deal with his lack of courage and to practice assertiveness. The frustration will continue because he never attacks the basic problem. The binge eating makes the person feel he cannot control the behavior pattern and therefore cannot control his life. Worse, the binge eating usually increases negative self-feelings.[2] Bingeing on a couple of pizzas and half a cake leads to feelings of guilt, embarrassment, and shame.

People who practice binge eating often have been shaped by families who do not address and express feelings in healthful ways. The parents nurture and comfort their children with food rather than engage in healthy exchanges of self-disclosure of feelings and potential solutions. Members of such families learn to eat in response to emotional needs and pain rather than hunger. Those who regularly practice binge eating may grow up nurturing others instead of themselves, avoiding their own feelings and taking little time for themselves. Not knowing how to satisfy their personal and emotional needs in more healthful ways, they turn to food.

People with binge-eating disorder may come from families with alcoholism or may have suffered sexual abuse.[27] Members of such dysfunctional families do not know how to deal effectively with emotions. They cope by turning to substances. Family members learn to cover up dysfunctional patterns for the alcoholic person and to nurture him or her at the expense of each other and their own needs.

For some people frequent dieting beginning in childhood or adolescence is a precursor to binge-eating disorder.[11] During periods when little food is eaten, they get very hungry and obsess about food. When allowed to eat more food or given permission to go off the diet, they feel driven to eat in a compulsive, uncontrolled fashion. The pattern of periods of strict dieting alternating with binge eating may continue into the future.

Help for the Binge Eater

Those with binge-eating disorder must learn to eat in response to hunger—a biological signal—rather than in response to emotional needs or external factors (e.g., the time of day or the simple presence of food). Counselors often direct binge eaters to record their perceptions of physical hunger throughout the day and at the beginning and end of every meal. These people must learn to eat to a prescribed amount of fullness at each meal. They also should avoid slimming diets because feelings of food deprivation can lead to more disruptive emotions and a greater sense of unmet needs. Diets are likely to encourage more intense problems with binge eating.

Since difficulty in identifying personal emotional needs and difficulty in expressing emotions are common predisposing factors in many binge eaters, these underlying problems must be addressed during treatment.[8] Binge eaters often must be helped to recognize their own buried emotions in anxiety-producing situations and then encouraged to share them. Learning simple but appropriate phrases to say to oneself can help stop bingeing when the desire is strong.

Self-help groups such as Overeaters Anonymous aim to help recovery from binge-eating disorder. Their treatment philosophy parallels that of Alcoholics Anonymous. Overeaters Anonymous attempts to create an environment of encouragement and accountability to overcome this eating disorder. Dietary goals typically range from avoiding restraint in eating to limiting binge foods. Some nutrition experts feel that learning to eat all foods—but in moderation—is an effective goal for binge eaters. This practice can head off the feelings of desperation and deprivation that come from limiting particular foods. There is no set answer, but diet extremism is not needed.

Many of the antidepressant medications mentioned previously in this chapter have been found to help reduce binge eating by decreasing depression. A medication called fenfluramine (Ponderal) has potential for decreasing the sensation of hunger and the intense drive to eat experienced by binge eaters.

BARYOPHOBIA

Some children and young adults who grow more slowly and have a shorter stature than normal may suffer from baryophobia (literally, "the fear of becoming heavy"). Decreased growth in children usually results from disease—commonly a hormonal or other metabolic abnormality. In the absence of a recognized disease in such children, the possibility of baryophobia should be investigated.

This disorder occurs when children are given the same low-fat, high-carbohydrate diet that adults follow.[13] Adults do this in an attempt to prevent children from developing obesity or heart disease later in life. Today's parents and caregivers, themselves frequently harassed by weight problems, may be determined that the children in their care will avoid such ordeals. Although well-intended, such severely restricted diets are detrimental for children because they don't supply enough energy to sustain an adequate growth rate. In young adults, low-energy diets may be self-imposed to avoid a perceived risk of obesity.

Since this disorder results largely from lack of appropriate nutrition information leading to poor food choices, nutritional counseling of caregivers and young adults is the most effective response. They need to be informed about the nutrient requirements and normal weight-gain patterns for the relevant age group. This counseling will show caregivers that including some sweets and medium-fat foods in a

baryophobia A disorder of young children and young adults characterized by stunted growth resulting from underfeeding in an attempt to prevent development of obesity and heart disease.

child's diet is appropriate (see Chapter 17). The diet can still minimize saturated fat and cholesterol intake, a more important focus in a diet designed to reduce the risk of heart disease. Supplying adequate carbohydrate, protein, and other nutrients is the key to promoting growth in both height and weight during childhood and the young-adult years, and it can be done in a healthful manner.[13]

CONCEPT CHECK

Bulimia nervosa is characterized by episodes of binge eating followed by purging, usually by vomiting. Vomiting is very destructive to the body, often causing severe dental decay, stomach ulcers, irritation of the esophagus, and blood potassium imbalances. Treatment using nutrition counseling and psychotherapy helps the patient to restore normal eating habits, to correct distorted beliefs about diet and lifestyle, and to develop healthful ways for coping with the stresses of life. Baryophobia in children and binge-eating disorder in adults are two recently recognized conditions that significantly affect people's eating behavior. The underlying causes of any eating disorder must first be determined, diagnosed, and treated before the abnormal eating practices can ultimately be corrected.

Preventing Eating Disorders

A key to developing and maintaining healthful eating behavior is to realize that some concern about diet, health, and weight is normal. It is also normal to experience variation in what we eat, how we feel, and even how much we weigh. For example, it is not abnormal to experience some minimal weight change (up to 2 to 3 pounds) throughout the day, and even more over the course of a week. A large weight fluctuation or ongoing weight gain or weight loss is a more likely indicator of a problem. If you notice a large change in your diet, how you feel, or your body weight, it is a good idea to consult with your physician. Treating physical and emotional problems early helps lead to peace of mind and good health.

We begin to form our opinions about food, nutrition, health, our weight, and our body image especially during puberty. Parents, friends, and professionals working with young adults should consider the following advice for preventing eating disorders:

- Discourage restrictive dieting, meal skipping, and fasting.
- Provide information about normal changes that occur during puberty.
- Correct misconceptions about nutrition, normal body weight, and approaches to weight loss.
- Carefully phrase weight-related recommendations and comments.
- Don't overemphasize numbers on a scale. Instead, primarily promote healthful behavior.
- Encourage normal expression of disruptive emotions.
- Encourage children to eat only when they're hungry.
- Teach the basics of proper nutrition and exercise in school and at home.
- Provide adolescents with an appropriate but not unlimited degree of independence, choice, responsibility, and self-accountability for their actions.
- Encourage coaches to be sensitive to weight and body-image issues among athletes.
- Emphasize that thinness is not necessarily associated with better athletic performance.

Our society as a whole can benefit from a fresh focus on healthful food practices and a healthful outlook toward food and weight.[18] Along with the technical articles listed in the References section, you can gain more insight into eating disorders from the following sources of less technical information:

CRITICAL THINKING

Tom, a high school teacher, is concerned about eating disorders. He wants to try to prevent young adults from falling into the deadly traps of anorexia nervosa and bulimia nervosa. What are some of the topics and issues he will discuss to counsel students in his health classes?

BOOKS

Arenson S: A substitute called food, ed 2, Blue Ridge Summit, PA, 1989, Tab Books.

Eades MD: Freeing someone you love from eating disorders, New York, 1993, Perigee Books/Putnam.

Freedman R: Body love: learning to like our looks and ourselves, Carlsbad, Calif, 1989, Gurze Books.

Hall L, Cohn L: Bulimia: a guide to recovery, Carlsbad, Calif, 1992, Gurze Books.

Kano S: Making peace with food, New York, 1989, Harper & Row.

Siegel M, Brisman J, Weinshel M: Surviving an eating disorder: perspectives and strategies for family and friends, Carlsbad, Calif, 1988, Gurze Books.

Tannehaus N: What you can do about eating disorders, New York, 1992, Lynn Sonberg Book Services.

Way K: Anorexia nervosa and recovery: a hunger for meaning, Binghamton, NY, 1993, Harrington Park Press.

ORGANIZATIONS AND SELF-HELP GROUPS

American Anorexia/Bulimia Association, Inc., 418 East 76th Street, New York, NY 10021 (phone: 212-501-8351).

Anorexia Nervosa and Associated Disorders, Inc., P.O. Box 7, Highland Park, IL 60035 (phone: 708-831-3438).

Anorexia Nervosa and Related Eating Disorders, Inc., P.O. Box 5102, Eugene, OR 97405 (phone: 503-344-1144). This nonprofit organization, which collects information about eating and exercise disorders, distributes information through booklets and a monthly newsletter. Staff lead workshops, self-help groups, and training programs for professionals. They also provide speakers.

National Eating Disorders Association (NEDO) at Laureatte Psychiatric Hospital, P.O. Box 470207, Tulsa, OK 74147 (phone: 918-481-4092). This organization publishes a quarterly newsletter appropriate for professional and personal use.

Summary

1. Anorexia nervosa is most common among high-achieving perfectionist girls from middle- and upper-class families marked by conflict, high expectations, rigidity, and denial. The disorder usually starts with dieting in early puberty and proceeds to the near-total refusal to eat. Early warning signs include intense concern about weight gain and dieting as well as abnormal food habits, such as cutting a pea in half before eating it and classifying foods as safe and unsafe. Anorexic persons become irritable, hostile, overly critical, and joyless; they tend to withdraw from family and friends. Eventually anorexia nervosa can lead to numerous physical effects, including a profound decrease in body weight and body fat, a fall in body temperature and heart rate, iron-deficiency anemia, a low white blood cell count, hair loss, constipation, low blood potassium, and the cessation of menstrual periods. Those with anorexia nervosa are physically very ill.

2. Treatment of anorexia nervosa includes increasing food intake to at least support basal metabolism and then to allow for gradual weight gain. Psychological counseling attempts to help patients establish regular food habits and to find means of coping with the life stresses that led to the disorder. Hospitalization may be necessary.

3. Bulimia nervosa is characterized by bingeing on up to 15,000 kcal at one sitting and then purging by vomiting, laxative use, exercise, or other means. Both men and women are at risk. Vomiting as a means of purging is especially destructive to the body; it can cause severe tooth decay, stomach ulcers, irritation of the esophagus, low blood potassium, and other problems. Bulimia nervosa poses a serious health problem and is associated with significant risk of suicide.

4. Treatment of bulimia nervosa includes psychological as well as nutritional counseling. During treatment, bulimic persons learn to accept themselves and to cope with problems in ways that do not involve food. Regular eating patterns are developed as these patients begin to plan meals in an informed, healthful manner.

5. The female athlete triad consists of disordered eating, amenorrhea, and abnormally low bone density, particularly in appearance-related and endurance sports. If not corrected, this disorder will eventually lead to decreased athletic performance and general health problems.

6. Binge-eating disorder, which is more widespread than either anorexia or bulimia, is most common among people with a history of frequent, unsuccessful dieting. Binge eaters typically either practice grazing (i.e., eating continually over extended periods) or bingeing without purging. Emotional disturbances are often at the root of this disordered form of eating. Treatment addresses deeper emotional issues, discourages food deprivation and restrictive diets, and helps to restore normal eating behaviors.

7. Baryophobia describes a condition in which children are underfed by caregivers in an attempt to limit risk of future disease, such as obesity or heart disease. Growth failure—in weight and height gains—can result if nutrient intake is not increased to appropriate amounts.

Study Questions

1. What, in your opinion, is a healthful attitude toward food and eating?

2. What are the typical characteristics of a person with anorexia nervosa? What may influence a person to begin rigid, self-imposed dietary patterns?

3. List the detrimental physical and psychological side effects of bulimia nervosa. Describe important goals of the psychological and nutrition therapy used to treat bulimic patients.

4. How might parents significantly contribute to the development of an eating disorder? Share an attitude that a parent or adult friend of yours displayed that may not have been conducive to developing a normal relationship to food.

5. Based on your knowledge of good nutrition and sound dietary habits, answer the following questions:
   a. How can repeated bingeing and purging lead to significant nutrient deficiencies?
   b. How can significant nutrient deficits contribute to major health problems in later life?
   c. A friend asks you, the nutrition expert, if it is okay to "cleanse" the body by eating only grapefruit for a week. What is your response?

6. How, in your opinion, has society contributed to the development of various forms of disordered eating? Provide an example.

7. List the three symptoms that compose the female athlete triad. What is the major health risk associated with amenorrhea in the female athlete?

8. How does binge-eating disorder differ from bulimia nervosa? Describe factors that contribute to the development and treatment of binge-eating disorder.

9. Explain the role of hypergymnasia in eating disorders. What is "debting"?

10. If you were a coach of an appearance-related or endurance sport, what steps would you take to prevent eating disorders among your athletes?

REFERENCES

1. ADA Reports: Position of the American Dietetic Association: Nutrition intervention in the treatment of anorexia nervosa, bulimia nervosa, and binge eating, Journal of the American Dietetic Association 94:902, 1994.

2. American Psychiatric Association: Diagnostic and statistical manual of mental disorders (DSM-IV), Washington, DC, 1994, The Association.

3. Beumont PJV and others: Excessive physical activity in dieting disorder patients: proposals for a supervised exercise program, International Journal of Eating Disorders 15:21, 1994.

4. Clark N: Counselling the athlete with an eating disorder: a case study, Journal of the American Dietetic Association 94:656, 1994.

5. Clark N: Athletes with amenorrhea, The Physician and Sports Medicine 21:45, 1993.

6. Comerci GD: Medical complications of anorexia nervosa and bulimia nervosa, Medical Clinics of North America 74:1293, 1990.

7. Emmons L: Dieting and purging behavior in black and white high school students, Journal of the American Dietetic Association, 92:306, 1992.

8. Fairburn CG and others: Cognitive-behavioral therapy for binge eating and bulimia ner-

vosa. In Fairbaurn CG, Wilson GT, editors: Binge eating, New York, 1994, Guilford Press.

9. Farley D: Eating disorders require medical attention, FDA Consumer, March 1992, p 27.

10. Gleaves DH, Eberenz KP: Sexual abuse histories among treatment-resistant bulimia nervosa patients, International Journal of Eating Disorders 15:227, 1994.

11. Grodner M: Forever dieting: chronic dieting syndrome, Journal of Nutrition Education 24:207, 1992.

12. Hetherington MM and others: Eating behavior in bulimia nervosa: multiple meal analyses, American Journal of Clinical Nutrition 60:864, 1994.

13. Lifshitz F: Children on adult diets: Is it harmful? Is it helpful? Journal of the American College of Nutrition 11:84S, 1992.

14. Lucas AR, Huse DM: Behavioral disorders affecting food intake: anorexia nervosa and bulimia nervosa. In Shils ME and others, editors: Modern nutrition in health and disease, Philadelphia, 1994, Lea & Febiger.

15. Marcos A and others: Evaluation of immunocompetence and nutrition in patients with bulimia nervosa, American Journal of Clinical Nutrition 57:65, 1993.

16. McClain CJ and others: Gastrointestinal and

nutritional aspects of eating disorders, Journal of the American College of Nutrition 12:466, 1993.

17. National Institute of Mental Health: Eating disorders, U.S. Government Printing Office, NIH Publication No 93-3477, Washington DC, 1993.

18. Neumark-Sztainer D: Excessive weight preoccupation, Nutrition Today 30:68, 1995.

19. Rock CL, Curran-Celentano J and others: Nutritional disorder of anorexia nervosa: a review, International Journal of Eating Disorders 15:187, 1994.

20. Rothschild R and others: A double-blind placebo-controlled comparison of phenelzine and imipramine in the treatment of bulimia in atypical depressives, International Journal of Eating Disorders, 15:1, 1994.

21. Ruff JC and others: Bulimia: dentomedical complication, General Dentistry, Jan/Feb 1992, p 22.

22. Skolnick AA: Female athlete triad risk for women, Journal of the American Medical Association 270:921, 1993.

23. Spitzer RL and others: Binge eating disorder: its further validation in a multisite study, International Journal of Eating Disorders 13:137, 1993.

24. Strubbe JH: Anorexia and bulimia nervosa. In Westerterp-Plantenga MS and others, editors: *Food intake and energy expenditure,* Boca Raton, Fla, 1994, CRC Press.

25. Telch CF and others: Obesity, binge eating, and psychopathology: are they related? *International Journal of Eating Disorders* 15:53, 1994.

26. Varner LM: Dual diagnosis: patients with eating and substance-related disorders, *Journal of the American Dietetic Association* 95:224, 1995.

27. Welch SL, Fairburn CG: Sexual abuse and bulimia nervosa: three integrated case control comparisons, *American Journal of Psychiatry* 151:402, 1994.

28. Weltzin TE and others: Serotonin and bulimia nervosa, *Nutrition Reviews* 52:399, 1994.

TAKE ACTION

Assessing your risk of having an eating disorder

The statements below are based on the primary diagnostic criteria for anorexia nervosa and bulimia nervosa listed in Table 11-1. Put an "X" in the space before statements that describe your characteristics and lifestyle. Respond as honestly as possible.

———— 1. You refuse to keep your body weight over a minimal normal weight for age and height.

———— 2. You intensely fear gaining weight or becoming fat, even though you are underweight.

———— 3. You feel fat even though you are quite thin.

———— 4. If you are female, you have missed at least three consecutive menstrual cycles.

———— 5. You have recurrent episodes of binge eating.

———— 6. You can't control your eating behavior during food binges.

———— 7. You regularly self-induce vomiting, use laxatives or diuretics, diet strictly or fast, or vigorously exercise to prevent weight gain.

———— 8. You engage in a minimum average of two binge-eating episodes a week.

———— 9. You are persistently and excessively concerned with your body shape and weight.

Questions 1 through 4 pertain to anorexia nervosa and 5 through 9 to bulimia nervosa.
Complete this activity by answering the following questions:

1. After having completed this checklist, do you feel that you might have an eating disorder or the potential to develop one?

_____

_____

2. Do you think some of your friends might have an eating disorder?

_____

_____

3. What counseling and education resources exist in your area or on your campus to help with a potential eating disorder?

_____

_____

4. If a friend had an eating disorder, what do you think would be the best way to assist him or her in getting help?

_____

_____

Eating Disorders: A Sociological Perspective

One of the many ways we evaluate ourselves is based on body image. We identify our body with our self and judge it as we think others see us, knowing that our appearance affects their opinions of us.

Early in life, we develop images of "acceptable" and "unacceptable" body types. Of all the attributes that constitute attractiveness, many people view body weight as the most important, partly because we can control our weight somewhat. Fatness is the most dreaded general deviation from our cultural ideals of body image, the one most derided and shunned, even among school children.[11]

Women in particular are likely to diet because they feel strongly about what is acceptable in both size and weight (Figure 11-8).[17] In general, though, most dieting women aren't technically obese. Rather, they diet to correct some perceived flaw or because they simply feel they should weigh less than they do now. Their general nature "to please" fosters this desire to look socially acceptable.

A Glamour magazine survey indicated that 80% of the 30,000 respondents were ashamed of their bodies. Those who were dissatisfied primarily wanted to weigh less and have smaller thighs, hips, buttocks, and waists, typical sites of greatest fat deposition in sexually mature women.

Changing Times

The "full-bodied" woman as a cultural ideal did not survive into the twentieth century in Western society, though it is still in fashion in many nonindustrialized countries in which a large body is a sign of wealth. In contrast, over the course of this century the "ideal" female body form in the United States has become thinner and thinner. A thin waist with modest hips is the overriding cultural "gold standard," at least as depicted by models. Our passion for thinness may have its roots in the Victorian era, which specialized in denying "unpleasant" physical realities, such as appetite and sexual desire. Flappers of the 1920s cemented a trend for thinness (Figure 11-9). Even as the ideal gradually moved toward a thinner, more angular body shape, the average weight among the general female population increased.

Researchers have linked this preference for a lean body type to the recent surge in eating disorders.[11] As the more full-figured woman (earth mother) was displaced by the ultrathin woman, the number of eating disorders increased, along with our society's preoccupation with obesity. It appears that the cultural pressures toward thinness are stretching the physiological capabilities of many women (and men). For example, researchers surmise that

CATHY

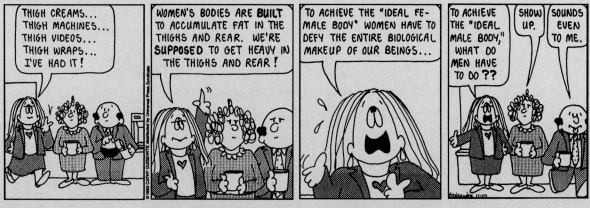

Figure 11-8 Cathy.

the theoretical body fat content of the "Barbie doll" would not allow for menstruation. Given the natural variability in human basal metabolism and genetic makeup, as well as Americans' easy access to food and increasingly sedentary lifestyles, it is no surprise that some of us gain weight. People predisposed to eating disorders for either biological or emotional reasons may be nudged "over the edge" by these social changes.[17]

Thinness As an Indicator of Competence

Unfortunately, many Americans today view obesity as a failure of control, willpower, competence, and productivity. At stake are social acceptance and even access to scarce resources, such as good jobs or an attractive spouse. Whether we like it or not, in today's society our appearance says a lot about us, even though the way we were raised and our genetic background are beyond our control. Some people simply are much more likely to become obese than others. Implicit in our societal attitudes is the notion that those who can't control themselves enough to stay slim are unlikely to be good at supervising employees, organizing their work day, and shouldering heavy responsibilities. Clearly, fat is out! A prevailing myth is that thin people are more competent, energetic, and forceful than obese people.

Mixed Messages and Social Trends

Despite the pressure for thinness, our society is filled with mixed messages. Half the advertisements in women's magazines may be for diets or show emaciated models; the other half, for tasty foods. Movie and television stars are almost always perfect physical specimens. Yet television advertisements encourage us to visit our local quick-service restaurant. There you can buy a hamburger, french fries, and milk shake, totaling about 1200 kcal—about the amount of energy our daily basal metabolism uses—without even leaving the car.

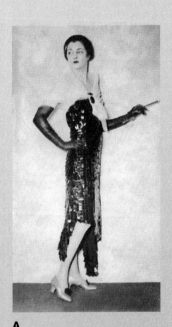 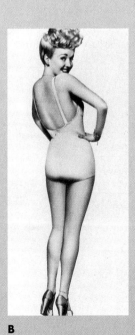 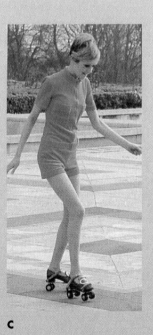 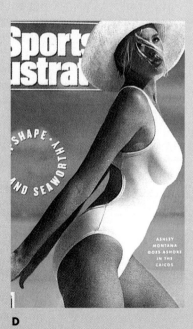

A   B   C   D

Figure 11-9 The changing views of desirable body weight. American society has imposed varying stereotypes for desirable body weight, especially for women. **A,** The svelte flapper of the 1920s. **B,** The "thin but curvaceous" look of the 1940s. **C,** Ultra-thin was in during the 1960s. **D,** Lean and well-toned physiques grace magazine covers of the 1990s.

In the past several decades, divorce, alcoholism in families, child abuse, school- and work-related stress, female employment, and crowded urban conditions have all increased. These changes in our family and social environments encourage children, adolescents, and adults alike to find a pressure-valve release. For many, that valve is food, setting the stage for development of an eating disorder.[17]

Internalizing the Thinness Ideal

Eating disorders are usually only a symptom of significant emotional trauma or psychological stress in a person's life. When psychiatrists are able to dig deeper, they find that eating disorders mask serious questions of self-worth, family struggles, and sometimes fears of puberty and the future. The real illnesses are not the eating disorders—though they eventually contribute to poor health—but, rather, the way people feel about themselves. And when people internalize the social value favoring thinness and can't meet that goal, their negative self-image is reinforced.[11]

As discussed in the chapter, those who suffer from anorexia nervosa or bulimia nervosa over an extended period are likely to develop significant health complications. The harm produced by milder, shorter periods of diet restriction is not clear. Evidence, however, suggests that even moderate diet restriction, if continued, increases the risk for various anemias, pregnancy complications, low-birthweight infants, and permanently reduced bone mass. As we mentioned, it also can impair growth in children and very young adolescents. The percentage of adolescents and young adults who significantly restrict food intake is not known. But at least two problems, iron-deficiency anemia and pregnancy complications, are significant problems in this age group.

Glimmers of Hope

Since eating disorders in part stem from certain societal values, changing these values might reduce the pressures predisposing some people to various types of disordered eating behavior. Feminists, for example, assert that true liberation means being free to find one's natural weight. Women who combine careers and motherhood are saying that they have more important things to worry about; fashion leaders are tolerating more curves; exercise programs are encouraging regular brisk walking, rather than mostly jogging and working out. Writers, therapists, and some registered dietitians are working to help women accept their bodies.

What is the difference between people who can accept themselves—even with a few more pounds than the glamorous people have—and those who chronically diet and feel dissatisfied? Perhaps it is the willingness to recognize that satisfaction with appearance comes from within, not from their image in the mirror or what someone else tells them. The challenge facing many Americans today is achieving a healthy body weight without excessive dieting. This means adopting and maintaining sensible eating habits, a physically active lifestyle, and realistic and positive attitudes and emotions, while practicing creative ways to handle stress.

CHAPTER TWELVE

W hen it comes to vitamins, we often hear, "If a little is good, then more must be better." Some people believe that consuming vitamins far in excess of their needs provides them with extra energy, protection from disease, and prolonged youth.[21] About 50% of adults in the United States take vitamin and mineral supplements. This helps fuel what has become a $3.5 billion industry.

In stark contrast, our total vitamin needs to prevent deficiency signs and symptoms are really quite small. In general, humans require a total of about 1 ounce (28 g) of vitamins for every 150 pounds (70 kg) of food consumed. Vitamins are found in plants and animals. Plants synthesize all the vitamins they need. Animals vary in their ability to synthesize vitamins. For example, guinea pigs and humans are two of the very few organisms that are unable to synthesize their own supply of vitamin C.

In this chapter we first briefly review some general properties of the vitamins. These vital nutrients are divided into two groups: the fat-soluble vitamins and the water-soluble vitamins. The bulk of this chapter then focuses on the functions and sources of the fat-soluble vitamins and human requirements for them. We describe the water-soluble vitamins in detail in the next chapter.

The Fat-Soluble Vitamins

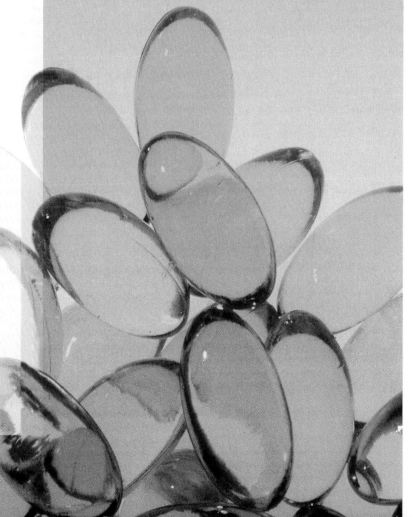

Nutrition Awareness Inventory

Answer these 15 statements about vitamins in general and fat-soluble vitamins in particular to test your current knowledge. If you think the answer is true or mostly true, circle T. If you think the answer is false or mostly false, circle F. Use the scoring key at the end of the book to compute your total score. Repeat this test after you have read the chapter, and compare your results.

1. **T F** If a vitamin is missing in your diet for 3 consecutive days, there is danger of developing deficiency signs and symptoms.
2. **T F** Vitamin K is excreted less efficiently than the other fat-soluble vitamins.
3. **T F** Some people don't need a dietary source of vitamin D to maintain their health.
4. **T F** Fat-soluble vitamins are generally lost more easily in cooking than are the water-soluble vitamins.
5. **T F** Most scientists believe that all the vitamins required for human health have been discovered.
6. **T F** Vitamin D improves calcium absorption.
7. **T F** Beta-carotene is an important precursor of vitamin D.
8. **T F** Intakes of vitamin A six to ten times the RDA over long periods of time may cause toxic effects.
9. **T F** Vitamin D can be considered a hormone.
10. **T F** Some foods can be fortified with vitamin D by exposure to ultraviolet light.
11. **T F** Vitamin E is an enzyme required in several energy-yielding reactions.
12. **T F** Vitamin K is important for blood clotting.
13. **T F** Antibiotic use can provoke a vitamin K deficiency.
14. **T F** Green vegetables are good sources of vitamin K.
15. **T F** Strength, quality, purity, and labeling of nutrient supplements are carefully controlled by FDA.

Vitamins: Vital Dietary Components

By definition, vitamins are essential organic (carbon-containing) substances needed in small amounts in the diet for normal function, growth, and maintenance of body tissues (organic micronutrients). Although vitamins themselves yield no energy to the body, they often facilitate energy-yielding chemical reactions. Vitamins A, D, E, and K dissolve in organic solvents, whereas the B vitamins and vitamin C dissolve in water. In addition, the B vitamins and vitamin K function as parts of coenzymes (i.e., molecules that help enzymes function).[8]

Vitamins are generally indispensable in human diets because they can't be synthesized in the human body, or their synthesis can be curtailed by environmental factors. Notable exceptions to a strict dietary need are vitamin D, which may be synthesized by the skin in the presence of sunlight; niacin, which may be synthesized from the amino acid tryptophan; and vitamin K and biotin, which may be synthesized by bacteria in the intestinal tract.[18,24]

Strictly speaking, for a substance to be classified as a vitamin, its absence from the diet for a defined period of time must produce deficiency signs and symptoms that—if caught in time—are quickly cured when the substance is resupplied. In addition to their use in correcting deficiency diseases, a few vitamins have also proved useful as medicinal agents in treating a limited number of nondeficiency diseases. These medical applications require administration of **megadoses** well above the RDAs for the vitamins. For example, megadoses of niacin are employed as part of serum cholesterol–lowering treatment for appropriately selected individuals. Other examples include the use of forms of vitamin D for psoriasis and of vitamin E for blood clotting disorders.[4,11] Nevertheless, at this time any claimed benefits from use of vitamin supplements, especially intakes in excess of 150% of the RDA, should be viewed critically because many unproved claims have been, and are continually, made.[17]

megadose Intake of a nutrient in excess of ten times of human need.

Both plant and animal foods supply vitamins in the human diet. Whether isolated from foods or synthesized in the laboratory, vitamins are the same chemical compounds and work equally well in the body. Contrary to claims in the health-food literature, "natural" vitamins isolated from foods are no more healthful than those synthesized in a laboratory. Some vitamins exist in several related forms that differ in chemical or physical properties. Vitamin E, for example, exists in eight separate forms.[11] These forms exist both in nature and in synthesized vitamin supplements. It is important to have enough of the specific vitamin forms that the body can use; we will point out these forms throughout the next two chapters.

HISTORICAL PERSPECTIVE ON THE VITAMINS

Long before any vitamins had been identified, certain foods were known to cure illnesses brought on by what we now recognize to be vitamin deficiencies. The ancient Egyptians, for example, treated night blindness with topical applications of juice extracted from liver, a rich source of vitamin A. Ancient Greeks also recommended consumption of cooked liver for this eye disorder, which was common at the time. As we'll see, vitamin A plays a critical role in vision.[28] Scurvy was common among sailors on the long sea voyages of the fifteenth and sixteenth centuries when few fruits and vegetables were available. British scientists eventually discovered that lime juice cured scurvy; after lemons and limes were included as a routine part of British sailors' diets, the incidence of scurvy declined greatly. We now know that this disease, marked by weakness, anemia, and open sores in the mouth, results from a deficiency of vitamin C. Native Americans in the United States had another treatment, pine needle extracts, to cure scurvy.

Modern vitamin research began in the early 1900s when Casimir Funk isolated a chemical substance he called "vitamine," a shortened form for "vital amine." We now know that many but not all vitamins are in fact amines, compounds that contain at least one carbon atom bonded to a nitrogen group ($-C-NH_2$). Funk's original name for these vital substances later was changed to vitamin.

"Fat-soluble A," discovered in 1913, was the first vitamin to be purified. The first vitamin to have its structure and chemical formula determined was thiamin, one of the B vitamins; this was achieved in 1937. During the 1930s, scientists also isolated vitamin C by extracting it from lemon juice. The last of the known vitamins to be discovered, vitamin B-12, was isolated in 1948. For the most part, as substances with suspected vitamin properties were discovered, they were designated with letters of the alphabet—A, B, C and so forth. When some of these suspected vitamins later were found to consist of more than one chemical compound, a number was added to distinguish the individual compounds (e.g., vitamin B-6 and vitamin B-12). A few suspected vitamins (e.g., vitamin G) eventually were shown not to be needed in the diet, and the letter designation was dropped.

Recognition of the vitamin nature of niacin—another B vitamin—was complicated by the fact that it can be produced in the body. During the 1920s, scientists found that diets high in protein foods could cure pellagra, a disease marked by scaly sores, diarrhea, and mental problems. Later they cured pellagra-like disease in dogs, called blacktongue, by administration of nicotinic acid, which today is called niacin. By the late 1940s, it was shown that the body could convert the amino acid tryptophan into niacin, thereby reducing the dietary requirement for niacin. Researchers eventually concluded that pellagra and blacktongue result from a deficiency of niacin, but that protein in the diet could compensate for the absence of dietary niacin.

Although some researchers still hope to discover one or more additional vitamins, we can be relatively confident that all vitamins needed by humans have been discovered. The ability of total parenteral nutrition (TPN) to support human life for years strongly supports the latter view. In this procedure patients receive intravenously a carefully formulated preparation containing all the nutrients, totally bypassing the gastrointestinal tract. Food is unnecessary. Those who receive protein, carbohydrate, fat, all the known vitamins, and the essential minerals in this manner can continue not only to live but also to build new body tissue, to have a baby, to heal wounds, and to combat existing diseases.

STORAGE OF VITAMINS IN THE BODY

Except for vitamin K, the fat-soluble vitamins are not readily excreted from the body.[24] In contrast, the water-soluble vitamins are generally lost from the body quite rapidly, partly because the water in cells dissolves these vitamins and flushes them out of the body via the kidneys. An exception is water-soluble vitamin B-12, which is stored much more readily than both the other water-soluble vitamins and the fat-soluble vitamin K. Because of the limited storage of many vitamins, they should be consumed in the diet daily, although an occasional lapse in the intake of even water-soluble vitamins generally causes no harm. An average person, for example, must consume no thiamin for 10 days or no vitamin C for 20 to 40 days before developing the first signs and symptoms of deficiency of these vitamins. The signs and symptoms of a vitamin deficiency occur only when that vitamin is lacking in the diet and body stores are essentially exhausted.

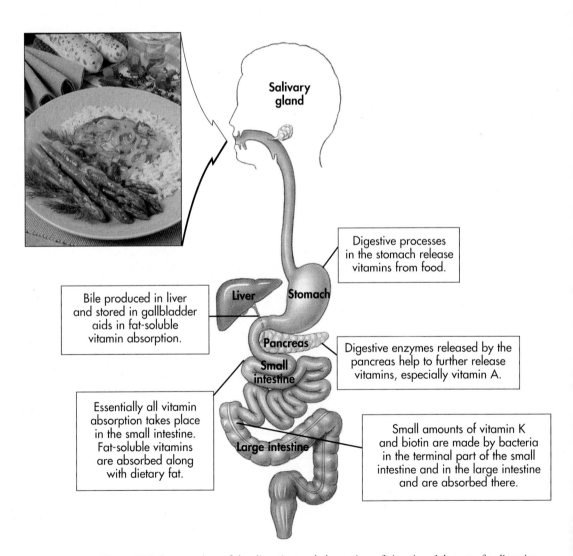

Salivary gland

Digestive processes in the stomach release vitamins from food.

Liver **Stomach**

Bile produced in liver and stored in gallbladder aids in fat-soluble vitamin absorption.

Pancreas

Small intestine

Digestive enzymes released by the pancreas help to further release vitamins, especially vitamin A.

Essentially all vitamin absorption takes place in the small intestine. Fat-soluble vitamins are absorbed along with dietary fat.

Large intestine

Small amounts of vitamin K and biotin are made by bacteria in the terminal part of the small intestine and in the large intestine and are absorbed there.

Figure 12-1 An overview of the digestion and absorption of vitamins. Adequate fat digestion and absorption are critical for the ultimate absorption of fat-soluble vitamins. Key participants in this process include bile, pancreatic enzymes, and a healthy small intestine absorptive surface.

VITAMIN TOXICITY

Because fat-soluble vitamins are not readily excreted, some can easily accumulate in the body and cause toxic effects. And while a toxic effect from an excessive intake of any vitamin is theoretically possible, toxicities of the fat-soluble vitamins A and D are the most frequently observed. Vitamin E and the water-soluble vitamins niacin, vitamin B-6, and vitamin C can also cause toxic effects, but only when consumed in very large amounts (15 to 100 times their RDA or more).[11] These four vitamins are unlikely to cause toxic effects unless taken in supplement (pill) form. In comparison, vitamins A and D can cause toxicity with long-term intake at just five to ten times their RDA.

Because regular use of a "one-a-day" type of multivitamin and mineral supplement usually yields less than two times the RDAs of the components, this practice is unlikely to cause toxic effects. But consuming many vitamin pills, especially highly potent sources of vitamin A and vitamin D, can cause problems. In the 1930s, consumption of cod liver oil and other fish oils, which contain high concentrations of vitamin A and vitamin D, was quite common and often led to toxicity symptoms. Today concentrated vitamin A and vitamin D supplements are widely available in grocery, drug, and health-food stores and still pose risks for toxicity when used inappropriately. See the Nutrition Perspective to find out whether you should take a vitamin and mineral supplement, and if so, how to do it safely.

MALABSORPTION OF VITAMINS

Vitamins consumed in foods must be absorbed efficiently from the intestine to meet body needs. If absorption of a vitamin is defective, people must consume larger amounts of it or they are likely to develop deficiency symptoms. As discussed on the next page, fat malabsorption resulting from various diseases is associated with malabsorption of the fat-soluble vitamins. Certain intestinal diseases also can lead to malabsorption of some B vitamins (e.g., folate).

Because recent research on a variety of nutrient supplements has revealed a lack of product quality, the USP (United States Pharmacopeia) designation is being extended to an increasing number of nutrient supplements. The USP standards designate strength, quality, purity, packaging, labeling, and acceptable length of storage of ingredients for drugs. The purpose of applying them to vitamin and mineral supplements is to establish professionally accepted standards for these products. Consumers who buy nutrient supplements should look for the USP label to ensure quality.

CONCEPT CHECK

In general, the fat-soluble vitamins—A, D, E, and K—are less readily excreted than are the water-soluble B vitamins and vitamin C. When a person ingests a vitamin-free diet, the first deficiency signs will be due to a lack of thiamin and will appear after about 10 days. This shows that even water-soluble vitamins persist to some extent in the body, so an occasional inadequate daily consumption is of no health concern. It is important, however, to regularly consume foods rich in both water-soluble and fat-soluble vitamins. Fat-soluble vitamins A and D pose the greatest risk of toxicity. Water-soluble vitamins known to show toxic effects when taken in supplement form are niacin, vitamin B-6, and vitamin C.

Absorption of the Fat-Soluble Vitamins

We begin our discussion of the individual fat-soluble vitamins—A, D, E, and K—by seeing how they are absorbed (Figure 12-1). You can see from the chemical structures of these vitamins, shown in Figure 12-2, that they are lipidlike molecules. Because these vitamins are absorbed along with dietary fat, adequate absorption of the fat-soluble vitamins depends on efficient fat absorption. This in turn depends on fat digestion mediated by bile salts and the enzyme lipase in the small intestine, as well as adequate absorptive capacity from a healthy intestinal wall. Under these conditions, about 40% to 90% of the fat-soluble vitamins consumed are absorbed when they are taken in RDA amounts.[11,23,26] Absorption efficiency generally falls with intakes greatly in excess of the RDA.

VITAMIN A FAMILY

β-carotene

2 molecules of retinal (vitamin A)

Retinol

Retinoic acid

VITAMIN D FAMILY

Cholecalciferol (vitamin D₃)

Action by liver and kidney to yield the final product

1,25 (OH)₂ vitamin D₃ (calcitriol)

VITAMIN E

α-tocopherol

VITAMIN K

Phylloquinone

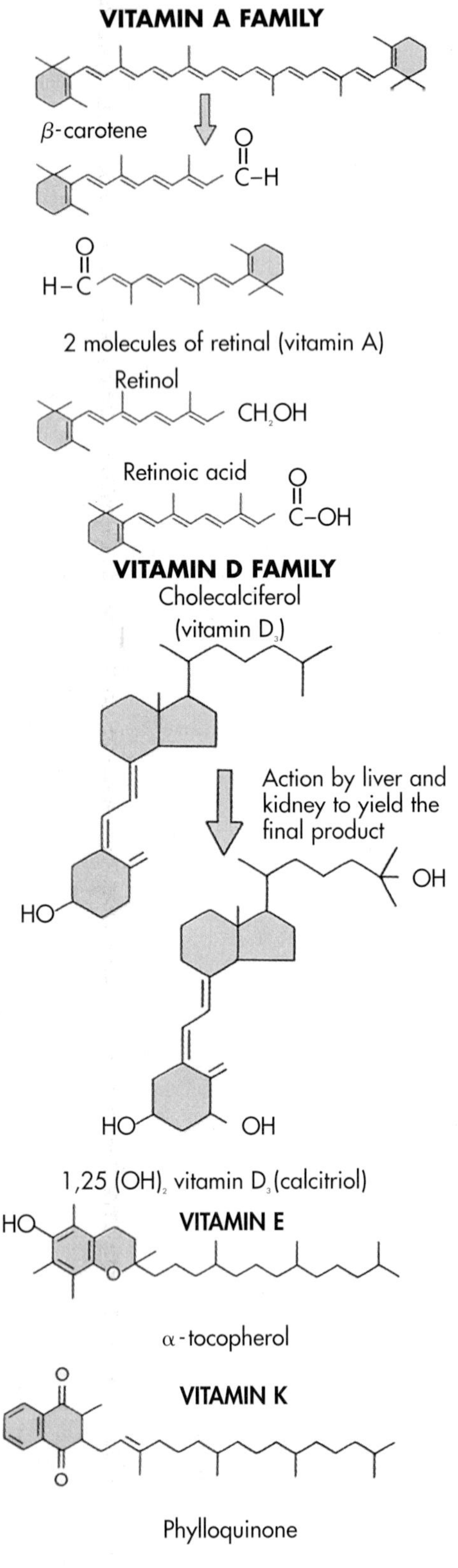

Figure 12-2

The fat-soluble vitamins: A, D, E, and K.

Once absorbed, fat-soluble vitamins are packaged and delivered to target cells throughout the body in a manner similar to that used for dietary fats—namely, by way of chylomicrons and other lipoproteins. Recall from Chapter 4 that as a chylomicron circulates in the bloodstream much of its triglyceride content is removed by body cells. What remains—the remnant—is taken up by the liver. This remnant contains the fat-soluble vitamins absorbed from the diet.[10] The liver can "repackage" fat-soluble vitamins with blood proteins for transport in the general circulation, or they can be stored in the liver for future use.

People with cystic fibrosis, celiac disease, Crohn's disease, or other diseases that hamper fat absorption also absorb fat-soluble vitamins poorly. Some medications also interfere with fat absorption. Unabsorbed fat carries these vitamins to the large intestine, where they are incorporated into the feces and excreted. People with such conditions are especially susceptible to vitamin K deficiency because body stores of vitamin K are lower than those of the other fat-soluble vitamins.[24] Vitamin supplements, taken under a physician's guidance, are the usual treatment for preventing vitamin deficiency associated with fat malabsorption.

Vitamin A

Americans are at little risk of developing a deficiency of vitamin A, since this vitamin is abundant in our food supply. But vitamin A deficiency constitutes one of the major public health problems in developing countries. Worldwide, vitamin A deficiency is the leading cause of nonaccidental blindness.[28] Children from impoverished nations in Africa, Asia, and South America are especially susceptible because their inadequate intake and diminished stores of vitamin A fail to meet the increased needs associated with rapid growth. Among the world's most destitute nations, hundreds of thousands of children become blind each year because they lack vitamin A; many die shortly thereafter because of infections.

Preformed vitamin A is present in animal foods as retinol, the alcohol form, and retinyl esters—compounds that have a fatty acid attached to the alcohol group of retinol. All these forms of vitamin A are derived only from animal foods or nutrient supplements. In the body, retinol is converted to retinal, an aldehyde form, and retinoic acid. Retinyl esters, which don't exhibit vitamin A activity as such, are broken down to yield retinol or retinoic acid. The three active forms of vitamin A—retinol, retinal, and retinoic acid—are collectively called **retinoids**.[26] Up to 90% of the dietary retinoids can be absorbed, again depending on the amount of fat in the diet. These mostly travel to the liver as part of the chylomicrons synthesized by the small intestine and enter the liver as part of the chylomicron remnant (see Figure 12-1).[26]

Although foods of plant origin contain no preformed vitamin A, they contain 600 or so pigments called **carotenoids,** some of which are convertible to vitamin A. Carotenoids are referred to as *provitamin A* and are the original source of all vitamin A in nature.[23] The yellow-orange pigment beta-carotene is the most common form of provitamin A (see Figure 12-2). Other important carotenoids include alpha-carotene, lutein, lycopene, zeaxanthin, and beta-cryptoxanthin. Many fruits and vegetables contain numerous different carotenoids. Once dietary carotenoids are consumed, some can be converted in the body to one of the retinoids, thereby supplying vitamin A activity. About 50 of the known carotenoids have the potential to be converted in this way.

Depending on the amount of fat in the diet, carotenoid absorption varies from 5% to 50%.[10] The lower values are seen when fat intake is less than about 20% of energy intake. In the intestinal cells most carotenoids that can yield vitamin A are split into two fragments, potentially yielding two molecules of vitamin A. Carotenoids can also be absorbed intact and deposited as such in adipose tissues, or they can undergo conversion to vitamin A (when possible) in the liver, after transport to this site by chylomicrons.[10]

The retinoids and provitamin A carotenoids are sometimes referred to collectively as *vitamin A.*

STORAGE AND TRANSPORT OF VITAMIN A

Under usual circumstances the liver contains more than 90% of the vitamin A in the body. Vitamin A is transported from this liver reserve to various target tissues when needed as retinol.[26] This attaches to a special retinol-binding protein in the liver for transport in the blood. The normal reserve in the liver is adequate for several months, explaining why the signs and symptoms of vitamin A deficiency take a long time to develop. Provitamin carotenoids that are not converted to retinoids in the liver travel from the liver to target tissues as part of the very-low-density lipoproteins (VLDLs).

Within target cells, intracellular retinoid-binding proteins direct the retinoids to specific enzymes that in turn provide control of metabolic processes, such as those related to growth and development.[26] In addition, these binding proteins protect the cell from the effects of "free" retinol or retinoic acid, which can be extremely damaging to cell metabolism.

FUNCTIONS OF VITAMIN A

Each of the three active forms of vitamin A performs important functions in the body: retinol is needed for reproduction; retinoic acid supports growth and allows cells to mature and differentiate; and retinal is crucial in night and color vision, perhaps the best-known role of vitamin A.[26]

The Visual Cycle

The sensory elements of the retina consist of specialized cells known as cones and rods. The cones are responsible for the visual processes occurring under bright lights, translating objects into color images. The rods are responsible for the visual processes that occur in dim light, translating objects into black-and-white images.

In the rods, the aldehyde form of vitamin A—retinal—combines with a protein, called opsin, to form rhodopsin (Figure 12-3). This is critical to the night vision capability of the rods. When light strikes rhodopsin in the retina of the eye, retinal undergoes a structural change (11-*cis*-retinal is converted to all-*trans*-retinal) and then detaches from the protein portion of the rhodopsin molecule, opsin. The free opsin assumes a new shape, leading to changes in the ion permeability of the cell membranes in the rods. The change in ion balance in these cell membranes stimulates nerve fibers, which in turn generates an electrical signal through the optic nerve. The optic nerve carries the message of black-and-white vision from the rod cells to the brain. This response to light of having rhodopsin break apart to retinal and opsin is referred to as the **bleaching process.**[14]

retinoids Collective term for the biologically active forms of vitamin A, including retinol, retinal, and retinoic acid.

carotenoids Red, yellow, and orange plant pigments, some of which can be metabolized to active vitamin A in the body. Those that yield vitamin A activity, such as beta-carotene, are called *provitamin A.*

See Appendix B for a description of *cis* and *trans* isomer forms.

bleaching process The process by which light depletes the rhodopsin concentration in the eye. This fall in rhodopsin concentration allows the eye to become adapted to bright light.

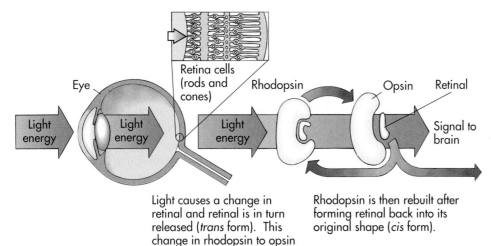

Light causes a change in retinal and retinal is in turn released (*trans* form). This change in rhodopsin to opsin and *trans* retinal in turn initiates a signal to the brain.

Rhodopsin is then rebuilt after forming retinal back into its original shape (*cis* form).

Some retinal is lost from cycle. This must be replaced by retinol from the bloodstream. It is converted to retinal in the eye.

Figure 12-3 Vitamin A participates in the visual cycle. Light (photons) produces changes in rhodopsin. This causes retinal to convert to a different form and simultaneously to separate from opsin. Opsin then changes shape, allowing the ion permeability of the retina membrane to change. This ion change signals "light" to the brain.

The light-induced bleaching process reduces the amount of rhodopsin in rods and also reduces the amount of related visual pigments in the cones. In bright light so much rhodopsin is broken down that not much is available to initiate signals to the brain. This allows the eyes to become "adapted" to bright light. When a person who has been in bright light enters a darkened room, his sensitivity to dim light is low and his vision is limited. Gradually, the ability to see increases because of a process called **dark adaptation,** which is linked to the increase in the amount of rhodopsin made in the rods that occurs in dark conditions.

The cells in the eye recover from a flash of light by first turning the all-*trans*-retinal formed during the bleaching process back into 11-*cis*-retinal and then resynthesizing rhodopsin. This series of actions constitutes the visual cycle. Not all retinal can be reused in this process: a certain amount is lost and must be replaced by retinol from the blood. Upon reaching the eye, retinol is converted to retinal (the form required for forming rhodopsin), allowing the rods to continue to provide night vision.[28]

If an adult's diet is deficient in vitamin A for many years, the vitamin A stores decrease. Because body stores are naturally lower in children, they are more likely to experience diminished retinol reserves.[23] When retinol in the blood is insufficient to replace the retinal lost during the visual cycle, the cells in the eye recover from flashes of light more slowly. This condition, called night blindness, reduces the ability of the eyes to quickly adapt to dim light following exposure to bright light.[28] A driver with night blindness, for example, would be temporarily blinded after the headlights from an oncoming car passed, taking much longer than normal to adapt to the dimmer light. An injection of vitamin A can cure night blindness in a matter of minutes!

Cones are less sensitive than rods to light. Thus when high-intensity light bleaches out the rods, the cones increasingly provide vision. The cones are also responsible for color vision and increased visual acuity. There are three types of cone cells. Each contains retinal plus one of three different proteins, responsive to either blue, green, or red light. Our perception of color depends on which cone cells are stimulated by visible light.[14]

Health and Maintenance of Cells

The epithelial tissues that cover external and internal body surfaces protect the body from all kinds of environmental contamination. (Skin and mucous membranes are examples of epithelial tissues.) Vitamin A as retinoic acid influences the way in which cells, such as **epithelial cells,** differentiate into mature forms.[26] It does so by stimulating expression of responsive genes, as we discuss in a later section on growth and development. This differentiation is very important for the maintenance of mucus-forming cells and the synthesis of various **mucopolysaccharides.** Thus retinoic acid is essential for the normal structure and function of epithelial cells.

Without vitamin A, mucus-forming cells deteriorate and no longer synthesize mucus, an essential lubricant used throughout the body. The eye, especially the cornea, is greatly affected by the loss of mucus, which lubricates the eye surface and washes away dirt and other particles that settle on the eye. The earliest clinical symptom of vitamin A deficiency is night blindness. Further deterioration of the eye results from bacterial invasion, as vitamin A plays an important role in resistance to infection. Conjunctival xerosis (abnormal dryness of the conjunctiva of the eye) and Bitot's spot (drying out of the eye and appearance of hardened epithelial cells) appear as vitamin A deficiency worsens. Irreversible changes in the cornea of the eye will ultimately develop with severe, prolonged vitamin A deficiency. The corneal ulceration and keratomalacia (softening of the cornea) result in scarring (Figure 12-4). The ultimate scarring may be barely detectable, or it could lead to loss of vision.[28] This sequence of changes in the eye—collectively known as **xerophthalmia** (dry eye)—causes blindness in millions of people worldwide. A recent study also suggests that deterioration of the retina more likely takes place when a person's diet is low in certain carotenoids (e.g., lutein and zeaxanthin) over an extended period of time.[27] Spinach and other leafy greens are good sources of these carotenoids.

dark adaptation The process by which the rhodopsin concentration in the eye increases in dark conditions. This in turn allows improved vision in the dark.

epithelial cells The surface cells that line the outside of the body and all external passages within it.

mucopolysaccharides Substances containing protein and carbohydrate parts; they are found in bone and body organs.

- - - - - - - - - - - - - -

Measuring serum vitamin A is one way to assess a person's status. However, this is an insensitive measure, since serum concentrations do not fall until vitamin A stores in the liver are very low.

- - - - - - - - - - - - - -

xerophthalmia A condition marked by dryness of the cornea and eye membranes that results from vitamin A deficiency and can lead to blindness. The specific cause is a lack of mucus production by the eye, which then leaves it more vulnerable to surface dirt and bacterial infections.

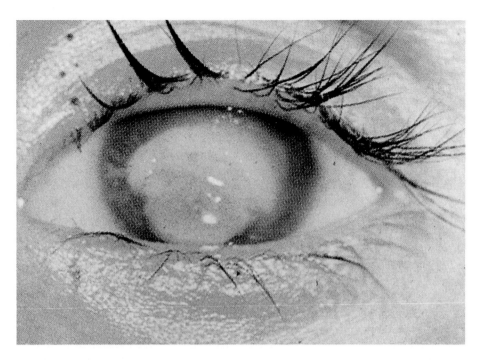

Figure 12-4 A vitamin A deficiency can eventually lead to blindness. Note the severe scar on this eye.

Vitamin A deficiency also produces skin changes referred to as **follicular hyperkeratosis.** Keratin is a normal component of the outer layers of skin, which serve to protect inner skin layers and reduce water loss through the skin. Skin constantly flakes off and so must be constantly replaced. During severe vitamin A deficiency, keratinized cells normally present only in the outer layers replace the normal epithelial cells in the underlying skin layers. Hair follicles also become plugged with keratin, giving a bumpy appearance and a rough texture to the skin.[10]

In a vitamin A deficiency, treatment with vitamin A can be given orally or intramuscularly.[23] A single large dose of vitamin A can meet the needs of a preschool child for up to 6 months. In many countries, deficiency of vitamin A is caused largely by the reliance on grains such as rice, wheat, and cassava, which are low in vitamin A, as basic staples and weaning foods. Carotenoid-containing fruits and vegetables are also disliked or avoided by many affected populations. Insufficient fat intake to allow for efficient carotenoid absorption then compounds the problem.

Resistance to Infection

Vitamin A has been called the anti-infection vitamin because of its role in helping the body combat bacterial, parasitic, and viral infections. Much remains to be learned about the action of vitamin A and resistance to disease. What is known is that many effects of vitamin A deficiency—insufficient mucus production in the eyes, intestinal tract, and lungs, deterioration of many types of cells, and reduced activity of some immune-system cells (e.g., T lymphocytes)—leave a person quite vulnerable to infections. That is why night blindness in children is accompanied by diarrhea, respiratory tract infections and corresponding morbidity, and increased risk of dying from measles.[12] Conversely, immune response to certain **antigens** increases when children deficient in vitamin A are supplemented with the vitamin.

Growth and Development

Vitamin A, specifically retinoic acid, is necessary for cellular differentiation, the process by which general precursor cells develop into a specific cell type that produces characteristic proteins.[26] During differentiation, specific portions of a cell's

---

In the United States, the leading cause of blindness in adults is diabetes; in children it is accidents.

follicular hyperkeratosis A condition in which keratin, a protein, accumulates around hair follicles.

CRITICAL THINKING

Stacy, a 3-year-old, has developed rough and scaly skin during the last year. After clinical evaluation of her condition and her food intake, her physician suspects that she has a vitamin A deficiency. He believes that she should start eating more foods rich in vitamin A. Stacy's mother is surprised at the doctor's advice. She remarks, "Doctor, there's nothing wrong with her eyes!" How can the doctor explain the diagnosis to Stacy's mother?

antigen Any foreign substance (e.g., proteins, bacteria, toxins) that can induce an immune response in the body. For example, egg protein is an antigen for people allergic to this protein. When such people eat eggs, they may develop skin reactions, shortness of breath, and headache.

nuclear receptor A site on the DNA in a cell where compounds (such as hormones) bind, leading to changes in gene expression and ultimately in the proteins produced by the cell. Cells that contain nuclear receptors for a specific compound are affected by that compound.

genetic material (DNA) are expressed, which means they are used to direct synthesis of proteins. Differentiated cells have specific roles within the various tissues of the body. In certain precursor cells, retinoic acid interacts with specific **nuclear receptors** present in the DNA, triggering differentiation of the cells. This function of vitamin A is particularly important in cellular differentiation in the developing embryo, such that embryos don't develop normally in laboratory animals deficient in vitamin A.[10] Thus these animals can't produce viable offspring.

Other types of growth are also enhanced by vitamin A. The development and maintenance of bone is especially dependent on adequate amounts of the vitamin. The synthesis of bone proteins and thus enlargement of bone is thought to require vitamins A and D. (See the later section in this chapter on vitamin D and Chapter 14 for more information about bone metabolism.)

Cancer Prevention

The ability of retinoids to influence cell development,[10] coupled with their ability to increase the activity of immune-system cells, could make them valuable tools in the fight against cancer, especially skin, lung, bladder, and breast cancer. Researchers have been encouraged by animal studies and also by the fact that most forms of cancer arise from cells that are influenced by vitamin A, namely, epithelial cells.

Cancer research with humans using various forms of vitamin A is now under way in research centers throughout the world. The results to date indicate that use of vitamin A supplements can lower the risk of breast cancer among women with very low intakes of dietary vitamin A.[19] However, most studies on prostate cancer indicate no protective effect from dietary vitamin A. The data from colon cancer studies are the same; vitamin A has little protective effect against this form of cancer. Because of the potential for toxicity, use of megadose vitamin A supplements to reduce cancer risk is currently not advised.

oxidizing agent Any substance capable of capturing an electron from (thus oxidizing) another compound (see Appendix B).

Carotenoids may help prevent cancer. The many double bonds present in some carotenoid molecules make them effective traps for the energy in highly reactive species of oxygen (singlet oxygen) and peroxides (such as H_2O_2), harmlessly releasing that energy as heat.[16] Singlet oxygen and peroxides are two of many **oxidizing agents** that can probably initiate the cancer process. By acting to block the effects of oxidizing agents, carotenoids are called antioxidants. Epidemiological evidence shows that regular consumption of foods rich in carotenoids decreases the risk of lung cancer, reproductive cancer, and oral cancer.[5] (Other benefits of antioxidants in the body are described later, in the section on vitamin E.)

However, a recent study from Finland failed to show a reduced incidence of lung cancer in male smokers who were given supplements of beta-carotene (and vitamin E) for 5 years. In fact, beta-carotene use increased the incidence of lung cancer by 18% compared with the control group.[3] One possible explanation for the absence of a benefit from beta-carotene supplements in this experimental study may be that the supplement was started too late in the course of the disease or that supplements are interfering with the metabolism of other antioxidants. In addition, something else in carotenoid-rich foods—other carotenoids, dietary fiber, various cancer-blocking chemicals (e.g., sulphoraphane, recently isolated from broccoli), or something not yet discovered—may confer the observed benefit of carotenoids seen in the epidemiological studies.

phytochemicals Compounds present in plants that influence production of certain enzymes involved in detoxifying carcinogens and removing them from the body. When consumed on a regular basis, some phytochemicals may help reduce the risk of cancer and heart disease.

Much more investigation is needed in this area before specific recommendations regarding carotenoids and cancer prevention—other than eating fruits and vegetables regularly—can be made.[5,31] It may be that certain **phytochemicals**, such as sulphoraphane, in fruits and vegetables are the actual protective agents. We discuss these compounds in the Nutrition Focus, and cancer in detail in Chapter 13.

Heart Disease Prevention

Carotenoids may play a role in preventing heart disease in persons at high risk, possibly linked to their antioxidant capability (see Chapter 4).[22] Until definitive studies are complete, many scientists recommend that we consume a total of at least

5 servings of fruit and vegetables per day as part of an overall effort to reduce the risk of heart disease.[15,29]

DIETARY SOURCES OF VITAMIN A AND CAROTENOIDS

Preformed vitamin A is found in liver, fish oils, fortified milk, and eggs. Margarine is fortified with vitamin A, but we don't eat enough to make it a significant source. Provitamin A carotenoids are mainly found in dark green and yellow-orange vegetables and some fruits. Carrots, spinach and other greens, winter squash, sweet potatoes, broccoli, mangoes, cantaloupe, peaches, and apricots are examples of such sources.[23] Two thirds of the vitamin A in the typical American diet comes from animal (preformed vitamin A) sources; the rest comes as provitamin A (Figure 12-5).

The major contributors of vitamin A—either the preformed or provitamin form—to American diets are liver, carrots, eggs, tomatoes, vegetable soup, milk, and greens. Among common foods, those having the highest nutrient density for vitamin A (μg/kcal) are carrots, liver, spinach and other greens, sweet potatoes, winter squash, romaine lettuce, broccoli, apricots, and nonfat and low-fat milk. Though rarely consumed in the United States, the oils from the livers of saltwater fish and marine mammals are extremely rich sources of vitamin A. Consumption of large amounts of such foods can even lead to symptoms of vitamin A toxicity.

Beta-carotene accounts for some of the orange color of carrots. In vegetables such as broccoli, this yellow-orange color is masked by dark-green chlorophyll pigments. Still, green vegetables contain provitamin A. Consuming a varied diet rich in green vegetables and carrots ensures sufficient sources for meeting vitamin A needs.[23]

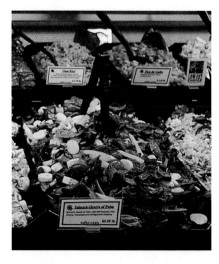

A regular intake of fruits and vegetables is advocated in the war against cancer.

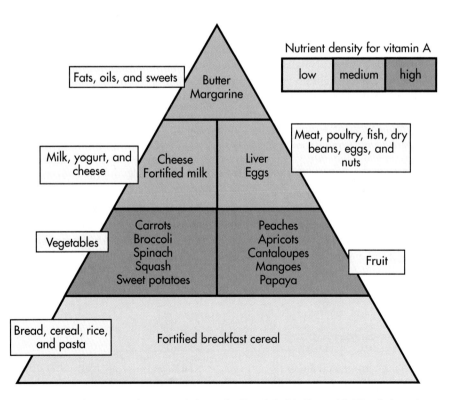

Figure 12-5 Food sources of vitamin A from the Food Guide Pyramid. The fruit and vegetable groups supply abundant carotenoids if they have an intense yellow-orange or green color. Some of these carotenoids yield vitamin A. Liver is the richest source of preformed vitamin A. Milk is often fortified with vitamin A. The background color of each food group indicates the average nutrient density for vitamin A in that group.

RETINOL EQUIVALENT (RE)

At one time, the amounts of most nutrients in foods were expressed in **international units (IUs).** These were usually based on the different growth rates exhibited by animals fed varying amounts of a specific nutrient or food. Today we can directly measure very small quantities of nutrients more precisely; consequently, milligrams (1/1000 of a gram) and micrograms (1/1,000,000 of a gram) have replaced international units as customary units of measure. Vitamin supplements may still display the older IU values.

For vitamin A, the current unit of measurement is the retinol equivalent (RE), which is basically 1 microgram (μg) of retinol. In this system, it is assumed that 6 μg of beta-carotene yield 1 μg of vitamin A activity and that 12 μg of other carotenoids yield 1 μg of vitamin A activity. The correction factors of 6 and 12 are estimates, based on incomplete knowledge, and primarily compensate for the poorer absorption of beta-carotene and other carotenoids compared with preformed vitamin A, as well as their incomplete conversion to the active form. The total RE value for a food is calculated by adding the actual weight of retinol and the adjusted equivalent weights of the provitamin A carotenoids present in the food.

Table 12-1 is a handy tool for converting amounts of vitamin A and carotenes expressed in one unit of measure into another unit of measure. For example, 3.3 IU of preformed vitamin A (retinol) equals 1 RE. Appendix N lists the carotenoid content of common plant foods.

RDA FOR VITAMIN A

The current RDA for vitamin A for adults is 1000 RE for men and 800 RE for women. (Throughout the next four chapters, refer to the inside cover for vitamin recommendations for other ages and to Appendix E for Canadian recommendations.) Average intakes for adult men and women in the United States meet the RDAs.[2]

Most adults in the United States have liver reserves of vitamin A that are three to five times greater than needed to provide for good health. Thus the use of vitamin A supplements by most people is completely unnecessary.

At present, there is no separate RDA for beta-carotene or any of the other provitamin A carotenoids. Some experts recommend a carotenoid intake of about 6 mg/day (10,000 IU/day).[5] Most Americans currently eat closer to 2 mg/day, since fruits and vegetables are not widely popular foods. The familiar "5 servings a day" goal for minimum total fruit and vegetable intake will probably yield the amount of carotenoids these experts recommend.

AMERICANS AT RISK FOR VITAMIN A DEFICIENCY

Deficient vitamin A status may be seen in preschool children who do not eat enough vegetables.[23] The urban poor, the elderly, and people with alcoholism or liver disease (which limits vitamin A storage) can also show diminished vitamin A status, especially with respect to stores. Finally, children and adults with severe fat-malabsorption syndromes, as in cases of celiac disease, chronic diarrhea, pancreatic insuf-

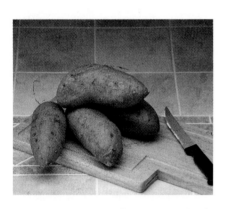

Sweet potatoes are rich in provitamin A carotenoids.

TABLE 12-1

Conversion values for vitamin A				
Compound with vitamin A activity	Micrograms	= RE	=	IU
Retinol	1	1		3.3
Beta-carotene	6	1		10
Other carotenoids (alpha-, delta-, etc.)	12	1		10
Mixture of both preformed and provitamin	—	1		5

ficiency, Crohn's disease, and cystic fibrosis, may also experience vitamin A deficiency.[23]

Parents and other caregivers often encourage their children to eat fruits and vegetables. Besides contributing to good food habits, this practice helps them obtain sufficient vitamin A. Adults are important role models for children, and adults can positively influence children's eating habits by eating as they want their children to eat.

VITAMIN A TOXICITY

Signs and symptoms of toxicity from excessive vitamin A—called **hypervitaminosis A**—can appear with long-term supplement use at just six to ten times the RDA (Figure 12-6).[23] Three kinds of vitamin A toxicity exist: acute, chronic, and **teratogenic.** Acute toxicity is caused by the ingestion of one very large dose of vitamin A or several large doses taken over several days (about 100,000 RE). The effects of acute toxicity are largely gastrointestinal upset, headache, blurred vision, and muscular incoordination. Once the dosing is stopped, these signs disappear. Extraordinarily large doses, about 12 g (12,000,000 RE), however, can be fatal.

Chronic toxicity, which is much more common than acute toxicity, results from ingesting excessive doses of vitamin A on a regular basis during a period of weeks to years. In infants and adults, there is a wide range of signs and symptoms: bone and muscle pain, loss of appetite, various skin disorders, headache, dry skin, hair loss, increased liver size, and vomiting. The treatment is simply to discontinue the supplement. Effects then decrease over the next few weeks to a month as blood concentrations fall to within a normal range. Permanent damage to the liver, bones, and eyes, as well as recurrent joint and muscle pain, however, can occur with chronic ingestion of excessive amounts of the vitamin.

A few individuals suffer effects of chronic vitamin A toxicity on relatively low daily intakes of vitamin A.[23] For example, intakes starting at just five times the adult male RDA (5000 RE) can provoke signs and symptoms. Such persons probably suffer from vitamin A intolerance, which seems to have a genetic basis and is often exacerbated by other clinical problems. These cases, although uncommon, are nonetheless worthy of note. In addition, the elderly as a group are more susceptible to toxic reactions than younger people.

hypervitaminosis Condition resulting from intake of excessive amounts of one or more vitamins.

teratogenic Tending to produce physical defects in a developing fetus.

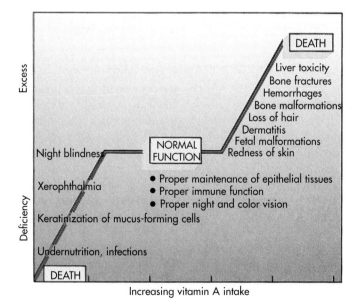

Figure 12-6 Consuming the right amount of vitamin A is critical to overall health. A very low (deficient) or a very high (toxic) vitamin A intake can produce damaging signs and symptoms and even lead to death. The severity of effects and the intake range vary among individuals.

The most serious and tragic effects of hypervitaminosis A are teratogenic, most notably birth defects. Vitamin A and its related **analog** forms, all-*trans*-retinoic acid (topical tretinoin to reduce wrinkling and acne) and 13-*cis*-retinoic acid (oral isotretinoin or Accutane used to treat acne), have been subjects of concern for years. Accutane causes spontaneous abortion and birth defects in experimental animals. The risk is significant for pregnant women taking large doses of Accutane for acne. Their offspring show congenital malformations of the head, probably because neural crest cells, which are important in the development of the head and brain, are known to be very sensitive to excess amounts of vitamin A. Women who expect to become pregnant are advised not to take medicinal forms of vitamin A that produce these effects. There appears to be no clear relationship between birth defects and excessive use of vitamin A as topical tretinoin.

Consuming carotenoids in huge amounts from foods does not readily result in toxicity in most people. Their rate of conversion into vitamin A (retinol), when possible, is relatively slow. In addition, the efficiency of carotenoid absorption from the small intestine decreases markedly as the oral intake increases. Thus nature protects us from any serious toxic effects from dietary carotenoids.

If someone consumes large amounts of carrots (in the form of carrot juice, for example) or if an infant eats a lot of winter squash, the resulting high carotenoid concentrations in the body can turn skin a yellow-orange color. The result is termed **hypercarotenemia,** or just carotenemia. (Recall that *hyper* means "high" and *emia* means "in the bloodstream.") The person appears to have jaundice but, unlike a true jaundice, the sclerae (whites of the eyes) are white (rather than yellow) and the liver is not enlarged. This carotenemia is generally thought to be harmless.

Some laboratory evidence suggests that when antioxidants like beta-carotene are consumed in very high amounts via supplements, they can cause disease. Recall that in the Finnish study mentioned earlier, the incidence of lung cancer was 18% higher in male smokers who took daily supplements of beta-carotene (20 mg) than in those who didn't take supplements.[3] However, another ongoing study involving 22,000 physicians who are taking either beta-carotene (50 mg) or a placebo every other day so far has revealed no ill effects. At present, use of beta-carotene supplements should be considered experimental, and as a lung cancer–prevention measure their use certainly does not substitute for stopping smoking. For now, the recommendation is to take no more than about 3 mg of beta-carotene (5000 IU) per day. That's the amount in most multivitamins that contain beta-carotene. The most cautious approach would be to take no carotenoid supplements at all and instead focus on food sources.

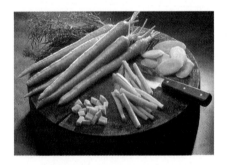

Foods rich in carotenoids pose little threat of vitamin A toxicity.

MEDICINAL USE OF LARGE VITAMIN A DOSES

In children, a single dose of 60,000 RE has been used for the possible prevention of vitamin A deficiency. This treatment, which causes mild, short-lived side effects in some children, is common medical practice in countries where the traditional diet is low in vitamin A. The dosage should last the child for 3 to 6 months.

In addition, evidence of vitamin A's role in immune processes has recently led researchers to examine supplementation as a treatment for childhood infection and disease.[28] In one study, administration of a single dose of 120,000 RE of vitamin A doubled the recovery rate in young children with measles. More interesting, the researchers found that vitamin A may greatly reduce infant susceptibility to infection, regardless of the child's status with respect to other nutrients.

Retinitis pigmentosa (RP) is an incurable eye disease that eventually leads to blindness. Consuming three times the RDA for vitamin A may postpone the inevitable decline for several years in people with the disease.

- - - - - - - - - - - - - -

Recently, derivatives of vitamin A have been put into creams (Retin-A) that manufacturers claim will reduce some effects of aging on the skin. Note that if the skin is already deeply wrinkled, these creams are ineffective. Limiting sun exposure (especially between 10 AM and 3 PM) and using sunblocks (sun protection factor 15 or higher) are much better preventive measures. Also keep in mind that there is no safe tan when it comes to protecting skin from damage.

- - - - - - - - - - - - - -

CONCEPT CHECK

Vitamin A has diverse functions, many of which are yet to be fully understood. Accumulating evidence suggests that binding of vitamin A to DNA can influence cell growth and differentiation. Vitamin A is important for maintaining vision and epithelial tissues and for ensuring proper function of the immune system. Vitamin A in the diet comes in two forms: retinoids (preformed vitamin A) and carotenoids (provitamin A). At present there is no definitive answer as to whether retinoids or carotenoids have specific anticancer properties. However, a diet that meets the RDA for vitamin A and contains plenty of carotenoid-containing fruits and vegetables is considered sound nutrition. Major food sources of vitamin A include liver, carrots, eggs, tomatoes, milk, and many vegetables. Americans most at risk for poor vitamin A status are preschool children and adults with alcoholism. Medicinal forms of vitamin A can be toxic, even at chronic dosages only about five to 10 times the RDA, especially during early pregnancy.

Vitamin D

The status of vitamin D as a vitamin is ambiguous because, in the presence of sunlight, skin cells are capable of synthesizing a sufficient supply of the vitamin from a derivative of cholesterol.[18] Since a dietary source is not required in this case, the vitamin is more correctly classified as a **prohormone** (i.e., a precursor of an active hormone). The prohormone form of vitamin D, whether synthesized in the body or obtained from the diet, is converted to the active form by specific enzymes in the liver and kidneys. The active form then is delivered to target organs, where it exerts its biological effects (Figure 12-7). Vitamin D is a generic term for both the provitamin (prohormone) and the active hormone form. Vitamin D achieves vitamin status because the diseases **rickets** and **osteomalacia** can be prevented and to some extent treated by consumption of vitamin D–rich foods.[9]

The amount of sun exposure individuals need to produce vitamin D depends on their skin color and their age: young, light-skinned people meet vitamin D needs through casual sun exposure, about 10 minutes per day on the face and hands. Dark-skinned people and the elderly need more sun exposure than light-skinned people. For example, African-Americans with very dark skin need about 10 times more sun exposure. People living in northern latitudes during the winter are at great risk of not making enough vitamin D because the prevailing sunlight under these conditions is less effective in promoting its synthesis. Anyone who does not receive enough sunshine to synthesize an adequate amount of vitamin D must have a dietary source of the vitamin.[18]

VITAMIN VERSUS PROHORMONE NATURE

The reason that the vitamin nature of vitamin D is emphasized more than its hormonal nature stems from early work on rickets. This disease was first described in England about 1650 and dubbed the "English disease." It spread throughout Europe in the years following, mostly due to the pall of coal smoke that blanketed Europe during the Industrial Revolution.

By the early 1900s it became increasingly clear to many physicians that sunlight had the power to prevent and cure rickets, as the disease was not seen in sunnier climates, such as in India. In 1919, a Berlin physician exposed four children with advanced rickets to the light from a mercury-vapor quartz lamp, which includes the ultraviolet wavelengths. He found that this exposure completely cured rickets within 2 months. In 1924, other researchers found that ingesting linseed, cottonseed, or yeast radiated with ultraviolet wavelengths also cured rickets.

In 1919, Sir Edward Mellanby also showed that a particular diet could cause rickets in dogs and that cod liver oil cured the condition. He hypothesized that a substance or "vitamine" in cod liver oil brought about the cure. The British Med-

prohormone Precursor of a hormone.

rickets A disease characterized by softening of the bones caused by poor calcium deposition. This deficiency disease arises in infants and children with a poor vitamin D status.

osteomalacia Softening of the bones that occurs in adults as the result of bone decalcification linked to inadequate vitamin D status.

- - - - - - - - - - - - -

Sunblock agents with an SPF of 8 or above reduce vitamin D synthesis in the skin. Use of these agents is recommended during prolonged sun exposure to reduce the risk of skin cancer. Such use is unlikely to result in low vitamin D status in children, as they undoubtedly spend some time each day in the sun without sunblock protection (e.g., during school recess or traveling to and from school). In addition, children often drink vitamin D–fortified milk. In contrast, elderly people should be sure to spend about 5 to 10 minutes each day in the sun without sunblock protection or seek a dietary source of vitamin D.

- - - - - - - - - - - - -

NUTRITION FOCUS

PHYTOCHEMICALS

Foods of plant origin contain a variety of substances that, unlike the vitamins and minerals, are not absolutely essential parts of the diet but still likely provide significant health benefits. Considerable research attention is now focused on the role of these substances, called phytochemicals (*phyto* means "plant"), in reducing the risks for certain diseases.[1] Since current vitamin and mineral supplements contain few or none of these potentially beneficial substances, they must be obtained from the diet.

Numerous epidemiological studies show reduced cancer risk among people who regularly consume fruits and vegetables.[29] This is true for cancer of the gastrointestinal tract, breast, lung, and bladder. Researchers surmise that the phytochemicals present in the fruits and vegetables can block the cancer process. We describe the cancer process in the Nutrition Perspective in Chapter 13. For now, realize that cancer develops over many years via a multistep process. If an agent such as a phytochemical can block any one of the steps in this process, the chances are reduced that cancer will ultimately appear in the body.

Other phytochemicals that have antioxidant capabilities have been linked to reduced risk of heart disease.[15] We have referred to various carotenoids in this regard in the chapter, but numerous other phytochemicals also have antioxidant properties.[1]

Currently, the pharmaceutical industry is experimenting with various phytochemicals in supplement form to be used in the prevention and treatment of disease. However, this work will involve only a few of the many potentially beneficial phytochemicals present in a diet that follows the Food Guide Pyramid recommendation of a total of at least 5 servings of fruits and vegetables a day. It will likely take many years for scientists to unravel the important effects of the myriad of phytochemicals in foods, and it is unlikely that all will ever be available in supplement form. For this reason, leading cancer researchers suggest that a diet rich in fruits and vegetables is the most reliable way to obtain the potential benefits of phytochemicals.[5,29]

Table 12-2 lists a variety of phytochemicals under study with their common food sources. Table 12-3 pro-

TABLE 12-2

Some phytochemicals currently under study

Phytochemical	Food source
Polyphenols (e.g., quercetin)	Onions, garlic, red wine, tea (especially green)
Indoles	Cruciferous vegetables*
Isothiocyanates (e.g., sulforaphane)	Cruciferous vegetables, especially broccoli
Carotenoids	Orange, yellow, and green vegetables; some fruits
Allyl sulfides	Onions, garlic, leeks, chives
Isoflavones (e.g., genistein)	Legumes (e.g., soybeans)
Monoterpenes (e.g., limonene)	Oils from citrus fruits; nuts, seeds
Phytic acid	Whole grains, legumes
Lignin	Seeds; some fruits and vegetables
Ellagic acid	Grapes
Caffeic acid, ferulic acid	Fruits
p-Coumaric acid, chlorogenic acid	Fruits and vegetables

*Cruciferous vegetables include bok choy, broccoli, brussels sprouts, cabbage, cauliflower, collards, kale, kohlrabi, mustard greens, rutabaga, turnip greens, and turnips.

Americans most at risk	Dietary sources	RDA	Toxicity symptoms

People in poverty, especially preschool children (still very rare)	Vitamin A:
	  Liver
	  Fortified milk
	Provitamin A:
	  Sweet potatoes
	  Spinach
	  Greens
	  Carrots
	  Cantaloupe
	  Apricots
	  Broccoli
		Females:
		  800 RE* (4000 IU†)
		Males:
		  1000 RE* (5000 IU†)
			Fetal malformations, hair loss, skin changes, pain in bones

Breast-fed infants, elderly shut-ins	Vitamin D–fortified milk Fish oils Sardines Salmon	5-10 µg (200-400 IU)	Growth retardation, kidney damage, calcium deposits in soft tissue

People with poor fat absorption (still very rare)	Vegetable oils
	Some greens
	Some fruits
		Females:
		  8 mg (alpha-toco-pherol equivalents)
		Males:
		  10 mg (alpha-toco-pherol equivalents)
			Muscle weakness, headaches, fatigue, nausea, inhibition of vitamin K metabolism

People taking antibiotics for months at a time (still quite rare)	Green vegetables Liver	60-80 µg	Anemia and jaundice

Summary

1. Vitamins are essential organic (carbon-containing) compounds needed for important metabolic reactions in the body. They are not a source of energy. Instead, they promote many energy-yielding and other reactions in the body, thereby promoting growth, development, and maintenance of various body tissues. Vitamins A, D, E, and K are fat soluble, while the B vitamins and vitamin C are water soluble. Fat-soluble vitamins are excreted less readily from the body and are less susceptible to cooking loss than are water-soluble vitamins.

2. Some fat-soluble vitamins pose a potential for toxicity. Vitamins A and D can readily accumulate in the body to toxic amounts. The water-soluble niacin, vitamin B-6, and vitamin C can also induce toxic signs and symptoms, but only at doses much higher than their RDAs.

3. Fat-soluble vitamins are absorbed along with dietary fat. They travel by way of the lymphatic system into the bloodstream, carried by chylomicrons, one type of lipoprotein. In disease states in which fat digestion is limited, fat-soluble vitamin status may be compromised, especially with vitamins E and K.

4. Vitamin A consists of a family of retinoid compounds: retinal, retinol, and retinoic acid. A plant derivative known as beta-carotene, along with some other carotenoids, yields vitamin A after metabolism by the intestine or liver. Vitamin A contributes to the maintenance of vision, the proper development of cells (especially mucus-forming cells), and immune function. Vitamin A is found in foods of animal origin, such as liver, fish oils, and fortified milk. Carotenoids are obtained from plants and are especially plentiful in dark green and orange vegetables and in some fruits. These contribute to protection from oxidizing agents for the body.

5. Americans at risk for poor vitamin A status are people exhibiting limited fat absorption and people with alcoholism. Vitamin A can be quite toxic when taken at just five to ten times the RDA. Certain forms of vitamin A taken during pregnancy are especially dangerous because they can lead to fetal malformations.

6. For most people, vitamin D is more correctly viewed as a hormone rather than a vitamin because sufficient amounts of it can be produced by the body. Provitamin D is synthesized in the skin from a derivative of cholesterol in a process that depends on ultraviolet light. With adequate sun exposure, no dietary intake of provitamin D is needed. The provitamin, whether produced in the skin or obtained from the diet, is metabolized in the liver and kidneys to yield calcitriol, the active hormonal form of vitamin D. Calcitriol is important for calcium absorption from the intestine, and with other hormones it helps regulate bone metabolism. Vitamin D is found in fish oils and fortified milk. Vitamin D can be very toxic when taken in supplement form, especially in childhood, when an intake just five times the RDA can be toxic. Anyone who feels a need to use a vitamin D supplement containing more than two times the RDA, such as an elderly person, should consult a physician first.

7. Vitamin E functions as an antioxidant. By donating electrons to electron-seeking compounds (oxidizing agents), it neutralizes their action. One group of electron-seeking compounds, known as free radicals, can cause widespread destruction both to cell membranes and to DNA. Vitamin E is one of several components in the body's defense system against oxidizing agents, which reduces damage to cells. Vitamin E is plentiful in plant oils. The more plant oils one consumes, the more vitamin E one needs, but this need is usually met by those same plant oils. Fish oils, in contrast, often contain little vitamin E. Use of megadose supplements of vitamin E by healthy adults to limit heart disease and cancer risk is a source of current scientific debate and an active area of research.

8. Vitamin K contributes to the body's blood-clotting ability by facilitating conversion of precursor proteins to active clotting factors, such as prothrombin, which take part in formation of clots. Some of the vitamin K absorbed each day comes from bacterial synthesis in the intestine; most comes from foods, primarily green leafy vegetables. Vitamin K is readily excreted in the body, but the usual daily intake from diet alone is about five times our needs.

Study Questions

1. Why is the risk of toxicity greater for fat-soluble vitamins than for water-soluble vitamins?
2. Why do the carotenoids pose much less of a threat for vitamin A toxicity than preformed vitamin A?
3. Explain how retinal functions in black-and-white and color vision.
4. How does vitamin A function in cellular differentiation? What form of vitamin A is active in this process?
5. How would you determine which fruits and vegetables displayed in the produce section of your supermarket likely provide plenty of carotenoids?
6. Elderly people residing in nursing homes are most likely to have a deficiency of which vitamin? Why? What signs and symptoms of this vitamin deficiency are common under these conditions?
7. What is the primary function of calcitriol? Discuss the specific mechanisms involved in this function.
8. Deficiencies of which fat-soluble vitamins are highly likely in children with inadequately treated or undetected cystic fibrosis?
9. Describe how vitamin E functions as an antioxidant.
10. What are the signs and symptoms of vitamin E deficiency in laboratory animals? Why are untreated preterm infants deficient in vitamin E, and what is the primary sign of this deficiency?
11. What is vitamin K's primary function in the body?
12. Why is it critical for a surgeon to know the vitamin K status of a patient before operating?

REFERENCES

1. ADA Reports: Position of The American Dietetic Association: Phytochemicals and functional foods, *Journal of the American Dietetic Association* 94:493, 1995.
2. Alaimo K and others: Dietary intake of vitamins, minerals, and fiber of persons ages 2 months and over in the United States: Third National Health and Nutrition Examination Survey, Phase 1, 1988-91, *Advance Data* 258(Nov 14):1, 1994.
3. Alpha-Tocopherol, Beta-Carotene Cancer Prevention Study Group: The effect of vitamin E and beta-carotene on the incidence of lung cancer and other cancers in male smokers, *New England Journal of Medicine* 15:1029, 1984.
4. Bikle DD: A bright future for the sunshine hormone, *Scientific American Science & Medicine* March/April 1995, p 58.
5. Block G, Langseth L: Antioxidant vitamins and disease prevention, *Food Technology* July 1994, p 80.
6. Bouillon R and others: Structure and function in the vitamin D endocrine system, *Endocrine Reviews* 16:200, 1995.
7. Chapuy MC and others: Vitamin D₃ and calcium to prevent hip fractures in elderly women, *New England Journal of Medicine* 23:1637, 1992.
8. Council on Scientific Affairs: Vitamin preparations as dietary supplements and as therapeutic agents, *Journal of the American Medical Association* 257:1929, 1987.
9. DeLuca HD: Vitamin D: 1993, *Nutrition Today*, Nov/Dec 1993, p 6.
10. De Luca LM and others: Retinoids in differentiation and neoplasia, *Scientific American Science & Medicine,* July/August 1995, p 28.

11. Farrell PM, Roberts RJ: Vitamin E. In Shils ME and others, editors: *Modern nutrition in health and disease,* ed 8, Philadelphia, 1994, Lea & Febiger.
12. Fawzi WW and others: Dietary vitamin A intake and the risk of mortality among children, *American Journal of Clinical Nutrition* 59:401, 1994.
13. Frei B: Reactive oxygen species and antioxidant vitamins: mechanisms of action, *American Journal of Medicine* 97(suppl 3A):5S, 1994.
14. Ganong WF: *Review of medical physiology,* ed 16, Norwalk, Conn, 1995, Appleton & Lange.
15. Gaziano JM: Antioxidant vitamins and coronary artery disease risk, *American Journal of Medicine* 97(suppl 3A):18S, 1994.
16. Halliwell B: Free radicals and antioxidants: a personal view, *Nutrition Reviews* 52:253, 1994.
17. Herbert V: The antioxidant supplement myth, *American Journal of Clinical Nutrition* 60:157, 1994.
18. Holick MF: Environmental factors that influence the cutaneous production of vitamin D, *American Journal of Clinical Nutrition* 61:638S, 1995.
19. Hunter DJ and others: A prospective study of the intake of vitamins C, E, and A and the risk of breast cancer, *New England Journal of Medicine* 329:234, 1994.
20. LaChance P: To supplement or not to supplement: is it a question? *Journal of the American College of Nutrition* 13:113, 1994.
21. Mertz W: A balanced approach to nutrition for health: the need for biologically essential minerals and vitamins, *Journal of the American Dietetic Association* 94:1259, 1994.

22. Morris DL and others: Serum carotenoids and coronary heart disease, *Journal of the American Medical Association* 272:1439, 1994.
23. Olsen JA: Needs and sources of carotenoids and vitamin A, *Nutrition Reviews* 52:S67, 1994.
24. Olsen RE: Vitamin K. In Shils ME and others, editors: *Modern nutrition in health and disease,* ed 8, Philadelphia, 1994, Lea & Febiger.
25. Porter DV: Dietary supplements: recent chronology and legislation, *Nutrition Reviews* 53:31, 1995.
26. Ross AC, Ternus ME: Vitamin A as a hormone: recent advances in understanding the actions of retinol, retinoic acid, and beta-carotene, *Journal of the American Dietetic Association* 93:1285, 1993.
27. Seddon JM and others: Dietary carotenoids, vitamins A, C, and E, and advanced age-related macular degeneration, *Journal of the American Medical Association* 272:1413, 1994.
28. Sommer A: Vitamin A: its effect on childhood sight and life, *Nutrition Reviews* 52:S60, 1994.
29. Voelker R: Ames agrees with mom's advice: eat your fruits and vegetables, *Journal of the American Medical Association* 273:1077, 1995.
30. Wallidus G and others: The effect of probucol on femoral atherosclerosis, *American Journal of Cardiology* 74:875, 1994.
31. Willett WC, Hunter DJ: Vitamin A and cancers of the breast, large bowel, and prostate: epidemiologic evidence, *Nutrition Reviews* 52:S53, 1994.

TAKE ACTION

Measuring your vitamin intake against the RDAs

This activity requires you to reexamine the nutritional assessment you did for Chapters 1 and 2. You recorded all the foods and drinks you consumed for 1 day and their quantities. Then you assessed your intake by recording the total amounts of nutrients you consumed. You were then asked to compare your nutrient intake to certain standards. Many of the standards you used were the 1989 RDAs found on the inside front cover of this book. Take your completed assessment and look at your intakes of vitamins A, E, C, B-6, B-12, and thiamin, riboflavin, niacin, and folate. Record these numbers in the table below. Next, record the RDAs for each of these nutrients from your assessment. Then, record the percentage of the RDA you consumed for each vitamin. Lastly, place a +, −, or = in the space provided, reflecting an intake higher than, lower than, or equal to the RDA.

VITAMIN	INTAKE	RDA	% OF RDA	+, −, =
A				
E				
C				
THIAMIN				
RIBOFLAVIN				
NIACIN				
B-6				
FOLATE				
B-12				

ANALYSIS

1. Which of your vitamin intakes equaled or exceeded the RDA?

_____

2. Which of your vitamin intakes were below the RDA?

_____

3. What foods could you eat to improve your dietary intake of vitamins in low amounts in your diet? (Review sources of certain vitamins in this chapter and the next.)

_____

_____

Vitamin Supplements: Who Needs Them?

Our opinions about vitamins have changed since the turn of the century, when Casimir Funk first coined the term from the words "vital amine." As you might have already noticed from some of the vitamin structures shown in this chapter, not all vitamins are actually amines, which contain a –C–NH$_2$ group. Although vitamins were at first just a curiosity, they soon became the subject of intense scientific scrutiny and research.

Today, vitamins are promoted as cure-alls by many health-food enthusiasts and consumed as supplements by about 50% of the American population. Supplements are big business; in fact, their sales more than tripled between the mid-1970s and mid-1990s, with current sales exceeding $3.5 billion.

Should you take a vitamin and mineral supplement? To answer that question, first look closely at your diet. Does it follow the Food Guide Pyramid outlined in Chapter 2, especially emphasizing low-fat and nonfat dairy products, lean meats, whole grains, leafy and dark green vegetables, fruits containing vitamin C, and some vegetable oil? If so, you are probably meeting your needs if you are a man. However, women with heavy menstrual flows still may need more iron. Second, do you regularly consume a fortified breakfast cereal? Most breakfast cereals are fortified with vitamins and minerals (Figure 12-16). However, one must consume any milk used in combination to get the full benefit, as some vitamins leak out into the milk.

Nutrition scientists generally agree that most people can obtain the vitamins and minerals they need if they eat a healthy diet, noting that dietary supplements are clearly no substitute for the vital components of a healthy lifestyle.[17,29] When people eat in moderation, choose balanced, low-fat, varied diets, and engage in regular physical activity, there is likely little need for supplements. Using Chapter 2 for guidance, improve your diet where needed. Only after that should you consider whether you still need a supplement. We advise discussing your plans with a physician, who may refer you to a registered dietitian.

People Most Likely to Need Supplements

Scientists from the American Institute of Nutrition and the American Society for Clinical Nutrition have suggested that the following vitamin and mineral supplementation should be considered for certain groups of healthy people:
- Women with excessive bleeding during menstruation may need extra iron.
- Women who are pregnant or breast-feeding may need extra iron, folate, and calcium.
- People with very low energy intakes need a range of vitamins and minerals.
- Some vegetarians may need extra calcium, iron, zinc, and vitamin B-12.
- Newborns, under the direction of a physician, need a single dose of vitamin K.

Individuals with certain medical conditions (e.g., vitamin-resistance diseases or fat-malabsorption syndromes) and those who use certain medications may require supplementation with specific vitamins and minerals under the direction of a physician. For example, patients taking thiazide diuretics often require extra potassium. The treatment of osteoporosis may include supplementation with vitamin D and calcium. Women who are able to become pregnant may need folate supplements if their diets do not provide enough, as deficient folate status increases the risk of certain birth defects (see Chapter 13).

Supplementation during illness and drug therapy especially needs to be directed by a physician because use of some vitamin and mineral supplements can cause harm by themselves, and may counteract the actions of certain medications. For example, vitamin B-6 can offset the action of L-dopa (used in treating Parkinson's disease). High intakes of vitamin E can inhibit vitamin K metabolism and, therefore, increase the action of oral anticoagulants, such as warfarin.[17] Conversely, high intakes of vitamin K reduce the action of oral anticoagulants.[24]

Which Supplement Should You Choose?

If you decide to take a vitamin and mineral supplement, which one should you choose? We suggest following the guidelines set forth by the Council on Scientific Affairs of the American

WHEATIES

Nutrition Facts
Serving Size 1 cup (30g)
Servings Per Container About 11

Amount Per Serving	Wheaties	with ½ cup skim milk
Calories	110	150
Calories from Fat	10	10

	% Daily Value**	
Total Fat 1g*	**1%**	**2%**
Saturated Fat 0g	**0%**	**0%**
Cholesterol 0mg	**0%**	**1%**
Sodium 210mg	**9%**	**11%**
Potassium 115mg	**3%**	**9%**
Total Carbohydrate 24g	**8%**	**10%**
Dietary Fiber 3g	**13%**	**13%**
Sugars 4g		
Other Carbohydrate 17g		
Protein 3g		

Vitamin A	25%	30%
Vitamin C	25%	25%
Calcium	6%	20%
Iron	45%	45%
Vitamin D	10%	25%
Thiamin	25%	30%
Riboflavin	25%	35%
Niacin	25%	25%
Vitamin B$_6$	25%	25%
Folic Acid	25%	25%
Phosphorus	10%	20%
Magnesium	8%	10%
Zinc	4%	8%
Copper	4%	4%

*Amount in Cereal. A serving of cereal plus milk provides 1g fat, <5mg cholesterol, 270mg sodium, 320mg potassium, 30g carbohydrate (10g sugars), and 7g protein.
**Percent Daily Values are based on a 2,000 calorie diet. Your daily values may be higher or lower depending on your calorie needs:

	Calories:	2,000	2,500
Total Fat	Less than	65g	80g
Sat Fat	Less than	20g	25g
Cholesterol	Less than	300mg	300mg
Sodium	Less than	2,400mg	2,400mg
Potassium		3,500mg	3,500mg
Total Carbohydrate		300g	375g

Figure 12-16 The amount of vitamin and mineral fortification in a typical breakfast cereal. Note that two of the four fat-soluble vitamins are included.

Medical Association. They recommend that a supplement contain no more than 50% to 150% of the adult Daily Values listed on the package (previously called U.S. RDAs) for vitamins A, D, E, and C, folate, thiamin, riboflavin, niacin, vitamin B-6, and vitamin B-12. The Council does not recommend that the supplement contain biotin or pantothenic acid (because deficiencies are so unlikely), nor vitamin K (because it can disturb oral anticoagulant therapy). For minerals, we suggest using the same guideline: 50% to 150% of the Daily Value listed on the package as an upper limit, or up to 100% of the estimated safe and adequate daily dietary intake for nutrients with no Daily Value (see the inside cover of this book). All of these guidelines are usually observed in a basic one-a-day type vitamin, but read the label to be sure. For example, the nutrient amounts in one tablet of a typical B-complex product can range from 33% of our needs for biotin to 6670% or more for thiamin. This is not what we consider a balanced formulation.

A balanced formulation in a multivitamin and mineral supplement is important. Balance will minimize the chance of vitamin and mineral competition as well as possible accompanying toxicity problems, such as the following:

- Excessive intake of vitamin C can cause overabsorption of iron and contribute to iron toxicity in susceptible people. Consuming excessive amounts of vitamin C also may inhibit copper absorption and decrease the ability of certain diagnostic tests to assess the development of diabetes or colon cancer.
- Large amounts of fish oil can lead to a decrease in blood clotting.
- Excessive zinc intake can inhibit iron and copper absorption.
- Excessive fluoride exposure during childhood may stain and even weaken the teeth (see Chapter 15).
- Large amounts of folate can mask signs and symptoms of a vitamin B-12 deficiency, thereby preventing the early diagnosis of a potentially life-threatening condition. Large doses of folate, approximately 100 times the RDA, can also inhibit the action of anticonvulsants. Patients with epilepsy who require anticonvulsant therapy jeopardize their health if they also consume large doses of folate supplements.

Furthermore, some nutrients produce toxic effects at intakes not much above their RDAs; these include vitamin A, vitamin D, and selenium.

The possibility of such interacting effects highlights the importance of discussing vitamin and mineral supplementation with a physician and registered dietitian. Only then can you appropriately evaluate whether supplementation is in your best interest. We will further discuss these and other potentially toxic effects of vitamin and mineral overuse in Chapters 13 through 15. For now, keep in mind that the amounts set by the Food and Nutrition Board for vitamins or minerals, as outlined in the RDA publication, are important for good health. But that does not mean that higher intakes will be safe or necessarily more beneficial.[21] In fact, the chances are great that as intakes increase, toxic signs and symptoms will eventually result.[17]

One consideration in choosing a supplement is the presence of superfluous ingredients, such as para-amino benzoic acid (PABA), hesperidin complex, inositol, bee pollen, and lecithin. These are not needed in our diets. The body can make adequate amounts of those that are used (e.g., lecithin); the others are pure and simple quackery (e.g., bee pollen). These extraneous substances are especially common in expensive supplements sold in health-food stores and by mail.

Surveys of people who use vitamin and mineral supplements find that they generally consume multivitamin and mineral preparations. About 60% of the supplement market consists of these. Iron, vitamins E and C, and calcium are the most common nutrients taken as a single supplement.

CRITICAL THINKING

Many vitamin supplements supply nutrients in amounts that exceed the Daily values listed on the label. Miguel believes that "more is better." How can you explain to him that the supplement he is about to start taking is "worse," since it contains amounts that exceed the Daily Values by ten times for many nutrients, including vitamin D?

Supplements Are Regulated Loosely by FDA

Note that unless FDA has evidence that a supplement is inherently dangerous or marked with illegal claims, it will not regulate it closely (see the section in Chapter 13 on folate for a major exception). FDA is in fact prevented from doing so by the Proxmire Amendment to the 1938 Food, Drug, and Cosmetic Act, along with follow-up legislation passed in 1994.[25]

Like foods, supplements can't carry disease-specific claims unless these assertions are backed by solid scientific evidence. However, supplements can make general claims about maintaining a healthy body, such as "vitamin A is important to maintain good vision." If so, supplement packages then must alert consumers that these claims have not been evaluated by FDA and that the supplements are not intended to diagnose, treat, cure, or prevent any disease.[25]

Currently, FDA has limited resources and has to act against manufacturers one at a time. Injuries are likely to occur before FDA can do anything to force a reformulation of an unsafe supplement. So Americans cannot rely on the federal government to protect them from vitamin and mineral supplement overuse. It is best to rely on the advice of physicians and registered dietitians for guidance.

A main concern of FDA currently is the array of substances other than vitamins and minerals that are found in some supplements, including enzymes, nucleic acids, and herbs and other botanicals. Little is known about some of these ingredients.

FDA officials insist that they have no plans to limit access to most supplements; they simply want to make sure that the products themselves are safe to use and, if manufacturers include health claims on the labels, that the claims are accurate. Note that some ingredients in herbal products contain chemicals that are naturally harmful, such as certain alkaloids. In other words, "natural" doesn't necessarily mean "safe."

Opinions Vary Concerning Supplements and Additional Food Fortification

In the future the RDAs for vitamins may be broadened to include one value sufficient to prevent known vitamin deficiency diseases and a higher value recommended to optimize the potential disease-preventing properties of some of these nutrients (e.g., the antioxidant vitamins). FDA and the National Academy of Sciences currently state that recommending supplements of antioxidant nutrients to the general public is premature. There is no consensus among knowledgeable scientists about whether healthy people who eat a varied diet should take vitamin and mineral supplements.

Scientists are also questioning whether further fortification of the American diet may be prudent, since many of us still do not follow the Food Guide Pyramid. If the diets of certain adults do not meet specific vitamin and mineral targets, should the federal government step in and make sure intakes of these nutrients increase by fortifying foods we already eat?[20] This worked in the 1940s when thiamin, niacin, riboflavin, and iron were first added to refined grains. In addition, the amount of vitamin E that some scientists would like us to consume daily (>100 IU) cannot be met with conventional food choices.

Would the overall health of the nation be improved if the government forced manufacturers to increase fortification of foods? Or would additional fortification lead to unbalanced nutrient intakes and in turn untoward effects? There is no consensus on this question. Consuming healthy, balanced diets is still the overriding theme—boring as it may sound to people seeking a simpler solution.[29]

CHAPTER THIRTEEN

The Water-Soluble Vitamins

A s defined in the previous chapter, vitamins are essential organic substances needed in very small amounts in the diet to support metabolism, growth, and maintenance of body cells.

The water-soluble vitamins discussed in this chapter include eight B vitamins and vitamin C. The B vitamins form coenzymes—organic compounds that enable certain enzymes to function.[13] As a group, the B vitamins are necessary for converting solar energy into cellular energy, transforming nutrients into characteristic cell structures, and creating various proteins, lipids, and carbohydrates. Vitamin C also participates in a wide variety of metabolic processes, although not in the form of a coenzyme.[22]

At the end of the chapter we briefly describe some "vitamin-like" compounds, which some people may require in their diets under atypical circumstances. These compounds currently are not classified as true vitamins because a healthy person does not require a dietary source of them and no specific deficiency disease results when they are absent from the diet.

1. **T F** The RDA for thiamin is set in proportion to the intake of dietary fat.
2. **T F** One of the richest sources of dietary thiamin is pork and pork products.
3. **T F** White rice is a good source of niacin.
4. **T F** Milk is an excellent source of riboflavin.
5. **T F** A deficiency in riboflavin suggests a simultaneous deficiency in thiamin, niacin, and vitamin B-6.
6. **T F** Elderly patients who exhibit megaloblastic anemia may have a vitamin B-12 deficiency.
7. **T F** The body can synthesize the vitamin niacin from the amino acid tryptophan.
8. **T F** A niacin deficiency causes severe skin inflammation.
9. **T F** Megadoses of nicotinic acid can lower serum cholesterol.
10. **T F** Alcohol decreases absorption of the vitamin folate.
11. **T F** Excessive supplementation with vitamin B-12 may mask a folate deficiency.
12. **T F** Vitamin B-12 is present only in animal foods.
13. **T F** A deficiency in vitamin C causes pinpoint hemorrhages in the skin.
14. **T F** Vitamin C contributes to iron absorption.
15. **T F** Vitamin C both prevents and cures the common cold.

Water-Soluble Vitamins: General Properties

For most of human history, diseases such as scurvy, beriberi, pellagra, and pernicious anemia caused enormous suffering. Early in this century, scientists began to recognize that these illnesses were caused by the absence of certain vital substances from the diet—now called the B vitamins and vitamin C. It was soon discovered that restoring these vitamins to the diet dramatically reversed these deficiency diseases if done before significant deterioration of the body took place.

The second vitamin to be discovered was designated vitamin B, according to the letter convention discussed in the last chapter. This water-soluble substance, which could cure beriberi, was initially thought to be a single chemical compound. When subsequent research showed that this substance actually consisted of several compounds, named the B vitamins, numbers were added to the letter to distinguish them (Figure 13-1). Of the eight B vitamins, only two are still commonly referred to by letter and number: vitamins B-6 and B-12. The others now are usually referred to by the following names: thiamin (previously B-1), riboflavin (previously B-2), niacin (previously B-3), pantothenic acid, biotin, and folate. The older designations are sometimes used on vitamin supplement labels.

In their **coenzyme** forms, B vitamins serve as carriers of specific ions or chemical groups, in turn allowing highly coordinated metabolic pathways in a cell to proceed (Figure 13-2).[13] All the eight B vitamins participate in energy metabolism; some also have other roles in the chemical reactions that take place within cells. Although vitamin C does not function as a coenzyme, it plays a role in the synthesis of several important compounds in cells.[22]

The B vitamins are present in foods in their coenzyme forms bound to specific proteins. After ingestion, the bound vitamin coenzymes are released in the stomach and small intestine. The free vitamins are then absorbed in the small intestine.

Typically about 50% to 90% of the B vitamins in the diet are absorbed. Once inside cells, the coenzyme forms of the vitamins are resynthesized. Health-food stores sell the coenzyme form of some vitamins, although they have no specific benefits to the consumer, since vitamins are not absorbed in this form.

Because they are water soluble, many of the B vitamins and vitamin C are more easily excreted from the body than the fat-soluble vitamins. Moreover, some of the

coenzyme A compound that combines with an inactive protein called an apoenzyme to form a catalytically active protein called a holoenzyme.

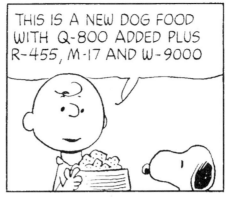
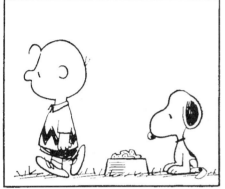

Figure 13-1 Peanuts.

Reprinted by permission of UFS, Inc.

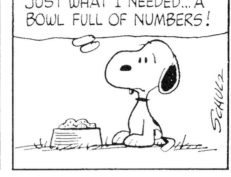

water-soluble vitamins are rather easily destroyed during cooking due to heat or alkalinity; all are subject to leaching into the cooking water. Retention of the B vitamins and vitamin C is greatest in foods that are prepared by steaming, stir-frying, microwaving, or simmering in minimal moisture.

B Vitamin and Vitamin C Status of Americans

The nutritional status of most Americans with respect to the B vitamins and vitamin C is generally good.[1] Typical diets in the United States contain plentiful and varied natural sources of these vitamins. In addition, many common foods are fortified with one or more of the water-soluble vitamins. In some countries of the Third World, however, deficiencies of the water-soluble vitamins are more common, and the resulting deficiency diseases pose significant public-health problems. (A detailed discussion of nutritional deficiencies worldwide is presented in Chapter 20.)

Despite the generally good B vitamin and vitamin C status of Americans, marginal deficiencies of the water-soluble vitamins may occur in some Americans and others in the western world, especially the elderly.[25] The long-term effects of such marginal deficiencies are as yet unknown, but increased risk of heart disease, cancer, and cataracts of the eye is suspected.[22,23,26] However, in the short run, in most people such a marginal deficiency likely leads only to fatigue or other bothersome and unspecific signs and symptoms.

With rare exceptions, healthy adults do not develop the more serious B vitamin and vitamin C deficiency diseases from diet alone. The exceptions are people with alcoholism. The extremely unbalanced diets of some people with alcoholism, in combination with alcohol-induced alteration of vitamin absorption and metabolism, create significant risks for some serious nutrient deficiencies.[17] We covered this topic in detail in the Nutrition Perspective in Chapter 7.

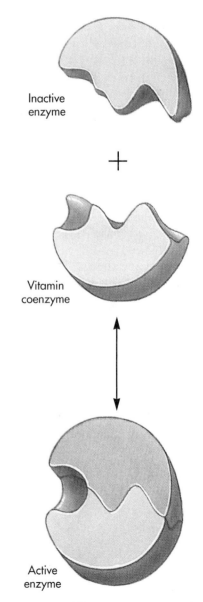

Figure 13-2 The enzyme-coenzyme interaction. The B vitamins form coenzymes, which are compounds that enable specific enzymes to function.

NUTRITION FOCUS

PRESERVING VITAMINS IN FOOD

Substantial amounts of vitamins can be lost from the time a fruit or vegetable is harvested until it is eaten. The water-soluble vitamins, particularly thiamin, vitamin C, and folate, can be destroyed with improper storage and overcooking. Heat, light, exposure to air, cooking in large amounts of water, and alkalinity are all factors that can destroy vitamins. The fresher the food, the less chance of nutrient loss.

In general, if a food is not to be eaten within a few days, freezing is the best method to retain nutrients. In fact, frozen vegetables and fruits are often better than supermarket "fresh" because frozen foods are generally processed immediately after harvesting. As part of the freezing process, vegetables first are quickly blanched in boiling water to destroy enzymes that would otherwise degrade the vitamins. "Fresh" foods often linger in the grocery store or at home for a matter of days or weeks before being eaten.

Below are some tips to aid in preserving the vitamins in food:

- Keep fruits and vegetables cool. Enzymes in foods begin to destroy vitamins once the fruit or vegetable is picked. Chilling reduces this process, so refrigerate these foods until they are consumed.
- Refrigerate foods in moisture-proof containers. Nutrients keep best at temperatures near freezing, at high humidity, and away from exposure to air.
- Avoid trimming and cutting fruits and vegetables into small pieces whenever possible. The greater the surface area, the more vitamin destruction by oxygen.
- Use the outer leaves of lettuce and other greens because these are higher in vitamins and minerals than the inner, tender leaves or stems. The skins of potatoes, apples, and carrots are also higher in vitamins and minerals than the center part.
- Cook vegetables by microwaving, steaming, or using a pan or wok with very small amounts of water or fat and a tight-fitting lid. The less contact with water and the shorter the cooking time, the more nutrients retained. Whenever possible, cook fruits or vegetables in their skins.
- Avoid reheating food, which reduces vitamin content.
- Don't add baking soda to water when cooking vegetables to enhance the green color. The alkalinity destroys vitamin C, thiamin, and other vitamins.
- Store canned foods in a cool place. To get maximum nutritive value from canned foods, serve any liquid packed with the food whenever possible. Canned foods vary in nutrients lost, largely because of differences in storage time and canning processes.
- Keep milk cold, covered, and away from strong light. Riboflavin is lost when exposed to ultraviolet light. Note, however, that pasteurization of raw milk does not destroy the main nutrients in milk products—protein, riboflavin, and calcium, among others.

Microwave cooking provides many advantages as far as preserving nutrients during cooking. When cooking vegetables in a microwave, little water is needed, in turn decreasing the amount of vitamins that can be lost into the surrounding fluid. Also, microwave cooking exposes food to heat for a shorter period than does a conventional oven or stove.

In the milling of grains, the seeds are crushed and the germ, bran, and husk layers are removed. This process leaves just the starch-containing endosperm, which is used to make flour, bread, and cereal products. Since the discarded fractions are rich in many nutrients, the time-honored milling process leads to loss of vitamins and minerals. In order to counteract this nutrient loss, bread and cereal products made from milled grains are enriched with three B vitamins—thiamin, riboflavin, and niacin—and with the mineral iron. This fortification, begun in the 1940s in the United States, has helped to protect Americans from the common deficiency diseases associated with a dietary lack of the added nutrients, but still leaves the products with less vitamin B-6, folate, magnesium, and zinc than that present in the whole grains. This is one reason nutrition experts advocate regular consumption of whole-grain products, such as whole-wheat bread, rather than just consuming enriched grain products.

Thiamin

The thiamin-deficiency disease **beriberi** is traditionally found among those populations in which polished (refined white) rice is a dietary staple. Brown rice, which has its bran and germ layers intact, is a good source of thiamin. White rice, with its bran and germ layers removed, is almost devoid of thiamin. Since thiamin is replaced during the enrichment process of rice and other grains in the U.S., as we just mentioned, beriberi is rarely diagnosed here.

The thiamin molecule consists of a central carbon atom to which is attached a six-member nitrogen-containing ring and a five-member sulfur-containing ring.[13] The name comes from *thio,* meaning "sulfur", and *amine,* referring to the nitrogen groups in the molecule. In modern spelling, the "e" is dropped from the word.

The chemical bond between each ring and the central carbon atom in thiamin is easily broken by prolonged exposure to heat (overcooked foods), thus destroying the function of the vitamin. This is also true if food is cooked in alkaline solutions (pH > 8.0). Sometimes baking soda is added to the water in which fresh green beans are cooked to retain their bright green color. This practice is not recommended.

beriberi The thiamin-deficiency disorder characterized by muscle weakness, loss of appetite, nerve degeneration, and sometimes edema.

Thiamin

Thiamin (red asterisk) has two phosphate groups added here to form the coenzyme thiamin pyrophosphate (TPP).

FUNCTIONS OF THIAMIN

Thiamin, like all other B vitamins, is biologically active in its coenzyme form as a functional part of an enzyme. Thiamin pyrophosphate (TPP) is the actual coenzyme form (Figure 13-3). A key type of reaction in which TPP participates is called a **decarboxylation** reaction, as a carboxyl group ($-\overset{\overset{\text{O}}{\|}}{\text{C}}-\text{OH}$) is removed from the substrate and released as carbon dioxide (CO_2).[13] An example is the conversion of pyruvate to acetyl-CoA during carbohydrate metabolism. The three-carbon pyruvate is decarboxylated, forming the two-carbon acetate molecule for entry into the citric acid cycle:

$$\text{pyruvate} \xrightarrow[]{\text{thiamin as TPP} \quad \text{CoA}} \text{acetyl-CoA}$$
$$CO_2$$

This conversion of pyruvate to acetyl-CoA is critical if aerobic metabolism of glucose is to be sustained (Figure 13-3). For a while, the body can bypass this reaction by using mostly fatty acids for fuel. But eventually the body will experience ill health if this metabolism of pyruvate cannot occur.

TPP also plays an active yet poorly understood role in nerve function. It is thought that TPP aids in the synthesis of neurotransmitters (such as acetylcholine), aids in the energy production needed by the highly active nerve tissue, and regulates nerve-impulse transmission.

Some cells possess an alternative metabolic pathway for carbohydrate, the hexose monophosphate shunt, which also requires TPP.[13] This pathway allows cells to make the five-carbon monosaccharides deoxyribose and ribose for DNA and RNA synthesis, respectively. In addition, TPP participates in reactions in which carbon dioxide is removed from some amino acids. Although thiamin functions in a variety of cellular metabolic pathways, its most important role is its link with carbohydrate metabolism.

Enzyme activities in red blood cells that require vitamins to function can be used to test vitamin status. The tests are categorized as functional or biochemical tests. Enzyme tests are available for thiamin (transketolase), riboflavin (glutathione reductase), and vitamin B-6 (aminotransferase) status.

THIAMIN-DEFICIENCY DISEASES

The classic thiamin-deficiency disease, called beriberi, has afflicted rice-eating populations for centuries. If little besides polished rice is eaten for weeks at a time, the disease develops.

Beriberi

In the Sinhalese language, which is spoken by inhabitants of Sri Lanka (Ceylon), the word beriberi means "I can't, I can't." This is because a thiamin deficiency affects the cardiovascular, muscular, nervous, and gastrointestinal systems. The signs and

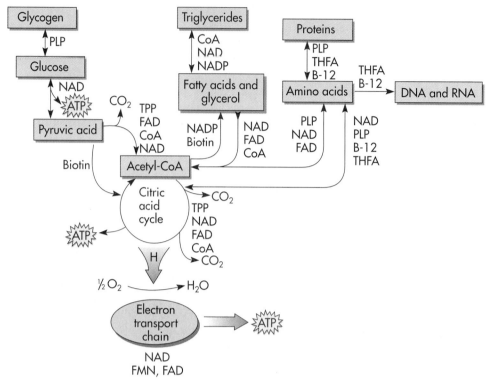

Figure 13-3 Many metabolic pathways, including those involved in energy metabolism, use coenzyme forms of the B vitamins: thiamin as TPP; riboflavin as FAD and FMN; niacin as NAD and NADP; pantothenic acid as CoA; and folate as THFA. Other, minor pathways associated with energy metabolism also exist but are not depicted.

symptoms of "dry" beriberi include weakness, nerve degeneration, irritability, loss of nerve transmission resulting in nervous tingling throughout the body, poor arm and leg coordination, and deep pain in the calf muscles. A person with "wet" beriberi often develops an enlarged heart, heart failure, and severe edema.

Bodily functions associated with brain and nervous action are often quick to show signs of a thiamin deficiency. This is because brain and nerve cells primarily use glucose for energy, converting pyruvate into acetyl-CoA and then pushing the acetyl-CoA through the citric acid cycle to eventually obtain ATP. The coenzyme TPP participates in these metabolic pathways. Nerve tissues are highly active and place great demands on pyruvate metabolism and the citric acid cycle to provide the energy they require.

Psychological disturbances, such as irritability, headache, fatigue, depression, and weakness, can be seen after only 10 days on a thiamin-free diet. This shows how minimally the human body retains thiamin. Thus it is best to consume ample thiamin from foods every day. Although the signs and symptoms of beriberi are due to a thiamin deficiency, they also often occur along with other B vitamin deficiencies. This association is found because different B vitamins are often present in the same foods, so a dietary deficiency of one B vitamin may mean that other B vitamins are deficient as well.[25]

Wernicke-Korsakoff Syndrome

Another thiamin-deficiency disease found mainly among people with alcoholism is called the Wernicke-Korsakoff syndrome. It is characterized by constant involuntary movement of the eyeball, paralysis of the eye muscle, staggering, and mental confusion. This is the picture you might imagine of a person in an uncontrollable drunken stupor, who obtains food energy primarily from alcohol and is simultaneously thiamin deficient.

When physicians see a person suffering from unexplained delirium in the emergency room, they must consider whether it may be caused by a thiamin deficiency related to alcoholism. The treatment is an injection of thiamin. Dietary supplementation will not suffice because thiamin is absorbed slowly, especially in a person with alcoholism.

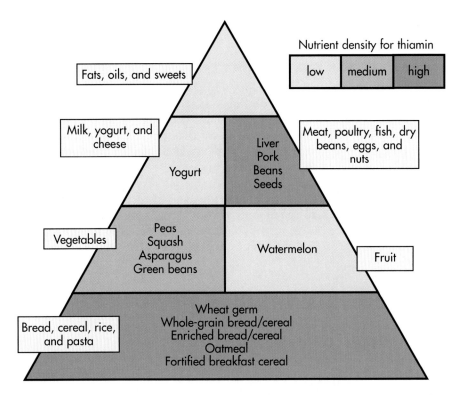

Figure 13-4 Food sources of thiamin from the Food Guide Pyramid. The meat, poultry, fish, dry beans, eggs, and nuts group and the breads, cereals, rice, and pasta group are especially good sources of this nutrient. The background color of each food group indicates the average nutrient density for thiamin in that group.

THIAMIN IN FOODS

Thiamin is found in a wide variety of foods, although generally in low amounts. Major individual contributors of thiamin to our diets are white bread and rolls, crackers, pork, hot dogs, luncheon meat, cold cereals, and orange juice. White bread, bakery products, and cereals are usually enriched with thiamin. They serve as important sources because people eat them so often.

Foods with a very high nutrient density for thiamin (mg/kcal) are pork products, sunflower seeds, legumes, wheat germ, and watermelon. Whole grains and enriched grains, green beans, asparagus, organ meats such as liver, peanuts and other seeds, and mushrooms also are good sources. However, aside from yeast and pork products, there is really no one especially nutrient-dense source of thiamin.

Many foods—especially meat, milk and milk products, seafood, and most fruits—contain very little thiamin. Eating a variety of foods in line with the Food Guide Pyramid pattern is the most reliable way to obtain sufficient thiamin from a diet (Figure 13-4). Some fish and shellfish contain an enzyme called thiaminase, which destroys thiamin. Fortunately, cooking destroys the thiaminase.

RDA FOR THIAMIN

The RDA for thiamin for adults is approximately 1.5 mg/day for men and 1.1 mg/day for women. (Throughout the rest of this chapter, refer to the inside cover for vitamin recommendations for other age groups and to Appendix E for Canadian recommendations.) The RDA is also expressed in terms of energy intake: 0.5 mg of thiamin per 1000 kcal, but no less than 1 mg/day even if a person is on a low-energy diet.

Average daily intakes for men and women—1.9 and 1.4 mg, respectively—exceed the RDA values.[1] Surplus dietary thiamin is rapidly excreted in the urine by the

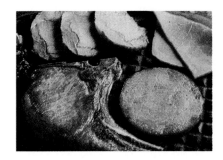

Pork is a good source of thiamin.

action of the kidneys, so there is no danger from excessive intake by the use of supplements.

AMERICANS AT RISK FOR THIAMIN DEFICIENCY

Some groups of people, such as the poor and elderly, may barely meet their needs for thiamin. A diet dominated by highly processed and unenriched foods, sugar, fat, and alcohol creates the potential for a thiamin deficiency.

People with alcoholism are at great risk for thiamin deficiency because absorption and use of thiamin are profoundly diminished by alcohol consumption. Furthermore, the low-quality diet that often accompanies severe alcoholism makes matters worse. Since there is limited thiamin storage in the body, an alcoholic binge lasting 1 to 2 weeks may quickly deplete already diminished amounts of the vitamin.

Hyperemesis gravidarum (commonly known as morning sickness) can lead to thiamin deficiency. Pregnant women who in the first trimester of pregnancy experience intense vomiting for more than 9 weeks or so deserve close scrutiny for thiamin status.

Riboflavin

A deficiency disease associated with an isolated lack of dietary riboflavin is rarely seen. Because riboflavin functions along with other B vitamins (e.g., vitamin B-6, niacin, thiamin, and folate) in numerous metabolic pathways, some symptoms ascribed to riboflavin deficiency are actually caused by failure of metabolic pathways associated with a lack of other nutrients. And as already noted, this assortment of B vitamins, such as riboflavin, thiamin, and niacin, is often found in the same foods.

The riboflavin molecule contains three linked six-membered rings with a ribitol (sugar alcohol) attached to the middle ring. The name comes from its yellow color (*flavin* means "yellow" in Latin). Riboflavin readily gains and loses electrons, so riboflavin exists in oxidized and reduced forms. Riboflavin is a component of two coenzymes: flavin mononucleotide (FMN) and flavin adenine dinucleotide (FAD).[13] The coenzyme forms are present in many foods; the free vitamin is found in milk and enriched grain products. All these forms can be used to meet the body's needs for riboflavin.

FUNCTIONS OF RIBOFLAVIN

FMN and FAD participate in many oxidation-reduction reactions in a variety of metabolic pathways (see Appendix B for a review of oxidation and reduction reactions). In both the citric acid cycle and the beta-oxidation pathway for catabolizing fatty acids, FAD accepts hydrogens (electrons), forming the reduced form, $FADH_2$. For example, FAD participates to allow succinate to be converted to fumarate in the citric acid cycle:

$$\text{succinate} \xrightarrow{\quad FAD \quad\quad FADH_2 \quad} \text{fumarate}$$

$FADH_2$ later donates the hydrogens to other acceptor molecules in the mitochondrial electron-transport chain. The other riboflavin coenzyme also functions in the electron-transport chain, shuttling between its oxidized form, FMN, and reduced form, $FMNH_2$. In all these examples, the coenzymes act first as electron and hydrogen ion acceptors and then as electron and hydrogen ion donors. When cells produce ATP by metabolizing glucose via aerobic pathways or by breaking down fatty acids, the riboflavin coenzymes play an indispensable role. Some vitamin and mineral metabolism also requires riboflavin. In addition, because of its link to glutathione peroxidase activity, riboflavin is suspected of having an antioxidant role in the body.[21]

RIBOFLAVIN DEFICIENCY

The signs and symptoms associated with a pure riboflavin deficiency (technically called **ariboflavinosis**) include inflammation of the tongue (glossitis), cracking of

CRITICAL THINKING

Gary has alcoholism and pays no attention to his diet. In addition to the detrimental effects on the liver, excess alcohol consumption can cause deficiencies in certain B vitamins. Explain why this can occur.

Riboflavin (oxidized)

Riboflavin (reduced)

For riboflavin, the italicized R denotes H in the free vitamin; phosphate in FMN; and an adenine dinucleotide in FAD. In the reduced form of riboflavin, the hydrogens are shown in red.

tissue around the corners of the mouth (cheilosis), seborrheic dermatitis (disease of the sebaceous glands of the skin), inflammation of the mouth (stomatitis) and throat, various eye and nervous system disorders, and confusion (Figure 13-5). The first evidence of a deficiency is inflammation of the mouth and tongue. The complete picture of a deficiency develops after approximately 2 months on a riboflavin-deficient diet (consuming one fourth of the RDA).

RIBOFLAVIN IN FOODS

One quarter of the riboflavin in our diets comes from milk and milk products. The milk, yogurt, and cheese group of the Food Guide Pyramid is the major contributor of riboflavin to the diet (Figure 13-6). Including dairy products in the diet is a good method for meeting riboflavin needs. The rest of riboflavin intake typically comes from enriched white bread, rolls, and crackers, as well as eggs and meats. Some people who consume minimal amounts of dairy products obtain considerable riboflavin from the liberal amounts of meat eaten.

The most nutrient-dense sources of riboflavin (mg/kcal) are liver, mushrooms, spinach and other green leafy vegetables, broccoli, asparagus, low-fat and nonfat milk, and cottage cheese.

Exposure to light (ultraviolet radiation) causes riboflavin to break down rapidly. To prevent this light-induced breakdown, paper and plastic cartons—not glass—are used in packaging riboflavin-rich foods, such as milk, milk products, and cereals.

RDA FOR RIBOFLAVIN

The RDA for riboflavin for adults is 1.4 to 1.7 mg/day for men and 1.2 to 1.3 mg/day for women. The RDA is based on 0.6 mg riboflavin per 1000 kcal intake, with a minimum of 1.2 mg/day. On average, daily intakes of riboflavin are slightly above the RDA: 2.3 mg and 1.7 mg for men and women, respectively.[1] Athletes at the outset of a training program may need extra riboflavin (about 1.5 times the

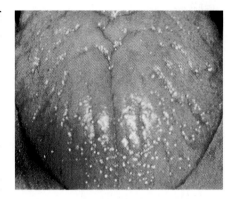

Figure 13-5 A painful, inflamed tongue (glossitis) can signal a deficiency of niacin, vitamin B-6, riboflavin, folate, or vitamin B-12. Often more than one deficiency is the cause. Since other medical conditions can also cause glossitis, further evaluation is needed before a nutrient deficiency can be diagnosed.

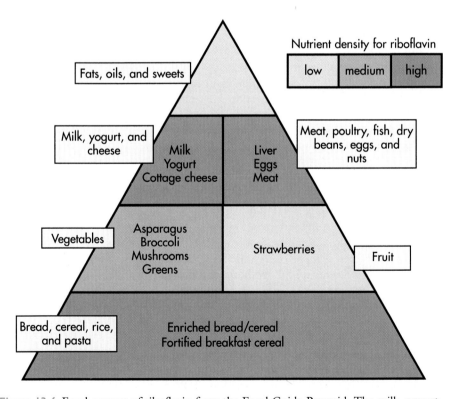

Figure 13-6 Food sources of riboflavin from the Food Guide Pyramid. The milk, yogurt, and cheese group and the meat, poultry, fish, dry beans, eggs, and nuts group are especially rich sources of this nutrient. The background color of each food group indicates the average nutrient density for riboflavin in that group.

The two coenzyme forms of niacin, NAD and NADP, contain nicotinamide linked to adenine dinucleotide or adenine dinucleotide phosphate, indicated by the italicized R. Both coenzymes undergo oxidation and reduction by loss or addition of an electron and a hydrogen (red).

Niacin status can be determined by measuring the amount of its breakdown product, N-methyl nicotinamide, in the urine. Low amounts suggest deficient status.

pellagra The niacin-deficiency disease characterized by inflammation of the skin, diarrhea, and eventual mental incapacity.

RDA), partly because of their increased use of fatty acids as fuel and of all the energy-yielding pathways. As we saw earlier, the riboflavin coenzymes are crucial to the operation of these pathways. The higher energy intakes typical of athletes should easily meet any additional riboflavin needs. There are no specific signs or symptoms that indicate riboflavin taken in megadoses causes toxicity.

AMERICANS AT RISK FOR RIBOFLAVIN DEFICIENCY

Although riboflavin deficiencies are rare, some people consume amounts that are barely adequate. Marginal intakes are most likely seen in those who do not consume milk or milk products. Such people would be wise to search for another plentiful dietary source of riboflavin, such as enriched breads and breakfast cereals. People with alcoholism risk a riboflavin deficiency because they often eat a very nutrient-deficient diet. Long-term use of phenobarbital may also compromise riboflavin status, as this drug leads to metabolic changes in the liver that increase breakdown of the vitamin.

Niacin

Signs and symptoms associated with **pellagra**—the niacin-deficiency disease—include inflammation of the skin after exposure to sunshine, diarrhea, dementia, and hallucinations. This pattern of disease has been described in humans since the fourteenth century.

The vitamin niacin actually exists in two forms—nicotinic acid (niacin) and nicotinamide (niacinamide). The molecule consists of a six-membered ring linked to a carboxyl group or amide group ($-\overset{O}{\overset{||}{C}}-NH_2$). In the body, both forms of the vitamin perform the functions attributed to niacin. The two coenzyme forms of niacin are nicotinamide adenine dinucleotide (NAD) and nicotinamide adenine dinucleotide phosphate (NADP).[13]

FUNCTIONS OF NIACIN

Like the coenzyme forms of riboflavin, the coenzyme forms of niacin, NAD and NADP, are active participants in oxidation-reduction reactions. The niacin coenzymes function in at least 200 different reactions in cellular metabolic pathways, especially those used to produce ATP. NAD participates in catabolic reactions, acting as an electron and hydrogen acceptor in glycolysis (conversion of glucose to pyruvate) and in the citric acid cycle. Under anaerobic conditions, the resulting reduced form, NADH, is used in converting pyruvate to lactate, thereby regenerating NAD:

$$NADH + H^+ \quad NAD$$

pyruvate - → lactate

Under aerobic conditions, NADH donates an electron and hydrogen to other acceptor molecules in the mitochondrial electron-transport chain.[13]

Synthetic pathways in the cell—those that make new compounds—often use NADPH, the reduced form of NADP. This coenzyme is important in the biochemical pathway for fatty acid synthesis. Cells that synthesize a lot of fatty acids (e.g., those in the liver and female mammary glands) have higher concentrations of NADPH than cells not involved in fatty acid synthesis (e.g., muscle cells).[13]

PELLAGRA

The first official record of the disease pellagra was made by the Spanish physician Casal in 1735. It was named *mal de la rosa*, or "red sickness." The typical redness appearing around the neck is today called "Casal's necklace." Later the disease was renamed *pellagra* (from Italian *pelle,* meaning "skin", and *agra,* meaning "rough").

Since almost every metabolic pathway uses either NAD or NADP, it is not surprising that a niacin deficiency causes widespread damage in the body. The effects of pellagra are known as the three "D's"—dementia, diarrhea, and dermatitis

(Figure 13-7). If the disease is not successfully treated, death (the fourth D) follows. Clinical evidence of pellagra develops in 50 to 60 days after instituting a niacin-deficient diet. Early symptoms include diminished appetite, weight loss, and weakness.

Pellagra is the only dietary deficiency disease ever to reach epidemic proportions in the United States. During the early 1900s, the incidence of pellagra increased dramatically in the southeastern region of the country, where corn—a poor source of naturally available niacin—was being increasingly used as a primary component of the diet. Over 10,000 Americans died of pellagra in 1915. From the end of World War I until the end of World War II, an estimated 200,000 Americans suffered from the disease. Many had such severe dementia they were forced to live out their lives in mental institutions.

Two discoveries were crucial to breaking the epidemic: in the 1920s, high-protein diets were found to prevent pellagra, and in the 1930s, insufficient niacin intake was shown to cause the disease. The introduction of niacin-enriched grains in 1941 and improved intake of dietary protein resulting from wartime prosperity led to the rapid disappearance of pellagra in the United States. The ability of high-protein diets to cure pellagra was finally explained in 1948, when researchers demonstrated that the amino acid tryptophan was converted into niacin in the body.[13] Pellagra is still found today throughout Southeast Asia and Africa among populations whose diets lack sufficient protein and niacin.

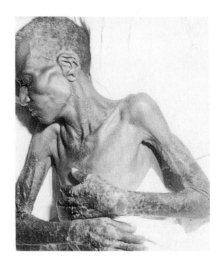

Figure 13-7 The dermatitis of pellagra. Dermatitis on both sides of the body (bilateral) is a typical symptom of pellagra. Sun exposure worsens the condition.

NIACIN IN FOODS

Most niacin in our diets comes from enriched white bread, rolls, crackers, and breakfast cereals. In the United States, these products are made from grains that have been fortified with niacin. Beef, chicken, and turkey also supply considerable niacin to typical American diets (Figure 13-8). Coffee and tea contribute a little

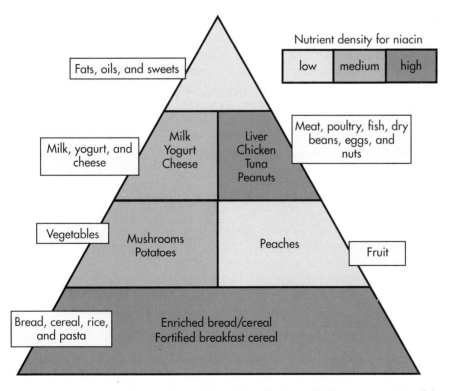

Figure 13-8 Food sources of niacin from the Food Guide Pyramid. The meat, poultry, fish, dry beans, eggs, and nuts group and the bread, cereal, rice, and pasta group are especially rich sources of this nutrient. The background color of each food group indicates the average nutrient density for niacin in that group. Some niacin is also supplied by synthesis of tryptophan within the body. Thus protein foods like milk yield niacin indirectly for the body.

niacin to some people's diets. Unlike some other water-soluble vitamins, niacin is very heat stable, and little is lost in cooking. The most nutrient-dense sources of niacin (mg/kcal) are mushrooms, wheat bran, tuna (as well as other fish), chicken and turkey, asparagus, and peanuts.

Besides the preformed niacin found in protein foods, each 60 mg of excess dietary tryptophan (leftover after protein synthesis) may be converted within the body to yield approximately 1 mg of niacin. This conversion requires participation of riboflavin and vitamin B-6 coenzymes. The number of milligrams of niacin supplied by dietary protein can be estimated by dividing the excess dietary protein intake (in grams) by 6. For example, if you consume 30 g of extra protein, your body will synthesize about 5 mg of niacin.

For most people, about half of niacin needs are supplied by the body's synthesis of niacin from tryptophan. Animal proteins (except gelatin) are especially rich in tryptophan. Since food composition tables list only preformed niacin, they underestimate the total niacin supplied by protein foods. For example, although eggs and milk lack niacin, they contain abundant tryptophan and thus indirectly contribute substantial amounts of niacin.

Considering the link between corn as a staple food and pellagra, you might be surprised to learn that the niacin content of corn is similar to that of rice and considerably higher than that of most other vegetables. However, the niacin in corn is marginally absorbed because it is tightly bound by a protein. Soaking corn in an alkaline solution such as lime water (calcium hydroxide dissolved in water) releases bound niacin, rendering it more usable by the body. Look for evidence of this form of processing on the label when you buy corn-meal products, such as tortillas. Because this practice was common among the native Indians of the American continent, they did not suffer from pellagra. Early Spanish explorers of the New World brought corn—a crop native to the Americas—back to Europe, but they were unaware of the importance of soaking corn in lime water. Thus as the use of corn as a staple spread in Europe, pellagra became widespread during the 1700s. In contrast, Spanish settlers in Latin America learned from the native Indians to soak corn meal in lime water before using it in cooking. The Hispanic populations descended from these settlers continued this practice and rarely suffered from pellagra, while other Americans who used untreated corn as a staple, often did. Currently, agricultural scientists are attempting to develop new strains of corn with improved tryptophan and niacin content.

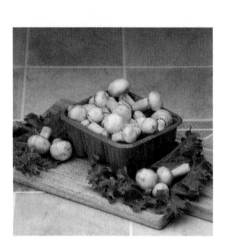

Mushrooms are a nutrient-dense source of niacin.

RDA FOR NIACIN

The RDA for niacin is expressed as niacin equivalents (NE) to account for niacin received preformed from the diet, as well as that synthesized from tryptophan. The RDA is based on 6.6 NE/1000 kcal in the diet, but not less than 13 NE/day for adults. For adult men, the RDA is 15 to 19 NE/day, and for adult women it is 13 to 15 NE/day.

Average daily intakes of niacin are 26 mg and 18 mg for men and women, respectively.[1] As long as one follows a varied diet, developing a niacin deficiency is highly unlikely. Aside from people with rare disorders of tryptophan metabolism, people with alcoholism are generally the only population group to show niacin deficiency, primarily because of an inadequate intake of foods rich in niacin.

MEDICAL USES AND TOXICITY OF NIACIN

In 1955 it was discovered that very large doses of nicotinic acid reduced serum cholesterol. Consuming 1.5 to 3 g of nicotinic acid per day—about 75 to 150 times the RDA—can decrease LDL and increase HDL. Unfortunately, niacin taken at this dosage may have serious side effects, including flushing of the skin, itching, nausea, and liver damage. Some people experience these symptoms at dosages as low as 250 mg/day. Because of the potential for side effects, nicotinic acid therapy must be supervised by a physician. Use of slow-release forms of nicotinic acid can lessen the side effects, or other medications can be prescribed to counteract the side effects.

CONCEPT CHECK

The B vitamins thiamin, niacin, and riboflavin function in various biochemical pathways used for the metabolism of glucose, amino acids, and fatty acids. Enriched grains are adequate sources of all three vitamins. Otherwise, pork is an excellent source of thiamin; milk is an excellent source of riboflavin; and protein foods in general are excellent sources of niacin. Deficiencies of all three vitamins can occur with alcoholism; of the three, a thiamin deficiency is the most likely. Only niacin leads to toxic effects when consumed in high doses.

Pantothenic Acid

A clinically recognized pantothenic acid–deficiency disease has not been reported in humans. However, a deficiency of this vitamin has been produced in humans by feeding them a semisynthetic diet devoid of pantothenic acid or by administering a pantothenic acid antagonist. Symptoms appear only after at least 9 weeks and include listlessness, fatigue, headache, sleep disturbances, nausea, tingling sensations in the hands, and abdominal distress.

A full-blown dietary deficiency of pantothenic acid may have occurred in World War II prisoners of war. Some prisoners in the Philippines and in Japan displayed a "burning foot" syndrome described as numbness and tingling in the toes and burning and shooting pains in the feet, in addition to other mental and neurological symptoms. The victims responded favorably to a preparation of pantothenic acid, but to no other B vitamin.

FUNCTIONS OF PANTOTHENIC ACID

Pantothenic acid is the essential component of coenzyme A (CoA). This coenzyme is formed when the vitamin combines with a derivative of ADP and the amino acid cysteine. Cysteine provides the sulfur atom, which is the "business end" of the coenzyme.[13]

Coenzyme A is essential for the production of ATP from the metabolism of carbohydrate, protein, and fat. The formation of acetyl-CoA allows the two-carbon acetate to enter the citric acid cycle by condensing with the four-carbon oxaloacetate to produce the six-carbon citrate. In another series of reactions acetyl-CoA condenses with carbon dioxide to begin synthesis of fatty acids:

$$CO_2$$

acetyl-CoA - - - - - - - - → malonyl-CoA - - → - - - → fatty acid

2 carbons   3 carbons

Pantothenic acid also forms part of a compound called the *acyl carrier protein*.[13] This protein attaches to fatty acids and shuttles them through the pathway designed to increase their chain length. Finally, pantothenic acid as coenzyme A also donates fatty acids to proteins in a process that can determine their location and function within a cell.

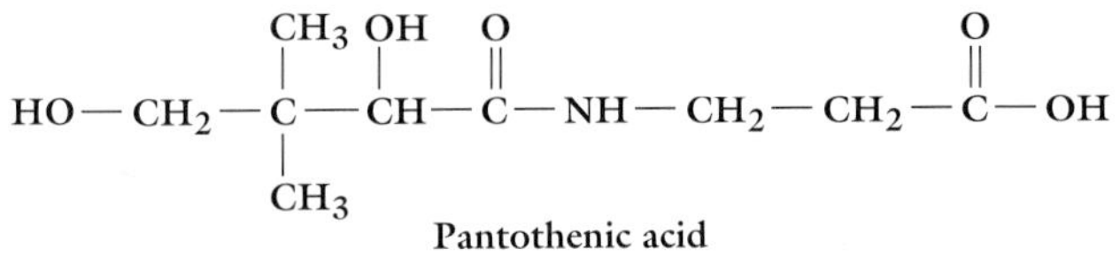

Pantothenic acid

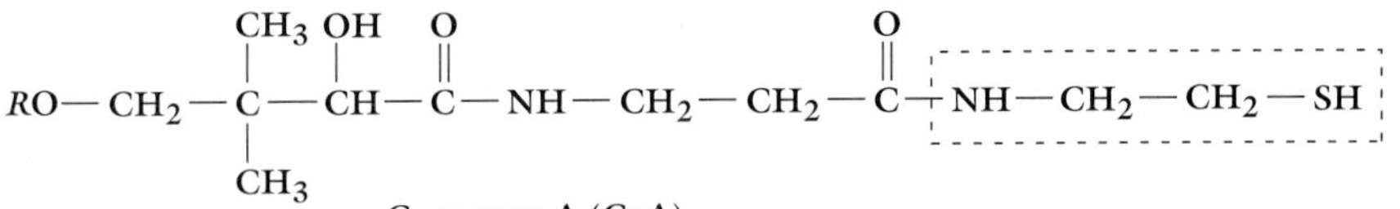

Coenzyme A (CoA)

Pantothenic acid is converted to coenzyme A by combining with a part of the amino acid cysteine (box) and with a derivative of adenosine diphosphate (ADP), indicated by the italicized R.

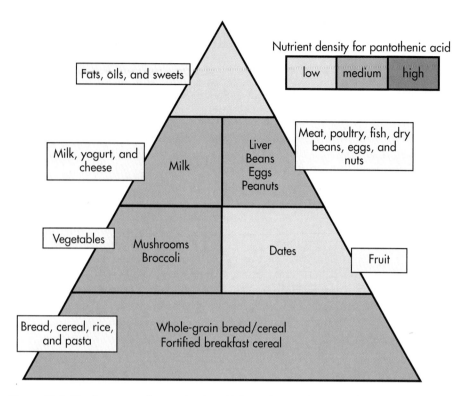

Figure 13-9 Food sources of pantothenic acid from the Food Guide Pyramid. No group includes especially rich sources of this nutrient. Pantothenic acid is scattered among the various foods we eat. The background color of each food group indicates the average nutrient density for pantothenic acid in that group.

PANTOTHENIC ACID IN FOODS

The Greek word *pantothen*, meaning "from every side," reflects the ample supply of pantothenic acid in foods (Figure 13-9). Common sources include meat, milk, and many vegetables.

Nutrient-dense sources of pantothenic acid (mg/kcal) are mushrooms, liver, peanuts, and eggs. Because pantothenic acid is not added to enriched grains, these products are not especially good sources of the vitamin.

ESADDI FOR PANTOTHENIC ACID

For adults, the estimated safe and adequate daily dietary intake (ESADDI) for pantothenic acid is 4 to 7 mg/day. Recall that an ESADDI is a range of acceptable intakes established by the Food and Nutrition Board for nutrients for which insufficient data are available to set RDAs (see Chapter 2). Current intakes of pantothenic acid by adults average about 6 mg/day.

A deficiency of pantothenic acid might occur in cases of alcoholism in which a very nutrient-deficient diet is consumed. However, the effects would probably be hidden among deficiencies of thiamin, riboflavin, vitamin B-6, and folate, so the pantothenic acid deficiency might go unrecognized. There is no known toxicity for pantothenic acid.

Biotin

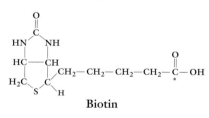

The vitamin biotin attaches to a protein by formation of a bond between its carboxyl group (red asterisk) and lysine in a protein, yielding the bound coenzyme form called biocytin.

Biotin is commonly found in two forms in foods: the free vitamin and the protein-bound coenzyme form, called biocytin. In the formation of biocytin, the carboxyl group of biotin forms a bond with the amino acid lysine in a protein.[13] Biotin is absorbed from the small intestine, whereas the biocytin form is not. The enzyme biotinidase, which is present in the small intestine, cleaves the bond linking biotin to a protein, releasing the free vitamin.

About 1 in 60,000 infants is born with a genetic defect that leaves them with very low amounts of biotinidase. Because these infants cannot break down biocytin to the absorbable free form, a biotin deficiency is likely to develop. If a deficiency is suspected, the infant is treated with 50 to 200 times the ESADDI for biotin.

FUNCTIONS OF BIOTIN

Biotin in its coenzyme form participates in numerous reactions involved in the metabolism of fat and carbohydrate.[13] It also participates in the entry of certain carbon skeletons from amino acids into the energy-yielding pathways, as well as in DNA synthesis.

The primary type of reaction catalyzed by biotin-containing enzymes involves addition of carbon dioxide to a substrate. An important example of such **carboxylation** reactions is the addition of carbon dioxide to the three-carbon pyruvate, yielding the four-carbon oxaloacetate:

$$CO_2$$

pyruvate - - - - - - - - → oxaloacetate - - - → - - - → glucose
3 carbons   4 carbons

This reaction, which occurs mainly in the liver, is an initial step in gluconeogenesis.

Biotin also aids in metabolism of the three-carbon fatty acids so that they can enter the citric acid cycle.[13] In addition, biotin-dependent enzymes are critical in preventing the depletion of key compounds of the citric acid cycle, such as oxaloacetate, as outlined above (see Chapter 7 for details). Without biotin, these compounds may not be sufficiently replenished, so the citric acid cycle could not run effectively. As a result, lactate (the anaerobic by-product of glycolysis) in the blood would rise, as aerobic glucose metabolism is slowed. It is postulated that increased lactate concentration within the central nervous system is the basis for the neurological disorders—depression, lethargy, hallucinations, and numbness of the extremities—that accompany a severe biotin deficiency.

Finally, the major regulatory enzyme in lipid synthesis contains biotin.[13] A person with a biotin deficiency shows signs similar to those of a person with an essential fatty acid deficiency—scaly inflammation of the skin and hair loss.

BIOTIN IN FOODS

The most nutrient-dense sources of biotin (μg/kcal) are cauliflower, egg yolks, liver, peanuts, and cheese. Most vegetables, fruits, and meats are generally deficient sources (Figure 13-10).

It is likely that intestinal synthesis of biotin by bacteria supplies at least part of our needs, as evidenced by the rather rare incidence of biotin deficiency. In fact, we excrete more biotin than we consume. However, questions remain about the actual bioavailability of the biotin synthesized by the intestinal flora, since this production takes place mostly in the large intestine, whereas biotin is most efficiently absorbed from the small intestine.

A protein called **avidin** in raw egg whites binds biotin and inhibits its absorption. Feeding many raw egg whites to animals leads to the classic "egg-white injury" deficiency disease. An occasional raw egg in eggnog is of no concern for this problem because it would take a regular daily consumption of 12 to 24 raw eggs to produce a biotin deficiency. Biotin deficiency resulting from consuming raw eggs has been reported, however, in people with alcoholism who eat as few as three raw eggs a day. These people probably existed on very deficient diets. The main concern about eating raw eggs for healthy people is the risk of food-borne illness caused by *Salmonella* bacteria, which may contaminate eggs (see Chapter 19).

avidin A protein found in raw egg whites that can bind biotin and inhibit absorption; cooking destroys avidin.

ESADDI FOR BIOTIN

The ESADDI for biotin is 30 to 100 μg/day for adults. Our food supply is thought to provide 100 to 300 μg/person/day. Biotin is relatively nontoxic. Large doses

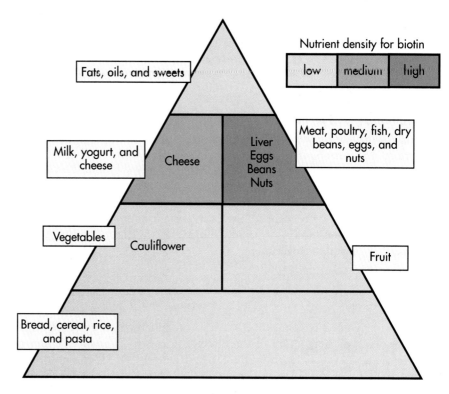

Figure 13-10 Food sources of biotin from the Food Guide Pyramid. The meat, poultry, fish, dry beans, eggs, and nuts group is a good source of this nutrient. The background color of each food group indicates the average nutrient density for biotin in that group. Some biotin for body use also arises from bacterial synthesis within the intestines.

have been given over an extended period of time to children without harmful side effects.

AMERICANS AT RISK FOR BIOTIN DEFICIENCY

If undetected, a lack of biotinidase leads to a severe biotin deficiency in infants. Signs and symptoms may appear within a few months of life, beginning with a skin rash and hair loss. Biotin-deficient individuals eventually develop convulsions and other neurological disorders, and infants and children experience impaired growth.

People on long-term anticonvulsant drug therapy run the risk of a biotin deficiency. Several of these drugs may directly inhibit intestinal uptake of biotin or block the action of biotinidase.

Vitamin B-6

In the early 1950s some infants fed commercial formulas in which the vitamin B-6 had been destroyed by oversterilization developed deficiency signs and symptoms, most notably convulsions and abnormal electroencephalograph (EEG) readings. The lack of sufficient vitamin B-6 remaining in these formulas likely was responsible for decreased synthesis of neurotransmitters by the infants. The problem was successfully treated with vitamin B-6. Today, formula manufacturers are much more aware of the importance of strict quality control with regard to all nutrients, including vitamin B-6.

Vitamin B-6 is actually a family of three compounds: pyridoxal, pyridoxine, and pyridoxamine. All three forms can be phosphorylated to the active vitamin B-6 coenzymes, the primary one being pyridoxal phosphate (PLP).[13] The generic name for the vitamin is B-6.

Vitamin B-6
(represented by pyridoxal)

Pyridoxal, one form of vitamin B-6, is converted to an active coenzyme—pyridoxal phosphate (PLP)—by addition of a phosphate group to the hydroxyl group, indicated by the red asterisk.

FUNCTIONS OF VITAMIN B-6

Vitamin B-6 is required for the activity of more than 100 different enzymes involved in carbohydrate, protein, and fat metabolism.

Metabolism of Amino Acids and Proteins

The most widespread function of vitamin B-6, as the coenzyme PLP, concerns metabolism of amino acids and other nitrogen-containing compounds, including transamination reactions (see Chapter 5 for a review). In *transamination* reactions, PLP aids in the transfer of an amino group from a donor amino acid to a receptor molecule, yielding the carbon skeleton of the original amino acid and a new amino acid[13]:

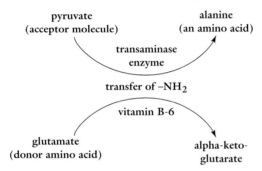

pyruvate
(acceptor molecule)

alanine
(an amino acid)

transaminase
enzyme

transfer of –NH₂

vitamin B-6

glutamate
(donor amino acid)

alpha-keto-
glutarate

If we didn't have the biochemical action of vitamin B-6, every amino acid would become "essential" (indispensable); that is, every amino acid would have to be supplied by the diet. Under normal circumstances, the human body can synthesize 11 of the 20 different amino acids needed to produce protein. None of the synthesis would be possible if vitamin B-6 were absent. Protein synthesis and overall cell metabolism is in turn impaired in a vitamin B-6 deficiency. As a facilitator of transamination reactions, vitamin B-6 is also involved in gluconeogenesis.

- - - - - - - - - - - - - - -
Vitamin B-6 status can be assessed by measuring the amount of coenzyme PLP in the blood.
- - - - - - - - - - - - - - -

Synthesis of Blood Cells

Vitamin B-6 is important for the synthesis of the hemoglobin ring structure, the oxygen-carrying part of the red blood cell.[13] The coenzyme PLP also aids in binding oxygen to hemoglobin. A **microcytic hypochromic anemia** resembling iron-deficiency anemia occurs with a vitamin B-6 deficiency (see Chapter 15). Vitamin B-6 is also necessary for the synthesis of white blood cells, major participants in the immune system.

microcytic hypochromic anemia An anemia characterized by small, pale red blood cells that lack sufficient hemoglobin and thus have reduced oxygen-carrying ability. It often is caused by an iron deficiency.

Carbohydrate Metabolism

Vitamin B-6 participates in glycogen breakdown and glucose production from amino acids (gluconeogenesis).[13]

Neurotransmitter Synthesis

The synthesis of many key neurotransmitters—serotonin, gamma-amino butyric acid (GABA), dopamine (DOPA), and norepinephrine—requires the action of vitamin B-6.[13] Because these neurotransmitters allow nerve cells to communicate with each other, a deficiency of vitamin B-6 results in neurological disorders, such as depression, headaches, confusion, and convulsions.

The link between vitamin B-6 and neurotransmitters suggested to some researchers that vitamin B-6 might be helpful in the treatment of **premenstrual syndrome (PMS).** This disorder appears in some women a few days before the menstrual period begins and is characterized by depression, irritability, anxiety, headache, bloating, and mood swings.[18] Researchers thought that increasing vitamin B-6 intake might increase the synthesis of serotonin, and in turn decrease the depression and confusion associated with premenstrual syndrome. However, vitamin B-6 has not turned out to be a reliable treatment for PMS. In addition, use of megadoses can also cause serious side effects (see the section on vitamin B-6 toxicity).

premenstrual syndrome (PMS) A disorder found in some women a few days before a menstrual period begins. It is characterized by depression, anxiety, headache, bloating, and mood swings. Severe cases are currently termed premenstrual dysphoric disorder (PDD).

Expert Opinion

Some Mysteries Surrounding Vitamin B-6

JIM LEKLEM, Ph.D.

Vitamin B-6 is one of the water-soluble micronutrients our body needs. Although it is a "micro" nutrient, this unique vitamin can be viewed as a "sleeping giant" in nutrition. Several new and some rediscovered areas of research are awakening a new view of vitamin B-6.

The water-soluble nature of this nutrient suggests that it is not retained or stored. In fact, recent studies have shown that the human body stores about 170 mg of vitamin B-6, with a majority in muscle tissue bound to glycogen phosphorylase enzyme in the active coenzyme form, pyridoxal phosphate (PLP). Because vitamin B-6 is stored, we would assume that in times of a dietary deficiency of vitamin B-6 these muscle stores are utilized. Research has shown that these stores are used in times of energy deficit. This is consistent with the role PLP plays in gluconeogenesis. In this process, PLP aids in the breakdown of certain amino acids such that their carbon skeletons are ultimately converted to glucose.

One of the areas where the interplay between energy needs and storage of vitamin B-6 may have a role is exercise. We have observed that vitamin B-6 metabolism is altered during exercise. Blood levels of PLP increase during exercise and then decrease significantly after exercise. There is also an increased excretion of the major metabolite of vitamin B-6 in trained as compared with untrained women. Similar loss of this metabolite also occurs with exercise as compared with no exercise in trained men. Based on this limited number of studies, athletes may need slightly more (5% to 7%) vitamin B-6 than persons who are sedentary.

Recent research has revealed a new and exciting role for vitamin B-6 as a possible modulator of steroid hormone action. Vitamin B-6, as PLP, interacts with steroid hormone receptor proteins in the body. As a result of this reaction of PLP with the receptors, hormone action is reduced. We must await further research to reveal to what extent the

action of these types of hormones is influenced by nutritional status of vitamin B-6 or by an excess intake of vitamin B-6, which could occur with use of vitamin B-6 supplements.

In some cases, vitamin B-6 supplements are consumed by people in an attempt to prevent certain disorders or to treat a given clinical condition. Premenstrual syndrome (PMS) and carpal tunnel syndrome, respectively, are two examples. Is vitamin B-6 effective for either of these syndromes? Of the 12 studies in which vitamin B-6 supplements have been used to treat PMS, only three found some beneficial effect. The remaining 9 studies found ambiguous or no positive effect of vitamin B-6. Until more well-controlled studies are conducted, it is not possible to conclude that vitamin B-6 supplements alleviate the symptoms of PMS.

Similarly, the benefit of using vitamin B-6 to treat carpal tunnel syndrome is open to question. This syndrome is thought to affect people whose jobs involve repetitive motion

---

Currently, a nutrition-related approach to treating PMS, whose cause is not well understood, is initially to recommend a nutrient-rich diet, especially with regard to calcium and magnesium; a decrease in alcohol, caffeine, and nicotine intake to decrease nervousness; a decrease in salt intake to decrease bloating; an increase in physical activity to stimulate relaxation; and adequate sleep.[18] If such therapy is not helpful, women with premenstrual syndrome should consult a physician, who may suggest trying various forms of antidepressant therapy. Women should definitely avoid the widely available PMS "cures" that are sold primarily in drug stores and through mail-order catalogues.

Other Important Roles

Vitamin B-6 participates in the conversion of the amino acid tryptophan to the vitamin niacin, as well as the synthesis of the amino acid methionine from homocysteine, which arises during methionine metabolism. Recall from Chapter 4 that ho-

that adversely impacts the carpal tunnel, an opening in the wrist through which tendons, nerves, and blood vessels pass. Of seven studies in which vitamin B-6 was used to treat this syndrome, five showed some modest improvement in certain symptoms. The one controlled study showed variable effect. Several of these studies were not double-blind, placebo-controlled trials; in addition, the criteria for improvement of symptoms varied among studies. Thus there is no strong evidence for a benefit of vitamin B-6, but a reduction in pain and other symptoms of carpal tunnel syndrome is possible. Because of potential toxicity, any therapy attempted must be supervised by a physician.

Vitamin B-6 supplementation has been suggested for prevention of coronary heart disease (CHD). Research in this area has centered on the effects of vitamin B-6 on cholesterol and lipid concentrations in the blood. Again no beneficial effect has been observed. The etiology (factors contributing to the disease) of CHD

is complex. A new player on the field is homocysteine, which is made in the body from the amino acid methionine. High blood concentrations of homocysteine are associated with an increased risk for CHD. Both vitamin B-6 alone and a combination of vitamin B-6, vitamin B-12, and folate have been found to reduce blood homocysteine. Whether such vitamin B-6 therapy (or combination vitamin therapy) will reduce the incidence of CHD must await further research.

A person's vitamin B-6 nutrition affects his immune system. In both men and women, and especially the elderly, low intakes of vitamin B-6 (less than 0.2 to 1.3 mg/day) have been shown to reduce immune response as determined by in vitro (i.e., test tube) methods. Of note was the finding that the reduced immune response occurred with vitamin B-6 intakes at or slightly below the current RDA.

While supplemental doses of vitamin B-6 may prove to be of benefit in some clinical conditions, maintenance of optimal vitamin B-6 status is a key to health and well-being. To ob-

tain optimal amounts of vitamin B-6 from foods, one should choose foods containing adequate amounts in a form that is highly available. In plant foods some vitamin B-6 is linked to glucose (pyridoxine glucose). This form of B-6 is poorly absorbed by both animals and humans. Animal foods do not contain glucose-linked vitamin B-6. Plant foods such as soybeans, peanuts, carrots, potatoes, wheat bran, and raisins contain 25% or more of their total vitamin B-6 in that form. In individuals who have a low intake of vitamin B-6, such as women and elderly persons, consumption of these foods at the expense of animal sources may adversely affect their vitamin B-6 status.

At the risk of being redundant, or of rousing the sleeping giant, meeting the RDA for vitamin B-6 from a variety of foods—both animals and plant sources—would be prudent.

Dr. Leklem, a professor in the Department of Nutrition and Food Management at Oregon State University, focuses his research efforts on vitamin B-6.

mocysteine produces a toxic effect on the cells that line the arteries, and in turn is linked to rapid development of atherosclerosis. Elderly people who under-consume vitamin B-6 and the vitamins folate and vitamin B-12 experience more heart disease and strokes than their better-nourished counterparts.[23] These three vitamins participate in homocysteine metabolism.

VITAMIN B-6 IN FOODS

Vitamin B-6 is stored in muscle tissues of animals, and thus meat, fish, and poultry are the best sources of this vitamin (Figure 13-11). Although vitamin B-6 in animal foods is often more readily absorbable than that in plant foods, whole grains also are good sources of vitamin B-6. However, vitamin B-6 is lost during refining of grains and is not one of the vitamins added during enrichment. The most nutrient-dense sources of vitamin B-6 (mg/kcal) are bananas, spinach, avocados, potatoes, fish, poultry, and sunflower seeds.

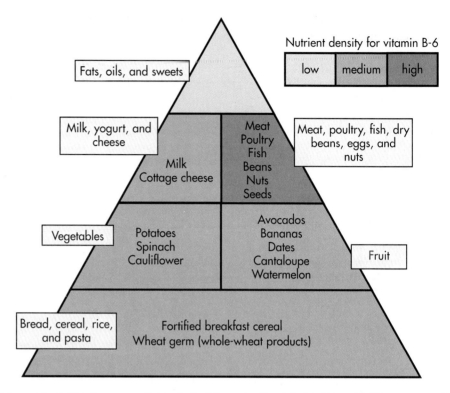

Figure 13-11 Food sources of vitamin B-6 from the Food Guide Pyramid. The meat, poultry, fish, dry beans, eggs, and nuts group is an especially rich source of this nutrient. The background color of each food group indicates the average nutrient density for vitamin B-6 in that group.

Vitamin B-6 is not stable under heat or alkaline conditions. Heat processing and other destructive processing technologies can reduce the vitamin B-6 content of a food by as much as 50%. Food composition tables listing vitamin B-6 sources often do not provide a complete picture of its availability because measuring this vitamin in foods is difficult.

RDA FOR VITAMIN B-6

The RDA for vitamin B-6 for adult men is 2 mg/day and for adult women is 1.6 mg/day. Because more vitamin B-6 is needed when more protein is consumed, the recommendation can also be expressed as 0.016 mg of vitamin B-6 per gram of protein consumed. The RDA values for vitamin B-6 are set to reflect the high protein intakes of Americans; the 2.0 mg value for men corresponds to a protein intake of 126 g—approximately twice the RDA for protein for adult men. Average daily consumption of vitamin B-6 is 2.0 mg for men and 1.5 mg for women, or just about equal to the RDA.[1]

Athletes may need slightly more vitamin B-6 because of their increased use of glycogen as a fuel (glycogen metabolism requires vitamin B-6), their increased use of amino acids for fuel, and their high protein intakes. Still, the protein foods in their diets should supply any extra vitamin B-6 needed.

AMERICANS AT RISK FOR VITAMIN B-6 DEFICIENCY

Vitamin B-6 deficiency is rare, but some elderly people have been found to exhibit signs of a deficiency. To study the effects of a deficiency, volunteers have consumed diets deficient in vitamin B-6. They became irritable and depressed, and experienced seborrheic dermatitis. Some of the subjects developed a peripheral nerve degeneration, cheilosis, glossitis, and angular stomatitis. These signs and symptoms are commonly seen in people with other B-vitamin deficiencies.

Numerous studies have shown that many adolescent and adult women have vitamin B-6 intakes below the RDA. However, since the vitamin B-6 values of many foods are not known, intake is probably greater. Routine multivitamin supplement use, which some women follow, probably also often makes up for the deficit. Moreover, the basis for the vitamin B-6 RDA assumes a daily intake of over 100 g of protein. Women, on average, consume only about 65 g of protein daily and thus will generally have lower needs for vitamin B-6 than the RDA suggests.

People with alcoholism are susceptible to a vitamin B-6 deficiency because acetaldehyde, a metabolite formed in ethanol metabolism, can displace the coenzyme form from enzymes, increasing its tendency to be destroyed. In addition, alcohol decreases the absorption of vitamin B-6 and decreases the synthesis of its coenzyme form. Cirrhosis and hepatitis (both of which may accompany alcoholism) also disable liver tissue from actively metabolizing vitamin B-6, which in turn decreases synthesis of its coenzyme form.

MEDICAL USES AND TOXICITY OF VITAMIN B-6

Carpal tunnel syndrome, a nerve disorder in the wrist, has been effectively treated with a daily dosage of 100 to 200 mg of vitamin B-6 for 3 months in some studies. No side effects were noticed. Pain diminished with vitamin treatment. However, other clinical trials demonstrate no therapeutic effect of vitamin B-6. Because of potential toxicity, any therapy must be supervised by a physician.[20]

Intakes of 2 to 6 g of vitamin B-6 per day for 2 or more months can lead to irreversible nerve damage, as can long-term intakes of 500 mg/day.[20] Use, or more appropriately misuse, of such high doses of vitamin B-6 have occurred among body builders and in women attempting to treat themselves for PMS. Symptoms include walking difficulties and hand and foot numbness. Some nerve damage in individual sensory neurons is probably reversible, but damage to the ganglia (where many nerve fibers converge) is probably permanent.

CONCEPT CHECK

Pantothenic acid and biotin both participate in metabolism of carbohydrate, protein, and fat. A deficiency of either vitamin is unlikely because pantothenic acid is found in a wide variety of foods and our need for biotin is partially met by synthesis from intestinal bacteria. Vitamin B-6 is important for protein metabolism, neurotransmitter synthesis, and other key metabolic functions. Headache, anemia, nausea, and vomiting can result from a vitamin B-6 deficiency. Animal protein sources and plant foods such as broccoli, spinach, and bananas are good sources of vitamin B-6. Doses of vitamin B-6 in excess of approximately 1000 times the RDA for a few months or 250 times the RDA for long-term use can cause nerve destruction.

Folic acid, also called folate monoglutamate, is the form absorbed in the intestine. Most of the folate in foods contains additional glutamate molecules linked to the carboxyl group, indicated by the red asterisk.

Folate

Two of the B vitamins, folate and vitamin B-12, produce a number of identical deficiency signs and symptoms when omitted from the diet.[10] These two water-soluble vitamins share a close relationship because of their biochemical interactions. For example, both vitamin B-12 and folate are responsible for DNA synthesis. We will explore the actions of folate first.

Because folate is needed for DNA synthesis, folate deficiency is induced during a common form of cancer therapy. The cancer drug methotrexate inhibits a key aspect of folate metabolism. When methotrexate is taken in high doses, it reduces DNA synthesis throughout the body by interfering with folate metabolism. This reduction in DNA synthesis can halt growth of cancer cells, but it also affects other rapidly proliferating cells, such as intestinal cells and red blood cells. Therefore typical side effects

Folic acid

Pteridine

Para-aminobenzoic acid

Glutamate

of methotrexate therapy are the same as for a folate deficiency (e.g., hair loss and diarrhea).

What we call folate today was known earlier as either folic acid or folacin. Today, the term folate is preferred because it encompasses the various forms of the vitamin found in foods. Only a few food forms are in folic acid configuration, but vitamin supplements often contain this form.

Folate consists of three parts: pteridine, *para*-aminobenzoic acid (PABA), and one or more molecules of the amino acid glutamic acid, or glutamate for short.[13] If only one glutamate molecule is present, it is designated folate monoglutamate. In food, about 90% of the folate molecules have 3 to 11 glutamates attached and are known as polyglutamates.

FOLATE ABSORPTION

In order to be absorbed, folate polyglutamates must be broken down to the monoglutamate form in the digestive process. The excess glutamates are removed by action of **conjugase** enzymes, which are present in the cells lining the small intestine.

conjugase An intestinal enzyme system that enhances folate absorption by removing glutamic acid molecules from polyglutamate forms.

About 70% to 85% of the monoglutamate form is absorbed. Alcohol is detrimental to folate absorption because it interferes with the action of the conjugase enzymes, as well as enterohepatic circulation of the vitamin (we discussed enterohepatic circulation in Chapter 6). Thus many people with alcoholism develop folate deficiencies.

About half of the body's total supply of folate is stored in the liver, most in the form of polyglutamates. Folate in excreted from the body through the bile and urine.

FUNCTIONS OF FOLATE

In the body's target cells, all forms of folate are readily converted to the basic coenzyme form, called tetrahydrofolic acid (THFA). There are actually five active coenzyme forms of THFA. These participate in metabolic reactions by accepting and donating single-carbon groups. Transfer of these single-carbon units is needed for the synthesis of DNA, metabolism of various amino acids and their derivatives, cell division, and maturation of red blood cells and other cells.[13]

- - - - - - - - - - - - -

THFA transfers the following single-carbon groups: methyl (–CH$_3$), formyl (–CH=O), methylene (–CH$_2$–), and methynyl (–CH=).

- - - - - - - - - - - - -

A crucial reaction requiring THFA is the transfer of a one-carbon methylene group (–CH$_2$–) to uridylate, forming thymidylate, an essential component of DNA and thus cell replication:

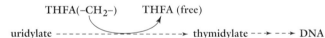

$$\text{THFA(–CH}_2\text{–)} \qquad \text{THFA (free)}$$

uridylate - - - - - - - - - - - - - - - - → thymidylate - - → - - → DNA

Another key compound whose biosynthesis depends on folate is *S*-adenosylmethionine (SAM), which is involved in the formation of neurotransmitters in the brain. Supplements of folate can improve the depressed state in some cases of mental illness.[10]

FOLATE DEFICIENCY

Folate deficiency generally results from low intakes; inadequate absorption, which often is associated with alcoholism; increased requirement, most commonly occurring in pregnancy; compromised utilization, typically associated with vitamin B-12 deficiency; and excessive excretion, linked to longstanding diarrhea.

Megaloblastic Anemia

As mentioned already, a deficiency of folate first affects cell types that are actively synthesizing DNA; such cells have a short life span and rapid turnover rate. Thus one of the first major folate-deficiency signs to appear is changes in the early phases of red blood cell synthesis, as these cells turn over every 120 days. Without folate, the precursor cells in the bone marrow cannot divide normally to become mature red blood cells because they cannot form new DNA. The cells grow larger because they can still synthesize enough protein and other cell components to make new

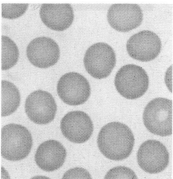

Normal blood cells. The size, shape, and color of the red blood cells show that they are normal. Mature red blood cells have lost their nuclei.

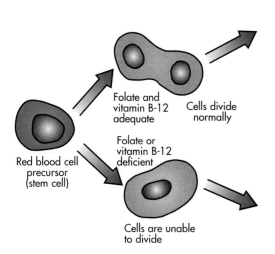

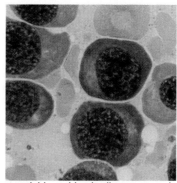

Megaloblastic blood cells are arrested at an immature stage of development. They still have their nuclei and are slightly larger than normal red blood cells.

Figure 13-12 Megaloblastic anemia occurs when blood cells are unable to divide, leaving large, immature red blood cells. Either a folate or vitamin B-12 deficiency may cause this condition. Measurements of serum concentrations of both vitamins are taken to help determine the cause of the anemia.

cells. Hemoglobin synthesis also intensifies. But when it is time for the cells to divide, they lack sufficient DNA for normal division. The cells thus remain in a large, immature form, known as **megaloblasts** (Figure 13-12). Unlike normal, mature red blood cells, megaloblasts retain the nucleus.

Megaloblasts may mature into abnormally large, fragile red blood cells, called **macrocytes,** which appear in the bloodstream. Since the bone marrow of a folate-deficient person produces mostly immature megaloblasts, few normal-size mature red blood cells (erythrocytes) arrive in the bloodstream. With fewer normal mature red blood cells present, oxygen-carrying capacity decreases, causing anemia. In short, the weakness and tiredness associated with a folate deficiency are caused by a form of anemia called megaloblastic anemia.[10]

Large, immature cells also appear along the entire length of the gastrointestinal tract during chronic folate deficiency. This change contributes to decreased absorptive capacity of the tract and a persistent diarrhea. White blood cell synthesis also is disrupted by a folate deficiency.

Because folate is stored in the body, it takes some time on a folate-free diet for a deficiency to be noticeable. For example, depending on their folate stores, individuals will show changes in red blood cell formation after 7 to 16 weeks on a folate-free diet. The large size of macrocytes causes an inevitable increase in mean corpuscular volume (MCV), which is a clinical measure of the average size of red blood cells. Physicians focus primarily on red blood cells in the initial diagnosis of a folate

megaloblast A large, nucleated, immature red blood cell that results from the inability of a precursor cell to divide when it normally should.

macrocyte An abnormally large mature red blood cell with a short lifespan.

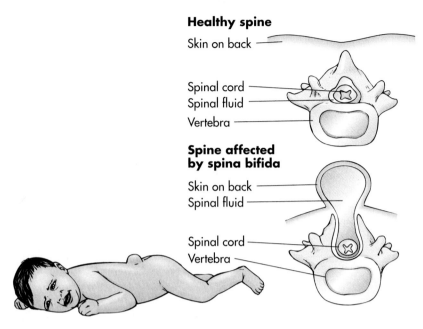

Figure 13-13 Neural tube defects result from a developmental failure affecting the spinal cord or brain in the embryo. Very early in fetal development, there is a ridge of neural-like tissue along the back of the embryo. As the fetus develops, this material differentiates into both the spinal cord and body nerves at the lower end, and into the brain at the upper end. At the same time, the bones that make up the back gradually surround the spinal cord on all sides. If any part of this sequence goes awry, many defects can appear. The worst is total lack of a brain (anencephaly). Much more common is spina bifida, in which the back bones do not form a complete ring to protect the spinal cord. Deficient folate status in the mother during the beginning of pregnancy increases the risk of neural tube defects.

deficiency because they are easy to examine. Other clinical signs and symptoms of folate deficiency include inflammation of the tongue and mouth, abnormal pigmentation of the skin, diarrhea, poor growth, depression and mental confusion, and problems in nerve function.

neural tube defect A defect in the formation of the neural tube occurring during early fetal development. This type of defect results in various nervous system disorders, such as spina bifida. Folate deficiency in the pregnant woman increases the risk that the fetus will develop this disorder.

Neural Tube Defects

A maternal deficiency of folate and a genetic predisposition have been linked to development of neural tube defects in the fetus (Figure 13-13).[27] These defects include spina bifida (spinal cord or spinal fluid bulge through the back) and anencephaly (absence of a brain). Between 2500 and 3000 infants are affected annually in the United States. Victims of spina bifida exhibit paralysis, incontinence, hydrocephalus, and learning disabilities. Children born with anencephaly die shortly after birth.

Some researchers have suggested fortification of foods (e.g., flour) to prevent neural tube defects. This suggestion is controversial because excessive folate intake can mask a vitamin B-12 deficiency. Because the metabolism and functions of folate and B-12 are linked, regular consumption of large amounts of folate can prevent the appearance of the primary early warning sign of vitamin B-12 deficiency—alteration in red blood cell formation. A lack of vitamin B-12, however, has other effects that may ultimately lead to paralysis and death. Thus early detection and treatment of a vitamin B-12 deficiency is critical. Considering the danger associated with overzealous folate intake, caution concerning folate supplementation is advised as scientists further evaluate the wisdom of adding folate to foods.[20]

FOLATE IN FOODS

The biological availability of folate varies with the source of the vitamin. The best sources from the standpoint of amount and availability are liver, fortified breakfast

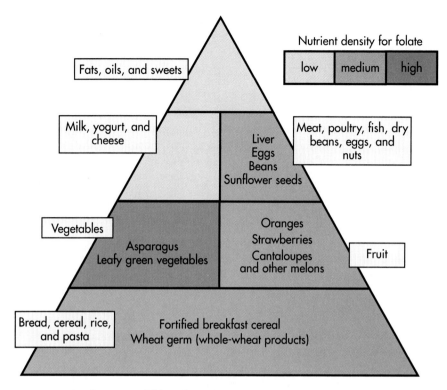

Figure 13-14 Food sources of folate from the Food Guide Pyramid. The vegetable group is an especially rich source of this nutrient. The background color of each food group indicates the average nutrient density for folate in that group.

cereals, legumes, and vegetables in general (the term *folate* is derived from the Latin *folium*, meaning "foliage"). Other, less rich sources of folate that contribute this vitamin to our diets include baked products (e.g., bread, rolls, and crackers), eggs, and oranges (Figure 13-14).

The most nutrient-dense sources of folate (µg/kcal) are spinach and other leafy greens, romaine lettuce, asparagus, broccoli, orange juice, wheat germ, liver, sunflower seeds, cauliflower, and cabbage.

Food processing and preparation can destroy 50% to 90% of the folate in food. Folate is extremely susceptible to destruction by heat, oxidation, and ultraviolet light. Consequently, it is important to eat fresh fruits and lightly cooked (or raw) vegetables on a regular basis. If vegetables must be cooked, this should be done quickly in a minimum amount of water—steaming, stir-frying, or microwaving. Vitamin C in foods helps protect folate from oxidative destruction. Highly refined and processed foods are not reliable sources of folate unless fortified, such as is the case for many refined breakfast cereals.

RDA FOR FOLATE

The RDA for folate for adults is 180 to 200 µg/day. Average daily folate intake in the United States is approximately 320 µg for men and 240 µg for women, somewhat above the RDA values.[1]

The Centers for Disease Control and Prevention, in conjunction with the U.S. Public Health Service, currently recommends that women of childbearing age consume 400 µg of folate per day to reduce the risk of neural tube defects in their offspring, as we discussed before.[26] The neural tube closes by the 28th day of gestation, a time when a woman would generally not know that she is pregnant. Hence the recommendation is that ample folate intake be instituted at least 1 month prior to conception.

AMERICANS AT RISK FOR FOLATE DEFICIENCY

Folate deficiencies sometimes appear in pregnant women. They need extra folate to meet an increased rate of cell division and thus of DNA synthesis in their own bodies and in the developing fetus. Today, prenatal care often includes vitamin and mineral supplements enriched with folate to compensate for the extra needs associated with pregnancy.

Young women in general often register low serum folate values. It is important for them to seek good sources of folate that they enjoy eating, and then eat those foods regularly.[19] Use of a balanced vitamin supplement is another option (see the Nutrition Perspective in Chapter 12). The elderly are also at risk for folate deficiency. Preliminary studies have linked low serum folate with severe vascular disease and heart disease (the homocysteine link discussed earlier), probably because of inadequate folate intake and absorption. Perhaps these people failed to consume sufficient amounts of fruits and vegetables because of poverty or physical problems, such as a lack of teeth. Finally, persons taking any of a long list of prescription drugs and those who smoke need to recognize that they have increased folate needs.[2]

TOXICITY OF FOLATE

Individuals with epilepsy who are treated with typical medications may experience resumption of seizures if given large amounts of supplemental folate. There are also several reports linking folate doses of 1 to 10 mg with hives, respiratory distress, redness of the skin, and itching. Smaller amounts of folate are considered nontoxic.

FDA limits the amount of folate in nonprescription vitamin supplements to 400 μg when no statement of age is listed on the supplement label. When age-related doses are listed, there can be no more than 100 μg for infants, 300 μg for children, or 400 μg for adults. Therefore consuming a large amount of folate would require ingesting many, many vitamin pills. FDA regulates potency of folate supplements because, as we saw earlier, consuming excessive amounts of folate can mask a vitamin B-12 deficiency.[10]

Vitamin B-12

What we call vitamin B-12 includes the free vitamin (cyanocobalamin) and two active coenzymes—methylcobalamin and 5-deoxyadenosylcobalamin. This vitamin has a complex structure containing the mineral cobalt.

All vitamin B-12 compounds are synthesized exclusively by bacteria, fungi, and algae. Animals such as cows and sheep obtain vitamin B-12 either from bacterial synthesis in their multiple stomachs (rumen) or from soil they ingest while eating and grazing. The only reliable source of the vitamin for humans is animal foods. Plants do not contain vitamin B-12, except for minor contamination of vegetable products by bacteria and soil.[10] The process of fermentation also contributes little vitamin B-12 to a food.

ABSORPTION, TRANSPORT, AND STORAGE OF VITAMIN B-12

Vitamin B-12 in food enters the stomach and is liberated from other materials by the digestive action of gastric juice. Within the stomach, free vitamin B-12 then binds with a substance called **R-protein.** The R-protein/vitamin B-12 complex travels to the small intestine, where pancreatic proteases (e.g., trypsin) release the vitamin B-12 from R-protein (Figure 13-15).

The free vitamin B-12 then binds to **intrinsic factor,** a glycoprotein produced by the stomach's parietal cells. The resulting intrinsic factor/vitamin B-12 complex travels to the terminal portion of the small intestine, the ileum, where it attaches to special receptor cells on the brush border. Cells within the ileum absorb vitamin B-12 and transfer it to a specific transport protein, transcobalamin II. This vitamin-protein complex enters the bloodstream and is taken up by the liver, bone marrow, and blood cells.[10]

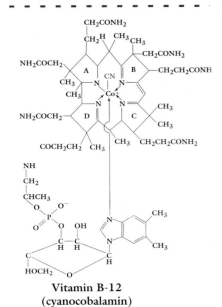

Vitamin B-12
(cyanocobalamin)

The cyanocobalamin form of vitamin B-12 is converted to the active coenzyme forms by replacement of the cyano group (red) with another group, such as a methyl group.

R-protein A protein produced by the salivary glands that enhances absorption of vitamin B-12, possibly by protecting the vitamin during its passage through the stomach.

intrinsic factor A substance present in gastric juice that enhances vitamin B-12 absorption.

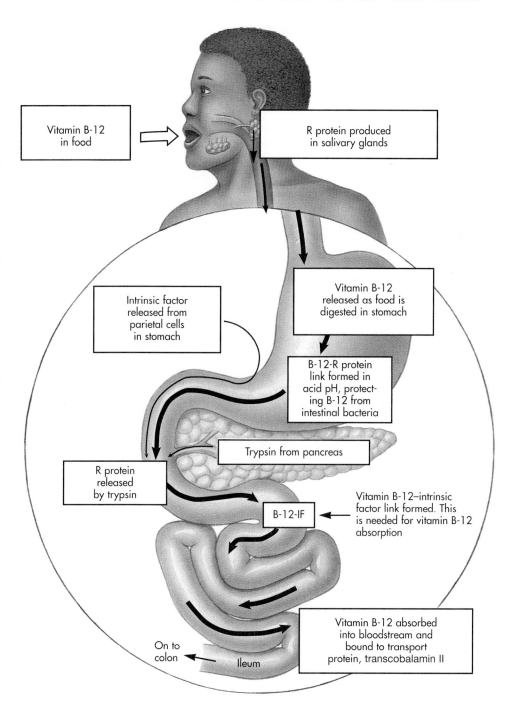

Figure 13-15 Absorption of vitamin B-12. Many factors and sites in the gastrointestinal tract participate. Defects arising in the stomach or small intestine can interfere with vitamin B-12 absorption, in turn causing pernicious anemia.

Microbial populations within the human large intestine are capable of producing vitamin B-12, but this synthesis occurs beyond the point at which the vitamin is absorbed. For this reason, we can't use the vitamin B-12 produced by these bacteria.

Depending on the body's need, approximately 15% to 70% of dietary vitamin B-12 is absorbed. Failure in any of the links found in the absorptive process reduces absorption to 2% or less of dietary vitamin B-12. Enterohepatic circulation is also important in conserving vitamin B-12 found in bile.

Absorption of vitamin B-12 can be disrupted by numerous defects, including the following:

- Absence or defective synthesis of R-protein, pancreatic proteases, or intrinsic factor
- Defective binding of the intrinsic factor/vitamin B-12 complex to receptor cells in the ileum
- Absence (or surgical removal) of part or all of the ileum or stomach
- Bacterial overgrowth of the small intestine
- Tapeworm infestation
- Use of certain antiulcer medications that significantly reduce acid production by the parietal cells (omeprazole [Prilosec]).

Three types of therapy are possible for patients diagnosed with a defect in vitamin B-12 absorption: monthly injections of vitamin B-12 to bypass the gastrointestinal tract, use of a vitamin B-12 nasal gel (nasal absorption does not require the intrinsic factor), or weekly ingestion of vitamin B-12 supplements in megadoses (300 times the RDA) that allow absorption by passive diffusion.

Ninety-five percent of all cases of vitamin B-12 deficiency among otherwise healthy people in the United States result from a defect in vitamin B-12 absorption, rather than from inadequate intake.

About 50% to 90% of the body's total supply of vitamin B-12 is stored in the liver. Stores range from 5 to 12 mg. In the body, vitamin B-12 is very stable and little is lost—just a small amount that escapes enterohepatic circulation of the bile. Since storage is so great, a single monthly injection of vitamin B-12 is sufficient to prevent a deficiency when absorption of dietary sources is significantly hampered.

FUNCTIONS OF VITAMIN B-12

Vitamin B-12 participates in a variety of reactions. Probably its most important function is in folate metabolism. Transfer of a methyl group ($-CH_3$) from the folate coenzyme THFA occurs in a two-step reaction involving vitamin B-12[13]:

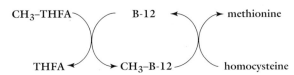

In the absence of vitamin B-12, THFA is trapped in the methyl-bound form, and the cell develops a shortage of enough of the other folate coenzymes to meet its metabolic needs. For example, shortage of the methylene form of THFA inhibits DNA synthesis, as we mentioned already. Thus a vitamin B-12 deficiency contributes to a secondary folate deficiency. And a deficiency of either folate or vitamin B-12 results in the same symptom, megaloblastic anemia. Measurement of serum folate and vitamin B-12 concentrations aids in determining which is the cause.[10]

Another vital function of vitamin B-12 is its role in maintaining the myelin sheath, which insulates nerve fibers. People with vitamin B-12 deficiencies show patchy destruction of the myelin sheath, especially in areas surrounding the nerves in the spinal cord. Although the actual cause of this destruction is unknown, alterations in the synthesis of either protein or lipid may diminish myelin formation. Whatever the cause, this destruction eventually causes paralysis and death.

A final function of vitamin B-12 is its ability to aid in rearranging carbon atoms in derivatives of three-carbon fatty acids so that they can eventually enter the citric acid cycle.[13]

PERNICIOUS ANEMIA

Researchers in mid–nineteenth century England noted a form of anemia that caused death within 2 to 5 years of initial diagnosis. They called this disease **pernicious anemia** (pernicious literally means "leading to death"). Clinically, this disease looked like a folate-deficiency anemia. In patients with either a folate or vitamin B-12 deficiency, many megaloblasts (abnormally large, immature blood cells) are seen in the blood, a hallmark of megaloblastic anemia. However, those with pernicious anemia stemming from a B-12 deficiency also experienced nerve degeneration, which was eventually fatal.

In the 1920s, researchers found that a vitamin B-12 deficiency could be cured by consumption of massive amounts of liver or concentrated water extracts of liver. In this case, the deficiency was caused by an absorption defect. If enough of the vitamin is ingested, it can be absorbed by simple diffusion, thereby overcoming the defective R-protein/intrinsic factor system.

pernicious anemia The anemia that results from the inability to absorb sufficient vitamin B-12; it is associated with nerve degeneration that can result in eventual paralysis.

As we noted previously, deficiency of vitamin B-12 and hence pernicious anemia is generally caused by diminished ability to absorb the vitamin. Before discovery and isolation of the vitamin in 1948, this condition was a death sentence. Today, once pernicious anemia is diagnosed, an injection of vitamin B-12 reverses the defects in red blood cell maturation and in some other clinical signs within 1 to 2 days.

Pernicious anemia and its accompanying nerve destruction most likely occurs after middle age. The average age of onset in Caucasians is 68 years; in African-Americans and Hispanics the disease typically appears about a decade sooner. As the stomach's parietal cells age, they lose their ability to synthesize the intrinsic factor needed for vitamin B-12 absorption. This failure likely arises from an autoimmune reaction; that is, people make white blood cells and other factors that attack their own parietal cells. Because parietal cells synthesize acid, pernicious anemia is often accompanied by a decrease in stomach acid production, a condition called **achlorhydria.**

Besides anemia, clinical signs and symptoms of pernicious anemia include weakness, a red and painful tongue, weight loss, anorexia, indigestion, diarrhea, and **paresthesia** in the extremities. Walking difficulties and mild dementia are common symptoms, along with mental slowness and memory loss. It generally takes about 3 years from the onset of the disease for symptoms of nerve destruction to develop. Unfortunately, significant nerve destruction often takes place before the anemia, which a physician can easily recognize, is seen, and this destruction is not reversible.[10]

Infants who are breast-fed by vegetarian or vegan mothers can develop vitamin B-12 deficiency accompanied by anemia and long-term neurological problems, such as diminished brain growth, degeneration of the spinal cord, and poor intellectual development. The problems may have their origins during pregnancy, when the mother is deficient in vitamin B-12. We noted in Chapter 5 that vegan diets supply little vitamin B-12 unless it is included as part of food choices enriched in vitamin B-12 or supplements are used.

achlorhydria A decrease in stomach acid primarily due to age-associated loss of acid-producing stomach cells.

paresthesia An abnormal spontaneous sensation such as of burning, prickling, and numbness.

VITAMIN B-12 IN FOODS

Important sources of vitamin B-12 include meat, poultry, seafood, and eggs (Figure 13-16). The most nutrient-dense sources of vitamin B-12 ($\mu g/kcal$) are organ meats (especially liver, kidneys, and heart), seafood, beef, eggs, hot dogs (they contain many organ meat scraps), and ham. A final source of vitamin B-12 is milk and milk products.

RDA FOR VITAMIN B-12

The RDA for vitamin B-12 for adults is 2 μg. On average, men consume 6 $\mu g/day$ and women consume 4 $\mu g/day$.[1] This high intake provides the average meat-eating person with 2 to 3 years' storage of vitamin B-12 in the liver. For people who eat animal foods regularly and can absorb vitamin B-12, a vitamin B-12 deficiency is highly unlikely.

It takes approximately 20 years of consuming a diet essentially free of vitamin B-12 for a person to exhibit nerve destruction caused by a deficiency. However, as mentioned before, it takes only approximately 2 to 3 years to see the same nerve destruction if a person develops an inability to absorb vitamin B-12. The difference arises mostly from the ability of the body to reclaim the vitamin B-12 it secretes into the small intestine via the bile if enterohepatic circulation is impossible.[10] Supplements of vitamin B-12 are virtually nontoxic.

AMERICANS AT RISK FOR VITAMIN B-12 DEFICIENCY

As we mentioned, vegans who eat no animal products should find reliable sources of vitamin B-12. Options include a vitamin supplement, fortified soy milk and breakfast cereals, and special yeast grown in media rich in vitamin B-12. Otherwise, a vitamin B-12 deficiency is possible. The elderly are at risk for developing pernicious anemia. Regular physical examinations should include an evaluation of red blood cell size, serum concentrations of vitamin B-12, and evidence of numbness

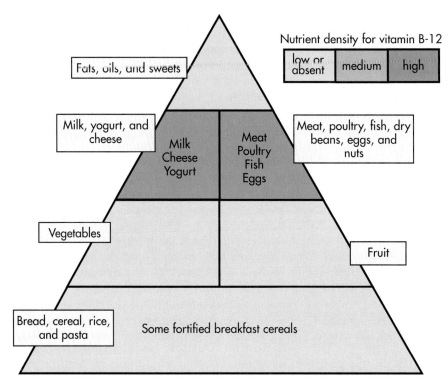

Figure 13-16 Food sources of vitamin B-12 from the Food Guide Pyramid. Animal products in the meat, poultry, fish, dry beans, eggs, and nuts group and the milk, yogurt, and cheese group are especially rich sources of this nutrient. The background color of each food group indicates the average nutrient density for vitamin B-12 in that group. Vegans need to supplement their diets with vitamin B-12 or consume foods fortified with vitamin B-12.

and tingling in the hands and feet. Infants who fail to thrive and exhibit anorexia and significant developmental regression should be examined for vitamin B-12 deficiency.

People who regularly consume excessive amounts of vitamin C supplements (just ten times the RDA) need to be aware of its effect on vitamin B-12. Although the exact mechanism has yet to be determined, vitamin C may be capable of reducing the food availability of vitamin B-12 by converting it to a biologically inactive form.[10]

CONCEPT CHECK

Folate is needed for cell division because it is essential for DNA synthesis. A folate deficiency results in megaloblastic anemia, as well as diarrhea, inflammation of the tongue, and poor growth—all signs of inadequate cell division. Folate is found in fresh vegetables and organ meats. It is important to emphasize "fresh" and "lightly cooked" with vegetables because much folate is lost during cooking. Folate deficiency is most commonly found in pregnant women, when needs are elevated, and in people with alcoholism, which interferes with absorption of folate. Vitamin B-12 is necessary for folate metabolism. Without dietary vitamin B-12, folate deficiency symptoms, such as megaloblastic anemia, develop. In addition, vitamin B-12 is necessary for maintaining the nervous system; paralysis can develop from a vitamin B-12 deficiency. Vitamin B-12 is found only in animal foods; meat eaters generally have a 3- to 5-year supply stored in the liver. However, vitamin B-12 absorption may decline in the elderly years. In this case a deficiency of vitamin B-12 is generally corrected by monthly injections of the vitamin.

Vitamin C

Vitamin C is found in all living tissues, and most animals are capable of synthesizing their own supply from glucose. Humans and other primates, guinea pigs, and a few birds, bats, and fish are unable to make their own vitamin C and therefore must obtain it from dietary sources. What is strange is that animals that synthesize vitamin C often make very large amounts. For instance, a hog produces 8 g/day, although we do not know how a hog benefits from this large amount. Incidentally, pork is not a good source of the vitamin, since it is lost in processing. This 8 g amount is over 130 times the human RDA of 60 mg. This RDA even appears to be quite generous; intakes as low as 10 mg/day can prevent scurvy, the vitamin C–deficiency disease. Why some animals make so much vitamin C, while a few other animals, including humans, appear to need so little, has fueled much controversy surrounding this vitamin.

Vitamin C exists in a reduced form, called ascorbic acid, and in an oxidized form, called dehydroascorbic acid. The two forms are interchangeable, and both are biologically active. Further oxidation of dehydroascorbic acid irreversibly converts it to diketogulonic acid, which has no vitamin C activity and is further metabolized to oxalic acid and other products.

ABSORPTION AND METABOLISM OF VITAMIN C

Absorption of vitamin C occurs in the small intestine by means of a specific energy-dependent transport system. The efficiency of the absorptive mechanism decreases at high intakes. About 80% to 90% of vitamin C is absorbed at daily intakes between 30 and 120 mg, whereas absorption efficiency drops to about 20% at intakes of 6 g/day. A common side effect of excessive vitamin C intake is diarrhea. The unabsorbed vitamin C remains in the small intestine, and its osmotic effect attracts water from the blood in sufficient quantities to cause diarrhea (see Chapter 14 for a review of osmosis). When megadoses of vitamin C are consumed, most of that absorbed from the body is eventually excreted in the urine as vitamin C itself or one of its close derivatives. Oxalic acid is a major breakdown product, or metabolite, when vitamin C intakes are moderate (about 100 mg/day).

FUNCTIONS OF VITAMIN C

Vitamin C performs a variety of very important cell functions. It does this primarily by acting as a nonspecific **reducing agent.** A reducing agent is a substance that donates electrons and in turn becomes oxidized. For example, vitamin C can donate electrons to metal ions, such as iron, in the oxidized state (e.g., ferric ion, Fe^{3+}), thus maintaining them in their reduced state (e.g., ferrous ion, Fe^{2+}).[22]

Collagen Synthesis

Vitamin C is required for formation of **collagen,** the fibrous protein that is a major component of **connective tissue**. Indeed collagen is found wherever tissues require strengthening, especially in those tissues with a protective, connective, or structural function. Collagen fibers are critical to the maintenance of bone and blood vessels and are essential in wound healing.

A collagen molecule consists of three polypeptide chains wound together to form a triple helix. Many of these triple-helical molecules associate side by side to form the collagen fibrils; these are stabilized by covalent bonds (cross-links) between the collagen molecules. The polypeptide chains constituting the starting structure of collagen contain many proline and lysine units. Synthesis of mature collagen depends on hydroxylation (addition of –OH groups) to these two amino acids, yielding hydroxyproline and hydroxylysine. Hydroxyproline is necessary for formation of stable collagen triple helices, and hydroxylysine plays a role in the cross-linking that stabilizes collagen fibrils.[13]

The role of vitamin C in collagen metabolism is to maintain the iron-containing enzymes that add hydroxyl groups to proline in the active form. For these enzymes to form hydroxyproline, their iron must be maintained in the reduced (ferrous)

Ascorbic acid (reduced)

Dehydroascorbic acid (oxidized)

Vitamin C undergoes reversible oxidation and reduction by loss or addition of two hydrogens (red).

reducing agent A compound capable of donating electrons (also hydrogen ions) to another compound (see Appendix B).

connective tissue The material that holds together the various structures of the body. Tendons and cartilage are composed largely of connective tissue. Connective tissue also forms part of bone and the nonmuscular structures of arteries and veins.

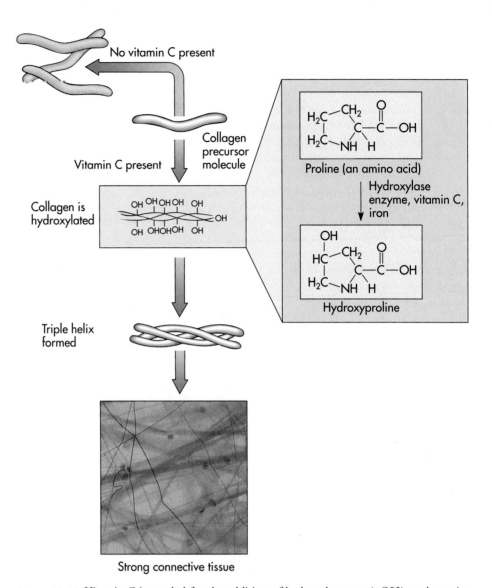

Figure 13-17 Vitamin C is needed for the addition of hydroxyl groups (–OH) to the amino acid proline in collagen molecules. Collagen is unique among body proteins because it contains large amounts of the amino acid hydroxyproline, which is necessary for formation of stable collagen fibers.

state, Fe^{2+}. The reducing action of vitamin C does this, and without this action, strong connective tissues made from collagen cannot be maintained (Figure 13-17).

Antioxidant Activity

Because of its ability to act as a reducing agent, vitamin C is one of the cell's water-soluble antioxidants. Vitamin C works with vitamin E as a pair of free-radical scavengers. (Recall that vitamin E is a fat-soluble antioxidant in the cell membrane.) Vitamin C also aids in reactivating oxidized vitamin E so that it can be reused.[22] In addition, vitamin C protects folate by stabilizing the coenzyme form of the vitamin in its reduced state. Finally, epidemiological studies suggest that vitamin C is effective in helping prevent certain cancers (e.g., esophageal, oral, and stomach cancers), heart disease, and cataracts in the eye, probably because of its antioxidant capabilities, but some researchers are skeptical about the true degree of these effects.[9]

Iron Absorption

The absorption of nonheme iron (iron primarily from plant foods) from the intestinal tract depends on its being in the reduced form. Vitamin C reduces the iron so it is more soluble in the slightly alkaline environment of the small intestine, and thus modestly improves iron absorption.[22] Vitamin C also counters the action of certain food components that inhibit iron absorption.

Synthesis of Other Vital Cell Compounds

Carnitine is a transport compound that moves fatty acids from the cytoplasm into the mitochondria for energy production. This process is especially important in muscle tissue. Biosynthesis of carnitine depends on vitamin C.

Norepinephrine is synthesized with the action of a copper-containing enzyme and vitamin C. The conversion of the amino acid tryptophan to the neurotransmitter serotonin requires vitamin C. Vitamin C is also necessary for biosynthesis of thyroxine (the thyroid hormone), epinephrine, bile acids, steroid hormones, and the purine bases used in DNA synthesis. The synthesis of all these compounds requires the addition of hydroxyl groups.

Immune Function

Vitamin C is vital for the function of the immune system, especially for the activity of certain cells (lymphocytes) in the immune system. In addition, vitamin C is used by chemical-detoxifying mechanisms in cells. Thus both disease states and drug use can increase the need for vitamin C.[22]

SCURVY

A deficiency of vitamin C prevents normal synthesis of collagen, thus causing widespread and significant changes in connective tissues throughout the body. The first signs and symptoms of scurvy, the deficiency disease, appear after about 20 to 40 days on a vitamin C–free diet and include weakness and pinpoint hemorrhages (petechiae) around hair follicles on the back of the arms and legs (Figure 13-18). These hemorrhages are the most characteristic sign of scurvy. In addition, there is bleeding in the gums and joints, a classic sign of connective tissue failure.[17] Other effects of scurvy include opening of previously healed wounds, bone pain, fractures, and diarrhea. Psychological problems such as depression are common in advanced scurvy.

VITAMIN C IN FOODS

Citrus fruits, potatoes, and green vegetables in general are good sources of vitamin C (Figure 13-19). The Food Guide Pyramid guideline of at least 5 servings/day of combined fruits and vegetables provides sufficient vitamin C. The major contributors of vitamin C to American diets are oranges and orange juice, grapefruit and grapefruit juice, tomatoes and tomato juice, fortified fruit drinks, tangerines, and potatoes. Although the isoascorbate (erythorbate) used as a food preservative in fruits and vegetables has no vitamin C activity, it does act as an antioxidant in the body.

The most nutrient-dense sources of vitamin C (mg/kcal) are green peppers, cauliflower, broccoli, cabbage, strawberries, papayas, romaine lettuce, oranges, and spinach and other greens.

Vitamin C is easily lost in processing and cooking. Juices are good foods to fortify with vitamin C because their acidity reduces vitamin C destruction. Vitamin C is very unstable when in contact with heat, iron, copper, or oxygen.

RDA FOR VITAMIN C

The RDA for vitamin C for adults is 60 mg. The current RDA publication suggests that cigarette smokers should consume 100 mg/day to overcome the rapid destruction of the vitamin in the lungs. Our food supply yields about twice the adult RDA (120 mg) of vitamin C per day. Approximately 80 mg is derived naturally from foods; the remainder comes from vitamin C added to foods. It is likely that nearly all nonsmoking Americans meet their daily needs for vitamin C, as men consume an average 120 mg/day and women consume 100 mg/day.[1] Advocates of increased vitamin C use often recommend intakes of 250 mg/day or more. Still, 250 mg/day

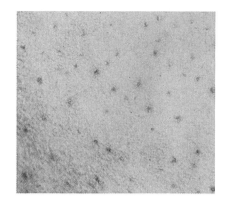

Figure 13-18 Pinpoint hemorrhages of the skin—an early symptom of scurvy. The spots on the skin are caused by slight bleeding into hair follicles. The person also will often show inadequate wound healing—all signs of defective collagen synthesis.

- - - - - - - - - - - - -

Vitamin C status is assessed by its concentration in white blood cells. A dietary history of limited fruit and vegetable consumption also suggests a deficiency.

- - - - - - - - - - - - -

Scurvy was the curse of sailors throughout the nineteenth century. On long sea voyages a captain often lost more than half of his crew to scurvy. From 1550 to 1857, more than 114 scurvy epidemics were reported in Europe. Soldiers in the U.S. Civil War died of scurvy. In 1740, Dr. James Lind, working aboard the HMS Salisbury, showed that citrus fruits—two oranges and one lemon a day—could cure scurvy. Fifty years after Lind's discovery, limes were added to the rations for British sailors to prevent scurvy. That is why the British today may be referred to as "limeys."

- - - - - - - - - - - - -

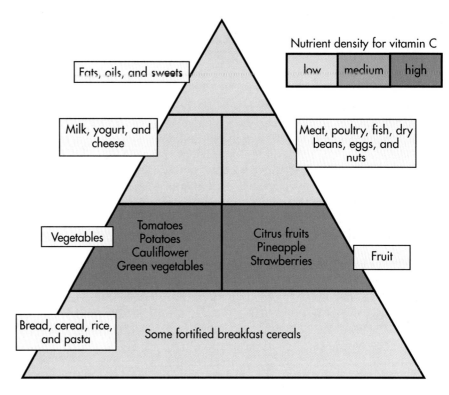

Figure 13-19 Food sources of vitamin C from the Food Guide Pyramid. The fruit group and the vegetable group are especially rich sources of this nutrient. The background color of each food group indicates the average nutrient density for vitamin C in that group.

is easily met by food intake, and data supporting the benefits of this dosage are sketchy.

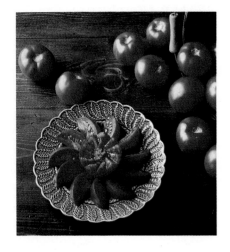

Tomatoes and tomato juice are major contributors of vitamin C to American diets.

AMERICANS AT RISK FOR VITAMIN C DEFICIENCY

Today vitamin C deficiency is most likely to occur in people with alcoholism or those addicted to other drugs, as they often consume a nutrient-poor diet.[17] Elderly men who eat very few fruits and vegetables are also susceptible to vitamin C deficiency. Studies show that about 20% of elderly men have low serum vitamin C. These men eat very few fruits and vegetables and are unlikely to take supplements. Men in general are more at risk of vitamin C deficiency compared with women because they are less apt to consume vitamin supplements.

People exposed to cigarette smoke generally have lower vitamin C status than nonsmokers.[24] Smokers may need as much as 200 mg of vitamin C daily in order to meet their needs and to maintain blood vitamin C equal to that of nonsmokers consuming the RDA. This is a troubling finding, since only about 25% of smokers consume even as much as the recommended 100 mg of vitamin C daily.

Worldwide, scurvy is associated with poverty. It is especially common in infants who are fed boiled milk (all forms of milk are poor sources of vitamin C) and not provided with a good food source of vitamin C or a supplement.

TOXICITY OF VITAMIN C

Vitamin C is probably not toxic to most healthy people when consumed in amounts less than 1 to 2 g/day, although this dosage causes destruction of some vitamin B-12 and enhances iron absorption. This second point is important to note, however, since some people suffer from hemochromatosis, a disease characterized by overstorage of iron (see Chapter 15). These people are actually harmed if an increased vitamin C intake increases their iron absorption and iron metabolism.[9] This is just one of many examples in which recommending a vitamin intake above the RDA can have conflicting results. Some people may benefit, whereas others may be injured.

Regularly consuming more than 1 to 2 g of vitamin C daily can cause stomach inflammation, diarrhea, oxalate kidney stones in people with a history of such stones, and possibly "rebound" or "withdrawal scurvy." At megadose intakes of vitamin C, the body is thought to develop enzyme systems that rapidly metabolize it. If individuals consuming high amounts of vitamin C abruptly reduce their intake to normal amounts, these enzyme systems take awhile to readjust; before they do, rebound scurvy is likely to develop. To avoid this effect, those with a history of high vitamin C intakes should slowly decrease the intake over a period of time.

Keep in mind that most vitamin C consumed in large doses escapes the body in the stool or urine. The body is totally saturated at intakes of about 150 mg/day.[5] In any event, maladies such as common colds are rarely severe enough, nor last long enough, to merit megadose vitamin C therapy. Consuming extra vitamin C may decrease a cold's severity and duration somewhat (about 1 day), so we see no reason to discourage people from drinking a few glasses of orange juice when they have a cold. However, double-blind studies provide no striking evidence that megadoses of vitamin C prevent or greatly decrease the severity or duration of a cold.

In addition, no credible evidence suggests that a dosage even as high as 10 g/day will cure colon cancer.[16] Early studies suggesting this role for vitamin C megadoses were too poorly controlled to be credible. If people with cancer want to experiment with large doses of vitamin C, they should alert their physician, primarily becaues high doses of vitamin C can change reactions to medical tests for diabetes or blood in the stool. Physicians may misdiagnose conditions when large doses of vitamin C are consumed without their knowledge.

• • •

Now that we have discussed the water-soluble vitamins, see Table 13-1 for a review.

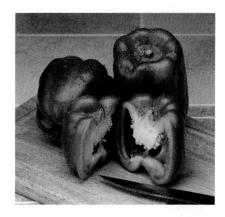

Green peppers are one vegetable source of vitamin C.

CRITICAL THINKING

Carlos just returned from a local mall and is excited because he saw an advertisement claiming that vitamin C will cure just about everything, from colds to heart disease. How would you explain to him vitamin C's main functions in the human body?

CONCEPT CHECK

Only guinea pigs, monkeys, some birds and fish, and humans need dietary vitamin C. It is used mainly in synthesis of collagen, a major connective tissue protein. A vitamin C deficiency causes scurvy, which is marked by many changes in the skin and gums, such as small hemorrhages, because of reduced collagen synthesis. Vitamin C also modestly improves iron absorption and is involved in the synthesis of certain hormones and neurotransmitters. Citrus fruits, green peppers, cauliflower, broccoli, and strawberries are good sources of vitamin C. As with folate, fresh or lightly cooked foods are the best sources, since loss of vitamin C in cooking can be high. At intakes greater than about 1 to 2 g/day, vitamin C can lead to diarrhea and overabsorption of iron. Such high dosages do not prevent the common cold or cure cancer.

Vitamin-like Compounds

The various vitamin-like compounds—choline, carnitine, inositol, taurine, and lipoic acid—are necessary to maintain normal metabolism in the body. They all can be synthesized by the body, but their biosynthesis often occurs at the expense of important nutrients, such as essential amino acids. The need for these compounds often increases during times of rapid tissue growth, as is the case with the premature infant.

There is no concern that deficiencies of these vitamin-like compounds exist in the average healthy adult. But more research is needed to clarify whether deficiencies might arise in certain disease states and whether the compounds should be included in infant formulas and total parenteral nutrition solutions. Presently, manufacturers often add these vitamin-like compounds to infant formulas.

TABLE 13-1

A summary of the water-soluble vitamins

Name and coenzyme	Major functions	Deficiency symptoms
Thiamin; TPP	Glycolysis, citric acid cycle, and hexose-monophosphate shunt activity; nerve function	Beriberi: nervous tingling, poor coordination, edema, heart changes, weakness
Riboflavin; FAD and FMN	Citric acid cycle and electron transport chain activity; fat breakdown	Ariboflavinosis: inflammation of mouth and tongue, cracks at corners of the mouth, eye disorders
Niacin; NAD and NADP	Glycolysis, citric acid cycle, and electron transport chain activity; fat synthesis, fat breakdown	Pellagra: diarrhea, bilateral dermatitis, dementia
Pantothenic acid; coenzyme A, acyl carrier protein	Citric acid cycle; fat synthesis, fat breakdown	Tingling in hands, fatigue, headache, nausea
Biotin; biocytin	Glucose production; fat synthesis; purine (part of DNA, RNA) synthesis	Dermatitis, tongue soreness, anemia, depression
Vitamin B-6, pyridoxine and other forms; PLP	Protein metabolism; neurotransmitter synthesis; many other functions	Headache, anemia, convulsions, nausea, vomiting, dermatitis, sore tongue
Folate; THFA	DNA and RNA synthesis; amino acid synthesis; red blood cell maturation	Megaloblastic anemia, inflammation of tongue, diarrhea, poor growth, mental disorders, birth defects
Vitamin B-12 (cobalamin, methylcobalamin)	Folate metabolism; nerve function	Megaloblastic anemia, poor nerve function
Vitamin C (ascorbic acid)	Collagen synthesis; hormone and neurotransmitter synthesis	Scurvy: poor wound healing, pinpoint hemorrhages, bleeding gums

Choline forms part of the natural emulsifiers called *lecithins*.

CHOLINE

Choline is widely distributed among plant and animal foods. Rich sources include lettuce, peanuts, liver, coffee, and cauliflower. So much choline occurs naturally that a dietary deficiency is quite unlikely. Choline is a very simple compound synthesized in the liver from the amino acid serine. Its synthesis depends on the action of vitamin B-6, vitamin B-12, and folate, as well as the amino acid methionine as a source of methyl groups ($-CH_3$). If there is inadequate dietary choline, the body can normally make up the deficiency by biosynthesis, provided there is plenty of protein in the diet to supply methionine, an essential amino acid.

Choline functions in several ways. The amino acid methionine can be regenerated after participating in certain metabolic reactions with the help of choline, which acts as a methyl donor in the process. Choline also forms part of several important cellular compounds, such as the neurotransmitter acetylcholine and the lecithins (also called phosphatidylcholines), which are naturally occurring emulsifiers present in lipoproteins, cell membranes, and bile.[13] The name choline comes from the French word *chole*, meaning "bile."

Test animals fed a choline-free diet develop a fatty liver and other choline-deficiency symptoms, suggesting that they cannot make enough choline to supply all their needs. Humans fed choline-deficient intravenous solutions have developed liver dysfunction similar to that seen in choline-deficient test animals. Normal human volunteers who consume a choline-free diet also develop liver abnormalities. These findings suggest that choline may be an essential nutrient for humans, al-

Deficiency risk conditions	Adult RDA or ESADDI	Dietary sources	Toxicity
Alcoholism, poverty	1.1-1.5 mg	Sunflower seeds, pork, whole and enriched grains, dried beans, peas, brewer's yeast	None possible from food
Possibly people on certain medications if no dairy products consumed	1.2-1.7 mg	Milk, mushrooms, spinach, liver, enriched grains	None reported
Severe poverty where corn is the dominant food; alcoholism	15-19 mg NE	Mushrooms, bran, tuna, salmon, chicken, beef, liver, peanuts, enriched grains	Flushing of skin at intakes >100 mg
Alcoholism	4-7 mg	Mushrooms, liver, broccoli, eggs; most foods have some	None
Alcoholism	30-100 μg	Cheese, egg yolks, cauliflower, peanuts, liver	Unknown
Adolescent and adult women; people on certain medications; alcoholism	1.6-2 mg	Animal protein foods, spinach, broccoli, bananas, salmon, sunflower seeds	Nerve destruction at doses 2 g/day or more for a few months or 500 mg per day for long-term use
Alcoholism; pregnancy; use of certain medications	180-200 μg	Green leafy vegetables, orange juice, organ meats, sprouts, sunflower seeds	None; nonprescription vitamin dosage is controlled by FDA
Elderly, due to poor absorption; vegans	2 μg	Animal foods, especially organ meats, oysters, clams (not natural in plants)	None
Alcoholism; elderly men living alone	60 mg	Citrus fruits, strawberries, broccoli, greens	Doses >1-2 g cause diarrhea and can alter some diagnostic tests; increased iron absorption can induce iron toxicity in some people

though further research is needed to confirm this.[28] In any case, we consume ample choline, about 600 to 1000 mg/day, to meet our needs.

The liver dysfunction associated with a lack of dietary choline differs from the fatty liver seen in people with alcoholism. Attempts to treat alcoholic fatty liver in humans with high doses of choline or lecithin have failed. Scientists have attempted to treat some neurological disorders, such as Alzheimer's disease and other forms of senile memory loss, with lecithin. Despite the highly active research in this area, it is still too early to say if persons with these problems can benefit from this type of therapy.

Daily doses of choline as high as 20 to 30 g have been administered, but with side effects such as "fishy" body odor, especially when choline itself, rather than lecithin, is used. Gastric distress, vomiting, and diarrhea may also result. There is some concern that such high megadoses of choline may also increase the risk of developing stomach cancer, since choline can be metabolized to compounds that form powerful carcinogens known as *nitrosamines*.

CARNITINE

Carnitine is a relatively simple compound that can be synthesized in the liver from the amino acids lysine and methionine. Human needs for carnitine are met from both animal foods and biosynthesis. Adults and children who are severely malnourished can have lower-than-normal concentrations of carnitine in their blood. An inadequate supply of protein (i.e., a lack of the amino acids needed for making carni-

Carnitine

tine) leads to abnormal fatty acid metabolism. There is speculation that people with cirrhosis may need carnitine from the diet to offset inadequate liver production.

Within the cell, carnitine transports fatty acids from the cytosol into the mitochondria, where the fatty acids are metabolized for energy. Carnitine also aids the mitochondria in removing excess organic acids, products of metabolic pathways.[13]

Meat and dairy products are the main sources of carnitine. We consume about 100 to 300 mg/day. Vegetarian diets are very low in carnitine because it is almost absent from plant foods. However, vegetarians show normal blood concentrations of carnitine. Consequently, it is doubtful that carnitine is necessary in the diet of healthy people. It may be considered a conditionally essential nutrient in times of recovery from disease, serious trauma, or preterm birth.

In addition, carnitine has displayed pharmaceutical usefulness in the removal of compounds that can build to toxic amounts in people with inborn errors of metabolism. Dosages approximately 10 times typical dietary intakes have also been shown to improve the condition of persons with progressive muscle disease and heart muscle deterioration.

INOSITOL

Of the nine possible isomers of inositol, only one—called myo-inositol—has nutritional implications for humans. The structure of inositol is related to that of glucose, from which it is synthesized in the body.

Much of the inositol in body cells occurs in phosphorylated forms, such as inositol triphosphate (IP_3), which is found free in the cell cytosol. Inositol is also incorporated into the phospholipids located in cell membranes.[13] These inositol phospholipids are important precursors of the eicosanoids, which have numerous hormone-like actions (see Chapter 4). Under certain conditions (e.g., binding of hormones), enzymes in the cell membrane act on the inositol phospholipids, releasing IP_3. This compound in turn mobilizes calcium ions (Ca^{2+}) from stores within cells. The resulting increase in the intracellular calcium concentration then leads to various cell responses in different tissues, such as the recognition and transfer of stimuli by nerve cells. This inositol-dependent function may explain why high concentrations of inositol phospholipids are found in brain tissue.

Both free inositol and inositol phospholipids are present in animal foods. Some plant foods (e.g., wheat bran) also contain inositol, mostly as part of phytic acid, a compound that binds minerals. The average American diet provides about 1 g of inositol per day, and another 4 g/day or more is synthesized in the kidneys.

The metabolism of inositol is altered by several medical conditions. The hyperglycemia associated with diabetes inhibits inositol transport. Abnormal inositol metabolism is also noted in multiple sclerosis, kidney failure, and certain cancers. Overall, it appears that inositol is an essential nutrient only in certain medical conditions.

TAURINE

Taurine is synthesized from the sulfur-containing amino acids methionine and cysteine. It is abundant in muscle, platelets, and nerve tissue. It is also attached to bile acids.[13] Although its mechanism of action is not understood well, taurine is involved in many vital functions. It is associated with photoreceptor activity in the eye, antioxidant activity in white blood cells, protection of pulmonary tissue from oxidation, central nervous system function, platelet aggregation, cardiac contraction, insulin action, and cell differentiation and growth.

Taurine is found only in animal foods. Americans consume about 40 to 400 mg/day. No clear cases of taurine deficiencies have been diagnosed in vegans, even though it is not found in plants, suggesting that synthesis by the body meets needs. Thus it appears that healthy people need not worry about consuming taurine.

Taurine supplementation may be of benefit to children with cystic fibrosis. They experience increased growth when treated with taurine, perhaps because of increased fat absorption from the action of taurine as part of bile. Preterm infants supplemented with taurine may also exhibit improved fat absorption.

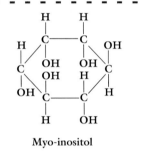

Myo-inositol

$$HO-\overset{\overset{\displaystyle O}{\|}}{\underset{\underset{\displaystyle O}{\|}}{S}}-CH_2-NH_2$$

Taurine

LIPOIC ACID

Lipoic acid is used in reactions in which a carbon dioxide molecule is lost from a substrate, as when pyruvate is converted into acetyl-CoA.[13] Health-food stores sell this compound, but the human body readily synthesizes lipoic acid.

$$CH_2-CH_2-CH-CH_2-CH_2-CH_2-CH_2-\overset{\overset{\displaystyle O}{\|}}{C}-OH$$

$$\underset{S-------S}{\vert\qquad\qquad\vert}$$

Lipoic acid

Bogus Vitamins

A variety of substances promoted by health-food enthusiasts as "vitamins" have no important role in human nutrition. Some may increase growth in less complex forms of life, so vitamin hucksters try to pass them off as necessary for humans (Figure 13-20).

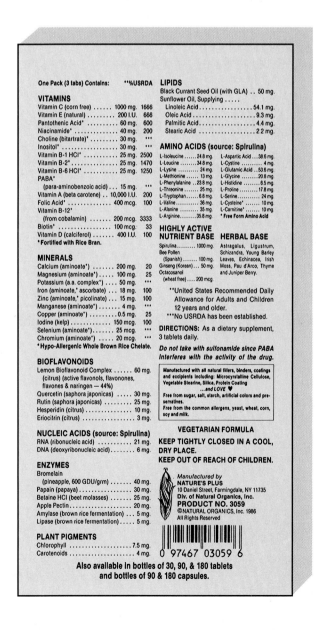

One Pack (3 tabs) Contains:		**%USRDA
VITAMINS		
Vitamin C (corn free)	1000 mg.	1666
Vitamin E (natural)	200 I.U.	666
Pantothenic Acid*	60 mg.	600
Niacinamide*	40 mg.	200
Choline (bitartrate)*	30 mg.	***
Inositol*	30 mg.	***
Vitamin B-1 HCl*	25 mg.	2500
Vitamin B-2*	25 mg.	1470
Vitamin B-6 HCl*	25 mg.	1250
PABA*		
(para-aminobenzoic acid)	15 mg.	***
Vitamin A (beta carotene)	10,000 I.U.	200
Folic Acid*	400 mcg.	100
Vitamin B-12*		
(from cobalamin)	200 mcg.	3333
Biotin*	100 mcg.	33
Vitamin D (calciferol)	400 I.U.	100
*Fortified with Rice Bran.		

MINERALS

Calcium (aminoate*)	200 mg.	20
Magnesium (aminoate*)	100 mg.	25
Potassium (a.a. complex)*	50 mg.	***
Iron (aminoate,* ascorbate)	18 mg.	100
Zinc (aminoate,* picolinate)	15 mg.	100
Manganese (aminoate*)	4 mg.	***
Copper (aminoate*)	0.5 mg.	25
Iodine (kelp)	150 mcg.	100
Selenium (aminoate*)	25 mcg.	***
Chromium (aminoate*)	20 mcg.	***
*Hypo-Allergenic Whole Brown Rice Chelate.		

BIOFLAVONOIDS

Lemon Bioflavonoid Complex ..... 60 mg.
(citrus) (active flavonols, flavonones, flavones & naringen — 44%)
Quercetin (saphora japonicas) ..... 30 mg.
Rutin (saphora japonicas) .... 25 mg.
Hesperidin (citrus) .... 10 mg.
Eriocitrin (citrus) .... 3 mg.

NUCLEIC ACIDS (source: Spirulina)

RNA (ribonucleic acid) .... 21 mg.
DNA (deoxyribonucleic acid) .... 6 mg.

ENZYMES

Bromelain
(pineapple, 600 GDU/grm) .... 40 mg.
Papain (papaya) .... 30 mg.
Betaine HCl (beet molasses) ...... 25 mg.
Apple Pectin .... 20 mg.
Amylase (brown rice fermentation) ... 5 mg.
Lipase (brown rice fermentation) .... 5 mg.

PLANT PIGMENTS

Chlorophyll .... 7.5 mg.
Carotenoids .... 4 mg.

LIPIDS

Black Currant Seed Oil (with GLA) .. 50 mg.
Sunflower Oil, Supplying .....
  Linoleic Acid .... 54.1 mg.
  Oleic Acid .... 9.3 mg.
  Palmitic Acid .... 4.4 mg.
  Stearic Acid .... 2.2 mg.

AMINO ACIDS (source: Spirulina)

L-Isoleucine	24.8 mg.	L-Aspartic Acid ... 38.6 mg.
L-Leucine	34.8 mg.	L-Cystine ..... 4 mg.
L-Lysine	24 mg.	L-Glutamic Acid ... 53.6 mg.
L-Methionine	13 mg.	L-Glycine ..... 20.8 mg.
L-Phenylalanine	23.8 mg.	L-Histidine ..... 6.5 mg.
L-Threonine	25 mg.	L-Proline ..... 17.8 mg.
L-Tryptophan	6.8 mg.	L-Serine ..... 24 mg.
L-Valine	36 mg.	L-Cysteine* ..... 10 mg.
L-Alanine	35 mg.	L-Carnitine* ..... 10 mg.
L-Arginine	35.8 mg.	* Free Form Amino Acid

HIGHLY ACTIVE NUTRIENT BASE — **HERBAL BASE**

Spirulina .... 1000 mg.   Astragalus, Ligustrum,
Bee Pollen   Schizandra, Young Barley
  (Spanish) ... 100 mg.   Leaves, Echinacea, Irish
Ginseng (Korean) ... 50 mg.   Moss, Pau d'Arco, Thyme
Octacosanol   and Juniper Berry.
  (wheat free) .... 200 mcg.

**United States Recommended Daily Allowance for Adults and Children 12 years and older.
***No USRDA has been established.

DIRECTIONS: As a dietary supplement, 3 tablets daily.

Do not take with sulfonamide since PABA interferes with the activity of the drug.

Manufactured with all natural fillers, binders, coatings and excipients including: Microcrystalline Cellulose, Vegetable Stearine, Silica, Protein Coating ...and LOVE ♥
Free from sugar, salt, starch, artificial colors and preservatives.
Free from the common allergens, yeast, wheat, corn, soy and milk.

VEGETARIAN FORMULA
KEEP TIGHTLY CLOSED IN A COOL, DRY PLACE.
KEEP OUT OF REACH OF CHILDREN.

Manufactured by
NATURE'S PLUS
10 Daniel Street, Farmingdale, NY 11735
Div. of Natural Organics, Inc.
PRODUCT NO. 3059
©NATURAL ORGANICS, Inc. 1986
All Rights Reserved

0 97467 03059 6

Also available in bottles of 30, 90, & 180 tablets and bottles of 90 & 180 capsules.

Figure 13-20 Health foods are noted for containing substances that are not vitamins. These include vitamin-like compounds, such as inositol.

The list of these pseudo-vitamins changes frequently. The following substances are among the more persistent of these bogus vitamins:

- *para*-aminobenzoic acid: This compound is part of folate but confers no benefit by itself. In fact, consumption of this compound in conjunction with sulfa antibiotics defeats the effect of the antibiotic.
- Laetrile: This cyanide-containing compound, wrongly labeled "vitamin B-17," is promoted as a cure for cancer, but FDA does not recognize it as a legitimate therapy.
- Bioflavonoids: These compounds, wrongly labeled "vitamin P," include rutin and hesperidin. They were originally thought to be more effective than vitamin C alone for treating fragile blood vessels in scurvy. Today, there is no recognized nutritional requirement for bioflavonoids, although they may enhance vitamin C absorption, and epidemiological evidence links consumption of foods rich in these substances with decreased risk from some cancers.
- Pangamic acid: This compound, wrongly labeled "vitamin B-15," has no link to nutrition and deserves no attention.

The hunt for additional compounds necessary for health will no doubt continue. As mentioned in the last chapter, since people have been maintained for years on parenteral feedings containing all the known essential nutrients without developing evidence of a nutrient deficiency, it is unlikely that any vitamin remains to be discovered. You can be sure that if a "new" compound has the potential to be a vitamin, the Food and Nutrition Board of the National Academy of Sciences will closely examine it. If it appears with the rest of the nutrients that have an RDA or ESADDI, you can be confident that the compound can be called a vitamin and is worth your attention.

CONCEPT CHECK

A variety of vitamin-like compounds are found in the body. They can be synthesized by cells using common building blocks, such as amino acids and glucose. Sometimes in disease states synthesis may not meet bodily needs, and therefore dietary intake can be crucial. The needs for dietary choline, carnitine, and taurine in certain conditions (e.g., in preterm infants or in total parenteral nutrition) are current areas of research.

Summary

1. Thiamin has a key role in carbohydrate metabolism. A deficiency will inhibit nervous system functions, primarily because nervous tissues use mostly carbohydrate for energy. Deficiencies are most likely to occur in people with alcoholism. Pork, dried beans, and enriched grains are excellent sources of thiamin.

2. Riboflavin participates in the metabolism of all energy-yielding nutrients because it plays key roles in the citric acid cycle, electron-transport chain, and fatty acid metabolism. An isolated deficiency will result in inflammation of the mouth and tongue, but it is quite unlikely that a riboflavin deficiency exists without a deficiency of other B vitamins. Dairy products and enriched grains are good sources of riboflavin.

3. Niacin is a key nutrient used in many pathways for metabolism of energy-yielding nutrients. A deficiency results in severe skin lesions, dementia, diarrhea, and eventually death. Alcoholism and the low quality of diets often consumed by those who drink excessively can lead to a deficiency. High niacin concentrations are found in the protein foods we commonly consume. The body can synthesize niacin from extra dietary intakes of the amino acid tryptophan.

4. Pantothenic acid participates in many aspects of cell metabolism, including fatty acid metabolism and the citric acid cycle. A deficiency of pantothenic acid is unlikely, since this vitamin is widely found in foods.

5. Biotin participates in synthesis of glucose production and fatty acids, and ushers the carbon skeletons of certain amino acids into the energy-producing pathways. A deficiency results in skin changes similar to an essential fatty acid deficiency. Biotin synthesis by intestinal bacteria probably suffices for some of our needs and adds to the biotin found in eggs, cheese, and peanuts.

6. Vitamin B-6 plays a vital role in protein metabolism, especially in the synthesis of nonessential (dispensable) amino acids. It also participates in the synthesis of neurotransmitters and performs other metabolic roles. Headaches, anemia, nausea, and vomiting result from a deficiency. Regular consumption of animal protein foods, cauliflower, and broccoli provides needed vitamin B-6. Megadoses of the vitamin cause destruction of nervous system tissues. Toxic effects may occur with doses of 1000 times the RDA for a few months or 250 times the RDA for a longer period.

7. Folate plays an important role in DNA synthesis. Signs of defective cell division, such as megaloblastic anemia, inflammation of the tongue, diarrhea, and poor growth, are seen in a deficiency. Pregnancy increases the demands for folate. A deficiency is most likely to occur with alcoholism. Excellent food sources are green leafy vegetables, organ meats, legumes, and fortified cereals. Since the amount of folate lost in cooking can be huge, dietary emphasis should be placed on lightly cooked vegetables. The federal government is considering fortifying flour with folate to reduce the chances of neural tube defects developing in the offspring of women deficient in folate during pregnancy.

8. Vitamin B-12 is needed for metabolizing folate and maintaining the insulation around nerves. A deficiency results in nerve destruction. Because of its relationship to folate, a deficiency of vitamin B-12 also results in the same type of megaloblastic anemia. Defective absorption of vitamin B-12 often occurs in the elderly. In such cases, monthly injections of the vitamin can be used. For others, a deficiency is unlikely because it is present in high concentrations in animal foods, which constitute a major part of our diets. Vitamin B-12 does not occur in plant foods except through minor soil contamination. Vegans need to find a supplemental source.

9. Vitamin C is needed mainly to synthesize collagen, a major protein used in building connective tissue. A vitamin C deficiency results in scurvy, which is evidenced by poor wound healing, pinpoint hemorrhages in the skin, and bleeding gums. Vitamin C also modestly enhances iron absorption and is needed for the synthesis of some hormones and neurotransmitters. Fresh fruits and vegetables, especially citrus fruits, are generally good sources. Since the amount of vitamin C lost in cooking is high, the dietary emphasis—as with folate—should be on fresh or lightly cooked vegetables. Deficiencies often occur in people with alcoholism and in elderly men whose diets lack enough fruits and vegetables. Megadoses of vitamin C often cause diarrhea and can lead to iron toxicity in some people.

10. A variety of vitamin-like compounds are found in the body. Cells synthesize them using common building blocks, such as amino acids and glucose. In disease states, synthesis may not meet needs, and therefore dietary intake becomes more critical. The use of choline, carnitine, and taurine supplementation for preterm infants and in total parenteral nutrition is currently being evaluated.

Study Questions

1. The need for certain vitamins increases as energy expenditure increases. Name two such vitamins and explain why this is the case.

2. Which two B vitamins have an endogenous source (originating within the body)? Describe how these vitamins are synthesized.

3. Explain why individual B vitamin deficiencies are rare in the United States. Which one of the eight B vitamins might be deficient in the American diet? Explain why.

4. Although folate is not known to have any toxic effects, FDA limits the amount that may be included in supplements. Why?

5. The vitamin C–deficiency disease scurvy is marked by significant signs and symptoms. Is it a good idea for Americans to take a great excess of vitamin C in an effort to avoid the possibility of a deficiency? Does the intake of vitamin C well above the RDA have any negative consequences?

6. What distinguishes the vitamin-like compound from the actual vitamins? Do their roles within the body warrant any special attention at all?

7. Draw a map of the energy-transformation pathways in the cell. Identify the sites where the B vitamins participate in specific reactions that eventually generate ATP.

8. Which vitamins are lost from cereal grains as a result of the "refining" process? By law, which vitamins are replaced in the subsequent enrichment process?

9. Name a water-soluble vitamin that has been employed as a drug for medical therapy. How does it achieve the results?

10. What factors enhance absorption of the B vitamins? What factors inhibit their absorption?

REFERENCES

1. Alaimo K and others: Dietary intake of vitamins, minerals, and fiber of persons ages 2 months and over in the United States, Third National Health and Nutrition Examination Survey, Phase 1, 1988-91, *Advance Data* 258 (Nov 14):1, 1994.

2. Brigden ML: A systemic approach to macrocytosis, *Postgraduate Medicine* 97:171, 1995.

3. Cline MJ: The molecular basis of leukemia, *New England Journal of Medicine* 330:328, 1994.

4. Collins A and others: Micronutrients and oxidative stress in the etiology of cancer, *Proceedings of the Nutrient Society* 53:67, 1994.

5. Gershoff SN: Vitamin C (ascorbic acid): new roles, new requirements? *Nutrition Reviews* 51 (Nov):313, 1993.

6. Greenwald P: Antioxidant vitamins and cancer risk, *Nutrition* 10:433, 1994.

7. Hankin JH: Role of nutrition in women's health: diet and breast cancer, *Journal of the American Dietetic Association* 93:994, 1993.

8. Hemila H, Herman ZS: Vitamin C and the common cold: a retrospective analysis of Chalmer's review, *Journal of the American College of Nutrition* 14:116, 1995.

9. Herbert V: Vitamin C supplements and disease—counterpoint, *Journal of the American College of Nutrition* 14:112, 1995.

10. Herbert VD: Folic acid and vitamin B-12. In Shils ME, and others, editors: *Modern nutrition in health and disease,* ed 8, Philadelphia, 1994, Lea & Febiger.

11. Hunter DJ, Willett WC: Diet, body build, and breast cancer, *Annual Review of Nutrition* 14:393, 1994.

12. Hwang H and others: Diet, *Helicobacter pylori* infection, food preservation and gastric cancer risk: are there new roles for preventative factors? *Nutrition Reviews* 52:75, 1994.

13. Lehninger AL and others: *Principles of biochemistry,* ed 2, New York, 1993, Worth.

14. Levine AJ: The genetic origin of neoplasia, *Journal of the American Medical Association* 273:592, 1995.

15. Machlin LJ, Sauberlich HE: New views on the function and health effects of vitamins, *Nutrition Today,* Jan/Feb 1994, p 25.

16. Moertel CG and others: High dose of vitamin C versus placebo in a treatment of patients with advanced cancer who have had no prior chemotherapy, *New England Journal of Medicine* 312:137, 1985.

17. Oeffinger KC: Scurvy: more than historical relevance, *American Family Physician* 48:609, 1993.

18. Parker PD: Premenstrual syndrome, *American Family Physician* 50:1309, 1994.

19. Picciano MF and others: The folate status of women and health. *Nutrition Today* 29:20, 1994.

20. Reynolds RD: Vitamin supplements: current controversies, *Journal of the American College of Nutrition* 13:118, 1994.

21. Rivlin RS, Dutta P: Vitamin B2 (riboflavin), *Nutrition Today* 30:62, 1995.

22. Sauberlich HE: Pharmacology of vitamin C, *Annual Review of Nutrition* 14:371, 1994.

23. Selhub J and others: Association between plasma homocysteine concentrations and extracranial carotid-artery stenosis, *New England Journal of Medicine* 332:286, 1995.

24. Tribble DL and others: Reduced plasma ascorbic acid concentrations in nonsmokers regularly exposed to environmental tobacco smoke, *American Journal of Clinical Nutrition* 58:886, 1993.

25. van der Beek EJ and others: Combinations of low thiamin, riboflavin, vitamin B$_6$ and vitamin C intake among Dutch adults (Dutch Nutrition Surveillance System), *Journal of the American College of Nutrition* 13:383, 1994.

26. Willett WC: Micronutrients and cancer risk, *American Journal of Clinical Nutrition* 59(suppl):1162S, 1994.

27. Williams RD: FDA proposes folic acid fortification, *FDA Consumer,* May 1994, p 11.

28. Zeisel SH, Blusztajn JK: Choline and human nutrition, *Annual Review of Nutrition* 14:269, 1994.

TAKE ACTION

Spotting fraudulent claims

I. Visit a health-food store and browse through its displays and magazines. Try to find as many statements about vitamins as you can that you consider fraudulent. List four of them below.

1. _____
   _____
   _____
   _____

2. _____
   _____
   _____
   _____

3. _____
   _____
   _____
   _____

4. _____
   _____
   _____
   _____

II. Then consult the most recent edition of the New York Times *Best Seller List. How many diet and nutrition books are big sellers? Look at one or two. Do they represent sound nutrition or are they mostly filled with quackery?*

_____
_____
_____
_____

Nutrition and Cancer

Cancer is currently the second leading cause of death for American adults and is projected to be the number one cause of early death in the next century, in part because as people live longer the risk of developing cancer increases. Cancer is actually many diseases; these differ in the types of cells affected and, in some cases, in the factors contributing to cancer development (Figure 13-21). For example, the factors leading to skin cancer differ from those leading to breast cancer. Similarly, the treatments for the different types of cancer may differ.

Cancer essentially represents abnormal and uncontrollable division of cells; if untreated or not treatable, it leads to death. Most cancers take the form of tumors, although not all tumors are cancers. A tumor is simply spontaneous new tissue growth that serves no physiological purpose. It can be benign, like a wart, or malignant, like most lung cancers. The terms *malignant tumor* and *malignant neoplasm* are synonymous with cancer.

Benign tumors are made up of cells similar to the surrounding normal cells and are enclosed in a membrane that prevents them from penetrating other tissues. They are dangerous only if their physical presence interferes with normal functions. A benign brain tumor, for example, can cause illness or death if it blocks blood flow in the brain. In contrast, a malignant tumor, or cancer, is capable of invading surrounding structures, including blood vessels, the lymph system, and nervous tissue. It can also spread, or **metastasize,** to distant sites via the blood and lymphatic circulation, thereby producing invasive tumors in almost any part of the body (Figure 13-22). A few cancers, such as leukemia, a form of cancer found in certain blood cells (leukocytes), don't produce a mass and so aren't properly classified as tumors. But since leukemic cells exhibit the fundamental property of rapid and inappropriate growth, they are still malignant and therefore represent a form of cancer.

Both genetics and lifestyle are potent forces that influence the risk for developing cancer.[3,6] Certain cancers tend to occur in some families more than in others. Thus persons within high-risk families are said to be genetically predisposed, or at risk for developing specific types of cancer. A genetic predisposition is especially important in development of colon cancer and some types of breast cancer. However, lifestyle is also a critical factor in most forms of cancer, as evidenced by the variation in cancer rates from country to country. The

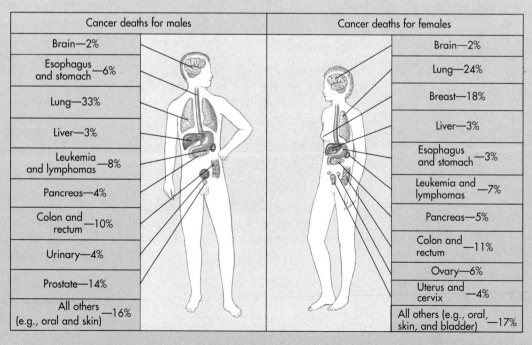

Cancer deaths for males			Cancer deaths for females
Brain—2%			Brain—2%
Esophagus and stomach—6%			Lung—24%
Lung—33%			Breast—18%
Liver—3%			Liver—3%
Leukemia and lymphomas—8%			Esophagus and stomach—3%
Pancreas—4%			Leukemia and lymphomas—7%
Colon and rectum—10%			Pancreas—5%
Urinary—4%			Colon and rectum—11%
Prostate—14%			Ovary—6%
			Uterus and cervix—4%
All others (e.g., oral and skin)—16%			All others (e.g., oral, skin, and bladder)—17%

Figure 13-21 Cancer is actually many diseases. Numerous types of cells and organs are its target. Note that about one third of all cancers arise from smoking.

Japanese, for example, have higher rates of stomach cancer than Americans, whereas Americans tend to have higher rates of colon cancer than the Japanese. When Japanese immigrate to the United States, their incidence of stomach cancer decreases but their incidence of colon cancer increases. In addition, women who have borne many children experience a reduced risk for endometrial cancer. Finally, people living in poverty show higher cancer death rates than middle- and upper-income groups, probably because of inadequate health care and deficient diets.[2]

Although we have little control over our genetic risks for cancer, we do have a great deal of choice in deciding which risks to take with respect to lifestyle, especially with regard to smoking, alcohol abuse, and nutrient intake (food choice). It is well established that one third of all cancers in the United States are due directly to tobacco use. About half of the cancers of the mouth, pharynx, and larynx are associated with heavy use of alcohol. A combination of alcohol use and smoking increases cancer risks even higher. In addition, it has become increasingly apparent that certain dietary factors either promote or inhibit cancer.[26] With diet, as with tobacco and alcohol use, imprudent choices today likely cause medical problems tomorrow.

Mechanisms of Carcinogenesis

To understand how cancer can be prevented, we first examine how cancer develops in the body. This process, termed *carcinogenesis,* involves multiple steps, starting with exposure of

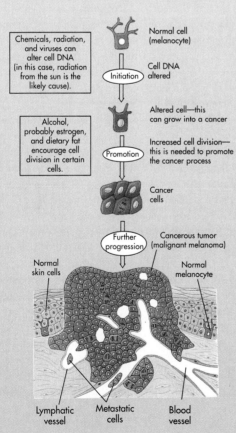

Figure 13-22 Progression from a normal skin cell to skin cancer through the initiation, promotion, and progression stages. The ball of cells is a developing tumor. As the mass of cells grows, it can invade surrounding tissues, eventually penetrating into both lymph and blood vessels. These vessels carry spreading (metastatic) cancer cells throughout the body, where they can form new cancer sites.

cancer initiation The stage in the process of cancer development that begins with alterations in DNA, the genetic material in a cell. This may cause the cell to no longer respond to normal physiological controls.

cancer promotion The stage in the cancer process when cell division increases, in turn decreasing the time available for repair enzymes to act on altered DNA and encouraging cells with altered DNA to develop and grow.

cancer progression The final stage in the cancer process, during which the cancer cells proliferate, forming a mass large enough to significantly affect body functions.

genotoxic carcinogen A compound that directly alters DNA or is converted in cells to metabolites that alter DNA, thereby providing the potential for cancer to develop.

mutation A change in the genetic material—the DNA—within a living cell. DNA, the main constituent of a cell's chromosomes, provides the coded instructions for the cell's activities. Many mutations are harmful, giving rise to cancers, birth defects, and hereditary diseases.

gene A portion of DNA that codes for, or provides the blueprint for, production of a single protein. The hereditary material in chromosomes includes thousands of genes coding for all the proteins needed by a cell.

oncogene A gene that codes for proteins that control cellular growth and development.

p53 gene A tumor-suppressor gene that can prevent inappropriate cell division.

a cell to a carcinogen, which triggers **cancer initiation.** Subsequent steps are **cancer promotion** and finally **cancer progression** (See Figure 13-22).

CANCER INITIATION AND GENOTOXIC CARCINOGENS

The initiation stage begins with alterations in regulatory or metabolically active regions of DNA, the genetic material in a cell.[3] As a result, the cell no longer responds to normal physiological controls on cell division. Initiation can develop spontaneously, or it can be induced by agents known as **genotoxic carcinogens.** The affected cell now can dictate its own rate of division and is not inhibited from doing so at the expense of surrounding cells. Alteration of DNA can occur within a few minutes to days. Among the genotoxic carcinogens that can initiate cancer development are radiant energy, chemical agents, and biological agents.

For example, radiation can alter DNA by cross-linking the double strands or breaking the strands into fragments. Damaging free radicals can also form as a result of radiation, and in turn alter DNA. As a practical example, various skin cancers often begin with overexposure to the sun. The altered skin cells may then begin to grow out of control.

Cancer can be induced by various chemicals, especially multi-ring chemicals, such as aflatoxin and benzo(a)pyrene. Aflatoxin, which is produced by molds present in peanuts and cereal grains, is a potent carcinogen for rats. For this reason, FDA regulates the amount of aflatoxin that can be present in peanut products (see Chapter 19). Rejecting moldy foods is one way to avoid possible carcinogens. Benzo(a)pyrene is formed as meat fat drips onto hot coals when foods are charcoal-broiled. If smoke containing the carcinogen penetrates the meat and the meat is consumed, benzo(a)pyrene is absorbed into the body.

Once inside body cells, these chemical carcinogens are converted to various metabolites by an enzyme system known as **cytochrome P-450.** Normally this enzyme system acts to convert compounds foreign to the body, called **xenobiotics,** into harmless, water-soluble metabolites, which are excreted. Because of the large array of xenobiotics present in food, water, and even air (tobacco smoke and other pollutants), the detoxifying activity of cytochrome P-450 is crucial for protecting the body from the potentially harmful effects of these substances. However, the action of cytochrome P-450 on aflatoxin, benzo(a)pyrene, and certain other chemicals produces highly reactive metabolites that are cancer initiators. These metabolites can attack DNA, RNA, and proteins. When the attack is on DNA, it leads to **mutations** and other genetic damage and may give rise to cancer. A few chemical carcinogens can also act directly on DNA without metabolic activation by cytochrome P-450.

Biological agents such as viruses can also initiate cancer development. Viruses contain RNA or DNA that they insert into target cells within the body. Alteration of the target-cell DNA by the viral information can transform a normal target cell into a malignant cell. When a virus invades a target cell, it in effect eventually adds **genes** to the target cell and/or alters the cell's existing genes. If the genes involved promote growth (so-called **oncogenes**), then the cell may begin to grow out of control. Human cells contain these growth-promoting oncogenes, constituting about 60 of the approximately 100,000 genes we have. Oncogenes are active during tissue growth but are turned off when growth is not indicated. If a virus turns on cell activity, an infected cell may be able to grow autonomously. However, at this stage other human genes, called tumor suppressors, may step in to prevent the abnormal growth. An important tumor-suppressor gene, *p53,* provides a check on inappropriate cellular division.[14]

If mutations cause the tumor suppressor to fail, this block against cancer development also fails. In addition, natural control of cell reproduction is destroyed. Mutations of tumor-suppressor gene *p53* have been linked to about half of all cancers. Overall, it may take one or more oncogenes plus the mutation of one or more suppressor genes for a tumor to develop.

To review, three basic agents can alter DNA: radiation, chemicals, and biological agents such as viruses. However, alteration of DNA does not necessarily mean cancer will develop. As we'll see, along with suppressor genes, some other substances also inhibit carcinogenesis.[27] In addition, special enzymes travel up and down the DNA double helix to repair breaks and correct defects.[4] About 99% of the time the repair enzymes find alterations caused by chemicals or radiation and correct them before the altered cell divides to begin its unrestrained growth. A key role of the *p53* tumor-suppressor gene is to allow time for that to take place before the next cell division.[14]

CANCER PROMOTION AND EPIGENETIC CARCINOGENS

The initiation stage of carcinogenesis, during which DNA is altered, is relatively short (minutes to days). In contrast, the promotion stage may last for months or years before the final stage, progression, appears. During the promotion stage the DNA alterations are "locked" into the genetic material of cells.

Anything that increases the rate of cell division decreases the chance that the repair enzymes will find the altered part of the DNA in time to do their work. Once a cell multiplies and incorporates its newly altered DNA into its genetic instructions, the repair enzymes can no longer detect the changes in DNA.

Compounds that increase cell division—called promoters, or **epigenetic carcinogens**—are thought to promote cancer either by decreasing the time available for repair enzymes to act or by encouraging cells with altered DNA to develop and grow.

These altered cells may develop and grow for 10 to 30 years before they become cancerous. We know this because increased lung cancer rates lagged about 30 years behind the increase in cigarette smoking that started in World War II. Common promoters are estrogen, alcohol, and probably high intakes of dietary fat.[7] Bacterial infections in the stomach are also suspected agents. Infections with *Helicobacter pylori* are associated with ulcers and may ultimately lead to stomach cancer.[12]

Studies with experimental animals have revealed that some substances, called antipromoters, can inhibit carcinogenesis during the promotion stage. Compounds present in cruciferous vegetables, onions, garlic, and citrus fruits—as well as vitamin A, vitamin D, and calcium—are thought to have antipromoter activity.[6,15,26] We discussed phytochemicals in general and their potential role in cancer prevention in the Nutrition Focus in Chapter 12. Cancer experts agree that a diet rich in fruits and vegetables is a key cancer-preventive measure.[6] Supplementation with individual nutrients, such as vitamin E and vitamin C, does not enjoy as much support, partly because this practice doesn't contribute phytochemicals, as food choices supplying these nutrients do.

CANCER PROGRESSION

The final stage in carcinogenesis begins with the appearance of cells that can grow autonomously (i.e., without normal controls on growth). During the progression stage these malignant, or cancer, cells proliferate, invade the surrounding tissue, and spread (metastasize) to other sites. Early in this stage, the immune system may find the altered cells and destroy them. Or the cancer cells may be so defective that their own DNA limits their ability to grow, and they die. If nothing impedes growth of cancer cells, one or more tumors eventually develop that are large enough to affect body functions, and signs and symptoms of cancer appear.

Diet and Cancer

Cancer quackery aside, a nutritious diet, as well as other factors related to lifestyle, can reduce the risk of cancer initiation and promotion.[4] For example, both obesity and physical inactivity are linked to an increased risk for many types of cancer.[11] Some food constituents may contribute to cancer development, whereas others have a protective effect (Table 13-2). We first discuss the association between fat/energy intake and cancer and then cover some of the food constituents that may reduce the risk for cancer.

CONTRIBUTION OF FAT AND ENERGY INTAKES TO CANCER RISK

Obesity is related to all major forms of cancer with the exception of lung cancer. This includes cancer of the breast, colon, **endometrium,** and **prostate gland.** The link probably occurs between adipose tissue and the synthesis of estrogen from other hormones in the blood. High concentrations of circulating estrogen in the blood are thought to promote cancer. A long-standing excess energy intake also may promote cancer. When animals are fed

epigenetic carcinogen A compound that increases cell division and thereby increases the chance that a cell with altered DNA will develop into cancer.

endometrium The membrane that lines the inside of the uterus. It increases in thickness during the menstrual cycle until ovulation occurs. The surface layers are shed during menstruation if conception does not take place.

prostate gland A solid, chestnut-shaped organ surrounding the first part of the urethra in the male. The prostate gland is situated immediately under the bladder and in front of the rectum. The prostate gland secretes substances into the semen as the fluid passes through ducts leading from the seminal vesicles into the urethra.

TABLE 13-2

Some food constituents suspected of having a role in cancer

Constituent	Dietary sources	Action
Possibly protective*		
Vitamin A	Liver, fortified milk, fruits, vegetables	Encourages normal cell development
Vitamin E	Whole grains, vegetable oil, green leafy vegetables	Antioxidant
Vitamin C	Fruits, vegetables	Antioxidant; can block conversion of nitrites and nitrates to potent carcinogens
Folate	Fruits, vegetables, whole grains	Encourages normal cell development
Selenium	Meats, whole grains	Part of the glutathione peroxidase antioxidant system
Carotenoids	Fruits, vegetables	Many are antioxidants; some may influence cell metabolism
Indoles, phenols and other plant substances	Vegetables, especially cabbage, cauliflower, brussels sprouts, garlic, onions, tea (especially green tea)	May reduce carcinogen activation
Dietary fiber	Whole grains, fruits, vegetables, beans	May bind carcinogens in the stool, decrease stool transit time, thus lowering risk of colon and rectal cancer
Calcium	Dairy products, green vegetables	Slows cell division in the colon, binds bile acids and free fatty acids
Omega-3 fatty acids	Cold-water fish	May inhibit tumor growth
Soy products		Phytic acid present may bind carcinogens in the intestinal tract; the genistein component may reduce growth and metastasis of malignant cells
Possibly carcinogenic		
Fats	Meats, high-fat milk and milk products, vegetable oils	Excessive body fat is linked to increased synthesis of estrogen and other sex hormones, which in excess may themselves increase the risk for cancer
Alcohol	Beer, wine, liquor	Contribute to cancers of the throat, liver, and bladder and possibly the breast. Increased cell turnover is the main mechanism
Nitrites, nitrates	Cured meats, especially ham, bacon, and sausages	Under very high temperatures will bind to amino acid derivatives to form nitrosamines, potent carcinogens
Multi-ring compounds: Aflatoxin	Formed when mold is present on peanuts and other grains	Multi-ringed compounds may alter DNA structure and inhibit its ability to properly respond to physiologic controls. Aflatoxin is linked to liver cancer; Benzo(a)pyrene is linked to stomach and other intestinal cancers
Benzo(a)pyrene	Charcoal-broiled foods, especially meats	

*Many of the actions listed for these possibly protective agents are speculative and have been verified only by animal studies.

diets high in fat or total energy, they tend to experience more cancers, especially in the colon and breast. The effect is most apparent when a carcinogen is used to deliberately initiate the cancer process, and the animals then are fed a high-fat or energy-rich diet. Fat and food energy are not considered initiators of cancer, but rather promoters.

The National Cancer Institute (NCI) believes there is a sufficient link between dietary fat and cancer, especially breast cancer, to encourage Americans to reduce fat intake. It recommends initially decreasing dietary fat to about 30% of total energy intake and eventually to 20% or less of total energy if the person is at high risk and can follow such a dietary pattern.

Some nutritionists, however, believe that the NCI has overreacted to the fat and cancer issue. Although epidemiological evidence does link fat and certain forms of cancer, the evidence is not strong. A stronger link actually exists between cancer and total energy in the diet. If rats or mice are treated with a carcinogen to promote either breast or colon cancer and then one group consumes a typical energy intake while a second group consumes a reduced energy intake, the group with the low energy intake will exhibit about a 40% reduction in tumor development. The amount of fat in the diet is not important, as long as energy intake is about 70% of the usual intake of the animals. Energy restriction is currently the most effective technique for preventing cancer in laboratory animals.

The mechanism behind this effect of total energy intake is probably hormonal. Production of the hormone ACTH is increased, and that of the sex hormones is decreased, with energy restriction. Also, corticosteroid production increases and prolactin production decreases with restricted feeding. This hormonal state inhibits tumor growth. The restricted diet may also lower estrogen production. As noted, this hormone likely promotes cancer. Slowing cell division is another possible mechanism, in turn allowing more time for any needed DNA repair.

Can we apply this evidence from animal studies to ourselves? We don't want to suffer from cancer, but very few of us want to eat only 70% of our usual energy intake. Despite the evidence of a strong link between some types of cancer and obesity, many Americans are still overweight and have not slimmed down to their desirable body weights. Further, it is very difficult to reduce dietary energy to 70% of usual intake. So while the data obtained from animal studies are interesting, nutritionists do not see any practical way to make recommendations on the basis of these studies. In addition, once cancer is present, energy restriction is no longer helpful.

CANCER-INHIBITING FOOD CONSTITUENTS

Many single nutrients may have cancer-inhibiting properties. These anticarcinogens include antioxidants, certain phytochemicals, and dietary fiber (Table 13-2).[26]

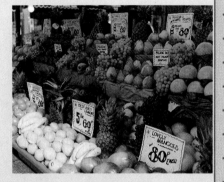

A diet rich in fruits and vegetables may reduce the risk of some forms of cancer.

The antioxidant activity of vitamin C and vitamin E helps to prevent formation of nitrosamines in the gastrointestinal tract, thus preventing formation of a potent carcinogen. Vitamin E also helps protect unsaturated fatty acids from damage by free radicals. Overall, carotenoids, vitamin E, vitamin C, and selenium function as or contribute to antioxidant systems in the body. These antioxidant systems help prevent the alteration of DNA by electron-seeking compounds.

In addition, phytochemicals from fruits and vegetables in some cases block cancer development. Numerous studies suggest that fruit and vegetable intake reduces the risk of cancers of the mouth, pharynx, larynx, esophagus, stomach, colon, rectum, bladder, and cervix. These foods are normally rich in carotenoids and vitamin C, plus dietary fiber and vitamin E. Inadequate vitamin D intake (coupled with little sun exposure) is suspected of fostering breast, colon, and prostate cancer. In sum, a diet that follows the Food Guide Pyramid, so that fruits, vegetables, whole grains, low-fat and nonfat dairy products, and some plant oils are eaten daily, is a rich source of anticarcinogens.

A current nationwide study is under way in the United States to reduce colon cancer risk. It employs a diet with fat at 20% of energy intake and 5 to 8 servings of fruits/vegetables per day. This diet also aims to provide about 30 g of dietary fiber per day.

In Chapters 3 and 6 the possible role of fiber in preventing colon cancer was introduced. Insoluble fiber decreases transit time so that the stool is in contact with the colon wall for a shorter period of time, thus reducing contact with carcinogens. Soluble fibers may bind bile acids and thus block some recycling of these by the body. Bile acids are thought to contribute to cancer risk by irritating the colon cells, in turn increasing cell division. In addition, dietary fiber (specifically the insoluble fiber content) may increase the binding and excretion of the sex hormones testosterone and estrogen from within the intestines. This is important because of the links between excessive amounts of sex hormones and certain types of cancer, specifically prostate and colon cancer. At the present time, the evidence regarding the importance of fiber in preventing colon cancer is still inconclusive. For now, the recommendation to consume 20 to 35 g a day is reasonable advice. Liberal use of whole grains, fruits, and vegetables should be sufficient to meet guidelines.

As we covered in the last chapter, cruciferous vegetables, onions, garlic, and various other plant foods contain cancer-inhibiting substances. These induce certain cellular enzymes that initiate a detoxification process for removing carcinogens from the body. Not all of the cancer-preventing chemicals in fruits and vegetables have been isolated, but candidates include those listed in Table 12-2.

Calcium is also linked to a decreased risk for developing colon cancer. As with fiber, the evidence is inconclusive. Some studies show that calcium decreases the growth of cells in the colon; therefore it probably decreases the risk of a genetically altered cell developing into a cancer. Calcium may also bind free fatty acids and bile acids in the colon, so they are less apt to interact with cells located there and induce cancer. We need more research before calcium can be promoted as a cancer-preventing agent. There are still, of course, many other important reasons for consuming the RDA for calcium (see Chapter 14).

The Bottom Line

Table 13-3 lists a variety of dietary changes that will reduce your risk for cancer. Start by making sure that your diet is moderate in energy and fat content and that you consume many fruits, vegetables, whole grains, beans, and low-fat or nonfat dairy products. In other words, follow the Food Guide Pyramid. In addition, remain physically active, avoid obesity, and moderate alcohol use. Until there is more definitive information about diet and cancer, that is all the diet-related advice we can offer.

Remember also that if a cancer is left untreated, it can spread quickly throughout the body. When this happens, it is much more likely to lead to death. Thus early detection is critical. Aids to early detection include the following warning signs:
- Unexplained weight loss
- A change in bowel or bladder habits
- A sore that does not heal
- Unusual bleeding or discharge
- A thickening or lump in the breast or elsewhere
- Indigestion or difficulty in swallowing
- An obvious change in a wart or mole
- A nagging cough or hoarseness

There are still other ways to detect cancer early. Colonoscopy examinations for middle-age and older adults, PSA (prostate-specific antigen) tests for men, and Papanicolaou tests (Pap smears) and regular breast examinations for women are recommended by the American Cancer Society.

CRITICAL THINKING

Joe is writing a report on cancer. One of the interesting facts he's discovered is that there may be a link between nutrition and certain forms of cancer. What evidence supports this hypothesis?

Moderation in consumption of char-broiled meat is advocated as part of a plan to reduce cancer risk.

TABLE 13-3

General dietary recommendations to reduce the risk of cancer*

1. Avoid obesity.
2. Reduce fat intake to 30% of total energy intake as a start. Then consider a reduction closer to 20% of total energy intake if at high risk, such as if there is much cancer in one's family history.
3. Eat more higher-fiber foods, such as fruits, vegetables, and whole-grain cereals.
4. Include foods rich in vitamins A, E, and C, as well as carotenoids, in the daily diet.
5. If alcohol is consumed, do not drink excessively.
6. Use moderation when consuming salt-cured, smoked, and nitrite-cured foods.

*The National Cancer Institute (U.S.) endorses all the above but warns not to exceed 35 g of dietary fiber intake.
The American Cancer Society endorses all the above, but sets no percentage for fat intake and adds a recommendation to include cruciferous vegetables in the diet (cabbage, broccoli, and brussels sprouts). These may decrease carcinogen activation.
The Canadian Dietetic Association generally endorses all of the above, but the specific language differs.

CHAPTER FOURTEEN

Water and the Major Minerals

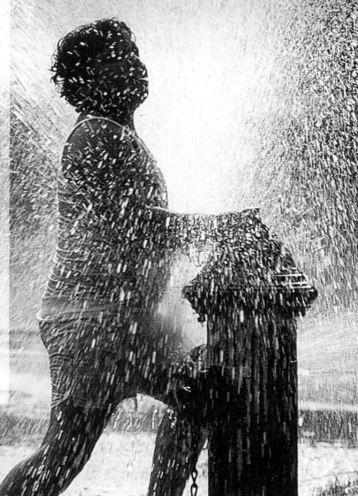

W ater—the most versatile medium for a variety of chemical reactions—constitutes the major portion of the human body.[1] Without water, biological processes necessary to life would cease in a matter of days. We operate on about 2 quarts (2 L) of water daily and must replenish it regularly because the body does not store water per se. We experience this constant demand for water as thirst. Many nutrients, including minerals, exist in the body dissolved in water. Because the functioning of minerals is related to the characteristics of water, we explore water and its roles in the body in this chapter.

Minerals, like water, are vital to health. As free atoms, they are considered inorganic because they are not bonded to carbon atoms. Minerals are key participants in body metabolism, muscle movement, body growth, and water balance, among other wide-ranging processes.[1] Some of the minerals found in our bodies—for example, vanadium and tin—may not be necessary to sustain human life. Nevertheless, we know that some mineral deficiencies can cause severe health problems. For this reason the study of minerals is critical to understanding human nutrition.

NUTRITION AWARENESS INVENTORY

Answer these 15 statements about water and the major minerals to test your current knowledge. If you think the answer is true or mostly true, circle T. If you think the answer is false or mostly false, circle F. Use the scoring key at the end of the book to compute your total score. Repeat the test after you have read this chapter, and compare your results.

1. **T F** Water is an electrolyte.
2. **T F** "Major" minerals are more important to health than "trace" minerals.
3. **T F** Vitamins often need minerals to help perform their metabolic functions.
4. **T F** Plant foods are usually the best sources of minerals.
5. **T F** You can survive longer without food than without water.
6. **T F** When water evaporates from your skin, you feel cooler because evaporating water takes heat energy with it.
7. **T F** An estimate of dietary water needs is 1 ml/kcal expended by the body.
8. **T F** You can never drink too much water.
9. **T F** Sodium is often added to processed foods.
10. **T F** Absorption of minerals is greatest when they are consumed in conjunction with high-fiber foods.
11. **T F** A preference for salty foods is partially learned.
12. **T F** Most foods in the same food group of the Food Guide Pyramid (e.g., the milk, yogurt, and cheese group) contain similar amounts of sodium.
13. **T F** Perspiration has a lower sodium concentration than blood.
14. **T F** Calcium supplements can prevent osteoporosis.
15. **T F** Alcohol intake is linked to hypertension, especially in African-Americans.

Water

To appreciate how minerals operate, the nature of water and its characteristics must be understood. Water serves as the base of operations for minerals and is the chief constituent of the human body.[11] An adult can probably survive about 8 weeks without eating food (depending on fat stores), but only a few days without drinking water. This is not because water is more important than the other nutrients, but because water as such is not stored in the body. Nor can we conserve water to a sufficient degree; regular intake is mandatory to compensate for daily losses if health is to be maintained.

The molecular structure of water is highly polar, as the positive charges tend to be located near the hydrogens and the negative charges near the oxygen:

δ denotes partial charge

Because of this, water can dissolve most substances, and in doing so enables minerals and other chemicals to react in the body. Water also lubricates joints and serves as a vehicle to transport minerals and other substances throughout the body. In addition, it is a key means of controlling body temperature and removing waste products.[11]

Water has several fascinating properties. It expands as it freezes, so that a jar full of water cracks after freezing. Water has a high heat capacity (**specific heat**), since water molecules are strongly attracted to each other. Therefore foods with high water content heat up and cool down slowly. In contrast, the molecules in fat are not strongly attracted to each other, and fats thus exhibit lower specific heat values than water. To illustrate this difference for yourself, compare the time it takes to heat water with the time it takes to heat butter in a microwave oven. Because water requires so much energy to change from a liquid to a gas, it forms an ideal medium for removing heat from the body. This will be discussed shortly.

specific heat The amount of heat required to raise the temperature of any substance 1° C compared with the heat required to raise the temperature of the same volume of water 1° C. Water has a high specific heat, meaning that a relatively large amount of heat is required to raise its temperature; therefore it tends to resist large temperature fluctuations.

FLUID AND ELECTROLYTES IN THE BODY

Since human life depends on water, it is not so surprising that we carry so much of it around within us. Looking only at the composition of our bodies, humans are not much more than an organized bag of seawater—fluid and **electrolytes.** Water accounts for between 50% and 70% of our body weight. Lean muscle tissue is composed of about 73% water.[11] At any given weight, the more body weight a person has, the less body water present. As fat content increases, the percentage of lean tissue (which is primarily water) at a given weight decreases in the body and thus total body water then drifts down toward 50%. Note that the water content of adipose tissues is negligible.

All of this water is strictly compartmentalized within the body. The presence of different fluid compartments and strict control of water movement throughout the body allow variations in electrolyte concentration and other conditions to exist in specific bodily locations.[13]

Intracellular and Extracellular Fluid

Water migrates in and out of body cells. When functioning inside cells, water is known as **intracellular fluid.** When outside cells, water is known as **extracellular fluid.** Extracellular fluid is further divided into **interstitial fluid**—water between cells—and **intravascular fluid**—water in the bloodstream (Figure 14-1).[11] Interstitial fluid forms an important transport link between tissue cells and the blood.

The ratio of intracellular to interstitial to intravascular fluid is about 25:14:3. Water shifts freely from one compartment to another. For example, if blood volume falls, water both inside and around cells can shift to the blood to increase blood volume. On the other hand, if blood volume increases, water can shift out of the blood into cells and the areas between them.[11]

Movement of Water and Ions

The body controls the amount of water in each compartment mainly by controlling the electrolyte concentrations in each compartment. In solution, electrolytes dissociate into charged particles called **ions.** Because of its polar nature, water is attracted to both positively charged and negatively charged ions. The slightly negative oxygen of water is attracted to positive sodium and potassium ions, and the slightly positive hydrogens of water are attracted to negative chloride and phosphate ions:

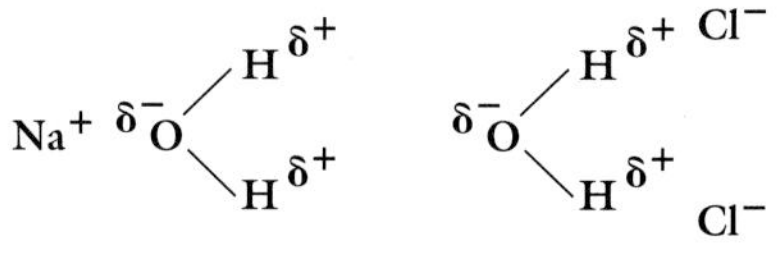

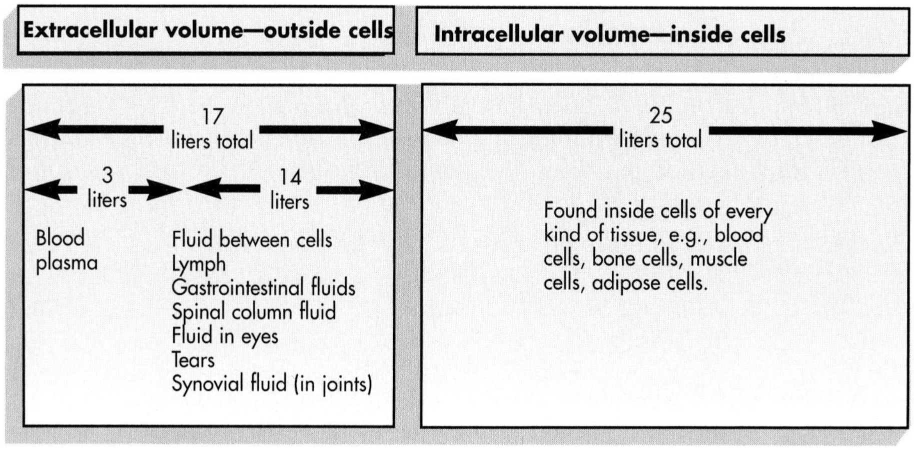

electrolyte A substance that dissolves into charged particles (ions) when dissolved in water and then is able to conduct an electrical current. The terms electrolyte and ion are commonly used interchangeably.

intracellular fluid Fluid contained within a cell.

extracellular fluid Fluid present outside the cells; it includes intravascular and interstitial fluids.

interstitial fluid Fluid between cells.

intravascular fluid Fluid within the bloodstream (that is, in the arteries, veins, and capillaries).

ion An atom or chemical group that carries a positive or negative charge. Important positive ions in cells are sodium (Na^+), potassium (K^+), magnesium (Mg^{2+}), and calcium (Ca^{2+}) ions. Important negative ions are chloride (Cl^-) and phosphate (PO_4^{3-}). Note that some ions carry multiple charges.

$$Na^+ \; {}^{\delta-}O \bigg\langle \begin{array}{c} H^{\delta+} \\ H^{\delta+} \end{array} \qquad {}^{\delta-}O \bigg\langle \begin{array}{c} H^{\delta+} \;\; Cl^- \\ H^{\delta+} \;\; Cl^- \end{array}$$

Extracellular volume—outside cells	Intracellular volume—inside cells
17 liters total ←3 liters→ ←14 liters→ Blood plasma / Fluid between cells, Lymph, Gastrointestinal fluids, Spinal column fluid, Fluid in eyes, Tears, Synovial fluid (in joints)	25 liters total Found inside cells of every kind of tissue, e.g., blood cells, bone cells, muscle cells, adipose cells.

Figure 14-1 The fluid compartments in the body.

osmosis Passive diffusion of a solvent (water) through a semipermeable membrane from a less concentrated solution to a more concentrated solution.

osmotic pressure The exerted pressure needed to keep particles in a solution from drawing liquid across a semipermeable membrane.

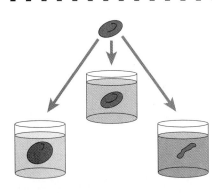

The effects of osmosis are easily demonstrated with red blood cells. When water is added to the fluid surrounding the cells, thereby diluting the fluid, water moves into the cells, causing them to expand. Conversely, when particles (e.g., ions) are added to the fluid, thereby concentrating it, water moves out of the cells, causing them to shrink.

Because of these interactions, most ions of biological importance are surrounded by a shell of water molecules. When ions move in and out of cellular compartments, their shell of water goes along with them. Thus by shifting electrolytes in and out of cellular compartments, the body can regulate the amount of water in each compartment. Where ions go, so goes water.

Much of the movement of body water results from the tendency of water to move across a semipermeable membrane so as to equalize the total particle concentration in the compartments on each side of the membrane. A semipermeable membrane is one through which water, but not particles, can pass. In the body, the particles are primarily electrolytes and the membranes are cell membranes. This passage of water (or other solvent), called **osmosis,** results in movement of water from a less concentrated to a more concentrated solution.[11]

Figure 14-2 (see next page) illustrates how osmosis works. When particles are added to the compartment on one side of a semipermeable membrane, this makes that compartment more concentrated than the other compartment. Since particles can't easily pass across the membrane, water moves by diffusion from the diluted compartment to the more concentrated compartment until their particle concentrations become identical. The term **osmotic pressure** refers to the amount of force needed to prevent dilution of the compartment containing the higher particle concentration. Examples of osmosis are sugar pulling fluid from strawberries, a salty salad dressing wilting lettuce, and red blood cells swelling or shrinking when put into solutions of different salt concentrations.

The movement of water across the membrane depicted in Figure 14-2 occurs by simple diffusion. Little of this actually occurs across cell membranes because of their high lipid content. Rather, certain proteins in cell membranes appear to act as "channels" through which water can move. In addition, cell membranes possess an extremely sophisticated gatekeeping system that makes them selectively permeable to many electrolytes as well as other compounds.[11] For example, a specific protein located in the membrane can pump potassium ions into a cell and sodium ions out (Figure 14-3). Energy is used by this sodium-potassium pump to move each of these ions against its concentration gradient. By use of such mechanisms in addition to osmotic processes, cells maintain their intracellular water volume and electrolyte concentrations within quite narrow ranges.

Positive ions, such as sodium and potassium, pair with negative ions, such as phosphate and chloride. Intracellular water volume depends primarily on intracellular potassium and phosphate concentration. Extracellular water volume depends primarily on the extracellular sodium and chloride concentration.

Besides balancing the electrolyte concentrations between the inside and outside of cells, the body must also balance electrolyte charges. If a negative electrolyte enters a cell, a positive electron must also enter the cell or another negative electrolyte must leave it.

FUNCTIONS OF WATER

Because of its unique chemical and physical characteristics, water plays several key roles in biological processes. Water functions in several ways in the body's chemical reactions: it serves as a solvent for many chemical compounds, it provides a medium in which many chemical reactions occur, and it actively participates as a reactant or product in some reactions.[11] For example, during digestion the enzyme maltase catalyzes the reaction between water and the disaccharide maltose, splitting maltose into 2 glucose molecules:

$$H_2O + maltose \xrightarrow{\text{maltase}} 2 \text{ glucose}$$

Temperature Regulation

One means by which the body loses fluid is perspiration—the evaporation of water through skin pores. Whether because of hard work, fever, exposure to heat, or merely normal metabolic reactions, an elevation of temperature within the body can

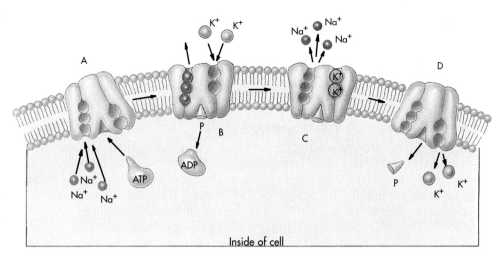

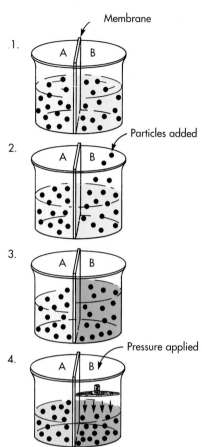

Figure 14-3 Schematic diagram of the sodium (Na^+) and potassium (K^+) pump cycle. *A,* Three Na^+ ions bind from inside the cell. *B,* The pump protein is activated by ATP. *C,* Activation causes a change of the protein form. This results in a decrease in the affinity of Na^+-binding sites and an increase in affinity of K^+-binding sites. The three Na^+ ions are then released to the outside of the cell. *D,* Two K^+ ions occupy the K^+-binding sites, and the pump protein releases the phosphate donated from ATP and returns to its original conformation. The affinity of the K^+-binding sites decreases, and that of the Na^+ sites increases. The K^+ ions are released to the cell. The pump is now ready to bind three Na^+ ions, and the cycle starts again.

Figure 14-2 A graphic representation of osmosis and osmotic pressure. *1.* An equal number of particles on each side allows equal amounts of water. *2.* Now additional particles are added to side B, but the particles cannot flow across the membrane. *3.* Water can flow across the membrane, so it flows to side B, where there are more particles. The volume of water becomes greater on side B, causing the particle concentrations on sides A and B to again become equal. *4.* If physical pressure (such as a pump) compressed the fluid on side B to restore its original volume, that pressure would equal the osmotic pressure exerted by the added particles.

be tolerated only within a very narrow range. As the amount of heat energy contained within the body increases, water in the surrounding tissues will absorb any excess heat energy. When the water absorbs sufficient heat energy, it will evaporate through the pores in the skin, in turn cooling the environment it leaves behind.[12] Each liter of perspiration lost represents approximately 600 kcal of energy lost from the skin and surrounding tissues.

Recall from Chapter 7 that about 60% of the chemical energy in food is turned directly into body heat. Only about 40% is converted to ATP energy, and almost all of that energy eventually leaves the body in the form of heat. If this heat could not be dissipated, the body temperature would rise enough to prevent enzyme systems from functioning efficiently. Perspiration is the primary way to prevent a rise in body temperature.

Removal of Waste Products

Water is an important vehicle for ridding the body of waste products. Most unwanted substances in the body are water soluble and can leave the body via the urine. In addition, liver metabolism converts some fat-soluble compounds into water-soluble compounds, so that they too can be excreted in the urine.

A major body waste product is urea, made from the amino groups ($-NH_2$) released during the breakdown of amino acids. The more protein eaten, the greater the necessity for excreting nitrogen (in the form of urea) in the urine. Likewise, the more sodium consumed, the more sodium excreted in the urine. Total urine production is primarily determined by protein and sodium chloride (salt) intake. Fluid output increases as the need to excrete more of these compounds increases. Limiting excess protein and sodium intakes reduces urine output—a useful practice, for example, in space flights.

A healthy urine volume totals at least 1 to 2 L (1 to 2 quarts) per day. More than that is fine, but less—especially less than 600 ml (2½ cups)—forces the kidneys to form a very concentrated urine. The high ion concentration of such a concentrated urine increases the risk of kidney stone formation in people susceptible to forming kidney stones. These stones are simply minerals and other substances that have precipitated out of the urine and eventually lodged in kidney tissues.

Humans tolerate hot, dry climates far better than they do hot, humid climates, because dry climates allow perspiration to evaporate, thereby cooling the skin. In hot, humid climates, not all perspiration can evaporate: some of it simply rolls off the skin or soaks into clothing. This perspiration does little to cool the body, so people just feel hot and sticky.

amniotic fluid Fluid contained in a sac within the uterus. This surrounds and protects the fetus during its development.

insensible losses Fluid losses that are not perceptible to the senses, such as losses from lungs, feces, and skin (an exception is heavy perspiration).

Other Functions of Water

Water helps form the lubricants found in knees and other joints of the body. It is the basis for saliva, bile, and **amniotic fluid.** Amniotic fluid acts as an important shock absorber surrounding the growing fetus. Electrolyte concentrations vary in each fluid compartment to accommodate specific needs, such as maintenance of a specific range in pH.

BALANCING WATER INPUT AND OUTPUT

The daily average water input and output for adults are summarized in Figure 14-4. For adults an estimated 1 ml of water is lost per kilocalorie expended. (Water needs of infants are reviewed in Chapter 17.) This works out to 2.4 L (10 cups) for an expenditure of 2400 kcal. Of this total output, about 1 L typically arises from water losses via the lungs (400 ml, or 1⅔ cups), feces (150 ml, or ⅔ cup), and skin (500 ml, or 2 cups). Since people are not normally aware of these water losses, they are called **insensible** water **losses.** The remaining water output is in the form of urine.

The loss of only 150 ml of water from feces per day is an incredible feat, considering that in addition to the 2000 ml of water (8 cups) added through the diet, about 8000 ml (33 cups) enters the gastrointestinal (GI) tract daily via secretions from the stomach, intestine, pancreas, and other organs.[11] Not too surprisingly, severe diarrhea (such as may be the result of viral or bacterial infections) can result in water losses as high as 1 L/hour.

On the input side, we consume about 1 L (4 cups) of water per day in various liquids (Figure 14-4). A fluid intake of about 8 cups per day is advocated by some

Water quality is a growing concern for many of us. People who have **AIDS** or other diseases that compromise function of the immune system (e.g., cancer, organ transplant therapy) are advised to boil tap water to rid it of potential *Cryptosporidium* (a parasite) contamination. Boiling for 1 minute is sufficient. Alternatively, one can purchase a water filter (call 800-673-8010 for a list of manufacturers). For most healthy Americans, water quality is satisfactory, but the water in some communities fails to meet EPA standards. Residents of these communities should also consider using a water filter. One's local water department can help in making this decision.

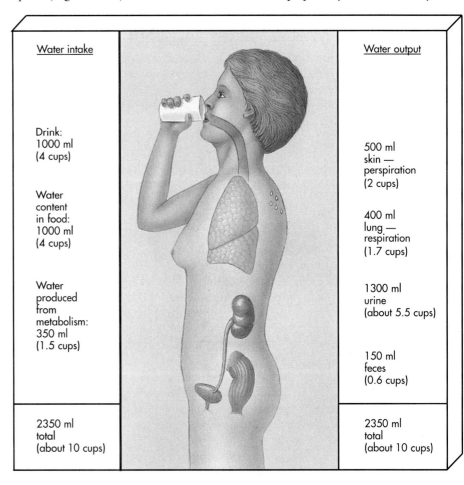

Figure 14-4 Water balance—intake versus output. We maintain body fluids at an optimum amount by adjusting water intake and output. Most water comes from the liquids we consume. Some comes from the moisture in more solid foods, and the remainder is manufactured during metabolism. Water output includes that lost via lungs, kidneys, skin, and bowels.

health authorities. Foods supply another liter of fluid, as many are primarily water (Figure 14-5). Finally, metabolism provides approximately 350 ml (1½ cups) of water, primarily as a by-product of energy transformation reactions. If we assume a fluid intake of 1 L, adding these other sources yields a total input of about 2.4 L (10 cups), a value close to estimates of water output (needs) based on a typical energy expenditure of 2400 kcal. If water input is greater or less than that needed to replace water losses, then the urine volume can be adjusted within certain limits to achieve water balance.

Thirst: Signal of Water Deprivation

If a person doesn't consume enough water, the hypothalamus in the unconscious brain signals to higher brain centers that the body needs water; as a result, the person feels thirsty. The sensation of thirst, however, is not a sensitive signal of fluid depletion and doesn't begin until somewhat after water losses have started to exceed intake. Moreover, thirst can be an unreliable signal and may not operate in people who are sick, elderly, or engaging in vigorous athletic events.[13] We have already mentioned in Chapter 10 that athletes should weigh themselves before and after training sessions to determine their rate of water loss and thus their extra water needs.

Children who are ill, especially those with fever, diarrhea, and increased perspiration, need to be reminded to drink plenty of fluid. Elderly people in general, and especially those in hospitals and nursing homes, should also be reminded to consume enough fluids, as well as have fluid intake and output monitored if necessary (see Chapter 18). Again, thirst alone is not a sufficient marker for fluid status. One other situation that demands extra fluid for the body is a long airplane flight: a traveler can lose approximately 1.5 L (6 cups) of water during a 3-hour flight. The dehumidified air in the airplane is so dry that excessive "insensible" perspiration and evaporation occur.

Water-Conservation Mechanisms

When the body registers a shortage of available water, fluid conservation increases. The pituitary gland releases **antidiuretic hormone (ADH).** This causes the kidneys to conserve water. As its name implies, ADH slows diuresis (urine flow).[11]

In addition, as fluid volume drops in the bloodstream, blood pressure falls. This fall initiates a sequence of events beginning in the kidneys. Signaled by highly sensitive pressure receptors, the kidneys release an enzyme called **renin.** Renin, in turn, activates a circulating blood protein called angiotensinogen to form **angiotensin I,** a polypeptide. Angiotensin I is converted to **angiotensin II,** which, among other effects, triggers the adrenal glands to release the hormone **aldosterone.** This hormone in turn signals the kidneys to retain more sodium and, therefore, more water (Figure 14-6).[13] Remember that water always follows electrolytes. Thus low blood pressure, through this roundabout measure using the kidneys, causes increased water conservation in the body.

The effectiveness of ADH and aldosterone in conserving body water is limited. Fluid is constantly lost via the insensible routes—feces, skin, and lungs. These losses, too, must be replaced. In addition, urine can become only so concentrated. Eventually, if fluid is not consumed, the body becomes dehydrated and can suffer ill effects, such as constipation and kidney stones. Even more serious effects can happen in athletes, notably heatstroke (see Chapter 10).[13]

Effects of Dehydration

By the time fluid losses equal 2% of body weight, a person will be thirsty. At a 3% loss of body weight, muscles undergo a significant drop in strength and endurance. Once body weight is reduced by 10% to 12%, heat tolerance decreases and the person feels very weak. At a 20% reduction, the person may lapse into a coma and die shortly thereafter.[13] The various effects of dehydration are outlined in Figure 14-7 (p. 495).

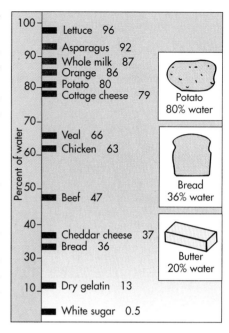

Figure 14-5 Water content of various foods as a percentage of total weight. Many foods consist primarily of water.

antidiuretic hormone (ADH) A hormone secreted by the pituitary gland that acts on the kidneys to cause a decrease in water excretion.

renin An enzyme formed in the kidneys in response to low blood pressure; it acts on a blood protein to produce angiotensin I.

- - - - - - - - - -

Alcohol inhibits the action of ADH. One reason people feel so weak the day after heaving drinking is that they are very dehydrated. Even though they may have consumed a lot of liquid in their drinks, they have lost even more liquid because alcohol has inhibited ADH. Caffeine also produces a diuretic effect on the body.

- - - - - - - - - -

aldosterone A hormone produced in the adrenal glands that acts on the kidneys, causing them to retain sodium and, therefore, water.

CRITICAL THINKING

Stacy has been working in the yard with her brother Tom. They have been busy mowing the lawn and pulling weeds since noon. Tom tells Stacy that he is feeling weak and has a headache. Stacy is concerned that her brother might be somewhat dehydrated. How can his symptoms be explained? How could Tom's risk of dehydration have been decreased?

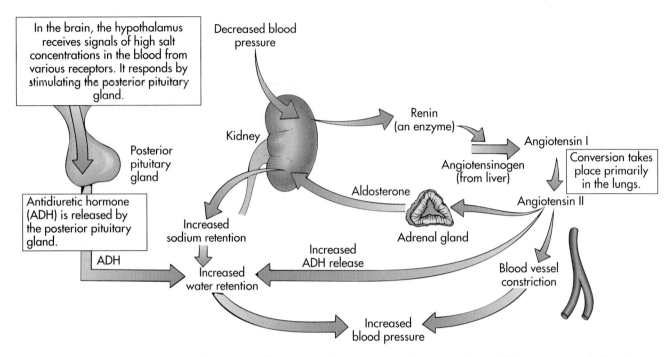

Figure 14-6 The renin-angiotensin system is one regulator of blood pressure. It functions with antidiuretic hormone to control blood pressure.

Water Intoxication

Strange as it may seem, water can be toxic if the amount of water taken in exceeds the kidneys' ability to excrete it. Water intoxication is most likely to occur if water intake is not accompanied by sufficient electrolytes. Healthy individuals, however, would have to drink a really excessive amount of water—approaching many liters (quarts) a day—before showing any signs of water intoxication.

People with certain diseases or mental disorders (e.g., schizophrenia) are most susceptible to water intoxication. If this occurs, the electrolyte concentration in extracellular fluids becomes dangerously diluted, causing water to enter cells from the extracellular fluid or causing potassium to leave cells. The imbalance in electrolytes and fluid content seen in various tissues in turn leads to headache, blurred vision, cramps, and eventually convulsions.

Water intoxication also can occur in infants fed large quantities of fluid low in electrolytes. This sometimes happens in newborns when first taken home if parents are not aware of proper care for newborns, during treatment for diarrhea, or as a result of feeding a formula that is too dilute (see Chapters 16 and 17).

CONCEPT CHECK

Since the body can neither readily store nor entirely conserve water, we can survive only a few days without it. Water functions as a solvent, a medium for chemical reactions, a thermoregulator, and a lubricant. Water constitutes 50% to 70% of body weight and is prevalent in lean tissue, intracellular and extracellular fluid, urine, and all other body fluids. For adults, water needs can be estimated as 1 ml/kcal expended. Thirst is the body's first sign of dehydration. If the thirst mechanism is faulty, as it may be during illness or vigorous physical activity, hormonal mechanisms also help conserve water. Excess fluid intake can be toxic.

Minerals: An Overview

Minerals are categorized based on the amount we need per day. Generally speaking, if we require 100 mg (¹⁄₅₀ of a teaspoon) or more per day of a mineral, it is consid-

NORMAL WEIGHT

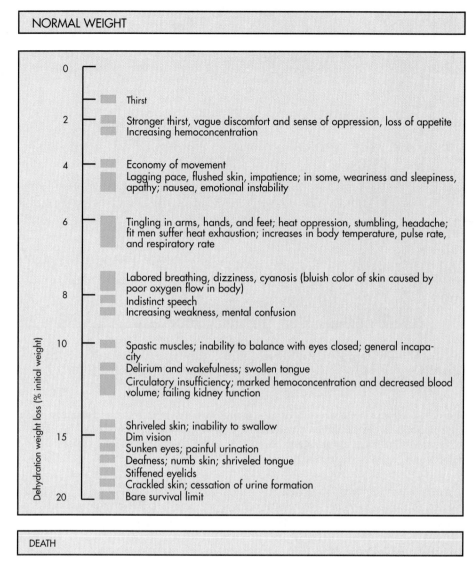

Figure 14-7 The effects of dehydration range from thirst to death, depending on the extent of body weight loss.

ered a **major mineral;** otherwise, it is considered a **trace mineral.** Using these criteria, calcium and phosphorus are major minerals and iron and zinc are trace minerals. However, although the total amount of all trace minerals in the body is less than 15 g (½ ounce), these nutrients are very important (Figure 14-8).

We discuss the roles and nutritional significance of the major minerals in this chapter and cover the trace minerals in the next. Before examining the properties of the individual major minerals, we consider some topics relevant to all the minerals.

FUNCTIONS OF MINERALS IN THE BODY

The various minerals exhibit a diverse array of metabolic roles. At all levels of human physiological organization—cellular, tissue, organ, and whole organism—minerals are critical to maintaining body functions.

Some minerals, such as magnesium and manganese, enable enzymes to function. Others are key components of important body compounds. For example, iodide is a component of the hormone thyroxine, and iron is a component of hemoglobin in the red blood cell. The ion forms of some minerals, such as sodium, potassium, calcium, and chloride, contribute to electrical balance throughout the body, aid in water balance, function in the transmission of nerve impulses and muscle contraction, and perform a multitude of other important roles. Finally, some minerals, such as

major mineral A mineral vital to health that is required in the diet in amounts greater than 100 mg/day.

trace mineral A mineral vital to health that is required in the diet in amounts less than 100 mg/day.

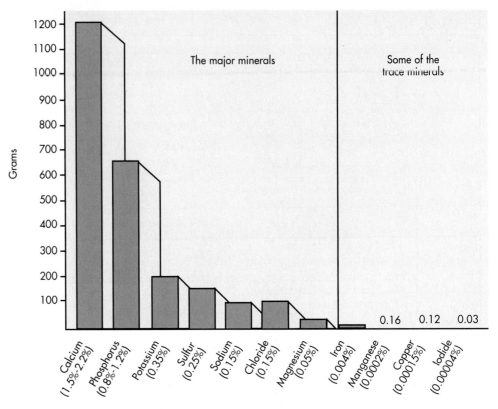

Figure 14-8 Approximate amounts of various minerals present in the average human body. The percent values in parentheses indicate the amounts as percentages of body weight. Other trace minerals of nutritional importance not listed include chromium, fluoride, molybdenum, selenium, and zinc.

calcium and phosphorus, have critical roles in the growth, development, and structural integrity of bones.[11]

MINERAL BIOAVAILABILITY

bioavailability The degree to which the amount of an ingested nutrient is absorbed and thus is available to the body.

Although we can obtain the entire gamut of minerals from dietary sources, variations in the **bioavailability** of minerals in different foods make it difficult to determine exactly how much in a specific food can be absorbed by the body. The bioavailability of a particular mineral—that is, its ability to be absorbed from the diet—depends on many factors. Thus the mineral values for a particular food listed in food consumption tables may not reflect the true contribution that food makes to our mineral needs. A significant factor determining the degree to which a mineral may be absorbed is the physiological need for that mineral at the time of consumption. Other factors are discussed below.

Mineral-Mineral Interactions

Many minerals have similar molecular weights and charges (valences). Magnesium, calcium, iron, and copper can exist in the 2+ valence state. Having similar size and the same charge causes these minerals to compete with each other for absorption, thereby affecting each other's bioavailability and metabolism.[27] Because of such interactions, individual mineral supplements should be taken only when specifically warranted, such as when a diet is chronically deficient in calcium. Still, despite the benefit in this instance, calcium supplements can reduce iron absorption. In this case, a calcium supplement should not be taken at meals that include the best iron sources, or the supplement should be taken between meals (see later discussion for more details).

We also know that the presence of a large amount of zinc in the digestive tract decreases copper absorption. If medically needed, oral zinc can even be used to minimize copper absorption. Such medical uses of mineral interactions are not typical, however, and generally they are not desirable.

Vitamin-Mineral Interactions

When consumed in conjunction with vitamin C, absorption of certain forms of iron improves. The vitamin D hormone calcitriol improves calcium absorption. Many vitamins require specific minerals to act as key components in their structure and function. For example, the thiamin coenzyme requires magnesium or manganese to function efficiently.[11]

Dietary Fiber–Mineral Interactions

Mineral bioavailability can be affected by nonmineral dietary substances as well. Phytic acid in grain fibers binds minerals, limiting their absorption, as does the oxalic acid in spinach and other vegetables. High-fiber diets—especially those rich in wheat bran—are known to decrease the absorption of iron, calcium, zinc, magnesium, and probably other minerals. In diets that contain more than 35 g of dietary fiber, decreased mineral absorption may occur to a problematic extent. We know very little about the long-term effects of very-high-fiber diets on mineral status in the body. Recognizing this, scientists are actively researching the area. We advise you not to over-consume dietary fiber—stick to the recommendation of up to 35 g/day, unless a physician recommends otherwise and provides close supervision.

If grains are leavened with yeast, as they are in bread, enzymes produced by the yeast can break some of the bonds between phytic acid and minerals. This increases mineral absorption. The zinc deficiencies found among some Middle Eastern populations can be attributed partly to low dietary zinc and partly to their use of unleavened breads. Phytic acid binds so much of the zinc from unleavened bread that little zinc is absorbed (see Chapter 15).

FOOD SOURCES OF MINERALS

Plant foods are good sources of trace minerals such as copper, molybdenum, selenium, and chromium; in general, however, the best dietary sources of many minerals are animal products, especially seafood. This is true mainly because minerals are more concentrated in animal tissues than in plant tissues. As an animal eats plants year after year, minerals from the plants concentrate in the animal's body tissues. Likewise, sea animals, such as clams, oysters, and shrimp, concentrate the minerals found in seawater as they take up copious amounts of sea water throughout their lives. Minerals in animal foods are also more bioavailable than those in plant foods because there are fewer mineral-binding substances in animal foods than in plant foods.

A diet devoid of animal products is very likely to be marginal in the major mineral, calcium, and in some trace minerals such as iron and zinc. A key exception is magnesium, which is far more plentiful in plant than in animal foods. Otherwise, some plant foods are good, but not excellent, sources of many minerals. Vegans need to be aware of this and regularly choose good plant sources of minerals (see Chapter 5).

MINERAL TOXICITY

Excess mineral intakes can easily lead to toxicity. As we cover each of the minerals in detail, it will become clear that toxicity is yet another reason to carefully consider the use of mineral supplements. Miners have suffered the ill effects of excessive mineral intake, especially of manganese. Selenium can also cause many toxic side effects (see Chapter 15). Mineral supplements exceeding 150% of the Daily Value on the label should be taken only under a physician's supervision, since toxicity and deleterious nutrient interactions are a distinct possibility.

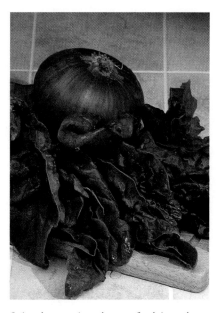

Spinach contains plenty of calcium, but only about 5% of it can be absorbed because of the vegetable's high concentration of oxalic acid. Usually, about 30% of calcium is absorbed from foods.

CONCEPT CHECK

Many minerals are vital to health, though our needs for some remain uncertain. The bioavailability of minerals depends on many factors, including a body's need for the mineral and the mineral's interaction with fiber as well as other minerals. Taking an individual mineral supplement can greatly affect the absorption and metabolism of others. Animal products are generally rich sources of minerals. Excess mineral intakes can easily lead to toxicity. This is another reason to carefully consider supplementation with any mineral.

Sodium

We both crave and hear warnings about sodium (Na) and its primary dietary source, table salt. This warning is partly justified, but some sodium intake is essential for health.

FUNCTIONS OF SODIUM

Almost all dietary sodium is absorbed. Its role within the body is primarily as the major positive ion (Na$^+$) in extracellular fluid. As such, it is one key for retaining water in that compartment, using the process of osmosis that we covered earlier. Fluid balance throughout the body depends partly on the various sodium concentrations found in body water compartments.[13] In addition, sodium participates in absorption of other nutrients (e.g., glucose) in the small intestine.

Sodium ions play a crucial role in conduction of nerve impulses.[11] Under resting conditions, when no impulses are being conducted, a small electric potential—called the resting potential—exists across the membrane of nerve cells, with the intracellular side having a negative charge and the extracellular side a positive charge.

Normally, the concentration of sodium ions is much higher outside cells than inside cells, whereas the concentration of potassium ions is much higher inside cells than outside cells. Certain stimuli can trigger opening of sodium channel proteins in the membrane of a nerve cell, allowing sodium ions (Na$^+$) to rush into a cell down the sodium concentration gradient. The movement of sodium ions causes reversal of the membrane potential, termed **depolarization.** This in turn triggers opening of other channel proteins through which potassium ions (K$^+$) move out of the cell down the potassium concentration gradient. The movement of potassium ions out of the cell returns the membrane potential to its resting value, and the nerve cell is ready to "fire" again. This temporary change in membrane potential that results, called the *action potential,* then moves along the length of a nerve, thus propagating the impulse.

Only a few sodium and potassium ions cross the membrane during a single action potential. After passage of numerous action potentials, however, the intracellular and extracellular concentrations of sodium and potassium ions would tend to become equal, thus abolishing the membrane potential. To prevent this, nerve cells employ the sodium-potassium pump discussed earlier (Figure 14-3). In a process requiring 1 ATP molecule, 3 Na$^+$ ions are pumped out of a cell and 2 K$^+$ ions are pumped in. The action of this pump thus maintains the usual ion concentrations inside (K$^+$ > Na$^+$) and outside (Na$^+$ > K$^+$) of nerve cells.[11]

SODIUM BALANCE IN THE BODY

A low-sodium diet coupled with high perspiration losses or diarrhea depletes the body of sodium. This state can lead to muscle cramps, nausea, vomiting, and dizziness and eventually to shock and coma. The kidneys are the major organs to respond to this depletion. They begin a variety of reactions that eventually triggers the release of the hormone aldosterone, as previously mentioned (Figure 14-6). Aldosterone then increases sodium retention by the kidneys.[13]

CRITICAL THINKING

Mrs. Massa has recently seen and heard a lot about the amount of salt (sodium) in foods. She has been surprised by the number of articles that advise the public to decrease the amount of salt in their food. If sodium is such a bad thing, Mrs. Massa wonders, why do you need to have any at all? How would you explain this to her?

depolarization Reversal of membrane potential, which triggers generation of the action potential in nerve and muscle cells.

To assess the sodium, potassium, chloride, magnesium, or phosphorus status of a person, blood concentrations can be measured. We will point out other methods, often more sensitive ones, when appropriate.

Sodium depletion is very unlikely, even when perspiration loss is high, because our diets contain ample sodium and the body stores considerable amounts of this nutrient. Only when weight loss from perspiration exceeds 3% of total body weight (or about 5 to 6 pounds) should sodium losses raise concern. Even then, merely salting foods is sufficient to restore body sodium for most people. Endurance athletes, however, may need to consume sports drinks during competition to avoid depletion of sodium and other electrolytes (see Chapter 10).

The concentration of sodium in perspiration (about 2 g/L) is only two thirds that in blood (about 3 g/L). The salty taste of perspiration on the skin is not caused by a high sodium concentration; rather, as perspiration evaporates from the skin, concentrated sodium is left behind.

SODIUM IN FOODS

About one third to one half the sodium we consume is added during cooking or at the table. Most of the rest is added during food manufacturing (Table 14-1). Most foods are naturally low in sodium; milk is one exception. The more "made-from-scratch" food choices in your diet, the more control you'll have over your sodium intake.

Major contributors of sodium to our diets (partly due to the frequency of consumption) are white bread, rolls, hot dogs, luncheon meats, cheese, soups, and spaghetti with tomato sauce. Other foods especially high in sodium are processed tomato-based products in general, salted snack foods, french fries, potato chips, sauces, and gravies (Figure 14-9).

You can't always rely on the salty taste of a food as an indicator of actual sodium content—tomato-based products are a prime example. Not too surprisingly, many condiments also contain large amounts of sodium, as salt makes many foods taste better.

When evaluating condiments, sauces, and seasonings, look first for the word *sodium*. The following are high in sodium: onion salt, celery salt, garlic salt, seasoned salt, baking powder, sea salt, salad dressings, pickles, soy sauce, steak sauce, barbecue sauce, meat tenderizer, baking soda, salt pork, brine, chili sauce, catsup, mustard, Worcestershire sauce, bouillon, monosodium glutamate (MSG), and relish.

TABLE 14-1

Increase in sodium content of foods during processing*

Food category	Sodium (mg)
Dairy products	
Fruited yogurt, ¾ cup	107
2% milk, 1½ cups	182
Cheddar cheese, 1¾ oz	307
American cheese food, 2 oz	548
Meats	
Beef roast, 1 oz	17
Beef jerky, ⅔ oz	540
Pork loin, 1 oz	22
Bacon, 2 pieces	202
Ham, 1½ oz	564
Vegetables	
Fresh peas, 1 cup	5
Frozen peas, 1 cup	139
Frozen peas in cheese sauce, ⅔ cup	205
Canned peas, 1 cup	372
Grain products	
Flour, ⅓ cup	1
Bread, 2 slices	286
Saltine crackers, 12	486

*All examples in a particular group contain the same amount of food energy.

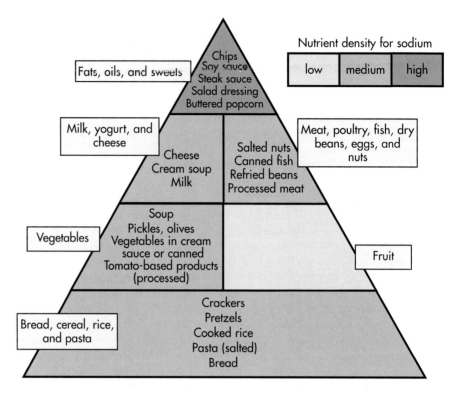

Figure 14-9 Food sources of sodium from the Food Guide Pyramid. All groups except fruit contain foods that are rich sources of this nutrient, most of which is added in food processing. The background color of each food group indicates the average nutrient density for sodium in that group. The salt shaker can add considerably more sodium, depending on use.

If we ate only unprocessed foods and added no salt, our sodium intake would be about 500 to 1000 mg/day. Since the actual intakes typical for Americans range from 3000 to 6000 mg (or more) per day,[2] food processing and cooking clearly contribute a considerable amount to our dietary sodium.

The actual sodium content of a food is listed on the Nutrition Facts panel of its label. In addition, various descriptive terms relating to sodium content may appear elsewhere on labels. Some terms defined by FDA are as follows[16]:

Sodium-free or *salt-free:* less than 5 mg of sodium per serving
Very low sodium: 35 mg or less per serving for servings greater than 30 g or 2 tablespoons. If the serving size is smaller, the standard is 35 mg or less of sodium per 50 g of food.
Low-sodium: 140 mg or less per serving if the serving is greater than 30 g or 3 tablespoons. If the serving size is smaller, the standard is 140 mg or less of sodium per 50 g of food.
Light in sodium: at least 50% less sodium per serving than average reference amount for the same food with no sodium reduction.
Reduced or less sodium: at least 25% less per serving than reference food.

See the Nutrition Perspective in Chapter 2 for further definitions.

Many medicines contain sodium, and they must be limited if dietary sodium is restricted. Similarly, when sodium is severely restricted, contributions from tap water (especially softened water) must be considered.

MINIMUM AND RECOMMENDED SODIUM INTAKES

The minimum sodium requirement for health is 500 mg/day for adults. (Throughout this chapter, see the inside cover for other age groups and Appendix E for Canadian recommendations. Chapter 2 reviews the concept of minimum requirements for health.) This is a generous amount considering that we really need only about 100 mg/day. Under FDA food-labeling rules, the Daily Value for sodium is 2400 mg. FDA established this value because it is consistent with recommendations and government reports that encourage reduced sodium intakes.[16]

Table salt is 40% sodium and 60% chloride. So an intake of 3 to 6 g of sodium per day corresponds to 7.5 to 15 g of salt (1½ to 3 teaspoons). Note that a teaspoon of salt contains about 2 g of sodium (a teaspoon of most dry substances equals approximately 5 g).

Most humans can adapt to various dietary salt intakes in terms of blood pressure regulation. However, for the approximately 10% to 15% of American adults who are sodium sensitive, high sodium intakes can contribute to hypertension (high blood pressure). For these people, diets lower in sodium (about 2 to 3 g, or about ½ teaspoon daily) often help in correcting the hypertension (see the Nutrition Perspective). Many scientific groups suggest that all adults should limit daily sodium intake to 2.4 to 3 g, mostly to limit the risk of developing hypertension in the future (Figure 14-10). The Dietary Guidelines recommend using salt and sodium only in moderation.

You can evaluate your sodium habits by completing the questionnaire in Table 14-2. The more checks in the "often" or "regularly" columns, the higher your dietary sodium intake. However, not all the habits in the table contribute the same amount of sodium. For example, many natural cheeses are relatively moderate in sodium, whereas processed cheeses and cottage cheese are much higher. You can choose to reduce your sodium intake by cutting back on those items for which you checked "often" or "regularly." You needn't suddenly eliminate foods from your diet. Rather, to moderate sodium intake, choose lower-sodium foods from each food group more often and balance high-sodium food choices with low-sodium ones. It is also important to pay attention to the sodium values listed on food labels. In addition, when eating out, avoiding foods commonly prepared with lots of sodium and asking to have sauces served on the side and then using only small amounts is a good idea.

Some experts, however, argue that there is no justification for the recommendation that salt intake be restricted in the general population to avert hypertension that may develop in the future. They suggest caution in issuing nationwide recommendations to reduce dietary sodium intake, preferring instead to provide advice on an individual basis, especially to people with hypertension who are also salt sensitive.[6] In addition, as we cover in the Nutrition Perspective, the possible contribution of inadequate intakes of potassium, calcium, and magnesium to hypertension also deserves consideration.

Many people who decide to lower their sodium intake eventually adapt to a low-sodium diet. Initially this may be easier with mixed dishes than with single foods, such as mashed potatoes.[1] Some foods in particular will taste quite bland, such as

Later in this chapter we note that sodium increases urinary calcium loss as it is excreted, providing another reason to control sodium intake.

BEETLE BAILEY

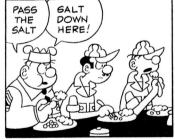
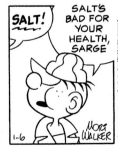
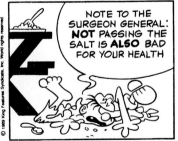

Figure 14-10 Beetle Bailey.

TABLE 14-2

Questionnaire for evaluating your sodium habits

	Rarely	Occasionally	Often	Regularly (daily)
How often do you:				
1. Eat cured or processed meats, such as ham, bacon, sausage, frankfurters, and other luncheon meats?	☐	☐	☐	☐
2. Choose canned or frozen vegetables with sauce?	☐	☐	☐	☐
3. Use commercially prepared meals, main dishes, or canned or dehydrated soups?	☐	☐	☐	☐
4. Eat cheese, especially processed cheese?	☐	☐	☐	☐
5. Eat salted nuts, popcorn, pretzels, corn chips, or potato chips?	☐	☐	☐	☐
6. Add salt to cooking water for vegetables, rice, or pasta?	☐	☐	☐	☐
7. Add salt, seasoning mixes, salad dressings, or condiments—such as soy sauce, steak sauce, catsup, and mustard—to foods during preparation or at the table?	☐	☐	☐	☐
8. Salt your food before tasting it?	☐	☐	☐	☐
9. Ignore labels for sodium content when buying foods?	☐	☐	☐	☐
10. Choose foods at restaurants with sauces, or foods that are obviously salty when dining out?	☐	☐	☐	☐

The more checks you have in the last two columns, the higher your dietary sodium intake.

Adapted from USDA Home and Garden Bulletin No. 232-6, April 1986.

unsalted cheese, but in time the threshold of the tongue's salt receptors will decrease, so they will respond to less salt. Overall, by slowly reducing dietary sodium and substituting garlic, oregano, lemon juice, and other herbs and spices, individuals can develop a flavorful diet that has only 2 to 3 g of sodium per day. Many newer cookbooks contain recipes for flavorful low-sodium foods. Except for yeast breads, omitting salt from food preparation can still yield an excellent product. For some people, this low-sodium approach to eating makes the difference between normal blood pressure and hypertension.

CONCEPT CHECK

Sodium is the major positive ion in the extracellular fluid. It is important for maintaining fluid balance and conducting nerve impulses. Sodium depletion is unlikely, since our diets have abundant sources and most sodium consumed is absorbed. The more foods we prepare at home, the more control we have over our sodium intakes. For adults the minimum sodium requirement for health is 500 mg/day. The average American consumes 3 to 6 g or more daily. About 10% to 15% of Americans are sensitive to sodium in the diet and may develop hypertension as a result of high sodium intakes. To try to correct this hypertension, they can limit sodium intake to about 2 to 3 g/day. Some scientific groups suggest that limiting sodium intake to this amount may reduce the risk for future hypertension in those who currently have normal blood pressure.

Potassium

Potassium (K) performs many of the same functions as sodium. Unlike sodium, which is found primarily outside cells as sodium ions (Na^+), potassium is found mostly inside cells as potassium ions (K^+). About 95% of the potassium in the body is in the intracellular fluid. Potassium participates in maintaining the body's fluid balance and works with sodium in conduction of nerve impulses, as discussed earlier.[11] Unlike sodium, which tends to raise blood pressure in some people, potassium is more associated with reducing blood pressure.[3] In addition, some of the enzymes that participate in energy metabolism function more efficiently when they are bound to potassium.

POTASSIUM DEFICIENCY

Although the body absorbs about 90% of the potassium consumed, we rarely add potassium to foods. For this reason, a potassium deficiency is more likely than a sodium deficiency. Potassium stores may be depleted in some disease states, such as long bouts of vomiting or diarrhea. A continually limited food intake, as may occur in alcoholism, can also result in a potassium deficiency.

Low blood potassium (hypokalemia) is a life-threatening condition. It often results in a loss of appetite, muscle cramps, confusion and apathy, and constipation. Eventually, the heart will beat irregularly, decreasing its capacity to pump blood.

POTASSIUM IN FOODS

Foods with the highest nutrient density for potassium (mg/kcal) are leafy greens (such as spinach), squash, asparagus, broccoli, cantaloupe, oranges and orange juice, potatoes, and legumes (e.g., lima beans, pinto beans, and kidney beans). Milk, whole grains, bananas, and meats are also good sources of potassium (Figure 14-11). Major contributors of potassium to the American diet include coffee, tea, milk, potatoes (french fries and other potato products), and orange juice.

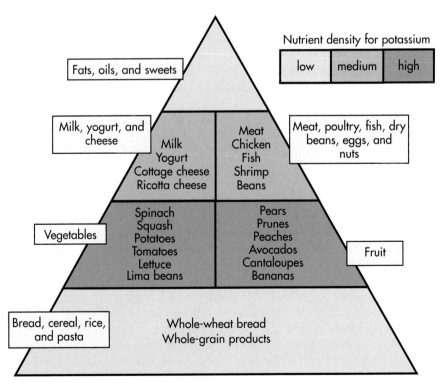

Figure 14-11 Food sources of potassium from the Food Guide Pyramid. The fruit group and the vegetable group are the best dietary sources of this nutrient, but it is widely distributed in foods. The background color of each food group indicates the average nutrient density for potassium in that group.

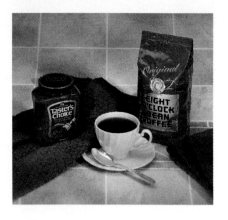

Coffee is a major contributor of potassium to the American diet.

The Daily Value for potassium used for food labels is 3500 mg. Information about a food's potassium content is required on the Nutrition Facts panel only if the food contains added potassium as a nutrient or if claims about this nutrient appear on the label. In all other cases, it is voluntary. Label descriptors for potassium and their definitions include the following[16]:

High-potassium: 700 mg or more per serving
Good source of potassium: 350 mg to 665 mg per serving
More or added potassium: at least 350 mg more per serving than reference food

MINIMUM POTASSIUM REQUIREMENT

The minimum potassium requirement for health for adults is 2000 mg (2 g) per day. Daily intakes in the United States average 2 to 3 g; women consume closer to the lower amount.[2]

AMERICANS AT RISK FOR POTASSIUM DEFICIENCY

People who take potassium-wasting diuretics, such as thiazides and furosemide, need to monitor their potassium intakes carefully. These medicines are used chiefly to control hypertension (see the Nutrition Perspective), but in the process they deplete body potassium, along with other electrolytes. Water follows the excreted electrolytes, eventually reducing blood volume and blood pressure. In such cases, high-potassium foods (e.g., fruits, fruit juices, and vegetables) are good additions to the diet. In more serious deficiencies, potassium chloride supplements may even be recommended by a physician.

Several other groups are at risk for potassium deficiency and need monitoring of blood potassium. The inadequate diet and frequent vomiting of those with anorexia nervosa or bulimia nervosa often lead to potassium deficiency. People on very-low-calorie diets (see the Expert Opinion in Chapter 9) or who just eat very little food are also at risk, as well as athletes undergoing heavy exertion. These people can avoid the detrimental side effects of low blood potassium by consuming potassium-rich food sources.

TOXICITY OF POTASSIUM

If the kidneys function normally, typical intakes of dietary potassium are not toxic. When the kidneys function poorly, potassium builds up in the blood, creating a condition called hyperkalemia. This inhibits heart function, causing slowed heartbeats. If untreated, this can be fatal, as the heart eventually stops beating.[11] Consequently, in cases of reduced kidney function, close control of potassium intake becomes critical.

Chloride

Chlorine (Cl) is a strong disinfectant that is commonly used in the gaseous form (Cl_2) to kill bacteria in public water supplies. Consequently most water-borne diseases are rare in America. Chlorinated water is generally harmless to humans in dilute concentrations, although a slight risk for rectal and bladder cancer is suspected. The federal government limits the amount of certain chlorination by-products that can be present in drinking water; a still greater reduction is possible but would be expensive for utilities to institute. It currently is unclear whether the slight decrease in cancer risk is worth the effort and expense.[7]

Some people find the taste of chlorinated water unpleasant. If you are such a person, or are concerned about the slight cancer risk, you can remove the chlorine from tap water by boiling it or by letting a large container filled with water stand uncovered overnight. In both cases the chlorine will evaporate, taking its characteristic flavor with it. Alternatively, you can install a filter on the household spigot from which you obtain your water. It should be designed to remove trihalomethanes, common chlorine by-products. Earlier in this chapter we provided a number to call for a list of water filter manufacturers.

FUNCTIONS OF CHLORIDE

Chloride (Cl^-), an ionic form of chlorine, is a major negative ion in the extracellular fluid. Chloride is a component of the hydrochloric acid produced by the parietal cells in the stomach and is also used during immune responses as white blood cells attack foreign cells. Nerve-impulse conduction also employs chloride.[11] Most of the body's chloride is excreted by the kidneys; some is lost in perspiration.

A chloride deficiency is unlikely because our dietary sodium chloride intake is so high. Frequent and lengthy bouts of vomiting, if coupled with a nutrient-poor diet, can contribute to a deficiency because stomach secretions contain chloride. In the late 1970s, not enough chloride was added to a brand of infant formula. Infants who consumed it suffered anorexia, weakness, growth failure, severe convulsions, and other health problems, clearly showing what can happen when the need for a nutrient normally abundant in our diets is not given adequate attention.

CHLORIDE IN FOODS

A few fruits and some vegetables are naturally good sources of chloride. However, most chloride comes from the addition of table salt (NaCl) to food. If we know a food's overall sodium content, we can predict its chloride content (sodium content × 1.5). Naturally occurring sodium or chloride doesn't significantly affect this calculation.

MINIMUM CHLORIDE REQUIREMENT

The minimum chloride requirement for health is 700 mg/day for adults. The average American probably consumes at least 7.5 g of salt daily, which yields 4.5 g (4500 mg) of chloride, a more than abundant intake of this nutrient.

TOXICITY OF CHLORIDE

The chloride ion itself may be an important part of the blood pressure–raising action of sodium. Together, then, the sodium and chloride components of salt are implicated in the genesis of some cases of hypertension. One research study suggested that a high intake of chloride ions, which tend to remain in the body, may trap positive sodium ions to balance the chemical charge. Whatever the exact mechanism, the implication for those with hypertension is the same: control salt intake and see if this helps the problem.

CONCEPT CHECK

Potassium is the main positive ion in intracellular fluid. Like sodium, potassium is vital to fluid balance and nerve impulse transmission. A potassium deficiency can be caused by inadequate intake, persistent vomiting, or use of certain diuretics. This in turn can lead to loss of appetite, muscle cramps, confusion, and heart arrhythmias. Leafy vegetables, melons, tomatoes, and potatoes are rich sources of potassium. A risk of toxicity accompanies impaired kidney function. Chloride is the major negative ion in extracellular fluid. It functions in digestion as part of hydrochloric acid, in nerve impulse transmission, and in immune system responses. Deficiencies are unlikely because dietary sodium chloride intake is so high.

Calcium

Calcium (Ca) is the most abundant mineral found within the body (see Figure 14-8). The body contains nearly 1200 g of calcium; this is about 40% of the total mass of all the minerals combined. Nearly 99% of this calcium acts to strengthen the teeth and bones. However, the remaining 1%, which circulates in the blood, is not to be discounted, as it plays important roles in the function of each cell.[11] Growth and bone development in laboratory animals are closely tied to calcium intake. This link is seen in humans, too, but we can probably better adapt to a low calcium intake.

ABSORPTION OF CALCIUM

Calcium absorption occurs primarily in the upper part of the small intestine (duodenum), because calcium requires a pH below 6 to stay in solution in an ionic state (Ca^{2+}). By the time the acidic stomach contents reach the duodenum, they have been partially neutralized by bicarbonate released from the pancreas but are still slightly acidic. This provides a suitable environment for calcium absorption. In addition, calcium absorption within the upper small intestine depends greatly on the active vitamin D hormone, calcitriol.[11] Because the intestinal contents become more alkaline as they pass along, calcium absorption is much less in the lower small intestine, although some still occurs.

In normal adolescents and adults consuming 400 to 1000 mg of calcium daily, absorption varies from about 20% to 40% of intake. An average value is 30%. The upper limit of absorption is seen in children during active periods of skeletal growth, when as much as 75% of dietary calcium intake may be absorbed. During pregnancy, absorption may be as high as 60% of intake. Young people in general tend to absorb calcium better than older people.[29] Postmenopausal women, in particular, exhibit very low absorption, as little as 20% of dietary calcium.

The female sex hormone estrogen plays a key role in the absorption of calcium, likely in part by allowing for increased synthesis and effectiveness of calcitriol. This in turn leads to increased calcium absorption. In women the blood concentrations of this crucial hormone plummet at menopause.[26] Fortunately, estrogen therapy (in a supplementary form of the hormone itself) can help treat the problem (see the Nutrition Focus).

Many cumulative factors enhance calcium absorption: the acidic environment of the upper small intestine; the vitamin D hormone (calcitriol) and parathyroid hormone; presence of glucose and lactose in the GI tract; and normal intestinal motility (flow).[5] Factors limiting calcium absorption include large amounts of phytic acid from dietary fiber (especially wheat bran); oxalic acid in spinach and some other vegetables; phosphorus in the diet; polyphenols (tannins) in tea; a vitamin D deficiency; menopause; diarrhea; rapid intestinal flow; some medications; and old age (Table 14-3).[24]

One problem in setting the RDA for calcium is predicting the extent to which calcium will be absorbed. The RDA is based on an estimated 30% to 40% absorption. Some people absorb calcium more efficiently than that, and others less effi-

TABLE 14-3

Factors influencing intestinal absorption of calcium

Factors favoring absorption	Factors hindering absorption
Acid nature of upper intestinal tract	Alkaline state in lower intestinal tract
Normal digestive activity and motility of intestinal tract	Large amounts of wheat bran
Dietary calcium and phosphorus in about equal amounts	Laxatives or any circumstances that cause diarrhea or rapid flow of intestinal contents
Vitamin D hormone (calcitriol)	Great excess of phosphorus, iron, or zinc in proportion to calcium
Need for higher amounts by the body, as during pregnancy	Phytic acid, oxalic acid, and unabsorbed fatty acids; they all bind calcium in the intestine
Low calcium intake	Vitamin D deficiency
Parathyroid hormone (increases active vitamin D synthesis)	Menopause
Lactose	Old age
Glucose	Polyphenols (tannins) in tea
	Certain medications, such as anticonvulsants

ciently. Less efficient absorption raises needs, but measuring an individual's calcium-absorption ability is a complex task.

Bone loss caused by insufficient calcium in the diet proceeds slowly. Only after many years are clinical signs apparent. By not meeting the RDA for calcium, some people, especially women, are likely setting the stage for future bone fractures.[15] But because we don't know how efficiently individuals absorb calcium, we often can't predict who is at high risk for bone loss and so for whom this poses a significant problem.

REGULATION OF BLOOD CALCIUM

Each cell has a critical need for calcium, as we will discuss. This is probably the reason humans have such excellent hormonal systems to control blood calcium. Normal blood calcium can be maintained despite a poor calcium intake. The bones, however, pay the price. This makes blood calcium a poor measure of calcium status.

As discussed in Chapter 12, when blood calcium falls, the parathyroid gland releases parathyroid hormone. This hormone, working with calcitriol, increases the kidneys' retrieval of calcium before it is excreted in the urine. Parathyroid hormone also helps to increase calcium absorption indirectly by increasing synthesis of calcitriol. In addition, parathyroid hormone, often working in conjunction with calcitriol, causes increased calcium release from bones by stimulating the activity of **osteoclasts** (bone-breakdown cells). In all these ways, then, parathyroid hormone acts to increase blood calcium (see Figure 12-8).[11]

When blood calcium is too high, release of parathyroid hormone falls. Then calcium loss from the kidneys increases. Calcitriol synthesis also decreases, and thus calcium absorption decreases. In addition, the thyroid gland secretes the hormone calcitonin, which decreases calcium loss from bones by inhibiting osteoclast activity. All these metabolic changes cause blood calcium to fall back toward the normal range.[11]

ROLE OF CALCIUM IN BONE STRUCTURE

The role of calcium in the structure and metabolism of bone is easily the most recognizable function of this mineral. To better understand the role calcium plays within bone structure, we must understand the varying degrees of structural sophistication found within bone and how this is maintained.

Microstructure of Bone

Despite its "dead" appearance, bone is very active metabolically. Bone contains two types of cells—osteoclasts and **osteoblasts**—that are integral to maintaining bones.[18]

Osteoclasts continually break down the structural network of bone in areas where bone is not needed. As noted, osteoclast activity is stimulated by parathyroid hormone, often in conjunction with calcitriol. Thus these bone cells are very active when a diet is deficient in calcium; their action releases calcium from the bone so it can enter the blood. Remember, a supply of calcium is vital to all cells, not just to bone cells.

Osteoblasts secrete a collagen protein matrix that forms the support structure of bone. They then secrete bone mineral, which strengthens the bone. This mineral matures and eventually approaches the composition of $Ca_{10}(PO_4)_6OH_2$, called **hydroxyapatite.**

Bone Remodeling

Bone turnover refers to a cycle of bone breakdown by osteoclasts followed by bone rebuilding by osteoblasts. The process is called **bone remodeling.**[18] In this way, bone is re-formed when necessary to respond to the physical demands placed on it. Before new bone can be built, the old bone in that area must be partially broken down.

During human growth, total osteoblast activity exceeds osteoclast activity, so we make more bone than we break down. In the first year of life, all bones in the body

hydroxyapatite A compound composed of calcium and phosphate that is deposited into the bone protein matrix to give it strength and rigidity.

bone remodeling A process by which bone is first absorbed by osteoclasts and then re-formed by osteoblasts. This process allows the body to form bone where needed, such as in areas of high mechanical stress.

are rebuilt. In the young adult, 15% to 30% of the skeleton is rebuilt each year, with more bone being built in areas put under high stress. A right-handed tennis player, for example, will build more bone in that arm than in the left arm.

Peak bone mass is developed in late adolescence, with limited accrual of additional bone mass between 20 and 30 years of age.[20] The adolescent growth spurt is a critical period for bone growth. That is when bone mass is increasing at the rate of about 8.5% per year. The ultimate amount of bone built by a person is clearly dependent on gender, race, familial patterns seen in the mother and father, and probably other genetically determined factors, such as vitamin D–receptor activity in the body. About 15% to 20% of people show diminished vitamin D–receptor activity, and this in turn likely compromises calcium metabolism and so bone maintenance.[22] In addition, men have higher bone mass values than women, and African-Americans have heavier skeletons than Caucasians. As a direct consequence, men and African-Americans have a lower risk of fractures than other populations. Slender, small-framed Caucasian and Asian women show the lowest bone mass values. Peak bone mass is also related to dietary intake of calcium and other nutrients.[15]

Macrostructure of Bone

Visual observation of the cross-sections of a bone reveals two primary bone structural types: **cortical bone** and **trabecular bone.** These interact within each bone to form quite an engineering marvel of strength (Figure 14-12).

The entire outer surface of all bones is composed of cortical (compact) bone, which is very dense. The shafts of long bones, such as those of the arm, are almost entirely cortical bone.

cortical bone Dense, compact bone that composes the outer surface and shafts of bones.

trabecular bone The spongy inner matrix of bone found primarily in the spine, pelvis, and ends of long bones.

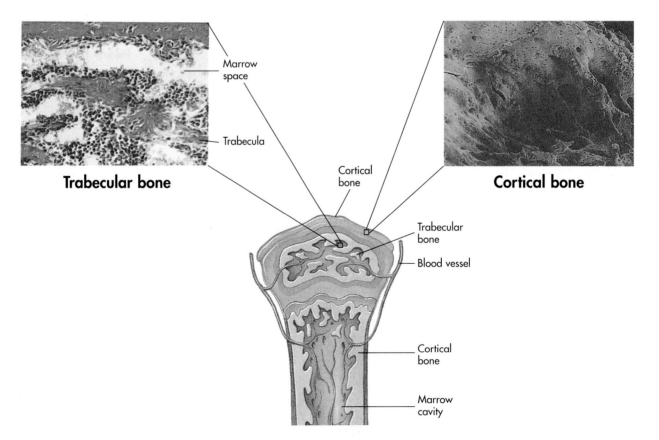

Trabecular bone

Marrow space

Trabecula

Cortical bone

Cortical bone

Trabecular bone

Blood vessel

Cortical bone

Marrow cavity

Figure 14-12 Cortical and trabecular bone. Cortical bone forms the shafts of bones and the outer mineral covering. Trabecular bone supports the outer shell of cortical bone in various bones of the body, as in the bone pictured.

Trabecular (spongy) bone is found in the ends of the long bones, inside the spinal vertebrae, and inside the flat bones of the pelvis. Trabecular bone forms an internal scaffolding network for a bone. It supports the outer cortical shell of the bone, especially in heavily stressed areas, such as joints.

Determinants of Bone Strength

Bone strength depends primarily on three factors: **bone mineral density,** rate of self-healing, and integrity of the trabecular support. The only factor that can be measured on intact bones within the body is bone mineral density. Clinically, although bone mineral density is helpful in predicting a person's risk for fracture, it is not sufficient.[26] Not all people with low bone mineral density suffer fractures, and some people with high bone mineral density do suffer fractures. In such cases, the other factors determining bone strength probably are critical.

Bone Mineral Density. Bone strength is determined partially by its density. The more densely packed the bone crystals are, the stronger the bone structure. Total bone mass refers to the weight of bone in the body, while bone mineral density reflects how densely packed the crystals are in a particular bone. The denser the bone, the stronger it is.

Bone Repair Rate. The next important determinant of bone strength is the rate at which the bone can heal itself. **Microfractures,** so small they cannot be seen on an x-ray or any type of bone scan, are constantly developing in bone. These microfractures must be knitted back together with collagen protein and bone crystal. Otherwise, they can accumulate and eventually allow for a major fracture.

Integrity of the Trabecular Bone Network. The third important element of bone strength is the trabecular bone network inside a bone. It is especially critical for the horizonal trabeculae to extend continuously—without breaks—between the areas of vertical trabeculae. Any break in either the horizontal or more vertical trabecular beams weakens the support system of a bone and increases the risk for bone fracture (refer again to Figure 14-12).

Osteoporosis

Failure to maintain enough bone mass in the body eventually results in **osteopenia** (from Greek *osteo* meaning "bone" and *penia* meaning "poverty"). Osteopenia can be caused by osteomalacia, the use of certain medications (such as glucocorticoids, antiseizure drugs, and thyroid hormones), and cancerous tumors. If these or similar causes are not present, the diagnosis is osteoporosis. Osteoporosis can be further classified as type I (postmenopausal), which appears in the years right after menopause, and type II (senile), which is found in people of advanced ages.[26]

Recall from Chapter 12 that in osteomalacia the bone is abnormal because it contains too little calcium.[11] In contrast, bone composition in osteoporosis is essentially normal. The bone may contain some extra sodium ions, but basically there is just less bone throughout the body. Because these bones have less substance, osteoporosis can lead to fractures in old age, distorted body shape, and loss of teeth (Figure 14-13).

OTHER FUNCTIONS OF CALCIUM

Although the role of calcium in bone formation and maintenance constitutes an obvious major function of this mineral, calcium is critical to at least four other processes in the body. These processes depend on the close hormonal regulation of blood calcium we mentioned earlier and occur without regard to dietary calcium intake.

Blood Clotting

Calcium ions participate in several reactions in the cascade that leads to formation of fibrin, the main protein component of a blood clot (see Figure 12-14). For example, the conversion of prothrombin to thrombin requires calcium. Without sufficient calcium in the blood, clots will not form.[11]

Researchers in Australia have uncovered what they think is one reason hip fractures are more common in Western countries than in the developing world. Because children in Western countries have higher average nutrient intakes than those in developing countries, they grow faster and to a greater extent. As a result, the part of the thigh bone that fits into the pelvis becomes quite long. The greater the length of this part, called the hip axial length, the more fragile this region of the hip is, and in turn the higher the risk for hip fracture, especially as bone mass decreases with advanced age. This suggests that people in Western countries especially must pursue strategies to avert hip fracture, notably in elderly years.

---

bone mineral density Total mineral content of bone at a specific bone site divided by the width of the bone at that site.

microfractures Small fractures, undetectable by x-rays or other bone scans, that may occur constantly in bones.

osteopenia Decreased bone mass resulting from cancer, hyperthyroidism, or other causes.

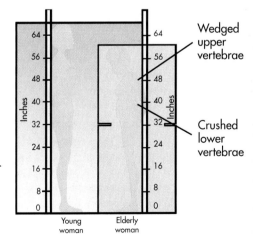

Figure 14-13 A loss of height and a distorted body shape are common signs of osteoporosis. Monitor your adult height changes to detect early osteoporosis.

CALCIUM AND OSTEOPOROSIS

Widespread advertising has made it almost impossible for women to ignore osteoporosis. Its crippling effect on elderly persons is now recognized as a major medical problem. The disease affects more than 25 million people in the United States, most of them women. Osteoporosis leads to approximately 1.5 million bone fractures per year, usually in the hip, spine, or wrist. About one third of all women experience osteoporosis-related fractures in their lifetimes.[26]

Scientific estimates of the physical activity and dietary patterns of humans living at the end of the Stone Age suggest that their calcium intake was twice that of contemporary humans and physical exertion was also greater than at present. Bony remains from that period also suggest that Stone Age humans developed a greater peak bone mass in young adulthood and experienced less age-related bone loss than do humans in the twentieth century. Does this tell us something?

The slender, inactive woman who smokes is most susceptible to osteoporosis, but any person who lives long enough can suffer from the disease, including men. About 25% of women over age 50 develop osteoporosis. Among people over 80 years old, osteoporosis becomes the rule—not the exception. The spine fractures commonly found in women with osteoporosis cause considerable pain and deformity and decrease physical ability (Figure 14-13); hip fractures are seen in both men and women with osteoporosis. Not only is this disease debilitating, it also can be fatal.[26] Between 12% and 20% of all elderly persons who suffer hip fractures eventually die from fracture-related complications.

BONE MINERAL DENSITY IS RELATED TO AGE AND GENDER

The question of how and why osteoporosis takes place is largely a matter of one's bone mineral density. Rapid and continual bone growth and calcification occur throughout the adolescent years.[20] Small increases in bone mineral density continue between 20 and 30 years of age. Women make less bone than do men, lose it at a faster rate, and tend to live longer. Thus women start their adult years with less bone and have a longer time in which to lose bone. Also, bone mineral density varies among young adult women; some have much denser bone than others, perhaps because they built more bone when they were young. Some women also may more easily adapt to lower-calcium diets. People who have developed more-dense

bone by early adulthood can sustain greater age-related bone loss with less fracture risk compared with those who have less-dense bone.

For women, bone loss begins about age 30 and proceeds slowly and continuously to menopause (approximately age 50).[26] It often speeds up at menopause and continues at a high rate for the next 10 years. By age 65 to 70, the rate of bone loss falls to about the same rate as before menopause. In men, bone loss is slow and steady from around age 30. Overall, this bone loss in both genders progresses without signs or symptoms.

ESTROGEN PLUS CALCIUM IS THE BEST APPROACH FOR REDUCING POSTMENOPAUSAL BONE LOSS

Hormone replacement therapy with estrogen (and often with added progestins) is widely recommended for women at menopause to prevent osteoporosis, especially if (1) they have no contraindications to use and (2) they fall in the lower third of bone mineral density values for their age.[26] Women with intermediate values who do not opt for estrogen treatment should have their bone mineral density values reevaluated at their physician's discretion, typically in 2 to 5 years. However, women postponing therapy should realize that alteration of the trabecular support system of the bone as a result of bone loss is currently a permanent phenomenon. No therapy can reverse this problem. Estrogen is also used to reduce the symptoms of menopause.

Estrogen replacement at menopause greatly slows further bone loss in women. Thus it is reasonable to assume that estrogen replacement therapy will significantly reduce the risk of osteoporosis and related fractures in women who begin treatment right after menopause and continue it for 20 years or so.

There are a number of ways that estrogen aids in bone maintenance. Some studies show that estrogen increases synthesis of the active vitamin D hormone, calcitriol. Estrogen also may increase the sensitivity of the intestine to calcitriol, in turn improving the action of this hormone to increase calcium absorption. In addition, estrogen may increase the sensitivity of the kidneys to parathyroid hormone, which in turn would lead to an increase in calcitriol synthesis. Finally, we know that there are receptors for estrogen on bone cells. Binding of estrogen to these receptors on osteoblasts in effect stimulates or inhibits synthesis of local factors that, respectively, decrease or increase activity of the bone-resorbing osteoclasts. As well, binding of estrogen to these receptors on osteoclasts may directly inhibit their function.[18]

Estrogen therapy is relatively safe for most women but still must be closely supervised by a physician. Resumption of menstruation with some forms of therapy is common, but subsides after a few years or so. A slight increased risk for certain forms of cancer, notably in the breast and endometrium (the latter if the woman has not had a hysterectomy), and gallbladder problems has been observed in women on estrogen therapy. Thus close monitoring is needed. Adding progestins to the regimen greatly reduces the endometrial cancer risk.

An additional benefit of estrogen replacement therapy is a significant reduction in the risk of heart disease. Heart disease risk climbs sharply after menopause. Estrogen blunts this change in part by lowering LDL and raising HDL, as we noted in Chapter 4. A direct beneficial effect of estrogen on the cells lining the blood vessels is also suspected, as well as other possible explanations for the effect. When the decreased risks for osteoporosis and heart disease are added together, estrogen replacement therapy ends up greatly improving the overall health risk profile for many women, especially those with many risk factors for osteoporosis or heart disease.[31] A woman and her physician should work together to see if that is true for her. The Women's Health Initiative trial, currently underway, is designed to help pinpoint the actual net benefit from estrogen replacement experienced by a wide variety of women, and in turn contribute to this decision making.

Some women cannot take estrogen because they have estrogen-sensitive breasts or uterine tumors. Other therapies, such as taking the active vitamin D hormone, calcitriol, certain bisphosphonate compounds, or the hormone calcitonin, are available and quite effective. But these treatments are still in experimental stages, more expensive, or more cumbersome than estrogen therapy.

The question that often arises is whether increasing calcium intake can substitute for use of estrogen or other medications in reducing bone loss in postmenopausal women. Overall, studies have found that taking as much as 2000 mg of extra calcium daily (equal to about 7 cups of milk) does not prevent bone loss in the spine, hip, or wrist after menopause as successfully as estrogen replacement does. Although such high intakes of dietary calcium do reduce bone loss in some areas, they are no more effective than just meeting the RDA in reducing the often significant loss of spinal bone that occurs in the 5 to 10 years immediately after menopause.

We noted that spinal fractures in women cause considerable pain and deformity and decrease physical ability. In addition, no reliable cure exists for osteoporosis. Therefore preventing these fractures is very important. Thus for most women at high risk for osteoporosis it is not a question of estrogen versus calcium. Rather, estrogen plus calcium probably constitutes the most effective treatment currently available. Also, as women not on estrogen therapy age 10 years beyond menopause, consuming 1500 mg of calcium and maintaining adequate vitamin D nutriture lead to less bone loss throughout the body than if not on this intervention. This therapy in turn led to a significant reduction in the risk of hip fracture in nursing home residents in a recent study.[8]

WILL A NUTRITIOUS DIET IN YOUTH HELP PREVENT OSTEOPOROSIS LATER?

Meeting at least the RDA for calcium from childhood through adolescence builds a stronger bone structure than does a lower calcium intake. The extent and importance of this difference in bone strength is currently under study. Some researchers think that the RDA for ages 11 through 24 for women is too low. Note that a recent NIH Consensus Conference on Optimal Calcium Intake recommended up to an additional 300 mg (to a total of 1500 mg/day) through age 24 in hopes that such higher calcium intakes will result in more bone being laid down compared with just following the RDA.[24] We will likely have the answer to this controversy from studies in progress, with results due about 1997.

ARE ALL WOMEN AT RISK FOR OSTEOPOROSIS?

We noted that about one third of all women experience osteoporosis-related fractures in their lifetimes. Some women just do not live long enough to suffer from osteoporosis. They may experience some bone loss, but their bones still remain reasonably strong throughout their lives. This is especially true of women who die before the age of 75 years.

Continued.

NUTRITION FOCUS

In addition, some women have much denser bone than others. They probably built more bone when they were young, so they can endure greater bone loss without experiencing more fractures. Actually, the reason for such variation in bone mineral density and fracture risk in women at any age still needs more research. However, scientists have identified numerous factors—including physical activity, calcium intake throughout life, and vitamin D–receptor activity in the body—associated with higher bone mineral density values in some studies (Table 14-4).[15,22,23] On the other hand, even more factors are associated with low bone mineral density values in women: a family history for osteoporosis; a lack of regular menstruation; premature menopause; use of certain

TABLE 14-4

Some factors associated with bone accretion/maintenance versus bone loss

Accretion/maintenance	Loss	
Normal menses	Lack of menses	Bed rest (months)
Estrogen replacement	Early menopause	Excessive wheat bran intake
African-American race	Glucocorticoid use	
Thiazide diuretics	Hyperparathyroidism	Anorexia nervosa
Physical activity	Hyperthyroidism	Inefficient vitamin D–receptor activity
Dietary calcium	Thyroid hormone replacement	
Vitamin D nutriture		Excessive sodium intake
Body weight	Factors made by white blood cells	Excessive caffeine intake
Overall adequate diet		Excessive phosphorus consumption if calcium RDA is not met
Efficient vitamin D–receptor activity	Alcoholism	
	Cigarette smoking	Excessive protein intake
Parents with large bone mass	Slender figure	

Transmission of Nerve Impulses to Target Cells

Earlier we examined the roles of sodium and potassium in conduction of nerve impulses. When an impulse reaches its target site, such as a muscle, other nerve cells, or a gland, the impulse is transmitted across the junction between the nerve and its target cells. In many nerves, arrival of action potentials at the target site stimulates an influx of calcium ions into the nerve from the extracellular medium. The rise in intracellular calcium ions then triggers release of neurotransmitters, which are responsible for carrying impulses to the target cells. Calcium also may influence the flow of other ions in and out of nerve cells.

In an entirely different process, nerves discharge spontaneously if insufficient calcium is available, leading to what is called hypocalcemic **tetany.** This condition is characterized by muscle spasms, as they receive continual nerve stimulation. Inadequate parathyroid hormone release or action is the typical cause of **hypocalcemia.**[11]

Muscle Contraction

The critical role of calcium in muscle contraction is most easily understood in the case of skeletal muscles. When a skeletal muscle is stimulated by a nerve impulse from the brain, calcium ions are released from intracellular stores within the muscle cells. The resulting increase in the concentration of calcium ions in a muscle cell is one factor, along with ATP, that permits the contractile proteins, actin and myosin,

tetany A state marked by sharp contraction of muscles and failure to relax afterward; usually associated with low blood calcium.

hypocalcemia Low blood calcium, typically arising from inadequate parathyroid hormone release or action.

medications (e.g., glucocorticoids, thyroid hormones, and antiseizure agents); excess dietary protein, caffeine, and sodium, which increase calcium loss in the urine; and prolonged bed rest.[14] We clearly can't focus only on calcium when discussing this disease—many factors are involved.

PROPER PLANNING HELPS PREVENT FRACTURES IN LATER LIFE

As women mature, different strategies for preventing osteoporosis are needed, based on the risk factors present. Young women should see a physician at any sign of irregular menstruation and should pursue an active lifestyle that includes sun exposure (to promote synthesis of vitamin D) and weight-bearing physical activity (to build/maintain muscle mass). Greater muscle mass linked to physical activity is associated with greater bone mineral density, as this keeps tension on bone.[23]

In young women, regular menstruation is the overwhelming key to bone maintenance, as evidenced by low bone mineral density in nonmenstruating female athletes and other women with irregular menstruation, such as in anorexia nervosa. Physical activity cannot prevent the bone loss associated with irregular menstruation. It is also important to at least meet the RDA for calcium, and possibly consume a bit more, as recommended by the recent NIH Consensus Conference on Optimal Calcium Intakes.[24]

Smoking and excessive alcohol intake work against bone strength. Smoking lowers estrogen in the blood in women, increasing bone loss. Alcohol is toxic to all cells, including bone cells. Alcoholism is probably a major undiagnosed and unrecognized cause of osteoporosis today. Moderation in caffeine, sodium, and protein intake is also advised. These are especially problematic when insufficient calcium is consumed.[14]

At menopause, women should discuss estrogen replacement therapy with a physician. They also need to accurately track their height. A decrease of more than 1 inch from premenopausal values is a sign that significant bone loss is taking place.

Elderly men and women need to stay physically active (if possible) and meet their RDA for calcium at the very least; a higher goal of 1500 mg/day is advocated by many researchers. As we mentioned, this most likely limits bone loss in some areas of the body, such as the hip. Elderly persons also need to minimize the risk for falls, especially by limiting their use of medications and alcohol, which might disturb coordination, and taking corrective measures if visual function is impaired.[9] Getting regular sun exposure and consuming food sources of vitamin D also are very important.

---

to interact. This leads to muscle contraction. Then, to allow for subsequent relaxation, the calcium ions are returned to intracellular stores, and the actin and myosin proteins can disconnect.[11]

Cell Metabolism

Finally, calcium ions help regulate metabolism in the cell by participating in the **calmodulin** system. When calcium enters a cell (often because of hormone action) and binds to the protein calmodulin, the resulting protein-calcium complex can regulate the activity for various enzymes, including those that synthesize glycogen.

calmodulin A cell protein that binds calcium ions. The resulting calmodulin–Ca^{2+} complex influences the activity of some enzymes in the cell.

Other Possible Health Benefits of Dietary Calcium

Dietary calcium may reduce the risk of colon cancer, especially in people consuming a high-fat diet. It appears that a high calcium content in the intestinal contents can bind free fatty acids and bile acids found there. These compounds, when unbound, tend to irritate the colon. The irritation may increase cell turnover and in turn increase the risk of cancer. Researchers analyzing the various studies in this area suggest that a daily dietary calcium intake of at least 1500 to 2000 mg is needed to reduce colon cancer risk.[32]

Calcium intakes of 800 to 1200 mg/day can decrease blood pressure, compared with intakes of 400 mg/day or less (see the Nutrition Perspective).[25] In addition, as we covered in Chapter 4, when people with elevated serum LDL consume a low-fat, low-cholesterol diet, supplementation with calcium at 1200 to 2200 mg/day further reduced LDL. Increasing calcium intake likely increases the fecal excretion of saturated fatty acids. This suggests that increasing calcium intake complements a serum cholesterol–lowering diet.

Research concerning the effectiveness of calcium in reducing colon cancer, high blood pressure, and serum LDL is relatively new. Practical dietary recommendations stemming from this research indicate that meeting the RDA or exceeding it somewhat may be beneficial for a variety of conditions, not just bone health.[24]

- - - - - - - - - - - -

A diet rich in calcium may also prevent pregnancy-induced hypertension, as we cover in Chapter 16.

- - - - - - - - - - - -

CALCIUM IN FOODS

Dairy products, such as milk and cheese, provide most of the calcium in American diets. The exception is cottage cheese because most calcium is lost during production. White bread, rolls, crackers, and other foods made with milk products are secondary contributors. Overall, about 50% of calcium intake in our diets comes from milk and milk products, with an additional 20% coming from milk and cheese used as food ingredients.

Foods with the highest nutrient density for calcium (mg/kcal) are leafy greens (such as spinach), broccoli, nonfat milk, Romano cheese, Swiss cheese, sardines, and canned salmon. However, much of the calcium in some leafy green vegetables, notably spinach, is not absorbed because of the presence of oxalic acid. This effect is not as strong, however, in kale, collard, turnip, and mustard greens. Overall, nonfat milk is the most nutrient-dense source of calcium because of its high bioavailability and low energy value, with some of the vegetables we noted following close behind (Figure 14-14). The new calcium-fortified versions of orange juice

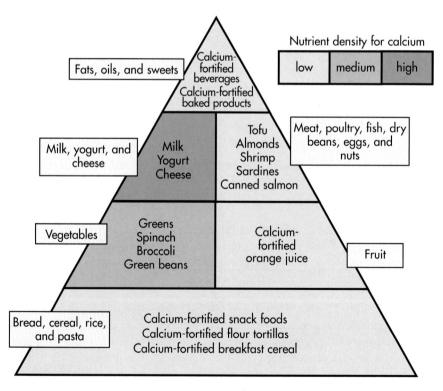

Figure 14-14 Food sources of calcium from the Food Guide Pyramid. The milk, yogurt, and cheese group includes the best dietary sources of this nutrient. The background color of each food group indicates the average nutrient density for calcium in that group. Additional calcium-fortified foods appear in stores each year and thus will add to the food sources currently listed for various groups.

and other beverages, as well as calcium-fortified bread, breakfast cereals, breakfast bars, and snacks, also follow as close competitors. Another good source of calcium is soybean curd (tofu) if it is made with calcium carbonate (check the label). Note that it is the bones in canned fish, such as salmon and sardines, that supply the calcium.

To review options for using dairy products in lactose intolerance, see Chapter 6.

One reason the Food Guide Pyramid contains a milk, yogurt, and cheese group is to supply calcium to the diet. In addition, this group provides protein, vitamin A, vitamin D, riboflavin, potassium, magnesium, and zinc. People who do not like milk can use products made with milk, such as chocolate milk, yogurt, cheese, and ice cream. All forms of milk, yogurt, and cheese allow about the same degree of calcium absorption. We hesitate to recommend either cheese or ice cream because they are usually high in saturated fat. However, some low-fat cheeses and ice milks are good calcium sources and have a low saturated-fat content.

Information about calcium is mandatory on food labels. The Daily Value for calcium used for food labels is 1000 mg. Allowable descriptive terms regarding calcium content have the following definitions[16]:

High-calcium: 200 mg or more per serving
Good source of calcium: 100 to 190 mg per serving
More or added calcium: at least 100 mg more per serving than reference food

CALCIUM SUPPLEMENTS

Calcium supplements can be used by people who don't like milk or cannot incorporate enough milk products, foods made with milk, or calcium-fortified foods into their diets. These supplements have become popular; sales increased 30% between 1991 and 1994 and now amount to about $250 million per year. Calcium carbonate has the highest concentration of calcium by weight (40%); calcium citrate has 21% calcium, and calcium phosphate has 8% calcium by weight. Other forms of calcium in supplements include calcium gluconate and calcium lactate.[17] With any supplement, it is important to read the label to see how much calcium is contained in each pill. In general, calcium supplements are absorbed more efficiently when consumed in doses of about 500 mg.

Some calcium supplements are poorly digested because they do not readily dissolve. To test a supplement for this, put one tablet in 6 ounces of cider vinegar. Stir every 5 minutes. It should dissolve within 30 minutes.

Calcium carbonate, the form commonly found in calcium-based antacid tablets, is the most common supplement used. People with ample output of gastric acid should take this supplement between meals. But those with low acid production should take a calcium carbonate supplement with meals, so that what little acid is produced during digestion can aid absorption. People with this problem also can use a supplement containing calcium citrate, which is acidic itself, between meals. The lower percentage of calcium in calcium citrate, however, requires using a greater number or size of pills, or consuming it in a tablet form that is designed to first be dissolved in water. Note that decreased output of gastric acid is common among elderly people.

We strongly suggest that those concerned about their calcium intake first try changing their diet, rather than use supplements, to improve their calcium status. Even though supplements are absorbed as well as milk calcium, many people have difficulty adhering to a supplement regimen. Regular food habits can likely be integrated more easily into a routine than can remembering to take several pills a day. In addition, it is difficult to consume an excess amount of calcium using foods. And calcium supplements themselves can reduce the absorption of other minerals (e.g., iron). In contrast, intakes of high-calcium food sources generally pose no such risk. Moreover, foods supply a natural balance of other minerals, in addition to calcium, thereby decreasing the likelihood of mineral imbalance.

Overall, taking 1000 mg of calcium daily in the form of calcium carbonate or calcium citrate is most likely safe, but people using a supplement should notify their physician of the practice.

Some calcium supplements pose a risk for lead toxicity. In Chapter 19 we note that lead produces an array of deleterious effects on the body, especially in children.

EXPERT OPINION

CALCIUM: AN UNDER-CONSUMED ESSENTIAL NUTRIENT

GREGORY D. MILLER, Ph.D., F.A.C.N.

Calcium is an essential nutrient responsible for a wide diversity of biological functions. These functions include structural support, cell adhesion, regulation of cell mitosis, blood clotting, nerve-impulse transmission, muscle contraction, and glandular secretion.

Calcium is the most abundant mineral in the human body, and 99% of it is contained within bones and teeth. The occurrence of the majority of calcium within the skeletal system underscores the importance of dietary calcium to bone health. By providing structural integrity to both trabecular and cortical bone, dietary calcium plays a critical role in reducing the risk of the bone-crippling disease osteoporosis. Consumption of an adequate calcium intake throughout life optimizes peak bone mass and minimizes bone loss later in life. Various government agencies and scientific organizations have concluded that a lifelong adequate intake of calcium is important for maintaining good bone health and may significantly reduce the risk of osteoporosis.

Dietary calcium has been demonstrated to reduce the risk of several types of cancer, including breast and colon cancer. Several possible mechanisms have been suggested. For example, dietary calcium directly decreases the hyperproliferation of cells—a state characteristic of early stages of cancer. Dietary calcium also forms insoluble soaps with fatty acids and bile acids in the intestine, thereby decreasing the ability of these agents to damage and induce hyperproliferation of intestinal cells.

Through its involvement in smooth muscle reactivity and the feedback regulation of calcitriol and parathyroid hormone, dietary calcium may reduce the risk of hypertension in a significant portion of the population. Calcium also appears to decrease blood pressure levels by preventing a sodium chloride–induced decrease in norepinephrine and by increasing serum calcitonin gene-related peptide, a protein that relaxes blood vessels. Salt-sensitive hypertensives, individuals with low calcium intakes, and pregnant women appear to benefit most from the blood pressure–lowering effects of dietary calcium. In 1993, for the first time, the Joint National Committee on Detection, Evaluation, and Treatment of High Blood Pressure recommended consuming an adequate level of calcium as one of the lifestyle modifications deemed important for reducing risk of and controlling hypertension.

A recent expert panel convened by the National Institutes of Health (NIH) examined the available scientific literature on calcium's many roles in reducing chronic disease risk with the intent of determining optimal calcium intakes. In developing its recommendations, this NIH panel focused primarily on the role of calcium in bone health. To optimize bone health and decrease the risk of osteoporosis, the panel recommended daily calcium intakes of 800 to 1200 mg for children 6 to 10 years; 1200 to 1500 mg for teenagers and young adults; and 1000 to 1500 mg for adult men and women. To reduce the risk of hypertension, the National High Blood Pressure Education Program Working Group recommends calcium intakes of 800 to 1200 mg/day. To reduce the risk of colon cancer, researchers recommend a daily intake of 1500 to 2000 mg of calcium. All these recommended calcium intakes exceed the RDAs for various ages.

Currently FDA has no standards for lead in food supplements. However, FDA does plan to regulate the lead content of supplements, including calcium, in the future. Until then, it is important to avoid bonemeal, the worst offender when it comes to lead. Tablet or liquid calcium supplements with the USP (United States Pharmacopeia) seal of approval are less likely than others to contain high concentrations of lead or other contaminants. When in doubt, contact the manufacturer concerning lead content.

RDA FOR CALCIUM

The RDA for calcium for adults is 800 mg/day. The current RDA extends the 1200 mg standard used in teenage years to 25, in hopes that these higher calcium intakes

Unfortunately, many Americans, especially young girls and women, fail to consume even the current RDA for calcium. According to the 1988-1991 National Health and Nutrition Examination Survey (NHANES III) data, after age 11 the average U.S. female fails to meet her RDA for calcium. These data are consistent with previous NHANES and Nationwide Food Consumption data. To achieve the optimal calcium intakes for bone health, the NIH panel recommends that foods naturally containing calcium be considered the preferred source of calcium and that calcium-fortified foods and supplements be considered additional sources.

Diets that are low in calcium tend also to be low in other essential nutrients, such as riboflavin, vitamin A, vitamin B-12, and potassium. Thus low calcium intake reflects poor dietary patterns. Research findings indicate that individuals who increase their calcium intake through foods, rather than pills, increase their intake of many other nutrients as well, including protein, carbohydrates, magnesium, phosphorus, potassium, vitamin C, vitamin D, thiamin, and riboflavin.

Milk and other dairy foods are the major source of dietary calcium in the United States, providing three quarters of the calcium available in the U.S. food supply. In addition to being good sources of calcium, milk and other dairy foods also contain substantial amounts of protein; vitamins A, B-6, and D; riboflavin; potassium; magnesium; and phosphorus. Research indicates that vitamin D is important for good bone health; vitamins A and D may help reduce some forms of cancer; and potassium and magnesium may help reduce the risk of hypertension. Many young girls and women tend to avoid dairy products because of their concerns related to fat and energy intake. However, recent studies have shown that adolescent girls and adults can consume 1400 mg of calcium per day mainly through dairy foods without negatively impacting weight gain, percentage of body fat, or blood lipids, while enhancing the nutrient quality of their diets.

Although calcium-fortified foods may be used to ensure adequate calcium intake, this approach may fail to improve overall nutrient intake to the same extent as consuming foods that naturally contain calcium. Calcium supplements should be used only as a last alternative to increasing calcium intake. The use of calcium supplements involves many inherent limitations: a higher potential for calcium over-consumption compared with calcium-containing foods, adverse interactions with other minerals, undesirable side effects (e.g., constipation, bloating), potential contamination with heavy metals, the need for a high degree of motivation, and failure to correct poor dietary habits.

Health professionals need to promote dietary patterns that can be easily implemented to close the gap between the current calcium intakes of Americans and the recommended levels. Until calcium consumption reaches recommended levels, Americans may expect to experience a growing incidence of calcium deficiency–related chronic diseases.

Dr. Miller is Vice President, Nutrition Technical Services, for the National Dairy Council. He has written and lectured extensively on the subject of diet and nutrition, especially with regard to calcium.

will contribute to building and maintaining a higher bone mass. There is reason to believe that this is a good idea. At 800 mg/day, young adults receive enough calcium to maintain bone, but some may not receive enough to keep building more bone.

A recent National Institutes of Health (NIH) Consensus Development Panel on Optimal Calcium Intake recommended even higher intakes of calcium than those specified by the RDAs (Table 14-5).[24]

CALCIUM INTAKE BY AMERICANS AT RISK OF CALCIUM DEFICIENCY

In the United States, average calcium intakes range from only approximately 600 to 800 mg/day for women and 800 to 1000 mg/day for men.[2] About 25% of women

TABLE 14-5

Recent recommendations for optimal daily calcium intakes
to reduce risk for osteoporosis

Age (years) or condition	Calcium intake (mg/day)
Children	
1-5	800
6-10	800-1200
11-24	1200-1500
Adults	
Women 25-50	1000
Women >50 (postmenopausal)	
Taking estrogen	1000
Not taking estrogen	1500
Women >65	1500
Men 25-65	1000
Men >65	1500

Adapted from NIH Consensus Development Panel on Optimal Calcium Intake: Optimal calcium intake, *Journal of the American Medical Association* 272:1909, 1994.

consume only about 300 mg/day. Thus dietary intakes of calcium by many women, especially young women, are well below the RDA, whereas intakes by most men are roughly equivalent to the RDA. The greater food consumption by men, to support their higher energy outputs, accounts for part of the difference. An easy way for women to increase calcium intake is to increase their physical activity and in turn their food consumption.

To estimate your calcium intake, use the rule of 300s. Give yourself 300 mg to account for calcium in the small amounts provided by a moderate energy intake from foods scattered throughout the diet. Add to that another 300 mg for every cup of milk or yogurt or 1.5 ounces (45 g) of cheese. If you eat a lot of tofu, almonds, or sardines, or drink calcium-fortified beverages, use food consumption tables to get a more accurate account of your calcium intake.

The rule of 300s underestimates calcium intake, especially in the case of vegans. It is important for vegetarians to focus on eating good plant sources of calcium as well as on the total amount of calcium ingested. Table 14-6 illustrates a vegan diet that provides about 975 mg of calcium.

TOXICITY OF CALCIUM

The major risk from taking excess calcium supplements is development of one form of kidney stones, as well as constipation and intestinal gas. Interestingly, daily intakes of about 1300 mg compared with about 500 mg or so may reduce risk for one form of kidney stones by binding oxalic acid in the small intestine, thus reducing the amount that ultimately enters the kidneys.[10] Oxalic acid is found in many kidney stones. However, greater intakes of calcium may increase risk of stone formation, especially in people who tend to form them. Thus experts suggest that calcium intake should not exceed 2000 mg/day, as a cautious estimate.[24] Any more could lead to excessive amounts of calcium in the urine. The body does absorb calcium less efficiently as calcium intake increases, but overzealous use of calcium supplements can overwhelm the control of absorption.

If calcium/antacid supplements and milk intake together become exceedingly high, a milk-alkali syndrome could result. In this condition, blood calcium climbs so high that calcium precipitates into tissues all over the body, causing local tissue death. Sticking to a daily limit of 2000 mg, however, poses no risk for developing this problem.

CRITICAL THINKING

Manuela is a vegan. She stopped eating meat and dairy products when she was 12 years old and is now in her mid-twenties. She wants to start a family but is concerned about whether she can obtain enough calcium from her diet to ensure her baby's health. She is also concerned that she may be at risk for osteoporosis. How can she consume enough calcium to meet her own and her baby's needs?

TABLE 14-6

Daily menu that meets calcium needs of an adult (age >24 years) following a vegan diet

Food choice	Energy (kcal)	Calcium (mg)
Breakfast		
1 cup orange juice (calcium-fortified)	110	300
1 bran muffin	125	60
Herbal tea	—	—
Lunch		
Sandwich:		
2 tbsp. peanut butter	190	10
2 tbsp. jam	110	10
2 slices whole-wheat bread	140	40
2 oatmeal raisin cookies	120	10
1 fresh peach	40	5
1 cup apple juice	120	15
Dinner		
2 bean burritos (no cheese)	500	135
2 cups romaine lettuce	20	40
½ tomato	10	5
2 tbsp. oil and vinegar dressing	140	5
1 cup sliced raw carrots	30	20
½ cup orange juice (calcium-fortified)	55	150
Snack		
Trail mix		
¼ cup almonds	200	100
¼ cup raisins	120	20
¼ cup chocolate peanuts	220	50
Totals	2250	975

For adolescents and young adults, the RDA of 1200 mg of calcium per day could be met by including snacks of calcium-fortified foods (e.g., certain ready-to-eat cereals and breads) or additional calcium-fortified beverages (e.g., soy milk).

CONCEPT CHECK

About 99% of calcium in the body is found in the bones. Aside from its critical role in bone, calcium also functions in blood clotting, muscle contraction, nerve-impulse transmission, and cell metabolism. Calcium requires a slightly acid pH and the vitamin D hormone, calcitriol, for efficient absorption. Factors that reduce calcium absorption include large amounts of dietary fiber (especially wheat bran), decreased estrogen in the bloodstream, and a great excess of phosphorus in the diet. Blood calcium is regulated primarily by parathyroid hormone and does not closely reflect daily intake or bone stores. Osteoporosis is bone loss with no outward cause. Women are particularly at risk for osteoporosis because they make less bone than men, lose it faster, and live longer. Dairy products are rich food sources of calcium. Certain calcium-fortified foods, such as beverages and bread, are rich sources as well. Supplemental forms, such as calcium carbonate, are well-absorbed by most people. However, supplements may interfere with the absorption of other minerals. Overzealous supplementation can also result in the development of one form of kidney stones.

Phosphorus

The body absorbs phosphorus (P) quite efficiently, about 70% of dietary intake. Because of its absorption and wide availability in foods, phosphorus poses less concern in diet planning than calcium.[4] The active vitamin D hormone, calcitriol, enhances phosphorus absorption, as it does for calcium. Excretion by the kidneys is primarily responsible for regulating the body content of phosphorus. In contrast, body calcium is regulated not only by excretion but also by changes in the rates of absorption.

FUNCTIONS OF PHOSPHORUS

Phosphorus plays many important roles in the body. It is a component of enzymes, adenosine triphosphate (ATP), cell membranes, and the bone mineral hydroxyapatite. Phosphorus also participates in pH control, especially inside cells. About 85% of phosphorus in the body is found in bone. The rest circulates freely in the bloodstream and operates within cells primarily in the form of phosphate ions (PO_4^{3-}).[11] No deficiency disease is currently associated with a deficient phosphorus intake. But low intakes may contribute to bone loss, especially in some elderly women.

PHOSPHORUS IN FOODS

Milk, cheese, bakery products, and meat provide most of the phosphorus in American diets (Figure 14-15). About 20% to 30% of dietary phosphorus comes from food additives, especially those found in baked goods, cheeses, and processed meats, as well as in soft drinks (about 75 mg per 12-ounce serving).

Foods with the highest nutrient density for phosphorus (mg/kcal) are wheat bran (in some breakfast cereals), nonfat milk, cheese, salmon and other fish, eggs, chicken and turkey, beef, and pork.

Phosphorus is one of the most difficult nutrients to limit in the diet, as is often needed in kidney disease, because it is found in so many foods.

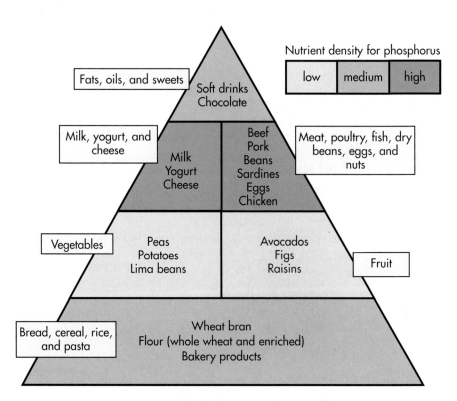

Figure 14-15 Food sources of phosphorus from the Food Guide Pyramid. The milk, yogurt, and cheese group, the bread, cereal, rice, and pasta group, and the meat, poultry, fish, dry beans, eggs, and nuts group are the best dietary sources of this nutrient. The background color of each food group indicates the average nutrient density for phosphorus in that group. Much phosphorus is also present in soft drinks.

RDA FOR PHOSPHORUS

The adult RDA for phosphorus is the same as that for calcium—800 mg/day. Adult intakes average about 900 to 1700 mg of phosphorus per day, with the lowest intakes found among the elderly.[2]

AMERICANS AT RISK FOR PHOSPHORUS DEFICIENCY

Marginal phosphorus status may be found in premature infants, vegans, people with alcoholism, elderly people consuming nutrient-poor diets, and those with long-standing diarrhea. People who use aluminum-containing antacids daily (usually part of the treatment for peptic ulcers, kidney failure, or kidney dialysis therapy) also are at risk for phosphorus deficiency. These types of antacids bind phosphorus in the small intestine. If a low dietary phosphorus intake is suspected, the diet's phosphorus content should be calculated.

TOXICITY OF PHOSPHORUS

If blood phosphorus is too high, the phosphate ions bind calcium, which leads to tetany and convulsions. Inefficient kidney function can cause such detrimentally high amounts. However, there is no known acute toxicity in healthy adults associated with phosphorus consumption. A chronic imbalance in the calcium to phosphorus ratio in the diet, resulting from a high phosphorus intake coupled with a low calcium intake, can contribute to bone loss, as this imbalance increases parathyroid hormone release.[4] This situation most likely arises when the RDA for calcium is not met, as can occur in adolescents and adults who regularly substitute soft drinks for milk, or otherwise under-consume calcium.

Magnesium

Magnesium (Mg) is present in the plant pigment chlorophyll, making plant foods a rich source of this mineral. We absorb about 30% to 40% of the magnesium in our diets, but absorption efficiency can increase to 80% when intakes of magnesium are low.[21] The active vitamin D hormone, calcitriol, may enhance magnesium absorption.

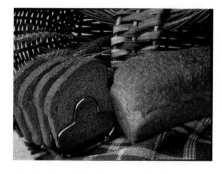

Whole-grain foods, such as bread, are good sources of magnesium.

FUNCTIONS OF MAGNESIUM

Bone contains 60% of the body's magnesium. We do not know if this magnesium is of functional significance or if it is just stored there. The rest circulates in the blood and operates inside cells in the form of magnesium ions (Mg^{2+}). Over 300 enzymes use magnesium as an activating co-factor. Without magnesium, many enzymes would function less efficiently. In addition, magnesium ions bind to ATP to form "active ATP." In this form, a magnesium ion bridges between the second and the last phosphate groups on the ATP molecule. Magnesium also contributes to potassium and calcium metabolism.[21]

Proper nerve, lung, and cardiac function require magnesium. Animals deficient in magnesium become very irritable. Eventually, if the deficiency becomes severe, the animals suffer convulsions and often die. In humans, a magnesium deficiency causes an irregular heartbeat, which is sometimes accompanied by weakness, muscle pain, disorientation, and seizures. However, a magnesium deficiency develops very slowly because we have large stores. A link between magnesium deficiency and sudden heart attacks has been observed, and its use in therapy for acute myocardial infarction is under investigation.[21] Adequate magnesium status also contributes to bone health. There is no test for magnesium deficiency that is both sufficiently accurate and available for use in routine clinical practice.

MAGNESIUM IN FOODS

Good food sources of magnesium are whole grains (wheat bran), broccoli, squash, beans, nuts, and seeds (Figure 14-16). One reason we continually emphasize the importance of whole grains and vegetables in the diet is that these foods are excel-

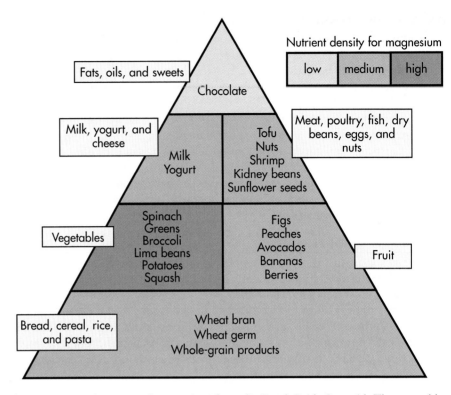

Figure 14-16 Food sources of magnesium from the Food Guide Pyramid. The vegetable group and whole-grain choices in the bread, cereal, rice, and pasta group are the best dietary sources of this nutrient. The background color of each food group indicates the average nutrient density for magnesium in that group.

lent magnesium sources. Dairy products, chocolate, and meats also contribute some magnesium to the diet.

Foods with the highest nutrient density (mg/kcal) for magnesium are spinach and other greens, wheat bran (in some breakfast cereals), broccoli, squash, shrimp, popcorn, sunflower seeds, nuts, kidney beans, and pork. "Hard" tap water often contains a high concentration of magnesium and so can be considered a food source.

RDA FOR MAGNESIUM

The adult RDA for magnesium is 350 mg/day for men and 280 mg/day for women. The Daily Value used for food labeling is 400 mg. Average daily intakes are about 300 to 350 mg for men and 220 to 250 mg for women.[2] We suggest women especially find some good food sources of magnesium that they like and eat them regularly.

AMERICANS AT RISK FOR MAGNESIUM DEFICIENCY

A magnesium deficiency is possible among people using thiazide diuretics, which increase magnesium excretion into the urine. In addition, heavy perspiration for weeks in hot climates and longstanding diarrhea or vomiting cause significant magnesium loss. Those with alcoholism are also at risk of a deficiency of magnesium because their dietary intake is likely to be inadequate and because alcohol increases excretion of this mineral in the urine. The disorientation and weakness associated with alcoholism is similar to that seen when blood magnesium is low. Excessive zinc intake (10 times the RDA) significantly reduces magnesium absorption and thus can be hazardous to magnesium status.[27] Presently, we have more questions than answers about the role of magnesium in human diseases, especially as this relates to bone health and critical illness.[21] The lack of an accurate and clinically practical measure of magnesium status complicates efforts to clarify the association of magnesium deficiency with specific disease states.

TOXICITY OF MAGNESIUM

Magnesium toxicity does not occur in healthy people who eat typical foods. Toxicity is associated with kidney failure because the kidneys primarily regulate blood magnesium. High blood magnesium leads to weakness, nausea, and eventual malaise. Elderly people are at particular risk, as kidney function may be compromised.

Sulfur

The minerals discussed so far function in the body primarily in the form of charged ions. In contrast, much of the sulfur (S) in the body occurs in nonionic forms as an integral component of organic compounds, such as the vitamins biotin and thiamin. Because the amino acids methionine and cysteine both contain sulfur, it also is present in proteins. Disulfide bridges form when the sulfur atoms in two cysteine residues bind to each other; these bridges stabilize the structure of many protein molecules (see Chapter 5). Ionic forms of sulfur, such as sulfate (SO_4^{2-}), participate in the acid-base balance in the body, are present in many substances found in the extracellular fluid, and play an important role in some drug-detoxifying pathways in the body.

We actually do not need to consume sulfur as such in our diets because proteins supply the sulfur we need. Sulfur is naturally a part of a healthful diet. Sulfur compounds are also used to preserve foods (see Chapter 19).

Oxygen

Oxygen (O) is in a class by itself: it is not a nutrient in a dietary sense but is still vital for sustaining life. We use oxygen for aerobic respiration at the last step of the electron-transport chain. In addition, some cellular metabolic reactions incorporate oxygen directly into compounds. About 21% of air is oxygen, a vital resource on which we all depend. All oxygen in the atmosphere either is produced by plants and microbes that perform photosynthesis or is released by chemical breakdown in rocks.

• • •

See Table 14-7 for a review of the major characteristics of water and the major minerals.

CONCEPT CHECK

Phosphorus absorption is quite efficient and is enhanced by the active vitamin D hormone, calcitriol. Urinary excretion mainly controls body content. Phosphorus aids enzyme function and is part of ATP molecules and cell membranes. No deficiency symptoms caused by an inadequate phosphorus intake have been reported. Good food sources include dairy products, baked goods, and meat. The RDA is met by most Americans. An excess intake of phosphorus can compromise bone health if sufficient calcium is not otherwise consumed. Magnesium is found mostly in plants, where it is a component of chlorophyll. Magnesium is required for proper nerve and cardiac function; it also acts as a co-factor for many enzymes. Good food sources of magnesium are whole grains (wheat bran), broccoli, squash, beans, nuts, and seeds. People using thiazide diuretics and people with alcoholism are at greatest risk of developing a deficiency. Magnesium toxicity is most likely in people with kidney failure. Sulfur is a component of certain vitamins and amino acids. It plays an important role in drug-detoxification and protein structure. The protein we consume supplies sufficient sulfur for the body's needs.

TABLE 14-7

A summary of water and the major minerals

Name	Major functions	Deficiency symptoms	People most at risk
Water	Medium for chemical reactions, removal of waste products, perspiration to cool the body	Thirst, muscle weakness, poor endurance	Infants with a fever, elderly persons, especially those in nursing homes, endurance athletes
Sodium	A major electrolyte of extracellular fluid; nerve-impulse conduction	Muscle cramps	People who severely restrict sodium to lower blood pressure (250-500 mg/day)
Potassium	A major electrolyte of intracellular fluid; nerve-impulse conduction	Irregular heart beat, loss of appetite, muscle cramps	People who use potassium-wasting diuretics or have poor diets, as seen in poverty and alcoholism
Chloride	A major electrolyte of extracellular fluid; acid production in stomach; nerve-impulse conduction	Convulsions in infants	No one, probably, as long as infant formula manufacturers control product quality adequately
Calcium	Bone and tooth strength; blood clotting; nerve-impulse transmission; muscle contraction; cell regulation	Inadequate intake increases the risk for osteoporosis	Women in general, especially those who constantly restrict their energy intake and consume few dairy products
Phosphorus	Bone and tooth strength; part of various metabolic compounds; major ion of intracellular fluid	Probably none; poor bone maintenance is a possibility	Elderly persons consuming very nutrient-poor diets; possibly vegans and people with alcoholism
Magnesium	Bone strength; enzyme function; nerve and heart function	Weakness, muscle pain, poor heart function	Women in general; people on thiazide diuretics
Sulfur	Part of vitamins and amino acids; drug detoxification; acid-base balance	None has been described	No one who meets his or her protein needs

*Values for calcium, potassium, and magnesium are RDAs. Values for other minerals are minimum requirements for health in adults.
†Just an approximation. It's best to keep urine volume greater than 1 L (4 cups) per day.

Summary

1. Many minerals are vital for sustaining life. For humans, animal products are typically the best sources of most minerals. Supplements exceeding 150% of the Daily Values for a mineral should be taken only under a physician's supervision, since toxicity and deleterious nutrient interactions are a distinct possibility.

2. Water constitutes 50% to 70% of the human body. Its unique chemical properties enable it to function as a solvent, a medium for chemical reactions, a thermoregulator, and a lubricant. For adults, daily water needs are estimated at 1 ml per kilocalorie expended.

3. Sodium, which supplies the major positive ion (Na$^+$) in the extracellular fluid, is vital in fluid balance and conduction of nerve impulses. It also participates in nutrient absorption. Our diets provide abundant amounts of sodium through processed foods and table salt. About 10% to 15% of the population is sodium sensitive and may develop hypertension by consuming excess sodium.

4. Potassium, which supplies the major positive ion (K$^+$) in the intracellular fluid, functions similarly to sodium in many cases. Fruits, vegetables, milk, and meats are good sources.

5. Chloride is the major negative ion (Cl$^-$) in the extracellular fluid. It functions in digestion as part of gastric hydrochloric acid and in nerve and immune function. Table salt added by us and food manufacturers supplies most of the chloride in our diets.

6. Calcium forms a vital part of bone structure and is also very important as a positive ion (Ca^{2+}) in blood clotting, muscle contraction, and nerve-impulse transmission. Calcium absorption is enhanced by stomach acid and calcitriol. Blood calcium is primarily regulated by the action of parathyroid hormone. Dairy products are important calcium sources.

7. Osteoporosis is defined as bone loss with no apparent cause. Women are particularly at risk and should maintain adequate calcium intake and perform regular phys-

RDA or minimum requirement*	Nutrient-dense dietary sources	Results of toxicity
1 ml per kcal expended†	As such and in foods	Probably occurs only in those with mental disorders: headache, blurred vision, convulsions
500 mg	Table salt, processed foods, condiments, sauces, soups, chips	Hypertension in susceptible individuals; some increase in calcium loss in the urine
2000 mg	Spinach, squash, bananas, orange juice, other vegetables and fruits, milk, meat, legumes, whole grains	Slowing of the heart beat; seen in kidney failure
700 mg	Table salt, processed foods, some vegetables	Hypertension in susceptible people when combined with sodium
800 mg (age >24 years) 1200 mg (age 11-24 years)	Dairy products, canned fish, leafy vegetables, tofu, fortified orange juice and other beverages, fortified bread and cereals	Very high intakes may cause kidney stones in susceptible people and reduce mineral absorption in general
800 mg (age >24 years) 1200 mg (age 11-24 years)	Dairy products, processed foods, meats, fish, soft drinks, bakery products	Hampers bone health in people with kidney failure; poor bone mineralization if calcium intakes are low
Men: 350 mg Women: 280 mg	Wheat bran, green vegetables, nuts, chocolate, legumes	Causes weakness in people with kidney failure
None	Protein foods	None likely

ical activity. Estrogen replacement at menopause is currently the most accepted way to stop significant adult bone loss in women.

8. Phosphorus aids the function of many enzymes and forms part of ATP molecules, numerous metabolites, and phospholipids in cell membranes. It is efficiently absorbed, and deficiencies are rare, although there is concern about the intake of some elderly women. Good food sources are dairy products, bakery products, and meats. Over-consumption can compromise bone health, especially if insufficient calcium is consumed.

9. Magnesium is the only mineral found mostly in plants, where it functions in chlorophyll. In humans, magnesium is important for nerve, lung, and heart function, as a co-factor for many coenzymes, and as well affects potassium and calcium metabolism. Good food sources are whole grains (bran), vegetables, nuts, and seeds.

10. Sulfur is incorporated into certain vitamins and amino acids. Its ability to bond with other sulfur atoms enables it to stabilize protein structure.

Study Questions

1. Approximately how much water do you need each day to stay healthy? Identify at least two situations that increase the need for water.

2. List three sources of water in the average person's diet.

3. Why are most minerals present in higher concentrations in animal foods than in plant foods?

4. How is water eliminated from the body? What physiological forces regulate this output?

5. Identify four factors that influence the bioavailability of minerals from food.

6. What is the relationship between sodium and water balance, and how is that relationship monitored as well as maintained in the body?

7. Within what physiological system do potassium, chloride, and calcium interact? What are the individual roles of these minerals in this system?

8. What might you tell a 12-year-old child about the importance of consuming enough calcium?

9. In terms of total amounts in the body, calcium and phosphorus are the first and second most abundant minerals, respectively. Name two ways in which phosphorus and calcium are alike and two ways in which they differ.

10. Describe the relationship between magnesium and the function/health of the cardiovascular system.

REFERENCES

1. Adams SO and others: Consumer acceptance of foods lower in sodium, *Journal of the American Dietetic Association* 95:447, 1995.

2. Alaimo K and others: Dietary intake of vitamins, minerals, and fiber of persons ages 2 months and over in the United States, Third National Health and Nutrition Examination Survey, Phase 1, 1988-91, *Advance Data* 258(Nov 14):1, 1994.

3. Alderman MH: Non-pharmacological treatment of hypertension, *Lancet* 344:307, 1994.

4. Anderson JJB, Barrett CJH: Dietary phosphorus: the benefits and the problems, *Nutrition Today*, March/April 1994, p 29.

5. Bronner F: Calcium and osteoporosis, *American Journal of Clinical Nutrition* 60:831, 1994.

6. Callaway W: Reexamining cholesterol and sodium recommendations, *Nutrition Today*, 29(Sept/Oct):32, 1994.

7. Cantor KP: Water chlorination, mutagenicity, and cancer epidemiology, *American Journal of Public Health* 84:1211, 1994.

8. Chapuy MC and others: Vitamin D_3 and calcium to prevent hip fractures in elderly women, *New England Journal of Medicine* 327:1637, 1992.

9. Cummings SR and others: Risk factors for hip fracture in white women, *New England Journal of Medicine* 332:767, 1995.

10. Curhan GC and others: A prospective study of dietary calcium and other nutrients and the risk of symptomatic kidney stones, *New England Journal of Medicine* 328:833, 1993.

11. Ganong WF: *Review of medical physiology*, ed 17, Norwalk, Conn, 1995, Appleton & Lange.

12. Gilman MW and others: Protective effect of fruits and vegetables on development of stroke in men, *Journal of the American Medical Association* 273:1113, 1995.

13. Greenleaf JE: Problem: thirst, drinking behavior, and involuntary dehydration, *Medicine and Science in Sports and Exercise* 24:645, 1993.

14. Harris SS, Dawson-Hughes B: Caffeine and bone loss in healthy postmenopausal women, *American Journal of Clinical Nutrition* 60:573, 1994.

15. Heaney RP: Nutritional factors in osteoporosis, *Annual Review of Nutrition* 13:287, 1993.

16. Kurtzweil P: Scouting for sodium and other nutrients important to blood pressure, *FDA Consumer* Sept 1994, p 18.

17. Levenson DI, Bockman RS: A review of calcium preparations, *Nutrition Reviews* 52:221, 1994.

18. Manolagas SC, Jilka RL: Bone marrow, cytokines, and bone remodeling, *New England Journal of Medicine* 332:305, 1995.

19. Marmot MG and others: Alcohol and blood pressure: the INTERSALT study, *British Medical Journal* 308:1263, 1994.

20. Matkovic V and others: Timing of peak bone mass in Caucasian females and its implication for the prevention of osteoporosis, *Journal of Clinical Investigation* 93:799, 1994.

21. McLean RM: Magnesium and its therapeutic uses: a review, *The American Journal of Medicine* 96:63, 1994.

22. Morrison NA and others: Prediction of bone density from vitamin D receptor alleles, *Nature* 367:284, 1994.

23. Nelson ME and others: Effects of high-intensity strength training on multiple risk factors for osteoporosis fractures, *Journal of the American Medical Association* 272:1909, 1994.

24. NIH Consensus Development Panel on Optimal Calcium Intake: Optimal calcium intake, *Journal of the American Medical Association* 272:1909, 1994.

25. Reusser ME, McCarron DA: Micronutrient effects on blood pressure regulation, *Nutrition Reviews* 52:367, 1994.

26. Riggs BL, Melton LJ: The prevention and treatment of osteoporosis, *New England Journal of Medicine* 327:620, 1992.

27. Spencer H, Norris C, Williams D: Inhibitory effects of zinc on magnesium balance and magnesium absorption in man, *Journal of the American College of Nutrition* 13:479, 1994.

28. U.S. Public Health Service: Blood pressure screening in adults, *American Family Physician* 50:1729, 1994.

29. Weaver CM and others: Differences in calcium metabolism between adolescent and adult females, *American Journal of Clinical Nutrition* 61:577, 1995.

30. Witteman JC and others: Reduction of blood pressure with oral magnesium supplementation in women with mild to moderate hypertension, *American Journal of Clinical Nutrition* 60:129, 1994.

31. Writing Group for the PEPI Trial: Effects of estrogen or estrogen/progestin regimens on heart disease risk factors in postmenopausal women, *Journal of the American Medical Association* 273:199, 1995.

32. Zimmerman J: Does dietary calcium supplementation reduce risk of colon cancer? *Nutrition Reviews* 51:109, 1993. See also the follow-up letter by Lipkin M (51:213, 1993).

TAKE ACTION

Working for denser bones

In the Nutrition Focus, you learned some significant information about the disease osteoporosis. This disease affects more than 25 million people in the United States. One third of all women experience fractures because of it. It leads to 1.5 million bone fractures per year. In addition, 12% to 20% of all elderly people who suffer hip fractures die from complications.

Osteoporosis is a disease you can do something about. Some risk factors cannot be changed, but others can. Let's see to what degree you are doing the things that can help prevent this debilitating disease. Answer "yes" or "no" to the following questions by placing an "X" on the appropriate line.

	YES	NO
1. Do you drink vitamin D–fortified milk regularly or obtain regular sun exposure on at least your face and hands to get enough vitamin D?	_____	_____
2. Do you regularly engage in weight-bearing physical activity (e.g., jogging, walking, etc.)?	_____	_____
3. If you are a woman, do you menstruate regularly?	_____	_____
4. Do you avoid smoking cigarettes?	_____	_____
5. Do you avoid regular consumption of large amounts of alcohol?	_____	_____
6. Based on your diet analysis from Chapter 2, did you meet your RDA for calcium on that day?	_____	_____

The more "yes" answers you have, the more you are actively doing to preserve your bone mineral density for the future. Also remember that this is not just a valuable consideration for women. If men plan to live well into their 80s and 90s, they too are at risk for osteoporosis.

Minerals and Hypertension

More than 50 million Americans suffer from a degree of hypertension that warrants therapy.[28] American Heart Association statistics show that hypertension kills about 31,000 people each year. A national health objective for the year 2000 is to increase to at least 90% the proportion of persons with hypertension who are taking action to help control their blood pressure.

Blood pressure is expressed by two different numbers. The higher number represents systolic blood pressure, which is the pressure in the arteries when the heart actively pumps blood. The second value is for diastolic pressure, which is the artery pressure when the heart is relaxed. Normal systolic blood pressure varies from 100 to 140 millimeters of mercury (mm Hg). Normal diastolic blood pressure varies from 60 to 90 mm Hg. A high diastolic pressure shows a strong relationship to various diseases, as does a high systolic pressure.[28]

Hypertension is defined as sustained high blood pressure, usually with systolic pressure exceeding 140 mm Hg or diastolic blood pressure exceeding 90 mm Hg. Most hypertension (90% to 95% of cases) has no apparent cause. It is called primary, or essential, hypertension. Kidney disease often causes the other 5% to 10% of cases, known as secondary hypertension.

African-Americans are more likely than Caucasians to develop hypertension and to do so earlier in life. As a result, they also suffer more from hypertension-related diseases. Unless blood pressure is measured periodically, development of hypertension is easily overlooked. Thus it's described as a "silent" disorder.[28]

A physician usually does not treat hypertension with medication until the diastolic blood pressure measures at least 95 mm Hg (or the systolic blood pressure reaches 160) on three or more occasions. Still, a diastolic value over 90 mm Hg is actually too high and deserves dietary and lifestyle interventions as a start.

Why Control Hypertension?

Hypertension needs to be controlled mainly to prevent heart disease, kidney disease, strokes, poor blood circulation in the legs, and sudden death. All these diseases are much more likely to be found in people with hypertension than in people with normal blood pressure. African-Americans are especially prone to developing kidney disease as a result. Smoking and elevated serum lipoproteins make these diseases even more likely in all races, and thus also deserve attention as a plan for hypertension therapy is instituted.

People with hypertension need to be diagnosed and treated as soon as possible, as the condition generally progresses to a more serious stage over time. Because of aggressive treatment of hypertension during the past 20 years, the average blood pressure values of hypertensive persons have fallen. The accompanying decrease in the number of strokes demonstrates the value of early, aggressive treatment of this condition. Interestingly, a recent study showed that a diet rich in fruits and vegetables also decreased stroke, even after accounting for the effects of blood pressure.[13] Have we convinced you by now to adopt such a diet?

Causes of Hypertension

A variety of factors affect blood pressure. Blood pressure usually increases as a person ages. Some increase is caused by atherosclerosis. As plaque builds up in the arteries, the arteries become less flexible and cannot expand. When vessels remain rigid, blood pressure remains high. Eventually the plaque begins to choke off blood supply to the kidneys, decreasing their ability to control blood volume, and in turn, blood pressure.

Obesity is often associated with hypertension, especially in women. High blood insulin associated with insulin-resistant adipose cells is one reason for this. Insulin increases sodium retention in the body and speeds atherosclerosis. Inactivity also is associated with hypertension. If an obese person can lose weight and engage in physical activity three to four times a week, blood pressure often returns to normal.[3] A weight loss of as little as 10 to 15 pounds can help. Often a minor change in lifestyle such as this can greatly reduce, or even eliminate, the need for medications.

Finally, the enzyme renin and some hormonelike compounds affect blood pressure (Figure 14-6). Medications are available to reduce the effect of the renin-angiotensin system.

Sodium and Blood Pressure

Sodium intake tends to increase blood pressure. The average American intake of 3 to 6 g per day (or more) can elevate blood pressure, particularly in those who are susceptible to the effect. However, only some Americans with hypertension are very susceptible to sodium-linked hypertension. So sodium in the diet is not a problem for everyone, even among people with hypertension.[6] Nevertheless, in populations that eat 1500 mg or less of sodium daily, hypertension is rare.

Groups of people who migrate from a developing to an industrialized nation and adopt a Western diet and lifestyle gradually attain the same risk of developing hypertension as people in the new country.[3] However, dietary changes would likely affect not only sodium intake, but also intakes of potassium, calcium, magnesium, protein, fat, dietary fiber, alcohol, and probably almost all other nutrients as well. Furthermore, changes in physical activity, obesity, psychosocial stresses (this is likely important because the norepinephrine released in response to stress reduces sodium excretion), and numerous other environmental factors make it impossible to single out any one factor as being causative. Although some scientific groups recommend that all people with hypertension reduce sodium intake, ideally dietary advice should be decided on an individual basis, once the response to treatment is verified.

If a person has hypertension, it is a good idea to reduce sodium. Approximately 2 to 3 g of sodium daily is the point at which sodium restriction usually improves hypertension. While an intake less than that may lower blood pressure even more, people find it very difficult to restrict sodium intake so severely for any length of time. Physicians usually resort to a combination of antihypertensive medications and a moderate sodium restriction (4 g daily) to help in patient compliance.

Calcium and Blood Pressure

Since 1983 there has been interest in whether calcium intake can affect blood pressure. Careful studies show that about 50% of people register slightly lower blood pressures when they consume at least the RDA for calcium per day, as compared with one third to one half that amount.[25] Systolic blood pressure is affected more than diastolic blood pressure. It is reasonable for a person with hypertension to experiment, in consultation with a physician, by increasing calcium intake to see if that produces a benefit.

Potassium, Magnesium, and Hypertension

Similarly to calcium, potassium supplementation has been shown to moderately decrease blood pressure in people currently consuming far below the recommended intakes. In addition, this effect of potassium supplementation is seen mostly in those people not on a sodium-restricted diet. Magnesium has been shown to be capable of lowering blood pressure at intakes about twice the RDA, but overall studies are inconsistent.[21,30]

Alcohol and Hypertension

In the United States, it is estimated that excess alcohol intake is responsible for about 10% of cases of hypertension, especially in middle-aged males and in African-Americans in general. As a result, it is an important cause of hypertension. Individuals who regularly consume more than 3 drinks per day show more hypertension than more moderate drinkers.[19] Because the hypertensive effects of regular consumption of even small doses of alcohol have been well documented, a prudent intake is 2 or fewer drinks per day for people with hypertension.

Preventing Hypertension

Many of the risk factors for hypertension are controllable, and appropriate lifestyle changes can reduce one's risk (Table 14-8). To prevent hypertension we recommend maintaining an active lifestyle and a healthy body weight.[3] Regular physical activity is a key component. Epidemiological evidence suggests that a low-sodium diet may lead to less hypertension in later life. You can decide if you want to restrict sodium in your diet now, or simply wait until hypertension develops. Hypertension does develop in many adults, especially in those with family histories of hypertension, but there are no studies to clearly guide the decision of when to restrict sodium in the diet. For many people, it probably takes decades of high sodium intake to lead to sodium-induced hypertension. Without a readily available test for sodium sensitivity, some scientists feel it is prudent for all adults to keep sodium intake to about 2 to 3 g/day. Limiting alcohol use is also very important. A reduction in stress adds to the list of preventive measures.

In addition, we suggest consuming a diet based on the Food Guide Pyramid, especially one rich in fruits and vegetables. This provides ample potassium and calcium, both of which help contribute to normal blood pressure values. Even if antihypertensive medications are still needed, a proper diet and lifestyle approach can often reduce the dosage, and in turn the expense and side effects of medications. Nutritional therapy is a key to treating hypertension.[3]

TABLE 14-8

A nutritional plan to minimize hypertension and stroke risk

1. Attain and maintain a desirable (healthy) body weight.
2. Incorporate regular physical activity into one's lifestyle (at least 3-5 times per week).
3. Meet the RDA for calcium, potassium, and magnesium.
4. Consume alcoholic beverages in moderation, if at all (1 or 2 drinks per day maximum).
5. Consume moderate to scant amounts of sodium.
6. Don't smoke.
7. Maintain blood lipoproteins in the normal range (see Chapter 4).

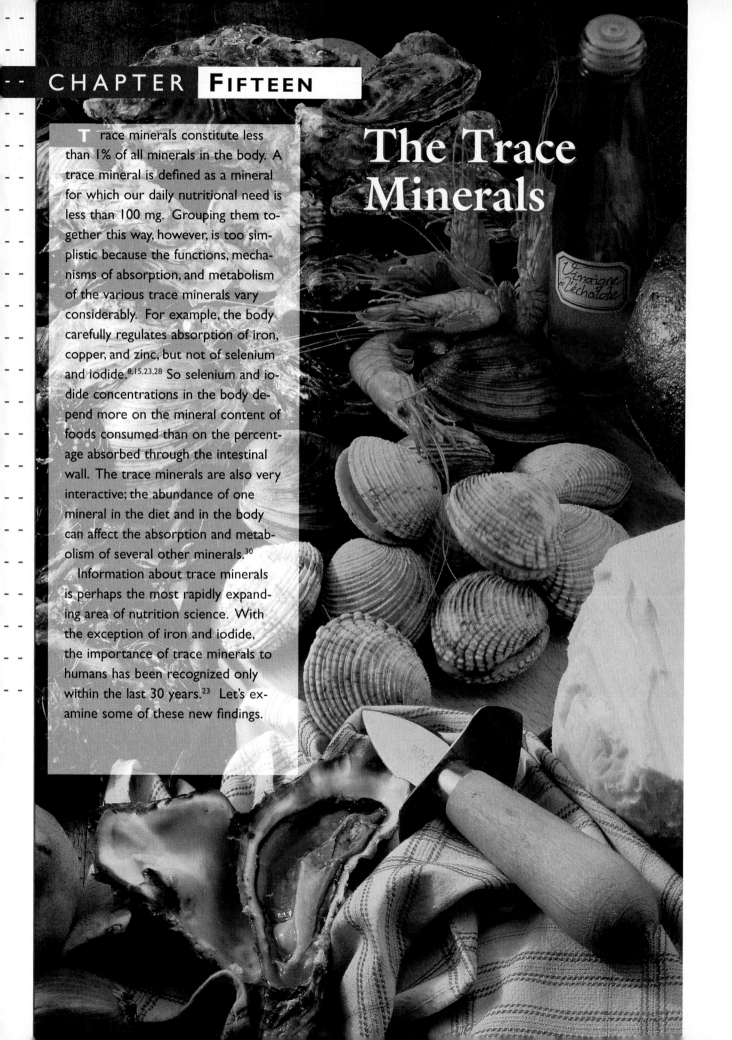

CHAPTER FIFTEEN

The Trace Minerals

T race minerals constitute less than 1% of all minerals in the body. A trace mineral is defined as a mineral for which our daily nutritional need is less than 100 mg. Grouping them together this way, however, is too simplistic because the functions, mechanisms of absorption, and metabolism of the various trace minerals vary considerably. For example, the body carefully regulates absorption of iron, copper, and zinc, but not of selenium and iodide.[8,15,23,28] So selenium and iodide concentrations in the body depend more on the mineral content of foods consumed than on the percentage absorbed through the intestinal wall. The trace minerals are also very interactive; the abundance of one mineral in the diet and in the body can affect the absorption and metabolism of several other minerals.[30]

Information about trace minerals is perhaps the most rapidly expanding area of nutrition science. With the exception of iron and iodide, the importance of trace minerals to humans has been recognized only within the last 30 years.[23] Let's examine some of these new findings.

Answer these 15 statements about trace minerals to test your current knowledge. If you think the answer is true or mostly true, circle T. If you think the answer is false or mostly false, circle F. Use the scoring key at the end of the book to compute your total score. Repeat this test after you have read this chapter, and compare your results.

1. **T F** Trace mineral deficiencies are often difficult to detect.
2. **T F** Some trace minerals can interfere with the absorption of other minerals.
3. **T F** Concentrations of trace minerals in plants usually depend on their concentrations in the soil in which the plants are grown.
4. **T F** Enriched grains contain less of many trace minerals than whole grains.
5. **T F** Iron is the only nutrient with a higher RDA for adult women than for adult men.
6. **T F** When consumed in excess, iron is easily excreted from the body.
7. **T F** Zinc is important to the growth of children.
8. **T F** Zinc nutritional status can be assessed using hair analysis.
9. **T F** High doses of zinc supplements can reduce immune function.
10. **T F** Copper plays a role in iron metabolism.
11. **T F** A copper deficiency could result from consuming too much zinc.
12. **T F** The ultimate source of most of our iodide intake is unprocessed foods.
13. **T F** Fluoride inhibits the metabolism and growth of the bacterium that causes dental caries.
14. **T F** Consuming excess chromium supplements is not dangerous, since there is little chance of chromium toxicity.
15. **T F** Because the terms *iron deficiency* and *anemia* are synonymous, they can be used interchangeably.

Trace Minerals

trace mineral A mineral vital to health that is required in a diet in amounts less than 100 mg/day.

Discovering the importance of each **trace mineral** to humans is a fairly recent and still unfolding drama that, in some cases, reads like a detective story. In 1961, scientists linked dwarfism in villagers in the Middle East to a zinc deficiency.[23] Other researchers recognized that an obscure form of heart disease in an isolated area of China was linked to a selenium deficiency.[15] In the United States, deficiencies of some trace minerals were first observed in the late 1960s to early 1970s when these nutrients were omitted in the preparation of synthetic formulas used in total parenteral nutrition.[23] Because research on trace minerals in humans is still in its infancy, our current understanding of trace mineral metabolism relies heavily on the knowledge gained from studies with farm and laboratory animals.

Not only are trace minerals needed in much smaller amounts than the major minerals, but the actual need for some trace minerals is still debatable. In Table 1-2 we listed nine essential trace minerals and eight possible ones. Demonstrating the essential nature of these latter nutrients is hampered by difficulty in measuring their amounts and by the rarity of naturally occurring deficiencies.[20] Before looking at each of the trace minerals, we discuss why research in this area is so complex.

DIFFICULTIES IN STUDYING TRACE MINERALS

Determining trace mineral needs is difficult because the body requires only minute amounts, and highly sophisticated technology is needed to measure such small amounts in both food and body tissues. Rigorous protocols often are required to produce a deficiency in animals. (All animal research referred to in this discussion was conducted with farm and/or laboratory animals.) The animals may need to be raised in ultraclean environments and have their diets carefully formulated from individual essential nutrients to ensure that no mineral contamination occurs. Stainless steel and plastic cages may also be needed so that the animals do not obtain any trace minerals, such as zinc, from chewing on the cages. Minerals must sometimes even be filtered from the air, and the water must be as free of minerals as possible.[20] In addition, glassware used for chemical analysis may need to be rinsed repeatedly in acid to eliminate trace mineral contamination; sometimes only plastic bottles are appropriate.[19]

In view of the difficulties encountered in experimentally producing most trace mineral deficiencies in laboratory animals, overt human deficiencies are unlikely, considering all the mineral sources in food, air, and water. However, some evidence is available indicating that marginal dietary intakes of certain trace minerals (e.g., iron, zinc, copper, and chromium) do occur, leading to mild undetected deficiencies in humans.[20,25,28,31] The lack of precise tests to pinpoint these deficiencies is the main reason there is concern, but not hard evidence.

Researchers generally like to use blood tests to assess mineral status because of the ease of obtaining blood. Unfortunately, the blood tests currently available for trace minerals are not reliable for every mineral under every circumstance. For instance, blood concentrations of the copper-containing protein **ceruloplasmin** are sometimes used to assess copper status, but these values can also be influenced by other than dietary factors.[28] Thus a researcher can't always tell what the true mineral status of a person really is. Indeed, the main factor limiting zinc research today is the lack of a sensitive measure of the zinc status of body tissues and fluids.[23]

SETTING NUTRIENT NEEDS FOR TRACE MINERALS

The difficulty in measuring trace mineral nutrition in humans makes setting their RDAs problematic. Most trace minerals have only an estimated safe and adequate daily dietary intake (ESADDI), not an RDA.

The primary method used to set trace mineral nutrient needs is the balance study. The same basic technique used for nitrogen balance studies works for minerals (see Chapters 2 and 5). Researchers try to determine the lowest mineral intake that meets all mineral losses from urine, feces, hair, skin, perspiration, menses, and so on. These studies are very expensive to perform. In addition, a balance study tells only the amount of dietary intake needed to maintain a specific **pool** of the mineral in the body, but this pool does not necessarily represent the amount needed to maintain good health.

There are further problems in establishing nutrient needs for trace minerals. Clinical signs and symptoms often appear only with severe deficiencies. We lack knowledge of the subtle physiological changes associated with most trace mineral deficiencies, so we cannot always detect people who are experiencing related ill health. They may consume just enough of a mineral to prevent obvious signs and symptoms from being expressed.[23]

A final complication is that trace minerals interact with each other. An overabundance of copper or iron in the digestive tract can interfere with absorption of the other minerals, such as zinc.[25] Thus, to set the RDA for zinc, nutrition scientists must estimate the amounts of copper and other minerals that will be consumed to predict how much zinc the body will actually absorb. Overall, quite a lot of scientific judgment must go into setting desired intakes for trace minerals.

TRACE MINERALS IN FOODS

The trace mineral content of plants depends primarily on the trace mineral concentration in the soil. Because soil concentrations of trace minerals vary greatly, the values of trace mineral contents of plant foods listed in food composition tables are sometimes misleading and of limited application. This is a less serious problem for foods of animal origin because animals eat a variety of plant products; in addition, some animals (especially cattle) are shipped from one area to another during their growth, processing, and finishing in a feed lot. Thus they generally consume foods grown under multiple soil conditions.

The bioavailability of trace minerals is another issue in planning diets. Even if a food is high in a particular mineral, it will not supply much to the body unless the mineral is absorbed well in the small intestine. Many factors found in foods inhibit mineral absorption. Mineral absorption from some plant sources can amount to only 3% to 6% of the total present. In general, animal sources of minerals are supe-

ceruloplasmin A blue, copper-containing protein in the blood that can remove an electron from Fe^{2+} (ferrous form) to yield Fe^{3+} (the ferric form). The Fe^{3+} form of iron can then bind with iron transport and storage proteins, such as transferrin.

pool The amount of a mineral or other substance stored within the body that can be easily mobilized when needed.

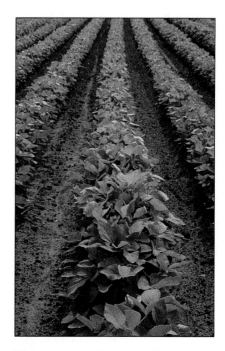

The trace mineral content of plant foods reflects the trace mineral concentration in the soil in which they were grown.

rior to plant sources because they show more efficient absorption.[7,23] Animal sources also often contain factors that enhance mineral absorption, even for those trace minerals supplied by plant foods in a meal.[7]

Throughout this book we repeatedly recommend eating a variety of foods. By doing so you can eat plants and animals that have derived nutrients from a variety of soils, and thus maximize your chances of consuming adequate amounts of trace minerals. In addition, with regard to most trace minerals, it is best to consume as many minimally processed foods as possible. Generally, the more refined a food, the lower its content of trace minerals. For example, during refining of wheat into white flour, the trace minerals iron, selenium, zinc, and copper are lost. Enrichment of white flour restores iron but not the other minerals.

Iron

Iron (Fe) is found in every living cell; total body content is about 5 g (about 1 teaspoon). The importance of iron for maintenance of health has been recognized for centuries. In 4000 BC, the Persian physician Melampus gave iron supplements to sailors to compensate for the iron lost from bleeding during battles. Today, iron-deficiency anemia is common worldwide.[31] In most developing nations about half of all children and women of childbearing age are estimated to suffer from iron deficiency; many of them have the more severe form of the disorder, iron-deficiency anemia.

ABSORPTION AND DISTRIBUTION OF IRON

The body uses several mechanisms to regulate iron absorption. Controlling absorption is important because the body cannot easily eliminate excess iron once absorbed. Iron absorption from foods typically varies from about 5% to 10% in healthy people and 10% to 20% in people with iron deficiency.[7] The extent of iron absorption depends on a variety of factors, the most important of which is the amount of current iron stores in the body (Table 15-1).[8]

Iron in foods occurs in several forms, which differ in their absorption by the body. Iron that is part of the **hemoglobin** and **myoglobin** molecules in animal flesh (about 40% of total iron present), called **heme iron,** is absorbed more than twice as efficiently as simple elemental iron, known as **nonheme iron.** Nonheme iron is also present in animal flesh, eggs, and milk, as well as in vegetables, grains, and other plant foods.

About 10% to 15% of iron in the American diet is heme iron, and usually about 20% is absorbed. Nonheme iron makes up the rest, and usually 2% to 20% is absorbed, with closer to the lower percentage being most typical.[7] Greater body needs are associated with greater absorption. Overall, the difference in absorption of heme and nonheme iron makes animal flesh (e.g., red meat and pork) a rich source of di-

---

Iron is the only nutrient for which adult women have a greater RDA than adult men.

---

hemoglobin Iron-containing protein in red blood cells that carries oxygen to the body tissues and some carbon dioxide away from the tissues. It is also responsible for the red color of blood.

myoglobin Iron-containing protein that binds oxygen (O_2) in muscle.

heme iron Iron provided from animal tissues primarily as a component of hemoglobin and myoglobin. Approximately 40% of the iron in meat is heme iron; it is readily absorbed.

nonheme iron Iron provided from plant sources and elemental iron components of animal tissues. Nonheme iron is less efficiently absorbed than heme iron, and absorption is also more closely dependent on body needs.

TABLE 15-1

Factors that affect iron absorption	
Increase	**Decrease**
Acid in the stomach	Phytic acid (in dietary fiber)
Heme iron	Oxalic acid
High body demand for red blood cells (blood loss, high altitude, physical training, pregnancy)	Polyphenols in tea and coffee
	Full body stores of iron
	Excess of other minerals (Zn, Mn, Ca)*
Low body stores of iron	Reduction in stomach acid
Meat protein factor (MPF)	Some antacids
Vitamin C	

*Especially when taken as supplements.

etary iron, considering both its iron content and the increased efficiency of absorption of the heme iron present.

Consuming heme iron and nonheme iron together increases nonheme iron absorption. A protein factor in meat, fish, and poultry also facilitates nonheme iron absorption. This factor appears to contain amino acids such as cysteine that bind iron to enhance absorption. Eating meat with vegetables and grain products generally improves the absorption of nonheme iron present in the meal.

Organic acids, such as vitamin C, modestly increase nonheme iron absorption by adding an electron to Fe^{3+} (the ferric form), yielding Fe^{2+} (the ferrous form).[14] Vitamin C then forms a complex, called a **chelate,** with Fe^{2+}, thereby enhancing absorption.

Ferrous iron is absorbed better than ferric iron because it crosses the mucus layer of the small intestine more readily to reach the brush border of intestinal absorptive cells. There, Fe^{2+} must then have an electron removed, re-forming Fe^{3+}, before it enters the absorptive cells. At the cell membrane of the brush border of the absorptive cells, Fe^{3+} binds to a receptor protein called membrane iron-binding protein, which finally transfers iron into the cell.[7]

Acid in the stomach also plays an important role in iron absorption by promoting the conversion of Fe^{3+} to Fe^{2+} and by solubilizing nonheme iron. The decreased production of stomach acid experienced by many elderly people can lower their iron absorption and ultimately their body stores of iron.

Heme iron follows a different absorptive process. It is likely absorbed directly into the absorptive cells after the globin (protein) fraction has been removed. Once inside the absorptive cells, the iron is released from the heme portion.[7]

Several dietary factors interfere with our ability to absorb iron. Phytic acid and other factors in grain fibers and oxalic acid in vegetables can all bind iron, reducing its absorption. A long-term concern about increasing dietary fiber intake above 35 g/day is the tendency for fiber components to bind iron (and other trace minerals), in turn decreasing absorption. Polyphenols, such as **tannins** found in tea and related substances found in coffee, also reduce iron absorption. People trying to rebuild iron stores are advised to reduce coffee and tea consumption, particularly at mealtimes. Finally, calcium supplements in amounts greater than 300 mg/day can reduce iron absorption.[30] Because of the ability of calcium to interfere with iron absorption, calcium supplements should be taken several hours before or after an iron-rich meal. If both calcium and iron supplements are used, they should not be taken at the same time of day.[9]

Because of the various influences on iron absorption, we can't easily estimate the amount of iron actually absorbed from individual foods. Rather, it is the overall composition of a meal and the needs of the person that largely determine the degree of absorption, and thus ultimately the amount of iron delivered to the body.[8]

Depending on body needs, some iron in the intestinal absorptive cells will be ushered directly into the bloodstream, where it is bound by the protein **transferrin.** The rest binds to apoferritin in the intestinal cells to form **ferritin.** Ferritin provides a short-term form of iron storage in intestinal cells. Eventually, the iron is either absorbed or sloughed off into the GI tract with the intestinal cell.

As noted already, the extent of iron stores in the body is the most important factor influencing iron absorption. When iron stores are adequate, all the iron-binding sites in transferrin are full (saturated) or nearly so. As a result, transfer of iron (especially nonheme iron) from the intestinal cells to the blood is inhibited, and much of the iron in these cells remains in the intestinal cells in the protein-bound form, ferritin. When intestinal cells are sloughed at the end of their 2- to 5-day life cycle, the iron returns to the GI tract and is excreted in the feces. On the other hand, when iron stores are low, transferrin in the blood readily binds more iron, shifting it directly from the intestinal cells into the blood or from ferritin stores in the intestinal cells into the blood. By this means—under normal circumstances—iron is absorbed only as needed.[8] This mechanism for resisting absorption of excess iron, primarily that in the nonheme form, is termed a "mucosal block" (Figure 15-1).

chelates Complexes formed between metal ions and substances with polar groups, such as proteins. The polar groups form two or more attachments with the metal ions, forming a ringed structure. The metal ion is then firmly bound and sequestered.

transferrin A protein that transports iron in the blood.

ferritin A protein compound that serves as the storage form of iron in the blood and tissues.

- - - - - - - - - - - -

The copper-containing blood protein ceruloplasmin removes an electron from Fe^{2+}, yielding Fe^{3+}, the form bound by transferrin. Thus copper metabolism and iron metabolism are closely linked. Eventually most of the iron in transferrin is deposited in the liver, forming ferritin.

- - - - - - - - - - - -

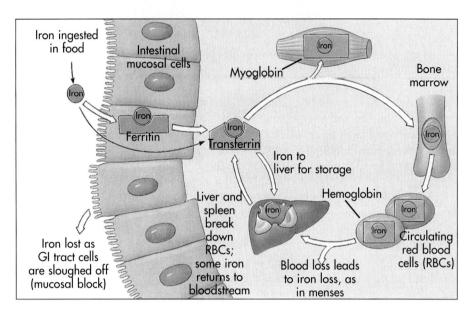

Figure 15-1 Iron absorption and distribution. Iron binds with a protein called apoferritin to form ferritin when stored in cells. If the intestinal absorptive cells are sloughed before iron is absorbed from them, the iron is not absorbed into the blood. This allows the body to control the absorption of iron, especially nonheme iron.

Almost all cells in the body have receptors for transferrin, so they can take up iron from the blood. About 70% of iron in the body ends up in the hemoglobin molecules in the red blood cells and myoglobin in muscle tissue (Figure 15-2). Some iron is stored in the bone marrow, and a small portion goes to other body cells or to the spleen and liver for storage in the form of ferritin. Each ferritin molecule can bind up to about 4000 iron atoms.[7] This sequestering of iron is important because free iron atoms are very reactive and could catalyze widespread cell destruction.[24] As the liver concentration of ferritin increases, associated with iron absorption in excess of needs, it is partly digested by the liver cells. The iron then forms a more insoluble product called **hemosiderin.**

As iron is needed, it can be mobilized from body stores and enter the blood. If dietary intake is inadequate, these iron stores become depleted. Only then do signs and symptoms of an iron deficiency appear.

FUNCTIONS OF IRON

Iron forms part of hemoglobin in red blood cells, myoglobin in muscle cells, and the cytochromes, which are components of the electron-transport chain in mitochondria. Iron also functions as a co-factor for some enzymes, including those involved in the synthesis of collagen and of various neurotransmitters (e.g., dopamine, epinephrine, norepinephrine, and serotonin). In addition, iron is needed for proper immune function and plays a role in drug-detoxification pathways.[7]

Hemoglobin molecules in red blood cells transport oxygen from the lungs to all cells and assist in the transport of some carbon dioxide (CO_2) from cells to the lungs for excretion. Bone marrow cells synthesize red blood cells when stimulated by **erythropoietin,** a hormone synthesized primarily by the kidneys. Erythropoietin is released in response to a decrease in oxygen concentration in the blood, blood loss, or binding of carbon monoxide (CO) to red blood cells. Erythropoietin targets the bone marrow to increase production of red blood cells.

As a red blood cell matures in the bone marrow, it expels its nucleus, which contains DNA, thus limiting the cell's lifespan (approximately 120 days). Without DNA, red blood cells can't direct new protein synthesis to replace worn-out cell parts, such as enzymes. Such a rapid cell turnover puts great nutrient demands on the body, and iron is one of the nutrients in greatest demand.[31]

hemosiderin An insoluble iron-protein compound in the liver. Hemosiderin stores iron when the amount of iron in the body exceeds the storage capacity of ferritin.

- - - - - - - - - - - -
A key attribute of iron is its ability to both take up and release oxygen atoms and electrons. This allows it to participate in carrying oxygen in the blood and in transferring electrons in the electron-transport chain of the cell mitochondria.
- - - - - - - - - - - -

erythropoietin A hormone that enhances the synthesis and release of red blood cells from bone marrow; it is produced mostly by the kidneys.

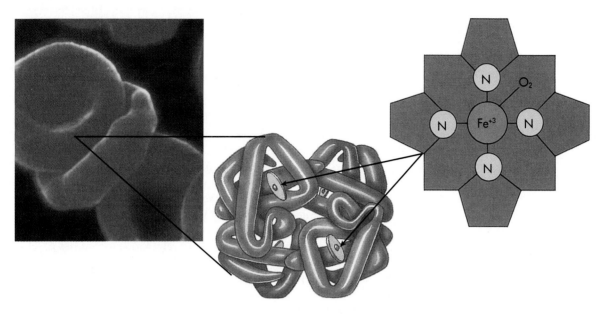

Figure 15-2 Most iron in the body is present in the hemoglobin molecules in the red blood cells. Iron gives hemoglobin the ability to carry oxygen.

REUTILIZATION AND LOSS OF IRON

Fortunately, the body conserves and reuses iron over and over again. As red blood cells die, macrophages in the liver, spleen, and other tissues release the iron from the red blood cells. The iron then attaches to transferrin in the blood and thus again becomes available either for storage as ferritin or ultimately for hemoglobin production. More than 90% of hemoglobin iron is recycled.[7]

Adult men lose about 0.9 to 1.2 mg of iron per day from the GI tract, urine, and skin. Women lose more iron because of menstrual blood loss. This varies among women, although each woman's menstrual blood loss generally is constant from month to month. When averaged over the entire month, iron losses for women are about 1.4 to 2.2 mg/day, depending on the amount of menstrual blood loss.[7]

IRON-DEFICIENCY ANEMIA

If neither the diet nor body stores can supply the iron needed for hemoglobin synthesis, red blood cell synthesis is reduced. Eventually, the number of red blood cells falls so low that the amount of oxygen carried in the blood is decreased. Such a person exhibits anemia, which is characterized by a decreased oxygen-carrying capacity of the blood. Although there are many types of anemia, the major type found worldwide is iron-deficiency anemia.[31]

Signs and Symptoms of Iron-Deficiency Anemia

In iron-deficiency anemia, the percentage of the total blood volume occupied by red blood cells, called the **hematocrit,** falls below 34% to 37%. The blood hemoglobin concentration also declines to less than 10 to 11 g/100 ml of blood. A variety of diseases can reduce hemoglobin and hematocrit values, but usually if both are reduced, the diagnosis is iron-deficiency anemia. Further evidence of anemia is a decreased volume of each red blood cell.[31]

In the United States, many women in their childbearing years have scant or no iron stores and thus are considered to be iron deficient. In most cases, their hemoglobin values remain normal and thus they do not experience iron-deficiency anemia. Such women, however, have no iron stores to draw from in times of illness, injury, or pregnancy.

Life stages during which iron-deficiency anemia often appears are infancy, the preschool years, and puberty for both males and females. The most common age for

Much anemia in the Mediterranean, Southeast Asia, and other parts of the world is due to a group of diseases called thalassemia. This genetic disease causes a person to synthesize incorrect forms of hemoglobin. The red blood cell then lacks the usual ability to carry oxygen.

hematocrit The percentage of total blood volume occupied by red blood cells.

iron-deficiency anemia is 6 months to 2 years. Women are also very vulnerable during childbearing years, when menses occurs. Anemia is often found in pregnant women, as will be discussed in Chapter 16. Up to about 6% of the total U.S. population is iron deficient, with about 7% to 12% of Americans in the high-risk categories actually having iron-deficiency anemia.[31]

During these critical life stages, the risk for iron-deficiency anemia is greatest either because growth, which is accompanied by increased blood volume and muscle mass, increases iron needs or because low energy intakes make it difficult to consume enough iron. Iron deficiency during pregnancy is especially dangerous because it significantly increases the risk of maternal and infant death, as well as preterm birth.[31]

Clinical signs and symptoms of iron-deficiency anemia include pale skin and brittle finger nails (sometimes spoon shaped), fatigue, weakness, difficulty breathing on exertion, inadequate temperature regulation, loss of appetite, and apathy. The fatigue is caused by insufficient synthesis of red blood cells and cytochromes because of the lack of iron. In early childhood, iron deficiency interferes with longitudinal growth, weight gain, and behavioral development. Behavior problems associated with childhood anemia are thought to be caused by interruptions in nerve impulse transmission.[7]

Inadequate iron stores can also decrease learning ability, work performance, and immune status, even before a person actually registers anemia. Keep in mind that many people with mild iron deficiency experience no obvious problems, other than vague symptoms of tiredness, headache, irritability, or depression. These people are iron deficient without showing signs or symptoms of anemia. It takes a long time for iron-deficiency anemia to develop. Overall, iron deficiency remains one of the most common and easily preventable nutrient deficiencies.[31] It is important to identify individuals experiencing the effects through regular physical examinations and to initiate treatment when needed. And of course, prevention is the best treatment.

Other Causes of Iron-Deficiency Anemia

In addition to the causes listed above, iron-deficiency anemia can be caused by chronic blood loss from heavy menses, ulcers, hemorrhoids, and colon cancer. Iron-deficiency anemia in men is usually linked to ulcers, colon cancer, or hemorrhoids.

The donation of 1 pint (0.5 L) of blood represents a loss of 200 to 250 mg of iron.[7] It generally takes several months to replace this iron. Most healthy people can donate blood two to four times a year without harmful consequences; generally women need the longer interval between donations to rebuild their iron status. As a precaution, blood banks first screen potential donors' blood for evidence of anemia.

In many developing countries a primary cause of iron-deficiency anemia is the inefficient absorption of iron from vegetable foods. The diets in these countries are largely vegetarian because meat is too expensive for most people to afford. Iron deficiency and anemia eventually affect the majority of individuals in such populations.[31]

Measuring Iron Status

The most sensitive measure of iron stores in the body currently available in healthcare settings is the concentration of ferritin in the blood. If ferritin is low, iron stores likely are low. Development of a measure of the amount of iron in the ferritin molecules is under way; this will be an even more sensitive measure of iron status.

As iron deficiency proceeds, the total iron-binding capacity of blood proteins increases. Many iron-binding sites on the blood proteins become free, leaving more room than usual for extra iron to bind. At the same time, the bone marrow, which synthesizes red blood cells, begins releasing immature red blood cell products called **free erythrocyte protoporphyrins (FEP).** As iron deficiency becomes more serious, hemoglobin and hematocrit values fall (Figure 15-3). The red blood cells will now be very small and pale. This blood picture is referred to as a **microcytic** (small

---

Consumption of clay and similar nonfood substances may lead to iron-deficiency anemia because clay can bind much of the iron in the GI tract. The practice of eating nonfood items, termed *pica,* is discussed in Chapter 16.

Blood loss caused by intestinal and blood-borne parasite infections is another common cause of anemia among poor populations, especially when people do not wear shoes. Parasites, such as hookworms, can easily penetrate the soles of the feet and legs and enter the bloodstream. Although hookworm disease has been largely eradicated through improved sanitation in the United States and other industrialized nations, it continues to plague more than one fifth of the world's population, mostly in tropical regions.[13]

---

free erythrocyte protoporphyrins (FEP) Immature red blood cells released from the bone marrow. An elevated blood FEP reflects a decreased ability to make red blood cells and suggests iron-deficiency anemia. Lead poisoning also raises blood FEP.

microcytic Describing red blood cells that are smaller than normal; literally, "small cell."

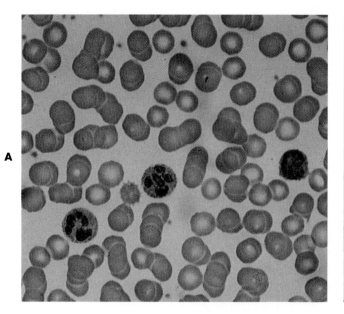
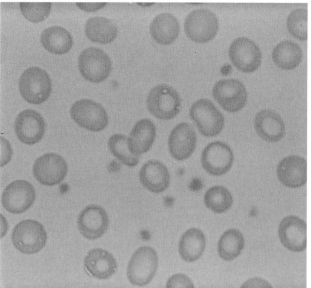

A

B

Figure 15-3 Iron-deficiency anemia. **A,** Normal cells; both cell size and color are normal. **B,** Iron-deficient cells; both cell size and color are decreased. The loss of color stems from the lower amount of the pigment hemoglobin. The stages of iron depletion in the body progress from (1) low serum ferritin to (2) low transferrin saturation to (3) an increase in free erythrocyte protoporphyrins to (4) microcytic hypochromic anemia.

cell) **hypochromic** (pale) anemia.[7] Only very severe cases of iron deficiency reach this point.

hypochromic Describing pale red blood cells lacking sufficient hemoglobin as a result of iron deficiency. Hypochromic cells have a reduced oxygen-carrying ability.

Treating Iron-Deficiency Anemia

To speed the cure of iron-deficiency anemia, medicinal forms of iron, such as ferrous sulfate, need to be ingested. A physician should also find the cause of the anemia so that it does not recur. A good diet may prevent iron-deficiency anemia, but medicinal iron is a better cure. This iron should be given to increase the hemoglobin and hematocrit values and to replace depleted iron stores. This treatment usually involves 325 mg of ferrous sulfate one to three times per day for 6 to 12 months, yielding about 180 mg of elemental iron per day. If the full dose upsets the stomach, a lower dose can be tried, with the time of treatment extended; the dose then can be increased as tolerance increases.[7]

IRON IN FOODS

Because much of the iron in animal foods is heme iron, the most bioavailable form, meats are the richest sources of iron. The major iron sources in American diets are animal foods, such as beef steaks, roasts, and hamburger (Figure 15-4). The next greatest sources are bakery products, including white breads, rolls, and crackers. Most of the iron in these products is elemental forms of iron added to refined flour as part of the enrichment process. Only about 5% of this iron consumed is absorbed.

Foods providing the highest nutrient density for iron (mg/kcal) are spinach, oysters, liver, peas, legumes, and beef. However, as we've seen already, neither the total iron content nor the nutrient density of individual foods is an accurate guide for choosing dietary sources of iron. Rather, the bioavailability of the iron present in a meal, which depends on its form and the presence or absence of factors that influence absorption, and the body's need for iron ultimately determine how much iron actually is delivered to the body.[8]

A common cause of iron-deficiency anemia in children is an over-reliance on milk, a very poor source of iron, and too little meat in their diets.[29] In the United States, a major contributor to decreasing rates of iron-deficiency anemia in preschool children has been the use of iron-fortified formulas and cereals in the Spe-

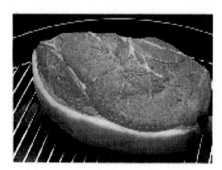

Red meat is a major source of iron in the American diet.

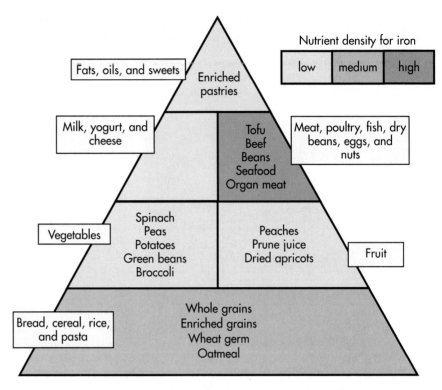

Figure 15-4 Food sources of iron from the Food Guide Pyramid. The meat, poultry, fish, dry beans, eggs, and nuts group and the bread, cereal, rice, and pasta group are the best dietary sources of this nutrient. The heme iron in the meat, poultry, fish, dry beans, eggs, and nuts group is especially well absorbed. The iron content of a food containing mostly nonheme iron is only an approximate measure of the amount delivered to body cells, as body need greatly influences the absorption of nonheme iron. The background color of each food group indicates the average nutrient density for iron in that group.

cial Supplemental Food Program for Women, Infants, and Children (WIC program; see Chapters 16 and 17).

Another source of iron is cooking utensils. When acidic foods, such as tomato sauce, are cooked in iron cookware, some iron from the pan is taken up by the food. The replacement of iron cookware with stainless steel and aluminum cookware in recent times likely has increased the risk for iron deficiency.

RDA FOR IRON

The body needs to absorb about 0.9 to 1.2 mg of iron daily for men and 1.4 to 2.2 mg daily for women.[7] The adult RDA for iron is 10 mg/day for men and 15 mg/day for women. (Throughout the rest of this chapter, consult the inside front cover for other age groups and Appendix E for Canadian recommendations.) The RDA values for iron are based on the assumption that about 10% to 15% of dietary iron is absorbed. If iron absorption exceeds that, less dietary iron is needed. On average, men consume 17 mg and women consume 12 mg of iron per day.[3]

The iron RDA was set higher for women primarily to account for menstrual blood loss. Women who menstruate more heavily and longer than "average" need even more dietary iron; those who have lighter and shorter flows may need less. The variation in menstrual blood loss makes it difficult to set an RDA for iron that is applicable to most women.

Analysis of daily dietary intakes recorded by a variety of women has shown that most women do not consume the RDA for iron (15 mg/day). Of course, not all women need this much iron, since the RDA is set high enough to meet the needs of nearly all women. Varying degrees of menstrual flow and wide differences in iron absorption (recall it varies with need) also complicate evaluation of dietary intakes

of iron. For instance, a person absorbing 20% of dietary iron could meet the RDA by consuming half as much iron as a person absorbing 10% of dietary intake.

People who find out they are not consuming the RDA for iron should be concerned but not alarmed. They are well advised to make dietary changes so they will meet the RDA. Whether persistent intakes somewhat below the RDA actually harm health is difficult to determine. Despite the availability of very sensitive measures of iron stores in the body, we lack the knowledge to translate this information into predictors of health status.[7]

AMERICANS AT RISK FOR IRON DEFICIENCY AND ANEMIA

As stated earlier, iron deficiency is most common when iron needs greatly exceed normal intake—such as during infancy and the preschool years, puberty, and women's childbearing years. Pregnancy and disease also increase iron needs and therefore the risk for deficiency. Repeated pregnancies pose a special challenge to women to maintain adequate iron stores.[7]

The American diet contains about 5 to 7 mg of iron per 1000 kcal. Thus men, who commonly have daily energy intakes of 2000 to 3000 kcal, generally meet their RDA for iron and achieve a good iron status. Most women, on the other hand, can't consume 3000 kcal daily and still maintain desirable weight. Thus they have difficulty consuming 15 mg of iron daily unless they include nutrient-dense forms of iron (e.g., fortified breakfast cereals and red meat) in their diets. If a change in diet does not suffice, a supplement should be used, under a physician's scrutiny. Inadequate iron stores and even iron-deficiency anemia are found among all social strata, not just among the poor. Vegans also should pay special attention to their intakes.

Athletes may incur a special type of anemia called **runner's anemia,** as we discussed in Chapter 10. Four possible factors contribute to it: high iron losses via increased perspiration, destruction of red blood cells (hemolysis) as they pass through the foot when it strikes the ground during exercise, the increase in blood volume associated with athletic fitness, and increased iron loss in the feces. Runner's anemia can decrease sports performance and so should be avoided. Athletes should have their blood hemoglobin and other indicators of iron status monitored to ensure adequate status.

runner's anemia A decrease in the blood's ability to carry oxygen found in otherwise healthy athletes. It may be caused by iron loss in perspiration and feces, red blood cell destruction due to the impact of the foot striking the ground during exercise, and increased blood volume.

TOXICITY OF IRON

Although not as common as iron deficiency, iron overload can be serious because it can easily lead to toxic symptoms.[7] Even a large single dose of iron of 60 mg can be life-threatening to a 1-year-old. Children are frequently victims of iron poisoning because iron pills and vitamin supplements containing iron are tempting targets on kitchen tables and in cabinets. FDA has proposed a rule that would require label warnings on iron supplements with 30 mg of iron or more per tablet, stating that iron may be lethal to children who ingest the product.

Smaller doses of iron (but still greater than what is needed) over a long period can also cause problems. A form of iron toxicity, for example, has been observed in an African tribe that brews beer in iron pots. Some people of Mediterranean descent have a type of anemia caused by increased destruction of red blood cells; low-dose iron therapy used to treat this disease can lead to toxicity symptoms.[7] Repeated blood transfusions can also lead to iron toxicity.

In addition, iron toxicity accompanies the genetic disease called hereditary **hemochromatosis.** People with hemochromatosis overabsorb iron. The disease is associated with a substantial increase in the activity of the membrane iron-binding protein present in hepatocytes and intestinal absorptive cells that we described earlier.[7] Thus this protein may play a critical role in the development of hemochromatosis. In those with this disease, the amount of iron in the body eventually builds up to dangerous amounts, especially in the blood and liver. Some iron is deposited in the muscles, pancreas, and heart. If not treated, the excess iron deposits contribute to severe organ damage, especially in the liver and heart. Diabetes, liver cirrhosis, and a bronze skin pigmentation are possible complications. Certain food-

CRITICAL THINKING

Tom is 13 years old and has taken up track in school. Every day for the last 6 weeks he has practiced after school for 1 or 2 hours. After taking his physical examination last week at his doctor's office, Tom was told that his low hemoglobin count indicates that he has anemia. Tom doesn't understand how this is possible, since he is eating normally and has not decreased his food intake at all. How can his doctor explain the diagnosis to him?

hemochromatosis A disorder of iron metabolism characterized by increased absorption, saturation of iron-binding proteins, and deposition of hemosiderin in the liver tissue.

borne microbes (*Yersenia enterocolotica* and *Vibrio vulnificus*) can also cause severe or fatal infections in persons with iron overload. The major causes of death from hemochromatosis are cirrhosis and liver cancer.[7]

Hereditary hemochromatosis is a recessive genetic disorder; that is, a person must carry two defective copies of a particular gene to develop the disease. People with one defective gene and one normal gene, called carriers, may also absorb excess dietary iron but not to the same extent as those with two defective genes. About 5% to 10% of white Americans of Northern European extraction are carriers of hemochromatosis. An estimated 0.25% to 0.4% of this population carries two defective genes and therefore has the potential for developing the disease.[11]

Carriers of hemochromatosis may be prime candidates for heart disease. As we noted in Chapter 4, excess iron in the blood may accelerate atherosclerosis in people with elevated LDL by contributing to oxidation of lipids in the LDL particles. This in turn allows LDL to be taken up more readily by scavenger cells in the blood vessels.[11] However, the importance of iron in stimulating atherosclerosis is still hotly debated.[24] Because of its relatively efficient absorption, dietary heme iron, such as that found in red meats, poses the greatest risk in this regard.[5,17] To put this research into perspective, a reasonable approach is for you to ask to be screened for iron overload at your next visit to a physician. If you show evidence of this it would be wise to undergo therapy, especially if you have high LDL as well.

There are several reliable screening tests for detecting iron overload. Elevated values for serum iron, ferritin, and transferrin saturation suggest its presence.[11] A more aggressive approach to screening for iron overload and hemochromatosis is likely to become common in the future. The advantage of screening and early detection is that appropriate treatment, such as frequent bleeding, can stop the disease process so that affected individuals can lead a healthier life. The first symptom of hemochromatosis often is arthritis-like symptoms, such as painful joints.[7]

Ideally, consent of a physician should precede any use of iron supplements.[11] Even when iron supplements are advised, there should be adequate follow-up so that supplementation does not go beyond what is necessary. Probably the only factor keeping many people with hemochromatosis and carriers of one gene from experiencing serious effects of the disease is that they consume such a low amount of iron.

CONCEPT CHECK

Iron absorption depends mostly on its form and the body's need for it. Absorption is affected by a "mucosal block," but excess iron intake can override the system, leading to toxicity. Iron absorption increases somewhat in the presence of vitamin C and decreases in the presence of large amounts of calcium and some components of grain fiber, such as phytic acid. Iron is most important in synthesizing hemoglobin and myoglobin, in supporting immune function, and in energy metabolism. An iron deficiency can cause decreased red blood cell synthesis, which can lead to anemia. It is particularly important for women of childbearing age to consume adequate iron, primarily to replace that lost in menstrual blood. Good sources include red meat, pork, liver, enriched grains and cereals, and oysters. Iron toxicity usually results from a genetic disorder called hemochromatosis. This disease causes overabsorption and accumulation of iron, which can result in severe liver and heart damage.

CRITICAL THINKING

Annie, Tom's friend, is taking a nutrition class at her university. She suggested that he consume some extra vitamin C every day. Tom is confused by this advice, since his doctor told him to increase the amount of iron in his diet, not the amount of vitamin C. How can Annie explain her recommendation to him?

Zinc

Although zinc (Zn) has been recognized as an essential nutrient in animals since the early 1900s, zinc deficiency was first recognized in humans in the early 1960s in Egypt and Iran.[23] The deficiency was determined to be the cause of growth retardation and inadequate sexual development in humans. Curiously, the zinc content was fairly high in their diets. However, the customary diet contained almost exclusively unleavened bread and little animal protein. Unleavened bread is very high in phytic acid and other factors that decrease zinc bioavailability. Yeast fermentation in the preparation of bread dough reduces the effect of phytic acid by tenfold. In addition, parasite infestation and the practice of eating clay also contributed to the initial cases of severe zinc deficiency observed in humans.[23]

In the United States, zinc deficiencies were first observed in the early 1970s in hospitalized patients receiving total parenteral nutrition.[25] Originally zinc was not added to the intravenous solutions, but the protein source in the solutions was based on milk protein or blood fibrin, which are naturally rich in zinc. When the solutions were later changed to include mostly isolated amino acids as the protein source, zinc-deficiency symptoms quickly developed. This source of protein is very low in zinc.

ABSORPTION OF ZINC

Like iron absorption, zinc absorption is influenced by the types of food ingested. About 10% to 35% of dietary zinc is absorbed from foods. The higher figure is more likely when animal protein sources are consumed, the body's zinc needs are elevated, and small amounts are consumed. The RDA for zinc is based on absorption of 20% of intake.[25]

Zinc absorption, despite extensive study, is not clearly understood, but probably involves a compound that works in the small intestine to help transport zinc into the intestinal cells. After entering the blood, zinc binds to blood proteins, such as albumin, and amino acids. About a third enters the liver; the remaining zinc is distributed throughout the body.

When zinc is absorbed into intestinal cells, it induces synthesis of **metallothionein,** a protein that binds zinc in much the same way that ferritin binds iron.[23] If zinc is not transferred to the blood from the intestinal cells within 2 to 5 days, it is sloughed off along with the cell and excreted. Thus a "mucosal block" works against overabsorption of zinc and iron, but much more so in the case of iron (Figure 15-5). If large doses of zinc are taken, they override the mucosal block. Luckily for overconsumers, zinc is also readily excreted via the pancreas into the intestinal tract and leaves the body by the feces, unlike iron.

Zinc intakes worldwide are generally low. Toasting cereals also reduces zinc absorption as it binds with flour constituents. Because most people worldwide rely on cereal grains for their sources of protein, energy, and zinc, finding adequate zinc sources and maintaining adequate zinc intakes is a problem.[23] And since zinc and iron are most available from the same foods, zinc and iron deficiencies occur together among similar populations of the developing countries. Therefore individuals with iron deficiency are also at very high risk for zinc deficiency.[25]

metallothionein A protein that binds and regulates the release of zinc and copper in intestinal and liver cells.

FUNCTIONS OF ZINC AND EFFECTS OF DEFICIENCY

Over 300 enzymes require zinc as a co-factor for optimal activity. Adequate zinc intake is necessary to support many bodily functions, such as[23]:

- nucleic acid synthesis and function (some factors that control expression of genes contain zinc-rich regions that bind DNA)
- protein metabolism, wound healing, and growth
- immune function (intakes in excess of the RDA do not provide any extra benefit to immune function)
- development of sexual organs and bone
- storage, release, and function of insulin
- cell membrane structure and function

Clinicians treating malnourished children observed that weight gain occurred much faster when the children consumed zinc supplements containing about three times the RDA. These findings highlight the importance of zinc for growth. Zinc is also important for behavioral development in infants.[23]

Two important enzymes that require zinc are carbonic anhydrase and alcohol dehydrogenase.[23] Carbonic anhydrase combines water (H_2O) and carbon dioxide

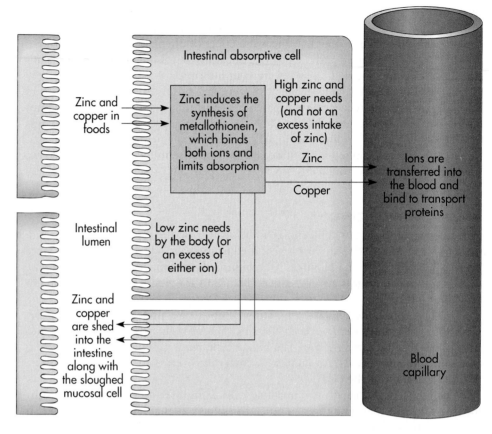

Figure 15-5 Zinc and copper absorption. Both minerals influence the absorption of the other. The effect is most obvious with excessive zinc intake, which greatly depresses copper absorption by inducing synthesis of metallothionein; this protein avidly binds copper. The short lifespan of the intestinal absorptive cells also influences absorption of these minerals, since any metallothionein-bound copper or zinc is sloughed off along with the intestinal cell into the intestinal tract.

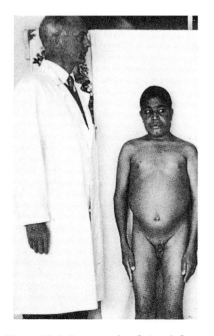

Figure 15-6 An example of zinc deficiency. An Egyptian farm boy, age 16 years and 49 inches tall, with dwarfism and inadequate sexual development associated with a zinc deficiency.

(CO_2) to form carbonic acid (H_2CO_3); this reaction is crucial for maintaining acid-base balance in the blood. Alcohol dehydrogenase breaks down alcohol.

Aside from inadequate growth, signs and symptoms of zinc deficiency include an acnelike rash, diarrhea, lack of appetite, fall in immune function, reduced sense of taste and smell, impaired appetite, hair loss, mental confusion, delivery of low birthweight infants by pregnant women, and inadequate sexual development in children and adolescents (Figure 15-6).[25] Reduced learning ability also may result, as zinc deficiency can be a cause of impaired neuropsychological function among infants and children, as is seen in iron deficiency. A persistent rash, especially in the presence of an inadequate diet, should prompt a clinician to evaluate zinc status in a person.

ZINC IN FOODS

In general, protein-rich diets are also rich in zinc. Americans get about 70% of their dietary zinc from animal foods. Lean meats—especially beef, other red meats, and shellfish—end up our best zinc sources because zinc from these animal sources is neither bound by phytic acid, nor so affected by local soil conditions.[25]

Foods with the highest nutrient density for zinc (mg/kcal) are oysters, wheat germ, crab, shrimp, beef and pork, liver, turkey, and legumes (Figure 15-7). Good plant sources of zinc, such as nuts, beans, and whole grains, can also deliver substantial amounts of zinc to body cells. Zinc is not part of the enrichment process, so refined flours are not a good source.

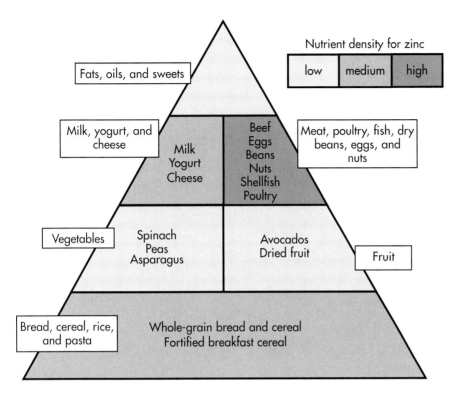

Figure 15-7 Food sources of zinc from the Food Guide Pyramid. The meat, poultry, fish, dry beans, eggs, and nuts group includes the best dietary sources of this nutrient. Some zinc is supplied by whole grains and fortified breakfast cereals from the bread, cereal, rice, and pasta group. The background color of each food group indicates the average nutrient density for zinc in that group.

RDA FOR ZINC

The adult RDA for zinc is 15 mg/day for men and 12 mg/day for women. The average adult intake of zinc is 15 mg and 9 mg daily for men and women, respectively.[3] Although some women may have marginal intakes, there is no evidence of widespread moderate or severe zinc deficiencies among otherwise healthy adult women or men. Strong homeostatic control of absorption and excretion can maintain persons in zinc balance even when intakes are somewhat lower than those furnished by typical diets of Americans. However, the long-term effects of marginal zinc intakes are not known.[25]

AMERICANS AT RISK FOR ZINC DEFICIENCY

Zinc deficiencies are most commonly found in hospital patients with severe malabsorption syndromes. Worldwide, protein-energy malnutrition is an important cause of zinc deficiency (see Chapter 20).[23] Sickle cell disease increases zinc needs by destroying massive numbers of red blood cells, which contain a significant amount of zinc. In addition, people with alcoholism or anorexia nervosa, elderly people, pregnant women, and vegans can be deficient in zinc because of either an inadequate overall nutrient intake or a diet low or lacking in animal foods.[25] Greater zinc intake in these people can sometimes increase their appetite and sense of taste. In the United States, symptoms of zinc deficiency have been observed in groups of middle-income and low-income children exhibiting inadequate growth. As we mentioned, supplementation with zinc can improve growth and appetite,[25] especially if the child is stunted for his or her age.

The link between zinc and appetite, taste acuity, wound healing, and immune response underscores zinc's importance in the diets of elderly people. Immune status is often depressed in elderly people. Because of poorly fitting dentures or low incomes, elderly people may not eat enough animal products. This reduces zinc intake.[25]

A rare disease, acrodermatitis enteropathica, results from an inherited inability to absorb zinc. Signs and symptoms in infants include rash, hair loss, depressed immune response, lack of appetite, and inadequate growth. This disease can be treated with supplements of zinc in amounts of about 30 to 45 mg/day, about 6 to 10 times the RDA for infants.[23]

Although many Americans likely have a marginal zinc status, we lack sensitive clinical measures for determining zinc status. The available clinical tests register a zinc deficiency only when body stores are very depleted. Assessment of zinc status is difficult because the amount of zinc in the blood does not reflect body stores, and no test using a zinc-containing enzyme is currently accepted.

TOXICITY OF ZINC

High zinc intakes, greater than about twice the RDA, inhibit copper absorption. Zinc does this by stimulating synthesis of the mineral-binding protein metallothionein. One study has shown that zinc supplements at approximately three to five times the RDA can reduce HDL by about 15%, perhaps by interfering with copper metabolism. That is disturbing for two reasons. First, low HDL is associated with an increased risk of developing heart disease (see Chapter 4). Second, it is common for people who take zinc supplements to consume this amount. Again, this shows why mineral supplements should not be consumed in excess of 1.5 times the Daily Value listed on the label except under close scrutiny of a physician. In fact, the RDA publication recommends not exceeding the RDA for zinc with supplements unless under close medical supervision. Zinc intakes over 100 mg/day also result in diarrhea, cramps, nausea, vomiting, and depressed immune system function, especially if intake exceeds 2 g/day.

Copper

Copper (Cu) is a part of certain enzymes, contributes to the activity of other enzymes, and aids in iron metabolism. About 10% to 55% of dietary copper is absorbed, with higher intakes associated with lower absorption. Copper is excreted primarily via the bile into the GI tract.

FUNCTIONS OF COPPER

Copper increases iron absorption by helping form a protein called ceruloplasmin (also known as ferroxidase). This compound mobilizes iron by accepting an electron from Fe^{2+} to form Fe^{3+}, the form that can cross the cell membrane of intestinal and other body cells. Thus ceruloplasmin enables iron to leave the intestinal cells and sites of iron storage in the liver and bind to the protein transferrin in the bloodstream.[28] The iron is then transported to cells in the bone marrow, where it is used in hemoglobin synthesis.

Copper is part of an enzyme that forms cross-links in collagen and elastin—connective tissue proteins. In laboratory animals with a copper deficiency, blood vessels rupture because collagen is not available to form the important connective tissue network needed to strengthen blood vessels (see Figure 13-17 for a review of collagen metabolism). The terminal enzyme in the electron-transport chain (cytochrome *C* oxidase) contains copper. This enzyme contributes to the formation of water from hydrogen and oxygen, in turn allowing for the formation of ATP.[28]

Copper is also part of enzymes that synthesize norepinephrine and dopamine, two neurotransmitters. In addition, copper-containing enzymes are needed in the formation and maintenance of myelin, the insulation material around nerves. One of the body's major scavengers for superoxide free radicals, the enzyme superoxide dismutase, also contains copper. (This is true for both the intracellular and extracellular forms of the enzyme.) Finally, copper participates in immune system function, blood clotting, and cholesterol metabolism.[28]

Signs and symptoms of copper deficiency include anemia, decreased numbers of white blood cells (specifically, the neutrophils), bone loss, and inadequate growth.[22] Frank copper deficiency has been linked to a form of heart disease in laboratory animals.[28]

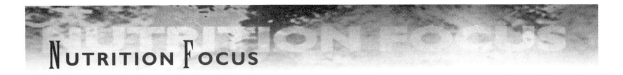

NUTRITION FOCUS

HAIR ANALYSIS: EXPERIMENTAL METHOD FOR TRACE MINERAL ASSESSMENT

For the last 20 years researchers have been experimenting with hair analysis as a way of assessing trace mineral status in the body. The technique is relatively simple: after a clump of hair is clipped close to the scalp, the 2 inches on the scalp end are removed and digested in acid. The amounts of trace minerals in the acid digest can be determined by sensitive analytical methods. To date, however, the results of hair analysis as an indicator of trace mineral status have been inconsistent and unreliable for several reasons.

Contamination of hair by air pollutants and treatment with shampoos, conditioners, dyes, and bleaches can substantially change the trace mineral content of hair. In the laboratory, slight changes in the method of washing and heating the hair before analysis can even make results from different laboratories difficult to compare. Only trained scientists with experience can produce reliable results.

Another problem is that the relationship between the trace mineral content of hair and that in the body is not well documented. And much more research is needed to determine whether small changes monitored by hair analysis actually reflect subtle changes in the body's trace mineral content. Thus the meaning of the results of hair analysis in terms of trace mineral status is often ambiguous.

Hair analysis is useful in establishing toxic levels of arsenic. It also may be a reliable method for measuring zinc status. At this time, however, no evidence supports the use of hair analysis for routine human nutrition assessment.

Commercial laboratories throughout America perform hair analysis. For about $25 to $50 they will analyze a hair sample and may send an impressive computer printout listing the mineral content of the hair. Some even list one's vitamin status based on the hair analysis, although there is no evidence that hair can predict vitamin status. The report may also predict the mineral status of the body and perhaps even include a few pages of health recommendations, including a catalog of supplements that will "restore" health.

A noted scientist sent samples of hair from two women to 13 commercial laboratories around the country. Reported results varied significantly from laboratory to laboratory for the same sample. Considering that scientists are having a difficult time determining the valid uses of hair analysis, it is improper for laboratories to offer this as a nutrition assessment tool for the average person. Reputable scientists suggest that hair analysis is still in the experimental phase and not ready for routine clinical applications.

COPPER IN FOODS

Copper is primarily found in organ meats (liver), seafood, cocoa, mushrooms, legumes, nuts, seeds, and whole-grain breads and cereals (Figure 15-8). It is not added in significant amounts to breakfast cereals, since it speeds fat breakdown in the product (Figure 15-9). Milk is also very low in copper.

Foods with the highest nutrient density for copper (mg/kcal) are oysters, lobster, liver, sunflower seeds, and various nuts. Food composition tables often list few values for copper, and even those values may not be reliable because soil conditions greatly affect the copper content of plant foods.

ESADDI FOR COPPER AND RISK FOR DEFICIENCY

Copper has an estimated safe and adequate daily dietary intake of 1.5 to 3 mg/day for adults. Our average intake is about 1 to 1.5 mg daily. Women generally have marginal intakes.[3] Even so, the copper status of adults in America appears to be fine.

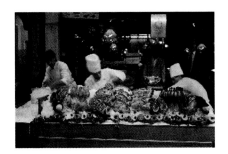

Seafood, especially oysters and lobster, is a rich source of copper.

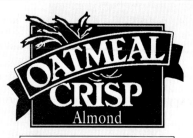

Nutrition Facts

Serving Size 1 cup (55g)
Servings Per Container About 8

Amount Per Serving	Oatmeal Crisp with Almonds	with ½ cup skim milk
Calories	230	270
Calories from Fat	50	50
	% Daily Value**	
Total Fat 6g*	**9%**	**9%**
Saturated Fat 0.5g	**3%**	**4%**
Cholesterol 0mg	**0%**	**1%**
Sodium 320mg	**13%**	**16%**
Potassium 150mg	**4%**	**10%**
Total Carbohydrate 39g	**13%**	**15%**
Dietary Fiber 3g	**12%**	**12%**
Sugars 11g		
Other Carbohydrate 25g		
Protein 6g		
Vitamin A	25%	30%
Vitamin C	25%	25%
Calcium	10%	25%
Iron	90%	90%
Vitamin D	10%	25%
Thiamin	25%	30%
Riboflavin	25%	35%
Niacin	25%	25%
Vitamin B$_6$	25%	25%
Folic Acid	25%	25%
Phosphorus	15%	25%
Magnesium	10%	15%
Zinc	25%	30%
Copper	8%	8%

*Amount in Cereal. A serving of cereal plus skim milk provides 6g fat (1g saturated), less than 5mg cholesterol, 380mg sodium, 360mg potassium, 45g carbohydrate (17g sugars), and 10g protein.

**Percent Daily Values are based on a 2,000 calorie diet. Your daily values may be higher or lower depending on your calorie needs:

		Calories:	2,000	2,500
Total Fat	Less than		65g	80g
Sat Fat	Less than		20g	25g
Cholesterol	Less than		300mg	300mg
Sodium	Less than		2,400mg	2,400mg
Total Carbohydrate			300g	375g
Dietary Fiber			25g	30g

INGREDIENTS: ROLLED OATS, RICE, ALMOND PIECES WITH FRESHNESS PRESERVED BY BHT, BROWN SUGAR, SUGAR, HONEY, SALT, CORN SYRUP, SUNFLOWER OIL, ARTIFICIAL AND NATURAL FLAVORS, CALCIUM CARBONATE.

VITAMINS AND MINERALS: IRON AND ZINC (MINERAL NUTRIENTS), VITAMIN C (SODIUM ASCORBATE), A B VITAMIN (NIACINAMIDE), VITAMIN B$_6$ (PYRIDOXINE HYDROCHLORIDE), VITAMIN A (PALMITATE), VITAMIN B$_2$ (RIBOFLAVIN), VITAMIN B$_1$ (THIAMIN MONONITRATE), A B VITAMIN (FOLIC ACID), VITAMIN D.

General Mills, Inc.
GENERAL OFFICES
MINNEAPOLIS, MINNESOTA 55440
Made in U.S.A.

© 1994 General Mills, Inc.

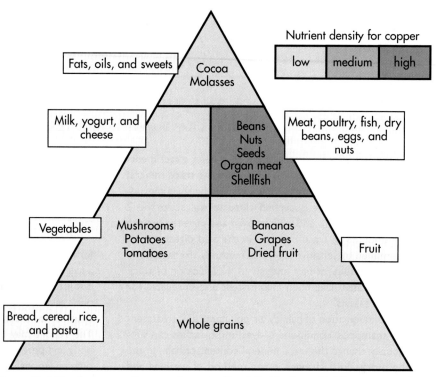

Figure 15-8 Food sources of copper from the Food Guide Pyramid. The meat, poultry, fish, dry beans, eggs, and nuts group includes the best dietary sources of this nutrient. Some copper is supplied by whole grains and fortified breakfast cereals from the bread, cereal, rice, and pasta group. The background color of each food group indicates the average nutrient density for copper in that group.

As with zinc, though, the absence of sensitive measures for copper status may result in some cases of marginal deficiencies being missed.

Among those at the greatest risk for a copper deficiency are preterm infants; infants recovering from undernutrition on a diet dominated by milk, which is an inadequate source of copper; people recovering from intestinal surgery, which reduces copper absorption; and people on long-term total parenteral nutrition if there is insufficient copper in the formula. Use of large doses of antacids also may bind enough copper in the intestine to cause a deficiency.[22]

A copper deficiency can result from overzealous supplementation of zinc, as we noted earlier, since excess zinc can hamper copper absorption (Figure 15-5). Zinc increases synthesis of the protein metallothionein, which binds both minerals—but particularly copper—in the intestinal cells, reducing future transfer of copper into the bloodstream.[23]

TOXICITY OF COPPER

Copper tends to cause vomiting at single doses greater than 10 to 15 mg. When copper is used to treat a deficiency, it must be given in divided doses to limit this effect. An inherited condition called Wilson's disease results in accumulation of copper in the liver, brain, kidneys, and cornea of the eye. If recognized early, treatment with agents that bind copper in the bloodstream and increase its excretion in the urine can prevent damage to these tissues and reduce the mental degeneration commonly seen in active cases. Ordinarily, excess copper is excreted through the bile by way of the gastrointestinal tract, but this does not happen in Wilson's disease.[28]

Figure 15-9 Breakfast cereals generally are better sources of iron and zinc than of copper. This is because adding copper would speed fat breakdown in the product.

CONCEPT CHECK

Similar to iron absorption, zinc absorption is partly regulated by a mucosal block. Animal protein sources, increased body needs, and small intakes lead to increased zinc absorption. Zinc functions as a co-factor for many enzymes and is important for growth, immune function, and sense of taste. Beef, seafood, and whole grains are good food sources of zinc. Copper functions mainly as part of enzymes and other compounds involved in iron metabolism, cross-linking of collagen, myelination of nerve cells, and neurotransmitter synthesis. A copper deficiency can result in a form of anemia and impaired immune function. Good food sources of copper are liver, seafood, legumes, nuts, and whole grains.

Selenium

Selenium (Se) exists in many ionic forms. Most selenium in foods is bound to derivatives of the amino acids methionine and cysteine. Because these substances are readily absorbed, the bioavailability of selenium is considerably higher than that of iron, zinc, and copper. About 50% to 100% of dietary selenium intake is absorbed. In addition, since no physiological mechanism appears to control selenium absorption, selenium has a definite potential for toxicity. Most selenium is excreted via the urine and feces.[15]

FUNCTIONS OF SELENIUM

Currently the best understood role for selenium is as a co-factor for a major form of the enzyme glutathione peroxidase. Selenium also plays a role in thyroid hormone metabolism and likely has other metabolic functions that have yet to be firmly established.[15]

Glutathione peroxidase participates in a system that metabolizes peroxides into less-toxic alcohol derivatives and water. In Chapter 12 we saw that peroxides tend to become free radicals, which in turn can attack and break down cell membranes, causing cell damage. As a co-factor for glutathione peroxidase, selenium is important for protecting heart cells and other cells against oxidative damage. Selenium also may aid immune function via activity of glutathione peroxidase.

Recall that vitamin E also functions to prevent attacks on cell membranes by free radicals. Thus vitamin E and selenium work together. Selenium participates in an enzyme system that prevents free-radical production by reducing peroxide concentration in the cell, and vitamin E can stop the action of free radicals once they are produced. So an adequate selenium intake spares some of the body's need for vitamin E, as it reduces the peroxide load in a cell (Figure 15-10).[15]

In Chapter 13 we discussed how electron-seeking compounds, especially free radicals, can alter DNA. Alterations in DNA are known to cause cancer. Because of selenium's ability to reduce free-radical production, adequate intake of this mineral may be important in preventing cancer. Laboratory animal studies in this area are conflicting; based on current knowledge, recommending selenium supplementation to prevent cancer in humans is speculation at best.

SELENIUM DEFICIENCY

The signs and symptoms of a selenium deficiency in animals and humans include muscle pain, muscle wasting, and cardiomyopathy, a form of heart disease. These same signs and symptoms are noted when there is insufficient selenium in total parenteral nutrition solutions. Farm animals in areas with low soil concentrations of selenium (e.g., New Zealand and Finland) and humans in some areas of China develop characteristic heart disorders associated with an inadequate selenium intake. A deficiency state associated with inadequate selenium intake is known as Keshan disease, named after an area in Northeast China where the soil is almost devoid of selenium and varying degrees of heart deterioration have been observed.[15] Although

---

An inherited condition known as Menkes' kinky hair syndrome is characterized by slow growth, brain degeneration, kinky white hair, and low blood copper. This condition results from a defect in copper absorption and incorporation into proteins, such as ceruloplasmin. Supplemental copper is given in an attempt to partially reverse this condition.[28]

We have now seen that the absence of many nutrients from the diet can lead to anemia:
- **Vitamin E deficiency can lead to hemolytic anemia (see Chapter 12).**
- **Vitamin K deficiency, especially coupled with use of antibiotics, can lead to blood loss and thus to hemorrhagic anemia (see Chapter 12).**
- **Vitamin B-6 deficiency can lead to microcytic anemia (see Chapter 13).**
- **Folate deficiency can lead to a megaloblastic anemia (see Chapter 13).**
- **Vitamin B-12 malabsorption can lead to megaloblastic anemia (see Chapter 13).**
- **An iron deficiency can lead to microcytic hypochromic anemia.**
- **A copper deficiency can lead, although rarely, to a secondary iron-deficiency anemia, as copper aids in iron metabolism.**

CRITICAL THINKING

Tammy read an article about antioxidants and their role in preventing free-radical damage to cells. When Tammy went to the drug store to take a closer look at such supplements, she saw that selenium was one of the antioxidants in the supplements. Why does selenium deserve consideration as an antioxidant?

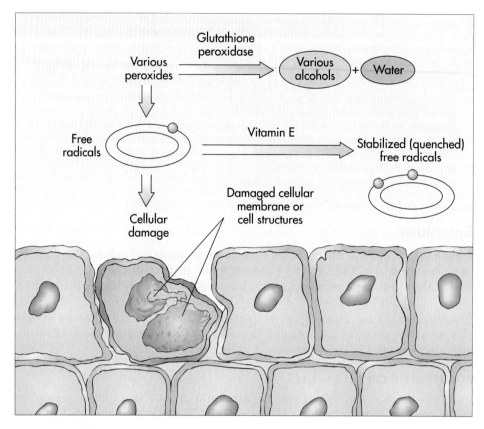

Figure 15-10 Selenium is part of the glutathione peroxidase system, which breaks down peroxides before they can form free radicals. This in turn spares some of the need for vitamin E, which is a major free-radical scavenger.

selenium is protective against development of the disease, selenium cannot correct the heart disorders once they have occurred.

SELENIUM IN FOODS

Fish, meat (especially organ meat), eggs, milk, and shellfish are good animal sources of selenium. Grains and sources of nuts and seeds grown in soils containing selenium are good plant sources (Figure 15-11).

Foods providing the highest nutrient density for selenium (μg/kcal) are tuna, whole-wheat bread, ham, eggs, oatmeal, white bread and related flour-based products, beef, and chicken.

Since we eat a varied diet supplied from many geographic areas, it is unlikely that selenium deficiency in the soil in a few areas will cause a selenium deficiency in our diets. But the difference in selenium content of foods grown throughout the United States makes it difficult to establish a general selenium value for any food, such as for bread.

RDA FOR SELENIUM

The RDA for selenium is 55 to 70 μg/day for women and men, respectively. American diets likely include enough selenium, since the average daily intake is about 110 μg.[15] Note that we do not have sensitive measures of selenium status and thus cannot accurately distinguish between a good and a marginal status.

TOXICITY OF SELENIUM

Excess selenium can be toxic. Daily intakes as low as 2 to 3 mg (just 35 times the RDA) can cause toxicity symptoms if taken for many months. These signs and symptoms include a garlicky odor of the breath, hair loss, nausea, diarrhea, fatigue, and changes in fingernails and toenails. Rashes and cirrhosis of the liver may also de-

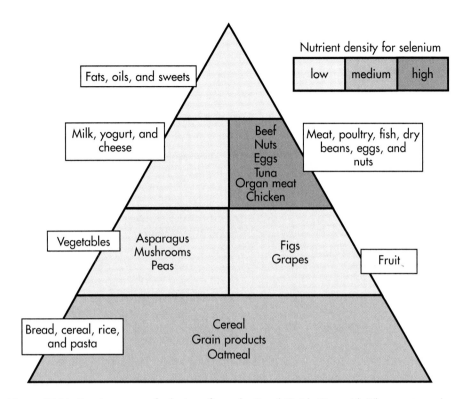

Nutrient density for selenium

| low | medium | high |

Fats, oils, and sweets

Milk, yogurt, and cheese

Beef
Nuts
Eggs
Tuna
Organ meat
Chicken

Meat, poultry, fish, dry beans, eggs, and nuts

Vegetables

Asparagus
Mushrooms
Peas

Figs
Grapes

Fruit

Bread, cereal, rice, and pasta

Cereal
Grain products
Oatmeal

Figure 15-11 Food sources of selenium from the Food Guide Pyramid. The meat, poultry, fish, dry beans, eggs, and nuts group and the bread, cereal, rice, and pasta group include the best dietary sources of this nutrient. The background color of each food group indicates the average nutrient density for selenium in that group.

velop. Because of the potential for toxic effects, FDA has limited supplemental selenium intakes in studies using humans to 200 µg/day.

Animals show selenium toxicity symptoms if they eat plants containing large amounts of selenium. Some plants naturally concentrate selenium from the soil. Birds who live in water polluted with selenium leached from nearby fields also have exhibited toxicity symptoms.

Iodide

Iodine (I_2), present in food as iodide (I^-) and other nonelemental forms, was linked to the presence of an enlarged thyroid gland (**goiter**) during World War I. Men drafted from the Pacific Northwest and the Great Lakes region of the United States had a much higher rate of goiter than men from other areas of the country. The soil in these areas is very low in iodide. During the 1920s, researchers in Ohio found that goiter could be prevented in children by feeding them low doses of iodide for an extended period. Following the lead of the Swiss, American companies began adding iodide to table salt. Use of iodized salt is the major method for correcting iodide deficiencies.[18]

Today, many nations, such as Canada, require iodide fortification of salt. In the United States, salt can be purchased either fortified or plain. Check for this on the label of a package of salt next time you are in a grocery store. By law, the label on a salt container sold in the United States must clearly state if iodide is present or not. Some areas of Europe, like northern Italy, have very low iodide concentrations in the soil but have yet to adopt the practice of fortifying salt with iodide. People in these areas, especially women, still suffer from goiter, as do people in areas of Latin America, Southeast Asia, and Africa. About one billion people worldwide are at risk of iodide deficiency, and approximately 20% of these people have goiter.[18]

Iodine (I_2), which is quite poisonous, can be used in a water solution as a topical antiinfective agent. The iodine ion (I^-) is the form of this trace mineral that is an essential nutrient. The term *iodine* is sometimes used in nutrition instead of iodide; to avoid confusion with this poisonous form, we use the term *iodide* exclusively.

goiter An enlargement of the thyroid gland, which can be caused by a lack of iodide in the diet.

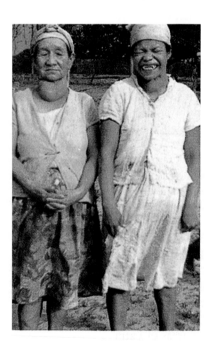

Structure of thyroxine.
Note that triiodothyronine lacks the iodide (I) indicated with a red asterisk.

thyroid-stimulating hormone A hormone that regulates the uptake of iodide by the thyroid gland and is secreted in response to a low blood concentration of circulating thyroxine.

cretinism Stunting of body growth and mental development during infancy and later development that results from inadequate maternal intake of iodide during pregnancy.

FUNCTIONS OF IODIDE

The thyroid gland actively accumulates and traps iodide from the bloodstream to support its hormone synthesis. The thyroid hormones thyroxine and triiodothyronine are synthesized from the amino acid tyrosine and iodide. These hormones help regulate metabolic rate and promote growth and development throughout the body, including the brain.

If a person's iodide intake is insufficient, the thyroid gland enlarges as it attempts to take up more iodide from the blood. The pituitary gland hormone that stimulates thyroid hormone production, **thyroid-stimulating hormone,** also stimulates the growth of the thyroid gland. Usually enough thyroxine is made to limit production of thyroid-stimulating hormone. However, in an iodide deficiency, insufficient thyroxine is produced to shut off synthesis of thyroid-stimulating hormone. The constant release of thyroid-stimulating hormone by the pituitary gland causes continual growth of the thyroid gland, eventually producing a greatly enlarged thyroid gland, or goiter (Figure 15-12).[18] A fall in metabolic rate and an increase in serum cholesterol are two other symptoms of thyroid hormone deficiency.

Goiter has been described in people as far back as 3000 BC, usually in women. Simple goiter is a painless condition, but if uncorrected it can lead to pressure on the trachea (wind pipe), which may cause difficulty in breathing. Treatment with iodide can result in a slow reduction in the size of the thyroid gland, although surgical removal of part of the gland may be required in severe cases.[18]

If a woman consumes an iodide-deficient diet during the early months of pregnancy, her infant may be born with short stature and develop mental retardation. Maternal iodide needs take precedence over fetal needs. The World Health Organization estimates that 20 million people in the world have varying degrees of preventable brain damage due to the effects of iodide deficiency on fetal brain development.[12] The retarded body growth is referred to as **cretinism.** Cretinism appeared in the United States before the program for iodide fortification of table salt began. Today, cretinism still appears in parts of Europe, Africa, Latin America, and Asia. In these areas, iodinated vegetable oil given orally or by injection is being used in an attempt to decrease iodide deficiency, in addition to fortification of salt with iodide.[12] Eradication of iodide deficiency is a goal of many health-related organizations worldwide.

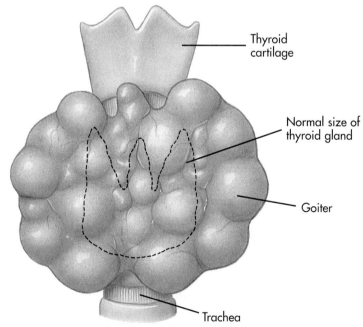

Figure 15-12 Goiter and cretinism in Bolivia. The mother on the left is goitrous, but otherwise normal. The daughter is goitrous, mentally retarded, deaf, and mute.

FOOD SOURCES OF IODIDE

Saltwater fish, seafood, iodized salt, molasses, and some plants contain various forms of iodide, especially the leaves of plants grown near the sea. Sea salt found in health-food stores, however, is not a good source, because the iodide is lost during processing. A half teaspoon (about 2 g) of iodide-fortified salt supplies the adult RDA for iodide. The actual amount of fortification in the United States is 76 μg of iodide per gram of salt.

The ocean is the source of most iodide naturally present in our diets. As ocean mist blows onto nearby land, iodide becomes part of the soil. Plants that grow in that soil accumulate the iodide.

Goiter is also associated with the consumption of **goitrogens.** Large amounts of these substances are found in raw turnips, cabbage, brussels sprouts, cauliflower, broccoli, rutabagas, and cassava, as well as other plants and even water-borne sources. Goitrogens inhibit iodide metabolism by the thyroid gland, and in turn inhibit thyroid hormone synthesis. However, goitrogens are not an important cause of goiter in developed countries, since they are destroyed by cooking and the foods they are found in do not often play an important role in the customary diets. They are, however, linked to the goiter in less developed parts of the world, especially where cassava is a dietary staple.[18]

goitrogens Substances in food and water that interfere with thyroid gland metabolism and thus may cause goiter if consumed in large amounts.

RDA FOR IODIDE

The RDA for iodide for adults is 150 μg/day. Probably the minimum intake to prevent goiter is 50 μg/day. Most Americans consume much more iodide than the RDA. Consumption is estimated to be about 170 to 250 μg/day (not including the iodide contributed from use of iodized salt at the table), with men consuming the higher amounts.

Such intakes of iodide are typical because it is used (1) as a sterilizing agent in dairies and restaurants, (2) as a dough conditioner in bakeries, (3) in food colorants, and (4) in iodized salt. So there is no need for concern about insufficient iodide intake in the United States and Canada unless dietary sodium intake must be kept below 500 mg/day. However, such low-sodium diets are rarely used today.

TOXICITY OF IODIDE

Iodide intakes up to 1 to 2 mg/day (6.5 to 13 times the RDA) appear to be safe. However, when very high amounts of iodide are consumed, thyroid hormone synthesis is inhibited, as in a deficiency. A "toxic goiter" results. Toxic goiter can appear in people who eat a lot of seaweed, since some seaweeds contain as much as 1% iodide by weight. Total iodide intake then can add up to 60 to 130 times the RDA. Manufacturers are working to reduce unnecessary iodide use in dairies, restaurants, and bakeries.

Fluoride

Dentists in the early 1900s noticed a lower incidence of dental caries in the southwestern United States, where the water naturally contained high concentrations of fluoride (F^-). Many people in these areas had small spots on the teeth, called **mottling,** due to deposits of fluoride; though discolored, these mottled teeth contained very few dental caries. After experiments showed that fluoride in the water did indeed decrease the rate of dental caries, controlled fluoridation of water in parts of the United States began in 1945 (see Chapter 3 for a review of the development of dental caries).

Those people who grew up drinking fluoridated water generally have 40% to 60% fewer dental caries than people who did not drink fluoridated water as children.[2] Dentists can provide fluoride treatments, and schools can provide fluoride tablets, but it is much less expensive and more reliable to simply put fluoride in a community's drinking water. Not all public or private water sources contain enough fluoride. When in doubt, contact your local water plant or have the water in your

Like chlorine, fluorine (F_2) is a poisonous gas. The fluoride ion (F^-) is the form of this trace mineral essential for human health.

mottling Discoloration or marking of the surfaces of teeth from exposure to excessive amounts of fluoride (fluorosis).

home analyzed for fluoride content. If the water doesn't contain the recommended amount—1 part per million parts of water (1 ppm, or 1 mg/L)—talk to your dentist about the best means for obtaining sufficient fluoride. About 80% to 90% of fluoride intake is absorbed.

FUNCTIONS OF FLUORIDE

fluorapatite A fluoride-containing, acid-resistant crystalline substance that is produced during bone and tooth development. Its presence in teeth helps prevent dental caries.

A dietary intake of fluoride during bone and tooth development aids the synthesis of **fluorapatite** crystals, rather than the typical hydroxyapatite crystals, described in Chapter 14. Fluoride taken internally, whether in drinking water or dietary supplements, strengthens developing teeth to resist decay. Fluorapatite crystals strongly resist acid, so teeth containing fluorapatite crystals are very resistant to dental caries. Fluoride also inhibits metabolism and growth of the bacterium that causes dental caries, and fluoride present in saliva directly inhibits tooth demineralization and enhances tooth remineralization.[2]

Fluoride applied to the surface of the teeth by dentists or from toothpaste adds additional protection against dental caries. Thus people of all ages benefit from the topical effects of fluoride, whether or not they consumed fluoridated water or fluoride supplements as children.[16] Dietary fluoride also improves growth rate in rats, but scientists are not sure if fluoride is actually necessary for growth in humans.

FLUORIDE IN FOODS

Tea, seafood, seaweed, and some natural water sources are the only good food sources of fluoride. Most of our fluoride intake comes from fluoride added to drinking water and toothpaste and from fluoride treatments performed by dentists.

ESADDI FOR FLUORIDE

The estimated safe and adequate daily dietary intake of fluoride for adults is 1.5 to 4 mg/day. The American Dental Association and the American Academy of Pediatrics recommend daily fluoride intakes of 0.25 mg through age 1 year, 0.5 mg for ages 2 and 3 years, and 1 mg after age 3 years and until the teenage years if the water supply is very low in fluoride; less is recommended as the fluoride concentration in the water increases (see *Pediatrics* 95:777, 1995). This range of intake provides the benefits of resistance to dental caries without causing mottling of the teeth. Typical fluoridated water contains about 0.2 mg per cup (contact the local water plant to find the specific amount in your water).

TOXICITY OF FLUORIDE

A fluoride intake greater than 6 mg/day can mottle teeth during their developmental stage. Children who consume large amounts of fluoridated toothpaste as part of daily tooth care are at greatest risk. Not swallowing toothpaste and limiting the amount used to "pea" size is the best way to prevent this problem.[2] High fluoride intake in adults does not cause mottling. When fluoride intakes reach 20 mg/day during tooth development, the tooth structure is weakened and can crumble. This is called **fluorosis** and appears in humans and other animals.

High doses of fluoride (≥ 20 mg/day) are being used experimentally in adults to treat severe osteoporosis, especially that seen in the spine. Such high fluoride dosages can cause significant side effects, such as stomach upset and bone pain. Ongoing research is attempting to establish a dose and duration of treatment that aid bone mass accretion and contribute to reduced fracture risk.[10]

CONCEPT CHECK

Selenium is important for the activity of glutathione peroxidase, an enzyme that reduces the concentration of peroxides, thus lessening the free-radical load in the body. In this way, selenium spares some of the need for vitamin E. A deficiency results in muscle and heart disorders. Organ meats, eggs, fish, and grains are good selenium sources; however, the selenium content in plants depends on the selenium concentration in the soil. A high selenium intake is potentially toxic. Iodide is vital in the synthesis of thyroid hormones. A prolonged insufficient intake will cause the thyroid gland to enlarge, resulting in goiter. Insufficient intake in pregnancy can lead to mental retardation in the offspring. The use of iodized salt has virtually eliminated this condition in the United States. Fluoride incorporated into teeth during development makes them resistant to acid and bacterial attack, in turn reducing development of dental caries. Fluoride also aids in remineralization of teeth once decay begins. Most of us receive adequate amounts of fluoride from that added to drinking water and toothpaste. A high fluoride intake during tooth development can lead to spotted, or mottled, teeth.

Chromium

The importance of chromium (Cr) in human diets has been recognized only in the past 20 years. There is much we do not understand about this mineral, but chromium deficiency may be related to diabetes in some individuals.

FUNCTIONS OF CHROMIUM

The most-studied function of chromium is the maintenance of glucose uptake into cells. Our current understanding is that chromium enters the cell and likely increases the number of insulin receptors or enhances the transport of glucose across the cell membrane.[20]

In both animals and man, a chromium deficiency is characterized by impaired glucose tolerance and elevated serum cholesterol and triglycerides. The mechanism by which chromium influences cholesterol metabolism is not known but may involve enzymes that control cholesterol synthesis. Chromium deficiency appears in people maintained on total parenteral nutrition not supplemented with chromium and in children with undernutrition.[20] Since sensitive measures of chromium status are not available, marginal chromium deficiencies may go undetected.

FOOD SOURCES OF CHROMIUM

Specific data regarding the chromium content of various foods are scant, and most food composition tables do not include values for this trace mineral. Egg yolks, whole grains (bran), organ meat, meat, mushrooms, nuts, and beer are good sources.[20] Yeast is also a source. Poor sources include fruits, vegetables, many seafoods, dairy products, highly processed foods, and drinking water. The amount of chromium in foods is closely tied to the local soil content of chromium. To provide yourself with a good chromium intake, regularly choose whole grains in preference to refined grains.

ESADDI FOR CHROMIUM

The estimated safe and adequate daily dietary intake of chromium is 50 to 200 μg/day. Average adult intakes in the United States are estimated at about 30 μg/day but could be somewhat higher. Marginal to low chromium intakes in the elderly may contribute to their increased risk for developing diabetes. Chromium intakes of less than 20 μg/day may be detrimental to a significant portion of the population that has marginally elevated blood glucose.[20]

Some research also shows that an intake at the high end of the ESADDI, or slightly above, may raise HDL. More studies are needed on this effect. Chromium

EXPERT OPINION

CHROMIUM: CHARLATANS' DELIGHT OR NUTRITIONISTS' CONCERN?

FORREST H. NIELSEN, Ph.D.

The general media and health-food or supplement industry, frequently with help from the scientific community, have reported on various nutrients in such a way that the American public is misguided, bewildered, or uncertain as to what to believe. Quite often, a nutrient bursts onto the scene and is touted everywhere as a therapeutic or prophylactic aid in preventing or alleviating some chronic disease; shortly thereafter, findings are reported that dispute these claims. Chromium, especially as chromium picolinate, is an element that currently fits into this category.

THE OPPOSING VIEWS

On one side are the zealots who claim that ingesting chromium, most often as a chromium supplement such as chromium picolinate, chromium nicotinate, or chromium-rich yeast, provides numerous beneficial effects. These include building muscle, losing weight as fat without dieting or exercising, and preventing diabetes, heart disease, and aging. Often concomitant with these claims is the statement that the dietary intake of chromium by a majority of Americans, maybe as many as 90%, is not adequate because it does not meet the lower limit of the ESADDI. On the other side are the disbelievers who state that there is no credible evidence to support most of these claims. The doubters note that even if chromium is an essential nutrient, chromium nutriture is an inconsequential concern for almost everyone.

With such polarized views, even scientists detached from the controversy have difficulty accurately assessing the nutritional importance of chromium. However, evidence accumulating since 1957 indicates that the true situation for chromium is somewhere between the extreme positions voiced by the zealots and the doubters.

EVIDENCE THAT CHROMIUM IS ESSENTIAL

There is a large amount of evidence supporting the view that chromium is an essential nutrient. For instance, humans on long-term total parenteral nutrition containing a low amount of chromium develop impaired glucose tolerance, or hyperglycemia, with glucose spilling into the urine, and a resistance to insulin action. These abnormalities can be reversed by chromium supplementation. Additionally, since 1966 a large number of reports from numerous research groups has described beneficial effects from chromium supplementation of subjects with degrees of glucose intolerance ranging from hypoglycemia to insulin-dependent diabetes. Beneficial effects of chromium supplementation on blood lipid profiles also have been reported.

Even with this evidence, chromium is not unequivocally accepted as being essential by all scientists, primarily for two reasons. First, it has been difficult to induce signs of chromium deficiency in experimental animals. Nutritional, metabolic, physiological, or hormonal stressors generally have to be employed to induce experimental animals to respond to chromium deprivation; in most cases, the responses have not been remarkable.

Second, a specific biochemical role has not been defined for chromium.

Despite the shortcomings of the evidence, chromium most likely is an essential nutrient for higher animals, including humans. Even the skeptics usually agree that chromium can be beneficial because of the positive findings on glucose and lipid metabolism in some individuals. Thus the major issue of debate concerning chromium is twofold: what is the extent of benefits, and who benefits from a luxuriant intake of chromium, which some people claim is best achieved by taking chromium supplements? Stated another way: what is the extent of the pathological consequences of chromium deficiency, and how common is chromium deficiency in the American population?

ADEQUATE CHROMIUM INTAKES

Although the ESADDI for chromium is 50 to 200 μg/day, consuming less than 50 μg/day does not mean that one would eventually become chromium deficient. For example, in one study 11 elderly women had an average chromium intake of 20.1 μg/day and 11 elderly men had an average intake of 29.8 μg/day; the range of intakes was 13.6 to 47.7 μg/day among the 22 subjects. Of these, 16 maintained equilibrium, four exhibited positive balance, and two exhibited slight and one exhibited severe negative balance. The one subject with severe negative balance ate a diet high in fiber, which may have influenced chromium absorption.

Several supplementation studies also suggest that chromium deficiency is not common. For example, in one study, chromium supplementation of 16 healthy, well-nourished elderly people did not change their glucose tolerance or blood insulin, cholesterol, and triglycerides. In a Finnish study, chromium supplementation for 6 months of 26 elderly subjects with persistent impaired glucose tolerance did not improve their glucose tolerance or blood lipid profiles; the mean daily intake of chromium in Finland is less than 30 μg.

Finally, in a study of chromium absorption, the percentage absorbed from the diet decreased from 2% of intake at dietary intakes of 10 μg/day to 0.5% at intakes of 40 μg/day; the percentage of absorption remained at 0.5% at dietary intakes up to 240 μg/day. The human body clearly has the ability to homeostatically control chromium status by adjusting absorption and excretion. It is likely that the increased percentage of absorption with decreased intake reflects this action; thus even when intake is less than 40 μg/day, balance is achieved.

The intake at which chromium is low enough to induce changes responsive to chromium supplementation is not well established. Moreover, because other substances in the diet influence absorption of chromium, the point at which chromium intake becomes inadequate depends in part on the other foods consumed. For example, vitamin C (ascorbic acid) and aspirin increase chromium absorption, while antacids decrease it. However, some data suggest that a chromium intake less than 20 μg/day is generally inadequate.

Based on dietary surveys, a significant number of Americans likely consume less than 20 μg/day. As a result, it is not surprising that many studies have identified some individuals who responded to chromium supplementation. However, a much larger number of individuals in most of these studies did not respond to chromium supplements. In other words, chromium apparently acts as an essential nutrient, not as a pharmaceutical agent. Thus, when chromium status is adequate, further supplementation has little or no effect on glucose and lipid metabolism, and therefore no effect on such things as body composition, weight loss, muscle building, or aging.

MISLEADING CLAIMS FOR CHROMIUM SUPPLEMENTS

The current promotion of chromium picolate as an ergogenic aid or weight-loss inducer provides a typical example of misleading use of research results by the health-food industry. The positive ergogenic findings that have come from the laboratory of the originator of chromium picolinate have been publicized. Several well-designed controlled studies, however, that have failed to duplicate these findings or have found only a few select individuals (possibly with initially low chromium status) whose body composition responded significantly to chromium supplementation have been ignored.

Likewise, weight-loss studies have not consistently shown positive results with chromium supplementation. Interestingly, one of the most successful studies in this regard used

high-fiber cookies and L-carnitine in addition to chromium in the weight-loss regimen. Thus other factors could have been influencing weight loss. In another touted study, some subjects lost more weight than others, which suggests that initial chromium status or some other factor influenced the response to supplementation. Even with some individuals responding significantly, the overall weight loss in this study, which required no change in diet with chromium supplementation, was small (2.8 pounds over a period of 10 weeks).

A REASONABLE APPROACH

Regardless of the uncertainties about chromium, substantial evidence exists suggesting that many individuals would benefit from an increased intake of chromium. The best and most enjoyable way of doing this is by eating a varied diet incorporating foods and beverages that are good sources of chromium. However, some individuals will insist upon taking a supplement for "insurance" or "peace of mind." For these people, a separate chromium supplement is unnecessary; a multivitamin-mineral supplement containing chromium will do.

Dr. Nielsen, the Center Director and Research Nutritionist at the USDA, ARS, Grand Forks Human Nutrition Research Center in Grand Forks, North Dakota, focuses his research efforts on the ultratrace elements. The opinions expressed are those of Forrest H. Nielsen; they do not represent or should not be construed as the official position or policy of the U.S. Department of Agriculture.

toxicity has been reported in people exposed to chromium in industrial settings and in painters using art supplies with a very high chromium content. Liver damage and lung cancer may result from such high intakes.

Manganese

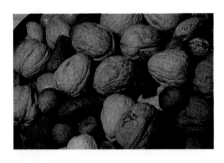

Nuts are a good source of manganese.

It is easy to confuse the mineral manganese (Mn) with magnesium (Mg). Their names are similar, and in a few metabolic pathways they can substitute for each other.

Manganese is a co-factor for certain enzymes, including pyruvate carboxylase, an important enzyme in carbohydrate metabolism.[20] Manganese is also important in bone formation. No manganese-deficiency symptoms have been observed in humans. Animals on manganese-deficient diets exhibit changes in brain function, bone formation, and reproduction. If human diets were low in manganese, these problems would probably appear in humans as well. As it happens, our need for manganese is very low, and our diets tend to be adequate in manganese if good food sources, which include nuts, oats and other whole grains, beans, tea, and leafy vegetables, are consumed.

The estimated safe and adequate daily dietary intake of manganese is 2 to 5 mg/day. Average intakes fall within this range.[20] Manganese toxicity has been seen in people working in manganese mines, and includes severe psychiatric abnormalities, hyperirritability, violence, hallucinations, and impaired control of muscles.

Molybdenum

xanthine dehydrogenase An enzyme containing molybdenum and iron that functions in the formation of uric acid and the mobilization of iron from liver ferritin stores.

Molybdenum (Mo) is notable for its interactions with iron and copper. In particular, high intakes of molybdenum inhibit copper absorption.

Several enzymes, including **xanthine dehydrogenase** and a related form, xanthine oxidase, require molybdenum. The oxidase form of the enzyme is produced from the dehydrogenase form during tissue injury. No molybdenum deficiency has been observed in people consuming a normal diet, though deficiency signs and symptoms have appeared in people on total parenteral nutrition. These symptoms include increased heart and respiration rates, night blindness, mental confusion, edema, weakness, and coma.[20]

Good food sources of molybdenum include milk and milk products, beans, whole grains, and nuts. The estimated safe and adequate daily dietary intake for molybdenum is 75 to 250 μg/day. Typical American intakes are 50 to 350 μg/day, with an average of close to 100 μg/day.[20] When laboratory animals consume high dosages of molybdenum, they develop evidence of toxicity, including anemia, weight loss, and decreased growth.

Trace Minerals of Questionable Status

Researchers are still trying to demonstrate a human need for numerous other trace minerals found in the body. Although at least some of these minerals may indeed be essential nutrients, we probably consume too much of them to suffer deficiencies. Moreover, even if truly essential, these minerals probably have relatively minor functions in the body. We briefly mention these trace minerals of questionable status because more research may clarify their importance to human health. If you have a concept of their roles in the body, you can put new research into perspective. And you can refute the need for widespread use of supplements of these trace minerals based on what we know now.

BORON

Boron (B) is an important growth factor for plants. In humans, boron may be involved in the metabolism of steroid (cholesterol-containing) hormones, such as the vitamin D hormone, calcitriol, and the estrogens, and is likely an essential nutrient.[19]

Good sources of boron include noncitrus fruits, leafy vegetables, nuts, and beans. Meat, fish, and dairy products are inadequate sources. Adults need about 1 to 10 mg/day. Daily human intakes vary widely, from about 0.5 to 3 mg/day.[20]

NICKEL

Plants and animals need nickel (Ni) for the activity of certain enzymes and perhaps for iron metabolism. Humans have never exhibited a deficiency of nickel when consuming a mixed diet. Good food sources of nickel include nuts, beans, grains, and chocolate. Researchers estimate that adults need about 100 to 300 μg of nickel per day.[20] Diets including rich sources of nickel supply much more than this, while more refined diets may just meet needs or supply slightly less.

VANADIUM

Vanadium (V) likely enhances the activity of some enzymes, especially those involved in sodium and potassium transport and in iodide metabolism. However, no clear role of vanadium in human metabolism has been verified. To produce a vanadium deficiency in animals, researchers need to use an ultraclean environment; even the air must be filtered. Good food sources of vanadium include shellfish, mushrooms, and grain products. Researchers estimate that adult vanadium needs are about 10 to 100 μg/day. Our dietary intakes are about 6 to 20 μg/day. Humans do not appear to run a risk for a vanadium deficiency.[20]

ARSENIC

Although arsenic (As) is a very poisonous compound, animals need it in small amounts to metabolize protein, amino acids (especially methionine), and taurine. Researchers estimate that adults need about 12 to 15 μg/day, about as much as the minimum amount adults generally eat. There is no known human deficiency of arsenic. Food sources include fish and grain products.[20]

OTHER POSSIBLE ESSENTIAL MINERALS

Animal data suggest that humans also need lithium (Li), silicon (Si), tin (Sn), cadmium (Cd), and cobalt (Co).[20] The human need for dietary sources of these minerals, however, has not been confirmed. Of course, cobalt forms part of vitamin B-12. Some researchers speculate that dietary cobalt may be used for synthesis of vitamin B-12 by bacteria in the human intestines, but no reliable evidence supports this idea. Adequate intake of vitamin B-12 itself is nutritionally more important than concern about cobalt intake.

• • •

See Table 15-2 to review what we have covered on trace minerals.

CONCEPT CHECK

Chromium may act to increase the action of the hormone insulin. The amount of chromium found in food depends on soil content. Whole grains, egg yolks, and meat are some of the better sources of chromium. Manganese is a component of bone and many enzymes, including those involved in glucose production. Since our need for it is low, deficiencies are rare. Good food sources of manganese are nuts, oats, tea, and beans. Molybdenum is a component of enzymes. Deficiencies have appeared only with total parenteral nutrition. Beans, milk and milk products, grains, and nuts are good sources of molybdenum. The needs for some other trace minerals—including boron, nickel, arsenic, and vanadium—have not been fully established in humans. These minerals are required in such small amounts that diets including a variety of foods and containing some plant protein and whole grains most likely supply adequate amounts.

TABLE 15-2

A summary of key trace minerals

Mineral	Major functions	Deficiency symptoms	People most at risk
Iron	Part of hemoglobin and other key compounds used in respiration; used for immune function	Low blood iron levels; small, pale red blood cells; low blood hemoglobin values	Infants, preschool children, adolescents, women in child-bearing years
Zinc	Co-factor for over 300 enzymes, including those involved in growth, immunity, alcohol metabolism, sexual development, and reproduction	Skin rash, diarrhea, decreased appetite and sense of taste, hair loss, poor growth and development, poor wound healing	Vegetarians, elderly persons
Selenium	Part of antioxidant system, glutathione peroxidase	Muscle pain, muscle weakness, heart disease	Unknown
Iodide	Part of thyroid hormone	Goiter; poor growth in infancy when mother is deficient during pregnancy	None in America because salt is usually fortified
Copper	Aids in iron metabolism; works with many enzymes, such as those involved in protein metabolism and hormone synthesis	Anemia, low white blood cell count, poor growth	Infants recovering from semi-starvation, people who use overzealous supplementation of zinc
Fluoride	Increases resistance to dental caries	Increased risk of dental caries	Areas where water is not fluoridated and dental treatments do not make up for a lack of fluoride
Chromium	Enhances blood glucose control	High blood glucose after eating	People on total parenteral nutrition and perhaps some elderly people with non–insulin-dependent diabetes
Manganese	Aids action of some enzymes, such as those involved in carbohydrate metabolism	None in humans	Unknown
Molybdenum	Aids action of some enzymes	None in humans	Unknown

Summary

1. Some trace mineral deficiencies are difficult to detect in humans and were first observed in small geographically isolated groups or in people nourished via total parenteral nutrition. Eating a variety of foods maximizes the chances of consuming adequate amounts of trace minerals. Consuming trace mineral supplements at doses greater than 1.5 times the Daily Value listed on the supplement label is potentially harmful, since so many questions remain regarding daily needs and interactions.

2. To account for iron losses in menstrual blood flow, iron is the only nutrient for which the RDA is set higher for adult women than for men. Iron absorption depends mainly on the form of iron present and the body's need for it, especially for nonheme iron; a mucosal block helps prevent over-absorption. Generally, heme iron from animal sources is better absorbed than the nonheme iron obtained primarily from plant sources. Consuming vitamin C and/or meat simultaneously with iron modestly increases nonheme iron absorption.

3. Iron is a critical component of hemoglobin, myoglobin, and the cytochromes. Iron is also a co-factor for some enzymes and is necessary for functioning of the immune system. A prolonged low iron intake can lead to decreased production of red blood cells and in turn reduced ability of the blood to carry sufficient oxygen. This condition, called iron-deficiency anemia, may result in fatigue and apathy, as well as decreased learning ability in children.

4. Foods rich in iron include beef, oysters, broccoli, and liver. Other sources are spinach and whole-grain and

RDA or ESADDI	Nutrient-dense dietary sources	Results of toxicity
Men: 10 mg Women: 15 mg	Meats, spinach, seafood, broccoli, peas, bran, enriched breads	Toxicity is seen in children who consume ≥60 mg in iron pills and in people with hemochromatosis; increased risk of heart disease suspected in people who overabsorb iron, especially if also have elevated LDL
Men: 15 mg Women: 12 mg	Seafood, meats, greens, whole grains	Reduced copper absorption; diarrhea, cramps, and depressed immune function
55-70 μg	Meats, eggs, fish, seafoods, whole grains	Nausea, vomiting, hair loss, weakness, liver disease
150 μg	Iodized salt, white bread, saltwater fish, dairy products	Inhibition of function of the thyroid gland
1.5-3 mg	Liver, cocoa, beans, nuts, whole grains, dried fruits	Vomiting; nervous system disorders
1.5-4 mg	Fluoridated water, toothpaste, dental treatments, tea, seaweed	Stomach upset; mottling (staining) of teeth during development; bone pain
50-200 μg	Egg yolks, whole grains, pork, nuts, mushrooms, beer	Caused by industrial contamination, not dietary excess
2-5 mg	Nuts, oats, beans, tea	Unknown in humans
75-250 μg	Beans, grains, nuts	Unknown in humans

enriched breads and cereals. However, iron from plant sources is generally not well absorbed. Iron toxicity usually results from a genetic disorder called *hemochromatosis*. This disease causes overabsorption and accumulation of iron, which can result in severe liver and heart damage.

5. Zinc functions as a co-factor for over 300 enzymes that are important for growth, development, immune function, wound healing, and taste sensation. A zinc deficiency results in inadequate growth, loss of appetite, inadequate mental function, reduced sense of taste and smell, fall in immune function, hair loss, and a persistent rash.

6. Zinc is best absorbed from animal sources, especially when body needs are high. A mucosal block in the intestinal cells approximately regulates zinc absorption,

in a manner similar to that of iron. Copper competes with zinc for absorption, especially when both are consumed as supplements. The most nutrient-dense sources of zinc are oysters, shrimp, crab, and beef. Good plant sources are whole grains, peanuts, and beans.

7. Copper is important for iron absorption and mobilization from body stores, collagen cross-linking, nerve cell myelination, and scavenging of free radicals. A copper deficiency can result in a secondary iron-deficiency anemia and rupture of blood vessels. Copper is found mainly in liver, cocoa, legumes, and whole grains. Milk is low in copper. Soil content greatly affects the copper content of plants.

8. The most-understood role of selenium is as a co-factor for glutathione peroxidase, whose action reduces the

production of free radicals. In this way, selenium reduces the need for vitamin E, which can scavenge free radicals once they are produced. Muscle pain, muscle wasting, and heart disease may result from a selenium deficiency. Meat (especially organ meat), eggs, fish, and shellfish are good animal sources of selenium. Good plant sources include grains and seeds from plants grown in selenium-rich soils. Selenium is potentially toxic because there is no physiological control of the amount absorbed. Symptoms of toxicity are a garlicky breath odor, hair loss, weakness, nausea, and vomiting.

9. Iodide forms part of the thyroid hormones. A lack of dietary iodide results in development of goiter and other metabolic problems, including stunted growth in childhood and mental retardation. Iodized salt is a good food source.

10. Fluoride incorporated into teeth during development makes them resistant to dental caries, and fluoride present in saliva aids in remineralization of damaged tooth surfaces. Most Americans receive the bulk of their fluoride from that added to drinking water and toothpaste.

11. Chromium likely contributes to insulin action. Meats and whole grains are good sources of chromium. Manganese and molybdenum contribute to the activity of various enzymes. Frank deficiencies are rarely seen for any of these three nutrients. The body's need for other trace minerals is so low that deficiencies are uncommon when a person consumes a mixed diet with some plant proteins and whole grains on a regular basis.

Study Questions

1. Minerals in the diet are likely to interact with each other. Provide two examples of such interactions involving trace minerals.

2. Describe how a "mucosal block" lessens the risk of developing an iron or zinc toxicity state.

3. Outline the histories of both iodide and fluoride in human nutrition from epidemiological observations to dietary intervention with fortified salt and water, respectively.

4. Describe the role of one trace mineral in immune function.

5. Discuss why research on trace mineral needs is so difficult, and define what a marginal deficiency state represents with respect to trace minerals.

6. Describe the signs and symptoms of iron-deficiency anemia.

7. Anemia can result from a dietary deficiency of any one of several nutrients. Identify three nutrients and the laboratory tests used to distinguish the various types of anemia.

8. Which trace minerals are lost from cereal grains when they are refined? Are any of these nutrients replaced by enrichment?

9. Which two factors most influence iron absorption from a meal? Describe why each is important.

10. Describe the chief function in the body of fluoride, copper, chromium, and manganese.

REFERENCES

1. Abbas AK, Lichtman AH, Pober JS: *Cellular and molecular immunology,* ed 2, Philadelphia, 1994, WB Saunders.
2. ADA Reports: Position of the American Dietetic Association: The impact of fluoride on dental health, *Journal of the American Dietetic Association* 94:1428, 1994.
3. Alaimo K and others: Dietary intake of vitamins, minerals, and fiber of persons ages 2 months and over in the United States, Third National Health and Nutrition Examination Survey, Phase 1, 1988-91, *Advance Data* 258(Nov 14):1, 1994.
4. Alexander JW: Specific nutrients and the immune response, *Nutrition* 11:229, 1995.
5. Ascherio A and others: Dietary iron intake and risk of coronary disease among men, *Circulation* 89:969, 1994.
6. Chandra RK: Effects of nutrition on the immune system, *Nutrition* 10:207, 1994.
7. Fairbanks VF: Iron in medicine and nutrition. In Shils ME and others, editors: *Modern nutrition in health and disease,* Philadelphia, 1994, Lea & Febiger.
8. Gavin MW and others: Evidence that iron stores regulate iron absorption—a setpoint theory, *American Journal of Clinical Nutrition* 59:1376, 1994.
9. Gleerup A and others: Iron absorption from the whole diet: comparison of the effect of two different distributions of daily calcium intake, *American Journal of Clinical Nutrition* 61:97, 1995.
10. Heaney RP: Fluoride and osteoporosis, *Annals of Internal Medicine* 120:689, 1994.
11. Herbert V: Everyone should be tested for iron disorders, *Journal of the American Dietetic Association* 91:1502, 1992.
12. Hetzel BS: Iodine deficiency and fetal brain damage, *New England Journal of Medicine* 331:1770, 1994.
13. Hotez PJ, Pritchard DI: Hookworm infection, *Scientific American,* June 1995, p 68.
14. Hunt JR and others: Effect of ascorbic acid on apparent iron absorption by women with low iron stores, *American Journal of Clinical Nutrition* 59:1381, 1994.
15. Levander OA, Burk RF: Selenium. In Shils ME and others, editors: *Modern nutrition in health and disease,* Philadelphia, 1994, Lea & Febiger.
16. Lokshin MF: Preventive oral health care: a review for family physicians, *American Family Physician* 50:1677, 1994.
17. Lynch SR: Overview of the relationship of iron to health, *Contemporary Nutrition* 19 (4,5), 1994.
18. Maberly GF: Iodine deficiency disorders, *Journal of Nutrition* 124:1473S, 1994.
19. Mastromatteo E, Sullivan F: Summary: International symposium on the health effects of boron and its compounds, *Environmental Health Perspectives* 102(suppl 7):139, 1994.
20. Nielsen FH: Chromium and ultratrace minerals. In Shils ME and others, editors: *Modern nutrition in health and disease,* Philadelphia, 1994, Lea & Febiger.
21. Nossal GJV: Life, death and the immune system, *Scientific American* 269(Sept):53, 1993.
22. Percival SS: Neutropenia caused by copper deficiency: possible mechanisms of action, *Nutrition Reviews* 53:59, 1995.
23. Prasad AS: Zinc: an overview, *Nutrition* 11:93, 1995.
24. Proulx MR, Weaver CM: Ironing out heart disease, *Nutrition Today* 30:16, 1995.
25. Sandstead HH: Is zinc deficiency a public health problem? *Nutrition* 11:87, 1995.
26. Shils ME: Magnesium. In Shils ME and others, editors: *Modern nutrition in health and disease,* Philadelphia, 1994, Lea & Febiger.
27. Shronts EP: Basic concepts of immunology and its application to clinical nutrition, *Nutrition in Clinical Practice* 8:177, 1993.
28. Turnlund JR: Copper. In Shils ME and others, editors: *Modern nutrition in health and disease,* Philadelphia, 1994, Lea & Febiger.
29. US Public Health Service: Anemia in children, *American Family Physician* 51:1121, 1995.
30. Whiting SJ: The inhibitory effect of dietary calcium on iron bioavailability: a cause for concern? *Nutrition Reviews* 53:77, 1994.
31. Yip R: Iron deficiency: contemporary scientific issues and international programmatic approaches, *Journal of Nutrition* 124:1479S, 1994.

TAKE ACTION

How does your trace mineral intake measure up?

To complete this activity, you must reexamine the nutritional assessment you did for Chapter 2. Based on that analysis of your nutritional intake for one day, fill in the values for your intake, the RDA or ESADDI, and the percentage of the RDA or ESADDI you consumed for each of the minerals listed in the table below. In the right-hand column, indicate whether your intake was higher than (+), lower than (−), or about equal to (=) the recommended intakes.

MINERAL	INTAKE	RDA OR ESADDI	% OF RDA OR ESADDI	+, −, =
Iron	_____	_____	_____	_____
Zinc	_____	_____	_____	_____
Selenium	_____	_____	_____	_____
Copper	_____	_____	_____	_____

Analysis

1. Which of your mineral intakes equaled or exceeded the RDA or ESADDI?

_____

2. Which of your intakes were below the standard for your age and gender?

_____

3. What foods or cooking practices could be emphasized or deemphasized to modify your weaknesses?

_____

_____

_____

_____

Nutrients and Immunity

Early humans were plagued by famine, infections, and death. Because of better nutrition, this tragic cycle is no longer a threat for many people.[4] Although good nutrition is crucial to proper functioning of the immune system, excess quantities of nutrients do not further boost immunity and can in some cases decrease it.[6] The complex, fascinating immune system is one of the most active areas of current biological research, in large part because the key to understanding and ultimately controlling AIDS (acquired immunodeficiency syndrome) depends on unraveling the mysteries of immunity.

The primary function of the immune system is to protect the body against foreign substances, called **antigens.** Antigens may be microorganisms, including disease-causing bacteria, viruses, fungi, and parasites (pathogens); toxins such as snake venoms; and substances called allergens (e.g., ragweed, certain foods and drugs) that trigger allergic reactions in some people. Immunity is the state of resistance to invasion by pathogens or other antigens.[1] We exhibit two types of immune responses: nonspecific immunity (also called natural or native) and specific immunity (also called acquired).[1] Because nonspecific immunity is initiated by antigens in general, it is innate. In contrast, specific immunity develops after exposure to particular antigens; such immunity is said to be acquired.

Nonspecific immune defenses are particularly important during first exposure to an antigen and early in the immune response. This type of immunity depends in part on the health of the skin and mucous membranes, which provide physical barriers to invaders, and on various secreted factors that are lethal to certain types of microbes. Certain **white blood cells,** called **phagocytic cells,** also provide nonspecific immunity, as they ingest and destroy large particulate antigens, including bacterial cells and parasites.[21]

Specific immunity depends on the ability of other white blood cells, the **lymphocytes,** to recognize and respond to a large number of specific, particular antigens. On first exposure to a certain antigen, this type of immune response is slower than the body's nonspecific defenses because it requires proliferation of the small number of cells that recognize the antigen. However, on second or subsequent exposure to the same antigen, specific immunity uses its "memory" capability to respond quickly and to a greater extent.[1]

Both defense systems work together as a well-orchestrated team, utilizing a variety of white blood cells.[21] Let's see how the various "bricks" in the body's edifice of immunity cooperate with each other to shield us, and which nutrients are crucial to our ability to resist disease (Figure 15-13).

antigen Any substance that stimulates one or more components of the immune system and induces a state of sensitivity and/or resistance to microbes or toxic substances; also, a substance that binds to a specific antibody. Antigens are recognized as "foreign" by the immune system.

white blood cells General term for blood cells that participate in immune responses; also called leukocytes. The five types of leukocytes are lymphocytes, monocytes, neutrophils, basophils, and eosinophils.

phagocytic cells White blood cells that can engulf microbes, other particulate antigens, and cellular debris and break down the ingested material; also called phagocytes.

lymphocytes A class of white blood cells responsible for antigen-specific immune responses. Lymphocytes generally comprise about 25% of all white blood cells.

Skin and Mucous Membranes: Physical Barriers to Microbes

Invading microbes have difficulty penetrating the skin, which forms an almost continuous barrier surrounding the body. If the skin is split by a wound or abrasion, however, bacteria and other microbes can easily penetrate it, gaining access to the body. Essential fatty acids, vitamin A, niacin, and zinc are particularly important for maintaining healthy skin.[27] Deficiencies of these nutrients may open the way for penetration of the skin by microorganisms.

Many pathogens gain entry to the body through the mucous membranes lining the internal cavities of the body and the eyes. However, several nonspecific defense mechanisms work to prevent invasion. Saliva, tears, and mucous secretions help wash away potential invaders. The cilia that cover the lining of the respiratory tract move in a synchronous fashion, propelling mucus-entrapped antigens out of the body. Certain cells in mucosal tissue also participate in specific immunity by producing **antibodies,** which can bind invading microbes, thus preventing them from crossing mucous membranes and entering the bloodstream.[1]

Vitamin A plays a crucial role in maintaining mucous membranes. If these membranes deteriorate, bacteria, fungi, and other microbes easily enter the body.[6] Recall that a common sign of vitamin A deficiency is bacterial infection of the eye. Production of antibodies to combat invaders in the intestine also falls if vitamin A and protein intakes are insufficient. This, combined with damage to intestinal cells, allows microbes to more easily enter the body,

antibody A protein produced by a type of lymphocyte that binds to a "matching" antigen and facilitates its removal from the body.

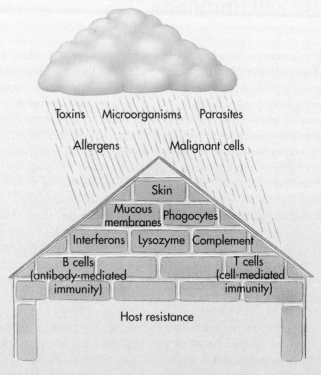

Figure 15-13 The immune system has many facets, "bricks," whose contributions to host resistance are influenced by nutrient intake.

leading to full-blown infection. Two common results are diarrhea and bacterial infections of the blood. In addition to vitamin A and protein, folate, various other vitamins (C, B-6, and B-12), copper, zinc, and other nutrients are needed for synthesis and maintenance of intestinal cells.[27]

Physiological Barriers That Inhibit Infection

Mucus, tears, and saliva contain the enzyme **lysozyme,** which can break down the outer layer of many bacteria, thus destroying them. In addition, secretions in the intestinal tract immobilize many microbes before they can penetrate mucous membranes.

Other contributors to nonspecific immunity are the **interferons.** These proteins are released by virus-infected cells and have a general antiviral effect on other cells, thus helping to prevent establishment of a viral infection.[21] Interferons also have antitumor activity and have shown promise for treating certain types of cancer.

A group of blood proteins forms the **complement** system, which contributes to both nonspecific and specific immune responses. Normally, complement proteins circulate in the blood in an inactive form. They can be activated in two ways: through a nonspecific pathway involving interaction with various constituents present on the surface of bacteria or through a specific pathway involving interaction with an antigen-antibody complex. Activation of the complement system leads to a series of reactions, generating a number of products that play roles in inflammation, clearing antigens from the body, and destroying microbes by cell lysis.[1]

Phagocytes: Multifunctional Nonspecific Defenders

Phagocytes are white blood cells that can engulf and destroy microbes and other particulate

interferons A group of proteins released by virus-infected cells that bind to other cells, stimulating synthesis of antiviral proteins that in turn inhibit viral multiplication.

complement A series of blood proteins that participate in a complex reaction cascade following stimulation by an antigen-antibody complex or the surface of a bacterial cell. Various activated complement proteins can enhance phagocytosis, contribute to inflammation, and destroy bacteria.

neutrophil The most common type of white blood cell, constituting 55% to 65% of their total number. Neutrophils, which are active phagocytes, form part of the body's early defense against infection by microbes.

macrophage Any large mononuclear phagocytic cell that is found in the tissues and is derived from a monocyte in the blood. Besides functioning as im-

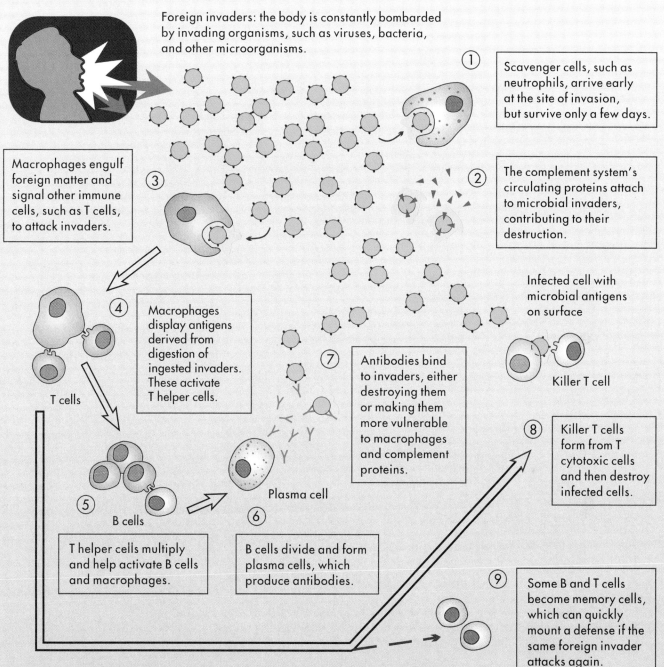

Foreign invaders: the body is constantly bombarded by invading organisms, such as viruses, bacteria, and other microorganisms.

① Scavenger cells, such as neutrophils, arrive early at the site of invasion, but survive only a few days.

② The complement system's circulating proteins attach to microbial invaders, contributing to their destruction.

③ Macrophages engulf foreign matter and signal other immune cells, such as T cells, to attack invaders.

④ Macrophages display antigens derived from digestion of ingested invaders. These activate T helper cells.

T cells

⑦ Antibodies bind to invaders, either destroying them or making them more vulnerable to macrophages and complement proteins.

Plasma cell

Infected cell with microbial antigens on surface

Killer T cell

⑧ Killer T cells form from T cytotoxic cells and then destroy infected cells.

⑤ T helper cells multiply and help activate B cells and macrophages.

B cells

⑥ B cells divide and form plasma cells, which produce antibodies.

⑨ Some B and T cells become memory cells, which can quickly mount a defense if the same foreign invader attacks again.

Figure 15-14 Biological warfare. The body commands a wide assortment of defenders to reduce the danger of infection and help guard against repeat microbial infections. The ultimate target of all immune responses is an antigen, commonly a foreign protein from a bacterium or other microbe.

ner if antibodies or certain complement proteins are bound to the surface of the invading microbe.[1]

After an antigen is taken up by a phagocyte, intracellular enzymes digest the ingested material. Macrophages that have interacted with antigens also secrete various enzymes into the area surrounding the microbe invasion or injury; this is one cause of the pain and swelling associated with inflammation.

Neutrophils and macrophages also have a second killing mechanism: they produce hydrogen peroxide and various free radicals, which are lethal to ingested microbes. Recent evidence shows that much of the antimicrobial activity of macrophages results from such toxic reactive products.[1] Because this activity may damage tissues in the vicinity, vitamin E and other antioxidants are important in sequestering the excess free radicals, thereby limiting the tissue damage.[27]

Macrophages have two other very important roles in the immune system. First, some of the antigen fragments that result from phagocytosis and digestion of microbes are transported to the surface of macrophages and "presented" to certain lymphocytes.[1] We'll see later that some lymphocytes recognize only an antigen when it is displayed by antigen-presenting cells. Second, after being activated, macrophages and other white blood cells secrete a variety of **cytokines.** These secreted protein factors exert numerous effects: some are directly toxic to foreign cells; others attract phagocytes to infected areas; still others activate and stimulate proliferation of lymphocytes.[1]

Neutrophils usually are the first white blood cells to enter infected tissues from the blood, but they often die after phagocytosing a single microbial cell. Soon **monocytes** in the blood also enter the area, grow larger, and are transformed into macrophages. Macrophages are responsible for most of the phagocytic activity in the late stages of an infection, including the removal of dead neutrophils and other cellular debris.[1]

Macrophages are also present in uninfected tissues, including the lymph nodes, liver, spleen, and lungs. As blood flows through the liver and spleen and lymph flows through the lymph nodes, these fixed (immobile) phagocytic cells can often destroy microbes before they replicate, as well as remove other dangerous materials and cellular debris.[1] Connective tissue also contains mobile defenses in the form of neutrophils and monocytes that scavenge for invaders and debris. These cells can squeeze through tiny spaces between cells to enter adjacent connective tissue.

Because neutrophils, monocytes, and macrophages live for only a few days, new ones must be continually produced in the bone marrow if the body's defenses are to perform well. Their constant synthesis requires a steady nutrient input: adequate amounts of protein, folate, and vitamins E, C, B-6, and B-12 are needed for general cell synthesis and, later, activity.[27] Zinc and vitamin A are required for overall development and growth of phagocytes, while copper is needed specifically for production of neutrophils.[22] Finally, production of toxic free-radical compounds depends on iron.

Lymphocytes: Generators of Specific Immunity

Now we turn to the lymphocytes, the cells responsible for the body's ability to recognize and respond to a particular antigen. There are two broad classes of lymphocytes: **B lymphocytes** (B cells) and **T lymphocytes** (T cells). Mature B cells are released from the bone marrow, and mature T cells are released from the thymus gland.[1] Both types of cells continually circulate in the blood and lymph tissues. B cells and T cells are produced constantly throughout the lifetime of an individual. However, production of T cells may slow down after adolescence, leading to reduced immune function in elderly people.

Roughly speaking, B cells and T cells are responsible for the two forms of specific immunity—antibody-mediated immunity and cell-mediated immunity, respectively. As we'll see, though, B and T cells work together; the full activity of each against an antigen depends on the other. Both types of lymphocytes have cell-surface receptors that recognize a single antigen (or small numbers of chemically related antigens). All the receptors on a given lymphocyte recognize the same antigen. B cells recognize antigens present in the circulation and extracellular spaces, while T cells are equipped to recognize antigens found inside cells.[1] Following stimulation by an antigen, B cells and T cells divide, generating other cells and releasing substances that ultimately lead to destruction of the antigen (Figure 15-14).

ANTIBODY-MEDIATED IMMUNITY

When a foreign antigen enters the body, it eventually encounters a B cell with a matching cell-surface receptor that binds the antigen. This interaction stimulates the B cell to undergo several divisions, finally yielding **plasma cells** and B **memory cells.**[21] The plasma cells then mass-produce and secrete antibodies that specifically interact with the original antigen and by various means act to eliminate it. Following the first exposure to an antigen, it normally takes a few days to weeks before enough antibodies are formed to effectively combat the

---

cytokines Proteins secreted by some antigen-activated white blood cells that generally (1) act to regulate various aspects of the immune response (the interleukins) or (2) lead to toxic injury to virus-infected cells (the interferons) or tumor cells (tumor necrosis factors).

monocyte A type of white blood cell, making up about 3% to 7% of the total number, that enlarges and develops into a macrophage after moving into tissues.

B lymphocyte (B cell) A type of white blood cell that recognizes antigens (e.g., bacteria) present in extracellular sites in the body and is responsible for antibody-mediated immunity. B cells originate and mature in the bone marrow and are released into the blood and lymph.

T lymphocyte (T cell) A type of white blood cell that recognizes intracellular antigens (e.g., viral antigens in infected cells), fragments of which move to the cell surface. T cells originate in the bone marrow but must mature in the thymus gland.

plasma cell An antibody-producing cell generated by the multiplication and differentiation of a B lymphocyte that has interacted with an antigen; a mature plasma cell can produce and secrete from 3000 to 30,000 antibody molecules per second.

memory cells Lymphocytes derived from B cells or T cells that have been exposed to an antigen; when exposed to the same antigen a second time, memory cells rapidly respond to provide immunity.

antigen. The body must rely on the nonspecific immune responses to hold infection in check during this period.

All antibodies belong to a group of structurally similar blood proteins called **immunoglobulins.** There are five major classes of immunoglobulins, denoted IgG, IgM, IgA, IgE, and IgD. All can interact with antigens, but they are specialized for different functions in the immune response and have different lifespans in the body (from a few days to about 3 weeks).[1]

The human body has an inherent capacity to recognize and respond to literally billions of different antigens.[1] Arrival of an antigen does not create this recognition capability; rather it simply accelerates formation of plasma cells that make the best-fitting antibody to combat a particular antigen. Thus even if an individual has never been exposed to a particular microbial invader, the chances are good that at least some B cells will have receptors that can bind to antigens on the surface of the microbe. Moreover, the B memory cells generated during the first (primary) response to a microbe serve as a data bank that can quickly respond if the body is invaded a second time by the same microbe.

CELL-MEDIATED IMMUNITY

The final component of the immune system are the T lymphocytes. One type of T cell, called a **T cytotoxic (T_c) cell,** often carries a cell surface marker termed CD^{8+} and is directly responsible for cell-mediated destruction of altered body cells, including virus-infected cells and tumor cells. The second major type of T cell, called a **T helper (T_H) cell,** often carries a CD^{4+} cell surface marker and is critical to activation of both B cells and T_c cells; thus both antibody-mediated and cell-mediated immunity depend on T_H cells.[1]

The antigen-specific receptors on T cells recognize only fragments of antigens that are complexed with certain proteins, termed **MHC molecules,** that are normally present on the surface of body cells.[1] For example, T_c cells can recognize fragments of viral proteins complexed with certain MHC molecules on the surfaces of virus-infected cells. Likewise, T_H cells recognize fragments of extracellular antigens complexed with other MHC molecules on antigen-presenting cells, such as macrophages. After these antigen-presenting cells take up an antigen, it is broken down and the resulting fragments associate with MHC molecules and move to the surface.[1]

Antigen-stimulated T_H cells proliferate and begin releasing a variety of cytokines, which can activate macrophages, stimulate development of B cells into plasma cells and their production of antibodies, and regulate the activities of other immune system cells. Activated T cells also generate T memory cells, which are available to speed the defense against a future attack by the same antigen.[1]

After a T_c cell interacts with an antigen-MHC complex on the surface of a virus-infected or tumor cell, it develops into a killer T cell. A cytokine secreted by activated T_H cells enhances formation of these killer T cells. Once formed, killer T cells interact with other target cells containing the same antigens, poking holes in the cell membrane and injecting substances that kill the target cells.[1]

The crucial role of T_H cells in immune responses is demonstrated by AIDS patients. As this disease progresses, the number of T_H cells, clinically called the CD^4 count, based on the CD^{4+} marker seen on the surface of many of these cells, plummets. Immune function then is reduced so much that **opportunistic infections** can take hold. Such infections occur in people with compromised immune systems. For instance, a usually harmless microbe called *Pneumocystis carinii* often infects people with AIDS, causing a type of pneumonia that rarely occurs in people with normal immune function.

NUTRIENTS AND SPECIFIC IMMUNITY

We've noted already the importance of nutrition to nonspecific immunity, particularly for the maintenance of healthy skin and mucous membranes and the steady production of phagocytes and other white blood cells. Likewise, many nutrients are crucial to specific immunity. A deficiency of vitamin B-6, for example, results in reduced stimulation of lymphocytes by antigens. Copper and zinc deficiencies lead to a decrease in the number of antibody-producing cells.[6]

immunoglobulins Proteins found in the blood that bind to specific antigens; also called antibodies. The five major classes of immunoglobulin play different roles in antibody-mediated immunity.

MHC molecules A large group of cell-surface proteins, present on body cells, referred to as the *major histocompatibility complex (MHC)*. Because many of these proteins are unique to each individual, they act as antigens when tissue from one person is transplanted to another person, triggering an immune response that results in graft rejection.

In the early 1970s, physicians began feeding patients with major body burns much sooner than they had in the past. This earlier feeding dramatically reduced the number of infections that burn patients suffered and thus greatly improved their chances of survival. A major reason for this improved survival is the earlier supply of nutrients to support immune function.

vaccine A preparation of antigenic material that is administered to induce long-term immunity against a pathogen; commonly killed or inactivated microbes are used as vaccines. Some vaccines consist of preformed antibodies, usually those that can neutralize a toxin; these provide only short-term protection.

In protein-energy undernutrition, lymphoid tissues atrophy and the thymus gland shrinks. As a result, production of T cells, which probably is most critical for effective immune responses, falls drastically. The amino acids arginine, glutamine, isoleucine, leucine, and valine appear to benefit the thymus gland and T cell activity most effectively.[4] The most important of these is arginine, which has a positive influence on the whole immune system. Deficiencies of vitamins A, B-6, C, and E, and folate, iron, and zinc also result in impaired cell-mediated immunity.[6]

Nutrition and Immune Function: A Recap and A Warning

Our normal ability to resist infection is clear evidence of how important nutrition is to immune status. By and large, common pathogens to which most people are exposed cause serious disease only in those who are severely malnourished. A good example is measles. Before use of the measles **vaccine** became common during the 1960s, most American children experienced this viral infection and recovered within a few days. Since these children had adequate nutrition, their immune systems quickly eliminated the measles virus. However, even today some 200,000 undernourished children, mostly in Third World countries, die every year from measles infection. Their immune systems are so debilitated from undernutrition that they can't win the battle against the virus.

A common clinical indicator of immune status is the white blood cell count, especially the number of T cells and B cells. When the lymphocyte count is low, infection is much more likely to lead to disease symptoms and even death. Thus poorly nourished people, whether in hospitals, nursing homes, or your neighborhood, often have not only poor liver and kidney function, but also impaired immune systems, making them susceptible to opportunistic infections.[27] Inadequate nutrient intake is especially detrimental to immune function among elderly people. Undernourishment also depresses the response to vaccines, including the flu vaccines that are given to many older Americans these days.

Although good nutritional status is associated with good immune status, an overabundance of certain nutrients can, paradoxically, actually harm the immune system. High intakes of total fat, omega-6 polyunsaturated fatty acids, and vitamin E have been implicated in decreasing immune response. Excess intakes of zinc (300 mg/day for 6 weeks) also reduce immune function, most probably because zinc interferes with copper absorption. The secondary copper deficiency then leads to decreased production of neutrophils. Excess iron can promote bacterial growth so much that the immune system can't keep up.

Clearly, eating a balanced diet helps maintain the health of all components of the immune system, which continuously protects us from environmental pathogens. But excessive intakes of individual nutrients do not provide more protection and may even harm certain aspects of immune function.[6] Researchers currently are investigating the ability of certain supplements (e.g., vitamin E, vitamin C, certain carotenoids, arginine, and vitamin B-6) to boost immune function.[4] At this time, however, no medical organization advocates use of single nutrients for this purpose. Any personal experimentation should be carefully considered and undertaken in consultation with a physician.

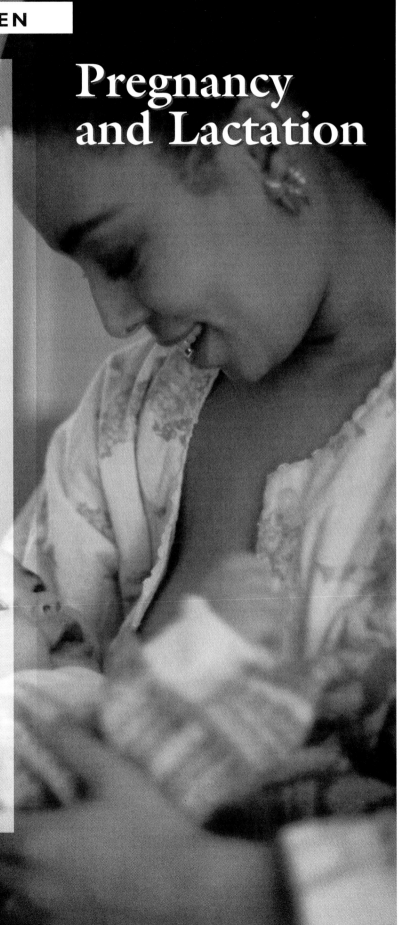

CHAPTER SIXTEEN

Pregnancy and Lactation

Pregnancy can be one of the most special times in a parent's life. It is also an especially important time for good nutrition to come into focus, as ideally the couple strives to do everything possible to turn the dream of a healthy infant into reality.[24]

The reality, however, is that the infant mortality rate in the United States is higher than that in 23 other industrialized nations.[5] The inadequate prenatal care received by about 20% of women, or the lack of any prenatal care, contributes substantially to this depressing statistic. Teenage mothers are at highest risk for receiving inadequate care. Overall, many lifestyle and nutritional choices can not only make pregnancy easier for a woman but can also increase the likelihood of her having a robust, lively newborn.[34]

Breastfeeding, whose popularity surged in the 1970s and 1980s, also provides many benefits to mother and child, one of which is forging a strong bond between them.[1] Even though nursing is a natural process, most women need education and encouragement to breastfeed successfully. Let's see what contributes to a healthy pregnancy and a satisfying period of breastfeeding for both mother and infant, in turn helping to make the parents' dreams of a healthy offspring become reality.

Nutrition Awareness Inventory

1. **T F** Infants weighing less than 5.5 pounds (2500 g) at birth are more likely to have medical problems than those weighing more than that.
2. **T F** The most crucial time for development of the human organism in utero is during the last 13 weeks of pregnancy.
3. **T F** Nutritional factors and length of gestation are more important than genetic factors in determining birthweight.
4. **T F** Energy needs are greater during pregnancy than in the nonpregnant state.
5. **T F** Most women should gain about 25 to 35 pounds during pregnancy.
6. **T F** In developed countries poor food choices by pregnant women are more common than low energy intakes.
7. **T F** Pregnant women know instinctively what to eat.
8. **T F** Mineral needs increase during pregnancy.
9. **T F** Pregnancy can precipitate a form of diabetes.
10. **T F** Breastfed infants suffer fewer respiratory infections than formula-fed infants.
11. **T F** A common barrier to breastfeeding is a lack of accurate information.
12. **T F** Mothers who must take medications should check with their doctors before making a decision to breastfeed.
13. **T F** The placenta is the site of oxygen and nutrient transfer from the mother to the fetus.
14. **T F** Most spontaneous abortions (miscarriages) occur during the first trimester of pregnancy.
15. **T F** Cow's milk can safely be substituted for human milk or formula when an infant is 2 to 3 months old.

Prenatal Growth and Development

The formation of the human organism begins when an egg and sperm unite to form the **zygote** (Figure 16-1). About 30 hours after the egg is fertilized, the zygote reproduces itself by dividing in half. The process of cell division then repeats many times. As the cluster of cells, commonly called the **conceptus,** drifts down the oviduct to the woman's uterus, several different kinds of cells emerge. The entire genetic code is passed to every cell, but each cell utilizes only a segment of the code to produce proteins. If this were not the case, there would be no different organs or body parts. For example, all cells carry genes that dictate hair color and eye color, but only the cells of the hair follicles and irises respond to that specific information.

On about the fourth day after fertilization, the conceptus, now about 64 to 128 cells and hollow, arrives in the uterus. By the tenth day, the conceptus implants into the uterine lining. Two weeks after conception the cell number has increased further and the conceptus is now termed an **embryo.** By day 35 of gestation the heart is beating, and although the embryo is only 8 mm (about 3/8 inch) long, the eyes and so-called limb buds, which ultimately form the arms and legs, are clearly visible. The embryo continues to grow, and the organ systems continue to develop. From about the end of the eighth week after conception to its birth about 32 weeks later, the developing offspring is known as a **fetus.**[34]

The mother nourishes her offspring in utero via a **placenta,** which forms in her uterus. The placenta serves to accommodate growth and development of the offspring throughout gestation (Figure 16-2).[34] Because women often do not suspect they are pregnant during the first few weeks after conception, many do not seek medical attention until about the first 2 to 3 months of embryonic development.

zygote The fertilized ovum; the cell resulting from union of an egg cell (ovum) and sperm until it divides.

conceptus A generic term for any developmental stage derived from the fertilized ovum (zygote) until birth. The conceptus includes the extraembryonic membranes, as well as the embryo or fetus.

embryo In humans, the developing in utero offspring from about the beginning of the third week to the end of the eighth week after conception.

fetus In humans, the developing in utero offspring from about the beginning of the ninth week after conception to birth.

placenta An organ that forms in pregnant women through which oxygen and nutrients from the mother's blood are transferred to the fetus and through which fetal wastes are removed. The placenta also releases hormones necessary

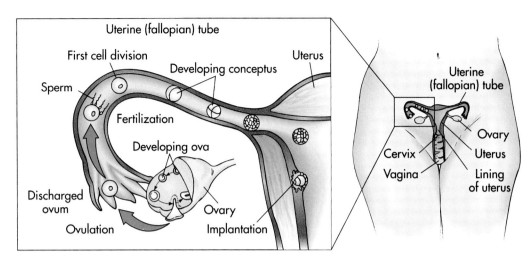

Figure 16-1 After ovulation, the discharged ovum first enters the abdominal cavity and then finds its way into the uterine (fallopian) tube, where conception, or fertilization, takes place. Sperm cells "swim" up the uterine tube toward the ovum. Fertilization most often occurs in the outer one third of the oviduct. The ovum also takes an active role in the process of fertilization by attracting and "trapping" sperm with special receptor molecules on its surface. As soon as the head and neck of one spermatozoon enter the ovum (the tail drops off), complex mechanisms in the egg are activated to ensure that no more sperm enter. The 23 chromosomes from the sperm combine with the 23 chromosomes already in the ovum to make up the 46 chromosomes of the conceptus.

Even without fanfare, the embryo grows and develops daily. For that reason, the health and nutritional habits of a woman both several years before pregnancy and while she is trying to become pregnant—or has the potential of becoming pregnant—are particularly important. For example, a history of anorexia nervosa or bulimia nervosa does not set the stage for a healthy pregnancy. While some aspects of fetal and newborn health are beyond our control, a woman's conscious decisions about social, health, and nutritional factors affect her infant's health and future.[5,10,24,27,30]

Good nutrition is especially critical during a woman's childbearing years. We know that deficiencies of certain nutrients (e.g., the vitamin folate) as well as use of certain medications, illegal drugs, and alcohol can all have detrimental effects on the

Although a mother's decisions, practices, and precautions during pregnancy contribute to the health of her fetus, she cannot guarantee fetal good health because some genetic and environmental factors are beyond her control.[16] Professionals should not foster an unrealistic illusion of control.

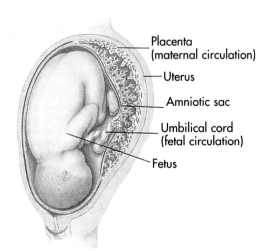

Figure 16-2 The fetus in relation to the placenta. The placenta is the organ through which nourishment flows to the fetus.

growing embryo even before a woman realizes she is pregnant.[10,15,27] Much research suggests that an adequate vitamin and mineral intake in the months before conception and during pregnancy may help prevent birth defects, such as neural tube defects, which have been linked to folate deficiency (see Chapter 13).[27] For these reasons, it is important for parents to be aware of the role nutrition plays in the development of a healthy infant *both* before and during pregnancy.[19]

The time to focus on good nutritional and other health habits, then, is before a woman becomes pregnant. Maternal nutrition should be a focus throughout the childbearing years—from **menarche** in childhood to menopause—to ensure that all women are in good health (including good nutritional status) at the time of conception. Good habits can then be carried into pregnancy, thereby providing optimal health and nutrition from before conception until birth.[19]

FIRST TRIMESTER OF PREGNANCY

For purposes of discussion, the duration of pregnancy—normally 38 to 42 weeks—is commonly divided into three periods called **trimesters.** Growth begins in the first trimester with a rapid increase in cell number (hyperplasia). This type of growth dominates embryonic and later fetal development. The newly formed cells then begin to grow larger (hypertrophy; see Chapter 8 to review these terms). Further growth and development then involve mostly hyperplasia with some hypertrophy.[34] By the end of 13 weeks—the first trimester—most organs are formed and the fetus can move (Figure 16-3).

At any stage of development an insult (injury) to the embryo or fetus caused by nutritional deficiencies, medications or illegal drugs, radiation, trauma, or other factors can alter or arrest the specific phase of growth and development in progress. Some effects—like cleft palate and missing limbs—can last a lifetime. The most critical time for **intrauterine** development is the first trimester, especially weeks two

menarche The onset of menstruation. Menarche usually occurs around age 13, 2 or 3 years after the first signs of puberty start to appear.

trimesters Three 13- to 14-week periods into which the normal pregnancy of 38 to 42 weeks is divided somewhat arbitrarily for purposes of discussion and analysis. Development of the embryo and fetus, however, is continuous throughout pregnancy with no specific physiological markers demarcating the transition from one trimester to the next.

intrauterine Within the uterus.

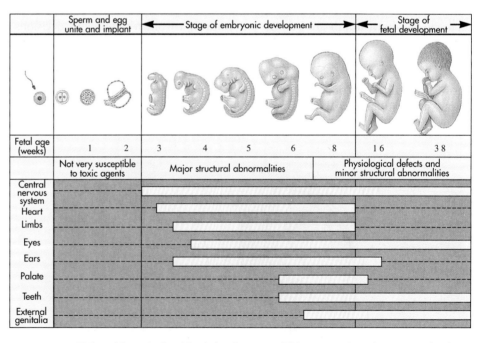

Figure 16-3 Vulnerable periods of fetal development. The most serious damage to the fetus from exposure to toxins is likely to occur during the first 8 weeks after conception. The lighter bars indicate the time of greatest risk to the organ. As the chart shows, however, damage to vital parts of the body—including the eyes, brain, and genitals—can also occur during the last months of pregnancy.

through eight. Most **spontaneous abortions** (miscarriages) occur during this period. An estimated one third of all pregnancies end in spontaneous abortion, often before a woman even realizes she is pregnant. Miscarriages usually result from a genetic defect or fatal error in embryonic or fetal development linked to environmental insults.[19]

During the first trimester, then, a woman must be especially careful to avoid substances that may harm the developing offspring. For example, a high vitamin A intake by the mother can result in serious **congenital** malformations. In addition, development is so rapid during the first trimester that if enough of a nutrient essential to development is not available, the growing embryo or fetus may be adversely affected even before the mother shows deficiency signs or symptoms. Even though many women experience loss of appetite and nausea during the first trimester, maintaining adequate nutrition is still extremely important.[34]

SECOND TRIMESTER OF PREGNANCY

By the beginning of the second trimester, a fetus typically weighs about 1 ounce. Arms, hands, fingers, legs, feet, and toes are fully formed. The fetus has ears and is beginning to form tooth sockets in its jawbone. During this phase of development organs continue to grow and mature, and a physician can detect a heart beat. Most bones will be distinctly evident throughout the body. Eventually the fetus begins to look more like an infant. It may suck its thumb and kick strongly enough to be felt by the mother.

THIRD TRIMESTER OF PREGNANCY

By the beginning of the third trimester, a fetus weighs approximately 2 to 3 pounds. An infant delivered after about 26 weeks of **gestation** and weighing more than 1 kg (2.2 pounds) is likely to survive if cared for in a nursery for high-risk newborns. Such infants, however, are deficient in mineral and fat stores that normally accumulate during the last month of gestation. These deficiencies and other medical problems complicate the neonatal care of infants born so early in gestation.[5] At 9 months, the typical fetus weighs about 7 to 8 pounds (about 3.5 kg) and is about 20 inches long (about 50 cm). There is an especially large soft spot on the top of the head (fontanelle) where the bones of the skull are growing together. It takes about 12 to 18 months after birth for that soft spot to close.

Defining a Successful Pregnancy

No generally accepted standards have been adopted by medical organizations to define a successful pregnancy. However, one common criterion is protection of the mother's physical and emotional health such that she can return to her prepregnancy health status. As for the infant, two widely accepted criteria are (1) a gestation period longer than 37 weeks and (2) a birthweight greater than 2.5 kg (5.5 pounds). Sufficient lung development, which is likely to have occurred by 37 weeks' gestation, is critical to survival of a newborn. The longer the gestation, the greater the ultimate birthweight and maturation, and hence fewer medical problems are likely to occur (Figure 16-4).[5]

Infants born before 37 weeks are called **preterm,** or premature. **Low-birthweight (LBW)** infants are those weighing less than 2.5 kg at birth. Most commonly LBW is associated with preterm birth. Full-term and preterm infants who weigh less than the expected weight for their duration of gestation, as the result of intrauterine growth retardation, are described as **small for gestational age (SGA).**[34] Thus a full-term infant weighing less than 2.5 kg at birth is SGA but not preterm, while a preterm infant born at 30 weeks' gestation most likely will have LBW but very often is not SGA. Infants who are SGA are more likely than normal-weight infants to have medical complications, including problems with blood glucose control, temperature regulation, and growth and development in the early weeks after birth.[34]

spontaneous abortion Any cessation of pregnancy and expulsion of the embryo or nonviable fetus as the result of natural causes, such as a genetic defect or developmental problem in the conceptus; also called *miscarriage*.

congenital Referring to conditions present at birth, regardless of their cause. Congenital abnormalities may result from (1) a genetic defect inherited from the parents, (2) damage or infection during intrauterine development, or (3) trauma during birth itself.

gestation The period of intrauterine development of offspring, from conception to birth; in humans, gestation lasts for about 40 weeks after the woman's last menstrual period.

preterm An infant born before 37 weeks of gestation; also referred to as *premature*.

low birthweight (LBW) Referring to any infant weighing less than 2.5 kg (5.5 pounds) at birth; most commonly results from preterm birth.

small for gestational age (SGA) Referring to any infant whose birthweight is less than the expected weight corresponding to the duration of gestation. A full-term newborn weighing less than 2.5 kg (5.5 pounds) is SGA. A preterm infant who is also SGA will most likely develop some medical complications.

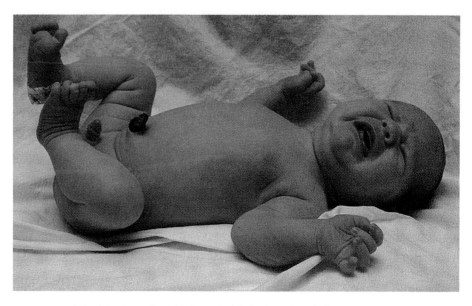

Figure 16-4 A healthy 1-week-old infant. At birth, American infants on average weigh about 7.5 pounds and are about 20 inches long.

Alexandra wants to have a baby. She has read that it is very important for the woman to be healthy during the pregnancy. However, Jane, her sister, tells her that actually before she becomes pregnant is the time to begin to assess her nutritional and health status. What information would Jane have given Alexandra?

Besides these minimal standards for a successful pregnancy, a newborn ideally should have the ability to grow, develop, learn, and eventually reproduce. Overall, prospective parents should strive to have an infant who is born healthy, on time, and with the mental, physical, and physiological capabilities to take advantage of all that life offers, while also protecting the mother's health (Figure 16-5).

Nutrition is one key to a successful pregnancy. This practice is vital during pregnancy to ensure the health of both the fetus and the mother. Fetal organs and body parts begin to develop very soon after conception. Again, the first trimester (13 weeks) is an especially critical period when inadequate nutrient intake or drug use can result in birth defects.[19]

For Better or For Worse®   by Lynn Johnston

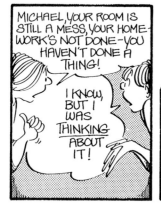
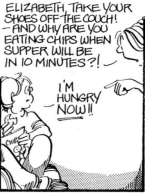
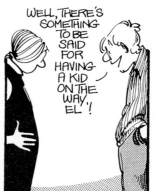
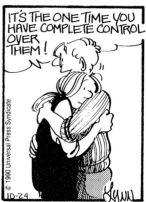

Figure 16-5 For Better or For Worse.

CONCEPT CHECK

Adequate nutrition is vital both before and during pregnancy to help ensure optimal health of both the fetus and the mother. Organs and body parts in the offspring begin to develop very soon after conception. The first trimester is a critical period when inadequate nutrient intake or alcohol and drug use can result in birth defects. During the second and third trimesters, organs continue to mature, and very rapid growth occurs. Nutritional insults during the last 7 months of pregnancy can also interfere with fetal growth and affect the newborn's ability to survive. Infants born after 37 weeks of gestation and weighing more than 2.5 kg (5.5 pounds) have the fewest medical problems at birth. To reduce the possibility of infant and maternal medical problems or death, those involved must be willing to take all steps necessary to allow the mother to carry her infant in the uterus for the entire 9 months. Good nutrition and health habits aid in this goal.

Nutrient Needs of Pregnant Women

Dietary advice given to pregnant women by the medical community has varied tremendously over the past century. In the 1950s, a common recommendation was that women restrict weight gain to between 15 and 18 pounds. Severe energy and sodium restrictions were at times also recommended to keep the infant small, in hopes of easing labor and avoiding complications. Few of these practices were based on sound scientific information; we know now that many of these recommendations are in fact harmful to the mother and fetus.

The first comprehensive scientific report about nutrition and pregnancy, titled *Maternal Nutrition and the Course of Pregnancy,* was issued in 1970 by the National Academy of Sciences. This document remains a landmark source of research information on the role of nutrition in human reproduction. The report was updated in 1990.[21] Both versions emphasize the increased nutritional requirements during pregnancy (not restrictions) and the importance of adequate weight gain and individual assessment and counseling of mothers-to-be (Table 16-1).

ENERGY NEEDS

Energy needs during the first trimester of pregnancy are essentially the same as during the nonpregnant state. During the second and third trimesters, however, the average pregnant woman requires an extra energy intake of approximately 300 kcal/day, although this amount is variable depending on the individual's energy output.[13] This extra 300 kcal needed daily is equivalent to just 2 cups of 2% milk and a slice of bread. Even though she may "eat for two," the pregnant woman must not double her normal energy intake. She cannot afford a "Big Mac" for herself and another for the fetus, even during late pregnancy. Many vitamin and mineral needs are increased by 20% to more than 100% during pregnancy, whereas energy needs during the second and third trimesters represent only about a 15% increase, based on an intake of 2000 kcal/day by nonpregnant women (Figure 16-6). Thus, in order to obtain the necessary vitamins and minerals without increasing her energy intake too much, a pregnant woman needs to seek high-quality, nutrient-dense foods to ensure the best possible health for her developing child.

If a woman is active during pregnancy, the energy she expends is added to any extra energy needed for pregnancy to balance her total energy use. The greater body weight of a pregnant woman requires a higher energy cost for activity. Physicians today recognize the benefits of physical activity and encourage women to continue most activities during pregnancy, except scuba diving, downhill skiing, weightlifting, and contact sports like hockey. Generally, activities that require jumping, jarring motions, or rapid changes in direction should be avoided because of joint instability, especially late in pregnancy. In addition, deep flexion or extension of

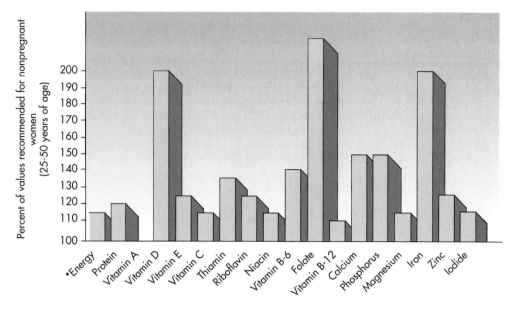

*Second and third trimesters only

Figure 16-6 Nutrient needs of pregnant women, expressed as percentage of the RDA for adult nonpregnant women. During pregnancy, women need higher amounts of most nutrients, with the exception of vitamin A, than at other times.

– – – – – – – – – – – –

The American College of Obstetrics and Gynecology suggests the following guidelines for physical activity during pregnancy:

1. **Do not allow heart rate to exceed 140 beats per minute.**
2. **Avoid exercising in hot, humid weather.**
3. **Discontinue exercise that causes discomfort or overheating.**
4. **Drink plenty of liquids, to avoid dehydration and overheating.**
5. **After about the fourth month, don't exercise while lying on your back.**
6. **Avoid an abrupt decrease in exertion. In other words, don't just stop and stand around after a hard workout; rather, continue exercising, but at a slow pace, gradually reducing pulse rate.**

– – – – – – – – – – – –

joints—particularly deep knee bends—should be avoided because connective tissue is lax during pregnancy. Still, walking, cycling, swimming, and light aerobics are appropriate for most pregnant women; they should simply stop when fatigued and not exercise to exhaustion or to the point of becoming overheated.[3] The latter has been linked to an increase in birth defects, especially during the first trimester.

Women with high-risk pregnancies, however, may need to restrict their physical activity. To ensure optimal health for both the mother and infant, a pregnant woman should first obtain advice regarding physical activity and possible limitations from her physician.

TABLE 16-1

Recommended weight gain in pregnancy based on prepregnancy body mass index (BMI)

BMI category*	Total weight gain†	
	(pound)	(kg)
Low (BMI <19.8)	28-40	12.5-18
Normal (BMI 19.8 to 26)	25-35	11.5-16
High (BMI 26 to 29)	15-25	7-11.5
Obese (BMI >29)	≤15	≤7

From National Academy of Sciences–Institute of Medicine, *Nutrition during pregnancy,* Washington, DC, 1990, National Academy of Sciences Press.
*See Chapter 8 to review the concept of body mass index (BMI).
†The listed values are for singleton pregnancies. For women of normal BMI who are carrying twins, the range is 35 to 45 pounds (16 to 20 kg). Adolescents within 2 years of menarche and African-American women should strive for gains at the upper end of the ranges; short women (<62 inches) should strive for gains at the lower end of the ranges.

RECOMMENDED WEIGHT GAIN

For women with a normal weight-to-height ratio, the prenatal diet should allow for approximately 2 to 4 pounds of weight gain during the first trimester and then a subsequent weight gain of 3/4 to 1 pound per week during the second and third trimesters. The total weight-gain goal is about 25 to 35 pounds (Table 16-1).[21] Although gaining this much weight concerns many women, it is an important goal for obtaining a good outcome of pregnancy. Adolescents and African-American women, who often have smaller infants, are strongly advised to aim for the higher weight gains in these ranges. Women carrying twins should gain 35 to 45 pounds.

For underweight women (body mass index <20), the recommended weight gain increases to 28 to 40 pounds. Adequate weight gain during pregnancy is particularly important in preventing low-birthweight infants among underweight women. For overweight women (body mass index between 26 and 29), the goal decreases to 15 to 25 pounds. Obese women (body mass index >29) should strive for the lower end of that weight gain recommendation.[21] It may be difficult for women who have a significant weight problem before pregnancy to understand the need to gain weight during pregnancy, but the goal of this weight gain is to help ensure a healthy infant.

Figure 16-7 shows why the weight-gain recommendation starts at 25 pounds for a woman at desirable weight. This total includes the total weight of the infant (8 pounds), placenta (1 pound), and amniotic fluid (2 pounds); the mother's increased uterus and breast tissue (6 pounds) and increased blood supply and other body fluids (4 pounds); and the increased fat (4 to 8 pounds) she needs to support pregnancy and lactation.[34]

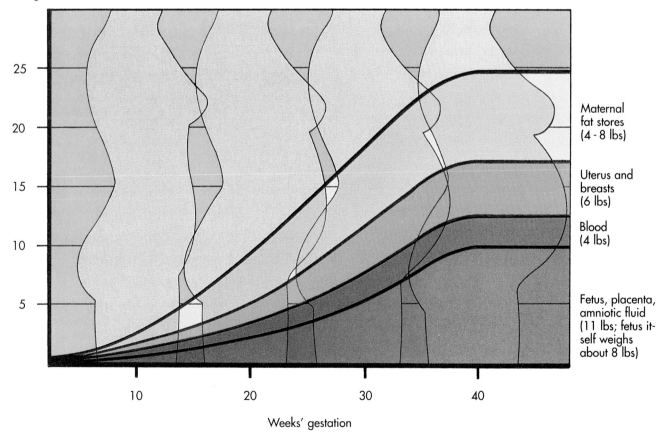

Figure 16-7 The components of weight gain in pregnancy. A weight gain of 25 to 35 pounds is recommended for most women. Note that the various components total about 25 pounds.

A weight gain of about 25 to 35 pounds has repeatedly been shown to yield optimal health for both mother and fetus.[21] This poundage, coupled with length of gestation of at least 38 weeks, should yield a birthweight of 3.5 kg (7.5 pounds). Energy deprivation leading to poor weight gain, such as is seen in famine conditions, is clearly linked to a poor pregnancy outcome.[34]

Weight gain during pregnancy needs regular monitoring such that it follows the pattern in Figure 16-7, especially in the teenage years. This weight gain provides the best indication that energy intake is adequate. Infant birthweights improve if the mother's weight meets the ranges just given. A prenatal weight-gain chart can be used to help assess how much the mother's food intake should be adjusted to promote adequate weight gain.[21] Appendix O contains such a chart. If a women deviates from the ideal weight-gain pattern, she should be counseled about appropriate corrective measures.

If her weight gain exceeds 2 pounds per week during the final two trimesters, a pregnant woman should not be encouraged to lose weight in order to get back on the curve. Rather, she should simply keep following her prenatal diet but avoid extra energy intake in order to slow the increase in weight and parallel the rise on the prenatal weight gain chart. In other words, the sources of the unneeded food energy should be found and then minimized. If a woman fails to gain as much weight as she should at a given point in pregnancy (e.g., <2 pounds per month in the final two trimesters), she should not be encouraged to gain the needed weight rapidly. Instead, she should slowly gain slightly more weight than the typical pattern to meet the charted line by the end of pregnancy.

During pregnancy, excess weight gain and poor food choices are more common than an inadequate intake. The focus needs to be both on a high-quality diet and on reasonable weight gain—neither should be ignored. In the United States, the problem often is how to limit weight gain appropriately—to about 25 to 35 pounds—to prevent the need for significant weight loss after pregnancy. Excessive weight gain increases risk for complications in pregnancy and encourages excess fetal growth, which can increase the risk for birth trauma. Multiple pregnancies with excessive weight gains can contribute to creeping obesity in women, especially in African-Americans. Loose, accommodating maternity clothes designed for comfort do not provide the usual feedback about weight gain, and fluid retention can likewise mask "true" weight gain during pregnancy. Thus careful monitoring by a health professional is desirable.[21]

PROTEIN NEEDS

During pregnancy the RDA for protein is increased by 10 g/day for women over age 24 and by about 15 g/day for those under age 24, for a total of 60 g/day. However, many nonpregnant women already consume this amount of protein per day and thus do not need to increase protein intake when they become pregnant. High-protein supplements are not recommended because they have been associated with an increased number of preterm infants and excessive fetal deaths.[34]

CARBOHYDRATE NEEDS

Carbohydrate needs for pregnant women are at least 100 g/day. This amount prevents ketosis, which may interrupt fetal development and brain maturation. Most nonpregnant women already consume about twice this amount each day.

VITAMIN NEEDS

Vitamin needs in general are increased during pregnancy, especially the need for vitamin D and folate (Figure 16-6).

Vitamin D

Calcium metabolism increases during pregnancy. To facilitate the absorption and distribution of calcium for forming fetal bones, the mother's RDA for vitamin D doubles to 10 μg/day. Pregnant women should get regular sunlight exposure. If that is impossible, such as in the winter months, and sufficient vitamin D–fortified milk is not consumed to make up the difference (4 cups [about 1 L] yields 10 μg), pregnant women, especially African-Americans, should consider a supplement containing 5 to 10 μg (200 to 400 IU).[30] The typical prenatal supplement contains this extra amount of vitamin D.

Folate

Because the synthesis of DNA requires folate, this nutrient is especially crucial during embryonic development. Ultimately both fetal and maternal growth in pregnancy depend on an ample supply of folate. Red blood cell formation, which requires folate, also increases during pregnancy. As a result of its role in DNA synthesis, folate breakdown also increases in pregnancy. Serious megaloblastic anemia can result if folate intake is inadequate during pregnancy (see Chapter 13). The RDA for folate more than doubles during pregnancy to 400 μg/day. This is a critical goal in the nutritional care of a pregnant woman and is advocated for women who have the potential to become pregnant as well.[27] As mentioned before, folate deficiency at conception and after has been associated with birth defects, specifically neural tube defects, such as spina bifida.

Some women have difficulty consuming sufficient folate from foods alone to satisfy their pregnancy needs. Recent studies show that some pregnant women consume only about the RDA for nonpregnant women. However, a woman can meet her needs by choosing folate-rich fruits and vegetables as outlined in the Food Guide Pyramid, as we show in a later section. Most breakfast cereals also provide folate via the fortification process. A prenatal vitamin and mineral supplement may also be used to meet the RDA for folate, especially for women with histories of inadequate folate intake, frequent or multiple births, folate-related anemia, or use of medications that increase folate needs. But normally, wise diet choices alone can suffice. Women who have previously given birth to an infant with a neural tube defect should consult with their physician about the need for folate supplementation; an intake of 4 mg/day is advocated but must be taken under a physician's supervision.[27]

Meeting folate needs during pregnancy may be problematic for women who have taken oral contraceptives for extended periods, as these inhibit folate absorption. A recent history of oral contraceptive use necessitates careful attention to folate intake during pregnancy. Ideally, the woman would begin a folate-rich diet (or take folate supplements) 4 to 5 weeks before conception.

MINERAL NEEDS

Although mineral needs generally increase during pregnancy, adequate intakes of iron, calcium, and zinc are particularly important for maternal and fetal health (Figure 16-6).

Iron

Much extra iron is needed for hemoglobin synthesis during pregnancy; the RDA doubles to 30 mg/day, especially in the second and third trimesters. Use of iron-fortified foods, such as breakfast cereals, is advocated. Eating foods rich in vitamin C along with nonheme iron–containing foods helps to increase iron absorption. Iron supplementation is routine during pregnancy in the United States, but its usefulness is under debate. This is partly because prepregnancy iron status varies considerably among women and because iron absorption increases during pregnacy.[28] Individual assessment of iron status is instead advocated, with treatment using medicinal iron only in women who show iron deficiency. Typical forms of iron supplements include ferrous sulfate, ferrous fumarate, and ferrous gluconate.

Currently the National Academy of Sciences still recommends that (1) all nonanemic pregnant women receive 30 mg of elemental iron daily during the sec-

In an effort to ensure that folate status is adequate in most women at the time of conception, FDA is considering the addition of folate to enriched flours, breads, rolls, buns, corn grits, corn meal, farina, rice, macaroni, and noodle products.

Some recent research suggests that fathers can contribute to a successful pregnancy by consuming adequate amounts of vitamin C, which is necessary for normal development of sperm.

ond and third trimesters of pregnancy and (2) anemic pregnant women receive 60 to 120 mg of elemental iron daily and also take a low-dose multivitamin-mineral preparation containing zinc and copper, but not at the same time during the day.[21] Iron interferes with absorption of these two minerals.

Severe iron-deficiency anemia in pregnancy may lead to preterm delivery, maternal complications or death during delivery, and increased risk for death of the offspring in the first weeks of gestation.[28]

Because iron supplements cause nausea, constipation, and decreased appetite in some people, women are advised to take these supplements between meals with liquids other than milk. Milk should not be consumed with a supplement, as calcium also interferes with iron absorption. Pregnant women also may wait until the second trimester to start iron supplementation; pregnancy-related nausea generally lessens by this time (see later section).

Calcium

Calcium is needed during pregnancy to promote adequate mineralization of the fetal skeleton and teeth and the health of the mother. Most calcium is required during the third trimester, when skeletal bones are growing most rapidly and teeth are forming.[25] However, extra calcium intake should start immediately after conception. The RDA for calcium for pregnant women of 1200 mg/day is the same as that for women ages 11 to 24 years and is 50% greater than the RDA for women over age 24 years. A recent NIH Consensus Conference on Optimal Calcium Intake recommended that calcium intake for pregnant women be increased to 1500 mg/day. The only practical food sources of calcium are foods in the milk, yogurt, and cheese group of the Food Guide Pyramid, calcium-fortified orange juice and other beverages, calcium-fortified bread, and various calcium-fortified snacks. Calcium supplements are advised if these options are not utilized. A prenatal supplement generally contains 200 mg of calcium.

Zinc

Zinc is an important mineral for supporting growth and development. The RDA for zinc is 15 mg/day for pregnant women, 25% higher than that for nonpregnant women. The extra protein foods in the diet of a pregnant woman should supply most of this zinc. Inadequate zinc status in pregnancy increases the risk for delivering a low-birthweight infant.[10]

VARIOUS CRAVINGS DURING PREGNANCY

Before moving on to diet planning for pregnant women, one very important misconception about pregnancy needs to be dispelled. Many people believe that mothers instinctively know what to eat and that their craving for pickles and ice cream is dictated by a natural desire to consume needed nutrients. These cravings are most common during the last two trimesters and could be related to hormonal changes in the mother or just to family traditions.

It remains an even greater mystery why some women crave nonfood items during pregnancy. The craving for and eating of items such as starch, ice, or clay, especially noted during pregnancy, is called **pica**.[34] This occurs more frequently among African-American women in the United States. This practice probably results more from cultural influences and learned behaviors than from a need for specific nutrients like iron and zinc. It also poses some health risks. Eating soil raises the risk of infections from parasites and can cause anemia as well as life-threatening blockages of the intestinal tract. Eating laundry starch should be discouraged because it contains toxic compounds, as do the wall plaster, mothballs, and toilet air fresheners consumed. Eating ice can break teeth.

Overall, although women may have a natural instinct to consume the right foods in pregnancy, humans are so far removed from living by instinct that relying on our desires is risky. Good nutritional counseling can focus food choices more reliably.[24]

CRITICAL THINKING

Steven and Mona have chosen pregnancy as their focus for a term paper on the human life cycle. They are preparing to write the paper by listing the important physiological changes that occur during pregnancy and the additional nutritional requirements necessary to support those changes. What should Steven and Mona include on their list and why?

- - - - - - - - - - -

If a pregnant woman finds herself with no desire at all for pickles and ice cream or frijoles and hot fudge, there is no need to panic: about one third of women experience no strong food cravings during pregnancy.

- - - - - - - - - - -

A Food Plan for Pregnant Women

Table 16-2 outlines one approach to an adequate diet during pregnancy based on the Food Guide Pyramid. It includes at least

- 3 servings from the milk, yogurt, and cheese group
- 3 servings from the meat, poultry, fish, dry beans, eggs, and nuts group
- 3 servings from the vegetable group
- 2 servings from the fruit group
- 6 servings from the bread, cereal, rice, and pasta group

Specifically, the servings from the milk, yogurt, and cheese group could include low-fat or nonfat versions of milk, yogurt, and cheese. These foods supply extra protein, calcium, riboflavin, and magnesium. Servings from the meat, poultry, fish, dry beans, eggs, and nuts group should include both animal and vegetable sources. Besides protein, the animal sources help provide the extra iron and zinc needed, and the vegetable sources help provide much of the extra magnesium needed during pregnancy.

The vegetable and fruit group servings provide a variety of vitamins and minerals. One serving from this combination should be a good vitamin C source, and one serving should be a green vegetable or other rich source of folate, such as spinach or orange juice. Selections from the bread, cereal, rice, and pasta group should focus on whole-grain and enriched foods.

Table 16-3 illustrates one daily menu based on the basic diet plan shown in Table 16-2. This daily menu supplies about 1800 kcal but still meets the extra nutrient needs associated with pregnancy. Women who need to consume more than this, and some do for various reasons, should add more servings from the fruit and vegetable groups and the bread, cereal, rice, and pasta group to the basic plan in Table 16-2.

TABLE 16-2

A basic food plan for pregnant and breastfeeding women based on the Food Guide Pyramid

Food group and single serving size	Key nutrients supplied	Number of servings
Milk, yogurt, and cheese: 1 cup; 1½ oz for cheese	Carbohydrate Protein Riboflavin Calcium	3*
Meat, poultry, fish, dry beans, eggs, and nuts: 2-3 oz of meat; 1 cup beans; 2 eggs; ½ cup nuts	Protein Thiamin Vitamin B-6 Iron Zinc	3
Vegetables: ½ cup cooked or ¾ cup raw	Carbohydrate Vitamin A Vitamin C Folate Dietary fiber	3 to 5
Fruits: Generally 1 piece	Carbohydrate Vitamin C Folate Dietary fiber	2 to 3
Bread, cereal, rice, and pasta: 1 slice or ½-¾ cup cooked	Carbohydrate B vitamins Iron Dietary fiber	6 to 11

*Four servings if a teenager.

TABLE 16-3

Sample 1800 kcal daily menu that meets nutritional needs of most pregnant and breastfeeding women*

Breakfast
1 hard-cooked egg
1 cup raisin bran cereal
½ cup orange juice
½ cup 1% milk

Snack
2 tbsp peanut butter
1 slice whole-wheat toast
½ cup plain low-fat yogurt
½ cup strawberries

Lunch
1½ cups spinach salad with 1 tbsp oil and vinegar dressing
½ whole tomato
1 slice whole-wheat toast
1½ oz provolone cheese

Snack
4 whole-wheat crackers
1 cup 1% milk

Dinner
3 oz lean hamburger, broiled
½ cup baked beans
1 hamburger bun
¾ cup cooked broccoli
1 tsp soft margarine
Iced tea (milk if a teenager)

*This diet meets the RDAs for pregnancy and lactation and supplies 24 mg of iron.

USE OF VITAMIN AND MINERAL SUPPLEMENTS BY PREGNANT WOMEN

Pregnancy, in particular, is not a time to self-prescribe vitamin and mineral supplements. The National Academy of Sciences supports the use of iron supplements, but no other vitamin or mineral supplements, during a routine pregnancy.[21] To meet the higher calcium intake recommended by a recent NIH consensus panel, however, some pregnant women may need to take a calcium supplement.

Although not necessarily recommended by these scientific organizations, specially formulated supplements for pregnant women are prescribed routinely by most physicians. They may do this because it is easier to prescribe supplements than to discuss diet changes. Also, some pregnant women are just not willing to change their diets to meet their increased nutrient needs, or they simply expect (or demand) this treatment. These prenatal supplements typically include the critical nutrients for pregnancy—iron, folate, vitamin D, and calcium—and many others, as well.

There is no evidence that prenatal supplements cause significant health problems in pregnancy, aside perhaps from the combined amounts of supplementary and dietary vitamin A (mainly during the first trimester). While generally unnecessary, prenatal supplements may contribute to a successful pregnancy for certain pregnant women, particularly poor women, teenagers, those with a generally deficient diet, and women carrying multiple fetuses.

PREGNANT VEGETARIANS

Women who practice either lacto-ovo vegetarianism or lacto vegetarianism generally do not face special difficulties in meeting their nutritional needs during pregnancy. Their major problem is meeting iron needs, similar to nonvegetarian pregnant women.

On the other hand, when a total vegetarian (vegan) becomes pregnant, she must carefully plan a diet that includes sufficient protein, vitamin D (or sufficient sun exposure), vitamin B-6, iron, calcium, and zinc, and also use a vitamin B-12 supplement. The basic vegan diet listed in Table 5-7 should be modified to include more grains, beans, nuts, and seeds to supply the needed extra amounts of some of these nutrients. Because iron and calcium are poorly absorbed from most plant foods, iron and calcium supplements are probably necessary, but should not be taken together to avoid competition for absorption.[21] The amounts provided by typical prenatal supplements should suffice to meet iron needs but not calcium needs. The prenatal supplement will also fulfill vitamin D needs if sufficient sun exposure does not take place.

CONCEPT CHECK

Energy needs increase by an average of about 300 kcal/day during the second and third trimesters of pregnancy. Weight gain should be slow and steady up to a total of 25 to 35 pounds for a woman at desirable weight. Protein, vitamin, and mineral needs all increase during pregnancy. Vitamin D, folate, iron, calcium, and zinc are nutrients of particular concern. A pregnant woman's diet should be varied and generally include more milk products and more specified fruits and vegetables (e.g., those rich in folate and vitamin C) than a prepregnancy diet. Prenatal supplemental vitamins and minerals are commonly prescribed but often are unnecessary, aside from the iron they supply.

Effects of Nutritional and Other Factors on Pregnancy Outcome

In the United States, about 12 of every 100,000 live births end in the mother's death. The infant mortality rate is even higher: for each 100,000 live births, about 850 infants die within the first year.[5] The infant death rate among African-Americans is more than double the rates among Caucasians and Hispanics in the United States. Based on the national statistics, the United States currently ranks 24th among industrial nations in terms of maternal and infant death rates. Such grim and discomfiting statistics can be attributed largely to the current high number of teenage pregnancies in this country and to inadequate prenatal care, as well as marginal nutritional status among poor pregnant woman.

American health professionals are expending considerable effort to reduce both infant and maternal deaths, focusing particularly on women most at risk for problems during pregnancy (Table 16-4). Good nutritional and health-related practices are two key factors in ensuring a successful pregnancy outcome.[21] We first review the nutritional demands of pregnancy, then describe some research findings demonstrating the importance of adequate maternal nutrition, and finally examine numerous lifestyle and medical factors that can adversely affect pregnancy.

NUTRITIONAL DEMANDS OF PREGNANCY

As we've discussed, the growth of the fetus and the changes in the mother's body that occur to accommodate the fetus require extra nutrients and energy. Although pregnancy is a normal process, the sizable changes in the mother's body pose nutritional stresses for her. Her uterus and breasts grow, the placenta develops, her total blood volume increases, the heart and kidneys work harder, and stores of body

In 1990 the hospital-related costs of caring for low-birthweight newborns totaled more than $2 billion, an average of $21,000 per child. Compare this with an average hospital-related cost of $2842 for a normal delivery and an average of $500 for preventive prenatal care.

TABLE 16-4

Women generally defined as nutritionally at risk during pregnancy
• Women who do not ordinarily consume an adequate diet • Women carrying more than one fetus • Women who use cigarettes, alcohol, or illegal drugs • Women whose children are closely spaced together • Women with lactose intolerance • Women who are underweight or overweight at conception or who gain inadequate or excessive weight during pregnancy • Adolescents (see Table 16-5) • Women who have poor knowledge about nutrition, who follow faddish food patterns, or who have insufficient financial resources to purchase adequate food

fat increase—all in preparation for birth and milk production.[34] The nutrients needed to support these maternal changes are in addition to the nutrient needs of both the growing fetus and the mother's own normal physiological functions. A pregnant adolescent, in particular, faces almost overwhelming nutritional demands and in turn needs close medical monitoring to ensure that her diet will allow for her growth and will also not cause nutrient deprivation for her fetus.

The specific effects on fetal development of either marginal nutrient and energy intakes during pregnancy or low maternal nutrient stores at conception are difficult to establish. Fetal growth and development clearly are retarded when the pregnant woman's diet supplies grossly insufficient energy (only 1000 kcal/day). Even on a less-than-optimal diet, a woman's body can adapt to the demands of pregnancy in a variety of ways, including increased absorption of some dietary nutrients. If the pregnant woman's diet is inadequate, the fetus can also draw on and deplete the maternal stores of some nutrients, such as iron and calcium. However, the ability of the fetus to survive intrauterine insult, including an inadequate supply of nutrients, without adverse effects is limited. Since maternal nutrient reserves cannot always insulate the fetus from dietary deficiencies, adequate maternal nutrition is necessary for normal fetal growth and development. Moreover, a successful pregnancy is one that not only results in a healthy infant but also maintains the health of the mother.[34]

Research shows that genetic background can explain very little of the observed differences in birthweight. Both environmental factors and nutritional factors, such as the length of gestation and mother's weight gain, are more important.[34] The worse the nutritional condition of the mother at the beginning of pregnancy, the more valuable a good prenatal diet and/or use of prenatal supplements will be in improving the course and outcome of her pregnancy.

ASSOCIATION BETWEEN ADEQUATE MATERNAL NUTRITION AND SUCCESSFUL PREGNANCY

We now know that inadequate maternal nutrition in the early months of pregnancy adversely affects the development and survival of the embryo, often leading to miscarriage. Inadequate nutrition in the second and third trimesters retards fetal growth, so a low-birthweight baby is likely. An unintended experiment during World War II demonstrated this second point. Parts of Russia and much of Holland were blockaded during this time period, and food supplies were quickly exhausted. The resulting undernutrition suffered by pregnant women in the second and third trimesters greatly reduced their infants' birthweight. The number of new pregnancies also fell as women's health status weakened. After the blockades were lifted, birthweights and the number of new pregnancies quickly rose again to prewar levels.[31]

At the same time, researchers working in Boston noticed that an adequate protein intake was associated with a greater success of pregnancy. It appeared that the mother's diet—not only during pregnancy but also preceding conception—contributed to the health of both mother and infant. Since women who could afford higher protein diets most likely obtained adequate prenatal health care, this latter factor probably also contributed to the well-being of these mothers and infants. Studies in Toronto subsequently showed that dietary supplements and nutritional counseling improved the health of pregnant women and yielded healthier infants. Rates of complications were also reduced.[34]

In the 1980s researchers in Great Britain reported that height and social class were better predictors of pregnancy outcome than dietary intake by itself. Of course, higher social class and better nutrition tend to be associated. A more recent study in Chicago supported the British results. This study also showed, however, that the risk for having a low-birthweight infant was greater among middle-class African-American women than among middle-class Caucasian women, a difference that possibly reflects the effects of previous generations of poverty. This finding again suggests that long-term nutritional intake is critical to successful pregnancy outcome.[19]

Numerous studies with laboratory animals have also highlighted the importance of maternal diet to pregnancy outcome. Food deprivation during pregnancy, for example, results in offspring with undersized organs, including the brain, which usually is very resistant to nutritional deprivation. In addition, the weight of the placenta is less than in animals receiving adequate nutrition; food-deprived pregnant animals also have fewer healthy offspring that survive the first weeks of life.[34]

OTHER FACTORS THAT ADVERSELY AFFECT PREGNANCY

In addition to nutrient intake per se, many other nutritional, medical, and lifestyle factors can adversely influence the health of the pregnant woman, fetal development and growth, and the condition of the newborn. Most of these are controllable; that is, they can be avoided or their effects mitigated. Organized efforts to reduce maternal and infant deaths in this country in large part focus on reducing these risk factors.

Low Socioeconomic Status

A constellation of characteristics—including poverty, inadequate health care, poor health-related practices, lack of education, and unmarried status—are commonly associated with low socioeconomic status. All of these characteristics are related to problems during pregnancy.

Closely Spaced Births

Siblings born in succession with less than a year between them are more likely to be born with low birthweight than those born further apart in age, especially by African-American women.[26]

Age under 18 Years

Young women continue to mature into physical adulthood for 5 years after menarche. Since the average age of menarche is 13 years in the United States, a woman under 18 years is not as physically ready to be pregnant as she will be later. Pregnancies under age 18 are high risk and need special monitoring (see the Nutrition Focus).[33] Overall, mothers who are between 25 and 34 years of age have the best pregnancy outcomes.

Obesity

Obese women are very susceptible to hypertension and diabetes during pregnancy and to surgical and other complications during delivery. These pregnancies require intense monitoring to reduce the potential risks for both the mother and the infant.

Inadequate Prenatal Care

Women who receive no prenatal care or delayed prenatal care may have undetected nutritional deficiencies that can deprive the fetus of needed nutrients, and/or may

The risks of low birthweight and preterm delivery increase modestly, but progressively, with maternal age. Given close monitoring, however, a woman over the age of 35 has an excellent chance of producing a healthy infant. Most women in this age group exhibit typical pregnancy-related problems, which usually are manageable.

have a poorly controlled chronic disease (e.g., hypertension or diabetes) that can increase the risk of fetal damage. Ideally, prenatal care should start at least 8 to 12 weeks *prior to* conception to maximize maternal health, and then continue at regular intervals during pregnancy to identify problems and begin immediate treatment if possible.[19] Today, about 20% of the pregnant women in the United States receive no prenatal care during the first trimester—a critical time to change habits.

Use of Legal and Illegal Drugs

The use of tobacco, alcohol, some medications, and illegal drugs (including marijuana)—singly or in combination—by a pregnant woman is likely to cause serious harmful effects in her infant. In developed countries, cigarette smoking is the most important factor associated with intrauterine growth retardation. Smoking is linked to low birthweight in the infant, especially when practiced in the third trimester, probably because nicotine constricts arteries, thus denying the fetus sufficient blood supply to carry needed oxygen.[34] Cigarette smoking during pregnancy also may increase the risk for birth defects, such as cleft lip and/or cleft palate, and fetal death. In addition, children whose mothers smoked during pregnancy appear to suffer more colds, asthma, and other respiratory problems than those whose mothers didn't smoke. Use of alcohol, the other common legal drug, by pregnant women can also adversely affect the fetus, as discussed in the Nutrition Perspective.[15]

Of the illegal drugs, fetal exposure to cocaine is the most troubling.[34] As cocaine use has become more common in recent years, the number of infants born to cocaine-using women has increased. Maternal use of cocaine during pregnancy has been linked to preterm birth as well as to an undersized head and body and several other physical malformations in the newborn. Exposure of the fetus to cocaine appears to disrupt development of its brain and nervous system and may reduce interactive behaviors and responses to environmental stimuli in the infant. Further studies and improved testing procedures are needed to assess the long-term developmental abnormalities in infants exposed to cocaine in utero.

Various surveys in recent years have given some idea about how many pregnant women use substances potentially harmful to the fetus. For instance, a 1989 study at a major Philadelphia hospital revealed that 15% of 852 pregnant women tested positive for cocaine or combinations of cocaine, marijuana, and narcotics. The percentage of drug users was about the same among private and publicly subsidized patients. Another study involving 36 hospitals located throughout the United States found that on average 11% of women used illegal drugs during pregnancy; the percentage reported from individual hospitals ranged from 1% to 27%. Based on a 1992 survey of approximately 67,000 maternity patients at California hospitals, an estimated 11% were found to have consumed alcohol and/or used an illegal drug within hours or days of delivery. These estimates of alcohol and illegal drug use are probably quite conservative because the urine tests in these studies only detect recent substance abuse. About 9% of the patients in the California study reported that they had recently smoked cigarettes.

Clearly, significant numbers of women smoke and/or use alcohol and other harmful drugs during pregnancy. Although the frequency of substance use tends to be higher among African-American women than other groups, infants adversely affected by these agents are found in all socioeconomic and ethnic groups. Thus the issue of substance use during pregnancy needs to be addressed with all women.[24] Needless to say, pregnant women should avoid these agents, which can have very detrimental short-term and long-term effects on their infants.

Prenatal Ketosis

The presence of ketone bodies in a pregnant woman's bloodstream likely is harmful to the growing fetus. The fetal brain is thought to metabolize ketone bodies slowly, resulting in impaired brain development. Since significant ketosis can develop after only 20 hours of fasting, pregnant women should avoid "crash" diets or fasting for more than 12 hours.

- - - - - - - - - - - - -
Women with acquired immune deficiency syndrome (AIDS) may pass the virus that causes this disease to the fetus during pregnancy or the birth process. About 1 in 3 infected newborns will develop AIDS symptoms and die within just a few years. Recent studies show that these odds of mother-infant transmission can be cut significantly if the woman begins taking the drug zidovudine (AZT) by the fourteenth week of pregancy. Thus screening pregnant women for AIDS and treating them with AZT is currently advocated.
- - - - - - - - - - - - -

Inadequate Weight Gain

Earlier we saw that a total weight gain of about 25 to 35 pounds during pregnancy is optimal for most women. Women who gain substantially less than this have an increased risk for delivering a low-birthweight infant.[21] Low-birthweight infants show a greater risk for infection, illness, disabilities, and death than normal-weight infants. In fact, 60% of all infant deaths occur in these infants. Preterm birth, inadequate diet during pregnancy, and some medical conditions in the mother (such as short stature and first pregnancy) are additional factors that increase the risk of delivering a low-birthweight infant. Reducing the number of low-birthweight infants will help reduce the total number of infant deaths.[5]

Caffeine Consumption

Research on the effects of caffeine consumption by pregnant women has yielded some provocative findings. Caffeine decreases absorption of iron, a key nutrient during pregnancy (as discussed earlier) and may reduce blood flow through the placenta. The risk of spontaneous abortion has been shown to increase in the first trimester and early in the second trimester with heavy caffeine consumption (>300 mg/day). About 2 to 3 cups of coffee per day contain this amount of caffeine (see Appendix M). In addition, as caffeine intake increases, so does the risk of delivering a low-birthweight infant. Heavy caffeine use during pregnancy may also lead to caffeine withdrawal symptoms in the newborn.[11] Although more research is needed, it is advisable to limit intake. No more than 2 cups of coffee and no more than 4 cups of caffeinated soft drinks per day during pregnancy, or when pregnancy is possible, is advocated. Limiting intake from tea, over-the-counter medicines, and chocolate is also important.[23] Some researchers advocate complete avoidance of caffeine during pregnancy.

Aspartame Consumption

Use of the alternative sweetener aspartame (NutraSweet and Equal), which contains the amino acid phenylalanine, should be avoided during pregnancy by women with phenylketonuria (PKU). People with this disease don't metabolize phenylalanine readily (see Chapter 5). Thus aspartame consumption by pregnant women with PKU can lead to high blood concentrations of phenylalanine breakdown products that can disrupt fetal brain development. However, the vast majority of women do not have PKU. It is unlikely that their offspring will be affected by aspartame use.[11] Some experts recommend cautious use of aspartame during pregnancy, but total abstinence is hardly warranted in this instance, based on our current knowledge. The variety of foods and beverages sweetened with aspartame can help satisfy a pregnant woman's taste for sweets without extra energy intake, leaving room for more nutritious foods.

Listeria Infection

Infection by the bacterium *Listeria monocytogenes* causes mild flulike symptoms, such as fever, headache, and vomiting, about 7 to 30 days after exposure. However, pregnant women, newborn infants, and people with depressed immune function may suffer more severe symptoms, including spontaneous abortion, meningitis, and serious blood infections. In these high-risk people, 25% of infections may be fatal.

Because unpasteurized milk, soft cheeses made from raw milk, and cabbage can be sources of listeria organisms, it is especially important that pregnant women and other people at high risk avoid these products. Consuming only pasteurized milk products and cooking meat, poultry, and seafood thoroughly to kill this organism are advised. It is unsafe to eat any raw meats. Chapter 19 covers food-borne illness, such as listeria infections, in more detail.

Toxoplasmosis is another infection that causes birth defects. Pregnant women can avoid exposure to the organism that causes toxoplasmosis by having someone else clean the cat's litter box, by avoiding contact with kittens or garden soil, and by not eating raw or undercooked meat.

Prenatal Care and Counseling

As we've stressed already, an adequate diet, early and consistent medical care, and appropriate counseling maximize the chances for a pregnant woman to give birth to

NUTRITION FOCUS

TEENAGE PREGNANCY

Surveys indicate that between about 10% and 13% of teenage girls become pregnant at least once by the age of 18, giving the United States the highest teenage pregnancy rate in the Western World—over twice that of England, France, or Canada.[32] According to one survey, 33% of teenage girls do not use any form of contraception during their first incident of sexual intercourse.

About half a million teenagers give birth in the United States each year, accounting for about 13% of all births. The teenage birth rate historically has been highest among African-Americans. In 1970, the birth rate for African-Americans age 15 to 19 was 141 per 1000, compared with 57 per 1000 Caucasians. In 1991, this disparity remained, with birth rates for African-American adolescents at 118 per 1000, compared with 43 per 1000 for Caucasian adolescents. Overall, minority teenagers with below-average academic skills and from families with below-poverty incomes are considerably more likely to become pregnant than other adolescent girls. Often these young mothers are the daughters of teenage mothers themselves.[32]

Teenage pregnancy poses special health problems for both the mother and child. To accommodate their normal growth even when not pregnant, teenagers need an extraordinary nutrient supply. Adolescent girls normally continue to grow taller for 2 years after they begin menstruating and to mature physically for 5 years. Teenage pregnancy adds the needs of the growing fetus to those of the growing mother. They both need considerable amounts of nutrients for their growing bodies.

Diets of teenagers—including those who are pregnant—vary greatly in nutritional adequacy. Many teenagers eat irregularly, skip meals, snack on foods with low nutrient density, and frequently follow restrictive diets. Many of them eat less than two thirds of the RDA for various vitamins and minerals.[2]

Pregnant teenagers frequently exhibit a variety of risk factors that can complicate pregnancy and pose a risk to the fetus (Table 16-5). For instance, teenagers are more likely than older women to be underweight at the beginning of pregnancy and to gain fewer than 16 pounds during pregnancy. Consequently, teenagers frequently give birth to preterm or low-birthweight infants; about 16% of low-birthweight infants are born to teenagers.[33] Additional complications, such as infant illness or even death, are tied to the teenage mother's day-to-day health practices.[32] If the mother leads a healthful life, she will be healthier and so too will her infant.

The specific needs of pregnant teenagers vary according to their own growth patterns, body build, and physical activity habits. This makes it difficult to predict their nutrient needs. Clinicians can evaluate the adequacy of their diet by checking for appropriate weight gain during pregnancy and for appropriate food choices. Teenagers should be regularly counseled concerning nutrition during their prenatal care. They need information about basic nutrition guidelines: the relationship between food and health, the kind and amount of food energy needed to support appropriate weight gain, how to select nutrient-rich foods, appropriate use of prenatal supplements, and preparation for breastfeeding or for using infant formulas. They also need to be made aware of the risks involved with smoking, drinking alcohol, and using drugs and medications not approved by their physicians.[2]

Programs specifically designed for pregnant teenagers are available in many communities. These typically provide information about community resources; many also offer clothing and supplies for the infant, food resources, transportation for prenatal checkups, and a supportive environment. Nonetheless, even when a teenager successfully delivers a healthy baby, the subsequent impact of parent-

"morning sickness," pregnancy-related nausea may occur at any time and persist all day. It is often the first signal to a woman that she is pregnant. To partially control mild nausea, pregnant women can try the following: avoid nauseating foods, such as fried or greasy foods; cook with open windows to dissipate nauseating smells; eat soda crackers, potato chips, or dry cereal before getting out of bed; avoid large fluid intakes early in the morning; and eat smaller, more frequent meals. Because the iron in prenatal supplements triggers nausea in some women, changing the type of supplement used may provide relief in some cases. If a woman thinks her prenatal

TABLE 16-5

Nutrition-related risk factors in teenage pregnancy

- Low pregnancy weight gain
- Low prepregnancy weight for height (or other evidence of inadequate nutrition)
- Smoking (mothers 18 to 19 years of age smoke more than do any other group of mothers)
- Excessive prepregnancy weight for height
- Anemia

Other risk factors suggested by health histories
- Unhealthy lifestyle (e.g., the use of drugs or alcohol)
- Unfavorable reproductive history
- Chronic diseases
- History of an eating disorder or excessive worry about maintaining a thin appearance

From ADA Reports: *Journal of the American Dietetic Association* 89:106, 1989.

hood on the mother's education and economic future is often devastating. Some teenage girls view early pregnancy as a quick route to a meaningful adult role. The reality of this adult role, however, may shock them. Few teenager mothers can successfully care for and support themselves and their children. Many young mothers end up foregoing the very education that would qualify them for better jobs, which might in turn permit them to adequately care for and support themselves and their children. Moreover, the vast majority of pregnant teenagers are unmarried and don't get married before the birth of their child. This further compounds the economic and social difficulties of the young mother and child.[32]

Given all the problems associated with teenage pregnancy and the subsequent situation of the young, often unmarried mother and her infant, many efforts are under way to reduce the rate of teenage pregnancy. This approach is currently receiving high priority by the federal government, especially as part of an overhaul of our nation's welfare programs. Three broad strategies for public interventions designed to reduce the problems associated with teenage pregnancy have been advocated: an emphasis on abstinence, more sex education and contraceptive services, and better support services for teenagers who become pregnant. Some politicians also advocate denying the teenager welfare payments, and in turn essentially requiring her to remain with her parents rather than set up her own household. We hope something will arise as an effective measure, as the current outlook for teenage mothers and their infants is often so bleak.[32]

supplement is related to morning sickness, she should discuss switching to another supplement with her physician.

Overall, whether it is broccoli or potato chips, if a food sounds good to a pregnant woman with morning sickness, she should eat it, and eat when she can, in turn striving to follow her prenatal diet. If the ability to follow her diet is greatly hampered, she should alert her physician of this and follow the advice given. Usually nausea stops after the first trimester, but in about 10% to 20% of cases it can continue throughout the entire pregnancy. In cases of serious nausea, the preceding practices offer little relief. Vitamin B-6 in amounts about 7.5 times the RDA then may be helpful, under a physician's supervision.[14] When appetite is severely reduced or vomiting persists, additional medical guidance is warranted. Hospitalization in turn may be needed if the mother exhibits significant dehydration and/or weight loss.

GESTATIONAL DIABETES

gestational diabetes A high blood glucose concentration that develops during pregnancy and returns to normal after birth; one cause is placental production of hormones that antagonize regulation of blood glucose by insulin.

Hormones synthesized by the placenta antagonize the action of the hormone insulin. This antagonism can precipitate **gestational diabetes,** often beginning in weeks 20 to 28, particularly in women who have a family history of diabetes and/or are obese. Gestational diabetes develops in about 3% of pregnancies. All pregnant women should have their urine or blood glucose concentration measured at about 20 weeks' gestation to monitor for developing diabetes. If diabetes is detected, a special diet and sometimes insulin injections are needed; regular physical activity is also helpful.[9] Although gestational diabetes often disappears after the infant's birth, it is linked to development of diabetes later in the mother's life, especially if she fails to maintain body weight in a desirable range. Proper control of both gestational diabetes and diabetes present in the mother before pregnancy is extremely important. If not treated, the fetus can grow quite large, often necessitating an early delivery and increasing the risk of birth trauma and malformations, as well as hypoglycemia in the infant at birth.

ANEMIA

physiological anemia The normal increase in blood volume in pregnancy that dilutes the concentration of red blood cells, resulting in anemia; also called *hemodilution.*

To supply fetal needs, the mother's blood volume expands to approximately 150% of normal, whereas the red cell mass expands only 20% to 30% above normal and does so more slowly than the increase in blood volume. This leaves proportionately fewer red cells in a pregnant woman's bloodstream. The lower ratio of red blood cells to total blood volume is a condition known as **physiological anemia** (or hemodilution) because it is a normal response to pregnancy. In response, the cut-off values for diagnosis of iron deficiency anemia are slightly lower than for nonpregnant women.[17]

In addition to this physiological cause, a woman with inadequate iron stores and/or inadequate dietary intake of iron or folate during pregnancy is likely to develop anemia for the same reasons discussed in Chapters 13 and 15. In this case, she may require more specific medical attention than simply following her prenatal diet and taking any supplement prescribed.[17] Sometimes physicians advise women to continue use of iron supplements after delivery to rebuild iron stores depleted during pregnancy, especially if they are breastfeeding the infant.

PREGNANCY-INDUCED HYPERTENSION

pregnancy-induced hypertension A serious disorder that can include high blood pressure, kidney failure, convulsions, and even death of the mother and fetus. Although its exact cause is not known, good nutrition (especially adequate calcium intake) and prenatal care may prevent or limit its severity. Mild cases are known as *preeclampsia;* more severe cases are called *eclampsia* (formerly called *toxemia*).

Pregnancy-induced hypertension is a serious disorder that develops in 5% to 7% of pregnancies. Mild forms are also known as *preeclampsia,* and severe forms are termed *eclampsia.* The condition resolves once the pregnancy state ends. There is no agreed-upon cause of the disorder, other than pregnancy itself. Current proposals include a high-fat diet and related altered prostaglandin synthesis, changes in sensitivity to angiotensin, and immunological reasons.[8] Early signs and symptoms include a rise in blood pressure, excess protein in the urine, and fluid retention. More severe effects, including convulsions, can occur in the second and third trimesters.

A sufficient diet, such as that outlined in Table 16-2, especially one supplying 1 to 2 g of calcium per day, may prevent or lessen the effects of pregnancy-related hypertension.[25] Additional studies on this disorder are under way. Bed rest and certain medications can also lessen mild effects, as may also a moderate sodium restriction. More severe effects, if not controlled, can lead to liver and kidney damage, and even death of the mother and fetus. Careful medical attention is needed; delivery of the infant is the only definite cure.[8]

CONCEPT CHECK

Heartburn, constipation, nausea and vomiting, edema, gestational diabetes, and anemia are possible discomforts and complications of pregnancy. Changes in food habits can often ease these problems. Pregnancy-induced hypertension, with high blood pressure and kidney failure, can lead to severe complications or even death of both the mother and fetus, if not treated. High calcium intake is linked to a reduced risk for pregnancy-induced hypertension.

Breastfeeding

Before 1900, infants who were not breastfed by their mothers were commonly breastfed by a "wet nurse." In those days, formula feeding was fraught with complications, primarily because people did not know the importance of sterilizing formulas against bacteria, nor much about the nutritional needs of infants. During the early 1900s, the technology of formula feeding improved. From the 1920s onward, especially during World War II, when many women worked in armament factories, more and more infants were fed formulas, mostly based on evaporated milk. Throughout the 1950s and early 1960s, interest in breastfeeding further waned. In the 1970s, breastfeeding enjoyed a resurgence, which has since leveled off.

Healthy People 2000, a federally sponsored program, has set a goal of 75% of women nursing their infants at time of hospital discharge, and 50% still nursing 6 months later. Recent surveys show, however, that only about 50% of American mothers now nurse their infants in the hospital, and at 6 months only 20% are still breastfeeding their infants. Clearly, American women have far to go to meet the Healthy People 2000 goal.

Women who choose to breastfeed usually find it an enjoyable and special time in their lives and in their relationship with their new infant (Figure 16-9). Bottle-feeding with an infant formula is also safe for infants, as we will discuss in the next chapter, but does not equal the benefits derived from human milk in all aspects. Note that if a woman doesn't nurse her child, breast weight returns to normal very soon after birth.

ABILITY TO BREASTFEED

In most cases, problems encountered in breastfeeding are due to a lack of appropriate information, as almost all women are physically capable of nursing their children.[22] Anatomic problems in breasts, such as inverted nipples, can be corrected during pregnancy. Breast size is no indication of success in breastfeeding and generally increases during pregnancy. Most women notice a pretty dramatic increase in the size and weight of their breasts by the third or fourth day of breastfeeding. These changes indicate that everything is going well. If these changes don't occur, a woman needs to speak with her physician.

Breastfed infants must be followed closely over the first few days of life to ensure that the process is proceeding normally. Monitoring is especially important with a mother's first child, as she will be inexperienced with the process of breastfeeding. Nowadays, mothers and healthy infants commonly are discharged from the hospital 1 to 2 days after delivery, whereas 20 years ago they stayed in the hospital for 3 to 4 days or longer. One result of such rapid discharge is a decreased period of infant monitoring by health-care professionals. Incidents have been reported of infants developing dehydration and blood clots soon after hospital discharge when breastfeeding did not proceed smoothly.

New parents generally need guidance about their infant's nutritional and other health-related needs by appropriate professionals for several weeks after hospital discharge. First-time mothers who plan to breastfeed should learn as much as they can about the process early in their pregnancy.[1] Interested women should learn the

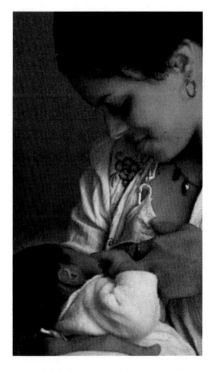

Figure 16-9 Breastfeeding fosters closeness between mother and infant. This is part of the process called bonding, an important component of the normal parent-child nurturing process. Bottle feeding also allows for this.

HUMAN MILK: THE ECOLOGICALLY SOUND WAY TO FEED AN INFANT

LINDA J. BOYNE, M.S., R.D., L.D.

Human milk is one of the world's greatest natural resources. It is unequaled as a source of nutrients for human infants and contributes to both the biological and emotional health of the mother-infant dyad. Human milk is environmentally beneficial, as it uses renewable resources and produces only biodegradable wastes. Nonetheless, human milk is an underutilized resource, as many mothers prefer to use modified cow's-milk formulas as the food of choice for their infants.

One major reason for the underutilization of human milk is lack of consistent and accurate information from health-care providers. Providers of health care often don't understand the process of lactation, nor the cultural factors that may affect a woman's decision on how to feed her infant. In addition, our society frequently erects barriers that discourage breastfeeding. Health-care facilities frequently have "necessary" routines or schedules that interfere with the initiation and/or establishment of a successful breastfeeding experi-

ence. Role models, particularly family members, are not available to many women.

Mothers should know that although breastfeeding is a "natural" process, it must be learned—by both the mother and the infant. Fortunately, infants are born with reflexes and instincts that help them. They are also born with adequate energy and fluid reserves on board to help them survive during this "learning" period.

It is important that health-care workers in contact with women be knowledgeable about the health, nutritional, and physiological aspects of appropriate infant feeding, the mechanics of breastfeeding, the psychosocial influences, possible difficulties that may occur, and how to overcome these difficulties. From early childhood into adolescence, boys, as well as girls, need to be positively oriented toward breastfeeding as a normal, accepted practice. Although knowledge is essential, a positive attitude toward breastfeeding and the advantages for the mother and her

infant are a must. This attitude is readily conveyed to the expectant family during prenatal counseling.

Mostly we tend to consider the advantages of breastfeeding to the infant. First, human milk is designed exclusively for human infants: it is bacteriologically safe and always fresh. Human milk provides the infant's first immunization by providing immunoglobulins (antibodies) to protect the infant from enteropathogens while his own immune system is gearing up. Human milk also ensures maturation of the gastrointestinal tract by providing the bifidus factor. Because of this bifidus factor, the development of diarrheal and respiratory diseases is considerably decreased, an especially important consideration in developing countries, where a safe water supply is often not available. Breastfeeding is an important contributor to reducing the risk for food allergies in infants, particularly in those with a positive family history of food hypersensitivities.

In addition to these immediate benefits to the infant, breastfeeding is

proper technique, what problems to expect, and how to respond to them. Overall, breastfeeding is a learned skill, and mothers need knowledge to nurse safely, especially the first time. Mothers-to-be may choose to stimulate their nipples by pulling, twisting, or rolling them between their fingers. This toughens the nipples in preparation for breastfeeding. Overall, familiarity with the process of breastfeeding builds the confidence and knowledge necessary for success.

PHYSIOLOGY OF LACTATION

During pregnancy, cells in the breast aggregate to form milk-producing cells called **lobules** (Figure 16-10). Hormones from the placenta stimulate these changes in the breast. After birth, increased maternal production of the hormone **prolactin** acts to maintain these changes in the breast and, in turn, enhances the ability to produce milk.

lobules Saclike structures in the breast that store milk.

prolactin A hormone secreted by a woman after giving birth that stimulates the synthesis of milk.

likely to help establish the habit of eating in moderation, thus reducing the possibility of obesity later in life. Only the infant really knows how much he eats; once he is finished the mother can't readily tell, and so won't be tempted to encourage more intake, as could be the case if a bottle-fed infant stopped feeding with an ounce or two of formula left. An infant's suckling at the mother's breast also contributes to proper development of the jaws and teeth, leading to better speech development and reducing the risk of developing otitis media (ear infections). Recent studies have shown that the risk of developing diabetes is also lower in children who were breastfed during infancy.

What are the advantages to a mother regarding breastfeeding her infant? Recovery from the pregnancy occurs earlier and more easily because oxytocin, a hormone involved in the let-down reflex, promotes the return of the uterus to its prepregnancy state and decreases the risk of postpartum hemorrhage. The risk

for ovarian cancer and premenopausal breast cancer has been found to be reduced in women who have breastfed their infants. If economic considerations are important, the cost of providing additional nutrients to the lactating woman is considerably less than providing commercial infant formula to her infant. In addition, psychological attachment (referred to as *bonding*) occurs more easily during the breastfeeding process. This latter consideration is, of course, important to both parties in the mother-infant dyad.

Health-care professionals should be able to provide consistent, accurate information about lactation and the breastfeeding process to mothers, fathers, and other support persons. They must be sure not to send mixed messages, such as providing literature that promotes breastfeeding but also advertises infant formulas. Is the literature portraying breastfeeding as a modest, discreet activity or one that may cause embarrassment to the mother and her partner? Health-care professionals must be

honest and inform the mother that there may be some pain when initiating breastfeeding. However, proper positioning of the infant, being sure that the infant is properly latched on, and helping the mother recognize when her infant is swallowing so that she will know he is indeed receiving her milk will aid in reducing the amount of pain that she may be fearful of experiencing. Parents also need to know what signs to look for that will reassure the mother that she is providing adequate nourishment for her infant, and as well how to provide adequate nourishment for herself.

Breastfeeding should be an enjoyable experience for both the mother and her infant, leading to a healthier life down the road for both parties.

Linda J. Boyne is an assistant professor in the Division of Medical Dietetics and an assistant professor in the Department of Pediatrics, College of Medicine, at The Ohio State University. She is a former chair of the Pediatric Nutrition Practice Group of the American Dietetic Association.

Suckling by the infant stimulates release of prolactin, which in turn stimulates milk synthesis. The longer the infant suckles, the more milk is produced. Thus milk production closely parallels infant demand—allowing for successful feeding of more than one infant. Demand is the driving force for milk production.[34]

Most protein found in human milk is synthesized by breast tissue. Some proteins, such as immune factors and enzymes, enter the milk directly from maternal circulation. Long-chain fatty acids, found as triglycerides in human milk, come primarily from the mother's diet. Short-chain fatty acids, also found as triglycerides in breast milk, are synthesized by breast tissue. The monosaccharide galactose is synthesized in the breast, while glucose enters from the maternal circulation. Together these monosaccharides form the disaccharide lactose, the primary carbohydrate in human milk.

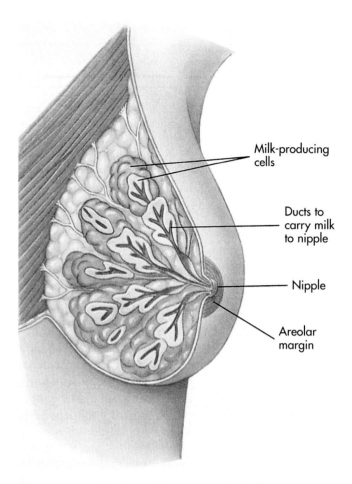

Figure 16-10 The anatomy of the breast. Many types of cells form a coordinated network to produce and secrete human milk.

Milk-producing cells

Ducts to carry milk to nipple

Nipple

Areolar margin

let-down reflex A reflex stimulated by infant suckling that causes the release (ejection) of milk from milk ducts in the mother's breasts.

- - - - - - - - - - - - - - -

Disposable diapers can absorb so much urine that it is difficult to judge when they are wet. A strip of paper towel laid inside a disposable diaper makes a good wetness indicator. Or cloth diapers may be used for a day or two to assess whether nursing is supplying sufficient milk.

- - - - - - - - - - - - - - -

THE LET-DOWN REFLEX

An important brain-breast connection—the **let-down reflex**—is necessary for successful breastfeeding (Figure 16-11). Suckling by the infant sends a signal to the mother's brain, which then sends a signal to the pituitary gland to release oxytocin; this hormone then travels to the breasts and induces them to "let down," or release, milk from storage sites. The milk is then transported to the nipple area and is available to the infant.[34] If the let-down reflex doesn't operate, little milk is available to the infant, who soon gets frustrated. The mother in turn may become upset and frustrated, further inhibiting the let-down reflex.

The let-down reflex is easily inhibited by nervous tension, a lack of confidence, and fatigue. Mothers should be especially aware of the link between tension and a weak let-down reflex. They need to find a relaxed environment where they can breastfeed.

After a few weeks, the let-down reflex becomes automatic. The mother's response can be triggered just by thoughts about her infant or by seeing or hearing another one. But at first the process can be a bit bewildering. Because she cannot measure the amount of milk the infant takes in, a mother may fear that she is not adequately nourishing the infant. As a general rule, a well-nourished breastfed infant should (1) have six or more wet diapers per day after the second day of life, (2) show a normal weight gain, and (3) pass one or two stools per day that look like lumpy mustard. In addition, softening of the breast during the feeding helps indicate that enough milk is being consumed. A mother who senses her infant is not

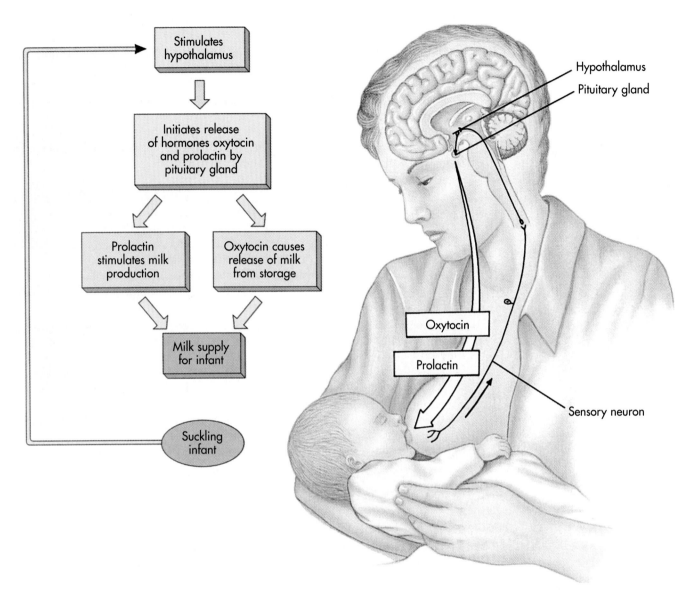

Figure 16-11 The let-down reflex. Stimulation of the nipple by the infant's suckling triggers nerve impulses to the hypothalamus. The hypothalamus then stimulates the posterior lobe of the pituitary gland to release oxytocin, which stimulates milk release from the breast and signals the anterior lobe to release prolactin, which stimulates additional milk production.

consuming enough milk should consult a physician immediately because dehydration can develop rapidly.

It generally takes 2 to 3 weeks to fully establish the feeding routine: infant and mother both feel comfortable, the milk supply meets infant demand, and initial nipple soreness disappears. Establishing the breastfeeding routine requires patience, but the rewards are great. The adjustments are easier if supplemental formula feedings are not introduced until breastfeeding is well established, after at least 3 weeks, but preferably not until after 2 to 3 months. Then a supplemental bottle or two of infant formula per day is fine.

Parents need not be concerned that breastfed infants grow a bit more slowly after about 3 months of age than formula-fed infants, based on increases in body weight. The infant's physician is the best judge of whether the rate of growth of the breastfed infant is satisfactory. Essentially the difference is of no consequence.

NUTRITIONAL QUALITIES OF HUMAN MILK

Human milk is very different in composition from cow's milk. Unless altered, cow's milk should not be used in infant feeding until the infant is 12 months old. Many authorities support this recommendation against using cow's milk until the infant is at least 1 year old, as it is too high in minerals and protein, does not contain enough carbohydrate to meet infant needs, and may trigger development of diabetes in infants with a genetic predisposition to the disorder (see Chapter 17 for a further discussion of this link to diabetes). In addition, the major protein in cow's milk, casein (composed mainly of β-lactoglobulin), is harder for an infant to digest than lactalbumin, the major protein found in human milk.[34]

Colostrum

colostrum The first fluid secreted by the breast during late pregnancy and the first few days after birth. This thick fluid is rich in immune factors and protein.

The first fluid made by the human breast is **colostrum.** This thick, yellowish fluid may leak from the breast during late pregnancy and is produced in earnest for a few days to a week after birth. Colostrum contains antibodies and immune-system cells (e.g., lymphocytes), some of which pass unaltered through the immature GI tract of the infant into the bloodstream. These immune factors and cells protect the infant from some gastrointestinal diseases and other infectious disorders, compensating for its own immature immune system during the first few months of life.[34] Various growth factors and other compounds in breast milk also contribute to the health of the infant.[6] One likely reason breastfed infants have fewer respiratory and intestinal infections than formula-fed infants is the presence of these immune factors, growth factors, and other compounds in colostrum and in breast milk.

meconium The first thick mucuslike stool passed after birth.

Lactobacillus bifidus factor A protective factor secreted in the colostrum that encourages growth of beneficial bacteria in the newborn's intestines.

Colostrum facilitates the passage of **meconium,** a stool produced during fetal life. One component of colostrum, the *Lactobacillus bifidus* **factor,** encourages the growth of *Lactobacillus bifidus* bacteria. These bacteria limit the growth of potentially toxic bacteria, such as *Escherichia coli*, in the intestine. Overall, breastfeeding promotes the intestinal health of the breastfed infant in this way and in other ways.[34]

Mature Milk

The composition of human milk gradually changes until several days after delivery, resulting in mature milk. This process takes place more quickly in women who have previously delivered at least one infant. Human milk is thin, almost watery, in appearance and often has a slight bluish tinge; it looks quite different from cow's milk. Mature breast milk has impressive nutritional qualities and is nearly a complete food for infants. Let's consider several of its constituents.

Proteins. Lactalbumin, the main protein in milk, forms a soft, light curd in the infant's stomach, easing digestion. The lactoferrin proteins bind iron, reducing the growth of iron-requiring bacteria, many of which cause diarrhea. The immunoglobulin proteins (antibodies) offer important immune protection. Human milk protein is noted for its relatively low concentration of the amino acid phenylalanine, which the infant has a limited ability to metabolize. Human milk also has a high concentration of taurine; this amino acid derivative is needed for synthesis of bile salts, which aid lipid digestion and may participate in functioning of the eye and brain.

Chapter 4 reviews the functions and metabolism of fatty acids, including docosahexaenoic acid.

Lipids. The lipids in human breast milk are high in linoleic acid and cholesterol, which are needed for brain development. It also contains long-chain omega-3 fatty acids, such as docosahexaenoic acid (DHA). This unsaturated fatty acid is used for synthesis of tissues in the brain, the rest of the central nervous system, and the eye.[18] Some evidence indicates that breastfed infants show greater visual acuity and better neurological development than infants fed formulas, none of which currently contain DHA. Researchers are currently determining the potential benefits of adding DHA to infant formulas. The long-term safety of this addition is under study.[12] Eventually, manufacturers may produce formulas for preterm and full-term infants with a fatty-acid composition equivalent to that of human milk, just as they have done for the protein and mineral content.

The fat composition of human milk changes in the course of each feeding. When an infant begins to nurse, the initial milk (called *fore milk*) released from the breast resembles skim milk; this milk represents about 60% of the total volume consumed in a feeding. After a period of nursing, the milk released (called *hind milk*), representing about 35% of the total volume, has a higher fat content, similar to that of whole milk. The final milk secreted, which is usually released after 10 to 20 minutes of nursing, is essentially like cream; this high-fat milk constitutes only about 5% of the total.[34] Infants need to nurse long enough (i.e., total of 20 or more minutes) to get the energy in this fat-rich milk to be satisfied between feedings and to grow well.

Lactose. Nearly all of the carbohydrate in human milk is lactose, which creates an acidic environment in the intestine by stimulating the growth of acid-producing bacteria. It also provides galactose for nerve sheath synthesis.

Vitamin D. Human milk contains some vitamin D. Nonetheless, an infant vitamin D supplement is commonly advised because sufficient sunlight exposure may not be available to produce vitamin D to compensate for any gap.

Iron. Although human milk is low in iron, about 50% of it is absorbed, compared with 2% to 30% for typical foods. The infant needs another source of iron by the age of 4 to 6 months.[34] By that time, the infant's iron stores, formed in utero, are probably depleted. Some researchers recommend iron supplements by 1 to 2 weeks after birth for breastfed infants.

Water. An infant that is exclusively breastfed will be adequately hydrated. A common question is whether breastfed infants need additional water to prevent dehydration if they are stressed by diarrhea, vomiting, fever, or high ambient temperatures. Providing up to 4 ounces of water a day from a bottle during hot weather to young breastfed infants is fine but generally is not really necessary. Note that greater amounts of supplemental water can lead to brain disorders, low blood sodium, and other problems, as we discuss in Chapter 17. For this reason, supplemental water generally should be given only under a physician's guidance. Overall, breastfeeding should suffice to meet an infant's fluid needs.

A Food Plan for Breastfeeding Women

For the most part, the nutrient needs of breastfeeding mothers are similar to those of pregnant women. However, nursing women need less folate and iron but more vitamin A, vitamin C, niacin, and zinc than they did during pregnancy. The basic food plan recommended for pregnancy is also appropriate during breastfeeding except that an additional serving from the milk, yogurt, and cheese group should be included (Table 16-2). This modification is especially important for teenagers who are breastfeeding. The NIH consensus panel that recently recommended a daily calcium intake of 1500 mg for pregnant women has made the same recommendation for breastfeeding mothers. Although some calcium is taken from the mother's bones for milk production, this bone-calcium loss appears to be replaced once nursing ceases.[29] Some researchers recommend that nursing mothers eat fish about twice a week, since the omega-3 fatty acids present in fish appear in her milk and are important for brain development in the infant, as we covered earlier. However, that recommendation is made to all adults, but not for the same reason (see Chapter 4).

A reasonable approach for a breastfeeding woman is to eat a balanced diet that supplies at least 1800 kcal/day, has a moderate fat content, and includes a variety of dairy products, fruits, vegetables, and grains.[22] It is important for the woman to drink fluids every time the infant nurses, as drinking to quench thirst encourages ample milk production. If a woman restricts her energy intake too severely, the quantity of milk also decreases. This is not a time to crash diet. Research also shows that more than two alcoholic drinks a day decreases milk output, as does smoking.

Milk production requires approximately 800 kcal/day. A breastfeeding woman generally needs a daily energy intake about 500 kcal higher than she needs when not nursing. A mother who continues to breastfeed beyond 4 to 6 months or performs much physical activity requires a higher energy intake. On the other hand, this ex-

Breastfeeding mothers should get their physician's permission before embarking on an exercise program. Breastfeeding women must also take care to drink plenty of fluids before and after workouts and should avoid exercising when fatigued.

tra energy allowance may be overly generous if a woman has gained too much weight during pregnancy.

The difference between the energy need for milk production and the typical recommended additional intake (800 vs 500 kcal) should result in slow loss of the 3 to 5-plus pounds of fat accumulated during pregnancy. This shows how practical the link is between pregnancy and breastfeeding, as fat laid down in pregnancy is readily mobilized, especially if breastfeeding continues for 6 months or more. Weight loss of 1 to 4 pounds per month is appropriate.[7] Milk output decreases at significantly greater rates of weight loss, as occurs with severe dieting when energy intake is less than about 1500 kcal/day.

Most substances that a nursing mother ingests are secreted to some extent into her milk. For this reason, caffeine intake should be limited or avoided and all medication use should be approved by a pediatrician. Some mothers believe that certain foods, such as garlic and chocolate, flavor the breast milk and upset the infant. If a woman notices a connection between a food she eats and later fussiness in her infant, she could consider avoiding that food. However, she might experiment again with it later. Infants become fussy for many reasons, and the suspected ingredient may not be the cause.

Some researchers, on the other hand, feel that the passage of flavors from the mother's diet into her milk affords an opportunity for the infant to learn about the flavor of the foods of its family long before solids are introduced. The researchers wonder whether bottle-fed infants may be missing significant sensory experiences that until recent times in human history were common to all infants.[20]

CONCEPT CHECK

Growing awareness by women of the benefits of breastfeeding has contributed to a resurgence in its popularity in the last 20 years. Almost all women have the ability to breastfeed. The hormone prolactin stimulates synthesis of milk by the breast tissue. Some components of human milk come directly from the mother's bloodstream. Infant suckling triggers a let-down reflex that releases the milk. The more an infant nurses, the more milk is synthesized. The nutrient composition of human milk is very different from that of cow's milk. Colostrum, which is released from the breast until about a week after birth, is very rich in antibodies, immune-system cells, and other factors that provide immunity to the infant. The fat content of mature breast milk increases as the infant nurses; after 10 to 20 minutes of nursing at each breast, the milk released resembles cream, being rich in both fat and energy. Breastfeeding women should follow a food plan similar to that for pregnant women except that they usually need to increase energy intake somewhat, depending on their weight gain during pregnancy, length of time nursing, and degree of physical activity.

Pros and Cons of Breastfeeding

As noted already, the vast majority of women are capable of breastfeeding, and infants benefit from it. Nonetheless, a woman's decision to nurse depends on a variety of factors, some of which may make breastfeeding impractical or undesirable for a woman. Mothers not wanting to breastfeed their infants should not feel they must do so. There are distinct advantages to breastfeeding, but none so great that a woman who decides to bottle-feed should feel she is significantly penalizing her infant.

BENEFITS OF BREASTFEEDING

Human milk is exquisitely tailored to meet the nutrient needs of infants for the first 4 to 6 months of life, with the possible exceptions of fluoride, iron, and vitamin D. Although formula feeding can be satisfying for the infant, mother, and the rest of the family (see Chapter 17), there are many physiological and practical advantages to breastfeeding.

Fewer Infections

Breastfeeding reduces an infant's general risk for infections. As previously mentioned, the immune factors present in human milk are particularly important in protecting breastfed infants from respiratory and intestinal infections. Ear infections are also reduced because infants don't sleep with a bottle in the mouth, as bottle-fed infants often do. While an infant sleeps with a bottle in his mouth, milk pools in the mouth and backs into the **eustachian tubes** and then into the middle ear. This creates a growth media for bacteria. Infant ear infections are a common problem that parents want to avoid to decrease discomfort for the infant and trips to the doctor, as well as to prevent possible hearing loss.

eustachian tubes Thin tubes in the middle ear that open into the throat.

Fewer Allergies and Intolerances

Breastfeeding reduces the incidence of allergies, especially in allergy-prone infants. Cow's milk contains a number of potentially allergy-causing proteins that are absent in human milk. Breastfeeding also avoids the possibility of infant intolerance of formulas. Formulas sometimes must be switched several times until caregivers find one on which the infant thrives.

Convenience and Cost

Breastfeeding frees the mother from the effort and expense involved in buying and preparing formula and washing bottles. Human milk is already "prepared" and sterile; it requires no measuring or mixing. The nursing mother thus has more time to spend with her infant. Breastfeeding is also less expensive than formula feeding, even when the cost of the extra food needed by the mother is considered.

BARRIERS TO BREASTFEEDING

A lack of role models, widespread misinformation, fear of appearing immodest, and working at an outside job all serve as barriers to breastfeeding. So do hospital routines established for the convenience of employees—not mothers and infants. Pregnant women should try to choose a hospital that is accommodating to breastfeeding.

Misinformation and Lack of Role Models

Probably the major barriers to breastfeeding are misinformation, such as the idea that it is hard to master, and lack of role models. If a woman is interested in breastfeeding, we suggest that she talk to women who have done it successfully. Experienced mothers can be an enormous help to the first-time mother. She should find a friend she can call on to ask questions. In almost every community a group called La Leche League offers classes in breastfeeding and advises women who have questions or may be having problems with the process. One can check the white pages of the telephone book or ask the local health department for the telephone number. The WIC program can also offer support and information, as can lactation consultants in hospitals or private practices.

Working at an Outside Job

Working outside the home often complicates plans to breastfeed. After 1 or 2 months of breastfeeding, a mother can readily express milk either by breast pump or by hand into a sterile plastic bottle or nursing bag to use in a disposable bottle system. Expressed breast milk must be kept sterile and chilled rapidly. There is a knack to learning how to express milk, but the freedom can be worth it. Then others can feed the mother's milk to the infant. Breast milk frozen for later use should not be thawed by microwaving, which may destroy immune factors present and create hot spots that can scald the infant's tongue and esophagus.

Some women can juggle both a job and breastfeeding, but others find it too cumbersome and decide instead to formula feed. A combination is possible: some breastfeedings, say early in the morning and at night, with formula feedings during the day. However, too many supplemental feedings decrease milk production. A schedule of expressing milk and using supplemental formula feedings is most successful if not initiated until after 1 to 2 months of exclusive breastfeeding. After 2 months, the infant is well adapted to breastfeeding and probably feels enough emotional security and other benefits from nursing that he or she is willing to drink both ways.[34]

The key time for breastfeeding is the first 2 to 3 months of an infant's life. Even just the first few weeks is beneficial. A longer commitment than 2 to 3 months is better, but the first few months are most critical. During that time, human milk provides the antiinfective properties needed until the infant's own immune system becomes fully operational. A working woman may find an infant day-care center close enough to her workplace that she can visit a few times during the day for feeding. Some businesses have day-care facilities on the premises that enable women to return to work and still breastfeed their children.

Social Reticence

Another barrier for some women is embarrassment when nursing a child in public. Our society historically has stressed modesty and frowned on baring breasts in public—even for so good a cause as nourishing infants. With appropriate clothing, it is possible to nurse quite discreetly.

Medical Conditions Precluding Breastfeeding

Breastfeeding may be ruled out by certain medical conditions in either the infant or mother. For example, infants with the disease galactosemia can't break down galactose, the major sugar in breast milk. They do not grow well if nursed, as well as experience vomiting and diarrhea. Ultimately if left untreated the infants develop liver disease, cataracts, and mental retardation. A special infant formula free of galactose must be used. Breastfeeding also may be detrimental to infants with phenylketonuria; the high concentration of phenylalanine in breast milk may overwhelm the impaired ability of these infants to metabolize this amino acid, leading to production of toxic products.

A mother who takes certain medications that pass into the milk and adversely affect the nursing infant may be advised by her physician to avoid breastfeeding. In addition, a woman who has a serious chronic disease (e.g., tuberculosis, AIDS or HIV-positive status, or hepatitis) or who is being treated with chemotherapy medications should not breastfeed.

ENVIRONMENTAL CONTAMINANTS AND BREAST MILK

Some women wonder whether breastfeeding is safe. Their concern about the concentration of some environmental contaminants in human milk is legitimate. The benefits of breastfeeding, however, are very well established, and the risks from environmental contaminants in milk are still largely theoretical. Thus it is probably best to operate with what we know works until sufficiently strong research data dissuade us.

A breastfeeding mother can observe several practices that will help reduce her risk of exposure to contaminants: (1) avoid freshwater fish from polluted waters; (2) carefully wash and peel fruits and vegetables; and (3) remove the fatty edges of meat, fish, and poultry. In addition, a woman should not try to lose weight rapidly while nursing, because contaminants stored in fat tissue will enter the bloodstream and ultimately the milk. If a woman questions whether her milk is safe, especially if she has lived in an area known to have a high concentration of toxic wastes or environmental pollution, she should ask her local health department for advice.

BREASTFEEDING OF PRETERM INFANTS

Feeding of preterm infants presents various difficulties. Bottle feeding of a preterm newborn typically requires a birthweight of about 1500 g (3.5 pounds) and a gestational age of 32 to 34 weeks. When human milk is the preferred form of nourishment, it must be expressed from the breast and usually fed through a tube. This type of feeding demands great dedication on the part of the mother. Fortification of the human milk with nutrients, such as calcium, phosphorus, sodium, and protein, may be needed to support the infant's rapid growth.[34] In some cases, special feeding problems may prevent use of human milk or necessitate some supplementation with infant formula. And sometimes total parenteral nutrition is the only option. Working as a team, the pediatrician, neonatal nurse, and registered dietitian guide the parents toward the most appropriate approach to feeding their preterm infant.

CONCEPT CHECK

Human milk supplies most of an infant's nutritional needs for the first 6 months, although supplementation with vitamin D, iron, and fluoride may be needed. Breastfeeding is less expensive and often more convenient than formula feeding. Compared with formula-fed infants, breastfed infants have fewer intestinal, respiratory, and ear infections and are less susceptible to allergies and food intolerances. Despite the advantages of breastfeeding, lack of role models, misinformation, and social reticence may dissuade a mother from breastfeeding. A combination of breastfeeding and formula feeding may be possible when a mother is regularly away from the infant. Breastfeeding is not desirable if a mother has certain diseases or must take medication potentially harmful to the infant. The preterm infant, depending on its condition, may benefit from consuming human milk.

Summary

1. Adequate nutrition is vital during pregnancy to ensure the well-being of both the infant and the mother. Poor maternal nutrition and use of some medications, especially during the first trimester, can cause birth defects. Growth retardation and altered development can also occur if these insults happen later in pregnancy.

2. Infants born preterm (before 37 weeks of gestation) or with low birthweight (<2.5 kg, or 5.5 pounds) usually have more medical problems at and following birth than normal infants.

3. A woman typically needs an additional 300 kcal/day during the second and third trimesters of pregnancy to meet her energy needs. Weight gain should occur slowly, reaching a total of 25 to 35 pounds in a normal-weight woman.

4. Protein, vitamin, and mineral needs increase during pregnancy. Extra servings from the milk, yogurt, and cheese group and the meat, poultry, fish, dry beans, eggs, and nuts group of the Food Guide Pyramid are recommended. Supplements of iron, in particular, may be needed. Folate nutriture should be adequate at the time of conception.

5. Pregnant teenagers require very careful prenatal and nutritional care. Complications of pregnancy are more common in teenagers than in more mature women be-

cause of their very high physiological demands and often compromised social and economic support.

6. Pregnancy-induced hypertension, gestational diabetes, heartburn, constipation, nausea, vomiting, edema, and anemia are all possible discomforts and complications of pregnancy. Nutrition therapy can often help minimize these problems.

7. Almost all women have the ability to nurse their infants. The nutrient composition of human milk is very different from unaltered cow's milk and much more desirable. Colostrum, the first fluid produced by the human breast, is very rich in immune factors. Mature milk is rich in the protein lactalbumin and in lactose.

8. Advantages of breastfeeding over formula feeding for the infant include fewer intestinal, respiratory, and ear infections and fewer allergies and food intolerances. Breastfeeding is also less expensive and may be more convenient for the mother than formula feeding. An infant can be adequately nourished with infant formula if the mother chooses not to breastfeed. Breastfeeding is not desirable if the mother has certain diseases or must take medication potentially harmful to the infant. Likewise, breastfeeding is not advised for infants with certain medical conditions, including some preterm infants.

Study Questions

1. What historical evidence established the importance of nutrition in pregnancy outcome?
2. Provide three key pieces of advice for a couple who are seeking to maximize their chances of having a healthy infant. Why did you single out those specific factors?
3. Outline current weight-gain recommendations during pregnancy. What is the basis for these recommendations?
4. How is the Food Guide Pyramid adapted to meet increased nutrient needs of pregnancy?
5. Why does teenage pregnancy receive so much attention these days? At what age do you think pregnancy would be ideal? Why?
6. Give three reasons why a woman should give serious consideration to breast-feeding her infant.
7. Describe the physiological mechanisms that stimulate milk production and release. How can knowing about these help mothers to nurse successfully?
8. What guidelines can a woman use to determine whether her breastfed infant is receiving sufficient nourishment?
9. How should the basic food plan suitable for pregnancy be modified during lactation?

REFERENCES

1. ADA Reports: Position of the American Dietetic Association: Promotion and support of breastfeeding, *Journal of the American Dietetic Association* 93:467, 1993.
2. ADA Reports: Position of the American Dietetic Association: Nutrition care for pregnant adolescents, *Journal of the American Dietetic Association* 94:449, 1994.
3. American College of Obstetricians and Gynecologists: ACOG issues recommendations on exercise during pregnancy and the postpartum period, *American Family Physician* 49:1258, 1994.
4. Buescher PA and others: Prenatal WIC participation can reduce low birth weight and newborn medical costs, *Journal of the American Dietetic Association* 93:163, 1993.
5. Centers for Disease Control: Infant mortality—United States, 1992, *Journal of the American Medical Association* 273:101, 1995.
6. Donovan SM, Odle J: Growth factors in milk as mediators of infant development, *Annual Review of Nutrition* 14:147, 1994.
7. Dusdieker LB and others: Is milk production impaired by dieting during lactation? *American Journal of Clinical Nutrition* 59:833, 1994.
8. Fadigan AB and others: Preeclampsia: progress and puzzle, *American Family Physician* 49:849, 1994.
9. Fagen C and others: Nutrition management in women with gestational diabetes, *Journal of the American Dietetic Association* 95:460, 1995.
10. Goldenberg RL and others: The effect of zinc supplementation on pregnancy outcome, *Journal of the American Medical Association* 274:463, 1995.
11. Hueston WJ and others: Common questions patients ask during pregnancy, *American Family Physician* 51:1465, 1995.
12. ISSFAL Board Statement: Recommendations for the essential fatty acid requirement for infant formulas, *Journal of the American College of Nutrition* 14:213, 1995.
13. King JC and others: Energy metabolism during pregnancy: influence of maternal energy status, *American Journal of Clinical Nutrition* 59:439S, 1994.
14. Kousen M: Treatment of nausea and vomiting in pregnancy, *American Family Physician* 48:1279, 1993.
15. Lewis DD, Woods SE: Fetal alcohol syndrome, *American Family Physician* 50:1025, 1994.
16. Lie RT and others: A population-based study of the risk of recurrence of birth defects, *New England Journal of Medicine* 331:1, 1994.
17. Lops VR and others: Anemia in pregnancy, *American Family Physician* 51:1189, 1995.
18. Makrides M and others: Fatty acid composition of brain, retina, and erythrocytes in breast- and formula-fed infants, *American Journal of Clinical Nutrition* 60:189, 1994.
19. McGanity WJ and others: Embryonic development, pregnancy, and lactation. In Shils ME and others, editors: *Modern nutrition in health and disease*, ed 8, Philadelphia, 1994, Lea & Febiger.
20. Mennella JA, Beauchamp GK: Early flavor experiences: when do they start, *Nutrition Today* 29:25, 1994.
21. National Academy of Sciences–Institute of Medicine: *Nutrition during pregnancy*, Washington, DC, 1990, National Academy of Sciences Press.
22. National Academy of Sciences–Institute of Medicine: *Nutrition during lactation*, Washington, DC, 1991, National Academy of Sciences Press.
23. Nehlig A, Debry G: Consequences on the newborn of chronic maternal consumption of coffee during gestation and lactation: a review, *Journal of the American College of Nutrition* 13:6, 1994.
24. Olson CM: Promoting positive nutritional practices during pregnancy and lactation, *American Journal of Clinical Nutrition* 59:525S, 1994.
25. Prentice A: Maternal calcium requirements during pregnancy and lactation, *American Journal of Clinical Nutrition* 59:477S, 1994.
26. Rawlings JS and others: Prevalence of low birthweight and preterm delivery in relation to the interval between pregnancies among white and black women, *New England Journal of Medicine* 332:69, 1995.
27. Rush D: Periconceptional folate and neural tube defect, *American Journal of Clinical Nutrition* 59:511S, 1994.
28. Scholl TO, Hediger ML: Anemia and iron-deficiency anemia: compilation of data on pregnancy outcome, *American Journal of Clinical Nutrition* 59:492S, 1994.
29. Sowers MF and others: Changes in bone density with lactation, *Journal of the American Medical Association* 269:3130, 1993.
30. Specker BL: Do North American women need supplemental vitamin D during pregnancy or lactation? *American Journal of Clinical Nutrition* 59:484S, 1994.
31. Susser M, Stein Z: Timing in prenatal nutrition: a reprise of the Dutch Famine Study, *Nutrition Reviews* 52:84, 1994.
32. US Public Health Service: Reducing teenage pregnancy increases life options for youth, *Prevention Report*, April/May 1994.
33. Wilcox A and others: Birth weight and perinatal mortality, *Journal of the American Medical Association* 273:709, 1995.
34. Worthington-Roberts B and others: *Nutrition in pregnancy and lactation*, St Louis, 1993, Mosby.

TAKE ACTION

Targeting nutrients necessary for pregnant women

In this chapter we mentioned that pregnant women may have difficulty meeting their increased needs for folate, vitamin D, iron, calcium, and zinc. List five foods rich in each of these nutrients next to the appropriate heading below. Refer to Chapters 12 to 15 if necessary.

NUTRIENT	FOODS	NUTRIENT	FOODS
Folate	_____	Calcium	_____
	_____		_____
	_____		_____
	_____		_____
	_____		_____
Vitamin D	_____	Zinc	_____
	_____		_____
	_____		_____
	_____		_____
	_____		_____
Iron	_____		
	_____		
	_____		
	_____		
	_____		

1. Foods rich in more than one of these nutrients would be especially valuable for pregnant women. Write on the line below any foods you listed above that are good sources of more than one of these clinical nutrients.

   _____

2. The RDAs for folate, vitamin D, iron, calcium, and zinc all increase considerably during pregnancy. For which of these nutrients can pregnant women usually obtain adequate intakes from dietary sources?

   _____

   Which of these nutrients are commonly taken in supplement form during pregnancy? Why might it be hard for pregnant women to meet their increased needs for these nutrients from foods alone?

   _____

   _____

3. Now design a diet you would like to follow that meets prenatal nutrient recommendations. Use the foods you selected in the above exercise to plan these meals. Try to show it to a pregnant woman. What insights have you gained?

   BREAKFAST: _____

   LUNCH: _____

   SNACK: _____

   DINNER: _____

   SNACK: _____

Fetal Alcohol Syndrome

Although much is known about diagnosing and treating some learning problems in children, many causes remain elusive. One particular question haunts many mothers: Did something happen while I was pregnant that created a learning disability in my child? This question leads directly to the topic of alcohol use during pregnancy, since alcohol is the most common damaging substance fetuses are exposed to.

Conclusive evidence shows that large amounts of alcohol harm the fetus, especially when associated with binge drinking ($\geq$ 5 drinks at one sitting). Binge drinking is especially perilous during the first 12 weeks of pregnancy as critical early development events take place in utero. Scientists don't know if pregnant women must eliminate alcohol use entirely to avoid risk of damage to the fetus. But until a safe level can be established, women are advised not to drink any alcohol during pregnancy or when there is a chance pregnancy might occur.[15]

When a pregnant woman drinks more alcohol than she can metabolize, the excess reaches the embryo (and at later stages the fetus), which has no means of detoxifying it. Women with chronic alcoholism produce children with a recognizable pattern of malformations called **fetal alcohol syndrome (FAS).** A diagnosis of FAS is based mainly on poor fetal and infant growth, physical deformities (especially of facial features), and mental retardation (Figure 16-12). The infant is frequently irritable and may develop hyperactivity and a short attention span. Limited hand-eye coordination is common. Defects in sight, hearing, and mental processing often then develop over time.[11]

The range of abnormalities from alcohol exposure varies from the severe effects associated with FAS to reduced birthweight, behavioral effects, growth retardation, and hampered learning ability in infants born to women who report only social drinking. The latter condition, termed *fetal alcohol effects (FAE)*, is not marked by telltale facial abnormalities. For this reason, parents may not suspect the presence of subtle defects caused by alcohol, even when they exist. FAE can devastate learning potential.

An estimated 6.7 per 10,000 infants born each year exhibit FAS; the incidence of FAS also has increased since the late 1970s. Many more infants are born annually with FAE. Alcohol use is in fact the leading cause of preventable birth defects and mental retardation in the United States and in the Western World as a whole.[15]

fetal alcohol syndrome (FAS) A group of physical and mental abnormalities in the infant that result from the mother's consuming alcohol during pregnancy.

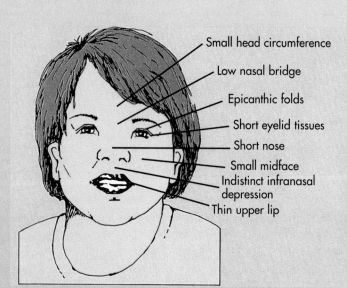

Small head circumference

Low nasal bridge

Epicanthic folds

Short eyelid tissues

Short nose

Small midface

Indistinct infranasal depression

Thin upper lip

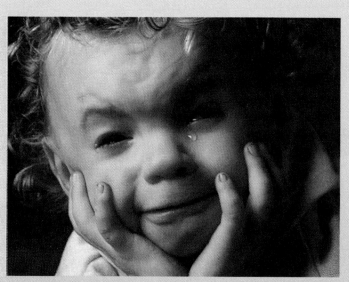

Figure 16-12 Fetal alcohol syndrome. Milder forms of alcohol-induced changes in the fetus and the infant are known as *fetal alcohol effects*. The facial features shown are typical of affected children. Additional abnormalities in the brain and other internal organs accompany fetal alcohol syndrome, but are not obvious from simply looking at the child.

Exactly how alcohol causes these defects is not known. One line of research suggests that alcohol, or acetaldehyde produced by metabolism of alcohol, causes faulty migration of cells in the brain during early stages of embryonic development. In addition, most likely inadequate nutrient intake, reduced nutrient and oxygen transfer across the placenta, altered eicosanoid metabolism, the cigarette smoking commonly linked to alcohol intake, drug use, and possibly other factors also contribute to the overall result. Furthermore, we do not know how much alcohol it takes to produce the effects. Again, for this reason many authorities—including the U.S. Surgeon General and the American Medical Association—believe it is best that mothers-to-be avoid alcohol altogether.

Abstinence is especially important during the first trimester, when key growth and development occur in utero. Alcohol reaches the fetal blood at the same concentration as the mother's blood within 15 minutes of her drinking. However, the effect on the fetus may be up to 10 times greater. For example, just one bout of binge drinking can arrest and alter cell division during critical phases of fetal development. The fetus then may develop an irreversible defect.

Physical damage to the embryo (and later the fetus) results more from first-trimester drinking because the basic structures of tissues and organs develop during this period. Emotional and learning problems stem more from third-trimester drinking because this is when critical further development of the brain occurs. And throughout the pregnancy alcohol interferes with growth in utero. Overall, mothers who drink at least one to two drinks a day throughout pregnancy are much more likely to have growth-retarded infants, and mothers who drink only in late pregnancy are more likely to give birth to preterm infants.[15]

Because alcohol has the capacity to adversely affect each stage of fetal development, the earlier in pregnancy that drinking ceases, the greater the potential for improved outcome. The best course is to consider alcohol an indulgence that must be eliminated from the time of conception until after pregnancy. One step in the right direction is the new congressionally mandated warnings about drinking during pregnancy that appear on all alcoholic beverage containers.

Pregnancy lasts only 9 months. In contrast, parents may spend a lifetime caring, often at great expense, for their offspring needlessly handicapped by FAS or FAE.

Pregnant women should recognize that many cough syrups contain alcohol. Cases have been reported of infants with FAS born to mothers who consumed generous amounts of such cough syrups but no other alcoholic beverages.[34]

CHAPTER SEVENTEEN

Infants, Children, and Teenagers

A s humans grow through their early years into adulthood, their needs for energy and nutrients change. Infants require concentrated sources of nutrients and energy to support their tremendous rate of growth and development.[26] As growth rate slows, children need to eat proportionately less. Childhood is a key time to establish healthy habits, including those related to food choice and physical activity.[23] Older family members make most decisions for children. Thus education designed to change the eating habits and overall health behavior of children must be directed simultaneously at the main caregivers, as they usually determine which foods are purchased and how these foods are prepared.

Later, teenagers sprout quickly during another growth spurt, amazing their elders with the sheer amount of food they can consume. Often their eating habits and lifestyles encourage eating on the run. Their typical hit-and-miss meal patterns challenge all meal planning that aims to meet their extra growth and nutrient needs.[26] In exploring these stages of life, we will look at the key roles various nutrients play and we will see how food habits can be tailored to meet those needs.

NUTRITION AWARENESS INVENTORY

1. T F Consuming a low-protein diet in childhood can greatly affect ultimate adult height.
2. T F An infant's length increases by 50% in the first year.
3. T F Brain growth is greatest during the teenage years.
4. T F Most obese infants become obese adults.
5. T F Infants have lower energy needs per pound than older children.
6. T F An infant's diet should be very low in fat.
7. T F Infants need solid food by 2 months of age.
8. T F Infants enjoy blander foods than do adults.
9. T F Atherosclerosis has been noted in children who have died in accidents.
10. T F Cow's milk fed during early infancy can increase risk for allergies later in life.
11. T F Iron-deficiency anemia often occurs in infants whose diets are composed mainly of cow's milk.
12. T F It is nutritionally important to put children on a schedule of three meals per day.
13. T F The two most common nutritional problems in childhood are obesity and iron-deficiency anemia.
14. T F Parents should carefully control the amount of food their children eat.
15. T F Acne can be avoided by limiting certain foods in the diet.

Human Growth and Physiological Development

During infancy a child's attitudes toward foods and the whole eating process begin to take shape. If parents and other caregivers practice good food habits and are flexible, they can lead a child into lifelong beneficial food habits.[29] Such an infant has a good chance of starting life with the nutrients needed to support brain and body growth spurts and of developing a willingness to try new foods. However, these physical and psychological advantages alone do not guarantee that a child will thrive.

Children additionally need specific attention focused on them; they need to grow in a stimulating environment, and they need a sense of security. Children hospitalized for growth failure gain weight more quickly when loving care accompanies needed nutrients.

For convenience, we often use the term *parents* in this chapter to refer generally to those who are raising children, including adults who are not a child's biological parents as well as single parents.

THE GROWING INFANT

It seems that all infants do is eat and sleep. There is a good reason for this. An infant's birthweight generally doubles within the first 4 to 6 months of life and triples within the first year. An infant typically increases in length by 50% during the first year. Such rapid growth requires both nourishment and sleep in abundance. Infants need concentrated sources of nutrients and energy to support their tremendous growth and development.[26]

During the first year of life, body water decreases from about the 75% of body weight typical of newborns to 60%, which is characteristic of adults. Also by 1 year of age an infant's body nitrogen content (and thus, protein content) has increased from 2% of body weight at birth to 3%, indicating that the infant has synthesized much new lean tissue.

THE GROWING CHILD AND ADOLESCENT

Beyond the first year, growth of the child is slower; it takes about 5 more years for the weight at 1 year to double. The child also continues to gain height continually

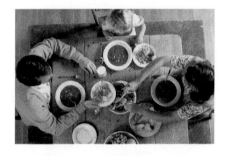

Parents and other caregivers can teach children lifelong beneficial food habits.

from the preschool through the teenage years. The rate of growth is not constant throughout these years; rather, spurts of growth, especially at adolescence, alternate with plateaus. Most girls begin the adolescent growth spurt between the ages of 10 and 13 years, whereas most boys begin it somewhat later, between the ages of 12 and 15 years. Nearly every organ in the body grows during this period of faster growth, which lasts about 3 years (Figure 17-1). Most noticeable are increases in height and weight and development of secondary sexual characteristics. Height gain is essentially complete by age 19, though increases of several inches may occur in the early 20s. Head size in proportion to total height shrinks from one fourth to one eighth during the climb from infancy to adulthood.[26]

The human body needs much more food to support growth and development than to merely maintain itself once growth ceases. When nutrients are missing at critical phases of growth and development, growth throughout the body slows and may even stop. Observations of Egyptian mummies have revealed that infants were about the same size in 300 BC as they are today, but adults were much smaller than adults today. Also, the suits of armor found in museum collections of the Middle Ages are too small to fit most modern adults. Such observations indicate that people living in these earlier periods generally ate nutrient-deficient diets that in turn were unable to support the growth we typically experience today.

In Third World countries today, about half the children are short and underweight for their ages. Inadequate nutrient intake—what we have called undernutrition—is at the heart of the problem. This condition occurs to a lesser extent in the United States, but nevertheless cannot be ignored, as about 14 million children here live in poverty (see Chapter 20). Undernourished children are simply smaller versions of nutritionally fit children. In poorer countries, after breastfeeding ceases, children are often fed a high-carbohydrate, low-protein diet. This diet supports some growth but does not allow children to attain their full genetic potential. To grow, children must consume adequate amounts of energy, protein, zinc, and other nutrients.[26]

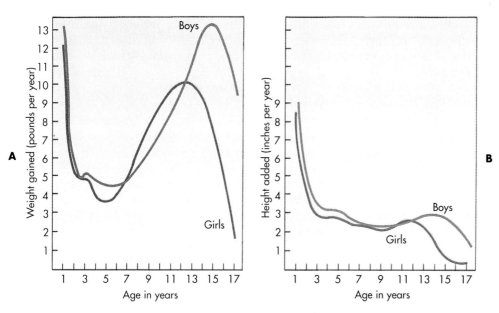

Figure 17-1 Growth rates. **A,** Average gains in weight for girls and boys. **B,** Average additions to height for girls and boys. The higher the line in any one year, the greater the amount of annual gain compared with that in other years. Large gains in weight occur in both infancy and puberty, whereas the very high length gain in infancy never is reached again. If graphs such as these were plotted in smaller time segments, they would appear as zig-zag lines, rather than smooth lines, reflecting short, periodic spurts in growth in the course of each year.

EFFECT OF UNDERNUTRITION ON GROWTH PROCESSES

In Chapter 16 we described growth as occurring first by cell division, or hyperplasia, followed by increase in the size of individual cells, or hypertrophy. The last stages of growth include both hypertrophy and hyperplasia, the relative mix depending on the organ system. For example, the liver exhibits much hyperplasia throughout life, whereas the muscles do not.

As with the fetus **in utero,** the long-term effects of nutritional problems in infancy and childhood depend on the severity, timing, and duration of the nutritional insult to cell processes. Probably the single best indicator of a child's nutritional status is growth. For instance, stunted growth in some children in the United States has been linked to mild zinc deficiencies. Improving the diets of these children, especially their zinc intakes, leads to improved growth. In clinical practice, the nutrient intake of infants who are not growing properly should be carefully assessed, as inadequate diet is a possible cause of poor growth in infants.[15]

Consuming an inadequate diet as an infant or child hampers the cellular hyperplasia that normally occurs during critical growth stages. Consuming an adequate diet later usually won't compensate for lost cellular hyperplasia because the high concentrations of hormones that trigger this process are then missing from the bloodstream. These hormones are present during the critical time when cells should be dividing, but their concentration in the bloodstream then falls. In addition, growth ceases in girls and boys when the skeleton reaches it final size. Growth plates at the ends of the bones, called **epiphyses,** fuse at different ages, beginning around 14 years of age in girls and 15 years of age in boys. Final stages of this process end at about 19 years of age in girls and 20 years of age in boys. Ultimate fusion prevents further linear bone growth. The failure of the skeleton to show catch-up growth after early bouts of undernutrition is another important reason why total growth of the body is hampered.[2] For example, muscles can increase in diameter later in life but can grow no longer than the bones that they are attached to allow.

For these reasons a 15-year-old Central American girl who is 4 feet 8 inches tall will never attain the adult height of a typical American woman even if she begins to eat better as a teenager. Girls experience their peak rate of growth before the onset of menstruation. Once the adolescent growth spurt ceases (in women this is about 2 years after they start menstruation), an adequate nutrient intake will help maintain health and lead to increased weight in part by allowing normal cellular hypertrophy. But growth lost because of inadequate cell hyperplasia generally cannot be reclaimed.

ASSESSING GROWTH AND DEVELOPMENT

Health professionals assess an infant's or child's increases in height and weight by comparing these measures with typical growth patterns recorded on charts. The typical charts contain seven percentile divisions, representing 90% of children (Figure 17-2).[2] A percentile simply represents the rank of the person among 100 peers matched for age and gender. Tony, for example, is at the ninetieth percentile height for age, meaning that of 100 boys of that age, he is shorter than 10 and taller than 89. A child at the fiftieth percentile is considered average. Fifty children will be taller than this child; 49 will be shorter.

Individual growth charts are available for both males and females, with ages ranging from 0 to 36 months (length, weight, and head circumference) and 2 to 18 years (height and weight). Length (height)-for-age, weight-for-age, and weight-for-length (height) can be plotted. Infants and children should have their growth assessed during regular health checkups. It takes 1 to 3 years for an infant to establish his or her own genetic percentile. Once this figure is established, such as length (height)-for-age, the child's measurement should then track along that percentile. If the child's growth does not keep up with his or her length (height)-for-age percentile, a physician needs to investigate whether a medical or nutritional problem is impeding the predicted growth.[15] Inappropriate weight gain—too little or too much—should also be investigated.

---

in utero "In the uterus"; in other words, during pregnancy.

epiphyses Ends of long bones. The epiphyseal plate—sometimes referred to as the *growth plate*—is made of cartilage and allows growth of bone to occur. During childhood the cartilage cells multiply and absorb calcium to develop into bone.

- - - - - - - - - - - -

Weight primarily reflects current nutrient intake. Height is a measure of long-term nutrient intake.

- - - - - - - - - - - -

- - - - - - - - - - - -

Because children under 2 to 3 years of age are measured while lying on their backs with their knees unflexed, the term *length* is used rather than *height*.

- - - - - - - - - - - -

BOYS: BIRTH TO 36 MONTHS
PHYSICAL GROWTH

NAME_____ RECORD #_____

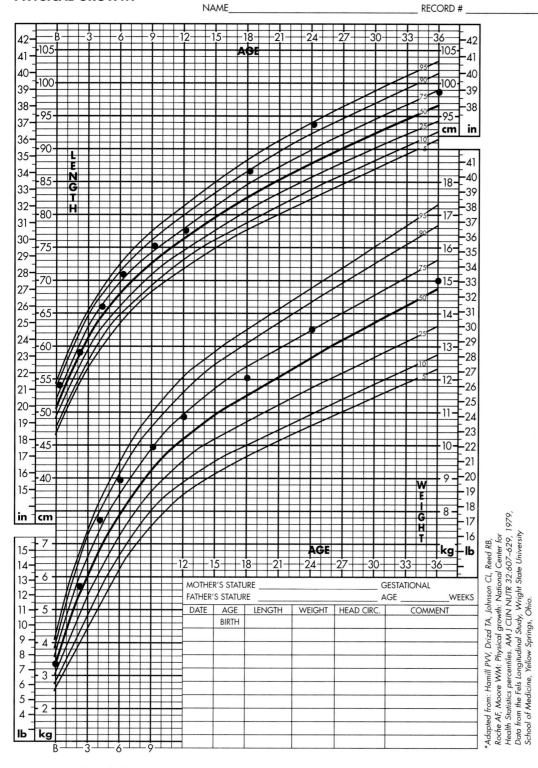

Adapted from: Hamill PVV, Drizd TA, Johnson CL, Reed RB, Roche AF, Moore WM: Physical growth: National Center for Health Statistics percentiles. AM J CLIN NUTR 32:607–629, 1979, Data from the Fels Longitudinal Study, Wright State University School of Medicine, Yellow Springs, Ohio.

Figure 17-2 Growth charts used to assess length (height) and weight in young boys. A certain weight and length (height) correspond to a percentile value, which is a ranking of the person among 100 peers. The growth pattern of Dr. Wardlaw's son is plotted to illustrate how this tool is used in clinical practice.

Infants born preterm may catch up in growth in 2 to 3 years. This requires that the child jump up in the percentiles. If this movement to higher percentiles occurs—especially in length (height)-for-age—it is usually no cause for alarm. On the other hand, jumping percentiles in weight-for-length (height) can be disturbing if the child approaches the 85th percentile. Generally a child at the 85th percentile for weight-for-length (height) is considered overweight. Above the 95th percentile, the child is considered obese.[26]

BRAIN GROWTH

The brain grows faster around the time of birth than at any other time of life. To accommodate this brain growth, an infant's head must be very large in proportion to the rest of the body. The rapid growth stops about 18 months of age, by which time the brain has reached more than 70% of its adult weight. The rest of the body eventually grows and ends up in a typical proportion to head-size. In early physical check-ups, a health professional usually measures the head circumference as another means of assessing growth, especially brain growth.[26] By age 10 many children have the brain weight of an adult.

The effect of nutrition on brain development and intelligence quotient (IQ) is difficult to determine because there is no easy way to separate the effects of nature from those of nurture. However, studies from Central America suggest that the amount of schooling a child receives is also important in ultimate IQ development.

ADIPOSE TISSUE GROWTH

Since 1970, researchers have speculated that overfeeding during infancy may increase the number of adipose (fat) cells. Today, we know that adipose cells can also increase in number as adulthood obesity develops (see Chapter 8). Restricting energy intake during infancy to limit adipose cell hyperplasia, however, may retard the growth of other organ systems, particularly the brain and nervous system. Thus restricting an infant's diet, especially fat intake, before 2 years of age is not recommended. Moreover, most obese infants become normal-weight preschoolers without excessive diet restriction. About 40% of energy intake from fat is recommended for infants. Without this fat intake, along with adequate intakes of other nutrients, infants are unlikely to attain their potential adult height.[26]

FAILURE TO THRIVE

Occasionally an infant does not grow much in the first few months, or growth begins to taper off. The diagnosis of failure to thrive can be defined as a deceleration of growth velocity in which at least two major percentile lines are crossed.[15] In the short term, a child with failure to thrive will drop in weight percentile before dropping in length and head circumference. Although the exact incidence of failure to thrive is not known, this problem is identified in 1% to 5% of children under 2 years of age who are admitted to a hospital.

Various physical problems may contribute to retarded growth in an infant: deficient development of the oral cavity, infections, heart irregularities, and persistent diarrhea associated with intestinal problems. However, more than half the infants who fail to thrive have no apparent disease. In these cases the main problem is poor infant-parent interaction, usually stemming from misinformation, no parent role model, or apathy about the child's welfare. In the absence of specific disease, failure to thrive often results from the parents' inexperience with infant care, rather than intentional negligence.[15]

Not only do infants need cuddling, they also respond to voices and eye contact, especially at feeding times. New parents need to appreciate the importance of these practices to their infant's well-being. Some parents also may be overcommitted to maintaining a lean infant in hopes of preventing future obesity, as we discussed in Chapter 11. The result, even though the intention was well-meaning, can be failure to thrive.

When clinicians encounter an infant who is failing to thrive, they must first determine whether the child is consuming enough energy. For infants, approximately 45 kcal/pound (95 kcal/kg) of body weight daily is adequate in early infancy. By 6 months of age, closer to 40 kcal/pound (85 kcal/kg) is recommended.[26] The clinician should make sure a breastfed infant is consuming sufficient milk; that is, the infant should be nursing about six to eight times a day for about 20 minutes a session and have six to eight wet diapers each day. The food and fluid intake of a breastfeeding mother should also be reviewed to make sure it supports sufficient milk production (see Chapter 16).

Failure to thrive is found primarily in infants, as food intake is limited to what caregivers provide. Because they are not wholly dependent on caregivers for food, children older than 2 years are less likely to experience this condition than infants.

CONCEPT CHECK

Growth occurs rapidly during infancy: birth weight doubles in about 4 to 6 months and triples within the first year. Lean tissue increases and the percentage of body water falls during the first year. Undernutrition in childhood can irreversibly inhibit growth and maturation so that an individual never attains his or her full genetic potential. Infant and child growth is assessed by tracking body weight, length (height), and head circumference over time. It is not desirable for infants to become obese, although no evidence strongly indicates that obese infants become obese adults. However, severe restriction of energy intake is not recommended for infants because it may slow growth of organ systems. When an infant does not grow properly, his or her failure to thrive may stem from physical disorders or inadequate care, including inappropriate feeding practices.

NUTRITIONAL NEEDS DURING INFANCY

Newborns receive needed nutrients by breastfeeding or formula feeding. Solid foods are usually not needed until after 4 to 6 months. Even after solid foods are added to the diet, human milk or formula form the basis of an infant's diet until about 1 year of age.[26] Because of the critical importance of adequate nutrition in infancy and the difficulties encountered in feeding some infants, we spend more time on this developmental period than on the later periods of childhood.

The nutrient needs of infants differ from those of adults in both amount and relative proportion (Figure 17-3). For example, infants require about 20% to 25% of the total energy and protein intakes of adults, whereas their needs for several vitamins and minerals are considerably higher relative to adults. Indeed, the RDA for vitamin D for infants exceeds that of adults 25 years or older. Then, as children get older, their nutrient needs generally increase even further.

Energy

As mentioned above, infants need about 40 to 45 kcal/pound (85 to 95 kcal/kg) of body weight daily to supply them with adequate energy. At 6 months of age this amounts to about 700 kcal daily for infants weighing about 16 pounds (7 kg).[26] Infants need an easy way to consume this amount of energy. The composition of either human milk or formula is ideal for meeting infants' energy needs during the first few months (Table 17-1). Both are high in fat and supply about 650 kcal/quart (700 kcal/L). After this initial period, the use of solid food along with human milk or formula can provide the additional energy needed as the infant gets older.[26]

The energy needs of infants are primarily driven by their rapid growth and high metabolic rate. The high metabolic rate is caused in part by their high ratio of body surface area to weight. More body surface allows more heat loss from the skin; the body must use extra energy to replace that heat.

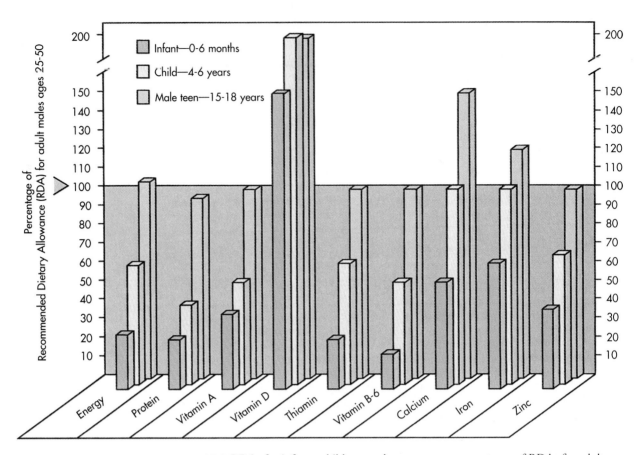

Figure 17-3 RDAs for infants, children, and teenagers as percentages of RDAs for adult males. Compared with adults, infants' relative energy needs are lower than are their needs for other nutrients, as illustrated by the different heights of the green bars. Thus infants need to obtain relatively larger amounts of nutrients from a smaller intake of food than do adults. This is also true of young children (yellow bars), but to a lesser extent.

Protein

The daily protein needs of infants range from 0.7 to 1 g/pound (1.6 to 2.2 g/kg) of body weight. Over 40% of total protein intake should come from essential amino acids. Both goals are satisfied by either human milk or formula.[26] Total protein intake should not exceed 20% of energy needs because the excess nitrogen and minerals supplied by high-protein diets would exceed the ability of an infant's kidneys to excrete the resulting metabolic waste products.

In the United States, protein deficiency in infants is unlikely, except when an infant's formula is diluted excessively with water or some other mistake in feeding practices occurs. Protein deficiency may also be induced by elimination diets used to detect food allergies. As foods are eliminated from the diet, infants may not be offered enough protein to compensate for the high-protein sources no longer present (see the Nutrition Perspective on food allergies and intolerances).[2]

Fat

Infants and children up to the age of 2 years should consume about 40% of their energy intake from fat. Current fat intakes in this age grouping range from 34% to 37% of energy intake.[19] More than 50% of energy intake from fat may lead to poor fat digestion. About half the energy supplied by both human milk and formula comes from fat. Essential fatty acids should make up at least 3% of total energy intake. Fat is an important part of the infant's diet because it is energy dense and vital to the development of the nervous system. As a concentrated energy source, fat helps resolve the potential problem of the infant's high energy needs and small

TABLE 17-1

Composition of human and cow's milk and infant formulas

Milk or formula	Energy (kcal/L)	Protein (g/L)	Fat (g/L)	Carbohydrate (g/L)	Minerals* (g/L)
Milk					
Human milk	750	11	45	70	2
Cow's milk, whole	670	36	36	49	7
Cow's milk, skim	360	36	1	51	7
Casein/whey-based formulas					
Similac	680	14	36	71	3
Enfamil	670	15	37	69	3
SMA	670	15	36	72	3
Carnation	670	16	34	73	3
Soybean protein–based formulas					
ProSobee	670	20	35	67	4
Isomil	680	16	36	68	4
Nursoy	670	18	36	69	4
Predigested protein					
Nutramigen	670	19	26	89	1
Alimentum	680	18	37	68	1
Transition formulas/beverages†					
Similac Toddler's Best	670	25	33	75	3
Enfamil Next Step	670	17	33	74	3
Carnation Follow-Up	670	17	27	88	3

*Calcium, phosphorus, and other minerals.
†For use after 6 months of age or later (see label).

stomach capacity. This is not an age to greatly restrict fat (nor cholesterol) intake (Figure 17-4).

Vitamins of Special Interest

Vitamin K is routinely provided by injection to all infants at birth. This dose lasts until the infant's intestinal bacteria are established and begin to synthesize vitamin K. Formula-fed infants receive the rest of the vitamins they need from the formula. Breastfed infants, especially dark-skinned ones, may require a vitamin D supplement if they are not exposed to much sunlight. (Sunlight exposure on human skin activates synthesis of vitamin D; see Chapter 12.) Breastfed infants whose mothers are total vegetarians (vegans) should receive a vitamin B-12 supplement. Infants who drink goat's milk, a practice that is not recommended, need a dietary supplement of folate because this milk doesn't supply a sufficient amount of this essential nutrient.

Minerals of Special Interest

The iron stores present in newborns generally are depleted by the time birthweight doubles, in 4 to 6 months. The American Academy of Pediatrics recommends that, to maintain a good iron status, formula-fed infants be given an iron-fortified formula from birth. Breastfed infants need solid foods, such as iron-fortified infant cereal, to supply extra iron at about 6 months of age. The need for iron is a major consideration in deciding when to introduce solid foods.[24] Some researchers recommend liquid iron supplements from birth or by 1 month of age for breastfed infants.

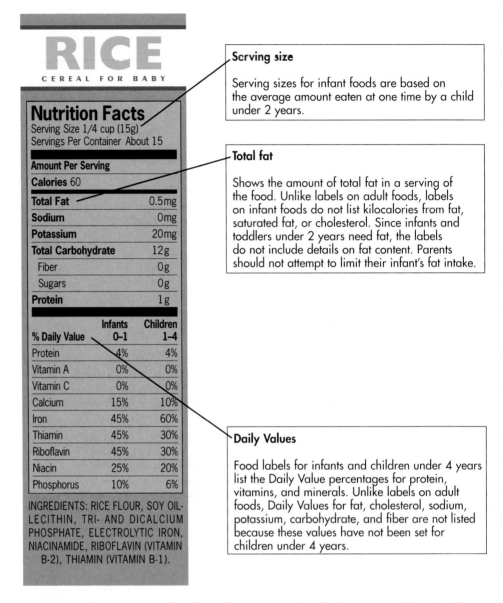

Serving size

Serving sizes for infant foods are based on the average amount eaten at one time by a child under 2 years.

Total fat

Shows the amount of total fat in a serving of the food. Unlike labels on adult foods, labels on infant foods do not list kilocalories from fat, saturated fat, or cholesterol. Since infants and toddlers under 2 years need fat, the labels do not include details on fat content. Parents should not attempt to limit their infant's fat intake.

Daily Values

Food labels for infants and children under 4 years list the Daily Value percentages for protein, vitamins, and minerals. Unlike labels on adult foods, Daily Values for fat, cholesterol, sodium, potassium, carbohydrate, and fiber are not listed because these values have not been set for children under 4 years.

Figure 17-4 The labels on infant foods, like those on adult foods, contain a Nutrition Facts panel. However, the information provided on infant food labels differs from that on adult food labels (see Figure 2-8 for a comparison).

Infants need adequate amounts of iodide and zinc to support growth. Human milk and formula adequately supply these needs when the infant's energy needs are met. In addition, some clinicians recommend fluoride supplements to aid tooth development for bottle-fed infants after six months of age if the water supply in the home does not contain fluoride.[14] Note that formula manufacturers use fluoride-free water in formula preparation. Parents should consult their dentist and/or pediatrician for advice on the need for fluoride for the infant.

Water

An infant needs about 2 ounces of water and other fluids combined per pound of body weight (about 125 to 150 ml/kg), which is equivalent to about 1.5 ml/kcal expended.[26] Infants typically consume enough human milk or formula to supply this amount. In hot climates, however, infants may need supplemental water. And any conditions that lead to water loss—diarrhea, vomiting, fever, and too much sun—often call for supplemental water.

Infants are easily dehydrated, a condition that has serious effects if not remedied. Dehydration can result in rapidly decreasing kidney function, and the infant may then require hospitalization for rehydration. Special electrolyte replacement solutions are available to treat dehydration. A physician needs to guide any use of these products.[20]

Too much supplemental water can be hazardous to infants. For example, it can lead to a low blood sodium concentration, which may be harmful to the brain and have other detrimental effects.[6] In some grocery stores, bottled water products marketed specifically for infants may be placed alongside infant formulas and electrolyte replacement solutions. This placement may give parents and caregivers the mistaken impression that bottled water products are an appropriate feeding supplement or substitute for infants; they are not and should not be used for such purposes. Generally, supplemental fluid should be limited to no more than about 4 ounces daily unless an infant's physician advises a greater intake because of disease or other conditions. Overall, extremes in fluid intake from water or formula—either too little or too much—can lead to health problems.

CONCEPT CHECK

Most nutrient needs in the first 6 months are met by human milk or formula. Breastfed infants may need vitamin D, fluoride, and iron supplements, and formula-fed infants may need fluoride supplements. Infants usually receive enough water from the human milk or formula they drink.

FORMULA FEEDING OF INFANTS

We discussed breastfeeding in detail in Chapter 16, including the immunological protection and other health benefits it provides. Let's now focus on formula feeding. The high standards of water purity and cleanliness in most American communities make formula feeding a safe and acceptable practice for most infants.

Composition of Formulas

Cow's milk must be altered for use as an infant food because of its high protein and mineral content and the nature of its fat, which is not easily digested by young infants (Table 17-1). Commercially altered forms of cow's milk, known as infant formulas, first became available in this country in 1931. Since 1980 infant formula manufacturers have been required to conform to strict guidelines for nutrient composition and quality set by federal law. Generally, infant formulas contain lactose and/or sucrose to meet carbohydrate needs, heat-treated **casein** and **whey** proteins from cow's milk to meet protein needs, and vegetable oils to meet fat needs.[26]

Today's formulas are much improved over earlier versions because the new heat-treated casein is easier to digest than the previously used natural forms of casein. Whey proteins are naturally easy to digest, so many formulas are supplemented with extra whey protein to bring the casein-to-whey ratio closer to that found in human milk.

Formulas contain vitamins and minerals in amounts suggested by the guidelines of the American Academy of Pediatrics. We recommend an iron-fortified formula. Parents should check the label on the formula container carefully, as not all formulas are iron fortified. Research shows that added iron does not lead to intestinal complaints, such as constipation, any more than nonfortified formulas do, though some people believe this misconception.

We mentioned in Chapter 16 that human milk is a rich source of an important omega-3 polyunsaturated acid called docosahexaenoic acid (DHA). DHA is used in the synthesis of tissues in the brain and the rest of the central nervous system, as well as in the eye in humans. Currently DHA is not added to formulas. Some can be

casein Proteins found in milk that form curds when exposed to acid and are difficult for infants to digest.

whey Proteins, such as lactalbumin, that are found in great amounts in human milk and are easy to digest.

made from the alpha-linolenic acid that may be present in formula, but it is not known whether this suffices to meet infant needs, particularly beyond 3 months of age. In the future, formula manufacturers may duplicate the lipid profile of human milk, thereby supplying this important polyunsaturated fatty acid to infants.[1]

Soy protein–based formulas are available for infants who can't tolerate (1) lactose (either sucrose or glucose polymers are substituted) or (2) the proteins found in cow's milk. If the soybean-based formula is not tolerated, the next step is to try using a predigested (hydrolyzed) protein formula, such as Nutramigen or Alimentum. A variety of other specialized formulas have been developed to meet the needs of preterm infants, infants with **allergies,** infants with higher energy needs, and infants with certain metabolic problems, such as phenylketonuria and galactosemia.[26]

A variety of new transition formulas/beverages for older infants and toddlers have recently been introduced (Table 17-1). Some of these products are intended for use after 6 months of age if the infant is consuming solid foods, while others are intended for use only with toddlers. These transition products are lower in fat than human milk or standard formulas; their iron content is higher than that of cow's milk, and their overall mineral content is generally more like human milk than cow's milk. According to the manufacturers, the advantages of these transition formulas/beverages over standard formulas for older infants and toddlers include reduced cost and better flavor. Parents should consult their pediatrician with regard to use of these products, which to date have seen little use.

Note that health-food stores often sell formula-type products that can lead unsuspecting parents into thinking they are providing their infants with a complete nutritional formula. Soy Moo, for example, a soy beverage sold in health-food stores, should not be confused with soy-based infant formulas. Unlike nutritionally complete infant formulas, this product and others like it lack some essential nutrients and can lead to severe nutritional deficiencies in infants. For example, a severely undernourished 5-month-old infant was admitted to Arkansas Children's Hospital in Little Rock with symptoms of heart failure, rickets, inflamed blood vessels, and possible nerve damage. The infant girl had been fed nothing but Soy Moo since she was 3 days old. Because of cases such as this one, parents should consult their physician for advice in choosing an appropriate infant formula.[26]

Preparation of Formula

In the 1950s, it was common to prepare a day's supply of bottles and then sterilize them in boiling water for about 30 minutes. Today, bottles are often prepared one at a time. Some infant formulas even come in a ready-to-feed form. These simply are poured into a clean bottle and fed immediately. Room-temperature formula is acceptable to many infants. Otherwise, to warm a bottle of formula, running hot water over it or placing it in a pan of simmering water briefly works. Note that infant formulas should not be heated in a microwave oven because hot spots may develop that can burn the infant's mouth and esophagus.

Powdered and concentrated fluid formula preparations are more commonly used than ready-to-feed varieties. All utensils used in preparing formula from these preparations should be washed and thoroughly rinsed. Powdered or concentrated formulas are poured into a bottle to which clean, cold water is added (following label directions) and then mixed. The formula is then warmed, if desired, and fed immediately to the infant. Hot water from the faucet should not be used to make formula, since it poses a risk for high lead content (see Chapter 19).

A convenient practice when using powdered formula is to measure out the correct amount of dry formula into a series of bottles to have on hand. When a bottle is needed, cold or warmed water is added and mixed; the formula is then ready for immediate use. Likewise, a whole can of concentrated formula (13 ounces of formula plus 13 ounces of water) can be made up and stored in the refrigerator in a clean, covered jar or pitcher. When feeding time comes, a caregiver need only fill a bottle with the diluted formula.

allergy A hypersensitive immune response that is triggered by foreign proteins (allergens) and is associated with various adverse effects on the body.

It is safe to refrigerate diluted formula for one day. However, formula left over from a feeding should be discarded because it will be contaminated by bacteria and enzymes in the infant's saliva. If well water is used, it should be boiled before making formula for at least the infant's first 3 months of life, and should also be analyzed for excessive concentration of naturally occurring nitrates, which can lead to a severe form of anemia.[26]

Feeding Technique

Because infants swallow a lot of air along with either formula or human milk, it is important to burp an infant after either 10 minutes of feeding or 1 to 2 ounces (30 to 60 ml) from a bottle, and again at the end of feeding. Spitting up a bit of milk is normal at this time. Once fed, the infant should be placed on her side, with a rolled-up blanket placed behind her back to support that position. In this position the infant has the least chance of choking on any milk it spits up. Infants should not be placed on their stomachs, as this sleeping position has been linked to the occurrence of sudden infant death syndrome.[2]

When the infant begins acting full, bottle feeding should be stopped, even if some milk is left in the bottle. Common cues that signal an infant has had enough include turning the head away, inattention, falling asleep, and becoming playful (Figure 17-5). Generally, the infant's appetite is a better guide than standardized recommendations concerning feeding amounts. As noted in the last chapter, breast-feeding infants usually have had enough to eat after about 20 minutes. Although it's difficult to tell how much milk breastfed infants are getting, they also give signs when full. By carefully observing bottle-feeding or nursing infants and responding to their cues appropriately, caregivers not only can be assured that the infants' energy needs are being met but also can develop a climate of trust and responsiveness.

SOLID FOODS

The time to introduce solid foods into an infant's diet hinges on four main factors: physical readiness and willingness to participate in the feeding process; nutritional need; physiological readiness; and decreased risk of allergies to proteins. Based on these criteria, the American Academy of Pediatrics recommends that solid foods not be introduced before 4 to 6 months of age. By this age most infants are ready to expand their culinary horizons and the body can safely handle solid foods. In general, a child starting solid foods should be drinking more than 32 ounces (1 L) of formula daily or breastfeeding more than 8 to 10 times within 24 hours. Most 6-month-old infants, and some 4-month-old infants, consume this much.

Factors Influencing When to Introduce Solid Foods

To understand why solid foods are not appropriate for very young infants, let's look more closely at those factors that determine the best time to introduce solid foods.[11]

Physical Ability and Feeding Skills Take Time to Develop. Three physical markers initially indicate that an infant is ready for solid foods: (1) the disappearance of the extrusion reflex (thrusting the tongue forward and pushing food out); (2) head and neck control; and (3) the ability to sit up with support. These usually occur around 4 to 6 months of age but vary with each infant.[26]

By 6 to 7 months, more specific skills begin to surface. Most infants have learned to grab and transfer objects from one hand to the other and thus can start to actively participate in feeding themselves (Table 17-2). They begin to handle finger foods with some dexterity, and the first teeth also generally appear at this age. Strips of dry toast offer hours of contented enjoyment and help soothe teething pain.

Nutritional Need Hinges on Iron Needs. Infant iron stores are exhausted by about 6 months of age. Breastfeeding infants and those fed formulas not supplemented with iron then need either solid foods or iron supplements to meet their iron needs.[24] Overall, addition of solid foods is most important for satisfying iron needs; before 4 to 6 months, solid food is not required to meet any other nutrient needs.

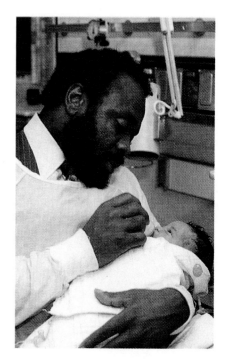

Figure 17-5 Careful attention during feeding allows the infant to signal the caregiver when the feeding should cease.

CRITICAL THINKING

Tatiana has been breastfeeding her baby since he was born 7 months ago. When she and her husband took the baby for his check-up, they were told that he was anemic. They were very surprised, since they thought that human milk contained all the nutrients the baby needed for the first year of life. How can you explain the baby's anemia?

TABLE 17-2

Typical progression of infant eating skills and solid-food introduction*

Age	Feeding skills	Oral motor skills	Types of food	Suggested activities
Birth- 4 months		Rooting reflex Sucking reflex Swallowing reflex Extrusion reflex	Breast milk Infant formula	Breastfeed or bottle-feed
5 months	Able to grasp objects voluntarily Learning to reach mouth with hands	Disappearance of extrusion reflex		Possible introduction of thinned cereal if baby not satisfied by breastfeeding or bottle-feeding
6 months	Sits with balance while using hands	Transfers food from front of tongue to back	Infant cereal Strained fruit Strained vegetables Egg yolk (if no family history of egg allergy)	Prepare cereal with formula or breastmilk to a semiliquid texture Use spoon Feed from a dish Advance to 1/3-1/2 cup cereal before adding fruits or vegetables
7 months	Improved grasp Can transfer objects from hand to hand	Mashes food with lateral movements of jaw Learns side-to-side or "rotary" chewing Tooth eruption	Infant cereal Strained to junior texture of fruits, vegetables, and meats	Thicken cereal to lumpier texture Sit in highchair with feet supported Introduce cup
8-10 months	Holds bottle without help Drinks from cup Decreases fluid intake and increases solids Coordinates hand-to-mouth movement		Juices (small amounts) Soft, mashed, or minced table foods	Begin finger foods like toast or crackers Do not add salt, sugar, or fats to food Present soft foods in chunks ready for finger-feeding
10-12 months	Feeds self Holds cup without help	Improved ability to bite and chew	Soft, chopped table foods Whole egg and whole milk (at 1 year of age)	Provide meals in pattern similar to rest of family Use cup at meals

From Queen P, Lang C: *Handbook of pediatric nutrition*, Rockville, Md, 1993, Aspen.
*This timeline is just an estimate, and individual infants may vary by several months from the ages given. A pediatrician should be consulted if caregivers are concerned about an infant's developmental progress. In general, there is no nutritional reason to begin introduction of solid foods before 4 to 6 months of age.

Physiological Capabilities Take Time to Develop. Before 3 months of age, infants can't readily digest starch, the primary storage carbohydrate in plant foods. As infants age, their bodies develop starch-digesting capabilities. Kidney function likewise is quite limited until about 4 to 6 weeks of age. Until then, waste products from high amounts of dietary protein or minerals are difficult to excrete.[26]

Reduced Risk of Allergic Reactions to Food Proteins Is an Important Consideration. An infant's intestinal tract readily absorbs whole proteins from birth until 4 to 5 months of age. Absorption of intact proteins during this period—especially proteins in cow's milk and egg whites—may predispose a child to future food allergies.[2] For this reason it is best to minimize the number of different types of proteins in infant diets, especially during the first 3 months of life. As the intestinal tract develops, dietary protein is broken down in the stomach and small intestine into small peptides and amino acids, which do not cause allergic reactions.

Researchers also suspect that early introduction of cow's milk into an infant's diet may set up an allergic-type reaction that increases the risk of insulin-dependent diabetes in infants generally susceptible to the disease.[31] Studies with laboratory animals suggest that proteins in cow's milk may trigger an immune-system attack against the pancreas, which is a key step in development of insulin-dependent diabetes. Because the proteins in infant formula are heat-treated and thus denatured, they don't pose the same risk of inducing an allergic reaction. Definitive research is still needed to clarify the possible link between early use of cow's milk and future allergy problems.[34] Nonetheless, the American Academy of Pediatrics advises against the use of any cow's milk during the first year of life, in part to reduce the risk of allergies and other health problems.

Why Feed Solid Foods Early in Life?

Many children are already eating solids by 2 months of age, even though only occasionally does a rapidly growing infant—one who consumes more than 32 ounces (1 liter) of formula daily—need solid foods before 4 months to meet nutrient needs. A common reason offered for introducing solid foods early, before 4 to 6 months of age, is that it helps the infant sleep through the night. However, many studies show that sleeping through the night is a developmental milestone for infants. It has nothing to do with how much food they eat before being put down for the night. Infants naturally begin sleeping through the night between the ages of 1 and 3 months. Girls reach this stage before boys. Filling them with cereal is not going to influence that process.

In addition, young infants have difficulty consuming much solid food. Attempts to push down solid foods have sometimes led to force-feeding with a feeder (a giant syringe) or to mixing infant cereal with milk and putting it in a bottle. Even if these are traditional practices in a family, there is no reason to continue them. The inconvenience alone should make one consider whether all the effort is worth it. Such early feeding of solid foods is unnecessary nutritionally, tedious, and possibly dangerous for infants because it increases the risk of allergies and choking or inhaling food when crying.[26]

How to Start Feeding Solid Foods

Before 6 months of age, the first solid foods should be iron-fortified cereals. Rice cereal is the best cereal to begin with because it is least likely to cause allergies. The cereal is mixed with expressed human milk or formula to a pastelike consistency. Early spoon feeding proceeds more easily if solid food is offered after a short period of nursing or formula feeding, which will partially satisfy the infant's hunger.

If solid foods aren't introduced until 6 months or later, selection of the initial food to feed is less critical. Some pediatricians suggest lean ground (strained) meats because they contain highly absorbable forms of iron. Although yogurt and cottage cheese are also well tolerated and their consistencies make them good candidates for early foods, note that they are not good sources of iron.

It is best to start with teaspoon amounts of pure solid foods—not mixtures—and increase the serving size gradually. Once a new food has been fed for 7 to 10 days without ill effects, another food can be added to the infant's diet.[2] Some experts feel 3 to 4 days is long enough to wait. The longer interval between starting new foods is primarily recommended for allergy-prone families, to ensure that the infant is not allergic to a new food. The next food added can be another type of cereal or perhaps a cooked and strained (blended) vegetable, meat, fruit, or egg yolk. Each feeding step builds on the last (Table 17-2).

Following introduction of a new food, it can take 7 to 10 days for signs of an allergy or intolerance to develop. Symptoms to look for are diarrhea, vomiting, skin rash, facial swelling, runny nose, or wheezing. If one or more of these symptoms appear, the suspected problem food should not be fed for several weeks and then reintroduced in a small quantity. If the problem continues, a physician should be consulted.[12]

Foods that commonly cause an allergic response in infants include egg whites, chocolate, nuts, and cow's milk. Use of mixed foods should be avoided until each component in a mixture has been introduced separately. Otherwise, if an allergy or

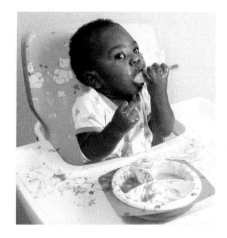

Early feeding attempts should be encouraged, even though they're messy.

intolerance develops, it will be difficult to identify the offending food. Fortunately, infants that exhibit sensitivity to one or more foods often outgrow them by late childhood (see the Nutrition Perspective.)[2]

A variety of strained foods is available for infant feeding. Check this out next time you are in a supermarket. Single-food items are more desirable than mixed dinners and desserts, which are less nutrient-dense. Most brands have no added salt, but some fruit desserts contain a lot of added sugar. It is best to introduce infants to a variety of foods so that by the end of the first year they are consuming many types of foods—dairy products, meats, fruits, vegetables, and grains.

As an alternative to commercial infant foods, plain foods from the table—vegetables, fruits, and meats—can be ground up in an inexpensive plastic baby food grinder/mill. Another option is to puree a larger amount of food in a blender, freeze it in ice-cube portions, store in plastic bags, and defrost and warm as needed. Careful attention to cleanliness is necessary. Infant foods made at home should be prepared before seasonings are added to please the taste of other family members. Infants do not notice the difference if salt, sugar, or spices are omitted.

During initial attempts to feed solid foods to infants, just getting the food into the mouth rather than all over the body proves to be a challenge. Caregivers must proceed slowly. For a period of time, solid foods should supplement—rather than replace—formula or human milk. It's best to let infants control the feeding situation, signaling when they are hungry and when they've had enough to eat. Self-feeding skills require coordination and can develop only if infants are allowed to practice and experiment. By age 7 to 8 months, infants should be able to push food around on a plate and begin to manipulate a drinking cup. Holding a bottle and self-feeding a cracker or piece of toast are also possible. Mastering these techniques helps infants develop self-confidence and self-esteem. Parents need to be patient and support these early feeding attempts, even though they appear inefficient and messy, as food is also used as a means to explore the environment. At around 10 months of age, infants earnestly practice self-feeding finger foods and drinking from a cup.[26]

To ease efforts in feeding solid foods, the following tips are helpful:

• Use an infant-sized spoon; a small spoon with a long handle is best.
• Hold the infant comfortably on the lap, as for breastfeeding or bottle-feeding, but in a little more upright position to ease swallowing. In this position, the infant expects food.
• Put a small dab of food on the spoon tip and gently place it on the infant's tongue.
• Convey a calm and casual approach to the infant. The infant needs time to get used to food.
• Expect the infant to take only two or three bites of the first meals.

By 8 months or so, juices and formula should be offered in a cup (Table 17-2). A heavy cup with a wide, flat bottom aids success. Drinking from a cup helps prevent nursing-bottle syndrome. This condition develops when an infant plays with a bottle for extended periods, allowing the carbohydrate-rich fluid to bathe the teeth. This fluid encourages growth of bacteria, which then produce acids that dissolve tooth structure. For this reason, an infant should never be put to bed with a bottle or placed in an infant seat with a bottle propped up. Both of these practices are likely to result in pooling of fluid in the mouth, increasing the likelihood of dental caries and ear infections (see Chapter 16 for the reason for the latter).

Getting an infant out of the bedtime-bottle habit is often difficult. But determined caregivers can either wince through a few nights of crying or can slowly wean the infant away from the bottle with either a pacifier or water (for a week or so).

By the end of the first year, most infants can eat with their fingers fairly efficiently, their ability to drink from a cup steadily improves, and the appearance of additional teeth makes chewing easier. These infants are usually crawling, and many are walking and self-feeding as well. While their attempts at eating by themselves are still erratic, such young children take great pride in doing more things independently. Fewer bottle feedings and/or breast feedings are necessary as drinking from

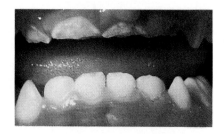

An extreme example of tooth decay caused by nursing-bottle syndrome. This child was probably often put to bed with a bottle. The upper teeth have decayed almost all the way to the gum line.

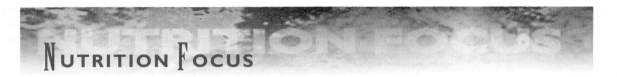

DIETARY GUIDELINES FOR INFANT FEEDING

In response to various controversies surrounding infant feeding, the American Academy of Pediatrics has issued a number of statements concerning infant diets. The following guidelines are based on these statements:

- **Build to a variety of foods.**
  For the first months of life, human milk is all an infant needs. When the infant is ready, start adding new foods one at a time. During the first year, the goal is to teach an infant to enjoy a variety of nutritious foods. A lifetime of healthy eating habits begins with this important first step.

- **Pay attention to your infant's appetite to avoid overfeeding or underfeeding.**
  Feed infants when hungry. Never force an infant to finish an unwanted serving of food. Watch for signs that indicate hunger or fullness.

- **Infants need fat.**
  While fat is the cause of many adult health problems, it is quite necessary for an infant. Fat is an excellent source of energy essential for growing infants. Fat also helps the brain and nervous system develop.

- **Choose fruits, vegetables, and grains, but avoid high-fiber foods.**
  Although many adults benefit from high-fiber diets, they are not good for infants. They are bulky, filling,

and often low in energy. The natural amounts of fiber and nutrients in fruits, vegetables, and grains are appropriate as part of a healthy infant diet.

- **Infants need sugars in moderation.**
  Sugars are an additional source of energy for active, rapidly growing infants. Foods such as human milk, fruits, and juices are natural sources of sugars and other nutrients as well. Foods that contain artificial sweeteners should be avoided; they do not contain the energy growing infants need.

- **Infants need sodium in moderation.**
  Sodium is a necessary mineral found naturally in almost all foods. As part of a healthy diet, infants need sodium for their bodies to work properly.

- **Choose foods containing iron, zinc, and calcium.**
  Infants need good sources of iron, zinc, and calcium for best growth in the first 2 years. These minerals are important for healthy blood, proper growth, and strong bones.

The recommendations in this chapter are consistent with these guidelines. In essence, there is no evidence that very restrictive diets during infancy have positive effects, although their hazards are well documented.

---

a cup becomes more frequent. The added mobility of walking should naturally lead to gradual weaning from the bottle or breast.[26]

Foods and Practices to Avoid during Infancy

For various reasons, several foods and feeding practices should be avoided in the initial stages after an infant starts eating solid foods. These include the following[26]:

- *Honey and corn syrup:* These products may contain spores of *Clostridium botulinum*. In the stomach these spores can develop into bacteria that cause the foodborne illness known as botulism. This disease is often fatal in children under 1 year of age (see Chapter 19).
- *Very salty and very sweet foods:* Since young children enjoy bland foods much more than adults do, there is no reason to load their food with salt and sugar.
- *Excessive amounts of formula or human milk:* After 6 to 8 months of age, solid foods should play the major role in satisfying the increasing appetite of infants; by this age they should not consume more than 40 ounces (1.2 L) of formula daily. The high proportion of solid foods is important because they are good

sources of iron, whereas human milk and low-iron formulas don't supply enough of this nutrient.[24] About 24 to 32 ounces (¾ to 1 L) of human milk or formula daily is preferable after 6 months of age, with solid foods supplying the rest of the nutritional needs.

- *Foods that cause choking:* Young children have a tendency to choke on certain foods. The worst offenders are hot dogs (unless finely cut into sticks, not coin shapes), grapes, meat chunks, raw carrots, peanuts, popcorn, and peanut butter. Caregivers should discourage young children from gobbling snack foods during playtime and should supervise their eating during all meals.

- *Cow's milk, especially low-fat and nonfat milk:* Cow's milk has a low iron content and contains many allergenic proteins, as we mentioned earlier. Both low-fat and nonfat cow's milk also contain large amounts of minerals relative to their energy content. For this reason, consumption of enough of these products to meet a major portion of the energy needs of young children could overwhelm the kidneys' ability to excrete the excess minerals. The low amount of fat supplied also might harm development of the nervous system. Recall that the American Academy of Pediatrics advises that children younger than 1 year not consume cow's milk. The group also advises that children under 2 years avoid low-fat and nonfat milk. After 2 years, children consume enough solid foods to meet their energy and fat needs and thus can drink 1% or 2% milk without danger of mineral excess.

- *Excessive amounts of apple or pear juice:* Because these juices contain the simple carbohydrates fructose and sorbitol, which are absorbed slowly, they can cause diarrhea when consumed in excessive amounts. Infants usually can safely consume 4 to 8 ounces of juice in the course of a day, with no more than 2 to 4 ounces given at a time. Diluting juices with an equal part water is a good idea. This reduces the fructose and sorbitol concentrations but needs to be started before an infant becomes accustomed to full-strength juices.

• • •

For a recap, infant feeding recommendations discussed so far include:

Breastfed Infants
- Breastfeed for 6 months or longer if possible. Then introduce infant formula if and when breastfeeding declines or ceases in infancy.
- Add iron-fortified cereal at about 6 months of age.
- Investigate the need for fluoride, iron, and vitamin D supplements.
- Provide a variety of basic, soft foods after 6 months of age, advancing to a varied diet (Table 17-3).

Formula-Fed Infants
- Use infant formula for the first year of life, preferably an iron-fortified type.
- Add iron-fortified cereal at about 6 months of age.
- Investigate the need for a fluoride supplement if water supply is not fluoridated.
- Provide a variety of basic, soft foods after 6 months, advancing to a varied diet (Table 17-3).

> **We noted earlier that egg whites also should not be fed to children before 1 year of age to help prevent the development of allergies.**

Concept Check

Infant formulas generally contain lactose or sucrose, heat-treated proteins from cow's milk, and vegetable oil. Formulas may or may not be fortified with iron. Sanitation is very important in preparing and storing formula. Solid food should not be added to an infant's diet until the child is both ready for and needs solid food, usually at about 4 to 6 months of age. The first solid food given can be iron-fortified infant cereal, with very gradual additions of other foods—one new food every week or so. Some foods to avoid in the first year include honey, cow's milk (particularly low-fat and nonfat milk), egg whites, very salty or sweet foods, and foods that may cause a child to choke.

TABLE 17-3

Sample daily menu for a 1-year-old child*

Breakfast

1-2 tbsp applesauce
¼ cup cheerios
½ cup whole milk

Snack

½ hard-cooked egg
½ slice wheat toast with ½ tsp margarine
½ cup orange juice

Lunch

1 oz roasted chicken
1-2 tbsp rice with ½ tsp margarine
1-2 tbsp cooked peas
½ cup whole milk

Snack

½ oz cheese
4 wheat crackers
½ cup whole milk

Dinner

1 oz hamburger (crumbled)
1-2 tbsp mashed potatoes with ½ tsp margarine
1-2 tbsp cooked carrots (cut in strips, NOT coins)
½ cup whole milk

Snack

½ banana
2 oatmeal cookies (no raisins)
½ cup whole milk

Nutrition analysis

Total energy (kcal)	1100
% energy from:	
Carbohydrate	40%
Protein	19%
Fat	41%

*This diet plan is just a start. A 1-year-old may need more or less food. In those cases, serving sizes should be adjusted. The milk can be fed by cup; some can be put into a bottle if the child has not been fully weaned from the bottle. The juice should be fed in a cup.

HEALTH PROBLEMS RELATED TO INFANT NUTRITION

Parents, other caregivers, and clinicians should be alert for a variety of potential health problems related to infant nutrition so corrective action can be taken quickly. In some cases, such problems stem from inappropriate feeding practices or inadequate nutrient intakes, including the following[26]:

- Diet providing insufficient iron
- Absence from the diet of an entire food group of the Food Guide Pyramid as solid foods are introduced and become the main source of nutrients
- Drinking raw (unpasteurized) cow's or goat's milk, which may be contaminated with bacteria or viruses
- Drinking goat's milk, which is low in folate
- Failure to begin drinking from a cup by 1 year of age

- Continuing to feed from a bottle past 18 months of age
- Intake of supplemental vitamins or minerals above 150% of the appropriate RDA
- Drinking much fruit juice before 6 months of age as a substitute for formula or human milk

Now let's look more closely at four common infant health problems that cause concern for caregivers. Parents and other caregivers usually need to consult with a physician in dealing with these conditions.

Colic

The first time an otherwise healthy, well-fed infant has a lengthy, unexplained crying spell, most parents panic. Crying episodes lasting 3 or more hours and unresponsive to typical remedies—such as feeding, holding, or diaper changes—are characteristic of infants who develop **colic.** Colic affects about 10% to 30% of all infants, so it is neither uncommon nor abnormal. Colicky infants typically cry during the late afternoon and early evening, and their nighttime sleeping is almost always disturbed by crying spells. The only good news is that colic usually goes away after a few months.[5]

Colic generally occurs in the absence of any physical abnormality in the affected infant. It tends to be most common in "temperamental" infants—those who are more sensitive, more irritable, more intense, less adaptable, and less soothable than average for their age. In addition, a lack of harmonious interaction between parents and their infant may contribute to the problem. Some researchers have speculated that immaturity of the central nervous system mechanisms in infants may be responsible for colic.

Parents state that colicky infants frequently pass gas rectally, clench their fists, draw up their legs, cry in the late afternoon and evening, hold the body straight, and want to be held. Parents can do several things to help reduce excessive crying. For instance, many infants tend to become quiet and alert when held snugly to the shoulder. Others can be settled down with movement, such as walking or rocking in an infant seat. For others, rhythmic sounds and pacifiers can be of some help.[5]

Breastfeeding of colicky infants should continue. A temporary decrease or cessation in consumption of dairy products by a breastfeeding mother may help reduce colic in her infant. Formula-fed infants with severe colic are sometimes helped by changing from a standard casein/whey–based formula to a soy-based or predigested protein formula (Table 17-1). In addition, physicians may prescribe certain medications to calm colicky infants and reduce gas build-up.

Caring for an inconsolable, colicky infant is stressful and frustrating for parents. Most parents benefit from the counsel and support of other adults during this trying period, which may last for several months. Sharing with others who have been through similar experiences can help parents improve their tolerance of stress and ability to cope, and increase confidence in their parenting abilities. Furthermore, to optimize their ability to be sensitive and responsive to their infant, parents need to be well rested and to have some time for themselves.[5]

Diarrhea

Diarrhea in infants results from various causes, including bacterial and viral infections. In the United States, about 500 infants die each year of simple dehydration resulting from diarrhea, and about 220,000 are hospitalized for this reason. To prevent dehydration, infants with diarrhea should be given plenty of fluids, as advised by a physician.[20] Specialized electrolyte-replacement fluids, such as Pedialyte, may be recommended. These contain glucose, sodium, potassium, chloride, and water.

Once diarrhea subsides, a bottle-fed infant may be switched to a soy-based, lactose-free formula for a few days. This allows time for the intestine to produce sufficient lactase enzyme to digest the large amount of lactose typically found in formulas. A breastfed infant should continue at the breast throughout the duration of the diarrhea.

colic Sharp abdominal pain that generally occurs in otherwise healthy infants and is associated with periodic inconsolable crying spells.

Milk Allergy

Cow's milk contains more than 25 proteins that can cause allergic reactions in infants. Although some of these proteins are inactivated by heating (scalding) milk, others are very heat stable. A "true" milk allergy develops in about 1% to 4% of formula-fed infants. Such infants may experience vomiting, diarrhea, blood in the stool, constipation, and other symptoms. If milk allergy is suspected, a formula-fed infant can be switched to a soy-based formula. In 20% to 50% of cases, however, use of soy formula provides only temporary relief because the soy protein eventually triggers an allergic reaction in some infants. In such cases, a predigested-protein formula will then be needed (Table 17-1). If the child is breastfeeding, the mother may experiment with eliminating cow's milk from her diet (see the Nutrition Perspective for details).[13]

Iron-Deficiency Anemia

Iron-deficiency anemia typically occurs in older infants who consume few solid foods and whose diets are dominated by cow's milk, which contains little iron. Iron stores are then quickly depleted by the daily need to synthesize new red blood cells. The best approach for preventing iron-deficiency anemia is to start an infant on iron-fortified cereals and meats at about 6 months and also to limit formula to 16 to 25 ounces (500 to 750 ml) daily at this time. Not only is cow's milk low in iron, but it can also cause intestinal bleeding in young infants. As mentioned earlier, cow's milk is not recommended during the first year of life; it's especially important that infants not consume cow's milk during the first 3 months. If anemia does develop, medicinal iron supplements are advised with a physician's guidance.[24]

FEEDING PRETERM INFANTS

Preterm infants are fed either a specially designed formula or human milk. As noted in Chapter 16, nutrients may be added to human milk to increase its protein, mineral, and energy content. Amino acids not normally needed in the diet (e.g. cysteine) may be essential for preterm infants. In addition, some vitamins—such as vitamin E, folate, and vitamin B-12—and vitamin-like compounds—such as carnitine—may be helpful additions to their diets.

Because many bacteria require iron to thrive, use of iron supplements with preterm infants may be delayed to reduce their risk of bacterial infections. Preterm infants must be fed immediately after birth, as their body stores of fat and glycogen are quite low. For example, the body of a preterm newborn may be only about 2% fat by weight, depending on gestational age, whereas a typical full-term infant's body composition is about 12% fat.[26]

CONCEPT CHECK

Colic is commonly associated with inconsolable crying. Switching to a formula made with soy or predigested proteins may reduce colic. It may also be helpful for breastfeeding mothers to decrease or avoid intake of dairy products, under a physician's guidance. Diarrhea requires additional fluids to prevent dehydration. Infants allergic to proteins in standard cow's milk formula can be switched to a formula containing soy protein or predigested protein. Introducing iron-containing solid foods at an appropriate time and avoiding use of cow's milk during the first year can generally prevent iron-deficiency anemia in infants.

Preschool Children

The rapid growth rate that characterizes infancy tapers off quickly during the subsequent few years. The average annual weight gain is only 4.5 to 6.5 pounds (2 to 3 kg), and the average annual height gain is only 3 to 4 inches (7.5 to 10 cm) be-

TABLE 17-5

Food plan for preschool and school-age children based on the Food Guide Pyramid

Food group	No. of servings	Approximate serving size*			
		Age 1-2	Age 3-4	Age 5-6	Age 7-12
Milk, yogurt, and cheese:	3	½-¾ cup or 1 oz	¾ cup or 1½ oz	1 cup or 2 oz	1 cup or 2 oz
Meat, poultry, fish, dry beans, eggs, and nuts:	2 or more	1 oz or 1-2 tbsp	1½ oz or 3-4 tbsp	1½ oz or ½ cup	2 oz or ½ cup
Vegetables:	3 or more	1-2 tbsp	3-4 tbsp	½ cup	½ cup
Fruit:	2 or more	1-2 tbsp or ½ cup juice	3-4 tbsp or ½ cup juice	½ cup or ½ cup juice	½ cup or ½ cup juice
Bread, cereal, rice, and pasta:	6 or more	½ slice or ½ cup	1 slice or ½ cup	1 slice or ¾ cup	1 slice or ¾ cup

Adapted from Food and Nutrition Service, US Department of Agriculture: *Meal pattern requirements and offer versus serve manual,* FNS-265, 1990.
*Use as a starting point. Increase serving size as energy yields dictate, but maintain variety in the diet by making sure all food groups are still appropriately represented.

nious family atmosphere is an important part of resolving many childhood feeding problems. In addition, parents must often be educated as to what to expect of a preschool child and what food-related goals to set (Table 17-4).[16] Let's consider some typical complaints and concerns of parents, the causes of the problems, and suggestions for correcting them.

• • •

"My child won't eat as much or as regularly as he did as an infant." This behavior is characteristic of preschoolers, since their growth rate slows after infancy and thus they don't need as much food. Parents often need reminding that a 3-year-old can't be expected to eat as voraciously as an infant, or to eat adult-size portions. Table 17-5 shows a general food plan, based on the Food Guide Pyramid, that is appropriate for preschool and school-age children. Note that until about 5 years of age, serving sizes in the vegetable group, fruit group, and meat, poultry, fish, dry beans, eggs, and nuts group can be estimated as 1 tablespoon per year of life.

Normal-weight children have a built-in physiological mechanism that adjusts hunger in relation to the needed food intake at each stage of growth.[4] If a child is developing and growing normally, is being provided with a variety of nutritious foods, and doesn't drink excessive amounts of milk, caregivers can be confident the youngster is meeting nutrient needs. Nagging and bribing a child to eat more is counterproductive, unpleasant for everyone, and not worth the effort. Parents should make nutritious food choices available, eat some themselves, and let the child decide the serving size.

Appetite also varies with degree of physical activity and general health. A common early symptom of illness is poor appetite. Picky eating also reflects preschoolers' striving toward independence and their strong desire to establish routines.[16] Asserting their own food preferences is a relatively easy way for children to do this.

Parents should recognize that food likes and dislikes change rapidly in childhood and are influenced by food temperature, appearance, texture, and taste. Sometimes children object to having foods mixed, as in stews or casseroles, even if they normally like the ingredients separately. Children are also easily distracted, so turning off the television and reducing other distractions during mealtimes is advised. The preschool years are also an important time for children to explore the world around them. Even good eaters are sometimes more interested in exploring than eating. There is room for occasional indulgences—a skipped meal or two or a tasty but less nutritious food. What matters most is not the occasional deviation, but instead the usual eating and lifestyle habits that children develop. Preschoolers are most likely

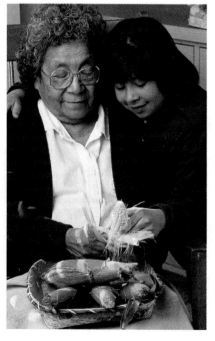

Children master their eating environments when adults provide opportunities to learn.

to establish good habits when adults give them opportunities to learn and support their exploration of the environment while discouraging inappropriate behavior.[16]

• • •

"My young daughter is always snacking but never finishes her meals." Because children have small stomachs, they often eat better when given six or so small meals each day rather than just three large meals. The practice of three meals a day is simply a social custom, convenient and appropriate for most adults, but without any special nutritional advantages. Indeed, when we eat is not nearly as important as what we eat.

Assuming that good dental care is observed, snacking is fine for children and typical for most. It's best to have a supply of nutritious snacks on hand (Table 17-6). Then, if a child gets hungry at midmorning or midafternoon, an acceptable snack is readily available to offer. Snacks at this time can tide them over until mealtime. Fruits and vegetables (fresh, frozen, or juice) and whole-grain breads and crackers are good snack choices.[7] Parents should make sure that appropriate snacks

TABLE 17-6

Ideas for nutritious snacks and beverages

Snack	Serving suggestion	Snack	Serving suggestion	Snack	Serving suggestion
Fresh raw vegetables	Serve with a dip of cottage cheese or yogurt blended with dried buttermilk dressing	Flour tortillas	Spread with refried beans or canned chili, sprinkle with grated cheese and broil; top with chili sauce	Popcorn	Serve plain or make three quarts and sprinkle with ¼ cup grated cheese and ½ tsp garlic or onion salt
Celery	Spread with peanut butter and sprinkle on raisins, shredded carrots, or finely chopped nuts	Ready-to-eat cereals	Use brands low in sugar and containing fiber; serve with raisins	Parfait	Make with yogurt, fruit, and granola
Bananas	Dip in sweetened yogurt or spread with peanut butter and roll in coconut, chopped nuts, or granola	Pita bread	Place sliced meat, cheese, lettuce, and tomato in open pocket	Gelatin	Add fruit or vegetable juice, vegetables, fruits, or cottage cheese
		English muffins or pita bread	Top with spaghetti sauce, grated cheese, and meats; broil or bake and cut in fourths	Frozen fruit cubes	Freeze puréed applesauce or fruit juice into cubes
Sliced apples or crackers	Serve with a dip of peanut butter, honey, nuts, raisins, and coconut	Potato skins	Sprinkle with shredded cheese, broil, and top with yogurt and bacon bits	Fruit fizz	Add club soda to juice instead of serving soft drinks
Bagels	Spread with cream cheese or peanut butter and top with chopped bananas, crushed pineapple, or shredded carrots	Canned chili	Heat and top with onions, lettuce, and tomato; use as dip for Italian or French bread, biscuits, or corn bread	Fruit shake	Blend milk with fresh fruit (bananas, berries, or a peach) and a dash of cinnamon or nutmeg
Quick bread or muffins	Make with carrots, zucchini, pumpkin, bananas, nuts, dates, raisins, lemons, squash, or berries	Kabobs	Make with any combination of the following: fruit, vegetables, and sliced or cubed cooked meat (remove toothpicks before serving)	Yogurt frost	Combine fruit juice and yogurt; add fresh fruit if desired
				Hot chocolate	Make hot chocolate or cocoa with milk chocolate and a dash of cinnamon
				Seeds	Shelled sunflower seeds
				Fish	Tunafish on crackers
				Canned soup	Cup of vegetable or minestrone; nice on a cold winter day

From National Meat and Livestock Board: *A food guide for the first five years,* Chicago.

EXPERT OPINION

HELPING CHILDREN TO EAT WELL

ELLYN SATTER, M.S., R.D. A.C.S.W.

Parents want their children to eat well and be healthy. Many worry that their children eat too much—or too little—or won't eat their vegetables or drink their milk. They feel guilty and responsible when children leave the table without eating—and angry when they come back 10 minutes later wanting a snack.

In some families, the dinner table becomes a battleground. Parents turn into reluctant food hustlers, insisting that children eat a regulation "four bites of broccoli before you can have dessert." Children gag. Adults feel pity and empathize. As one sensitive mother observed, "When you don't want to eat something, it feels as if it grows in your mouth." Nonetheless, this perceptive mother feels obligated to insist that her son eat his vegetables.

How many bites of broccoli does it take to earn dessert? How do you get yourself out of the position where you have to make such ridiculous rules?

RESPECT THE CHILD'S CAPABILITY

Children have built-in motivators to eat. They get hungry, they are inter-ested in eating, they have hearty appetites for good food, and they are interested in survival. But the way they operate with eating can fool you. Children are wary of new food: If it's new, they often don't like it.

But children do work to master new foods and new eating skills in the same way that they work to master other skills. They see new foods, taste them (needing as many as 15 or 20 attempts), and eventually learn to like them. Keep in mind that a taste is just a taste, and not necessarily a swallow. Toddlers put foods into their mouths, sample them for flavor and texture, and take them out again.

Unfortunately, to adults, these attempts at mastery look very much like rejection. While children are learning to like the new foods, the adults get anxious and try to hurry them along. It doesn't work. Bribing backfires. Researchers find that pre-schoolers who are rewarded for eating a new food are less likely to go back to it later than preschoolers who are allowed to approach the food on their own. In addition, food rewards produce a negative side effect: children who get dessert for eating their vegetables learn to like the dessert more and the vegetables less. Giving a reward for eating a new food is not a good idea; it gives the child the clearest of messages that you don't expect her to learn to like the new food. So she won't.

Children naturally eat a variety of foods. An internal process called *sensory-specific satiety* ensures that they will tire of even favorite foods and eat something different. Adults have the same tendency, but they ignore it. They override their appetites and eat because the food is good for them, or because they paid for it, or to keep from getting hungry later.

Children know how much they need to eat. They respond to their internal sense of hunger and fullness more strongly than adults do, and they eat the right amount of foods for proper growth. Unlike most adults, they stop when they are full rather than when the food is gone. Their food intake fluctuates considerably from meal to meal and from day to day. This is alarming to many parents, who often try to train this sensitivity out of their children by encouraging them to eat past satiety or restraining them when they eat heavily.

are available if their children are in day-care centers or other child-care arrangements. Since snacking is normal, caregivers need to plan ahead so that children don't load up on chips, candy, cookies, sugared soft drinks, and the like.

• • •

"My child never eats vegetables." Most people dislike some foods, and children are no exception. Preschool children who find vegetables unappealing can be encouraged to try just one bite at first. Children eventually learn that they can eat a little of a food without first gagging, choking, and yelling, "Oh gross!" As we discussed already, with repeated exposure to unfamiliar or disliked foods in appropri-

Whether these tactics succeed depends on the determination of the parent—and the child. Some children submit to parental controls. Others fight back. Children whose parents attempt to overfeed them may be revolted by food and may tend to undereat when they get the chance. Children whose parents attempt to underfeed them may become preoccupied with food and overeat when they get the chance.

PROVIDE APPROPRIATE SUPPORT

So what are parents to do? They can only provide a variety of attractive, wholesome foods in pleasant surroundings and approach feeding in a positive way. They can't force children to eat.

Maintain structure. Children eat best and are more likely to learn to like a variety of foods if they have regular meals and snacks at predictable times and aren't allowed to panhandle between times. Consistent eating times help children to come to the table hungry and, therefore, they are more likely to accept the food.

Prepare a variety of foods, then let the child pick and choose from what's available. A meal should include a main dish, a fruit or vegetable, and a starchy food, such as potato or rice. Don't limit the menu to foods the child readily accepts, and don't be a short-order cook.

Let the child learn from mistakes. If a toddler gets down from the table having eaten nothing and comes around 5 minutes later begging for a cookie, tell him, "Nothing until snack time." He may feel frustrated, but if you hold firm, the next time he may take his meal more seriously.

MAINTAIN A DIVISION OF RESPONSIBILITY IN FEEDING

It all boils down to what I call a "division of responsibility in feeding." The parents are responsible for what their child is offered to eat and for setting up a pleasant eating environment. The child is responsible for deciding how much or even whether he eats. Children master their eating when adults provide opportunities to learn, give support for exploration, and limit inappropriate behavior.

Kids have their own ways of learning and eating, so over the short term it can look as if they are doing poorly. But children will eat, and they will learn to like a variety of foods, and they will grow appropriately. Just don't hold your breath.

Ellyn Satter, a family therapist and specialist in eating disorders, is the author of How to Get Your Kid to Eat ... But Not Too Much, *Palo Alto, Calif, 1987, Bull Publishing.*

ate settings, most children eventually grow to like them. Again, forcing or bribing does not foster acceptance of particular foods.

Children need to develop independence and identities separate from their parents. In other words, children have to choose for themselves—a practice that should be encouraged. Parents could designate a section of the refrigerator or cupboard as a "kids' shelf." This way parents can monitor eating habits of their children while still letting them make their own selections, such as with vegetable snacks.

No one food is an essential part of a diet. Hunger is still the best means for getting preschool children to eat. It may work to feed them vegetables at the start of a meal, when they are hungriest, or to offer new foods—including vegetables—with familiar ones. A platter of raw or lightly cooked carrots, broccoli, green and red peppers, cabbage, and mushrooms eaten as a snack with friends can do a lot to remedy a vegetable problem. A 4- or 5-year-old child can safely consume raw vegetables without fear of choking. Nutritious dips sell vegetables to many children. Vegetables may acquire more appeal when children help prepare them.

• • •

"How do I know whether my child is eating a healthful diet?" If preschool and school-age children generally eat according to the food plan outlined in Table 17-5 and regularly gain in height and weight, they are following a nutritious diet. Serving sizes in the various food groups increase with age as energy needs and appetite increase. Among the nutrients that deserve special attention during childhood are calcium, iron, zinc, and vitamins A, B-6, and C.[26] These nutrients should be readily supplied if a child's diet includes choices from all the food groups.

Many 2-year-olds prefer peculiar foods, and parents need not worry about this. A child may switch from one specific food focus (often called a jag) to another with equal intensity. If the caregiver continues to offer choices, the child will soon begin to eat a wider variety of foods again, and the specific food focus will disappear as suddenly as it appeared, or will change to a new one.

Major scientific groups, including the American Dietetic Association and the American Society for Clinical Nutrition, do not recommend vitamin and mineral supplements for healthy children. It is better to emphasize a healthy assortment of foods. However, a nutrient supplement up to 150% of the Daily Value standards may be needed when a child is ill, especially if the illness persists. Studies show that most parents offer children conservative amounts of supplemental vitamins and minerals, so toxicity is unlikely. Still, the practice of giving supplements is often unnecessary, especially given today's typical highly fortified breakfast cereals, which children often eat.

NUTRITION-RELATED CONDITIONS IN PRESCHOOL CHILDREN

Three nutrition-related problems found in preschool children are iron-deficiency anemia, constipation, and dental caries. Proper diet can correct or relieve these conditions substantially.

Iron-Deficiency Anemia

The highest incidence of iron-deficiency anemia occurs in infants and toddlers between the ages of 6 and 24 months. However, this condition is found in some preschool children. It can lead to poor stamina, decreased resistance to disease, and reduced learning ability.[24]

Overall, the incidence of childhood anemia currently is quite low in the United States, partly because many parents feed their young children iron-fortified breakfast cereals. In addition, the Special Supplemental Food Program for Women, Infants, and Children (WIC), sponsored by the federal government, deserves credit. This program emphasizes the importance of iron-fortified formulas and cereals and distributes them—along with nutrition education—to low-income parents of infants and preschool children considered to be at nutritional risk.

The best way to prevent iron-deficiency anemia in children is to regularly feed them foods that are adequate sources of iron. Iron-fortified breakfast cereals and a few ounces of lean meat are convenient means of adding more iron to a child's diet. The high proportion of heme iron in many animal foods allows the iron to be more readily absorbed than the iron from plant foods. Consuming a vitamin C source along with the less readily absorbed iron in plants and supplements will aid absorption.

Constipation

Although constipation may be associated with disease, some young children experience constipation that is unrelated to any medical condition. When presented with a constipated child, a physician first has to rule out a medical cause, such as intestinal blockage. Treatment generally consists of first evacuating the bowels, generally with an enema. Promotion of regular bowel habits then follows, with laxative use as directed by the physician. Several months to years of supportive intervention may be required for effective treatment.[18]

Dietary interventions include eating more dietary fiber and drinking more fluids. Foods to emphasize for dietary fiber are fruits, vegetables, whole-grain breads and cereals, and beans.[21] The current daily dietary fiber goal for children between ages 3 and 13 years is the child's age plus 5 g. After that age typical adult recommendations are appropriate (see Chapter 3). Fluid recommendations are 5 cups per day for toddlers, and up to 9 cups per day for older children.

Dental Caries

A good diet goes a long way in reducing the risk for dental caries in young children. We mentioned earlier that infants are prone to nursing-bottle syndrome, which can lead to excessive tooth decay. The following tips can help reduce dental problems in infants and children:

- Begin oral hygiene when an infant's first tooth appears.
- Seek early pediatric dental care.
- Drink fluoridated water.
- Use fluoridated toothpaste twice daily.
- Snack in moderation.
- Have a dentist apply tooth sealants if needed.

Chapter 3 provides a fuller description of diet and dental health. If needed, that discussion will aid in putting this list of recommendations into perspective.

MODIFYING CHILDHOOD DIETS TO REDUCE FUTURE DISEASE RISK

We've discussed in earlier chapters the role of diet in development of heart disease and hypertension and the recommendations concerning diet, to reduce the risk for these diseases. Parents sometimes wonder whether similar diet modifications are appropriate and beneficial during childhood.

Restrictive Low-Fat Diets Are Not Recommended

The American Academy of Pediatrics does not recommend low-fat diets (below 30% of total energy intake) for young children. Experts do recommend screening for high serum cholesterol in children from families with histories of early heart disease, and then treating children who have high serum cholesterol with appropriate diet and drug therapy when needed, as discussed in Chapter 4.[30] The diet needs to be carefully planned so that it still provides an adequate overall nutrient intake. Currently, children consume about 33% of their energy intake from fat and about 13% of their energy intake from saturated fat.[19]

The early stages of plaque build-up linked to eventual heart disease are already present in many children. Thus, although highly restrictive low-fat diets are not advised for children, they certainly should not consume excessive amounts of fat. Currently many authorities recommend that from the age of 2 until linear growth ends, total fat intake should gradually fall to no more than 30% of energy intake, with saturated fat supplying no more than 10% of energy intake. The Food Guide Pyramid, with its emphasis on bread, cereal, rice, and pasta, is a good guide for achieving this intake pattern (Table 17-5).

Moderation is the best strategy, as very restrictive diets can be detrimental to overall nutrient intake and growth in children. Instead of restrictive diets, which are appropriate for adults who are obese or have high serum cholesterol, children need to consume adequate energy for growth while building good eating habits that they can carry into the teenage years. This can be achieved by limiting the amount of high-fat, nutritionally empty foods eaten each day and increasing consumption of lean meats, beans, fruits, vegetables, and breads and cereals.[33] Children can be en-

We mentioned earlier that a cow's milk allergy may also lead to constipation. This possibility should be investigated by the physician.

couraged to make some easy diet changes: bagels rather than doughnuts, nonfat frozen yogurt rather than ice cream, 1% or 2% milk rather than whole milk, fruit rather than crackers and cheese for snacks, and air-popped popcorn rather than chips.

Overall, the focus should be on total fat intake, not whether a specific food is high in fat. No food need be eliminated, but only moderated. Children also need ample opportunity for physical activity.[23]

Moderate Sodium Intake Is Preferable for Children

Available scientific evidence neither confirms nor refutes the notion that children who eat less salt will be less likely to develop future hypertension than other children. However, if children become accustomed to moderate amounts of salt in their food, they will be unlikely to eat very salty foods as adults because the taste for salty foods is largely acquired. So moderate sodium consumption by children does establish a healthy habit, which may be especially important if they later develop hypertension and need to reduce sodium intake even further.

VEGETARIANISM IN CHILDHOOD

Vegetarian diets pose several risks for young children. These include the possibility of developing iron-deficiency anemia, a deficiency of vitamin B-12, and rickets. During the first few years of life, children may not consume enough energy when following a bulky vegetarian diet. But these known pitfalls are easily avoided by informed diet planning (see the Nutrition Perspective in Chapter 5). Diets for children who eat totally vegetarian fare should especially focus on protein, vitamin D (or regular sun exposure), vitamin B-12, calcium, iron, and zinc content.[27]

CONCEPT CHECK

The rapid growth rate of an infant's first year slows during the toddler and preschool years (ages 1 to 5). As a child's appetite decreases, adults need to serve nutrient-dense foods and allow the child to decide how much to eat. Sudden shifts in food preferences are to be expected. Snacking is fine if attention is given to the selection of healthful foods and good dental hygiene. Vitamin and mineral supplements are usually not needed, as a food plan following the Food Guide Pyramid should meet nutrient needs. Children need plenty of iron-rich foods to prevent iron-deficiency anemia. Adequate dietary fiber and fluid help prevent constipation. Developing heart-healthy habits after the age of 2 years is good health insurance, but highly restrictive diets are not appropriate during childhood. Diets for children who eat totally vegetarian fare should emphasize protein, vitamin D (or regular sun exposure), vitamin B-12, calcium, iron, and zinc content.

School-Age Children

In general, the nutritional concerns and goals applicable to school-age children are the same as those we've discussed in relation to preschoolers. The Food Guide Pyramid continues to be a good basis for diet planning, with an emphasis on moderating fat intake and ensuring adequate iron and calcium intake. The only difference is that serving size increases as energy needs increase (Table 17-5). Now we'll look at several nutritional issues of particular concern during the school-age years.

BREAKFAST, FAT INTAKE, AND SNACKS

Once children enter school, their eating patterns are less flexible and consumption of regular meals—especially breakfast—becomes an important focus. Some research suggests that the energy and nutrients consumed during breakfast help children perform better during the school hours by increasing their attention and motivation.

The test scores, as well as sports performance, of youngsters who regularly eat breakfast are generally better than those of children who tend to skip breakfast. This finding makes sense because breakfast replenishes depleted carbohydrate stores in the liver. Other researchers, however, question the influence of eating breakfast on learning and motivation. They claim that students who are motivated and perform well are likely to eat breakfast, not that eating breakfast is likely to improve motivation and performance. Despite this chicken-and-egg conundrum, we advise providing breakfast to all school-age children, as it gives a nutrient-rich start to the daily diet.

Breakfast menus need not be limited to traditional fare. A little imagination can spark the interest of the most reluctant child. Instead of conventional breakfast foods, parents can offer leftovers from dinner, pizza, spaghetti, soups, yogurt with trail mix on top, chili, or sandwiches for starters.

Currently, the typical lunch served in school lunch programs contains 38% of total energy as fat. Based on current nutritional trends and changes in guidelines, the fat content of school lunches is expected to decrease to 30% of energy over the next few years.[25]

There is general agreement that diets of school-age children should include a variety of foods from each major group, while not necessarily excluding any specific food because of its fat content. Overemphasis on fat-reduced diets during childhood has been linked to an increase in eating disorders and encourages an inappropriate "good food," "bad food" attitude.

Steering children toward healthful foods, in school and at home, is likely to be more successful if they are exposed to nutrition education. Such education can help children understand why eating a proper diet will make them feel more energetic, look better, and work more efficiently. A recent survey of schoolchildren highlights the need for nutrition education. On the day of the survey, 40% of the children ate no vegetables, except for potatoes or tomato sauce; 20% ate no fruits; and 75% snacked at least twice. Some 36% of the students ate at least four different types of snack foods. Clearly, the diets of many school-age students can stand general improvement, with selection of nutritious snacks deserving particular emphasis (Table 17-6).

POSSIBLE ADVERSE EFFECTS OF SUCROSE ON CHILDREN

Some researchers have suggested that sucrose affects behavior, especially in children. They claim sucrose creates an excited, even antisocial state, which may lead to violence and disruptive behavior. However, almost all researchers and health authorities find that sucrose itself is not the villain. Studies show that the behavior of children is similar whether they consume sucrose or aspartame, and aspartame is a protein and not a sugar.[32] In addition, no adequate evidence supports the hypothesis that reactive hypoglycemia caused by sucrose consumption commonly causes violent behavior. If there is a villain, it is probably the excitement or tension surrounding high-sucrose foods (such as is seen at parties and during Halloween) or the extra attention a child receives when put on a relatively sucrose-free diet. Thus recommendations to lower the amount of sucrose in children's diets in hope of preventing or treating behavioral problems for most affected children are at best premature.

This does not, however, mean that children should have unlimited access to sugar. If energy intake from sugar replaces intake of essential nutrients, problems of undernutrition may result. Overall, the recommendation stated in the Dietary Guidelines for Americans to use sugar in moderation applies to children as well as adults.

CHILDHOOD OBESITY

In the United States, about 25% of school-age children place above the 85th percentile in weight-for-height and are considered overweight,[28] and the incidence of this disorder is currently increasing. In the short run, ridicule and embarrassment

CRITICAL THINKING

Tim refuses to eat breakfast before school. He doesn't like cereal, toast, or any of the other usual breakfast foods. What can Tim's parents do to ensure that he eats nutritious foods before leaving for school? They have read that children who eat a nourishing breakfast are more alert and tend to have higher test scores. Does any research support this idea?

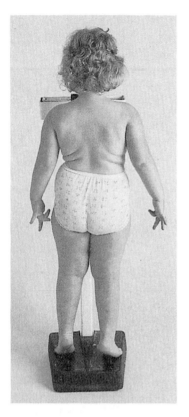

Figure 17-7 Children who are obese, like this young girl, often face a battle against obesity for the rest of their lives. Early childhood represents an ideal time to intervene with moderation in energy intake and ample opportunities for physical activity.

are the main consequences of such obesity (Figure 17-7). Significant health problems associated with obesity, such as heart disease, diabetes, and hypertension, usually do not appear until adulthood. Unfortunately, about 40% of obese children (and about 80% of obese adolescents) become obese adults. Significant weight gain generally begins between ages 5 and 7 years or during the teenage years.[8] Childhood obesity should not be ignored because the chances are great that an obese school-age child will become an obese adult.[10] The sooner corrective measures are taken, the more likely they are to succeed.

Causes of Obesity in Children

Current research indicates that there are many potential causes of childhood obesity. Recall the nature versus nurture discussion in Chapter 8. Some infants are born with lower metabolic rates; they use energy more efficiently and, in turn, have an easier time saving energy intake for fat storage. Thus childhood obesity is linked to heredity. Children presenting for obesity treatment also show a high prevalence of sibling (50%) and maternal (63%) obesity.

Research shows a moderate relationship between the number of hours a child spends watching television and playing video games and obesity.[23] The television generation now glues itself to the tube for an average of 24 hours a week, including hours of advertisements for high-fat and sugar-laden foods; many children spend another 10 or so hours playing computer and video games. In addition, excessive snacking, little physical activity (especially in girls), parental neglect, lack of safe areas to play, latch-key conditions, and high-fat/high-energy food choices most likely contribute to childhood obesity. Fundamentally, obesity results from an imbalance between energy input and output. For many children, a low amount of physical activity, rather than excessive energy intake, may be the primary culprit leading to obesity.[10,23]

Treating the Obese Child

The initial approach in treating an obese child is to assess how much physical activity he or she engages in. If a child spends much free time in sedentary activities (such as watching television or playing video games), more physical activities should be encouraged. Getting the family together for a brisk walk after dinner and finding an after-school sport the child enjoys are two good ideas. An increase in physical activity won't just happen; parents need to plan for it.

Moderation in energy intake is important, especially limitation of high-fat and high-energy foods and sugar-laden carbonated beverages. More nutrient-dense foods should be the primary focus. A diet containing 30% of energy intake as fat can support normal growth and development during childhood, provided that the foods selected follow the Food Guide Pyramid.[32]

Resorting to a weight-loss diet is usually unnecessary. Changing habits should be the emphasis in the short run.[9] Children have an advantage over adults in dealing with obesity: their bodies can use stored energy for growth. Thus, if weight gain can be moderated, increase in height may reduce the amount of stored fat, yielding a desirable weight-to-height ratio. This is one reason treating obesity in childhood is so desirable. Further growth can contribute to success.

Sometimes weight loss is necessary if a child will still be obese after attaining ultimate adult height. This is especially appropriate after the adolescent growth spurt. Weight loss should be gradual, perhaps ½ pound per week. If weight loss is necessary in younger children, the child should be watched closely to ensure that during this weight loss the rate of growth is normal. It is important that the child's energy intake not be so low that gains in height diminish.

Behavior modification adds a third important component to treating childhood obesity. One underlying environmental cause of obesity can be parents' attitudes and behaviors toward their child's eating. A heavy parental hand in overly restricting or controlling the child's food intake may lead to struggles around eating that actually interfere with a child's ability to eat sensibly. Obese children often need to find a new way to relate to foods, especially snack foods. An important family rule could be that children are allowed to eat only while sitting at the meal table or in the kitchen. Parents choose the foods, and the child chooses how much to eat (see the Expert Opinion). Eating only at the meal table or in the kitchen could stop endless hours of snacking in front of the television and makes all family members more conscious of when they are eating. It might also help to put portions on plates rather than allow snacking to go on indefinitely, as often happens when children eat directly from a full box of crackers or cookies.

The self-esteem of a child is quite fragile. Obesity itself affects the child's psyche. Humiliation does not work; it only makes the child feel worse. Support, admiration, and encouragement of the child's efforts at weight control are more effective and should be emphasized. Parents should also realize that by denying a child favorite foods, they do not necessarily deny love. The child can have treats, such as candy, in small amounts—just not a whole bag. Often parents and overweight children need to develop new ways of relating—ways that do not involve food and obesity.[28]

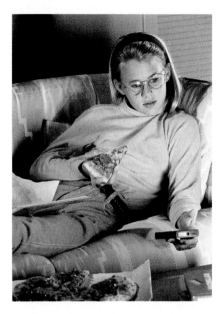

Environmental influences, such as watching television and snacking, are among the factors that can eventually lead to childhood obesity.

CONCEPT CHECK

The school-age child is advised to follow the Food Guide Pyramid, moderating choices high in fat and simple sugars. Breakfast is an important meal to refuel the body for a new school day. Attention to regular physical activity and healthy diet should help prevent childhood obesity and build a desirable lifestyle pattern for later life.

Teenagers

We noted before that most girls begin a rapid growth spurt between the ages of 10 and 13 years, and most boys grow more between the ages of 12 and 15 years.[26] Nearly every organ in the body grows during these periods of faster growth, which last about 3 years. Most noticeable are increases in height and weight and development of secondary sexual characteristics. Girls usually begin menstruating (reach menarche) during this growth spurt, and they grow very little beyond 2 years after menarche. Early-maturing girls may begin their growth spurt as early as ages 7 to 8, whereas early-maturing boys may begin growing by ages 9 to 10.

During the growth spurt, girls gain about 10 inches (25 cm) in height and boys gain about 12 inches (30 cm). From about age 10 years, girls also tend to accumulate both lean and fat tissue, whereas boys tend to gain mostly lean tissue. The adolescent growth spurt provides about 50% of ultimate adult weight and 15% of ultimate adult height (Figure 17-1). Skeletal growth during adolescence accounts for approximately 45% of final adult bone mass.

Fortunately, as the growth spurt begins, teenagers begin to eat more. If teenagers choose nutritious foods, they can take advantage of their increased hunger and easily satisfy their nutrient needs. As with younger children, the Food Guide Pyramid provides the basis for meeting these nutrient needs (Table 17-7).

NUTRITIONAL PROBLEMS AND CONCERNS OF TEENAGERS

Some teenagers have a difficult time evaluating their weight status. Girls especially may view themselves as too fat even when they in fact fall within a range for healthy weight. In Chapter 11 we discussed a major potential nutritional problem in the adolescent years that can result from this misperception—eating disorders, including anorexia nervosa and bulimia nervosa. Another significant health problem—alcoholism—also may have its roots in the teenage years (see the Nutrition Perspective in Chapter 7 for details). Here we look at several more common nutritional problems experienced by many teenagers.

TABLE 17-7

Food plan for teenagers based on the Food Guide Pyramid*

Food category	Minimum number of daily servings†
Milk, yogurt, and cheese (preferably low fat or nonfat)	3
Meat, poultry, fish, dry beans, eggs, and nuts	2-3
Vegetables	3-5
Fruit	2-4
Bread, cereal, rice, and pasta (preferably whole grain; otherwise, enriched or fortified)	6-11
Fats, oils, and sweets	Use sparingly

*Here we define "teenager" as a person who has added height in the past year and is at least 12 years old. This food plan is applicable through age 24 years.
†Use same serving sizes as for adults (see Table 2-1).

Inadequate Calcium Intake by Girls

Many teenage girls do not drink milk at all or drink it infrequently. These girls most probably, then, do not consume enough calcium to allow for maximum mineralization of bones through their early twenties. Young women who do not consume enough calcium likely are sowing the seeds for future osteoporosis, as we discussed in the Nutrition Focus in Chapter 14.

The RDA for calcium for both males and females between ages 11 and 24 years is 1200 mg/day, compared with 800 mg/day for school-age children. A recent NIH Consensus Conference on Optimal Intake of Calcium increased the calcium goal further, to 1500 mg/day. Unfortunately, only about 1 in 6 teenage girls consumes the RDA for calcium.

Drinking soft drinks in place of milk contributes to inadequate calcium intakes by many teenagers. Because soft drinks are rich in phosphorus, this practice produces an imbalance in the intakes of calcium and phosphorus, a pattern that does not promote optimal bone development. Three servings from the milk, yogurt, and cheese group per day are recommended for all teenagers and young adults until age 24.

Iron-Deficiency Anemia

During the adolescent growth spurt between 11 and 18 years of age, iron needs are increased over those of early childhood. For boys, the RDA for iron is set at 12 mg/day, mostly to sustain their rapidly enlarging lean body mass. For girls, the RDA is 15 mg/day, to offset their additional menstrual losses that begin during this time.

Iron-deficiency anemia sometimes appears in girls after they start menstruating and in boys during their growth spurt. Up to about 10% of teenagers have low iron stores or related anemia. Teenagers who strive to forge an identity by adopting dietary patterns unfamiliar to their families—vegetarianism, for example—may not know enough about the alternative diet pattern to keep from developing health problems, such as iron-deficiency anemia.[27] All teenagers need to choose good food sources of iron, such as lean meats, whole grains, and enriched grains. Teenage girls with heavy menstrual flows likely are at the greatest risk for iron-deficiency anemia. Eating good sources of iron, and perhaps regularly consuming an iron supplement, is especially important for these girls. Iron-deficiency anemia can produce fatigue and decreased ability to concentrate and learn, and generally is not favorable to an active, enjoyable lifestyle.[26] School performance and athletic performance eventually may suffer (see Chapter 10 for discussion of sports anemia).

Acne

About 80% of teenagers suffer from acne, making this one of the most common problems of these years. Eating nuts, chocolate, and pizza is commonly thought to make acne worse, but scientific studies have failed to demonstrate a strong link between any dietary factor and acne. Teenagers are simply warned to avoid "trigger foods," assuming that planning a well-balanced diet is still possible. Since acne naturally waxes and wanes, teenagers fall easy prey to notions relating it to various dietary factors.

The immediate cause of acne is overactivity by **sebaceous glands,** which are small saclike structures surrounding hair follicles in the skin. The activity of these glands is stimulated by certain hormones called **androgens,** especially testosterone, the primary male sex hormone. For this reason, acne usually does not appear until puberty, when production of the sex hormones increases dramatically.[22] Although women produce some androgens, men produce much higher amounts of these hormones. Thus acne tends to be more severe and last longer in men than women. However, some women may produce relatively large amounts of androgens and as a result may experience serious acne. Many women suffer premenstrual acne flare-ups that are prompted by the release of progesterone after ovulation. Women using high-progesterone birth control pills also may develop acne.

One medication dermatologists sometimes prescribe for acne is tretinoin, which is sold under various trade names (e.g., Retin-A). A derivative of vitamin A, tretinoin is rubbed onto the skin once nightly.[22] It is highly effective for treating blackheads and modestly effective for treating pimples. Scientists do not know exactly how tretinoin works, but research suggests that it both pushes out the plugs in the ducts beneath the skin and helps prevent their re-formation. The combination of benzoyl peroxide in the morning and tretinoin at night is often a very effective therapy for acne.

Accutane, another vitamin A derivative, offers exciting possibilities for treating serious acne (see Chapter 12 for additional discussion). This prescription oral medication appears to change development of sebaceous glands so they produce less **sebum,** leading to a decrease in the number of acne lesions.[22] The medication is especially helpful in treating cases resistant to antibiotic therapy. Because Accutane poses a high risk for serious birth defects, sexually active girls who use this medication must practice effective birth control.

Teenagers should not self-medicate with vitamin A itself in hopes of curtailing acne. Instead they should rely on advice from their physician. It is the derivatives of vitamin A—not the vitamin itself—that are helpful, and these are available only by prescription. Recall as well that excessive dosages of vitamin A can be toxic, so self-medication would also likely be a hazardous choice.

A CLOSER LOOK AT TEENAGERS' DIETS

Teenagers consume about 34% of energy intake as fat and 13% of energy intake as saturated fat. These values exceed the recommended goals of 30% and 10% of energy intake from these two energy sources, respectively. Teenage boys consume about 335 mg of cholesterol per day, more than the recommended daily intake of 300 mg. In contrast, teenage girls consume only about 205 mg of cholesterol per day.[19] In addition to low intakes of calcium and iron, mentioned already, some teenagers—especially girls—consume inadequate amounts of vitamins A and C and zinc.

Fear of excessive weight gain causes some young girls to limit their energy intake, thus restricting their available food options. Busy schedules, part-time jobs, athletics, and social activities may also interfere with regular mealtimes and adequate nutritional intake. Many teenagers skip breakfast, often depriving themselves of sufficient energy intake and nutrients. The increased responsibility for purchasing and preparing food assumed by today's teenagers, who frequently lack sufficient knowledge to make healthy food choices, also contributes to their risk for nutrition-related problems. If their food choices consist primarily of french fries, soft drinks, and

sebaceous glands Small glands surrounding hair follicles on the face, ears, back, chest, eyelids, and other areas. Blockage of a duct in a sebaceous gland by small particles can lead to an infection and local pressure, resulting in an acne lesion.

androgens A general term for hormones that stimulate development in male sex organs; testosterone is one example.

sebum Secretion of the sebaceous gland consisting of waxes and various triglycerides.

pastries, little room is left for foods that are rich nutrient sources. For instance, only about 15% of teenagers consume a total of five fruits and vegetables per day—an important diet-planning goal for all children and adults.

To optimize performance, adolescents in competitive sports may also try to lose body weight by using diuretics, laxatives and diet pills, starvation, and enhanced sweating. These extreme weight-loss measures can impair both performance and health. A more realistic approach to diet and physical performance is needed (see Chapter 10).

Fad diets are popular in the teenage years, most notably among girls. Chapter 9 reviews these diets and also provides some better advice for weight-conscious teenagers.

Some teenagers embrace vegetarian diets, which can be a nutritious option if properly planned. Because vegetarianism is an odd, unfamiliar practice for many parents, they are unable to adequately evaluate their child's food choices. The potential for low intakes of certain nutrients—particularly iron, calcium, and vitamin B-12—on vegetarian diets can be avoided by following the advice in the Nutrition Perspective in Chapter 5.[27]

HELPING TEENAGERS CHOOSE A MORE NUTRITIOUS DIET

Teenagers face a variety of upheavals in their lives. They seek independence, experience identity crises, desire peer acceptance, and worry about physical appearance. All these concerns influence food choice, and advertisers take advantage of them when promoting a vast array of food products—candy, gum, soft drinks, and snacks—targeted toward the teenage market.

Most teenagers rarely relate today's food habits to tomorrow's health concerns. The future is a hazy, distant time for them. They figure that when and if the time comes, they can easily change poor habits later; there is no hurry about developing healthful food habits. Part of teenagers' aversion to nutritious diets is their mistaken belief that healthful food habits mean they have to avoid favorite, often high-fat, foods. However, rather than eliminating tasty fatty foods, small portions of such foods can complement larger portions of more nutritious ones. A plain hamburger with a garden salad (minimize the amount of regular dressing or use a low-fat variety) and small order of french fries plus low-fat or nonfat milk incorporates this approach.

Overcoming the Teenage Mindset

One strategy for working with teenage boys is to stress the importance of nutrition for physical development—especially muscular development—and for fitness, vigor, and health. With teenage girls, one approach is to help them understand how to choose nutrient-dense foods that lead to better health while maintaining appropriate weight. It can be explained that beauty is based on the glow of health, something that sick people often do not have. Generally the most effective approach with teenagers is to focus on the benefits they can reap right now from a healthful diet, rather than stressing the possible future health hazards associated with a less healthful diet.

Parents can also do their part by having nutritious foods available—for instance, keeping a fruit salad or cut-up vegetables and low-fat dip in the refrigerator. In addition, parents can insist that teenagers come to the table at mealtime.

Snacking and Quick-Service Eating by Teenagers

As with younger children, what teenagers eat is more important than when or where they eat. Snacks supply one fourth to one third of daily intakes of energy and major nutrients for many teenagers (Figure 17-8). Key reasons for teenage snacking and frequent use of quick-service restaurants include the opportunity to get out and socialize with friends, accessibility, hunger, and celebrating a special event. By choosing wisely from the menu and eating in moderation, teenagers can eat at quick-service restaurants and still consume a very healthy diet. Snacks and quick-ser-

Clinicians who work with teenagers, including physicians, registered dietitians, and nurses, need to be prepared to discuss and deal with a variety of concerns: sports nutrition, eating disorders, use of steroids, and drug and alcohol abuse. Except for substance abuse, these topics usually are not a concern when working with older adult clients.

vice restaurants in and of themselves are not the problem; poor food choices are. Unfortunately, a recent Gallup poll has found just what you might expect—that teenagers snack mostly on potato and corn chips, cookies, candies, and ice cream. Many teenagers could easily improve their diets by developing a taste for the more nutritious snacks described in Table 17-6.

• • •

Poor dietary habits formed during teenage years often continue into adulthood, giving rise to an increased risk of chronic diseases, such as heart disease, osteoporosis, and some types of cancer. Getting this message across to teenagers is an important and challenging task for parents and health professionals.

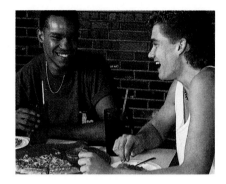

Figure 17-8 The teenage years are noted for snacking and eating at quick-service restaurants. With proper food choices, teenagers can have healthful diets while still enjoying snacks and socializing at their favorite hangouts.

CONCEPT CHECK

The final period of rapid growth occurs during the teenage years, when numerous psychological, social, and physical changes occur rapidly. Girls generally start the adolescent growth spurt earlier than boys. The Food Guide Pyramid should direct meal planning during these critical years. Common nutrition-related problems and concerns include inadequate calcium intake in girls; iron-deficiency anemia; fad dieting; acne, which tends to be worse in boys; and high intakes of saturated fats, often as the result of poor choices of snacks and menu items at quick-service restaurants. Teenagers usually are not very concerned about the risk of future health problems stemming from poor food habits. They are more susceptible to information focusing on the current benefits—fitness, vigor, weight control, appearance—of making nutritious food choices.

Summary

1. Growth is very rapid during infancy; birthweight doubles in about 4 to 6 months, and length increases by 50% within the first year. Adequate intake of nutrients—especially of energy, protein, and zinc—is critical to normal growth of infants. Undernutrition can cause irreversible changes in growth and development. Growth in infants and children can be assessed by measuring body weight, length (height), and head circumference over time.

2. Nutrient needs in the first 6 months can be met by human milk or iron-fortified formula. Supplementary vitamin D and iron may be needed by breastfed infants during the first 6 months, and many infants may need supplemental fluoride.

3. Infant formulas generally contain lactose or sucrose, heat-treated proteins from cow's milk, and vegetable oils. Formulas may or may not be fortified with iron. Sanitation is very important when preparing and storing formula.

4. Most infants do not need solid foods before about 4 to 6 months of age. The appropriate time for introducing solid foods depends on several factors: need for greater nutrient intake than can be supplied without solid food; ability of the intestinal system to digest most foods; an infant's physical ability to control tongue thrusting and to participate in the feeding process; and reduction in the risk of developing food allergies.

5. The first solid food given should be iron-fortified infant cereals or ground meats. Other single foods can be added gradually, at the rate of about one each week. Some foods to avoid giving infants in the first year include honey, low-fat cow's milk, very salty or sweet foods, egg whites, or foods that may cause choking.

6. Introducing iron-containing solid food at the appropriate time and not offering cow's milk until 1 year of age generally prevent iron-deficiency anemia in late infancy.

7. Because of children's slower growth rate during the preschool years, use of nutrient-dense foods and appropriate serving sizes is important to nutritious diet planning during this period. Again, consumption of iron-rich foods, such as lean red meats, helps to avert development of iron-deficiency anemia. Preschoolers should be given some leeway in determining serving size and should be encouraged to try new foods. Highly restrictive diets designed to reduce the risk of heart disease or hypertension are not recommended for preschoolers or older children.

8. A large proportion of obese children and adolescents become obese adults, with all the associated health risks. Obese infants, in contrast, are less likely to become obese children and later adults. Often insufficient physical activity is more important than excessive food intake in causing childhood obesity. Both increased physical activity and an adequate diet that supports growth are critical for obese children. Parents can provide healthful food choices but let the child control portion size. When dealt with early, childhood obesity may correct itself as the child continues to grow in height.

9. During the adolescent growth spurt, both boys and girls have increased needs for iron and calcium. Inadequate calcium intake by teenage girls is a major concern because it can set the stage for development of osteoporosis later in life. Teenagers generally should watch their intake of high-fat foods, especially snacks and quick-service foods, which they often consume in abundance.

Study Questions

1. List two factors that limit "catch-up" growth in adulthood when a nutrient-deficient diet has been consumed throughout childhood.

2. Outline the procedures for preparing various types of infant formula: powdered, concentrated, and ready-to-feed.

3. Describe how you would assess whether an 8-month-old infant is consuming a healthful diet.

4. Outline three key factors that help determine when to introduce solid foods into an infant's diet.

5. List three reasons why preschoolers are noted for "fussy" eating. For each, describe an appropriate parent response.

6. Why should obesity in childhood be discouraged? What three factors are likely to contribute to this problem in a typical 6-year-old child?

7. Compare the guidelines for infant feeding summarized in the Nutrition Focus with the Dietary Guidelines for children over 2 and adults discussed in Chapter 2. Which guidelines are similar? Do any contradict each other? If so, what would be the reason(s)?

8. Describe three pros and cons of snacking. What is the basic advice for healthful snacking from childhood through the teenage years?

9. Which two nutrients are of particular interest in planning diets for teenagers? Why does each deserve to be singled out?

10. In the teenage years, which nutrient generally most deserves an "in moderation" warning? Briefly describe why this is so.

REFERENCES

1. Agostoni C and others: Effects of diet on the lipid and fatty acid status of full-term infants at 4 months, *Journal of the American College of Nutrition* 13:658, 1994.

2. Behrman RE and others: *Nelson essentials of pediatrics,* ed 2, Philadelphia, 1994, WB Saunders.

3. Birch LL: Children's preferences for high-fat foods, *Nutrition Reviews* 50:249, 1992.

4. Birch LL and others: Effects of a nonenergy fat substitute on children's energy and macronutrient intake, *American Journal of Clinical Nutrition* 58:326, 1993.

5. Cary WB: The effectiveness of parent counseling in managing colic, *Pediatrics* 94:333, 1994.

6. Centers for Disease Control and Prevention: Hyponatremic seizures among infants fed with commercial bottled drinking water—Wisconsin, 1993, *Journal of the American Medical Association* 272:996, 1994.

7. Cross AT and others: Snacking patterns among 1,800 adults and children, *Journal of the American Dietetic Association* 94:1398, 1994.

8. Dietz WH: Critical periods in childhood for the development of obesity, *American Journal of Clinical Nutrition* 59:955, 1994.

9. Emmons L: Predisposing factors differentiating adolescent dieters and nondieters, *Journal of the American Dietetic Association* 94:725, 1994.

10. Guo SS and others: The predictive value of childhood body mass index values for overweight at age 35 years, *American Journal of Clinical Nutrition* 59:810, 1994.

11. Hendricks KM, Badruddin SM: Weaning recommendations: the scientific basis, *Nutrition Reviews* 50:125, 1992.

12. Kennedy E, Goldberg J: What are children eating? Implications for public policy, *Nutrition Reviews,* 53:111, 1995.

13. King C: Cow's milk intolerance, *Maternal and Child Health,* April 1995, p 125.

14. Klish WJ and others: Fluoride supplementation for children: interim policy recommendations, *Pediatrics* 95:777, 1995.

15. Leung AKC and others: Assessment of the child with failure to thrive, *American Family Physician* 48:1432, 1993.

16. Leung AKC, Robson MLM: The toddler

who does not eat, *American Family Physician* 49:1789, 1994.

17. Lloyd T and others: Calcium supplementation and bone mineral density in adolescent girls, *Journal of the American Medical Association* 270:841, 1993.

18. Loening-Baucke V: Management of chronic constipation in infants and toddlers, *American Family Physician* 49:397, 1994.

19. McDowell MA and others: Energy and macronutrient intakes of persons ages 2 months and over in the United States: Third National Health and Nutrition Examination Survey, Advanced Data No. 255, October 24, 1994.

20. Meyers A: Modern management of acute diarrhea and dehydration in children, *American Family Physician* 51:1103, 1995.

21. Nicklas TA and others: Dietary fiber intake of children and young adults: the Bogalusa Heart Study, *Journal of the American Dietetic Association* 95:209, 1995.

22. Nguyen QH and others: Management of acne vulgaris, *American Family Physician* 50:89, 1994.

23. Obarzanek E and others: Energy intake and physical activity in relation to indexes of body fat: the young girls National Heart, Lung, and Blood Institute Growth and Health Study, *American Journal of Clinical Nutrition* 60:15, 1994.

24. Oski FA: Iron deficiency in infancy and childhood, *New England Journal of Medicine* 329:190, 1993.

25. Pannell DV: Why school meals are high in fat and some suggested solutions, *American Journal of Clinical Nutrition* 61:245S, 1995.

26. Pipes PL: *Nutrition in infancy and childhood*, St Louis, 1993, Mosby.

27. Saunders TAB, Reddy S: Vegetarian diets and children, *American Journal of Clinical Nutrition* 59(suppl):1176S, 1994.

28. Schlicker SA and others: The weight and fitness status of United States children, *Nutrition Reviews* 52:11, 1994.

29. Sullivan SA, Birch LL: Infant dietary experi-ence and acceptance of solid foods, *Pediatrics* 93:271, 1994.

30. US Public Health Service: Cholesterol screening in children, *American Family Physician* 51:1923, 1995.

31. Virtanen SM and others: Diet, cow's milk protein antibodies and the risk of IDDM in Finnish children: Childhood Diabetes in Finland Study Group, *Diabetologia* 37:381, 1994.

32. White JW, Wolraich M: Effect of sugar on behavior and mental performance, *American Journal of Clinical Nutrition* 62:242S, 1995.

33. Writing Group for the DISC Collaborative Research Group: Efficacy and safety of lowering dietary intake of fat and cholesterol in children with elevated low-density lipoprotein cholesterol, *Journal of the American Medical Association* 273:1429, 1995.

34. Working Group on Cow's Milk Protein and Diabetes Mellitus: Infant feeding practices and their possible relationship to the etiology of diabetes mellitus, *Pediatrics* 94:752, 1994.

TAKE ACTION

Getting young Bill to eat

Bill is 3 years old, and his mother is worried about his eating habits. He absolutely refuses to eat vegetables, meat, and dinner in general. Some days he eats very little food, although he wants to snack often. His mother discourages snacking because she thinks Bill should eat a formal lunch and dinner to get the nutrients he needs. Mealtime is a battle. Bill complains that his mother wants him to eat everything on his plate even though he isn't hungry. Each day he drinks 5 or 6 glasses of milk, the one food he really likes.

When his mother prepares dinner, she makes plenty of vegetables, boiling them until they are soft, hoping this will appeal to Bill. Bill's dad waits to eat his vegetables last, regularly telling his family that he eats them only because he has to. Bill saves his vegetables until last and usually gags when his mother orders him to eat them. Bill has been known to sit at the dinner table for an hour until the war of wills ends. Bill's mother serves casseroles and stews regularly because these are her best dishes. Bill likes to eat breakfast cereals, fruit, and cheese and regularly asks for these foods as snacks. However, his mother tries to deny his requests so he will have an appetite for dinner.

Analysis

1. List four mistakes Bill's parents are making that contribute to his poor eating habits.

_____

_____

_____

2. List four strategies they might try to promote good eating habits in Bill.

_____

_____

_____

Food Allergies and Intolerances

A dverse reactions to foods—indicated by sneezing, coughing, nausea, vomiting, diarrhea, hives, and other rashes—are broadly classed as food allergies (also called hypersensitivities) or **food intolerances.** Allergies involve responses of the immune system designed to eliminate foreign proteins, called **allergens.** The symptoms experienced by susceptible people, such as rapid increase in heart rate and shortness of breath, are the result of this battle. In contrast, the signs and symptoms of food intolerances do not result from a true allergic reaction. Rather, food intolerances are caused by an individual's inability to digest certain food components or by the direct effect of a food component or contaminant on the body. Let's examine each process, first allergies and then intolerances, so you can learn how to reduce the risk of becoming a victim of the food you eat.

Food Allergies: Symptoms and Mechanism

Allergic reactions to foods are quite common and occur more frequently in females than males. The incidence of food allergies is highest during infancy and young adulthood. Experts estimate that about 2% of adults and from 2% to 8% of children are allergic to certain foods. Three types of reactions may occur following ingestion of problem foods by susceptible people:
- *Classic*—itching, reddening skin, asthma, swelling, choking, and a runny nose
- *Gastrointestinal*—nausea, vomiting, diarrhea, intestinal gas, bloating, pain, constipation, and indigestion
- *General*—headache, skin reactions, tension and fatigue, tremors, and psychological problems

Any reaction that is milder than these distinct allergic ones is referred to as a **food sensitivity.**[2]

Allergic reactions vary not only in the body system affected but also in their duration, ranging from seconds to a few days. A generalized, all-systems reaction is called **anaphylactic shock.** This severe allergic response results in lowered blood pressure and respiratory and gastrointestinal distress. It can be fatal. A person who is extremely sensitive to a food may not be able to touch the food or even be in the same room where it is being cooked without responding to it. Although any food can trigger anaphylactic shock, peanuts, tree nuts (walnuts, pecans, etc.), shellfish, milk, eggs, soybeans, wheat, and fish are the most common culprits. For a small number of people, avoiding foods like peanuts or shellfish is a matter of life and death.[2]

About 95% of food allergies are caused by milk, eggs, nuts (especially peanuts), seafood, soy products, and wheat. Other foods frequently identified with adverse reactions include meat and meat products, corn, fruits, and cheese. These foods contain acidlike proteins, usually with a molecular weight between about 18,000 and 40,000, that stimulate production of IgE immunoglobulins in susceptible people. As we discussed in the Nutrition Perspective in Chapter 15, the immune response to many foreign proteins (antigens) involves production of IgG antibodies belonging to the G class of immunoglobulins. Normally, production of IgE antibodies is quite low except in response to parasitic infections.

The signs and symptoms of food allergies result from overproduction of IgE antibody following exposure to an allergen. When a susceptible person is exposed to an allergen for the first time, specific antibodies of the IgE class are formed. These attach to specialized cells, called **mast cells,** which are located primarily in the GI tract. No allergic reaction occurs as the result of this initial encounter. However, if the person is exposed to the same allergen subsequently, the allergen binds to its specific IgE antibodies on mast cells. This association triggers a series of events within a mast cell leading to release of **histamine,** serotonin, and other chemical factors. These factors then cause the signs and symptoms associated with an allergy. Histamine, for example, interacts with receptors on various target cells, causing contraction of smooth muscle, increased permeability and relaxation of blood vessels, nasal secretions, itching, and changes in dilation of the airways.

food intolerance An adverse reaction to food that does not involve an allergic reaction.

allergen A foreign protein, or antigen, that induces excess production of IgE antibodies; subsequent exposure to the same protein leads to allergic symptoms. While all allergens are antigens, not all antigens are allergens.

food sensitivity A mild reaction to a substance in a food that might be expressed as slight itching or redness of the skin.

anaphylactic shock A severe allergic response that results in lowered blood pressure and respiratory and GI tract disorders. It can be fatal.

mast cells Cells that contain histamine and are responsible for some aspects of allergic and inflammatory reactions.

histamine A small mediating chemical produced by mast cells that causes a variety of effects on the body, including contraction of smooth muscles, increased nasal secretions, relaxation of blood vessels, and changes in relaxation of airways.

We noted in Chapter 6 that food proteins are normally degraded in the intestinal system into amino acids, which are then transported across the wall of the GI tract (see Figure 6-12). Although derived from foreign proteins, absorbed amino acids cause no adverse reactions and are metabolized by the body. To trigger an allergic reaction, a food protein must instead cross the intestinal wall intact and interact with the immune system.

You might well ask how allergens can do this given the effectiveness of the body's digestive system. Various evidence indicates that large protein particles can gain access to the immune system by passing through gaps between intestinal cells and then entering the lymph system or capillaries. Eventually these particles are transported via the bloodstream to various body sites, where they can trigger an allergic reaction, as occurs when they bind to IgE antibodies on mast cells. Interestingly, people with food allergies appear to be somewhat deficient in production of IgA antibodies by cells associated with mucous membranes, including the intestinal lining. IgA antibodies are particularly important in preventing bacteria and viruses from invading the body through mucous membranes, but they also hamper passage of intact allergens across these membranes.

Testing for a Food Allergy

Diagnosis of a food allergy can often be a difficult task. It requires the advice of a skilled physician. The first step in determining whether a food allergy is present is to record in detail a history of symptoms, time from ingestion to onset of symptoms, most recent reaction, quantity and nature of food needed to produce a reaction, and the food suspected of causing a reaction. A family history of allergic diseases can also help, as allergic reactions tend to run in families. A physical examination may reveal evidence of an allergy, such as inflammation in the nasal cavity, skin diseases, and asthma; various diagnostic tests can rule out other conditions (Table 17-8).[2]

Perhaps the best laboratory test for determining which compounds a person is allergic to is the RAST test. This test estimates the blood concentration of IgE that binds certain food-borne antigens. Skin tests can also be used; a drop of antigen is placed on the skin where it has been scratched or punctured. If a person is allergic to the test antigen, a red eruption will develop.

TABLE 17-8

Assessment strategies for food allergies	
History:	Includes description of symptoms, time between food ingestion and onset of symptoms, duration of symptoms, most recent allergic episode, quantity of food required to produce reaction, suspected foods, and allergic diseases in other family members
Physical examination:	Look for signs of an allergic reaction (rash, itching, intestinal bloating, etc.)
RAST test:	Determine presence of IgE antibodies in blood that bind to antigens tested
Elimination diet:	Establish a diet lacking the suspected offending foods and stay on it for 1 to 2 weeks or until symptoms clear
Food challenge:	Add back small amounts of excluded foods one at a time, as long as anaphylactic shock is not a possible consequence

elimination diet A restrictive diet that systematically tests foods that may cause an allergic response by first eliminating them for 1 to 2 weeks and then adding them back one at a time.

cytotoxic test An unreliable test to define food allergies that involves mixing whole blood with food proteins.

CRITICAL THINKING

Irene and Chris had a baby 11 months ago. At the last check-up, the doctor told them to start feeding the baby some new solid foods. After 5 days of eating a new food, the baby woke up with a runny nose and vomiting. The doctor told them to stop giving the baby that particular food. How can the doctor justify his recommendations?

The American Academy of Allergy and Immunology has a 24-hour toll-free hotline (800-822-2762) to answer questions about food allergies and to help direct people to specialists who treat the problem.

---

prognosis A forecast of the course and end of a disease.

The next step is to eliminate from the diet for 1 to 2 weeks all tested compounds that appear to cause allergic symptoms, plus all other foods suspected of causing an allergy based on the person's food history.[13] The person generally starts out eating foods to which almost no one reacts, such as rice, vegetables, non-citrus fruits, and fresh meats and poultry. If symptoms are still present, the person can more severely restrict the diet or even use special formula diets that are hypoallergenic.

Once a diet is found that causes no symptoms, called an **elimination diet,** foods that are known not to trigger anaphylactic shock can be added back one at a time. Doses of 1/2 to 1 teaspoon (2.5 to 5 ml) are given at first. The amount is increased until the dose approximates usual intake. This should be done using a double-blind approach (see Nutrition Perspective in Chapter 1), especially when there is a psychological component to the reaction or when symptoms are vague or ill-defined. Dried foods can be encapsulated and then given to the person. Any reintroduced food that causes symptoms to significantly appear is identified as an allergen for the person.[2]

A bogus method to test for food allergies is the **cytotoxic test.** In this case, food proteins are mixed with whole blood or serum, and then the number of white blood cells broken during the subsequent reaction between the proteins and the blood is counted. This method is quite unreliable in predicting food allergies. We recommend that anyone with a possible food allergy consult a physician-allergist, rather than rely on a pseudoscientific method such as cytotoxic testing.

Treatment of Food Allergies

Once potential allergens are identified, the best treatment is to avoid them, especially for people with zero tolerance. Careful reading of food labels is essential for many allergic people and advisable for all. A major challenge for the clinician treating a person with a food allergy is to make sure that what remains in the diet can still provide essential nutrients. The small food intake of children permits less leeway in removing offending foods that may contain numerous nutrients. A registered dietitian can help guide the diet-planning process to ensure that what remains of the food choices still meets nutrient needs, or to guide supplement use if that is necessary.

If an allergy-prone woman is pregnant or breastfeeding, she should avoid offending foods—like eggs and peanuts—because antigens can cross the placenta during pregnancy. Antigens will also be secreted in her milk. She should work with her physician and registered dietitian to make sure an adequate diet is still consumed. In addition, when food allergies run in the family, women are advised to breastfeed their infants exclusively for 6 months. Human milk contains factors that may play a role in maturation of the small intestine. Formula-fed infants, especially those on formulas based on cow's milk, have a greater risk for developing allergies. Breastfeeding thus should continue for as long as possible, preferably to 1 year.[13]

The **prognosis** for food allergies that first appear before 3 years of age is good. About 80% of young children with food allergies outgrow them within 3 years. Parents should be made aware of this and certainly not assume the allergy will necessarily be long-lived. Food allergies diagnosed after 3 years of age, however, are often more long-lived, but not always. In these cases about 33% of people outgrow their food allergies within 3 years. For others, the condition may be prolonged; some food allergies can last a lifetime. Periodic reintroduction of offending foods can be tried every 6 to 12 months or so to see whether the allergic reaction has decreased.[2] If no symptoms appear, tolerance to the food has developed.

Food Intolerances

Food intolerances are adverse reactions to food that do not involve allergic mechanisms. Generally, larger amounts of an offending food are required to produce symptoms of an intolerance than to trigger allergic symptoms. Common causes of food intolerances include the following:

• Constituents of certain foods (e.g., red wine, tomatoes, pineapples) that have a druglike activity, causing physiological effects, such as changes in blood pressure

- Certain synthetic compounds added to foods, such as sulfites, food-coloring agents, and monosodium glutamate (MSG)
- Food contaminants, including antibiotics and other chemicals used in the production of livestock and crops, as well as insect parts not removed during processing
- Toxic contaminants resulting from ingestion of improperly handled and prepared foods containing *Clostridium botulinum, Salmonella* bacteria, or other food-borne microbes (see Chapter 19)
- Deficiencies in digestive enzymes, such as lactase (see Nutrition Focus in Chapter 3)

Nearly everyone is sensitive to one or more of these causes of food intolerance, many of which produce GI tract symptoms.

Sulfites, which are added to foods and beverages as antioxidants, cause flushing, spasms of the airways, and a loss of blood pressure in susceptible people. Wine, dehydrated potatoes, dried fruits, gravy, soup mixes, and restaurant salad greens commonly contain sulfites. A reaction to MSG may include an increase in blood pressure, numbness, sweating, vomiting, headache, and facial pressure. MSG is commonly found in Chinese food and many processed foods (e.g., soups). A reaction to tartrazine, a food-coloring additive, includes spasm of the airways, itching, and reddening skin. Tyramine, a derivative of the amino acid tyrosine, is commonly found in "aged" foods, such as cheeses and red wines. This natural food constituent can cause high blood pressure in people taking monoamine-oxidase inhibitor medications, which may be prescribed for mental depression.

The basic treatment for food intolerances is to avoid specific offending components. However, total elimination often is not required because people generally are not as sensitive to compounds causing food intolerances as they would be to allergens. For instance, a slight amount of sulfites in a glass of wine may be tolerable, whereas a large amount from a chef's salad may cause a reaction.

Chapter 19, on food safety, covers food-borne illness resulting from bacterial contamination of foods and presents additional information on natural food constituents and additives that can cause adverse reactions.

Food Additives and Hyperactivity in Children: A Possible Link?

In 1973, Dr. Benjamin Feingold suggested that food additives could cause hyperactivity in some children. This condition is now considered part of the attention-deficit hyperactivity disorder (ADHD). Feingold theorized that children who are allergic to aspirin-like medications would also be allergic to certain food additives that have aspirin-like chemical structures. Although this proposal stimulated much research, the results generally have not supported a strong or predictable association between the consumption of food additives and hyperactivity in children.

Today ADHD is seen in up to 9% of school-age children; boys are affected four to six times more frequently than are girls. The initial identification of hyperactive children commonly occurs when they enter nursery or elementary school. Teachers report that these students are uncontrollable, easily distracted, and unable to sit still; fail to finish assignments; act impulsively; bother other children; and, especially, intrude into other children's activities. Psychological testing can be used to further characterize the behaviors and reasons behind them.[2]

Not only is the diagnosis of ADHD surrounded by some controversy, but research on the association between diet and hyperactive behavior is also confounded by many pitfalls. For example, when parents give a hyperactive child a special additive-free diet, they are likely to pay more attention to the child and his behavior. If the child's disruptive behavior subsequently decreases, it's unclear whether the diet or the extra attention or the combination should get the credit. In addition, an additive-free diet is likely to be more nutrient rich than a typical diet for children because it contains more whole foods and fewer processed foods. Again, it is difficult to know whether behavior changes in a hyperactive child on such a diet result from eliminating additives or adding more nutrients.

The only definitive way to study this relationship is to use a double-blind protocol. A child would be given an additive-free food and then later a food full of additives. Neither the parents, the child, nor the researchers should know what is in the food. After the child has consumed the foods, the researchers score the child's behavior.

This procedure is much too cumbersome to be used in a school system or by a private pediatrician. Thus many suspected cases of food additive–linked hyperactivity are not tested in a definitive scientific manner. This is a real problem because diets used for hyperactive children may eliminate more than just food additives. Some popular approaches eliminate nutrient-rich foods, such as milk, fruits, and some grain products. The more limited the diet, the greater the risk of nutrient deficiencies and poor growth.

If an additive-free diet follows the Food Guide Pyramid and actually improves a child's attention span and behavior, there is no reason not to employ it. Eliminating food colors from the diet has no harmful effect as such. However, a physician should agree that special diet restrictions are worth trying. Even then, diet changes must be handled carefully. In addition, a child should not be singled out as different from his or her peers and shouldn't end up feeling deprived as a result of dietary restrictions. Finally, a hyperactive child should not be encouraged in the belief that diet completely determines his or her behavior. A child's attitudes, feelings, and personality traits all influence behavior. Parents who look for excuses for a child's behavior may often find it easiest to blame inappropriate behavior on something concrete, like food.

Will anything actually help the hyperactive child? Time is a very important therapy; hyperactivity may decrease as a child matures, but it can also linger through adulthood. When hyperactivity contributes to true ADHD, behavior therapies (especially to reinforce structure in the child's life), frequent opportunities for physical activity, and stimulant medications (Ritalin, for example) can be used to treat the problem. The advice of a pediatrician skilled in the diagnosis and treatment of this disease should be sought.[2]

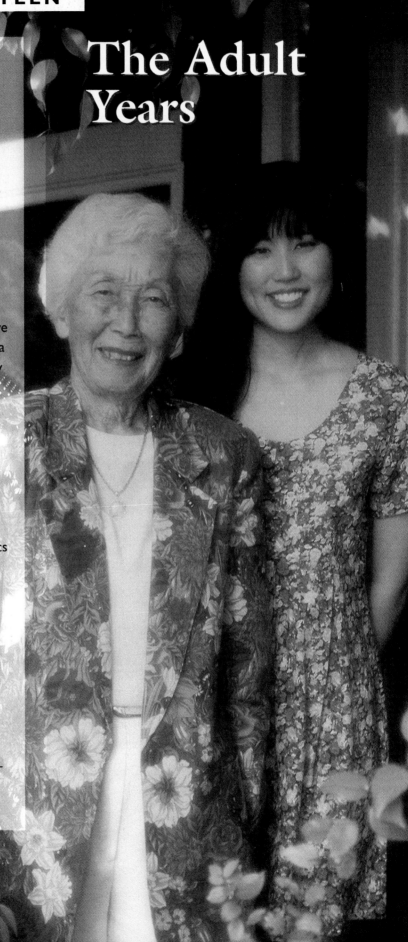

CHAPTER EIGHTEEN

The Adult Years

E ating is one of our great pleasures. Guided by common sense and moderation, eating well is also a means to good health. Most of us want a long, productive life, free of illness. Yet many people from early middle age onward suffer heart disease, strokes, diabetes, osteoporosis, or other chronic disease. We can slow the development of, and in some cases even prevent, these diseases by pursuing a diet that works against them.[27] This action is most profitable if begun early and continued throughout adulthood. We serve ourselves best, as individuals and as a nation, by striving to maintain vitality even in the later decades of life.[33] This concept was first explored in Chapters 1 and 2. We discuss it again in this chapter as we address the special nutritional needs of elderly people.

Your current day-to-day health practices can significantly influence your future health. Although genetics does play a role, many health problems that occur with age are not inevitable; they result from disease processes. Much can be learned from healthy elderly people whose attention to diet and physical activity, along with a little luck, keeps them active and vibrant.[25] Thus, as we noted in the Nutrition Focus in Chapter 2, successful aging should be the goal. Age quickly or slowly—it is partly your choice.

NUTRITION AWARENESS INVENTORY

NUTRITION AWARENESS

Answer these 15 statements about nutrition for adults and the elderly to test your current knowledge. If you think the answer is true or mostly true, circle T. If you think the answer is false or mostly false, circle F. Use the scoring key at the end of the book to compute your total score. Repeat this test after you have read this chapter, and compare your results.

1. **T F** The maximum age at which people die has increased dramatically in the last century.
2. **T F** Adults should aim to spend at least 30 minutes in moderate physical activity each day.
3. **T F** Medication taken by the elderly can cause nutritional problems.
4. **T F** The greatest nutritional problem for many Americans is overeating.
5. **T F** The health-care needs of people over age 65 account for more than half the health-care costs in the United States.
6. **T F** Optimal diets can stop the aging process.
7. **T F** The senses of taste and smell usually increase with age.
8. **T F** Older people often lose their desire for liquids.
9. **T F** Vitamin B-12 absorption often decreases in elderly people.
10. **T F** The most frequent intestinal problem in the elderly is constipation.
11. **T F** Excessive intake of vitamin A supplements can cause bone pain and hair loss in the elderly.
12. **T F** Delayed wound healing should alert a clinician to examine the protein, zinc, and vitamin C intakes of an elderly person.
13. **T F** An active lifestyle helps to maintain muscle and bone mass.
14. **T F** Dietary recommendations made by the American Heart Association could, if followed, substantially reduce serum cholesterol in everyone.
15. **T F** People over 65 years of age are quite similar in physical capabilities.

Adulthood

life expectancy The average length of life for a given group of people.

compression of morbidity Delaying the onset of disabilities caused by chronic disease.

Although most of us wish for long life, we do not like the thought of failing health in old age. And rightly so! A long life can be enjoyable if it is productive and relatively free of illness. Rather than suffer the ravages of heart disease, obesity, strokes, diabetes, osteoporosis, and other chronic diseases from age 40 or 60 years until death, we should strive to be as free of disease as possible and enjoy vitality throughout even our last decade. The focus here is not necessarily on living longer, but on living healthier. **Life expectancy** is at a record high of 75.8 years for the general population in the United States today, although the span of healthy life is only 64 years. Many people spend the majority of these years in a healthy, productive body—what better goal to have?

Striving to have the greatest number of healthy years and the fewest years of illness is often referred to as **compression of morbidity**.[25] In other words, a person tries to compress significant sickness related to aging into the last few years—or months—of life. An example of this concept is illustrated for heart disease in Figure 18-1. Of the three lines shown, the line on the left depicts rapid deterioration in health; symptoms of heart disease appear by about age 40, and death occurs at about age 60. In addition, between the ages of 40 and 60 years, symptoms of heart disease, and therefore disability, are present.

A healthier lifestyle follows the middle line. Here, heart disease is postponed so that the first symptoms are not apparent until age 60; severe symptoms occur at age 80, with death following a few years later. The line on the right is ideal. Disease progresses so slowly that symptoms do not appear during a person's lifetime; therefore the disease process never hampers activities.

Aging is a natural process; body cells age no matter what health practices we follow. But to a considerable extent you can choose how quickly you age throughout your adult years (Table 18-1). In light of the many studies showing the ability even to reverse atherosclerosis, we can say that the rate at which you age is partly your choice.

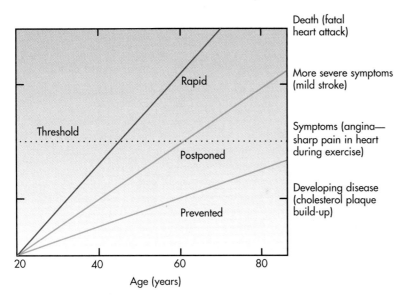

Figure 18-1 Compression of morbidity. The goal is to postpone illness until the final days of life. Heart disease is used as an example. The line on the left shows rapid deterioration in health status, in which symptoms of heart disease appear by about age 40 and death occurs at about age 60. In addition, between the ages of 40 and 60 years, symptoms of heart disease—and therefore disability—are present. A healthier lifestyle follows the middle line pattern. Here, heart disease is postponed so that the first symptoms are not apparent until age 60; severe symptoms occur at age 80, with death following a few years later. The line on the right is the ideal: the disease progresses so slowly that symptoms do not appear during the lifetime, and therefore the disease process never hampers life's activities.

Although there is little doubt of the benefits of a healthy lifestyle, scientists have also found a strong genetic component to longevity, as well as to certain diseases (see Chapter 1).[20] Studies of families, and of twins in particular, provide strong evidence for genetic control of human longevity. Identical twins tend to die at similar ages and of similar causes. Since identical twins have exactly the same genetic information, this implies that longevity is at least partially hereditary.

Still, many adults in America today are doing what is within their control to achieve a healthy lifestyle, such as a healthful diet and a regimen of regular physical activity. Coupled with avoidance of tobacco products, limitation of or other adaptation to stress, adequate sleep, adequate fluid intake, and consultation of health-care professionals on a regular basis, these actions contribute to a healthful, long life.[33]

Overall, the key to maximizing health throughout life is to establish harmony between the physical, mental, psychological, and social states. There is no general formula for this ideal; each of us must juggle and balance personal goals with opportunities and obstacles encountered. In addition, people who practice health promotion and disease prevention may not necessarily live longer—because of heredity, accidents, or other things outside of their control—but they probably live healthier lives. Thus the quality of the life lived is enhanced.

A DIET FOR THE ADULT YEARS

One diet approach that optimizes long-term nutritional health emphasizes low-fat and nonfat dairy products, some lean meats, plant proteins, a rich variety of fruits and vegetables, and generous amounts of whole-grain breads and cereals. The Food Guide Pyramid in Chapter 2 is a blueprint for this diet.[33]

To further refine these food choices, recall also from Chapter 2 the latest Dietary Guidelines issued by the USDA/DHHS. The U.S. Surgeon General, the American Heart Association, the American Dietetic Association, the American Medical Association, the National Cancer Institute, the National Academy of Sciences, and the World Health Organization have added recommendations to the framework of the

Nutrition expert **Dr. Irwin Rosenberg** recently provided his "bottom line" for a healthy lifestyle: "Research has shown no better way to slow or even reverse the progress of aging itself and of all the age-related degenerative conditions than through the combination of aerobic and strength-building exercise and a balanced, nutritious diet."[27]

TABLE 18-1

What to expect from adequate nutrition and good health habits

Diet

Eating enough essential nutrients and meeting energy needs help prevent:
  Birth defects and low birthweight in pregnancy
  Stunted growth and poor resistance to disease in infancy and childhood
  Poor resistance to disease in adulthood
  Deficiency diseases, such as cretinism (lack of iodide), scurvy (lack of vitamin C), and anemia (lack of iron, folate, or other nutrients)
Eating enough calcium helps:
  Build bone mass in childhood and adolescence
  Prevent some adult bone loss, especially in elderly years
Obtaining adequate intake of fluoride and minimizing sugar intake helps prevent:
  Dental caries
Eating enough dietary fiber helps prevent:
  Digestive problems, such as constipation, and likely some forms of intestinal cancer
Eating enough vitamin A and carotenoids may help reduce:
  Susceptibility to some cancers
  Degeneration of the retina (intake of carotenoids specifically)
Moderating energy intake helps prevent:
  Obesity and related diseases, such as diabetes, hypertension, cancer, and premature heart disease
Limiting intake of sodium helps prevent:
  Hypertension and related diseases of the heart and kidney in susceptible people
Moderating intake of saturated fat helps prevent:
  Premature heart disease
Moderating intake of essential nutrients by using vitamin and mineral supplements wisely, if at all, prevents:
  Most chances for nutrient toxicities

Physical activity

Adequate, regular physical activity helps prevent:
  Obesity
  The major form of diabetes (NIDDM)
  Premature heart disease
  Some adult bone loss
  Loss of muscle tone

Lifestyle

Minimizing alcohol intake helps prevent:
  Liver disease
  Fetal alcohol syndrome
  Accidents
Not smoking helps prevent:
  Lung cancer and other lung disease

In addition, minimum use of medication, no illicit drug use, adequate sleep, adequate fluid intake, and limiting stress provide a more complete approach to good nutrition and health.

Dietary Guidelines.[33] Following is a summary of the advice provided by these Dietary Guidelines, with additional comments from various health-related organizations.

1. **Eat a variety of foods.** Most groups specifically suggest variety and moderation in food choices. In addition, limit protein intake to no more than twice the RDA and do not take nutrient supplements in quantities greater than 150% of the Daily Values listed on the label in any one day. Everyone should also at least meet the RDA for calcium, especially women.

2. **Balance the food you eat with physical activity; maintain or improve your weight.** Use the middle ranges of the Metropolitan Life Insurance Table as a standard or use a Body Mass Index (BMI) of 20 to 25 for ages under 35, and 21 to 27 for ages over 35 (see Chapter 8). Note, however, that some researchers advocate the lower BMI range for all adults, recommending against weight gain during aging. Nevertheless, it is important to balance food intake with regular physical activity to avoid substantial weight gain in adulthood that can lead to obesity.[33]

   For those trying to lose weight, the recommended rate of weight loss is 1 to 2 pounds a week once an interval of weight maintenance has been demonstrated (see Chapter 9). To do this, increase physical activity and eat low-fat, nutrient-rich foods: more fruits, vegetables, and grains; less sugar and fewer alcoholic beverages.

3. **Choose a diet with plenty of grain products, vegetables, and fruits.** Choose at least five or more servings of vegetables and fruits daily. This recommendation enjoys the most overwhelming support of nutrition experts.[35] Add to that six or more servings of a combination of bread, cereals, rice, and pasta daily, many of which are whole-grain varieties. These food choices should meet the goal of 20 to 30 g of dietary fiber per day. The current U.S. average for dietary fiber intake is closer to 16 g/day.

   Since there are several kinds of dietary fiber, each with a different chemical structure and biological effect, it's best to include a variety of fiber-rich foods (see Chapter 3 for details).

4. **Choose a diet low in fat, saturated fat, and cholesterol.** Limit fat intake to 20% to 30% of total energy intake and saturated fat to no more than one third of total fat intake ($\leq$ 10% of total energy intake). A common dietary cholesterol limit is 200 to 300 mg/day.[33] (The average American consumes 12% of total energy as saturated fat and about 300 mg of cholesterol per day.) Choose lean meat, fish, poultry, and dry beans and peas as protein sources; use nonfat or low-fat milk and milk products; limit eggs to 3-4 per week; limit intake of dairy fats, hydrogenated fats, and other fats and oils high in saturated fat; trim fat off meats; broil, bake, or boil instead of frying; and aim for moderate or scant consumption of breaded or deep-fried foods.

5. **Choose a diet moderate in sugars.** Some authorities recommend that simple sugars supply no more than 10% to 15% of total energy intake. As noted in Chapter 3, 15% of energy intake corresponds to about 75 g of simple sugars per day, or about 15 teaspoons. American adults eat about 80 g of simple sugars daily. This 80 g is made up mostly of simple sugars added during food processing and cooking. This total intake of sugars corresponds to about 18% of total energy intake.

6. **Choose a diet moderate in salt and sodium.** Limit sodium intake to 2.4 to 3 g per day. This is the amount of sodium contained in 6 g (3 teaspoons) of salt (40% of salt is sodium). To do this, especially limit the amount of salt in cooking and avoid adding it to food at the table. In addition, only very small amounts of salty, highly processed, salt-preserved, and salt-pickled foods should be eaten. The average person eats 4 to 7 g of sodium per day. A sodium restriction of 2.4 to 3 g/day requires a great change in food habits for many of us. It means not eating processed (lunch) meats, salted snack foods, most canned and prepared soups, most types of cheese, and many tomato-based processed foods on more than an occasional basis.

Appendix E reviews diet planning guidelines issued by the Canadian government for Canadians.

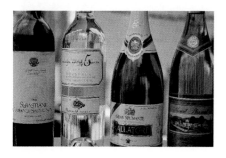

Alcoholic beverages are high in food energy and low in or devoid of essential nutrients.

7. **If you drink alcoholic beverages, do so in moderation.** A moderate alcohol intake consists of 2 or fewer servings of 12 ounces of beer, 5 ounces of wine, or 1½ ounces of distilled spirits (80 proof) per day. Women are advised to strive for no more than 1 serving a day, as they are more sensitive than men to alcohol-related cirrhosis of the liver. If you are concerned about excess energy intake and want a nutritious diet, keep in mind that alcoholic beverages are energy-rich and low in or devoid of essential nutrients.

Beyond these overall recommendations, aim for moderate use of salt-cured, smoked, and nitrate-cured foods because they likely increase the risk of certain forms of cancer. Obtain adequate fluoride to promote dental health. Finally, women of childbearing age especially need to eat iron-rich foods, primarily to avoid developing iron-deficiency anemia.

This group of guidelines provides a good general focus for diet planning. The practices recommended can accommodate many cultural dietary patterns, as we show in the Nutrition Perspective. They are broad enough to allow you to include all the foods you enjoy in an eating plan—you just may have to eat some foods less frequently than others and/or in smaller portions, depending on your health needs and preferences. Moderation, rather than elimination, is the overriding consideration with food choice.

ARE ADULTS FOLLOWING THESE DIET RECOMMENDATIONS?

In general, American adults, both young and old, are trying to follow many of the diet recommendations listed. Since the mid-1950s we have consumed less saturated fat as more people substitute nonfat and low-fat milk for cream and whole milk. We eat more cheese, however, which is usually a concentrated form of saturated fat. Since 1963 we have eaten less butter, fewer eggs, less animal fat, and more vegetable fats and oils and fish. These changes generally follow the recommendations to reduce the intake of saturated fat and cholesterol and instead emphasize unsaturated fat. Today, animal breeders are raising much leaner cattle and hogs than in 1950, which helps. Our demand for chicken, a relatively lean source of animal protein, has skyrocketed.

Other aspects of the average U.S. diet are more mixed. Nutrition surveys from the early 1980s (the most comprehensive to date) show that the major contributors of energy to the adult diet are white bread, rolls, and crackers; doughnuts, cakes, and cookies; alcoholic beverages; whole milk and beverages made with whole milk; and hamburgers, cheeseburgers, and meatloaf. If the trend in diets were truly toward decreasing alcohol, sugar, and saturated fat and increasing dietary fiber, these foods could hardly appear at the top of the list.

FRANK & ERNEST® by Bob Thaves

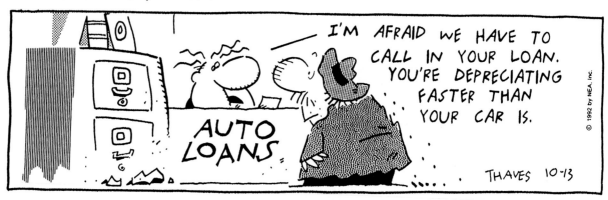

Figure 18-2 Frank & Ernest.

A list following our suggestions for improvement would stress low-fat and non-fat milk, whole-wheat bread and whole-grain cereals, lean meat and tuna, peanuts and kidney beans, and oranges and broccoli. What would your list look like?

Your task, as an adult, is to pinpoint your lifestyle practices most likely to cause illness and chronic disease and to change those specifically. You began that process in Chapter 1. Whether needed changes include switching to raisin bran cereal, rice, spinach pasta, fish, chicken, asparagus, and bok choy and walking every day is up to you. These practices all provide a means of promoting and maintaining nutritional and overall health.

A lifestyle that includes at least 30 minutes of moderate physical activity each day, combined with a sensible diet, can reduce the risk of premature development of almost all the chronic diseases adults face, including those that may develop in the elderly years.[19,24] To have physical activity significantly contribute to longevity, however, a recent study suggests that it must be fairly vigorous. This would include walking briskly at 4 to 5 mph for 45 minutes a day, 5 days a week. Jogging or playing tennis at least an hour 3 times a week also qualifies.[17]

The overriding consideration should be quality and length of life and the impact dietary changes might have on them (Figure 18-2). Now is the time to design and begin to practice this plan. Adulthood, and the sooner the better, is a key time to learn more about your risk factors for chronic diseases and do something about each one where possible.[27]

A NOTE OF CAUTION

Not all nutrition and health researchers agree with the blanket guidelines set by major health and science institutions, as noted in Chapter 2. Some scientists do not think that general recommendations for the public can be justified for sugar, sodium, and cholesterol. Rather, they believe these recommendations need to be individualized.

Although it can be argued that individualized dietary recommendations for such nutrients as sodium are best, that approach is too costly for the nation and therefore impractical. General recommendations can be made if they benefit most people while not hampering the health of others. Not all people will benefit equally from following the general recommendations—for example, a reduction in sodium intake—but no one will be harmed. The dietary change may cause some inconvenience, and perhaps for some people require new eating habits. Nevertheless, we should all consider the general dietary recommendations, personalizing the advice when possible under the guidance of our health-care advisors.[19]

HEALTH OBJECTIVES FOR THE UNITED STATES FOR THE YEAR 2000

Health promotion and disease prevention became a public health strategy in the United States in the late 1970s. One part of this strategy is *Healthy People 2000,* a report issued in 1990 by the U.S. Department of Health and Human Services' Public Health Service. This report consists of national health promotion and disease prevention objectives for the nation for the year 2000 and assigns each of the objectives to appropriate federal agencies to address.

Healthy People 2000's nutrition-related challenges address the following[18]:

- Iron-deficiency anemia (degree of progress currently unclear)
- Stunted growth in infants and children (progress is being made)
- High fat intake (progress is being made, especially by women)
- Obesity (we are currently losing this battle)
- Elevated LDL (progress is being made)
- High sodium intake (degree of progress currently unclear)
- Low calcium intake (mixed findings on progress to date)
- Low complex carbohydrate and dietary fiber intakes (no data on progress to date)
- The need for more home-delivered meals for elderly people (no data on progress to date)

CRITICAL THINKING

The "fountain of youth" remains a mystery. Many people believe a source exists that can stop the aging process, allowing youth to remain. However, Neil, a history student, asserts that the fountain of youth is not a place or a particular thing, but rather is a combination of diet and lifestyle. How can he justify this claim?

- A relative lack of breastfeeding, poor general nutrition knowledge, and the lack of nutrition education (mixed findings on progress to date)

The main objective of *Healthy People 2000* is to promote healthful lifestyles and reduce preventable death and disability in all Americans.

Concept Check

Compression of morbidity, delaying symptoms of and disabilities from chronic disease for as many years as possible, is a worthwhile goal. A basic plan to promote health and prevent disease includes eating a balanced, varied diet, performing regular physical activity, abstaining from smoking, limiting or abstaining from alcohol intake, and limiting or learning ways to deal with stress more effectively. More specific dietary guidelines direct people to eat a variety of foods; maintain healthy weight; choose a diet low in fat, saturated fat, and cholesterol; choose a diet with plenty of vegetables, fruits, and grain products; use sugars only in moderation; use salt and sodium only in moderation; and, if you drink alcoholic beverages, do so in moderation. Recommendations to pay particular attention to iron and calcium intake for women are also included, as well as warnings against abusing nutrient supplements. Some scientists believe that these guidelines do not necessarily constitute an individual "prescription." *Healthy People 2000* is a federal agenda aimed at disease prevention and health promotion for all Americans.

Nutrition in the Elderly Years

How long do your family members generally live? Of those who died early in adulthood, can you pinpoint some causes? Do you plan to live longer than your parents did or will? How long will that be? Some basic statistics can help you predict the latter.

LIFESPAN

lifespan The potential oldest age a person can reach.

Lifespan refers to the maximal number of years humans live. As far as we know, this hasn't changed much in recorded time. The longest human life documented to date is 120 years.[25] In contrast, the domestic dog has a lifespan of 20 years, and a rat, 5 years.

LIFE EXPECTANCY

Life expectancy is the time an average person born in a specific year, such as 1995, can expect to live. Life expectancy in America is currently 71.1 years for men and 78.3 years for women. Worldwide, the highest average life expectancy is 82 years for women and 76 years for men in Japan. Researchers suggest that a diet based on rice, fish, vegetable protein sources, and limited meat contributes to this record longevity.[7]

Life expectancy hasn't always been this long; for primitive humans it was about 30 to 35 years. It increased to 49 years in medieval England and remained so until the turn of this century. During the last 80 years, life expectancy for nearly all people has increased, mainly because of changes in the principal causes of death.

At the turn of this century, infectious diseases such as pneumonia, influenza, and tuberculosis commonly caused death. Vaccines and antibiotics have tremendously lowered rates of death from disease. The decline in infant and childhood deaths, coupled with better diets and health care, has allowed more people to age first into maturity and then into elderly years. Now the principal causes of death in Western societies are related to heart disease and cancer (Table 18-2).[33]

Historically, the trend in America has been toward an ever-older population. During colonial times, half the population was over 16 years of age. By 1990, half was over 33. By 2050, half could be over 43, and approximately 20% of the entire U.S. population will be 65 years and older, twice as many as reach 65 years today

> Although life expectancy has increased since 1900, the maximum lifespan of a human hasn't changed much throughout recorded time.

TABLE 18-2

Changes in leading causes of death during this century in the United States

Chronic diseases, rather than infectious diseases, are now the major killers.

Rank	Cause of death	Percentage mortality*
1900		
1	Pneumonia and influenza	12
2	Tuberculosis	11
3	Diarrhea and enteritis	8
4	Heart disease	8
5	Cerebrovascular disease (stroke)	6
6	Nephritis	5
7	Accidents	4
8	Cancer	4
9	Diphtheria	2
10	Meningitis	2
1992		
1	Heart disease	29
2	Cancer	26
3	Cerebrovascular disease (stroke)	5
4	Chronic obstructive pulmonary disease and allied conditions	4
5	Accidents and adverse effects†	6
	Motor vehicle accidents	3
	All other accidents and adverse effects	3
6	Pneumonia and influenza	3
7	Diabetes	2
8	Acquired immunodeficiency syndrome (AIDS)	2
9	Suicide	2
10	Homicide and legal intervention	2

*Percentage of all deaths in that year.
†3% for motor vehicle accidents; 3% for all other accidents.

(Figure 18-3). This age, 65 years old, is an arbitrary dividing line for the beginning of the elderly years because a person of that age can generally qualify for full retirement benefits. But the timing of the elderly years for each of us varies with health and independence. Some people are quite healthy and independent at age 65, whereas others are disabled and greatly dependent on assistance for activities of daily living.[12]

The group age 85+ years is the fastest growing segment of the older population. Given current mortality rates, 55 percent of girls and 35 percent of boys should live long enough to celebrate their 85th birthdays. Between 1986 and 2050, the population age 85+ years is expected to increase from about 1% to more than 5% of the total U.S. population. This is the first time in history our society will need to deal with such a large elderly population. The associated expense will be enormous if a large percentage need special care because of ill health.[25]

THE "GRAYING" OF AMERICA

The "graying" of America poses some problems. Today, while people older than 65 account for 13% of the U.S. population, they account for more than 25% of all prescription medication used, 40% of acute care hospital stays, and 50% of the federal health budget. More than 80% of elderly people have nutrition-related problems, such as heart problems, diabetes, hypertension, osteoporosis, and obesity (Table 18-3). Compression of morbidity, as suggested at the beginning of this chapter, is an important goal for controlling health-care costs in the future, since the increase

EXPERT OPINION

EXPERT OPINION

WHAT SHOULD I EAT TO LIVE LONGER?

DAVID M. KLURFELD, Ph.D.

The fountain of youth emanates, according to popular culture, from a proper diet. This rosy view stems, in part, from the dietary recommendations made to reduce the risk of chronic disease. Implicit in the recommendations is the promise of longer life—but how long and for whom?

Cardiovascular disease and cancer account for almost three fourths of all deaths in affluent societies. One reason is that many causes of premature death—infection, poor sanitation, and accidents—have been dramatically allayed. This change translates into a life expectancy at birth in the United States of about 76 years. At the same time more people are overweight and health-care costs are a greater percentage of the economy than in any other country, so we have lots of room for improvement.

In spite of our highly publicized "killer diet," deaths from heart disease, stroke, and cancer unrelated to tobacco have all declined markedly over the last 25 years. We don't know for sure why this drop oc-

curred, but it has been attributed, in part, to less use of tobacco and reductions in hypertension and serum cholesterol, along with better medical care. These changes in risk factors point to the multiple causes of both heart disease and cancer. In addition, since many environmental factors interact with genetic predisposition to disease, it is incorrect to attribute most of the risk for chronic disease to diet alone.

Many estimates of dietary contribution to the risk of cancer are made by default; that is, cancers that are not traceable to other risk factors are often lumped together as being caused by diet. The National Academy of Sciences' 1989 Report on Diet and Health concluded that "the data are not sufficient . . . to quantify the contribution of the diet to overall cancer risk or to determine the amount of reduction in risk that might be achieved by dietary modification." Nevertheless, this committee and others have proposed a low-fat, high-complex-carbohydrate diet to reduce cancer risk. They point out

that in Mediterranean countries death rates for diet-associated cancers are half those in the United States. But do these people live longer or enjoy better health? There is a conspicuous lack of good data to decide this. The only dietary change effective in reducing many types of cancer and increasing lifespan in animals is energy restriction. Reduction of energy intake, when all nutrient requirements are met, results in physiologically younger animals. We don't know why this works, nor whether it is effective in people.

Can we reduce cardiovascular disease by dietary means with some degree of certainty? Probably, according to epidemiologic and animal data. But epidemiology offers only leads; it cannot prove cause and effect. Today there's little controversy over increased risk of heart disease with elevated serum cholesterol. What is debated is at what point dietary or drug treatments should begin. And although the consensus recommendation is to reduce cholesterol below 200 mg/dl, some argue

in the elderly population alone will require more total health-care services. The more independent, healthy years we live, the less we burden our health-care system, which will have increasing difficulty accommodating a burgeoning elderly population.[25]

WHAT ACTUALLY IS AGING?

The process of aging is still a mystery. It is also difficult to design a model for it because so often disease speeds the process. But diseases that commonly accompany old age, osteoporosis and atherosclerosis, for example, are not an inevitable part of aging. Some people do just die of "old age," and not as a direct result of a chronic disease. In and of itself, aging is not a disease.

One view of aging describes it as processes of slow cell death beginning soon after fertilization. When we are young, aging is not apparent because the major meta-

that this is too modest a target, while others contend that it's an unnecessary one. Still, the slope of heart disease versus serum cholesterol is quite steep at concentrations over 250 mg/dl, but shallow near 210 mg/dl. So, much less benefit is derived from lowering average cholesterol values. However, some individuals showed regression of coronary disease when exercise was combined with very-low-fat (10%) diets. The Multiple Risk Factor Intervention Trial (MRFIT) data show the lowest mortality at average serum cholesterol values. These results, and those from most other studies, indicate that a reduction in high serum cholesterol is of benefit in preventing heart disease but not in prolonging life.

There's a strong statistical correlation of gross national product, telephones, flush toilets, and other signs of wealth with the incidence of cancer and heart disease because life expectancy is longer in more affluent countries. Chronic disease is much more common among older individ-

uals. Populations that can afford to eat a lot of fat, sugar, and salt do so because these three dietary components are what people think make food taste good. Americans have been told to follow a low-sodium diet even though only a minority are hypertensive and only some of those are salt sensitive. In addition, there is also substantial evidence implicating adequate potassium, calcium, and magnesium intake in controlling blood pressure, but this evidence often goes unreported.

A potential explanation for the lack of uniformity in response to dietary factors is that perhaps only some of the population shows elevated serum cholesterol from eating saturated fat and only some people are genetically predisposed to colon cancer, while a fortunate few are destined to live long, healthy lives no matter what rules they violate. This observation does not discount the importance of nutrition in longevity but suggests that recommendations for dietary modification should not be blanket public health policies. In-

stead dietary guidelines need to be made on an individualized basis— that is, for those who are at increased risk for specific diseases because of family history or the presence of other risk factors. This conclusion should not be taken to mean that diet is unimportant. A high rate of consumption of fruits, vegetables, and whole grains is associated with less obesity, intestinal disorders, heart disease, and cancer.

Reasoning that diet modification can't hurt may satisfy some, but it's certainly not scientific. The burden of proof should fall on those who suggest major dietary changes rather than on those who question the efficacy of those changes. Although what is written today will surely be outdated in the future, there are two nutritional rules that make sense over time: (1) eat a variety of foods, and (2) consume all foods in moderation. Boring, perhaps, but advice one can take to heart.

Dr. Klurfeld is Professor and Chairman of the Department of Nutrition and Food Science at Wayne State University.

bolic activities are geared toward growth and maturation. We produce plenty of active cells to meet physiological needs. During late adolescence and adulthood the body's major task is to maintain cells. But, inevitably, cells age and die. Eventually as more cells die the body cannot adjust to meet all physiological demands. Body functioning begins to decrease, but organs usually retain enough **reserve capacity** that the body shows no outward disease for a long time.[25] Although no symptoms appear, subclinical disease may develop, and if the disease is allowed to progress unchecked, organ function and then body function eventually deteriorate noticeably.

The aging process is clearly illustrated by changes that many people experience in the function of the enzyme lactase. For some people, lactase activity in the small intestine falls during childhood. Generally, however, clear symptoms of a significant decline in activity—gas and bloating after milk consumption—do not appear until adulthood.[12] Although lactase output decreases in these cases, generally be-

reserve capacity The extent to which an organ can preserve essentially normal function despite decreasing cell number or cell activity.

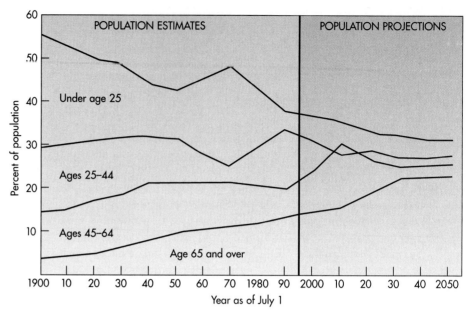

Figure 18-3 Trend in age distribution of U.S. population (including armed forces overseas), 1900 to 2050. The United States population has never before had so many elderly people.

TABLE 18-3

Selected diseases associated with aging				
	Rate of occurrence per 1000 people			
Chronic condition	**Total**	**45-64 years**	**65-74 years**	**75+ years**
Arthritis	131	280	460	508
Hypertension	124	265	408	395
Hearing impairment	91	149	261	381
Heart condition	83	137	291	339
Visual impairment	35	46	72	136
Deformities or ortho- pedic impairment	121	175	191	198
Diabetes	26	55	98	92
Diverticula of intestines	8	15	36	45
Asthma	37	32	47	26

ginning about 2 years of age, enough enzyme is produced to digest lactose until adulthood.

Cells age probably because of automatic cellular changes and environmental influences. Even in the most supportive of environments cell structure and function inevitably decline. Eventually, cells lose their ability to regenerate the internal parts they need, and they die.[25] As more and more cells in an organ system die, organ function decreases. After about age 14 months human brain cells are continually lost, but we have enough reserve capacity to maintain mental function throughout life. **Kidney nephrons** are also continually lost. In some people this loss leads to eventual kidney failure, but most of us maintain sufficient kidney function throughout life. Again, in aging, there is first a reduction in reserve capacity. Only after that is exhausted does actual organ function noticeably decrease.

kidney nephrons Units of kidney cells that filter wastes from the bloodstream.

HYPOTHESES ABOUT THE CAUSES OF AGING

Although the causes of aging remain a mystery, many hypotheses have been promoted to explain it[3]:

Errors occur in copying the genetic blueprint (DNA)—Some of these errors are spontaneous, while others arise from degradative processes induced by chemicals and radiation. Once sufficient errors in DNA copying accumulate, a cell can no longer synthesize the major proteins needed to function, and therefore it dies. There is a genetically determined ability to combat this type of damage.[25] Gene variants that give rise to unusually efficient resistance to damage could contribute to lifespan by slowing the rate at which cells experience lethal damage.

Mutations in mitochondrial DNA also may play a major role in aging. Mitochondrial DNA contains templates for synthesizing various compounds used in protein synthesis. This type of DNA has a much greater mutation rate than does nuclear DNA. A marked increase in mitochondrial DNA mutations has been demonstrated to occur in the human brain and heart with advancing age.[20]

Connective tissue stiffens—Parallel collagen protein strands, found mostly in connective tissue, chemically bond and crosslink to each other. The bonding decreases flexibility in key body components, altering organ function. Skin wrinkles and joints and arteries stiffen. The bonding may also restrict nutrients from entering cells.

Toxic products build up—Breakdown products of lipids called **lipofuscin** may act as intracellular sludge, hampering normal metabolic processes by clogging cells.

Electron-seeking compounds damage cell parts—Electron-seeking free radicals can break down cell membranes and proteins. One way to prevent some damage from these compounds is to consume adequate—not excessive—amounts of vitamins E and C, selenium, and carotenoids. In contrast, it's not effective to consume enzymes designed to break down the damaging compounds, such as **superoxide dismutase.** Ingested enzymes are themselves broken down during digestion before they can act in the body.[23] Despite that, some health food stores sell superoxide dismutase, as noted in Chapter 12.

Hormone function changes—The hormone known as dehydroepiandrosterone (DHEA), produced by adrenal glands (located on top of the kidneys), circulates at extremely high concentration in young adults and falls sharply after the age of 25. By age 70, DHEA concentration is 10% of what it was at age 25. This change has led to speculation that DHEA decline plays a role in aging. However, the physiological function of this steroid hormone is unclear, and long-term effects of using products containing this hormone are also unknown. Research is ongoing.[20] FDA has not approved use of DHEA, so marketing it to the public is illegal in the United States. Even if current research on DHEA produces promising results, it will be at least another year or two before it is ready for government evaluation. Then FDA approval could take years.

A fall in growth hormone concentration is also being investigated as a potentially treatable hormonal cause of aging. Growth hormone is secreted by the pituitary gland and stimulates protein synthesis in cells, such as muscle cells, as well as produces various other effects in the body. Replacing growth hormone has wide-ranging, unpredictable effects and is very costly. Studies so far support the hypothesis that growth hormone–related loss of lean body mass plays a role in aging. However, once treatment with growth hormone in adults is stopped, gains in lean body mass are lost. The risks and benefits of this treatment probably will be known within 2 or 3 years, but it could take another 5 to 10 years to determine the best dosage. Growth hormone therapy has also been associated with significant adverse effects that may limit its clinical usefulness in the elderly.[20] These include carpal tunnel syndrome and possibly hypertension and diabetes-like symptoms. FDA has not approved growth hormone treatment for prevention of the effects of aging. Growth hormone administered to older people with protein-energy undernutrition has demonstrated positive effects on nitrogen retention and suggests this approach may be useful in severely undernourished older people.

lipofuscin (ceroid pigments) Lipid breakdown products in cells. Those compounds have fluorescence, and in that way can be detected in aged cells, such as the eye, the heart, and the brain.

superoxide dismutase An enzyme that can quench (deactivate) a superoxide negative free radical ($\cdot O_2^-$).

Testosterone concentration declines with age. This decline in testosterone is linked to a decline in muscle strength. Animal studies have also suggested that testosterone may improve memory retention. These studies support the concept that a subgroup of older males may benefit from testosterone therapy. Postmenopausal women, especially those who have undergone surgical menopause, may also be candidates for testosterone therapy if estrogen therapy alone does not reduce related symptoms. Note that these are some side effects with use; treatment is still in the experimental phase.[14]

Finally, production of melatonin by the pineal gland (located in the center of the brain) declines after puberty. Melatonin is best known for its ability to induce sleep; laboratory animal studies suggest that it may also slow the aging process. FDA has not yet approved use of melatonin, but there is great interest in its use as a sleeping aid. It is not currently available in a pure form. The melatonin sold in health-food stores can be of questionable quality. Leading researchers note that little is known about the long-term effects of melatonin treatment on humans, but there is evidence that it reduces ovulation in women. Overall, it is premature to take melatonin preparations in the hope of slowing the aging process until it is shown to be safe and effective for this purpose.

The immune system loses some efficiency—The thymus gland (located in the upper chest) is a major component of the immune system, as noted in Chapter 15. During adolescence, the thymus gland reaches its maximal size, and by age 50 it is barely visible. The immune system itself runs a somewhat parallel course. It is most efficient during childhood and young adulthood, but with advancing age it is less able to recognize and counteract foreign substances, such as viruses, that enter the body. As we age, then, the immune system's ability to detect and destroy developing cancer cells decreases, allowing them to multiply autonomously.

Nutrient deficiencies, particularly of protein, vitamin B-6, and zinc, hamper immune function, in turn making matters worse for the aging body. Maintaining an adequate nutrient intake, especially in the elderly years, is crucial for immune function.[6,8]

Autoimmunity develops—**Autoimmune** reactions occur when white blood cells and other immune bodies fail to distinguish between substances normally present in the body and invading foreign antigens. White blood cells and other immune bodies then begin to attack body tissues in addition to foreign antigens. Many diseases, including some forms of diabetes and arthritis, involve this autoimmune response.

Death is programmed into the cell—Each human cell can divide only about 50 times. Once this number of divisions occurs, the cell automatically succumbs. This degradation occurs by design, likely as a way for the body to regulate cell number. Programmed cell death plays one of its most important roles in the maturation of cells used for immune function.

Glycosylation of proteins—Blood glucose, especially when chronically elevated—as occurs in poorly controlled diabetes—attaches to various blood and body proteins. This decreases protein function and can encourage immune system attack on such altered proteins.[20] Eventually cell health declines.

Most likely, aging results from an interaction of these events and changes. Even very healthy people have a shortened life expectancy if they are exposed to sufficient environmental stress, such as radiation and certain chemical agents, for example, industrial solvents. Because cell aging and diseases like cancer are aggravated by environmental factors, it makes good sense to avoid such risks as excessive sunlight exposure and hazardous chemicals. Again, as we have stressed, we have some control over how quickly we age.

CAN DIET STOP THE AGING PROCESS?

No diet can stop aging, but research shows that raising laboratory animals after weaning on low-energy diets—about two thirds the energy they normally con-

---

autoimmune Immune reactions against normal body cells; self against self.

- - - - - - - - - - - -

As the number of possible cell divisions increases, so does lifespan. The Galapagos tortoise, whose cells divide about 140 times, has a lifespan of perhaps 200 years.

- - - - - - - - - - - - -

sume—greatly slows aging. Animals on these lean rations live about 50% longer than control groups allowed to feed **ad libitum** (at their pleasure) and show much lower rates of cancer.[16] Scientists have found this to be true for mice, hamsters, spiders, fish, and mollusks, and are optimistic that it may work in monkeys. A study of this possibility is currently under way in monkeys.

ad libitum At one's desire or pleasure.

The key is to restrict only energy intake, not other nutrients. Humans living in semistarvation conditions do not live longer than typical Western World life expectancy; their diets are low in energy but also low in protein, many vitamins, and many minerals.

It is not clear how a low-energy diet increases the lifespan of animals. Hormonal or immune system changes may be involved. Less insulin release, for example, could reduce cell turnover, a factor associated with aging. Delaying puberty may also play a key role. Lessening DNA damage, leading to reduced activity of cancer-causing genes, is also suggested as a mechanism. The ability of cells to repair damaged DNA could also be affected by energy intake. It is clear that the animals grow more slowly, and this may affect their tendency to develop disease. Overall, it is likely that several of these mechanisms come into play when animals are underfed. Still other reasons for the longer life expectancy are possible.[16]

The extended life expectancies gained from reduced feeding may actually be equal to the natural lifespans of animals in the wild. Perhaps what we see in laboratory animals is an acceleration of the aging process caused by *ad libitum* diets (and so overfeeding). Might well-fed Western humans again look to long-lived rural people for the fountain of youth? However, severe energy restriction, especially for infants and young children, is dangerous. We must wait for further research before applying this idea to humans, especially because some processes of aging seen in rats and mice differ from those in humans. Even so, will people be willing to give up cheeseburgers and fries for lighter fare to have an unknown number of additional years of life? For many of us the deferred benefit of a longer, healthier life is overshadowed by the immediate pleasure of a high-fat diet.

Clearly, we should consider striking a balance between immediate gratification and a pleasant long-term future. It is not just longevity, but quality of life lived, that is worth serious consideration.

With regard to vitamins, some scientists suggest that adults each day should consume from 250 to 1000 mg of vitamin C; from 100 to 800 IU of vitamin E; and from 10 to 50 mg of beta carotene as a means of preventing chronic age-related disease.[34] However, as we noted in Chapter 12, agencies including FDA and the National Academy of Sciences say such a recommendation to the general public is premature, based on the available supporting evidence.

CONCEPT CHECK

While lifespan has not changed, life expectancy has increased dramatically over the past century. In many societies this means an increasing proportion of the population is, and will be, over 65 years of age. Sidestepping continually rising healthcare costs and maximizing satisfaction with life require postponing and minimizing chronic illness. Aging begins early in life and probably results from both automatic cellular changes and environmental influences. Some popular hypotheses of aging suggest these possible causes: errors in DNA replication accumulate, connective tissue stiffens, lipid by-products build up, electron-seeking free-radical compounds break down cell parts, hormonal and immune systems don't function well, and autoimmune responses and high blood glucose damage key body compounds. Diet can play a role in slowing some of these processes. Medical therapies to do so are also in experimental phases.

Effects of Aging on the Nutritional Status of Elderly People

Elderly people vary more in health status than do people in any other age group. This means that chronological age is not very useful in predicting physical health (physiological age).[12] Among people age 65 and over, some are totally independent, healthy people, whereas others are frail and require almost total care. To predict the nutritional problems of an elderly person, it is necessary to know the extent of physiological change caused by aging (Figure 18-4) and whether the person shows early warning signs and symptoms of long-term nutrient deficiency. As we examine how aging affects body systems and how these changes affect nutritional health, we suggest ways to lessen the health risks and parallel changes in diet to counteract problems.

DECREASED APPETITE AND FOOD INTAKE

Decreases in body weight are common in adults age 65 to 90, as they may not eat enough to meet energy needs. This poses a problem for the elderly because it increases the risk of nutrition-related illness, especially when the concentration of the serum protein albumin falls below about 4 g/100 ml. A more typical albumin concentration is about 4 to 5 mg/dl.

There are many possible causes of inadequate food intake in the elderly. Researchers suspect that biological origins, such as changes in the neuroendocrine factors that influence feeding, account for some of this (see Chapter 8 for a review of these factors). When older men are underfed in metabolic ward settings, they do not later increase food intake to compensate for reduced food consumption when given the opportunity.[26] Changes in taste and smell also may be important.[28] In addition, social aspects play a role in reduced food intake. Many elderly people live alone, which is associated with less food consumption than when eating with others.

Declining weight needs to be addressed if health is to be maintained in the elderly years.[21] Significant weight loss in elderly people, sometimes termed the "dwindles," increases risk of death. It may also indicate ongoing illness and reduced tolerance to medication, or simple withdrawal from life itself.

In any event the reason for weight loss needs to be investigated and, ideally, treated. When assessing weight in elderly people, it is a good practice to compare present weight with the previous year's weight.[12] A loss of 5% or more in a month

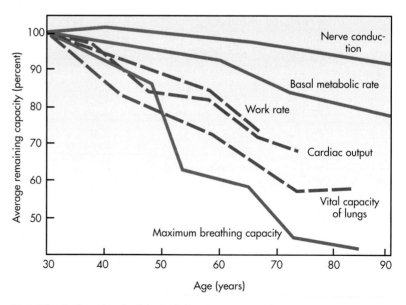

Figure 18-4 The declines in physiological function seen with aging. The decline in many body functions is seen primarily in sedentary people.

or 10% or more in 6 months indicates potential trouble. Even in apparently healthy older individuals, successful weight maintenance may require an increased conscious control over food intake relative to younger individuals.[26]

THE SENSES OF TASTE AND SMELL

Sensitivity to taste and smell often decreases with age. The loss begins around age 60 and becomes more pronounced after age 70. This results from effects of aging on the cells that sense taste and smell, as well as from use of certain medications and medical therapies.[28] Stronger seasonings may be required to make foods taste good; other foods may require equivalent nutrient substitution or changes in preparation if they no longer taste good. In the elderly an inadequate diet, most notably a zinc deficiency, can also contribute to a loss of taste. Therefore a change in taste or smell should never be dismissed simply as a characteristic of old age. Some causes can be remedied.

Variety in the diet helps compensate for the decrease in taste and smell.[28] Food companies also are filling a niche in the marketplace—using a variety of flavor enhancers they make foods tastier for elderly people.

DENTAL HEALTH

Total loss of teeth is common in 55% of those over age 85, in 44% of those age 75 to 84, and in 30% of those age 65 to 74.[10] Attention to dental hygiene and dental care throughout life greatly lessens this risk. Gum disease is also common and promotes tooth loss. Replacement dentures enable some to chew normally, but many elderly people, especially men, have denture problems. A puréed diet is not necessarily the remedy. Solving individual dietary needs requires identifying foods that need to be modified in consistency and those that can be eaten in a typical state. When people have problems chewing, nutrient-dense snacks like yogurt, bananas, and peanut butter can help. Sometimes just allowing extra time for chewing and swallowing encourages more eating.

THIRST

Elderly people often partially lose their sense of thirst, and in turn don't drink enough fluids. In addition, there is diminished activity of antidiuretic hormone and aldosterone. Total body water also falls with aging. Together these changes make elderly people more likely to become dehydrated, a condition that leads to confusion and sometimes to hospitalization.[10]

It is important for elderly people to consume enough fluids, and if necessary, they should be monitored to ensure they do so, especially when ill and during hot weather. An approximate fluid recommendation is the same as for younger adults, 1 ml/kcal expended. This works out to about 8 cups (2000 ml) of fluid daily. A glass of water at every meal provides a good start toward meeting fluid needs. The total amount of water needed must be adjusted if diuretics are used or fluid is lost through other routes, such as through an **ostomy** (a surgically created opening in the body). Some important signs of dehydration, other than confusion, include dry lips, sunken eyes, swollen tongue, increased body temperature, decreased blood pressure, constipation, decreased urine output, and nausea.[10]

THE GASTROINTESTINAL TRACT

The main gastrointestinal problem for elderly people is constipation (see Chapter 3 for a review of this problem). Complaints associated with constipation include decreased frequency of bowel movements, painful defecation, hard stools, or a feeling of incomplete evacuation. To keep the intestinal tract performing efficiently, elderly people generally need to consume more dietary fiber than they did in their youth.[12] The goal is approximately 10 to 13 g/1000 kcal in the diet, but generally no more than 35 g on a daily basis.

Eating nuts, vegetables, beans, and whole grains regularly provides enough dietary fiber. Generally there is no need to use fiber supplements. Elderly persons

---

- - - - - - - - - - - -

Incontinence, the inability to control the muscle responsible for retaining urine, affects up to 20% of the elderly living at home and about 75% of those in nursing homes. The embarrassment of having to wear diapers causes many to avoid fluids (resulting in dehydration and constipation) and to become socially isolated.

- - - - - - - - - - - -

ostomy A surgically created short circuit in intestinal flow where the end point usually opens from the abdominal cavity rather than the anus; for example, a colostomy.

should also drink more fluid to transport fecal masses that form from dietary fiber intake.

Physical activity likewise helps keep things moving smoothly. In addition, the person should go to the bathroom as soon as the urge is felt. Delaying the process promotes constipation. Because medication can induce constipation, a physician should be consulted if constipation might be related to a medication.[15] If mineral oil is taken as a laxative, it should always be used with caution, and not at mealtimes because it binds fat-soluble vitamins and limits their absorption.

As noted earlier, lactase production frequently decreases with age. Several options for people with lactose intolerance are listed in Chapter 3.

Acid production in the stomach slows with age, usually associated with a reduced synthesis of intrinsic factor. These two changes can contribute to poor absorption of vitamin B-12 and eventually to pernicious anemia and other health problems. Anyone with an unexplained neuropsychiatric problem should be tested for vitamin B-12 deficiency. Neuropsychiatric problems commonly occur before vitamin B-12–related anemia is seen, and there is a limited time during which intervention is effective. Thus those responsible for the care of older individuals need to be vigilant with regard to the diagnosis of early vitamin B-12 deficiency. Oral supplementation with crystalline vitamin B-12 helps those in the early stages of gastric atrophy, but routine intramuscular injections are needed when the condition progresses to lack of intrinsic factor.[1]

Less stomach acid also hampers iron absorption. Other conditions that affect the body's iron status occur with regular use of aspirin, which frequently causes blood loss in the stomach, and use of antacids, which may bind iron. Ulcers, hemorrhoids, and colon cancer can also cause blood loss and in fact are the most common causes of anemia in the elderly. Careful attention to iron status is especially needed in these cases.

LIVER, GALLBLADDER, AND PANCREAS

With age, the liver functions less efficiently. When there is a history of significant alcohol consumption, fat build-up in the liver accounts for some decline. If cirrhosis develops, the liver functions even less efficiently (see the Nutrition Perspective in Chapter 7). When liver function deteriorates, many medications can't be efficiently detoxified. Alcohol abuse is a problem among a small but significant group of older individuals who may continue alcohol abuse from earlier in life or develop heavy drinking patterns and alcoholism later in life. The latter sometimes arises from the loneliness and social isolation of retirement or loss of a spouse. Alcohol-related sickness is high in older people, so the health consequences of this excess are considerable. Also, elderly people are more likely to take chronic medications that potentiate alcohol's effects.[15] The possibility for vitamin A toxicity also increases from the effects of liver disease. Elderly people, especially those with liver disease, should be warned not to take excessive amounts of vitamin A because toxic effects can easily result, causing malaise, headache, bone pain, liver dysfunction, and a decrease in white blood cell count.

The gallbladder also functions less efficiently as we age. Gallstones may dam up the bile to be secreted through the gallbladder, causing it to pool and back up into the liver instead. Gallstones can also interfere with fat digestion by allowing less bile into the small intestine. A low-fat diet or even surgery may be necessary.

Although the digestive function of the pancreas may decline with age, the pancreas has a large reserve capacity. A sign of a failing pancreas is high blood glucose, which occurs under several different conditions. Glucose instead may circulate primarily in the blood, rather than being taken up by cells, because the pancreas secretes less insulin or because cells resist insulin action—especially the enlarged adipose cells in obese people. Another cause can be insufficient chromium intake. Where appropriate, improved nutrient intake, regular physical activity, and weight loss can improve insulin action and blood glucose regulation.

KIDNEY FUNCTION

The kidneys filter wastes more slowly as they lose nephrons. As noted in Chapter 5, kidneys deteriorate more often in people who have regularly eaten excessive protein, and in some cases, excess energy (inferred from studies on laboratory animals). However, clinical signs and symptoms of this decline occur in only a subset of the elderly. The deterioration, when present, significantly decreases the kidneys' ability to excrete the products of protein breakdown. People whose decreased kidney function causes urea, a main by-product of protein metabolism, to accumulate in the blood need to limit protein intake under a physician's guidance to help compensate for this change.

IMMUNE FUNCTION

The immune system often operates less efficiently with age, starting after age 25. The change is quite variable among people of a specific age bracket. Consuming adequate protein, vitamins such as vitamin B-6, and zinc helps maintain the health of the immune system.[8] Recurrent sickness and delayed wound healing are warning signs of a deficiency, especially of protein and zinc, usually caused by eating too little food in general or too few animal protein sources. Older people may eliminate meat from their diet because it's too hard to chew or just doesn't taste good. Animal proteins are an excellent source of zinc. Nutrient supplements can help with vitamin B-6 and zinc intake if dietary intake is marginal.[6] On the other hand, overnutrition is equally harmful to the immune system. For example, obesity and excessive fat, iron, and zinc can suppress the immune system.

LUNG FUNCTION

Lung efficiency declines somewhat with age, and is especially pronounced in elderly people who have smoked and continue to smoke tobacco products. Breathing becomes shallower, faster, and more difficult as the number of lung **alveoli** decreases. Smoking often leads to emphysema and/or lung cancer. The decrease in lung efficiency contributes to a general downward spiral in body function; breathing difficulties limit physical activity and endurance and frequently discourage eating. These changes eventually cancel other efforts to maintain overall health.

Along with not smoking, exercise helps prevent lung problems. Nonsmokers need not lose their capacity to breathe deeply as long as sufficient aerobic exercise is part of their regular routine.[24] Otherwise, merely walking can demand the cardiopulmonary exertion of a marathon pace.

HEARING AND VISION

Hearing and vision both decline as we age. Approximately 4% of people under 45 years of age and 29% of those 65 years or over have a handicapping loss of hearing. Hearing impairment occurs mainly in members of industrial societies with urban traffic, aircraft noise, and loud music.

Degenerating eyesight is frequently caused by **macular degeneration.** The macula is a small area of the retina of the eye that distinguishes fine detail. As the macula degenerates, visual acuity declines. Increasing the consumption of foods rich in carotenoids, in particular dark green, leafy vegetables, such as kale, collard greens, spinach, swiss chard, mustard greens, and romaine lettuce, decreases the risk of developing macular degeneration. These vegetables are rich in lutein and zeaxanthin, two carotenoids found in the portion of the eye subject to damage from age-related macular degeneration. The outer retina, rich in polyunsaturated fatty acids, may be altered adversely by free radicals and, consequently, may be protected by carotenoids that block this damage. Scientists speculate that by accumulating in the retina and filtering short-wavelength (blue) light that may damage it, these carotenoids leave both the retina and the macula less vulnerable to oxidative degeneration.[29]

Cataracts are another common reason for declining sight. Recall from Chapter 13 the potential role of antioxidants, such as vitamin C, in reducing risk of cataracts

alveoli Small air sacs in the lungs.

macular degeneration Failing visual acuity and blindness caused by degeneration of the macula, a small area of the retina of the eye that distinguishes fine detail. Increasing the consumption of foods rich in carotenoids, in particular dark green, leafy vegetables, decreases the risk of developing macular degeneration.

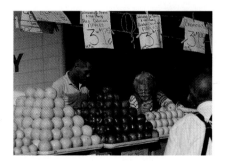

Deteriorating vision can hamper a person's ability to get to a grocery store, purchase nutritious foods, and prepare them at home.

in the eye. This provides another reason for adults to consume a diet rich in fruits and vegetables.

A decline in vision can affect a person's ability to physically get to a grocery store, locate the foods desired, read labels for nutritional content, and prepare the foods at home. Elderly people may also avoid social contacts because they can't hear. Such changes may make people afraid to socialize, be active, or take care of important routines of daily life, such as shopping and correctly following directions for use of medications. If so, family members and others need to step in to help as appropriate.[12]

DECREASE IN LEAN TISSUE

Some muscle cells shrink and others are lost as muscles age; some muscles lose their ability to contract as they accumulate fat and collagen. Lifestyle greatly determines the rate of muscle mass deterioration. As you might predict, an active lifestyle tends to maintain muscle mass, whereas a very inactive one encourages its loss.[4] Ideally this activity should include some weight training throughout life. The latter reduces muscle loss in elderly people.[13]

Overall, physical activity increases muscle strength and mobility, improves mental outlook, eases daily tasks that require some strength, improves sleep, and slows bone loss. But in one study, when older adults stopped their weight-training program, any gains in muscle strength were quickly lost.[13] This illustrates the importance of regular physical activity throughout life.

Elderly people can seek out programs to begin strength and aerobic training at community recreation centers or the local YMCA or YWCA, after receiving a physician's approval. Most of these organizations have qualified trainers who can help set up a program. Dumbbells are inexpensive and thus are ideal for performing weight training at home. Recall that Chapter 10 provides some general advice on this topic, including advice for warm-up, stretching, and cool-down activities.

Physical activity is also desirable for elderly people because it allows them to eat more food by raising energy expenditure, thereby increasing their chances of consuming adequate amounts of nutrients. Overall, much of what we associate with aging in terms of physical health is a direct result of longstanding sedentary lifestyles.[4]

INCREASE IN FAT STORES

As lean tissue decreases with age, the body often takes on more fat. Much of this results from minimal physical activity. As we noted earlier, some researchers feel that some extra fat stores in the elderly may be fine, while others recommend against fat gain through adulthood. However, obesity is not desirable, especially in android distribution, because it can raise blood pressure and blood glucose, as well as make it more difficult to walk and to perform daily tasks.

CARDIOVASCULAR HEALTH

The heart often pumps blood less efficiently in elderly people, usually because of a longstanding history of insufficient physical activity. Poor heart conditioning allows fatty and connective tissues to infiltrate the heart's muscular wall. This decline in **cardiac output** is not inevitable with aging and does not occur to as great an extent among elderly people who remain physically active.

cardiac output The amount of blood pumped by the heart.

Heart attack and stroke, the major causes of death in all adults, are caused primarily by atherosclerosis and high blood pressure.[22] With age, atherosclerotic plaque accumulates in the arteries, reducing their elasticity, constricting blood flow, and consequently elevating blood pressure.

The main way to limit the build-up of atherosclerotic plaque is to keep LDL and the total cholesterol to HDL cholesterol ratio in the desirable range (see Chapter 4). New evidence shows that even a diet very low in fat can cause some plaques to shrink. Other studies used diet and medication or surgery (to remove part of the intestine) to lower serum cholesterol, which, in turn, reduced the size of plaques in the arteries supplying the heart. This suggests that a heart-healthy diet is more important during adult and early elderly years than previously thought. Consuming sufficient vitamin B-6, folate, and vitamin B-12 is also important to avoid elevated blood homocysteine, an additional risk factor for heart disease.[30]

There is much controversy surrounding treatment for elevated LDL in people over ages 70 to 75. If these people adhere to extremely restrictive diets limited in fat and energy to the point that they can't keep up their weight, or if their diets lack variety, they may become undernourished. This may be a worse predicament for them than having high serum LDL. So treating elevated LDL in an elderly person who has other ills like chronic lung disease and **dementia,** which are likely to shorten life as well as hamper its quality, is probably inappropriate. But if a healthy 70-year-old with a likely 10 to 15 years of living ahead has both elevated LDL and evidence of heart disease, an eating and exercise plan is probably in order to reduce the chance of heart attack.[11] Overall, the pros and cons of different treatments to reduce heart disease need to be weighed carefully before they are advocated for an elderly person. Discussion probably should be the first step, in which both a person's overall health and quality of life are considered.[32] Note that the advisability of fat restrictions for the very old (those older than 85 years of age) for the amelioration of chronic disease is questionable. Dietary modifications should be made instead to respond to the current disease state, such as the presence of diabetes or failing kidney function.

Hypertension is heavily implicated in both stroke and heart attack in the elderly.[22] Blood pressure can be lowered in most people by severe sodium restriction. A limit of 2 g of sodium helps many people with hypertension, but that is a difficult diet to plan and follow. Alternatively, a mild sodium restriction (not to exceed 4 g of sodium daily), while effective for salt-sensitive people, is not so helpful by itself for those who are not salt sensitive, but does aid the action of medications used to treat hypertension. (The Nutrition Perspective in Chapter 14 reviews the effects of other nutrients and lifestyle interventions on blood pressure.)

We can do much to prevent heart attack and stroke just by balanced eating, walking briskly and otherwise performing regular physical activity, controlling blood pressure, not smoking, and maintaining a desirable weight. Regular physical activity and a diet rich in fruits and vegetables are also associated with fewer strokes as adults age.

BONE HEALTH

In Chapter 14 we discussed the decline in bone density associated with aging. Recall that bone loss in women occurs especially after menopause. Bone loss in men is slow and steady from middle age throughout the elderly years. Estrogen replacement at menopause is the most reliable treatment to lessen bone loss in women. For elderly women not taking estrogen, increasing calcium intake to 1500 mg/day helps maintain bone density in some types of bones, such as the hip. The same was advised for elderly men by the recent NIH Consensus Report on Optimal Calcium Intake. Currently many elderly people fail to meet this recommendation.

Other measures to prevent bone loss can be started earlier and continued throughout life—maintaining adequate vitamin D nutriture, not smoking, and drinking alcohol moderately or not at all (refer to the Dietary Guidelines). It should be noted that underweight women are at especially high risk for developing osteoporosis. Performing weight-bearing exercises also helps sustain bone.

For adult women at menopause who are at high risk or who may have osteoporosis, medical treatment should be considered—estrogen replacement therapy, active vitamin D hormone (calcitriol) therapy, bisphosphonate, or calcitonin therapy—administered with a physician's guidance (see Chapter 14).

Very severe osteoporosis limits the ability of elderly people to exercise, shop, prepare food, and live normally. They eat less and get fewer nutrients.

A plan to limit falls should also be instituted. Falls may be caused by the side effects of medication, by gait and balance disorders, by impaired vision, or by environmental hazards. Protective hip padding can reduce the risk of fracture in indi-

dementia General persistent loss of or decrease in mental function.

viduals who fall. Typical measures to take around the home to reduce the risk of falling include:

- remain as physically active as possible
- remove clutter and clear pathways
- secure carpets and stair treads
- remove loose electrical cords
- replace or repair unstable furniture
- do not wax floors
- increase lighting, especially at night
- use a cane, walking stick, or walker if needed to maintain balance
- install grab bars in bathroom (tub, shower, toilet)
- use nonskid bathmats
- store personal items and frequently used items at eye level or below
- do not rise quickly after eating or sitting for a period of time if dizziness is experienced; begin instead to rise up slowly.

Many elderly people may suffer from hidden osteomalacia, a condition that occurs primarily when there is not enough sun exposure and therefore lessened vitamin D synthesis in the skin. When they can't get regular sun exposure—during the winter or when they are homebound—elderly people need a source for 10 to 20 micrograms (μg) (400 to 800 IU) of vitamin D per day.[5] Both fortified milk products and a vitamin supplement can be used to meet this goal.

OTHER FACTORS THAT INFLUENCE NUTRIENT NEEDS IN ELDERLY PEOPLE

Medication and old age often go together. Medications can improve health and quality of life, but some of them also profoundly affect nutrient needs at all ages, including the elderly years (Table 18-4). Forty-five percent of the elderly population regularly takes multiple prescription drugs; many drugs affect appetite or absorption of nutrients.[5] Often elderly people take several medications for long periods. They should make sure to work with their physician and pharmacist to coordinate all medication taken. Pharmacists can advise when to take drugs—with or between meals—for greatest effectiveness.

Drug-related nutritional problems include: (1) increased need for potassium when certain types of diuretics augment excretion by the body; and (2) changes in appetite caused by antidepressant agents or certain antibiotics. Blood loss from long-term use of aspirin or aspirin-like medication strains iron reserves and can lead to anemia. People who must take one or more medications for more than just a few weeks should closely watch their diets, eat nutrient-dense foods, and possibly take nutrient supplements to counteract effects of certain medications. A physician should guide this last practice, as some supplements can interfere with the function of certain medications. For example, vitamin K can reduce activity of oral anticoagulants (see Chapter 12).

About 15% of elderly people experience significant depression. That—combined with isolation and loneliness as family and friends die, move away, or become less mobile—frequently contributes to apathetic eating and weight loss in older people. People living alone (especially men) do not necessarily make unwise food choices, but they often consume less energy, in part from skipping meals. About one third of all elderly persons not in nursing homes live alone. Depression can be a downward spiral in which poor appetite produces weakness that leads to even poorer appetite (Figure 18-5). In elderly people, the resulting poor nutritional state can produce further mental confusion and increased isolation and loneliness.[10]

Nutrition has a role in preserving mental function in elderly people. Specific nutritional deficiencies of thiamin, niacin, vitamins B-6 and B-12, and folate, as well as excessive alcohol use, cause well-recognized central nervous system disorders.[3] The subtle effects of consuming minimal food energy, leading to semistarvation, are often overlooked. Alcohol abuse may be overlooked as well. In addition, as mentioned

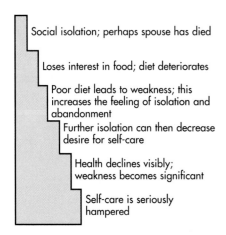

Social isolation; perhaps spouse has died

Loses interest in food; diet deteriorates

Poor diet leads to weakness; this increases the feeling of isolation and abandonment

Further isolation can then decrease desire for self-care

Health declines visibly; weakness becomes significant

Self-care is seriously hampered

Figure 18-5 The decline of health often seen in elderly persons. This decline needs to be prevented whenever possible.

TABLE 18-4

Potential drug-nutrient interactions for some commonly used drugs

Drug	Use	Nutrient	Potential side effect
Digoxin	Antiarrhythmic	Potassium, calcium, magnesium	Drug toxicity more likely if potassium is deficient
Antacids (Maalox)	Reduce stomach acidity	Calcium, vitamin B-12, and iron	Decreased absorption from altered gastrointestinal pH
Anticoagulants (Coumadin)	Prevention of blood clots	Vitamin K	Poor utilization
Antihistamines (Benadryl)	Treatment of allergies and nausea; as local anesthetic	—	Weight gain
Beta-blocker (propranolol, Inderal)	Decrease hypertension	Cholesterol*	Some can increase serum cholesterol
Aspirin	Antiinflammatory, pain reduction	Iron	Anemia from blood loss
Cathartics (laxatives)	Induce bowel movement	Calcium, potassium; vitamins A, D, E, and K with mineral oil	Poor absorption
Cholestyramine	Reduces blood cholesterol	Vitamins A, D, E, and K	Poor absorption
Cimetidine (Tagamet)	Treatment of ulcers	Vitamin B-12	Poor absorption
Colchicine	Treatment of gout	Vitamin B-12, carotenoids, and magnesium	Decreased absorption from damaged intestinal mucosa
Corticosteroids (prednisone)	Antiinflammatory	Zinc / Calcium	Poor absorption / Poor utilization
Furosemide (Lasix)	Potassium-wasting diuretic	Potassium, sodium, and magnesium	Increased loss
Isoniazid (INH, Neomycin)	Tuberculosis / Antibiotic	Vitamin B-6 / Fat, protein, sodium, potassium, calcium, iron, and vitamin B-12	Poor utilization / Decreases pancreatic lipase, binds bile salts, and so interferes with absorption
MAO inhibitors (Parnate)	Antidepressant	(Tyramine in aged foods)	Hypertension caused by poor tyramine metabolism
Phenobarbital	Sedative; treatment of epilepsy	Vitamin D and folate	Reduced metabolism and utilization
Phenytoin (Dilantin)	Treatment of epilepsy	Vitamin D, folate, vitamin B-12, vitamin K	Reduced metabolism and utilization
Tricyclic antidepressants (Elavil)	Antidepressant	—	Weight gain from appetite stimulation

Modified from Chernoff R: Aging and nutrition, *Nutrition Today,* p 4, March/April 1987.
*Not a nutrient.

earlier, an inadequate fluid intake may lead to dehydration and, in turn, to confusion (Table 18-5).

Mental illness can lead to a diminished nutritional state, but the extent to which subtle nutritional deficiencies can lead to a poor mental state is not as clear cut. It is important to prevent overt nutrient deficiencies, especially those mentioned previously.

Overall, elderly people should keep active, physically and mentally, stay involved in life, and make use of the accumulated wisdom and experience of years. A long and healthy life for almost everyone means that age, far from implying disengagement, can become a time to get even more involved.[25] This, along with nutrient intake, supports mental function.

Lastly, other social circumstances can lead to problems. In today's mobile society, in which the extended family may not be close at hand, there may be no one to assist with the daily needs of the elderly, including shopping for and preparation of

CRITICAL THINKING

Maria is interested in helping the elderly and works as a volunteer at a retirement community. She has noticed that many of the residents have decreased appetites and less keen senses of taste and smell. In addition, depression seems to be common among the residents. How can Maria explain these observations?

TABLE 18-5

Warning signals for poor nutritional status

Obesity	Advanced age (>80 years)
Recent unplanned weight change of	Dry mouth
± 3 kg (7 lb)	Frequent nausea/vomiting
Chewing/swallowing difficulties	Diarrhea/constipation
Diminished appetite	High alcohol intake
Recent surgery	Side effects of medication, especially
Illness lasting longer than 3 weeks	with long-term and multiple usage
Lung disease	Frequent skipped meals or fluids
Diabetes	Limited food stores
Physical disability that affects shop-	Widespread food avoidance
ping for or eating food	Little use of fruit, fruit juices, and
Lack of sunlight exposure	raw or freshly cooked vegetables
Recent loss of spouse	Low budget for food
Depression/loneliness/social isolation	Limited nutritional knowledge
Mental confusion	

meals. Transportation may be difficult. Many elderly people are no longer able to drive, do not have ready access to public transportation, and may not have the stamina to get to the bus stop, take the bus, get to the final destination, and reverse the process. Even if it were physically possible to complete this process, how many would be strong enough to carry the groceries home?

Some older Americans are too proud to ask for assistance, having been independent all of their lives. Asking for assistance may seem like being on the "public dole." Many are afraid of asking for help in meal preparation for fear of losing their independence or being victimized by those they hire.

Concept Check

Nutritional problems of the elderly are related to both the presence of chronic diseases and the normal decrease in organ function that occur with time. All these organ systems and functions can decrease as we age: appetite; sense of taste, smell, thirst, hearing, and sight; digestion and absorption; liver, gallbladder, pancreas, kidneys, lungs, heart; and the immune system. In addition, muscle mass (largely due to inactivity) and bone mass gradually decrease. Diet changes and regular physical activity can often help reduce the impact of these results of aging.

Meeting the Nutrient Needs of the Elderly

The RDAs for nutrients and energy include a category for both men and women who are 51 years of age and older. Because the lifestyle of an active 70-year-old person differs considerably from that of a 90-year-old nursing home resident, this wide age range in the RDAs is likely to be problematic.[5] The recommendations for energy intake assume an active lifestyle, a characteristic the RDA committee supports. Note also that the nutrient recommendations for the elderly have largely been projected from studies of young adults.

DO THE RDAs INCREASE IN THE ELDERLY YEARS?

Only during the last few years has much research focused on this question. Because the RDAs apply only to healthy people, many elderly people—for example, those who have ulcers or are heavy aspirin users—are not covered by RDAs. Indeed it is particularly tricky to evolve RDAs valid for most older people because many of them are ill and/or regularly take medication.

NUTRITION FOCUS

ALZHEIMER'S DISEASE

Alzheimer's disease has become a dreaded reality for many people approaching old age. Many of us have had first-hand experience as loved ones have been "lost" to this form of progressive dementia. Although it seems a disease of our times, it has been around for quite a while.

In 1907 Dr. Alois Alzheimer documented several cases of what seemed to be early senility. Typical symptoms of the disease included personality changes, unreasonable fears, explosive outbursts, depression, and general forgetfulness. Today the disease Dr. Alzheimer first described affects about 4 million people in the United States, including about 45% of all people over the age of 85 and 50% of all people in nursing homes.[20]

More reports of Alzheimer's disease surface very day. Is this a disease of modern society, or has it always been around but undiagnosed? Old age is often accompanied by a general decline in mental function. What makes Alzheimer's disease different is that it can be diagnosed specifically by the presence of specific protein deposits and tangled masses of nerves in areas of the brain that are linked to memory and thinking.[31] However, this type of diagnosis can be done only at autopsy, and so it is difficult to know precisely how many cases of dementia in old age are actually Alzheimer's. Clinical assessments can and should be made by an experienced physician. Because more is known about the typical course of the disease, clinical methods have recently become more reliable in differentiating between Alzheimer's disease and other causes of dementia.

CAUSES AND PHYSICAL EFFECTS

In general terms, Alzheimer's disease is best described as a progressive brain disorder marked by an inability to remember, reason, or understand what is going on. Age is the primary risk factor. Scientists propose causes, including altered cell development, altered brain proteins, and unidentified blood-borne agents.[31] Research over the last few years suggests that a specific apolipoprotein, called *apolipoprotein E-4,* increases the risk of developing Alzheimer's disease.[31] It is thought that this compound interferes with the growth and maintenance of nerve cells. Many people have the E-2 or E-3 variant of this apolipoprotein. If the E-4 gene is inherited from both parents, the risk of Alzheimer's disease is about nine times greater in the offspring than if neither gene is E-4. Researchers note, however, that it is premature to test individuals for

presence of the E-4 variant, as this provides no guarantee the person will or will not develop the disease. It is merely a risk factor. Still, there is some interest in developing medications that may compensate for the presence of E-4. Other risk factors under investigation include less educational and occupational attainment, as well as loss of estrogen at menopause in women.

In people with Alzheimer's disease, aluminum is highly concentrated in abnormal protein accumulations in the brain, but this high amount of aluminum is more likely an effect than a cause of the disease. Evidence supporting this is that people mining aluminum develop cancer from aluminum toxicity but typically don't develop Alzheimer's disease. Accordingly, a role for aluminum in the neuropathology of Alzheimer's disease remains speculative at present. Whether there are other, yet unknown, causes of Alzheimer's disease remains to be discovered, but this is likely.

Alzheimer's disease is a progressive disorder. Its course has been described as four stages, although these can vary in duration and intensity with individuals. Generally it (1) begins as forgetfulness and fatigue, (2) develops into confusion, depression, delusion, hostility, anxiety, and short-term memory loss, (3) advances to long-term memory loss and problems in communication, perception, and maintenance of bodily functions, and (4) may conclude with the individual becoming bedridden and completely dependent. Wandering is a frequent reason people with Alzheimer's disease are put in nursing homes. Death in Alzheimer's disease is frequently attributable to bacterial infection or to pneumonia associated with accidental food inhalation.

TREATMENT

The environment of the person with Alzheimer's disease needs to be safe, with attention paid to risks such as wandering or forgetting about food cooking on a stove. Establishing routines is also helpful, along with regular physical activity. Today, medical treatment of Alzheimer's disease is usually limited to the use of antidepressants and other drugs that target related symptoms of the disease. A new medication currently in use is tacrine (Cognex), a drug that may slow the brain's breakdown of acetylcholine, a major neurotransmitter used in sending nerve messages. Side effects currently limit its usefulness to a subset of patients. It also is not a cure for the disease,

NUTRITION FOCUS

and it does not significantly deter disease progression. In Alzheimer's disease, the decreased amount of neurotransmitter activity appears to relate strongly to the degree of memory impairment.

Therapies currently under clinical investigation range from the use of aspirin and other antiinflammatory agents to overlapping doses of potent, synthetically produced brain chemicals. But, to prevent a disease, its causes need to be understood. And unfortunately, we don't yet know as much as we need to about Alzheimer's disease.

NUTRITION CONSIDERATIONS

The main nutrition goal for people with this disease is a healthful diet that maintains body weight. Forgetfulness may lead to irregular eating habits with associated weight loss. Because one characteristic of Alzheimer's disease is the death of cells that secrete acetylcholine, scientists once thought that a diet that provided choline and the related compound lecithin might correct this deficit. However, studies have found this to have no effect on Alzheimer's patients.

Abnormal food behavior, such as gorging, is often seen early in the course of Alzheimer's disease. A craving for sweets may lead to a temporary weight gain that can be managed by offering lower-energy snacks and meals. At the other extreme, there is often a partial or complete refusal to eat. Frequent, small meals and nutrient-dense snacks using favorite foods when possible may encourage more regular eating. People who are still leading reasonably independent lives may not be able to shop or to remember to eat meals. Congregate feeding programs and home-delivered meals may be helpful during the early stages of disease. Keep in mind that by the time the disease has been diagnosed, some people have already developed nutritional problems.

With the progression of the disease, there is more confusion and distractibility. At this stage it is wise for others to oversee food planning and mealtimes. Measures should be taken to control distractions—such as television, radio, children, pets, and the telephone—that can disrupt a meal for someone with Alzheimer's disease. Others should monitor food temperatures because people with Alzheimer's disease may ignore discomfort and burn themselves. Tough or crunchy foods that may easily cause choking should be avoided.

For those still capable of self-feeding, assistance devices should be used when appropriate: roller-rocker knives, bowls, plate guards, a damp washcloth under the plate to prevent skidding, cups with tops, flexible straws, and large bibs. These are available at medical supply houses. As people with Alzheimer's disease become less able to manage eating by themselves, it becomes more of a challenge to those trying to feed them. They may hold food in the mouth, forget how to eat or swallow, spit out food, and play with and then refuse food.

All of us need to pay attention to dietary recommendations to promote and maintain health. People with Alzheimer's disease may not be able to do this on their own. In later stages of this disease people may not be attuned to their needs. The responsibility for providing good nutrition ultimately falls to family, health-care providers, and nursing home staff. The fastest-growing segment of the population is made up of people age 85 and older. Thus, in the future, Alzheimer's disease could have devastating consequences for America's already strained health-care system. The disease also takes an immense emotional toll on people with Alzheimer's disease and their family members.

Ten warning signs of Alzheimer's disease
1. **Recent memory loss that affects job performance**
2. **Difficulty performing familiar tasks**
3. **Problems with language**
4. **Disorientation to time and place**
5. **Faulty or decreased judgment**
6. **Problems with abstract thinking**
7. **Misplacing things**
8. **Changes in mood or behavior**
9. **Changes in personality**
10. **Loss of initiative**

To find out more about Alzheimer's disease, call the Alzheimer's Association at (800) 272-3900, or the National Institute on Aging's Alzheimer's Disease Education and Referral Center at (800) 438-4380.

Researchers have suggested that the current RDAs for healthy elderly people are probably too high for vitamin A; a bit too low in protein (for active people); too low for vitamins D, B-6, and B-12; and about right for the other vitamins.[3] For most minerals, the RDAs are likely about right or a bit generous.[37] The "about right" category suggests that we lack evidence to make a more definitive statement (Table 18-6). There is, however, concern that the RDA for calcium should be increased to help slow the acceleration of bone loss suffered by elderly women and men. As we just mentioned, 1500 mg/day was recently recommended for both genders by an NIH Consensus Conference on Optimal Calcium Needs.

Still, a well-planned diet that follows the Food Guide Pyramid can meet all nutrient needs for elderly people within about 1600 to 1800 kcal, except for probably 1500 mg of calcium (see Table 2-2). That would take at least four servings from the milk, yogurt, and cheese group—a recommendation that most elderly people would find difficult to meet. Calcium-fortified foods and calcium supplements can help when necessary (see Chapter 14 for details.)

If a 1600 to 1800 kcal diet plan represents too much food energy, a special attempt should be made to regularly choose some nutrient-fortified foods, like ready-to-eat breakfast cereals. Nutrient supplements are another possibility. In that case supplement use should complement nutritious food choices and focus on the nutrients just mentioned. Also, too much of some supplements can lead to toxicity. Between about 35% and 70% of elderly people regularly take supplements, some in potentially toxic amounts. If supplements are necessary, the elderly person should work closely with a physician or registered dietitian to determine which nutrients to include and the least amounts that are necessary. For example, the possibility of vitamin D deficiency is easily assessed by asking about the intake of vitamin D–fortified milk and the availability of regular sun exposure.

CRITICAL THINKING

Jorge is studying nutritional guidelines for the elderly. As a geriatric nurse, he wants to make sure he knows the RDAs of the nutrients his patients need. The NIH Consensus Conference on Optimal Calcium Intake suggests raising the calcium RDA for the elderly to 1500 mg/day. Jorge agrees with this recommendation and has to justify it to his superior at the hospital. How can he do so?

- - - - - - - - - - -

Elderly women need less iron because they no longer menstruate. However, chronic ulcers, hemorrhoids, and aspirin use may necessitate an increased iron intake.

- - - - - - - - - - -

TABLE 18-6

Comparing the current RDAs for the elderly to projected needs based on recent research		
Nutrient	**Differing needs of elderly vs. RDA**	**Reason for differing needs**
Protein	1.0-1.25 g/kg vs 0.8 g/kg	• Help blunt loss in lean body mass • Possibly lower efficiency of dietary protein utilization
Vitamin A	Caution with supplement use is advised	• Increased absorption because of changes in lining of small intestine
Vitamin D	10-20 μg vs 5 μg (400-800 IU vs 200 IU)	• Limited exposure to sunlight • Reduced dermal synthesis • Reduced kidney conversion to active hormone
Vitamin B-6	No amount set	• Blood concentrations fall with age • Blunted response to intake
Vitamin B-12*	3 μg vs 2 μg	• Fall in gastric acid reduces absorption • If intrinsic factor synthesis is inadequate, vitamin B-12 injections are recommended
Calcium	1500 mg vs 800 mg	• Absorption falls, especially in women after menopause • Slows bone loss in nonvertebral bone, such as in hip region

From reference no. 3.
*Some scientists argue that the RDA is adequate, and attention should instead be paid to screening the elderly for low serum vitamin B-12 concentration. They feel increasing the amount consumed by 1 μg will not help, as the fall in vitamin B-12 status results from a profound decrease in absorption. Instead, regular intramuscular injections are needed to maintain vitamin B-12 status once gastric atrophy is in advanced stages.

PLANNING A DIET FOR ELDERLY PERSONS

To supply energy needs for males age 51 years and older, the current RDA suggestion is 2300 kcal; for females, the recommendation is 1900 kcal. (These values are based on a 170-pound, 68-inch tall man and a 143-pound, 63-inch tall woman.) Studies show that elderly men eat closer to 1800 to 2100 kcal, whereas women eat about 1300 to 1600 kcal. Thus diet plans for elderly persons should focus on nutrient density. A good practice is to decrease sugar and fat consumption to increase the diet's nutrient density and to make sure dietary fiber intake is adequate.[27] In addition, some protein should come from lean meats to help meet vitamin B-6 and zinc needs, two nutrients of special concern.

Fluid needs are 1 ml/kcal expended, or about 8 cups (2 L) per day. A high-fiber diet especially requires attention to fluid needs.[10] Fiber intake should be slowly increased up to about 35 g a day, with each serving of fiber accompanied by a glass of water (or other fluid).

Singles of all ages face logistical problems with food: purchasing, preparing, storing, and using food with minimal waste is challenging. Economy packages of meats and vegetables are normally too large to be useful for a single person. Many singles live in small dwellings, some without kitchens and freezers. Gearing a diet to accommodate a limited budget and facilities and a single appetite requires special considerations.[12] Following are some practical suggestions for diet planning for singles:

- If you own a freezer, cook large amounts, divide into portions, and freeze.
- Buy only what you can use; small containers may be expensive, but letting food spoil is also costly.
- Ask the grocer to break open a family-sized package of wrapped meat or fresh vegetables and separate it into smaller units.
- Buy only several pieces of fruit—perhaps a ripe one, a medium-ripe one, and an unripe one—so that the fruit can be eaten over a period of several days.
- Keep a box of dry milk handy to add a nutritious punch to recipes for baked foods and other foods for which this addition is acceptable.

Nutritional deficiencies and protein-energy undernutrition have been identified among some elderly populations, particularly those in nursing homes or long-term care facilities and those who are hospitalized.[21] This increases the risk for many diseases, including bed sores (pressure ulcers), and compromises recovery from illness and surgery.[2] Feeding sick, infirm, and/or mentally confused people is time-consuming and demanding work that requires special training. Friends, relatives, and health personnel should look for poor nutrient intake in all elderly people, including those who live in nursing home settings. About 40% of adults now age 65 will spend some time in a nursing home. Family members have a unique opportunity to make sure nutrient needs of elderly people are met by looking for weight maintenance based on regular, healthful meal patterns. If problems arise in instituting a healthful diet, registered dietitians can offer professional and personalized advice.

Surveys show that the majority of elderly people like most vegetables, despite misconceptions that older people do not like broccoli (because it forms gas) or tomatoes (because they contain too much acid). By the time we reach adulthood, our eating habits reflect regional tastes, social class, ethnic group, and life experiences. There is no generic food list for elderly persons.

Overall, good nutrition benefits elderly people in many ways. It delays the onset of some diseases; improves management of some existing diseases; hastens recovery from many illnesses; can increase mental, physical, and social well-being; and often decreases the need for and length of hospitalization. Thus a good nutritional intake should be a vital part of the health maintenance program for elderly people.[12] A variety of strategies can promote healthful eating in the elderly years (Table 18-7). These should focus on presenting nutritious, tasty foods in a pleasant, friendly environment.

TABLE 18-7

Guidelines for healthful eating in later years

- Eat regularly; small, frequent meals may be best. Use nutrient-dense foods as a basis for each menu.
- Find out which convenience foods and labor-saving devices can be of help.
- Try new foods, new seasonings, and new ways of preparing foods. Don't use just convenience foods and canned goods.
- Keep some easy-to-prepare foods on hand for times when tired.
- Have a treat occasionally, perhaps an expensive cut of meat or a favorite fresh fruit.
- Eat in a well-lit or sunny area; serve meals attractively; use foods with different flavors, colors, shapes, textures, and smells.
- Arrange things so food preparation and clean-up are easier.
- Eat with friends, relatives, or at a senior center when possible.
- Share cooking responsibilities with a neighbor.
- Use community resources for help in shopping and other daily care needs.
- Stay physically active.
- If possible, take a walk before eating to stimulate appetite.
- When necessary, chop, grind, or blend hard-to-chew foods. Softer, protein-rich foods can be substituted for meat when poor dental function limits normal food intake. Prepare soups, stews, cooked whole-grain cereals, and casseroles.
- If eating movements are limited, cut the food ahead of time, use utensils with deep sides or handles, and obtain more specialized utensils if needed.

COMMUNITY NUTRITION SERVICES FOR ELDERLY PEOPLE

Health-care advice and services for elderly persons can come from clinics, private practitioners, hospitals, and health maintenance organizations. Home health-care agencies, adult day-care programs, adult overnight-care programs, and **hospice** centers (for the terminally ill) can supply day-to-day care. Professionals in the above-mentioned organizations can help identify elderly people whose health needs may require extra attention. Figure 18-6 shows a valuable screening tool, based on the acronym "DETERMINE."

Nutrition programs for those age 60 and over offer congregate meal programs, which provide lunch at a central location, and home-delivered meals (often known as Meals-on-Wheels if sponsored by local private or public agencies) (Figure 18-7). Federal commodity distribution is available in some areas of the United States to low-income elderly people. Food stamps can also aid elderly persons whose incomes are below the poverty level. Food cooperatives and a variety of clubs and social organizations provide additional aid.

Congregate meal programs and home-delivered meals are funded partially by the U.S. government under Title III of the Older Americans Act and through volunteer community efforts (Figure 18-8). The federal government sets specific standards for home-delivered meals and for those served in congregate feeding centers. The meals are designed to provide one third of the RDA. The basic meal pattern is 3 ounces of meat or meat alternative, 2½ cups of fruit or vegetable, 1 slice of bread or alternative, 1 teaspoon of butter or margarine, 1 cup of milk, and ½ cup of dessert. Foods rich in vitamins A and C are emphasized. The social aspect often improves appetite and general outlook.

Many eligible elderly people are missing meals and are poorly nourished simply because they don't know of available programs. Irregular meal patterns and weight loss, often because of difficulties in preparing food, are warning signs that undernutrition may be developing.[12] An effort should be made to identify and inform poorly nourished people of community services.

hospice A facility offering care that emphasizes comfort and dignity in death.

- **Disease**
- **Eating poorly**
- **Tooth loss or mouth pain**
- **Economic hardship**
- **Reduced social contact and interaction**
- **Multiple medications**
- **Involuntary weight loss or gain**
- **Need for assistance with self care**
- **Elder at an advanced age**

A Nutrition Test For Older Adults

Here's a nutrition check for anyone over age 65. Circle the number of points for each statement that applies. Then compute the total and check it against the nutritional score.

1. The person has a chronic illness or current condition that has changed the kind or amount of food eaten. (2 points)

2. The person eats fewer than two full meals per day. (3 points)

3. The person eats few fruits, vegetables, or milk products. (2 points)

4. The person drinks 3 or more servings of beer, liquor, or wine almost every day. (2 points)

5. The person has tooth or mouth problems that make eating difficult. (2 points)

6. The person does not have enough money for food. (4 points)

7. The person eats alone most of the time. (1 point)

8. The person takes three or more different prescription or over-the-counter drugs each day. (1 point)

9. The person has unintentionally lost or gained 10 pounds within the last 6 months. (2 points)

10. The person cannot always shop, cook, or feed himself or herself. (2 points)

Nutritional score:

0–2: Good. Recheck in 6 months.

3–5: Marginal. A local agency on aging has information about nutrition programs for the elderly. The National Association of Area Agencies on Aging can assist in finding help; call (800) 677-1116. Recheck in 6 months.

6 or more: High risk. A doctor should review this test and suggest how to improve nutritional health.

(Modified from the Nutrition Screening Initiative, 1010 Wisconsin Avenue, NW, Suite 800, Washington, DC 20002.)

Figure 18-6 A nutrition checklist for elderly people.

Studies have found that congregate and home-delivered meal programs can positively influence the nutritional status of otherwise homebound people, especially in cases of poverty and with people of minority groups (where poverty is more often seen). Still, congregate meal programs provide at most one meal a day and usually not every day of the week. So if people come to depend on them exclusively, they eat too few meals. The problem with home-delivered meals is that the one or two meals delivered may never be eaten, and if not eaten on delivery and left at room temperature, they may become unsafe to eat later. Thus though these programs help elderly people, even more help is often needed.

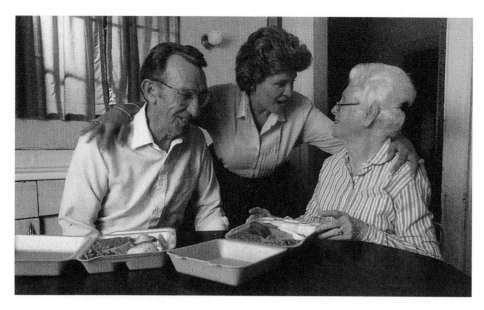

Figure 18-7 The home-delivered meals program is a gift of nutrition and caring from a community to its elderly citizens.

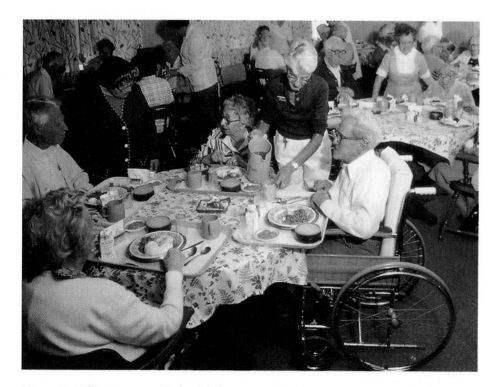

Figure 18-8 Congregate meals for elderly persons. Sites in many communities in the United States provide nutritious meals and an opportunity for socialization among elderly people.

CONCEPT CHECK

Specific nutrient requirements for elderly persons are only now being extensively studied. Diet plans for elderly persons should be modified for decreased physical abilities, presence of drug-nutrient interactions, possible depression, and economic constraints. Particular attention should be paid to the opportunity for sun exposure and intake of the vitamins D, B-6, folate, and B-12, as well as the minerals calcium and zinc, and dietary fiber. A nutrient-dense diet helps to meet these needs. In the United States, many nutrition services—such as congregate and home-delivered meals—are available to help the elderly population obtain a healthful diet.

Summary

1. Compression of morbidity means delaying symptoms of and disabilities from chronic disease for as many years of life as possible. Good nutritional habits, especially following the Food Guide Pyramid and the Dietary Guidelines for Americans, play a role in this process.

2. A basic plan for health promotion and disease prevention includes eating a proper diet that focuses on a variety of foods and moderation in fat intake, performing regular physical activity, consuming an adequate amount of fluids, abstaining from smoking, and limiting alcohol intake.

3. The 1990 Dietary Guidelines for Americans recommend that individuals eat a variety of foods; balance the food you eat with physical activity to maintain or improve your weight; choose a diet with plenty of grain products, vegetables, and fruits; choose a diet low in fat, saturated fat, and cholesterol; choose a diet moderate in sugars; choose a diet moderate in salt and sodium; and, for those who drink alcoholic beverages, do so in moderation. In addition, specific recommendations to reduce cancer risk emphasize moderation in use of cured and smoked meats. Fluoride use can minimize risk of dental caries.

4. Scientists disagree as to the best diet recommendations for the general public. Genetic background, medical condition, and other lifestyle practices influence a person's optimal diet. An overall emphasis on variety in the diet, control of body weight, moderation in total fat and saturated fat intake, consumption of ample fruits and vegetables, and moderation in alcohol intake has wide support.

5. While maximum lifespan has not changed, life expectancy has increased dramatically over the past century. This has resulted in an increasing proportion of the population over 65 years of age. Health-care costs associated with this trend are increasing, making the goal of compression of morbidity very important.

6. Aging probably begins before birth. This aging likely results from automatic cellular changes and environmental influences, such as DNA damage, free-radical reactions, hormonal changes, and alterations in immune function.

7. Nutritional problems of the elderly are related to the presence of chronic disease and to normal decreases in organ function that occur with age. These include loss of teeth, a reduction in senses of taste and smell, changes in gastrointestinal tract function, and deterioration in heart and bone health.

8. Specific nutrient requirements for the elderly are only now being extensively studied. Diet plans should be based on the Food Guide Pyramid, with consideration for present health problems, decreased physical abilities, presence of drug-nutrient interactions, possible depression, and economic constraints. Specific nutrients, such as protein, vitamin D, vitamin B-6, folate, vitamin B-12, zinc, and calcium, along with dietary fiber, often deserve special attention in diet planning.

9. Alzheimer's disease is a progressive and irreversible brain disorder. Its causes are only beginning to be understood. It differs from other types of senile dementia in that the brain tissue accumulates abnormal protein plaques and tangled nerves (observable by autopsy). Nutritional health for people in advanced stages of disease is often complicated by special feeding problems.

Study Questions

1. Describe the concept of compression of morbidity. How does this concept relate to the purpose of the many nutrition and health guidelines discussed in this chapter?

2. Currently there is a debate about the appropriateness of issuing recommendations for specific nutrient intakes, such as for sodium, to the general public. Describe the pros and cons of general dietary recommendations.

3. Define the term *reserve capacity* of organs and describe how it tends to hide the early effects of aging.

4. Describe two hypotheses proposed to explain the causes of aging and note evidence for each in your daily life experiences.

5. List four organ systems that can decline in function in the elderly years, along with a diet/lifestyle response to help cope with the decline.

6. Defend the recommendation for regular physical activity during adult and elderly years, including some weight training.

7. How do nutrition needs of elderly people differ from those of younger people? How are their needs similar? Be specific.

8. What three resources in a community are widely available to aid elderly people in maintaining nutritional health?

9. Describe some early warning signs of Alzheimer's disease and note some of the nutrition implications as this disease advances.

10. List four warning signs of undernutrition in the elderly that are part of the acronym "DETERMINE." Briefly justify the inclusion of each.

REFERENCES

1. Allen LH and others: Vitamin B-12 deficiency in elderly individuals: diagnosis and requirements, *American Journal of Clinical Nutrition* 60:12, 1994.

2. Allman RM and others: Pressure ulcer risk factors among hospitalized patients with activity limitation, *Journal of the American Medical Association* 273:865, 1995.

3. Ausman LM, Russell RM: Nutrition in the elderly. In Shils ME and others, editors: *Modern nutrition and health and disease*, Philadelphia, 1994, Lea & Febiger.

4. Blair SN and others: Changes in physical fitness and all-cause mortality, *Journal of the American Medical Association* 273:865, 1995.

5. Blumberg J: Nutrient requirements of the healthy elderly—should there be specific RDAs? *Nutrition Reviews* 51:S15, 1994.

6. Bodgen JD and others: Daily micronutrient supplements enhance delayed hypersensitivity skin test responses in older people, *American Journal of Clinical Nutrition* 60:437, 1994.

7. Campbell TC and others: Diet and chronic degenerative diseases: perspectives from China, *American Journal of Clinical Nutrition* 59:1153S, 1994.

8. Chandra R: Nutrition and immunity in the elderly, *Nutrition Reviews* 53:S80, 1995.

9. Chapuy MC and others: Effect of calcium and cholecalciferol treatment for three years on hip fractures in elderly women, *British Medical Journal* 308:1081, 1994.

10. Chernoff R: Meeting the nutritional needs of the elderly in the institutional setting, *Nutrition Reviews* 52:132, 1994.

11. Corti MC and others: HDL cholesterol predicts coronary heart disease mortality in older persons, *Journal of the American Medical Association* 274:539, 1995.

12. Dwyer J: Strategies to detect and prevent malnutrition in the elderly: the nutrition screening initiative, *Nutrition Today* 29:14, 1994.

13. Fiatarone MA and others: Exercise training and nutritional supplementation for physical frailty in very elderly people, *The New England Journal of Medicine* 330:1769, 1994.

14. Flieger K: Testosterone: key to masculinity and more, *FDA Consumer*, p 27, May 1995.

15. Kirk JK: Significant drug-nutrient interactions, *American Family Physician* 51:1175, 1995.

16. Kritchevsky D: Caloric restriction and experimental tumorigenesis, *Nutrition Today*, p 25, Jan/Feb 1993.

17. Lee I and others: Exercise intensity and longevity in men, *Journal of the American Medical Association* 273:1179, 1995.

18. Lewis CJ and others: Healthy People 2000: report on the 1994 nutrition progress review, *Nutrition Today* 29:6, 1994.

19. Miller AB: Dietary advice and competing risks, *Nutrition* 11:57, 1995.

20. Morley JE and others: Major issues in geriatrics over the last five years, *Journal of the American Geriatrics Society* 42:218, 1994.

21. Mowe M and others: Reduced nutritional status in an elderly population (>70 y) is probable before disease and possibly contributes to the development of disease, *American Journal of Clinical Nutrition* 59:317, 1994.

22. Mulrow CD and others: Hypertension in the elderly: implications and generalizability of randomized trials, *Journal of the American Medical Association* 272:1932, 1994.

23. Napier K: Unproven medical treatments lure elderly, *FDA Consumer*, p 33, March 1994.

24. Pate RR and others: Physical activity and public health: a recommendation from the Centers for Disease Control and Prevention and the American College of Sports Medicine, *Journal of the American Medical Association*, 273:402, 1995.

25. Perls TT: The oldest old, *Scientific American*, p 70, Jan 1995.

26. Roberts SB and others: Control of food intake in older men, *Journal of the American Medical Association*, 272:1601, 1994.

27. Rosenberg IH: Keys to a longer, healthier, more vital life, *Nutrition Reviews* 52:S50, 1994.

28. Schiffman S: Changes in taste and smell: drug interactions and food preferences, *Nutrition Reviews* 52:S11, 1994.

29. Seddon JM and others: Dietary carotenoids, vitamins A, C, and E, and advanced age-related macular degeneration, *Journal of the American Medical Association* 272:1413, 1994.

30. Selhub J and others: Vitamin status and intake as primary determinants of homocysteinemia in an elderly population, *Journal of the American Medical Association* 270:2693, 1993.

31. Selkoe DJ: Deciphering Alzheimer's disease: molecular genetics and cell biology yield major clues, *The Journal of NIH Research* 7:57, 1995.

32. Stone NJ: The 75-year-old patient with hypercholesterolemia: to treat or not to treat? *Nutrition Reviews* 52:531, 1994.

33. U.S. Public Health Service: Nutrition in adults, *American Family Physician* p 1485, May 1, 1995.

34. Voelker R: Recommendations for antioxidants: how much evidence is enough? *Journal of the American Medical Association* 271:1148, 1994.

35. Willett WC: Diet and health: what should we eat? *Science* 264:532, 1994.

36. Willett WC: Mediterranean diet pyramid: a cultural model for healthy eating, *American Journal of Clinical Nutrition* 61:14025, 1995.

37. Wood RJ and others: Mineral requirements of elderly people, *American Journal of Clinical Nutrition* 62.493, 1995.

TAKE ACTION

Helping the elderly eat better

People usually eat meals with families or loved ones throughout their lifetimes. As people are reaching even older ages, many of them are faced with living and eating alone. In a study of the diets of 4400 older Americans, one man of every five living alone and over age 55 ate poorly. One of every four women between the ages of 55 and 64 years followed a low-quality diet. These inadequate diets contribute to deteriorating mental and physical health. Consider the following example of the living situation of an elderly person:

Neal, a 70-year-old man, lives alone in a house in a suburban area. He lost his wife 1 year ago. He doesn't have many friends; his wife was his primary confidante. His neighbors across the street and next door are friendly, and Neal used to help them with yard projects in his spare time. Neal's health has been good, but he has had trouble with his teeth recently. His diet has been limited, and in the last 3 months his physical and mental vigor has deteriorated. He has been slowly lapsing into depression, and so keeps the shades drawn and rarely leaves his house. Neal keeps very little food in the house because his wife did most of the cooking and shopping and he just isn't very interested in food.

If you were one of Neal's relatives and learned of Neal's situation, what six things could you do or suggest to help improve his nutritional status and mental outlook? Look back into the chapter to get some ideas.

1. _____

2. _____

3. _____

4. _____

5. _____

6. _____

NUTRITION PERSPECTIVE

Ethnic Influences on the American Diet

Over the centuries, peoples of various cultures have migrated to new locations. Typically, migrants keep some traditional dietary habits, or *foodways,* change some habits, and abandon others. As people migrate and mingle with those of other cultures their cuisines tend to mingle as well. Changes in affluence and technology also affect dietary habits, some for better and some for worse.

In this Nutrition Perspective we will examine how the cuisines of various cultures have affected the American diet. Examining the nutrition attributes of a number of ethnic diets will help you to understand that no single cuisine is either completely healthful or unhealthful. The trick to finding healthful food is to evaluate individual dishes carefully. Let's look at six cuisines that contribute to food "American style."

Native Americans

The size and varied geography of the American continent meant that different foods were available to people living in different locations. Some of these people were hunter-gatherers, depending on wild vegetation and wild game for subsistence. Others learned to grow vegetable crops. Depending on where they lived, Native American groups cultivated early forms of such plant foods as tomatoes, sweet potatoes, squash, vanilla, and cocoa. They also hunted whatever wild game was available. Their diets tended to be low in sodium and fat and high in dietary fiber. In the far North, populations subsisted on fish, sea mammals, other game, and a few plants, such as seaweed, willow leaves, and berries.

Recent studies have shown that the diseases that affected these societies differed significantly from the diseases common in American society. For example, Alaskan natives who still eat the traditional diet have heart disease rates lower than those in the general United States population. Younger generations of Alaskan natives, however, who usually do not eat the traditional diet, have developed heart disease at rates similar to those in the U.S. population in general. These and other studies indicate that as societies become more uniform, so too do disease patterns.

Mexican-Americans

When Spanish colonists arrived in what is now called Latin America, they brought foods, flavors, and cooking techniques that they combined with locally available foods. Several cuisines developed from those combinations, influenced also by the arrival of other groups. Thus the Cuban cuisine combined native foods with those of both Spanish and Chinese immigrants, whereas the Puerto Rican cuisine combined native foods with Spanish and African contributions. In Mexico, the Spanish influence mingled with that of local Native American cuisines.

The Mayans, Aztecs, and other populations in Mexico grew corn, beans, and chili peppers; these were the basis of Mexican cuisine. They also grew such fruits as avocados, papayas, and pineapples. By the end of the fifteenth century, wheat, chickpeas, melons, radishes, grapes, and sugar cane had been brought to the New World. Rice, citrus fruits, and some kinds of nuts came soon afterward. The Spanish also introduced beef, lamb, and chicken. Native inhabitants had previously eaten mostly fish and wild game. Spices such as cinnamon, black pepper, cloves, thyme, marjoram, and bay leaves were introduced and also became part of the cuisine.

Mexican cuisine today shows regional variety. In southern Mexico, savory sauces and stews and corn tortillas reflect the native heritage. The Gulf states are renowned for delicious seafood dishes prepared with tomatoes, herbs, and olives, whereas Yucatan cuisine follows Mayan tradition, with such specialties as wild turkey and fish flavored with lime juice. Fresh produce adds color, flavor, and nutrition to authentic Mexican dining. Markets in the United States are now beginning to offer some of these plant foods, such as chayote, squash, jicama root, plantains, and cactus leaves and fruit.

Today, true Mexican cooking bears little resemblance to the dishes usually found in "Mexican" restaurants. Usually it is neither oily nor heavy and is based primarily on rice and beans.

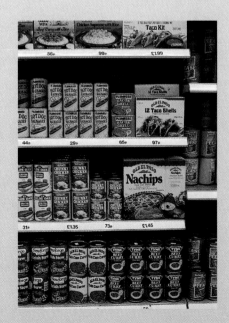

Adaptations of traditional Mexican foods are available in most local supermarkets.

Restaurant Mexican food tends to use larger portions of meat, as well as adding portions of high-fat sour cream, guacamole, and cheese to many dishes. To lower your fat intake in such a restaurant, order a bean burrito without cheese. Or have a bean or meat taco with a soft (unfried) shell. Fajitas can also be constructed with low-fat ingredients. Order such fried dishes as tortilla chips, chimichangas, or enchiladas infrequently.

European-Americans

Immigrants from Western Europe are responsible for the "meat-and-potatoes" presentation of traditional American home cooking. The first large group of settlers from Europe—the English, French, and Germans—brought their traditional foodways with them. As all cooks and cultures must do, these immigrants adapted to the foods available in the regions in which they settled. Native Americans shared new foods that are now staples of the American diet: corn and corn products such as popcorn and hominy, some kinds of squash, and tomatoes.

However, because the new immigrants often settled in regions of the "new land" that most closely resembled their homes in Europe, they were able to grow many familiar foods and retain many of their traditional foodways. One of these foodways involved the way food is presented.

A sizeable portion of meat arranged with vegetables and potatoes in separate portions on a plate is the European pattern, compared with other cuisines in which a mixture of starch, vegetables, and a much smaller portion of protein (such as a stir-fry) is more typical. The meat on the "American" dinner plate may be, for example, sausage or roast beef, the potatoes may be boiled or mashed, and the vegetable may be sauerkraut or green peas. Whatever the choices, the Western European pattern is still followed by many in this country.

This traditional pattern provides abundant protein and nutrients from dairy and meat products. However, the protein also contains saturated fat, and the large portions of protein and starch may mean that insufficient amounts of whole grains, vegetables, and fruits are eaten. Try a smaller portion of skinless chicken breast, accompanied by a plain baked potato with the skin and a hearty portion of green beans or broccoli, for example. This combination of foods follows the traditional pattern while allowing for more healthful food choices.

African-Americans

Involuntary immigrants to the New World, people from West Africa struggled to survive under harsh conditions. Their ability to adapt familiar foodways to new conditions became a lasting influence on today's American cuisine.

The "soul food" of African-Americans is the basis of the regional cuisines of the American South. Many understand "soul food" to consist mainly of barbecued meat, fried chicken, sweet potatoes, and chitterlings. In fact, true soul food includes a wide range of dishes created by African-American cooks. They used traditional methods and foods brought from Africa, such as yams, okra, and peanuts, as well as what was available in the New World. African-American women, cooking for their families, created dishes that they often adapted for the plantation owner's table as well, creating the basis of Southern cuisine. The combination of these African-American foodways with Native American, Spanish, and French traditions produced the Cajun and Creole cuisines enjoyed today in Louisiana and throughout the nation.

Pork and corn products were the basis of soul food. The plantation owner ate the better parts of the pig. As with other foods, slaves learned to make the less desirable parts of the pig, such as entrails, feet, ears, and head, palatable. Corn was ground for corn bread. Unrefined yellow cornmeal was mixed with water and lard to make "hoecake," baked on a hoe blade by cooks who had neither ovens nor cooking utensils for their own use. The plantation owner probably ate white cornbread made from refined cornmeal.

Among other dishes still considered soul food staples are greens, usually cooked with a small portion of smoked pork. The greens used include collards, mustard, turnip, or dandelion greens, and kale. Black-eyed peas, first brought to the New World by slaves, are also cooked with pork. Sweet potatoes and yams were and remain basic soul foods; sweet potato pie is the soul food equivalent of pumpkin pie.

Today's traditional African-American cuisine has both nutritional benefits and deficits. The variety of fruits, vegetables, and grain products used provides ample vitamins, minerals, and dietary fiber. For instance, African-Americans in general consume more cruciferous vegetables, and fruits and vegetables containing vitamins A and C than do Caucasian Americans. However, cured pork products contribute undesirable levels of sodium as well as saturated fat. Traditional reliance on frying, especially with lard, also adds fat to the diet. Boiling vegetables for long periods depletes water-soluble vitamins. Dairy products may not be used enough, especially by older people who follow traditional dietary customs. This avoidance is based in part on the difficulty many African-American adults experience in digesting lactose; see Chapter 3 for details.

Chinese-Americans

Known for its variety, the average Chinese diet provides about 70% of energy as carbohydrate, 15% as protein, and 15% as fat. This is similar to the proportions recommended by some Western nutritionists and cancer experts. Over 200 different vegetables are used in Chinese cuisine; bok choy and other forms of Chinese cabbage are perhaps the most widely eaten vegetables in the world. In the southeastern coastal region of China, home of the Cantonese cuisine, the number of dishes may be as high as 50,000.

China is a huge country, with varying climates and many regional cuisines. Rice is the core of the diet in southern China, whereas in the temperate North, wheat is used in noodles (China is the original home of pasta), bread, and dumplings. Popular dishes include hot pots (stews containing many ingredients) and stir-fried mixtures of vegetables and small amounts of meat or fish cooked in a lightly-oiled, very hot pan.

Chinese immigration to America began with the California gold rush in the middle of the nineteenth century. Chinese workers brought with them food preparation methods that tend to preserve nutrients, as well as a variety of sauces and seasonings, such as ginger root, garlic, rice wine, scallions, and sesame seeds and oil. Although many of the traditional foodways have been preserved, North American restaurant versions of Chinese cuisine, whether Cantonese, Szechuan, or Mandarin, are usually not authentic. Chinese-American restaurant food is often prepared with far more fat than in true Chinese cooking, which tends to use flavorful but fat-free sauces and seasoning. The restaurant versions of Chinese dishes also contain much larger portions of protein.

However, choosing a healthful meal in a Chinese-American restaurant is still possible. Select dishes that are not deep-fat fried (such as egg rolls or batter-coated meats or seafood). Choose at least one vegetable dish instead of a meat entrée. Leave most of the sauce behind by eating Chinese style. Lift the food from the sauce and place it on top of a mouthful of rice, which in China is the basis of the meal. Limit the amount of soy sauce you sprinkle on the rice. (Even in China, health authorities are now calling for a cut in salt intake and a switch from saturated to unsaturated fats.)

Italian-Americans

Authentic Italian cuisine, like Chinese cuisine, is more diverse than most Americans realize. Foods of different regions reflect Italy's varied geography and climate. Northern Italy, the more affluent part of the country, is the principal producer of meat and dairy products, such as butter and cheese. Rice dishes such as risotto are popular there. Fish is more important in regions near the sea, and lighter foods, such as fresh vegetables prepared with herbs, garlic, and olive oil, are characteristic. The poorer regions south of Rome, as well as the island of Sicily, have a diet rich in grains, vegetables, dried beans, and fish, with little meat or oil. Compared with Northern Italians of the same class, Southern Italians eat less beef, veal, chicken, and butter, and more bread, pasta, vegetables, fruit, and fish.

Pasta is the heart of the Italian diet. Italians eat six times more of this simple wheat and water product than do North Americans, although Americans have also learned to love this

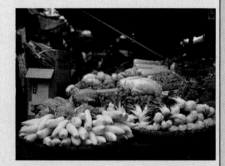

The Chinese diet is known for its variety—over 200 different vegetables are used in Chinese cuisine.

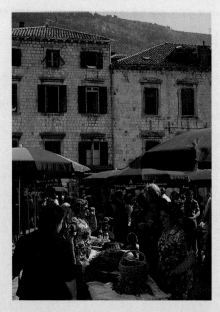

A Yugoslavian market. Many Eastern European cuisines have influenced the American diet.

nutritious dish. Pasta in America, however, often means spaghetti, with a tomato-based sauce that includes meatballs or sausage. In contrast, Italians eat pasta in a variety of shapes and with a variety of sauces, often excluding meat.

Most of the Italian-American cuisine found in restaurants offers foods more common to the North of Italy, including veal, cheese, and cream and pesto sauces for pasta. Pizza, a Southern Italian dish, is the exception, and it is fast becoming the most frequently consumed food in the United States. Pizza in this country is served on a variety of flour crusts topped with anything from high-fat meats such as pepperoni to vegetables or even fruit, combined with a variety of cheeses, tomatoes, and oregano for seasoning. Purists in Naples, however, insist that classic pizza consists only of a thin crust, tomato, basil, and mozzarella cheese.

Although some components of the Italian diet contain substantial amounts of saturated fat, nutritionists now know that other compounds, such as pasta, olive oil, and vegetables, contribute to good health. Healthy choices in an Italian-American restaurant might include a pasta dish with fresh tomato sauce, rather than cheese-laden Alfredo sauce, and an entrée of fish and vegetables cooked with wine, olive oil, and herbs. Limiting the cheeses and meats offered on the antipasto tray, and avoiding fried foods such as veal Parmigiana, are also wise moves.

Ethnic Diets and Present Trends

Only six ethnic diets have been described here; see Table 18-8 for a summary of their advantages and disadvantages. Many other cuisines have also influenced the American diet, and

TABLE 18-8

The world's fare has influenced the American diet

The following is a brief summary of healthful attributes and shortcomings of the ethnic diet influences covered in this Nutrition Perspective.

	Advantages	Shortcomings
Native American; Alaskan Native	Variety of seafood, lean wild game; early Native Americans ate variety of vegetables, berries, leaves	High fat content of some meat/seafood; low in calcium
Hispanic-American	Excellent variety of vegetables, legumes, fruits; high in dietary fiber	Traditional Hispanic diet may fall short in calcium; Mexican-American restaurants serve much high-fat fare, rich in sour cream, cheese, and guacamole
European-American	Abundant sources of protein, iron, calcium from meat and dairy groups	Less variety from vegetables, fruits, legumes; high in fat
African-American	Good variety of vitamin A and carotenoid-containing vegetables; high fiber. Many variations including Cajun, Creole dishes	Traditional meats high in fat. May fall short in calcium
Chinese-American	Excellent variety of vegetables, grains; cooking methods retain nutrients in foods	Some sauces are high in salt and fat
Italian-American	Varies regionally—some regions provide excellent variety of seafood; overall high grain intake, good vegetable and fruit variety	Italian-American restaurants often serve many foods made with high-fat cheese, sauces, and meats; likely low in calcium

new arrivals continue to bring their traditions and foodways to this country. For example, recent social upheavals have increased the immigration of Russians and other Eastern European peoples to the United States. On the other side of the world, continuing unrest in southeast Asia has brought peoples from that area here. Restaurants serving traditional Russian or Thai fare, for instance, are now offering new foodways to those willing to experiment.

The growing American concern with healthful eating as well as growing interest in ethnic cuisines is shown by the recent publicity surrounding the "Mediterranean Diet." This is a cuisine based on food choices like those traditionally found in the simple cuisines of Greece and southern Italy. In 1994, components of this diet were arranged into a pyramid analogous to the USDA Food Guide Pyramid by representatives from the Harvard School of Public Health, the World Health Organization's Regional Office for Europe, and the nonprofit Oldways Preservations & Exchange Trust (Figure 18-9).

The Mediterranean pyramid allows 25% to 35% of total fat in the diet, compared with the typical recommendation of not more than 30%. However, it recommends consuming the type of fat consumed in the Mediterranean region: olive oil. The plan recommends that very small portions of red meat be eaten only a few times a month, and also suggests regular physical activity and modest alcohol intake (wine, preferably red wine) with meals. Eggs and sweets are to be used sparingly as well.

This alternative pyramid was developed because some nutrition scientists have for some time observed much lower rates of heart disease and certain forms of cancer in Mediterranean populations than in America. These nutritionists also believed that Americans were not sufficiently aware of the significant role diet may play in disease processes.

However, the Mediterranean pyramid falls short in some areas. Like the Food Guide Pyramid, it recommends a generous base of grains, fruits, vegetables, and legumes. In contrast, it does not limit fat to the same extent. Olive oil is not rich in saturated fats, but like all fats it is a concentrated source of energy, and obesity is a major public health problem in the United States. The whole-milk cheese and yogurt included in the Mediterranean pyramid contain high amounts of saturated fat, which contributes to heart disease. Recommending reduced-fat varieties of dairy products would improve the plan. Calcium intake is likely to be low in this plan, because low-fat or nonfat milk are omitted. Architects of the plan suggest that calcium supplements be used to meet this shortfall.

Many Americans do consume diets of high-fat convenience foods that offer little variety. The first steps to a better diet should be made away from that pattern and toward the bottom of either pyramid. However, we believe that using the Food Guide Pyramid is still a good way to begin getting the balance and variety in fruits, vegetables, and whole grains that Americans should strive for in their diets. The food choices provided in the Food Guide Pyramid allow for limiting red meat consumption, if that is desired. Undoubtedly, observations included in the Mediterranean diet pyramid, such as the use of red wine with meals and the risks of red meat consumption with respect to colon cancer, are worth further study.

Using research also begun many years ago, still other scientists suggest that a healthful diet consists of the inexpensive traditional dishes based on grains, fruits, and vegetables that form the backbone of a number of ethnic cuisines. These are precisely the dishes that people abandon as they become affluent and seek convenience. Simple foods prepared in simple ways have fed most of humanity for virtually its entire existence. As we turn toward a new century, some Americans are rediscovering the simple foods of their respective pasts, learning to enjoy a variety of cuisines, and finding how each cuisine can contribute to a healthier American diet.

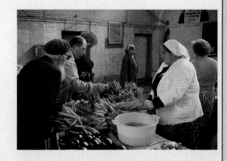

A Russian produce market. Russian immigrants have brought their traditional foodways with them to America.

Consider the following suggestions if you want to begin following a more Mediterranean diet:
- **Plan meals ahead of time in order to have better control over food intake.**
- **Switch to olive oil as a main source of fat. For a less expensive option, canola oil has about the same fatty acid profile, but it does not qualify as the typical Mediterranean fat.**
- **Reduce intake of butter and margarine.**
- **Add bread in abundance to each meal.**
- **Begin or end most meals with a salad.**
- **Add more vegetables and different vegetables to meals.**
- **Cut down on the amount of meat consumed.**
- **Substitute wine in moderation for other alcoholic beverages.**
- **Include desserts only occasionally.**

Figure 18-9 Battle of the pyramids—which pattern best meets your nutrient needs and palate?

A, The USDA Food Guide Pyramid. This plan suggests forming a diet primarily from breads and other starches, fruits, and vegetables. It allows small amounts of fats, oils, and sweets. Following this pyramid results in most fat in the diet coming from the 2 to 3 daily servings of the meat, poultry, fish, dry beans, eggs, and nuts group, and the milk, yogurt, and cheese group.

B, The traditional healthy Mediterranean Diet Pyramid. This plan is based on longstanding eating habits in southern Italy, Crete, and Greece. The base of the diet comes from bread and grains, fruits and vegetables, and beans and potatoes. Red meat is consumed sparingly—moderate amounts of fish and poultry are preferred. Wine may be included with meals. A recommendation for regular physical activity is also made. Most of the fat in this plan comes from olive oil. Cheese and yogurt supply some fat and some calcium.

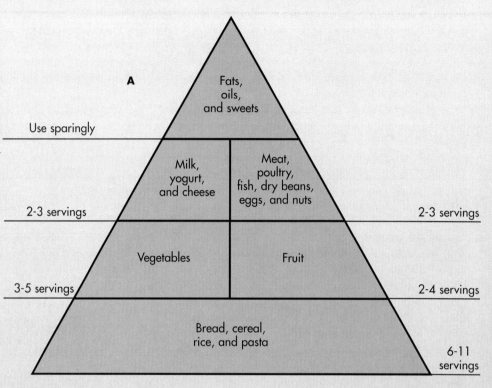

A

Fats, oils, and sweets

Use sparingly

Milk, yogurt, and cheese

Meat, poultry, fish, dry beans, eggs, and nuts

2-3 servings

2-3 servings

Vegetables

Fruit

3-5 servings

2-4 servings

Bread, cereal, rice, and pasta

6-11 servings

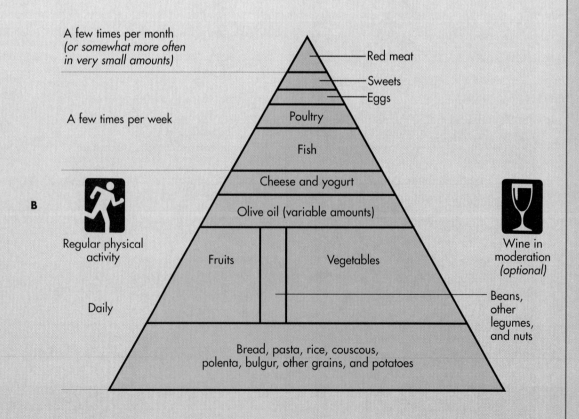

B

A few times per month *(or somewhat more often in very small amounts)* — Red meat

— Sweets

— Eggs

A few times per week — Poultry

Fish

Cheese and yogurt

Olive oil (variable amounts)

Regular physical activity

Wine in moderation *(optional)*

Fruits

Vegetables

Beans, other legumes, and nuts

Daily

Bread, pasta, rice, couscous, polenta, bulgur, other grains, and potatoes

CHAPTER NINETEEN

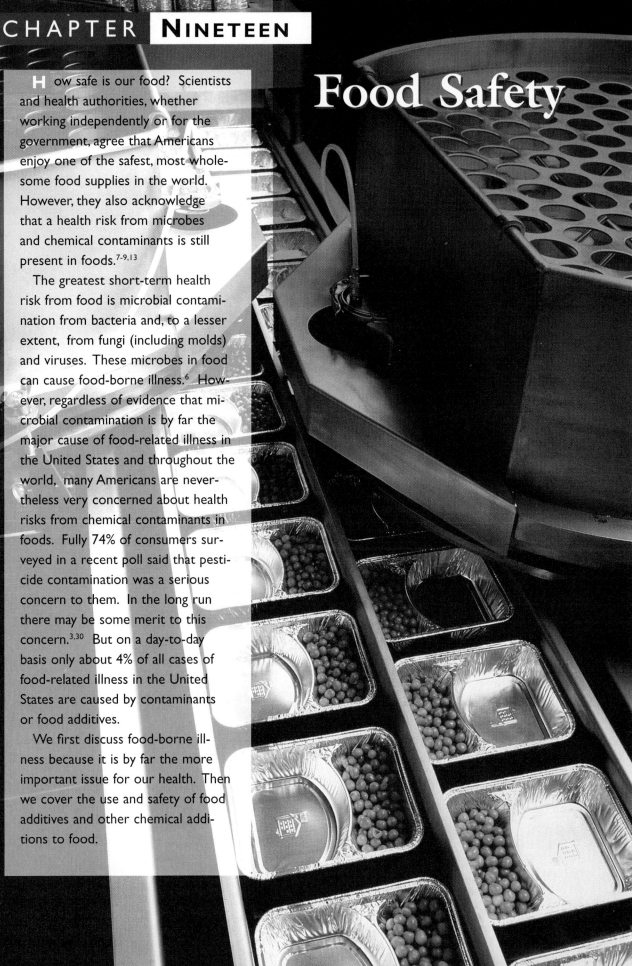

Food Safety

H ow safe is our food? Scientists and health authorities, whether working independently or for the government, agree that Americans enjoy one of the safest, most wholesome food supplies in the world. However, they also acknowledge that a health risk from microbes and chemical contaminants is still present in foods.[7-9,13]

The greatest short-term health risk from food is microbial contamination from bacteria and, to a lesser extent, from fungi (including molds) and viruses. These microbes in food can cause food-borne illness.[6] However, regardless of evidence that microbial contamination is by far the major cause of food-related illness in the United States and throughout the world, many Americans are nevertheless very concerned about health risks from chemical contaminants in foods. Fully 74% of consumers surveyed in a recent poll said that pesticide contamination was a serious concern to them. In the long run there may be some merit to this concern.[3,30] But on a day-to-day basis only about 4% of all cases of food-related illness in the United States are caused by contaminants or food additives.

We first discuss food-borne illness because it is by far the more important issue for our health. Then we cover the use and safety of food additives and other chemical additions to food.

NUTRITION AWARENESS INVENTORY

NUTRITION AWARENESS

Answer these 15 statements about food safety to test your current knowledge. If you think the answer is true or mostly true, circle T. If you think the answer is false or mostly false, circle F. Use the scoring key at the end of the book to compute your total score. Repeat this test after you have read this chapter, and compare your results.

1. **T F** In the United States many people suffer a bout of food-borne illness each year.
2. **T F** You can usually tell from a food's taste, odor, or appearance if that food poses a risk for food-borne illness.
3. **T F** Imported food does not pose a risk for food-borne illness because of careful inspection on entry into this country.
4. **T F** Synthetic (man-made) chemicals are more harmful to health than those that occur naturally.
5. **T F** Exposure to oxygen causes some foods to spoil.
6. **T F** Food can be preserved by reducing its water content.
7. **T F** Most kinds of bacteria can cause food-borne illness.
8. **T F** Most food-borne illness microbes thrive at temperatures between 40° F and 140° F (4° C and 60° C).
9. **T F** Symptoms of food-borne illness include diarrhea.
10. **T F** Victims of food-borne illness receive some immunity against future attacks.
11. **T F** Chickens are a common source of *Salmonella* infection.
12. **T F** Botulism is a very deadly form of food-borne illness, and the bacterium that causes it is present in soil.
13. **T F** *Clostridium botulinum,* the bacteria that cause botulism, grow only in the absence of air.
14. **T F** Eating raw shellfish, or any raw animal product, can lead to serious health problems.
15. **T F** Aside from the alcohol present, alcoholic beverages are free of toxic compounds.

Food-Borne Illness

food-borne illness Sickness caused by ingestion of food containing toxic substances produced by microorganisms.

A t the turn of the century, conditions in Chicago's meat-packing industry were sickening. Moldy, spoiled meat was commonly doused with borax to cover up the smell, and glycerine was added to make it look fresh. Upton Sinclair outraged the American public with his first-hand account of these deplorable conditions in *The Jungle,* published in 1906. Increasing public pressure forced the passage of the first Food and Drug Act later that year. Federal inspection then began to safeguard the public from worm-infested and diseased meat. Food preparation standards also generally improved. Indeed, we have come a long way.

Still, diarrhea cases caused by **food-borne illness** are common today. Estimates are that up to about 1 in 8 Americans is afflicted each year. This food-borne illness costs the United States economy up to 23 billion dollars annually in medical expenses and lost productivity and leads to about 9000 deaths.[8] Thus microbes in food remain a considerable health risk.[24,31]

Food-borne illness generally leads to a brief yet distressing episode of diarrhea, similar to traveler's diarrhea. It generally presents no real long-term health risk for the average person, but for many it can be more serious. Some people especially suffer greatly from food-borne illness, including:
- infants and children
- the elderly
- those with liver disease or diabetes
- cancer patients
- pregnant women
- people taking immunosuppressant agents

- people with gastrointestinal disease, including previous gastric surgery, and reduced amounts of gastric acid (e.g., from antacid use or **achlorhydria** [decreased gastric acidity])
- acquired immunodeficiency syndrome (AIDS) patients

These more serious bouts of food-borne illness can be lengthy and lead to food allergies, seizures, blood poisoning (from toxins or microbes in the blood), or other illness.[24,31] Susceptible individuals are at highest risk during the warmest months of the year, as heat encourages microbial growth. In turn there is a need to take extra care at this time of year to thoroughly cook meat, fish, and poultry, and especially seafood such as oysters.

Because much of food-borne illness results from unsafe handling of food at home, we each bear some responsibility for preventing it. It is generally not possible to tell from taste, smell, or sight that a particular food poses a risk for food-borne illness. The main exception to this rule is the uncommon *Bacillus subtilis*, which causes "off flavors" in pastry items. So your last case of diarrhea actually may have had a food-borne cause, as the symptoms often include that, as well as vomiting, fever, and weakness.

WHY IS FOOD-BORNE ILLNESS SO COMMON?

People may long for the days when they could eat rare hamburgers without fear. What has changed to cause a seemingly sudden increase of dangerous microbes in food such as this?

In the past, people contracted tuberculosis from milk and typhoid fever from water and seafood. Today, the risk of food-borne illness is still high, but of a different sort. This is because, in addition to consumers' mishandling food, social trends have added new causes. First, there is greater consumer interest in eating foods of animal origin raw or undercooked. In addition, a larger part of the population receives medication that suppresses their ability to combat food-borne infectious agents. Also, there is a continuing increase in the elderly population. We noted earlier that these two groups of people are at greater risk of food-borne illness.[24]

The food industry is also increasing where possible the shelf life of products. A longer shelf life at room temperature allows more time for bacteria in food to multiply. Some bacteria grow even at refrigeration temperatures, for example, *Listeria* and *Yersinia*. Partially cooked, and some fully cooked, products pose a special risk because refrigerated storage may only slow—not prevent—bacterial growth. FDA and other federal agencies are working hard to reduce this problem.[29]

The risk of illness from food-borne microbes has also increased as more centralized kitchens outside the home prepare foods. With so many two-income families, people are looking for convenient, easily prepared foods. Supermarkets have responded to the demand and become major food processors over the past decade. They now offer a variety of prepared foods from specialty meat shops, salad bars, and bakeries. Entrées can be served immediately or reheated. The foods are usually prepared in central kitchens or processing plants and shipped to individual stores. If a food product is contaminated in the central kitchen or processing plant, patrons of stores over a wide area can suffer food-borne illness.[16] Extra handling also adds to contamination problems, but the foods look so "sterile" in their plastic wrapping that consumers may forget they carry risks for food-borne illness.

The centralization of food production by the food processing industry also adds to the risk of food-borne illness. For example, a malfunction in a dairy plant in 1985 resulted in 16,284 confirmed cases of *Salmonella* bacteria infections and at least two deaths from contaminated milk. In 1987, lettuce shredded in a Texas plant and then placed in large plastic bags was the cause of the largest *Shigella* bacteria outbreak ever reported in the United States. At least 347 people fell ill. The nutrients released when the lettuce was shredded, coupled with the moist environment provided by the plastic bags, allowed growth and reproduction of the organism. In 1993 at least four people died and 700 became ill in Washington and surrounding western states

Food contamination presents a unique risk to the elderly, whose possibly poor eyesight and reduced senses of smell and taste make it harder to spot spoiled food or dirty utensils. Their reduced appetite can lead to a weakened immune system. The elderly face further risks because their stomachs may be low in acid, which destroys harmful bacteria, and because of poor blood circulation, which can prevent antibodies from reaching sites of infection.

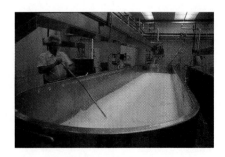

If food is contaminated in a central kitchen, like this cottage cheese processing plant, patrons of stores over a wide area can suffer food-borne illness.

after eating at a chain of quick-service restaurants. The source of the problem was undercooked hamburger contaminated with the bacterium *Escherichia coli 0157:H7*.[2] The hamburger came from a central plant in California. Recently, ice cream made in Minnesota and carried in a contaminated tank truck was blamed for thousands of suspected cases of *Salmonella* infection in at least 30 states.[16] In Minnesota alone, about 2500 people reported getting sick after eating the ice cream. Overall, the growth of large-scale food production technologies has introduced new and different food-borne risks.

Still another cause of increased food-borne illness in America is greater consumption of ready-to-eat foods imported from foreign countries. In the past, food imports were mostly raw products processed here under strict sanitation standards. Now, however, we import processed foods, such as cheese from France and shrimp and other seafood from Asia, some of which are contaminated.[6]

Finally, more cases of food-borne disease are reported now because we are more aware of the role of various players in the process. Every decade the list of microorganisms suspected of causing food-borne illness expands.[11] In addition, physicians now show greater recognition of the possibility that "stomach complaints" may have a food-borne cause. As well, laboratories have improved diagnostic capabilities for detecting the causative organisms. Furthermore, we now know that food, besides serving as a good growth medium for some microorganisms, simply transmits many others as well.[22]

Seafood especially is being scrutinized much more than in the past by FDA as a source of food-borne illness. New FDA regulations require for the first time that the seafood industry keep detailed records of safety procedures and label all shellfish to show where it was caught. These are important advances in the seafood industry, which before received less regulatory scrutiny than the purveyors of beef, poultry, and other meats. FDA provides a seafood hotline to answer consumers' questions and for them to report suspected illness related to consumption: (800) FDA-4010 or (202) 205-4314 (in the Washington, D.C., area).

Food Preservation—Past, Present, and Future

For centuries, salt, sugar, smoke, fermentation, and drying have been used to preserve food. Ancient Romans used sulfites to disinfect wine containers and preserve wine. In the age of exploration, European adventurers traveling to the New World preserved their meat by salting it.

Many preservation methods work on the principle of reducing the amount of **free water** in food. Salts and sugar reduce free water by binding it, and drying drives off free water. A measure of the free water in a food is known as its **water activity.** Most bacteria need a water activity greater than 0.9 to grow. Yeasts can grow at water activity above 0.8, and molds grow at water activity above 0.6. The water activities of typical foods are listed in the margin. This list shows why bacteria are a problem in eggs and meat but not in jam. You can also see that, unless properly treated and stored, dried fruits can still support the growth of molds.

Some foods with high water activity would be greatly altered by a decrease in their free-water content. In these cases, selected bacteria are used to ferment (pickle) or "spoil" the food. Pickles, sauerkraut, yogurt, and wine are all examples of this type of processing. The fermenting bacteria or yeasts make acids and alcohol, which minimize the growth of other microbes. The acid produced is helpful in preventing the growth of *Clostridium botulinum,* a potential problem in many canned foods.

Today, we can add **pasteurization,** sterilization, refrigeration, freezing, canning, chemical preservatives, and **irradiation** to the list of food-preservation techniques. Food irradiation is the newest of these.[19,21] In 1986, FDA approved the use of food irradiation for the preservation of spices, potatoes, and grains. Approval was then extended to include poultry, pork, fruits, and vegetables. The high-energy radiation used produces free radicals that can destroy cell membranes, break down DNA, and

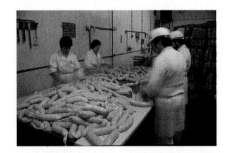

The growth of large-scale food-production technologies has introduced unique risks for food-borne illness.

free water The water not bound to the components in the food, making it available for microbial use.

water activity A measure of the amount of free water in a food. Most bacteria need a water activity greater than 0.9 to grow, while molds can grow with water activity as low as 0.6.

Foods	Water activity
fruits and vegetables	0.97
eggs	0.96
meats	0.96
cheese, bread	0.96
jam	0.85
honey	0.75
dried fruit	0.70

link proteins. The radiation used does not make the food radioactive. By altering DNA, enzymes, and proteins, irradiation can prevent the growth of microorganisms, parasites, and insects without creating much heat in the food product.[19] Thus it is referred to as *cold sterilization.*

Proponents claim that food irradiation is a safe and effective means of preservation that extends the shelf life of foods, destroys microorganisms, slows the rapid ripening of harvested produce, and reduces the need for pesticides, some of which are harmful.[21] However, researchers have also shown that irradiation can cause unpleasant flavors, off colors, and changes in texture. In addition, decreases in thiamin, vitamin A, and vitamin E content of foods have been detected after irradiation.

To date, consumer acceptance of food irradiation in the United States remains very low. Certain consumer groups continually try to block its use. Continued attempts to employ this technology are likely, but whether the public will accept it as it does canning (which also originally met with skepticism) is still in question. Worldwide, countries such as Japan, France, Italy, and Mexico use food irradiation technology.[21] When food is irradiated, it must carry the label shown in the margin. However, note that if irradiated spices are incorporated into another food, there is no requirement that the "second-generation" food carry the irradiation label.

Another new method of food preservation, **aseptic packaging,** simultaneously sterilizes the product and the package separately, filling the package without recontaminating the product, and sealing it so that microbes cannot enter. Liquid foods, such as fruit juices, are especially easy to process in this manner. With aseptic packaging, boxes of milk and juices can remain untainted on supermarket shelves, free of microbial growth, for many years. This method of food preservation has the advantages of producing a product at a lower price, with lighter weight and excellent flavor qualities. It is widely used in Europe and becoming increasingly common in the United States.

A Closer Look at Food-Borne Illness

Microbiological research has clearly demonstrated that specific toxins produced by bacteria and other microbes cause food-borne illness. These organisms do so in two ways: (1) directly, by invading the intestinal wall and releasing **endotoxin,** as do *Salmonella* organisms, or (2) indirectly, by producing an **exotoxin,** as does the *Staphylococcus* bacterium. Many different types of microorganisms cause food-borne illness, especially bacteria such as *Bacillus, Campylobacter, Clostridium, Escherichia, Listeria, Vibrio, Yersinia, Salmonella,* and *Staphylococcus.*[25]

Because each teaspoon of soil contains about two billion bacteria, we are constantly at risk for bacteria-caused illness. Luckily, only a small number of all bacteria actually pose a threat. Determining which microbe has caused food-borne illness depends on identifying the clinical features of the outbreak, the incubation period for the symptoms to appear, and the food source.

GENERAL RULES FOR PREVENTING FOOD-BORNE ILLNESS

The Centers for Disease Control and Prevention has estimated that 85% of all food-borne illness could be avoided if people took proper precautionary steps at home. Improper final storage and preparation of food in the home or in a restaurant can undo all the safety precautions implemented up to that point by farmers, food processors, and grocers.

Following are important rules to greatly minimize the risk for food-borne illness. It is a long list; there are simply many risky habits that need to be addressed.

Purchasing Food

• Select frozen foods and perishable foods, such as meat, poultry, or fish, last when shopping. Always have these products put in separate plastic bags so that drip-

International label for noting prior irradiation of the food product.

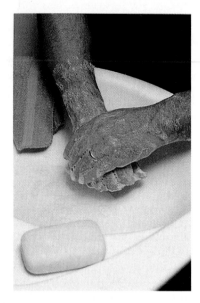

Washing hands thoroughly with hot water and soap should be the first step in food preparation.

CRITICAL THINKING

Jon wants to buy a cutting board for his new kitchen. He's been looking at all of the possibilities: plexiglass, plastic, and wood. How would you advise him so that he can minimize the risk of any food-borne illness from his food preparation?

- - - - - - - - - - - -

The microwave has one food safety disadvantage. It sometimes leaves cold spots in food, where bacteria can survive. To avoid risks:

- **Stir and rotate food at least once or twice for even cooking.**
- **Observe the standing time called for in a recipe or package directions. During the standing time, food finishes cooking as heat is distributed throughout the product.**
- **Use the oven temperature probe or a meat thermometer to check that food is done. Insert it at several spots.**

- - - - - - - - - - - -

pings don't contaminate other foods in the shopping cart. Then don't let groceries sit in a warm car; this allows bacteria to grow. Get the perishable foods home and promptly refrigerate or freeze.

- Don't buy or use food from flawed containers that leak, bulge, or are severely dented, nor buy or use food from jars that are cracked or have loose or bulging lids. Do not taste or use food that has a foul odor, or any food that spurts liquid when the can is opened; the deadly *Clostridium botulinum* toxin may be present.
- Purchase only pasteurized milk and cheese. This is especially important for pregnant women because very toxic bacteria, such as *Listeria,* and viruses that can harm the fetus thrive in unpasteurized milk.[29]

Preparing Food

- Thoroughly wash hands with hot, soapy water before and after handling food. It is especially important when handling raw meat, fish, poultry, or eggs.
- Make sure counters, cutting boards, dishes, and other equipment are thoroughly cleaned and rinsed before use. Be especially careful to use hot, soapy water to wash countertops, cutting boards, utensils, and other pieces of equipment that have come in contact with raw meat, fish, poultry, and eggs as soon as possible to remove *Salmonella* bacteria that may be present.
- If possible, cut foods to be eaten raw on a clean cutting board reserved for that purpose. Then clean this cutting board using hot, soapy water. If the same board must be used for both meat and other foods, cut the raw items before cutting any potentially contaminated items, such as meat.

  USDA recommends cutting boards with unmarred surfaces that are made of easy-to-clean, nonporous materials, such as plastic, marble, or glass. If a wooden board is preferred, it should be reserved for a specific purpose; for example, set it aside for cutting raw meat and poultry. Then keep a separate board for chopping produce or slicing bread to avoid the possibility of these products picking up bacteria from raw meat. Note that many foods are served raw, so any bacteria clinging to them are not destroyed.

  Furthermore, USDA recommends that all cutting boards, plastic or wood, be replaced when they become streaked with hard-to-clean grooves or cuts, as these may harbor bacteria. In addition, both wood and plastic boards should be sanitized once a week in a solution of two teaspoons chlorine bleach per quart of water. Flood the board with the solution, let it sit a few minutes, and then rinse thoroughly.

- When thawing foods, do so in the refrigerator for 1 to 3 days, under cold running water, or in a microwave oven. Never let frozen foods thaw unrefrigerated all day or night. Also, marinate food in the refrigerator.
- Avoid coughing or sneezing over foods, even when you are healthy. Cover cuts on hands with a sterile bandage. This helps stop *Staphylococcus aureus* from entering food.
- Carefully wash fresh fruit and vegetables under running water to remove dirt and bacteria clinging to the surface. Use a vegetable brush for potatoes if the skin is to be eaten. People became ill recently from *Salmonella* that was introduced from melons used in making a fruit salad. The bacteria were on the outside of the melon.
- Completely remove moldy portions of food or don't eat the food. When in doubt, throw the food out. Mold growth is prevented by properly storing food at cold temperatures and using the food within a reasonable length of time.
- Use refrigerated ground meat and patties in one to two days and frozen meat and patties within 3 to 4 months.

Cooking Food

- Cook food thoroughly, especially beef, fish, and pork (160° F [71° C]), poultry (180° F [82° C]), and eggs (until the yolk and white are hard). Cooking destroys most food-borne bacteria, while freezing only halts growth. A good general precaution is to eat no raw animal products. Most chickens are contaminated by *Salmonella,* which is killed by thorough cooking (white flesh, not pink). Undercooked pork can allow infection by the parasite that causes trichinosis.[28] USDA answers questions about safe use of animal products (phone: 800-535-4555, 10 AM to 4 PM weekdays, Eastern time).

Seafood also poses risk of food-borne illness. Properly cooked fish should be opaque or dull, firm, and flake easily. If it's translucent or shiny, it's not done.

Raw fish dishes, such as sushi, can be safe for most people to eat if they are made with very fresh fish that is commercially frozen and then thawed. The freezing is important to eliminate potential health risks from parasites. FDA recommends that the fish be frozen to an internal temperature of $-10°$ F for 7 days. If you choose to eat uncooked fish, purchase the fish from reputable establishments that have high standards for quality and sanitation. People at high risk for food-borne illness that we listed at the outset would be wise to avoid raw fish products (Figure 19-1).

Many people, especially people with liver disease, fall ill each year from eating raw shellfish. Clams and oysters can contain *Vibrio vulnificus,* which can cause severe food-borne illness.[24]

- Cook stuffing separately from poultry (or wash poultry thoroughly, stuff immediately before cooking, and then transfer the stuffing to a clean bowl immediately after cooking). Make sure the stuffing reaches 165° F (74° C). Again, *Salmonella* is the major concern with poultry.
- Once a food is cooked, consume it right away, or cool it to 40° F (4° C) within 2 hours. If it is not to be eaten immediately, in hot weather (85° F and above) make sure this cooling is done within 1 hour. Do this by separating the food into as many shallow pans as needed to provide a large surface area. Be careful not to recontaminate cooked food by contact with raw meat or juices from hands, cutting boards, dirty utensils, or in other ways.
- Serve meat, poultry, and fish on a clean plate, never the same plate that was used to hold the raw product. For example, when grilling hamburgers don't put cooked items on the same plate that was used to carry the raw product out to the grill.
- Cook food completely at the picnic site, with no partial cooking ahead.

Storing and Reheating Cooked Food
- Keep hot foods hot and cold foods cold. Hold food below 40° F (4° C) or above 140° F (60° C) (Figure 19-2). Food-borne illness microbes thrive in more moderate temperatures (60° to 110° F [16° to 40° C]). Some microbes can even grow in the refrigerator. Again, do not leave cooked or refrigerated foods, such as meats and salads, at room temperature for more than 2 hours (or 1 hour in hot weather) because that provides microbes an opportunity to grow. Store dry food at 60° F to 70° F (16° C to 21° C).
- Reheat leftovers to 165° F (74° C); reheat gravy to a rolling boil to kill potential *Clostridium perfringens* bacteria present. Stopping at a good eating temperature is not good enough to kill sufficient bacteria.
- Make sure the refrigerator stays below 40° F (4° C). Either use a refrigerator thermometer or keep it as cold as possible without freezing milk or lettuce.

• • •

Microbes that cause food-borne illness commonly enter food through cross-contamination and grow in temperatures favorable to them. A recent example comes from a large gathering where turkey franks were contaminated with *Listeria monocytogenes.* When the franks were later added to a salad, it too became contaminated, causing food-borne illness.

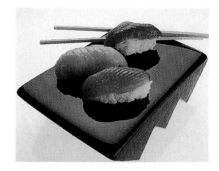

Figure 19-1 Sushi, like all raw fish or meat dishes, is a high-risk food. Animal foods should be cooked thoroughly before eating for maximum protection from food-borne illness. If you choose to eat uncooked fish, purchase fish from reputable establishments that have high standards for quality and sanitation. People at high risk for food-borne illness would be wise to avoid these products.

Safe Handling Instructions

This product was prepared from inspected and passed meat and/or poultry. Some food products may contain bacteria that could cause illness if the product is mishandled or cooked improperly. For your protection, follow these safe handling instructions.

Keep refrigerated or frozen.
Thaw in refrigerator or microwave.

Keep raw meat and poultry separate from other foods. Wash working surfaces (including cutting boards), utensils, and hands after touching raw meat or poultry.

Cook thoroughly.

Keep hot foods hot. Refrigerate leftovers immediately or discard.

Current safe handling instructions issued by USDA for meat and poultry products.

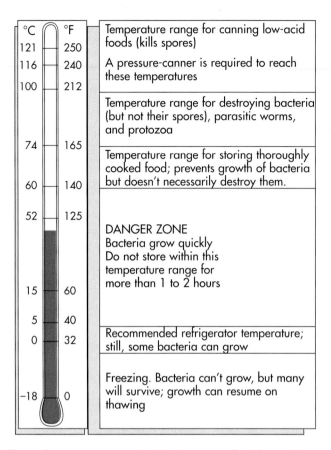

Figure 19-2 Effects of temperature on microbes that cause food-borne illness.
(Adapted from *Temperature guide to food safety: food and home notes,* No. 25, Washington, DC, June 20, 1977, USDA.)

The World Health Organization's Golden Rules for Safe Food Preparation
1. **Choose foods processed for safety.**
2. **Cook food thoroughly.**
3. **Eat cooked foods immediately.**
4. **Store cooked foods carefully.**
5. **Reheat cooked foods thoroughly.**
6. **Avoid contact between raw and cooked foods.**
7. **Wash hands repeatedly.**
8. **Keep all kitchen surfaces meticulously clean.**
9. **Protect foods from insects, rodents, and other animals.**
10. **Use pure water.**

Overall, it is important to practice sanitary food-handling procedures when preparing any food. And as one final precaution, watch for safe food-handling techniques when you eat out. Check that foods in a salad bar are iced; custard and pudding pies are chilled; hot foods served on a hot food bar are in fact hot; and vending machines are checked regularly, especially those containing sandwiches and milk. Send back any meat, poultry, seafood, or fish that does not appear thoroughly cooked. Keep track of how long cooked foods or salads have been sitting on the buffet table and avoid anything there for 2 hours or more. Food stored and served in dormitory cafeterias should be properly handled.

TREATMENT OF FOOD-BORNE ILLNESS

To offset the effects of diarrhea, drink a lot of fluids. To prevent further contamination, thoroughly wash hands before handling or eating food until the diarrhea disappears. Bed rest speeds recovery. A fever of 102° F (39° C) or greater, blood in the stool, and dehydration from frequent vomiting or diarrhea (a symptom of dehydration is dizziness when standing) deserves a physician's evaluation, especially if these persist for more than 2 or 3 days. In cases of suspected botulism, a physician should be consulted immediately because use of an antitoxin may speed recovery.

USDA specifies three particular situations in which it is vital for consumers to report incidents of food-borne illness to the local health department:
- If the food in question was eaten at a large gathering
- If the item came from a restaurant, delicatessen, sidewalk vendor, or kitchen that serves large numbers of people
- If the suspect food was a commercial product, such as some kind of canned goods or a frozen, packaged item

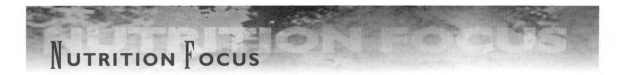

Nutrition Focus

Protecting the United States Food Supply

A variety of federal, state, and local agencies in the United States monitor food safety. The history of the food laws they enforce is listed in Table 19-1. Some of the agencies involved are:

- **United States Department of Agriculture (USDA).** This agency enforces standards for wholesomeness and quality of grains, produce, meat, poultry, milk, and eggs produced in the United States through inspection and grading. As part of this effort, more than 7000 inspectors visually examine the carcasses of more than 120 million animals a year in an effort to keep obviously diseased meat from going to market. USDA also routinely monitors animal foods for antibiotics. Once the food product leaves the field and enters into food production and distribution, FDA takes over for all foods containing less than 2% meat or poultry. Foods containing more remain under USDA jurisdiction. USDA now requires companies to put a "Safe Handling Label" on meat and poultry products (see page 703). The labels explain how to properly handle, cook, and store these products. USDA is planning a national consumer awareness campaign on safe food handling practices.

- **Bureau of Alcohol, Tobacco, and Firearms.** This agency is responsible for enforcing laws first enacted in 1935 that cover the production, distribution, and labeling of most alcoholic beverages. This agency and FDA sometimes share responsibility in cases of adulteration, or when an alcoholic beverage contains food or color additives, pesticides, or contaminants.

- **Environmental Protection Agency (EPA).** This agency regulates pesticides based on laws passed from 1947 through 1974. EPA must approve all pesticides before they are sold in the United States. It determines the safety of new pesticide products and sets allowable limits for pesticide residue in foods. This limit is not necessarily the maximal safe amount of a pesticide in a food; EPA sets limits no higher than needed for a product's intended use. These amounts are then enforced by FDA. EPA also establishes water quality standards, including those for drinking water.

TABLE 19-1

Some key U.S. food laws
1906: **Pure Food and Drug Act and Federal Meat Inspection Act**—This most importantly defined adulterated foods: those foods containing "any added poisons or other added deleterious ingredient which may render such article injurious to health."
1938: **Federal Food, Drug, and Cosmetic Act**—This provided for exemptions and safe tolerances for substances that, although not desirable in foods, were either necessary in production or unavoidable.
1958: **Food Additives Amendment (and the Color Additives Amendment of 1960)**—These made it necessary for manufacturers to demonstrate the safety of a new food additive before approval by FDA. The 1958 act also included the Delaney Clause: "No additive shall be deemed to be safe if it is found to produce cancer when ingested by man or animals, or if it is found after tests which are appropriate for the evaluation of the safety of the food additive to induce cancer in man or animals."
1990: **Nutrition Labeling and Education Act**—This law expanded the number of foods required to contain a nutrition label and formalized rules for label descriptors, such as "lite." It also set standards for health claims on foods, such as whether a food can lower the risk of heart disease.

Primarily from Expert Panel on Food Safety and Nutrition: *Food Technology*, p 73, Jan 1992.

NUTRITION FOCUS

- **Food and Drug Administration (FDA).** This agency is responsible for ensuring the safety and wholesomeness of all foods sold in interstate commerce (except for meat and poultry, which are primarily under USDA jurisdiction). Follow their actions by reading *FDA Consumer.*

  FDA is primarily responsible for the regulation of seafood and has been putting more resources toward this task. FDA has about 350 inspectors to monitor seafood processing plants and imported seafood, oversee the National Shellfish Sanitation Program, sample and test seafood products, enforce labeling requirements, and provide education on seafood issues. FDA works with individual states to implement these regulatory programs.

  FDA also sets standards for specific foods and enforces federal regulations for labeling, food and color additives, food sanitation, and the safety of foods. The agency inspects food plants, imported food products, and mills that make feeds containing medications or nutritional supplements for animals destined for human consumption. Over 90,000 businesses are inspected each year; about half are food-related businesses.

  FDA acts primarily when the public health is endangered, for example, when proper medical care is being discouraged in favor of quackery. It regulates products, not people. FDA cannot control what people say, just what is on a product's label and how it is promoted. FDA gives low priority to products that are simply economically deceptive.

  To monitor foods for contaminants, FDA routinely samples items of dietary importance, such as produce. Foods suspected of containing illegal residues receive a more intensive evaluation. An important part of FDA's safety sampling is a "market basket" study of foods that typify the American diet. Four times a year, identical purchases of 234 foods, including processed foods, are analyzed for pesticide residues, radioactive elements, toxic metals, and other undesirable substances. Imported foods with illegal residues can be refused entry into the country.

  Traditionally, FDA does not regularly inspect food-processing plants. It relies instead on its "Good Manufacturer's Procedures" plan that food processors and manufacturers are expected to follow. FDA inspectors may visit a specific food-processing establishment only infrequently. The agency relies on consumer complaints to alert it to potential dangers, then it researches these in greater detail. There just isn't enough staff at FDA to carefully inspect all instances where federal regulations must be adhered to.

- **Centers for Disease Control and Prevention (CDC).** A branch of the Department of Health and Human Services, CDC becomes involved as a protector of food safety, including responding to emergencies when food-borne diseases are a factor. CDC surveys and studies environmental health problems. It directs and enforces quarantines, and it administers national programs for prevention and control of vector-born diseases (diseases transmitted by a host organism) and other preventable conditions.

- **National Marine Fishery Service.** This agency is part of the Department of Commerce. It is responsible for overseeing fisheries management and harvesting. It provides a voluntary program for inspection and grading of fish products. Its guidelines closely match regulations for which FDA has enforcement authority.

- **State and local government.** States inspect restaurants, retail food establishments, dairies, grain processing plants, and other food-related establishments within their borders. States have the primary responsibility for milk safety. FDA provides guidelines to state and local governments for regulating dairy products and restaurants.

- **Foreign governments.** Governments of at least 40 nations are now partners with the United States in ensuring food safety through agreements that cover 24 food products, including shellfish. International cooperation in food inspection and regulatory standards is expanding.

  Again, the limited budgets of government enforcement agencies at all levels limit the number and thoroughness of inspections. So individuals must assume some responsibility for these protective activities themselves. We must remain alert in cases of apparent abuse and contact the appropriate government agency. Finally, we must promote safe food practices in our daily lives.

CONCEPT CHECK

Bacteria and the toxins they produce pose the greatest risk for food-borne illness. In the past, the addition to foods of sugar, salt, and smoke, as well as drying, were used to prevent the growth of microorganisms. Today, we know that cleanliness, keeping hot foods hot and cold foods cold, and cooking foods thoroughly offer additional protection from food-borne illness. Treat all raw animal products, any cooked food, and raw fruits and vegetables as potential sources of food-borne illness. Symptoms of an attack are diarrhea, vomiting, abdominal bloating, and headache. Treatment generally requires only bed rest and extra fluids.

Microbes That Cause Food-Borne Illness

We noted that finding the agent that caused food-borne illness requires some detective skills. Determining the agent depends on knowing the food source, the incubation time for symptoms, the types of symptoms, and the duration of illness associated with an outbreak (Table 19-2).

Let's now look at the characteristics of the major "problem" microbes individually. One general rule: When you exhaust the possibilities, the cause of the illness is probably a virus.

BACTERIA POSE THE GREATEST RISK FOR FOOD-BORNE ILLNESS

Bacteria are extremely simple structures. They contain only one chromosome and lack mitochondria, endoplasmic reticulum, and lysosomes. Enzymes of the electron transport chain are located in the cell membrane. Many bacteria are enclosed in a carbohydrate-like capsule, which protects them and aids their adherence to tissues. Some bacteria can survive harsh environmental conditions through spore formation. In the spore state, bacteria can remain stable for months or years.

Most bacteria derive nutrients from organic material, producing enzymes that digest complex organic molecules. Bacteria living in the presence of oxygen are called *aerobes*, while those living in the absence of oxygen are called *anaerobes*. Those that prefer free oxygen but can live in its absence are called *facultative anaerobes*.

Certain bacteria can thrive in almost freezing temperatures, while others thrive in very high temperatures. The optimum temperature for most disease-causing bacteria is about 98° F (body temperature; 37° C). Many bacteria produce toxins.

Staphylococcus aureus (S. aureus)

The bacterium *Staphylococcus aureus (S. aureus)* causes 20% to 40% of cases of food-borne illness each year. While growing in food, this microbe produces an endotoxin that, once ingested, causes nausea, vomiting, diarrhea, headaches, and abdominal cramps. Thus illness caused by the bacterium is classified as bacterial intoxication. Symptoms usually develop within 2 to 6 hours of eating the contaminated food.[25] The person rarely dies, but develops no immunity against future attacks. Bed rest and fluids are generally the only treatment, and recovery takes place usually within 2 to 3 days.

S. aureus bacteria live mainly in the nasal passages and in sores on the skin. These microbes enter food when food handlers sneeze and cough over food or expose food to open skin sores. Once in food it begins to grow. *S. aureus* prefers a temperature near 100° F (38° C). It multiplies rapidly and can release enough exotoxin to cause illness in about 4 hours. The toxin is heat stable, so cooking the food at this point kills the bacteria but does not inactivate the toxin. The contaminated food neither appears or tastes unusual, nor has a detectable odor.

Common foods associated with intoxications from *S. aureus* are custard, ham salad, egg salad, cheese, seafood, cream-filled pastries, and milk. Whipped cream standing at room temperature for hours is a typical source of *S. aureus*. Keeping

TABLE 19-2

Organisms that cause food-borne illness: their sources, symptoms, and prevention

Organism	Source	Symptoms	Prevention methods
Bacteria			
Staphylococcus aureus	Found in nasal passages and in cuts on skin. Toxin is produced when food contaminated by bacteria is left for extended time at room temperature. Meats, poultry, egg products, tuna, potato and macaroni salads, and cream-filled pastries pose greatest risk.	Onset: 2-6 hours after eating. Diarrhea, vomiting, nausea, and abdominal cramps. Mimics flu. Lasts 24-36 hours. Rarely fatal.	• Sanitary food-handling practices. • Prompt and proper refrigeration of foods. • Keeping cuts on skin covered.
Salmonella	Found in raw meats, poultry, eggs, fish, unpasteurized milk, and products made with these items. Multiplies rapidly at room temperature. The bacteria themselves are toxic.	Onset: 5-72 hours after eating. Nausea, fever, headache, abdominal cramps, diarrhea, and vomiting. Can be fatal in infants, the elderly, and the sick.	• Sanitary food-handling practices. • Thorough cooking of foods. • Prompt and proper refrigeration of foods. • Avoiding cross-contamination.
Clostridium perfringens	Found throughout the environment. Generally found in meat and poultry dishes. Multiply rapidly in anaerobic conditions when foods are left for extended time at room temperature, such as in the center of stew or gravy. The bacteria themselves are toxic.	Onset: 8-24 hours after eating (usually 12 hours). Abdominal pain and diarrhea. Symptoms last a day or less, usually mild. Can be more serious in older or ill people.	• Sanitary handling of foods, especially meat and meat dishes, gravies, and leftovers. • Thorough cooking and reheating of foods. • Prompt and proper refrigeration.
Clostridium botulinum	Found throughout the environment. However, bacteria produce toxin only in a low-acid, anaerobic (oxygen-free) environment, such as in canned green beans, mushrooms, spinach, olives, and beef. Honey and corn syrup may carry spores.	Onset: 12-36 hours after eating. Neurotoxic symptoms include double vision, inability to swallow, speech difficulty, and progressive paralysis of the respiratory system. OBTAIN MEDICAL HELP IMMEDIATELY. BOTULISM CAN BE FATAL.	• Using proper methods for canning low-acid foods. • Avoiding commercial cans of low-acid foods that have leaky seals or are bent, bulging, or broken. • Destroying toxin after can or jar is opened by boiling contents hard for 20 minutes, but discarding if toxin is suspected (off odors are a sign).
Campylobacter jejuni	Found on poultry, beef, and lamb, and can contaminate the meat and milk. Chief food sources are raw poultry and meat and unpasteurized milk.	Onset: 2-5 days after eating, or longer. Diarrhea, abdominal cramping, fever, and sometimes bloody stools. Lasts 2-7 days.	• Thorough cooking of foods. • Sanitary food-handling practices. • Avoiding unpasteurized milk.
Listeria monocytogenes	Found in soft cheeses and unpasteurized milk. Resists acid, heat, salt, and nitrate well.	Onset: 7-30 days. Fever, headache, vomiting, and sometimes more severe symptoms. May be fatal.	• Thorough cooking of foods. • Sanitary food-handling practices. • Avoiding unpasteurized milk.
Yersinia enterocolitica	Found throughout nature; carried in food and water. They multiply rapidly at both room and refrigerator temperatures. Generally found in raw vegetables, meats, water, and unpasteurized milk.	Onset: 2-3 days. Fever, headache, nausea, diarrhea, and general malaise. Mimics flu and appendicitis. May cause gastroenteritis in children.	• Thorough cooking. • Sanitizing cutting instruments and cutting boards before preparing foods to be eaten raw. • Avoiding unpasteurized milk and untreated water.
Escherichia coli (*0157:H7* and other strains)	Undercooked beef, especially ground beef. Fruits, vegetables, and yogurt are also sources.	Onset: 2-4 days. Bloody diarrhea, abdominal cramps, kidney failure.	• Thorough cooking, especially of beef. • Avoiding unpasteurized milk, untreated apple cider.

TABLE 19-2

Organisms that cause food-borne illness: their sources, symptoms, and prevention—cont'd

Organism	Source	Symptoms	Prevention methods
Viruses			
Hepatitis A virus	Found in shellfish harvested from contaminated areas and foods that are handled a lot during preparation and then eaten raw.	Onset: 30-60 days. Jaundice, fatigue. May cause liver damage and death.	• Sanitary handling of foods. • Use of pure drinking water. • Adequate sewage disposal. • Thorough cooking of foods.
Norwalk, human rota-virus	Found in the human intestinal tract and expelled in feces. Contamination occurs: (1) when sewage is used to enrich garden/farm soil (2) by direct hand-to-food contact during the preparation of meals (3) when shellfish-growing waters are contaminated by sewage	Onset: 1-7 days. Severe diarrhea, nausea, and vomiting. Respiratory symptoms. Usually lasts 4-5 days, but may last for weeks.	• Sanitary handling of foods. • Use of pure drinking water. • Adequate sewage disposal. • Adequate cooking of foods.
Parasites			
Trichinella spiralis	Found in pork and wild game.	Onset: weeks to months. Muscle weakness, fluid retention in face, fever, flulike symptoms.	• Thorough cooking of pork and wild game.
Anisakis	Found in raw fish.	Onset: 12 hours. Stomach infection, severe stomach pain.	• Thorough cooking of fish.
Tapeworms	Found in raw beef, pork, and fish.	May cause abdominal discomfort, diarrhea.	• Thorough cooking of all animal products. • Avoiding raw fish dishes, such as sushi.
Fungi			
A group of toxic compounds (mycotoxins) produced by molds, such as aflatoxin B-1 and ergot	Found in foods that are relatively high in moisture. Chief food sources: beans and grains that have been stored in a moist place.	May cause liver and/or kidney disease.	• Checking foods for visible mold and discarding those that are contaminated. • Properly storing susceptible foods.

these and other foods above 140° F (60° C) or below 40° F (4° C) prevents the bacterium's growth, thus preventing production of its toxin. Susceptible foods should never be left between these temperature extremes for more than 1 to 2 hours. To further prevent this type of food-borne illness, hand cleanliness and sanitation are important, as are directing coughs and sneezes away from food and covering infected skin with sterile bandages when handling food. Food-borne infections caused by this microbe are most common during the summer months and at holiday time.

Salmonella

There are over 2000 types of *Salmonella*, which have been isolated from poultry, reptiles, livestock, rodents, birds, and humans. All types of *Salmonella* can be killed by normal cooking. Yet *Salmonella* are responsible for about 60% of cases of food-borne illness.

Salmonella are commonly found in animal and human feces and enter food via infected water, contaminated cutting boards, contaminated meat products, cracked eggs, and actual bits of feces in food.[25] Ingesting the live bacteria with subsequent release of an endotoxin causes the illness, which is classed as a food-borne infection. FDA calculates that *Salmonella*-related illness costs more than $10 billion a year in medical care and lost work time in the United States.

Symptoms of a *Salmonella* infection are the same as those of *Staphylococcus* intoxications, but take 5 to 72 hours to develop. Again, bed rest and fluids is the only treatment, and recovery usually occurs within 2 to 3 days. Fatalities are rare.[25]

The disease occurs when the microorganism has an opportunity to multiply to a high density in a food, such as eggs, chicken, meat (and meat products), and custard made with contaminated eggs (Figure 19-3). More than a third of raw chickens are contaminated. Even fruits like melons may harbor *Salmonella* on the rind. Washing fruit before preparation minimizes the *Salmonella* risk from this source. Undercooked foods pose a special risk, as thorough cooking kills *Salmonella* bacteria.

Recent research indicates not only that cracked eggs pose a risk for *Salmonella* infection, but also that strains of the bacteria occasionally exist inside an intact egg, especially if it has been at room temperature for a few hours. In September 1993, health authorities were notified about an outbreak of acute intestinal disease among people who attended a cookout at a psychiatric treatment hospital in Jacksonville, Florida. Eleven of the 12 people who became ill had eaten homemade ice cream made with raw eggs and served at the cookout. Testing of a sample of ice cream showed *Salmonella* present.

To be safe, eggs should be simmered 7 minutes, poached 5 minutes, or fried 3 minutes on each side until the yolk is not runny and the white is firm. Raw eggs should not be used in salads or sauces. Hollandaise sauce, often warmed at low heat, is a significant threat. In October 1993, 23 people who consumed an entrée served with hollandaise or bearnaise sauce fell ill from a *Salmonella* infection. If raw eggs are needed in a recipe that doesn't involve cooking, commercial egg products that have been pasteurized are the safest alternative.

Most outbreaks of *Salmonella* infection can be traced to mistakes in food handling (Figure 19-4). *Salmonella* bacteria need about 8 hours to reproduce enough to cause illness. Observing the temperature precautions for *Staphylococcus* organisms also prevents *Salmonella* bacteria growth.

FDA warns us not to consume homemade ice cream, eggnog, and mayonnaise if made with unpasteurized, raw eggs because of the risk of *Salmonella* food-borne illness. Commercial forms of these products are safe because the egg products used have been pasteurized, which kills *Salmonella* bacteria. In addition, commercial mayonnaise contains enough acid to prevent bacterial growth.

Calvin and Hobbes   by Bill Watterson

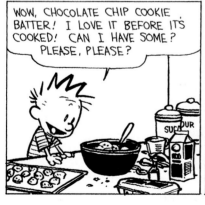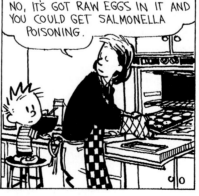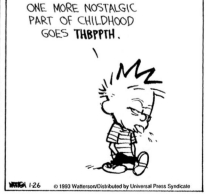

Figure 19-3 Calvin and Hobbes.

Salmonella poses a great risk for cross-contamination of foods. In November 1986, five residents of a Windsor, Connecticut, nursing home died and 25 others became ill from *Salmonella*. Health officials suspect that a blender used to purée food had previously been used to mix raw eggs and had not been properly cleaned.

Risk of *Salmonella* infection can be minimized by keeping hands and utensils clean when preparing foods; scrubbing cutting boards with a chlorinated cleanser after contact with raw meat or poultry; cooking animal products thoroughly (including eggs); storing foods in temperatures either hot or cold enough to prevent bacterial growth; and marinating meats in the refrigerator. Although acid in a marinade slows bacterial growth, it does not stop it. Finally, do not thaw foods on the kitchen counter.

Clostridium perfringens (C. perfringens)

Clostridia are widely dispersed in soil and water (particularly when contaminated with feces) and in the normal GI tracts of animals, including humans. They cause a variety of diseases, including food-borne illness. Their survival in adverse environmental conditions arises from their ability to form spores.

C. perfringens grows rapidly under favorable conditions. During this time the exotoxin that causes the illness is produced. *C. perfringens* is called the "cafeteria germ" because most food-borne outbreaks of this organism are associated with the food-service industry or with events where large quantities of food are prepared and served. Symptoms of the illness resemble those caused by *Salmonella:* abdominal cramps and watery diarrhea, but without fever or vomiting. Symptoms occur within 8 to 24 hours after consuming a food product contaminated with a large amount of the bacteria.[25] Again, bed rest and fluids is the only treatment, and recovery occurs usually within a few days.

C. perfringens is an anaerobic bacterium. The spores it produces are quite resistant to heat. Foods stored in deep serving dishes are especially fertile media for bacterial growth because the centers are isolated from air and stay warm. At moderate temperatures, spores germinate and become bacteria, multiplying quickly to disease-causing amounts.

C. perfringens organisms are often found in cooked beef, turkey, gravy, dressing, stews, and casseroles. The best way to prevent their growth is to maintain proper holding temperatures and to divide large leftover portions into shallow pans. The latter treatment exposes more food to air, reducing the anaerobic conditions, and also aids cooling. Be especially careful to cook meats completely and cool them rapidly in small, shallow containers. Thoroughly reheat leftover meat as described earlier before serving. Always bring leftover gravy to a rolling boil. Store cold cuts and sliced meats in the refrigerator and serve them cold.

Clostridium botulinum (C. botulinum)

C. botulinum bacteria can cause fatal food-borne illness via production of a potent nerve toxin. This anaerobic microbe is present in the soil and is therefore probably present as a bacterium or spore in all foods. The bacteria release the deadly exotoxin as they grow in food. The toxin binds to nerve endings and prevents release of a neurotransmitter. When transmission of certain nerve impulses is blocked, weakness and paralysis result.[25] The death rate, which depends on the amount of toxin consumed, is about 10% if modern medical therapies are employed.

Symptoms of botulism appear within 12 to 36 hours of consuming contaminated foods. These include vomiting, abdominal pain, double vision, and dizziness. Death occurs from respiratory failure as nerve function is profoundly diminished. Diarrhea does not occur. Survivors recover within 10 days. Normally, bed rest is the only therapy. Sometimes, treatment for botulism requires intensive care, including mechanical ventilation; the early administration of antitoxin is recommended. Still, ultimate recovery may be slow. Although botulism receives much public attention, few cases are reported each year in the United States.

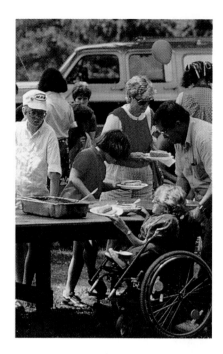

Figure 19-4 A picnic is a likely target for food-borne illness. Keeping hot foods hot and cold foods cold is one key to minimizing the risk of food-borne illness at picnics. The warm days of summer make this especially important.

CRITICAL THINKING

Diana had a party at her house for her son's birthday. After cleaning up after the kids went home, she realized she had forgotten to put away the potato salad and coleslaw, and decided to discard it. However, her husband Tim wanted her to just refrigerate it. "After all," he reasoned, "it was only left out for a couple of hours." Why was Diana right in wanting to throw the leftover unrefrigerated food away?

roast beef, although unpasteurized milk, untreated apple cider, salad greens grown in cow manure, cantaloupe, dry-cured salami (because it is not cooked during processing), and contaminated water have also been implicated. After an incubation period of 2 to 4 days, the disease normally lasts 4 to 10 days.

Symptoms include severe abdominal cramps, bloody diarrhea, and kidney failure. *E. coli* infection should be suspected in any case of bloody diarrhea. We noted earlier that in 1993 at least 4 people died and 700 became ill in Washington and surrounding western states after eating at a chain of quick-service restaurants. The source of the problem was undercooked hamburger contaminated with *E. coli 0517:H7*. Cooking meat until it is gray or brown in color and juices run yellow to clear (no pink color left) and then avoiding recontamination are important ways to prevent this type of food-borne illness.[11] Cider that is not pasteurized or that does not contain preservatives can be heated to a slow simmer until steam rises from the pan before serving or refrigerating.

Food-borne illness caused by the *Shigella* bacterium is a common childhood disease of youngsters in day-care centers, nurseries, and custodial institutions. The infection is transmitted by the fecal-oral route, primarily by way of the hands, and to a lesser extent by food and water. Symptoms include abdominal cramps, diarrhea, fever, and bloody stools.[14] There are carriers of *Shigella* who show no effect but represent a potential threat to all who are in their care. Recently, 407 adults who ate at one restaurant were infected with *Shigella*. In September 1994 a cruise was cut short when more than 600 people developed shigellosis and one person died. Handwashing and sanitary food production offer the best protection.

Infection from *Vibrio vulnificus (V. vulnificus),* a newly identified bacterium, has been linked to eating raw seafood, especially raw oysters.[24] *V. vulnificus* causes a serious infection that can be fatal in about 45% to 75% of cases, especially in people with liver disease and compromised immunity. Since 1992, 17 people in Florida have died of *V. vulnificus* infection after eating raw oysters. Eating any raw or lightly (partially) cooked seafood poses a high risk, especially that harvested from the Gulf Coast from April through October. Symptoms include diarrhea, fever, weakness, blood infection, and other serious health problems. Prompt treatment is needed. Cooking destroys this organism.

V. cholerae causes a severe form of GI tract infection. Sources of *V. cholerae* are human carriers and infected shellfish. The disease is spread by contaminated water and food. Cholera is usually seen in countries with poor sanitation. Foreign travel and raw seafood, particularly raw shellfish, have accounted for all but a handful of the cholera cases in this country during the past decade. Handwashing after defecating is vital to reducing risk. The disease occurs 2 to 3 days after ingesting contaminated food or water. Symptoms include vomiting and severe watery diarrhea, which can lead to dehydration and cardiovascular collapse. The death rate can be as high as 60%. Treatment consists of replacement of fluids and electrolytes.

VIRUSES

Viruses do not metabolize, grow, or move by themselves. Instead, they reproduce within a living host cell, and thus cannot grow in food once it is harvested or slaughtered. Viruses consist of a protein coat surrounding a nucleic acid core of either DNA or RNA. They have no cell wall. Upon entering a host cell, a virus takes over the cell's metabolic "machinery" and causes it to reproduce the virus' genetic material. Generally the host cell dies in the process and bursts open, releasing new viruses into the surrounding medium. Many viruses cause disease in humans.

Because viruses cannot multiply in foods, they must enter in sufficient amounts through bits of feces that contaminate food. A well-known example is the hepatitis A virus, although this route accounts for only a small percentage of the total number of hepatitis A infections. This food-borne agent most often thrives because of unsanitary food handling by carriers of the virus in restaurants. People have also contracted hepatitis A infections from eating raw or undercooked shellfish—clams, oysters, mussels—harvested from waters contaminated with raw or improperly treated sewage. Symptoms include intestinal problems, weakness, fatigue, jaundice, and sometimes even development of serious liver disease requiring hospitalization. Because symptoms of hepatitis A infection do not usually occur until about 1 to 2 months after eating contaminated food, the source is difficult to identify.

Raw clams and oysters are especially risky foods because they are filter feeders, a process that concentrates viruses and toxins present in the water as it is filtered for food. Consumption of these raw shellfish means consumption of live viruses and bacteria, too. It is important to buy oysters and clams only from the most reliable sources. By law, shellfish offered for sale must come from licensed beds, but they may not. So be careful when you either purchase these foods or harvest them yourself. Check with the local health department if you question the safety of waters in an area.

Proper handwashing by food service personnel is especially important in restaurants, day-care centers, hospitals, and other institutions to lessen hepatitis outbreaks. Chlorination of drinking water is a reliable means of destroying the virus.

Norwalk viral infections usually cause mild illness, with nausea, vomiting, diarrhea, weakness, abdominal pain, loss of appetite, headache, and fever. The virus is found in water and foods, and shellfish and salads are most often implicated, though cooking destroys the virus.[17] Norwalk viruses are probably responsible for about 30% to 40% of all cases of viral intestinal infection in adults. The infection is typically found in nursing homes. Recently, outbreaks caused by contaminated ice occurred in Pennsylvania and Delaware. Another recent outbreak was attributed to an infected bakery worker who stirred a vat full of buttercream frosting with his bare hand and arm. Washing hands thoroughly before preparing food can help prevent the spread of the Norwalk virus.

Rotaviruses are another important cause of diarrhea, mainly in children. Symptoms appear in 1 to 7 days. Day-care centers are common sites for infections. Thorough, regular handwashing is a necessary and important practice at these sites, especially after diaper changing.

PARASITES

Parasites that enter the body through the intestinal tract include some single-celled protozoans, flukes, nematodes, roundworms, and tapeworms. In the United States, the parasite most apt to be in the food supply is *Trichinella spiralis*.[28] This tiny organism may be present in raw and undercooked pork and pork products, such as sausage. Trichinosis is rare today, probably because people realize that pork must be cooked thoroughly to kill the nematode worm that causes it, and modern sanitary feeding practices have reduced *Trichinella* in hogs. About a hundred cases of trichinosis per year are reported in the United States. However, other cases may be unreported. In addition to pork, bear meat and other raw meats are potential sources. It is seldom found in commercial meat.

This infection begins with the consumption of meat containing the **larvae.** The larvae are released during digestion in the small intestine. Within 2 days the larvae develop into adult nematodes. New larvae are then produced and move into the blood via the intestinal mucosa. The blood carries the larvae to muscle fibers, where they become resident.

In early stages, trichinosis is difficult to diagnose. The symptoms in mild cases develop over weeks to months and are usually thought to be flu. If enough larvae are present, muscle weakness, fever, and fluid retention in the face may eventually result. Greater numbers of larvae usually mean more severe symptoms. Thoroughly cooking meat, especially pork, destroys the larvae.

Anisakis is a roundworm parasite found in larval form in raw fish. They invade the stomach or intestinal tract, causing mild or serious effects. The infection is difficult to diagnose and cannot be treated. A stomach infection is characterized by sudden onset of violent pain within 12 hours of eating raw fish. The larvae may penetrate the stomach lining.[26] Serious stomach pain can continue until the larvae are surgically removed. The fresher the fish, the less likely this disease will occur because

larvae An early developmental stage in the life history of some organisms, such as parasites.

larvae move from the fish's stomach to the tissues only after the fish is dead. Thoroughly cooking fish or freezing it for at least 72 hours are reliable methods for eliminating the threat of *Anisakis* disease. Consumption of raw or slightly cooked fish increases the risk for infection.

Recent problems with contaminated water in metropolitan Milwaukee were traced to a microscopic parasite few people had ever heard of before—*cryptosporidium*.[26] This parasite is found in many species of birds and animals, and in their feces. Consumption of food contaminated with the parasite can cause cryptosporidiosis, a rare but potentially serious disease. Recent outbreaks have occurred at public swimming pools and from raw apple cider. Fecal contamination was suspected in both cases. Symptoms include severe diarrhea, dehydration, nausea, fever, and abdominal cramps. Unknown as a human disease until 1976, cryptosporidiosis is now considered one of the foremost causes of diarrhea in the world, especially among children.

As with many other intestinal infections, people can contract the disease by ingesting food or water contaminated with fecal material. Safe food-handling practices and good personal hygiene, especially handwashing, can lower infection rates. Pasteurization and common water treatment procedures render the parasite noninfective. People with weakened immune systems (AIDS and cancer patients, for instance), infants, and the elderly are particularly susceptible to these infections.

OTHER RISKS FROM SEAFOOD

Scombroidosis results from an acute allergic reaction to eating spoiled fish. Fish typically implicated are tuna, mackerel, and mahi mahi. An affected person develops facial flushing, itching, intestinal upset, and headache within 10 to 60 minutes of consumption. The illness is caused by a toxin found in the flesh of the spoiled fish. Improperly refrigerated fish poses a special problem, and cooking does not destroy the toxin. So it is important to carefully refrigerate and use fresh fish soon after purchase, especially those varieties mentioned above.

Paralytic shellfish poisoning occurs when toxins produced by microscopic algae, called *dinoflagellates,* are consumed. These toxins are associated with the phenomenon known as a *red tide,* which is actually an explosive growth of the dinoflagellates in water. Symptoms, such as respiratory difficulty, appear within 4 hours. It is important that shellfish are harvested in clean waters, uncontaminated by sewage, industrial waste, and high amounts of toxic dinoflagellates. An outbreak in Guatemala in 1985 killed 26 people.

Ciguatera fish poisoning is not a major contributor to the overall incidence of food-borne disease, but it is still by some estimates the most common illness associated with fish consumption in the United States.[18] About 90% of cases occur in Hawaii and southern Florida. Ciguatera poisoning comes only from certain species of fish—notably grouper, snapper, amberjack, and barracuda—that live in warm waters near coral reefs. The toxin is produced by tiny one-celled plants that live on the reefs. The plants are eaten by small fish, which in turn are eaten by the larger fish that humans consume.

Researchers have documented an outbreak of ciguatera in California traced to frozen fillets shipped from Florida. Similar outbreaks have occurred in Vermont, Virginia, and Illinois, among other states. The symptoms tend to start in the GI tract within 6 hours after consumption of contaminated fish. Then, following a bout of diarrhea accompanied by abdominal pain, nausea, and perhaps vomiting, neurological problems begin, including tingling in the mouth, palms, and soles of the feet, aches throughout the body, and quite often the sensation that hot items are cold and cold items hot. This last symptom is considered the most definitive. The disease lasts from several weeks to several months or longer. There is as yet no test for ciguatera toxicity. It can be diagnosed only by its symptoms.

There is no way to tell if fish is contaminated before it is eaten and no way to "kill" the ciguatera toxin; it is not destroyed by heating or freezing. Furthermore, medication cannot "cure" the illness. It can only relieve symptoms, and not in all cases.

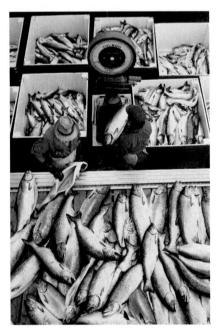

Fresh fish should be carefully refrigerated and used soon after purchase.

Food safety experts advise staying away from potentially contaminated fish. The easiest way to exercise that caution is not to eat grouper, snapper, amberjack, moray eel, or barracuda from Caribbean waters.[18] Small fish pose less risk. The larger the fish, the greater the chance that it has accumulated much toxin because of its relatively long life.

FUNGI

Fungi are mostly multicellular organisms. Those of concern in food safety do not infect people, but mushrooms may be intrinsically toxic, and molds growing on foods may produce toxins called **mycotoxins.** Fungi possess cell walls, a nucleus, and a nuclear membrane. They live on dead or decaying organic matter, living together with other organisms either in mutual advantage or as parasites. Fungi can grow as single cells, like yeasts, or as multicellular filamentous colonies, as with molds. They cannot synthesize their own food. Fungi digest their food outside their cell walls and absorb the simpler organic substances for use within the cell.

Most fungi are molds that consist of long branched threads called *hyphae*. Hyphae form a tangled mass of filaments called *mycelium*. The mold often seen on bread is the mycelia of fungi.

Fungi require moisture to grow and can obtain water from the medium on which they live or from the atmosphere. When the atmosphere becomes dry they can go into a resting state or form spores. They can live in a pH range of 2 to 9. They can grow in concentrated salt and sugar solutions. They thrive over a wide temperature range, even in the refrigerator. As spores, fungi can be scattered by the wind or carried by animals. When an airborne spore lights on an appropriate target, such as a ripe peach, the spore germinates and begins to grow, producing the typical mold observed on spoiled fruit.

The best-known mycotoxins are the aflatoxins, produced by *Aspergillus flavus*.[25] Aflatoxin B-1 causes cancer in animals; thus human exposure is regulated by FDA. The foods most often contaminated with aflatoxins are tree nuts (for example, walnuts and pecans), peanuts, corn, wheat, and oil seeds, such as cottonseed. FDA considers aflatoxins unavoidable contaminants on foods and therefore has set practical limits for aflatoxins in food and animal feed.

Cooking and freezing halt fungal growth but do not eliminate mycotoxins already produced. Moldy food should not be eaten, or at least not without discarding the moldy portion and much of the surrounding area. Again, when in doubt, throw the food out. Mold growth is prevented by properly storing perishable foods at cold temperatures and using it within a reasonable length of time.

mycotoxins A group of toxic compounds produced by molds, such as aflatoxin B-1, found on moldly grains.

CONCEPT CHECK

To prevent food-borne intoxication from *Staphylococcus* organisms, cover cuts on hands and avoid sneezing on foods. To avoid *Salmonella* infection, separate raw meats, especially poultry products, from cooked foods. Then thoroughly cook meat and poultry products to destroy any *Salmonella* bacteria present. To avoid intoxication from *Clostridium perfringens*, rapidly cool leftover foods and thoroughly reheat them. To avoid intoxication from *Clostridium botulinum*, carefully examine canned foods. Overall, don't allow cooked food to stand for more than 1 to 2 hours at room temperature. For other causes of food-borne illness, precautions already mentioned generally apply as well. In addition, carefully handle raw animal products so that their juices do not contaminate other foods; thoroughly cook all foods, especially fish and other seafood; consume only pasteurized dairy products; wash all fruits and vegetables; and thoroughly wash your hands with soap and water before and after preparing food, and after using the bathroom.

Food Additives

By the time you see a food on the market shelf it has usually had substances added to it to make it more palatable or to increase its nutrient content or shelf life.[10] Manufacturers also add some substances to foods to make them easier to process. Other substances may have found their way by accident into the foods you buy. All these extraneous substances are known as additives, and although some are beneficial, others can be harmful. All purposely added substances must be evaluated by FDA. Appendix P provides a comprehensive list of food additives and their uses in foods.

WHY ARE FOOD ADDITIVES USED?

Limiting food spoilage is the main reason for most additive use. Food additives, such as potassium sorbate, are used to maintain the safety and acceptability of foods by retarding the growth of microbes implicated in food-borne illness.[10]

Additives are also used to combat some enzymes that lead to undesirable changes in color and flavor in foods, but do not cause anything as serious as food-borne illness. This second type of food spoilage occurs when enzymes in a food react with oxygen—for example, when apple and peach slices darken or turn rust color as they are exposed to air. Antioxidants are a type of preservative that retards the action of oxygen-requiring enzymes on food surfaces. These preservatives include vitamins E and C and a variety of sulfites.

Without the use of some food additives, it would be impossible to produce and distribute massive quantities of foods safely. Despite consumer concerns about the safety of food additives, many have been extensively studied and proved safe when FDA guidelines for their use are followed.

INTENTIONAL VERSUS INCIDENTAL FOOD ADDITIVES

Food additives are classified into two types: those that are **intentionally** (directly) added to foods and those that have **incidentally** (indirectly) entered foods as contaminants. Both types of agents are regulated by FDA. Currently, more than 2800 different substances are intentionally added to foods. As many as 10,000 other substances enter foods as contaminants. This includes substances that may reasonably be expected to enter food through surface contact with processing equipment or packaging materials.

THE GRAS LIST

In 1958, all food additives used in the United States and considered safe at that time were put on a **generally recognized as safe (GRAS)** list.[13] Congress established the GRAS list because it felt manufacturers did not need to prove the safety of substances that were already generally regarded as safe by scientists. As is still the case, FDA was assigned responsibility for proving that a substance did not belong on the GRAS list.

Since 1958 some substances on the list have been reviewed. A few, such as cyclamates, failed the review process and were removed from the list. Recently the additive red dye #3 was banned because it is linked to cancer.[15] Many chemicals on the GRAS list have not yet been rigorously tested, primarily because of expense. These chemicals have received a low priority for testing, mostly because they have long histories of use without evidence of harm and/or because their chemical structures do not suggest they are potential health hazards.

ARE SYNTHETIC CHEMICALS ALWAYS HARMFUL?

Nothing about a natural product makes it inherently safer than a synthetic (man-made) product. Many synthetic products are simply laboratory copies of chemicals that also occur in nature (see the discussion in Chapter 20 on biotechnology for some examples). And although human endeavors contribute some toxins to foods, such as synthetic pesticides and industrial chemicals, nature's toxins are often even more potent and prevalent. Some cancer researchers suggest that we ingest at least 10,000 times more (by weight) natural toxins produced by plants than we do man-

---

Because food spoilage is an ongoing process, when buying products, especially perishables, check the product date for safety. Four types of dates are commonly used. The pack date is the day the product was manufactured. The pull or sell date indicates the last date the product should be sold. It allows some time for storing food at home before eating. Check the expiration date on foods stored at home because that is the last date the food can safely be consumed. Last, baked goods may have a freshness date, indicating that the product may safely be eaten for a short time after the date but may not taste the same.

---

intentional food additives Additives knowingly (directly) incorporated into food products by manufacturers.

incidental food additives Additives that appear in food products indirectly, from environmental contamination of food ingredients or during the manufacturing process.

generally recognized as safe (GRAS) A list of food additives that in 1958 were considered safe for consumption. Manufacturers were allowed to continue to use these food additives, without special clearance, when needed in food products. FDA bears responsibility for proving they are not safe and can remove unsafe products from the list.

made pesticide residues. This comparison doesn't make man-made chemicals any less toxic, but it does lend perspective.

Consider the familiar food additive baking powder, which is a leavening agent used to make the batter rise in cakes, pancakes, and other quick breads. When manufacturers list potassium acid tartrate, sodium aluminum phosphate, or monocalcium phosphate on cake mix labels, they are referring to baking powder by its chemical names. Baking soda can be listed by its proper name, sodium bicarbonate, just as ordinary table salt could be called sodium chloride. The question should not be whether a food additive, such as salt, is a chemical (because all foods are in essence simply an organized grouping of atoms), but rather whether the chemical additive is safe to use.

Vitamin E is often added to food to prevent rancidity of fats. This chemical is safe when used within certain limits. However, high doses have been associated with health problems, such as inhibition of vitamin K metabolism. Thus even well-known chemicals can be toxic in some circumstances and at certain concentrations.

TESTING FOOD ADDITIVES FOR SAFETY

Food additives are tested under FDA scrutiny for safety on at least two animal species, usually rats and mice. The test chemical is administered in food or water, or it is delivered to the stomach through a tube. Scientists determine the highest dose of the additive that produces **no observable effects** in the animals, such as significant mortality. High doses are needed to reduce the cost and length of the tests. Still, these doses are proportionately much higher than humans are ever exposed to. The maximal dosage is then divided by at least 100 to establish a margin of safety for human use. The rationale for reducing the no observable effects level by a 100-fold margin is that humans are assumed to be at least 10 times more sensitive to food additives than laboratory animals and any one person might be 10 times more sensitive than another.

This very broad margin of safety essentially ensures that the food additive in question causes no deleterious health effects in humans. In fact, many synthetic chemicals are probably more harmless at these low doses than some natural compounds found in apples or celery. Other terms used to express this margin of safety concept are *tolerance, allowable level,* and *acceptable level.*

One important exception applies to the schema for testing intentional food additives: if an additive is shown to cause cancer, even though tested at very high doses, no margin of safety is allowed. The food additive cannot be used because it would violate the **Delaney Clause** in the 1958 Food Additives Amendment. This clause prohibits intentionally adding to foods a compound that was introduced after 1958 that causes cancer. Evidence for cancer can come from either laboratory animal or human studies.

Recently, the value of animal cancer tests has been questioned. Research suggests that when rats are fed massive doses of chemicals, as they typically are in the tests, it may be the dose itself, rather than the chemical action, that causes cancer. The scientific community is currently debating which is the best method for testing additives to evaluate cancer risk in humans. The question boils down to how to test chemicals efficiently and how to apply data obtained from laboratory animals to humans. Nevertheless, we are left with our current approach of banning intentional food additives that cause cancer until a better method is established.

Incidental food additives are another matter altogether. FDA cannot simply ban various industrial chemicals, pesticide residues, and mold toxins from foods, even though some of these contaminants can cause cancer. These products are not purposely added to foods—they are present whether we like it or not. FDA sets an acceptable concentration for these substances. Basically, it establishes a cancer safety margin of 1 million, which means that a substance found in a food cannot contribute to more than one cancer case during the lifetimes of 1 million people. If a higher risk exists, then the amount of the compound in a food must be reduced until the guideline is met. However, if the compound is a pesticide, causes cancer,

no observable effects level (NOEL) This corresponds to the highest dose of an additive that produces no deleterious health effects in animals.

- - - - - - - - - -

Some definitions here might help you:

toxicology	The scientific study of harmful substances
safety	The relative certainty that a substance won't cause injury
hazard	The chance that injury will result from use of a substance
toxicity	The capacity of a substance to produce injury or illness at some dosage

- - - - - - - - - -

Delaney Clause This clause to the 1958 Food Additives Amendment of the Pure Food and Drug Act in the United States prevents the intentional (direct) addition to foods of a compound that has been shown to cause cancer in animals or humans.

HOW SAFE IS THE AMERICAN FOOD SUPPLY?

JOHN N. HATHCOCK, Ph.D.

Today those who take too seriously every scary headline about pesticides, food additives, and bacterial contamination are apt to feel that practically anything they eat may lead to dire consequences. On one hand, we are told to eat more fruits, vegetables, fish, and poultry, and on the other, we are warned that these foods may contain dangerous substances. Within a recent short period, we were alarmed by reports that poisons in apples, grapes, fish, poultry, and eggs could make us ill, even violently so. Often one set of claims contradicted another, leading to widespread confusion. How can we distinguish between extremist claims and the truth?

THE CONCEPT OF SAFETY

What is a safe food supply? To a nutritionist, it is a food supply available in quantity and at prices allowing easy selection of a variety of diets that provide good nutrition without excessive intakes of specific food components, such as fats. To a toxicologist, it is a food supply that allows easy selection of a variety of diets that don't generate significant hazard because of toxic components.

Absolute safety is the total absence of hazard. Because of the logical and statistical nature of the evidence, proof of absolute safety would require proof of a negative—that something cannot occur. The science of toxicology never allows such a proof. It does provide evidence that supports the conclusion that almost all foods in the American food supply usually provide adequate safety. "Usually" and "adequate" may seem like hedge words, but really they are not; they simply recognize that proof of absolute safety is not possible and that, occasionally, some particular foods may not be adequately safe. Why don't we strive for "always" in safety? There are three reasons: (1) it's not possible; (2) there are trade-offs that make it unwise, that is, actions taken to decrease one type of risk may generate another; and (3) maximum reduction in many types of risk would be prohibitively expensive.

TRADE-OFFS IN FOOD SAFETY

Cooking improves food safety. Safety is improved because microbes are killed, reducing food spoilage and food-borne infection. On the other hand, cooking may produce mutagenic and carcinogenic chemicals in very small quantities, usually through heat destruction of fat or protein. Although these chemicals are produced in only trace quantities, some of them may cause more risk of cancer than the worrisome pesticides and food additives.

The safety of food additives, such as sodium nitrite, has been widely questioned in the popular press and by some scientists. Nitrite has antibacterial properties that help protect against the growth of the bacteria that cause botulism, a disease that can quickly cause death. Nitrite also contributes color and flavor to some foods. No responsible scientist can say that the use of nitrite is perfectly safe. It can react with naturally present amines and other essential substances to produce

and has a concentration in finished foods much greater than that allowed for use on crops, then generally its use in that crop will be banned by the Delaney Clause.

Currently some politicians and scientists want to see such a "one in a million" standard applied to all pesticide contamination. This in effect would mean canceling the Delaney Clause in the case of pesticides. Proponents claim that smoking cessation programs and educating the public about the dangers of a high-fat diet are vastly more important in terms of fighting cancer than pesticide residues in foods. Still, it's unlikely that the proposal will easily make it through Congress. Consumer groups have criticized the plan as too lax; food industry lobbyists have called it

nitrosamines. Many nitrosamines cause cancer in experimental animals. With only this in mind, it may seem logical to avoid all nitrite-containing foods, but that is not the case. The first reason relates to the protective action of nitrite against botulism. The second is that such avoidance would have little effect on exposure to nitrite. Most nitrite in the human body does not come from food additives. Instead, nitrates normally present in vegetables are converted by bacteria in the mouth and intestine to nitrite. This vegetable source provides most of the nitrite to which people are exposed (approximately 75%, depending on the particular dietary pattern).

Many foods, especially those containing polyunsaturated oils, have synthetic antioxidants (such as BHA, BHT, and propyl gallate) added to prevent rancidity. Some products formed when fats undergo oxidative rancidity have toxic effects, possibly including risk of cancer and accelerated aging. The safety of these synthetic antioxidant food additives has been questioned in relation to reports that BHT can have cancer-enhancing effects under some exper-

imental conditions. These reports indicate that bladder cancer increases but liver cancer decreases in experimental animals also treated with certain chemical carcinogens. Under other experimental conditions, treatment with synthetic antioxidants decreases the effects of chemical carcinogens. Overall, the evidence indicates that the synthetic antioxidants are more likely to decrease risk of cancer in humans than to increase it.

Nevertheless, if synthetic antioxidants have any adverse effects, why not replace them with a natural antioxidant, such as vitamin E? The replacement of all other antioxidants by vitamin E is not desirable for several reasons. Vitamin E is not as effective as synthetic antioxidants. Such replacement would dramatically increase intake of vitamin E, and if intakes become high enough, questions about the safety of high intakes of vitamin E would arise. Furthermore, vitamin E as a food antioxidant is more expensive than synthetic antioxidants.

CONCLUSIONS

The familiar advice to eat a variety of foods to ensure nutritional adequacy

also makes sense for avoiding excessive intakes of any particular substance. Certainly, eating a variety of foods increases the probability that a variety of contaminating chemicals will be consumed in small quantities. The common fear that such multiple exposure will dramatically enhance toxicity of those substances is not well founded. Actually, just the opposite is likely. Often one substance enhances our ability to metabolize and detoxify others, thereby decreasing risk of toxicity rather than increasing it.

Overall, the American food supply is outstandingly safe. Occasional exceptions, such as contamination with microbes or their toxins, can make certain foods unsafe. Absolute safety of food is impossible, but the greatest dietary risks are associated with too much food, too much fat, and too much sodium, rather than with chemical contaminants.

Dr. Hathcock is a senior scientist with FDA. No official support or endorsement by the Food and Drug Administration is intended or should be inferred.

unacceptable. The Nutrition Perspective in this chapter covers this issue in more detail.

OBTAINING APPROVAL FOR A NEW FOOD ADDITIVE

Today, before a new substance can be added to foods, FDA must approve its use. Besides rigorously testing an additive to establish its safety margins, manufacturers must give the FDA information that (1) identifies the new additive, (2) gives its chemical composition, (3) states how it is manufactured, and (4) specifies laboratory methods used to measure its presence in the food supply at amounts of intended use.

Manufacturers must also offer proof that the additive accomplishes its intended purpose in a food, that it is safe, and that the amount present is no higher than needed. Additives cannot be used to hide defective food ingredients, such as rancid oils, to deceive consumers, or to replace good manufacturing practices. A manufacturer also must establish that the ingredient is necessary for producing a specific food product.

COMMON FOOD ADDITIVES

A list of food additive categories appears in Table 19-3, some of which serve the general function of preservatives: acidic or alkaline agents, antioxidants, antimicrobial agents, curing and pickling agents, and **sequestrants.** Let's look at some of the specific categories of additives to understand exactly why these are used and to learn more about the specific substances employed.

Acidic or Alkaline Agents. Acids have many uses in foods. As flavor-enhancing agents they impart a tart taste to soft drinks, sherbets, and cheese spreads. As preservatives they inhibit microbial growth. As antioxidants they prevent discoloration and rancidity. They also adjust acid and base balance. Such addition of acids during food processing increases the margin of protection against botulism in naturally low-acid vegetables, such as beets.

Alkaline products, such as sodium hydroxide, can alter the texture and flavor of foods, including chocolate. In processing, alkaline products are sometimes used to produce a milder flavor by neutralizing the acids produced during fermentation.

Alternative Sweeteners. Currently, saccharin, aspartame (Nutrasweet), and acesulfame (Sunette) are the only alternative sweeteners used in foods (see Chapter 3 to review all three). All are used to reduce the energy content of foods while supplying sweetness.

Anticaking Agents. By absorbing moisture, such compounds as calcium silicate, ammonium citrate, magnesium stearate, and silicon dioxide keep table salt, baking powder, powdered sugar, and other powdered food products free flowing. These agents prevent the caking and lumping that make powdered or crystalline products hard to use.

Antimicrobial Agents. Sodium benzoate, sorbic acid, and calcium propionate are common preservatives.[10] Sorbic acid is a potent inhibitor of molds and fungal growth. Calcium propionate, a natural component of some cheeses, inhibits mold growth.

Antioxidants. This type of food preservative helps delay food discoloration from oxygen exposure, such as occurs when potatoes are diced. It also helps keep fats from turning rancid. Two widely used antioxidants are BHA (butylated hydroxy-

sequestrants Compounds that bind free metal ions. By so doing, they reduce the ability of ions to cause rancidity in foods containing fat.

Today, sugar, salt, corn syrup, and citric acid constitute 98% of all additives (by weight) used in food processing.

TABLE 19-3

Food additive categories		
Anticaking agents	Formulation aids: carriers, binders, fillers, plasticizers	lants, filter aids, crystallization inhibitors
Antimicrobial agents		
Antioxidants		
Color and adjuncts	Fumigants	Propellants
Conditioners	Humectants	Sequestrants
Curing and pickling	Leavening	Solvents and vehicles
Dough strengtheners	Lubricants and release agents	
Drying agents	Nonnutritive sweeteners	Stabilizers and thickeners
Emulsifiers	Nutritive sweeteners	
Enzymes	Oxidizing and reducing agents	Surface active agents
Firming agents		Surface-finishing agents
Flavor enhancers	pH control	
Flavoring agents	Processing aids: clarifying, clouding, catalyst, floccu-	Synergists
Flour treating		Texturizers

anisole) and BHT (butylated hydroxytoluene).[10] Despite some public concern to the contrary, these do not cause cancer and in fact might help prevent it. Vitamin E and related compounds also serve as antioxidants.

Sulfites also are widely used antioxidants in foods.[10] Sulfites are actually a group of sulfur-based chemicals—sulfur dioxide, sulfur gas, sodium and potassium bisulfite, and sodium and potassium meta bisulfite. After ingesting sulfites, people who are very sensitive to them may have difficulty breathing or may vomit, as well as develop hives, diarrhea, abdominal pain, cramps, and dizziness. Often these people already have asthma.[20,32] FDA now limits the use of sulfites on raw fruits and vegetables—an action directed mainly at salad bars. Potatoes currently are not covered by such regulation. FDA also prohibits the use of sulfites in foods that are important sources of thiamin, such as enriched flour, because sulfites destroy the nutrient. In addition, FDA requires manufacturers to declare the presence of sulfites on labels of packaged foods containing at least 10 parts per million of sulfites. Labels on wine bottles often carry a sulfite warning.

Colors. Color additives do not improve nutritional qualities, but they can make foods more appealing. Sources include extracts of plant products and synthetic varieties using petroleum distillates as the starting ingredients.[15] Food colorings cannot be used to deceive consumers—for example, by covering blemishes; to conceal inferiority; or to mislead people in any way. Although colorings are arguably unnecessary additives, manufacturers have satisfied FDA that color is "necessary" for the production of certain foods. The most popular colors are FD&C red No. 40 and FD&C yellow No. 5.

Controversy has surrounded the use of some food colors. Some red dyes have raised concerns, and some have been banned. Currently, the safety of tartrazine (FD&C yellow No. 5) is disputed. It has caused allergic symptoms such as hives, itching, and nasal discharge in sensitive individuals, especially in people allergic to aspirin. FDA requires manufacturers to list all forms of synthetic colors on the labels of foods that contain them. Pigments extracted from plant sources are exempted from specific description on food labels.[15]

Curing and Pickling Agents. Nitrates and the related form nitrites are used as preservatives, especially to prevent growth of *Clostridium botulinum*. Sodium and potassium nitrates and nitrites are used to preserve meats, such as bacon, ham, salami, and hot dogs (Figure 19-5). Nitrates and nitrites have been used for centuries, in conjunction with salt, to preserve meat. An added effect of nitrates is their reaction to myoglobin pigments in meat to form a bright pink color. This gives the characteristic appearance to ham, hot dogs, and other cured meats.

Nitrate consumption from both cured foods and natural vegetables has been associated with the synthesis of nitrosamines in the stomach. Some nitrosamines are cancer-causing agents, particularly for the stomach and esophagus. The actual risk appears to be low, however, except for people who secrete little stomach acid (some elderly people, for example). A slightly increased risk for childhood leukemia and brain tumors is also suspected, but the data are preliminary in nature.[23]

FDA surmises that consumers take for granted a margin of microbial safety gained from nitrite use in cured meats. People often serve these meats cold or at least underheated. Consequently, government agencies have chosen not to ban nitrate or nitrite use in foods, but rather to change manufacturing practices to lower amounts of preformed nitrosamines and suggest moderation in use of these food products. And much progress has been made in this area during the last 25 years.

The addition of vitamin C (sodium ascorbate) to cured meats, such as bacon, is one way to reduce the amount of nitrosamines formed in foods. This is a common manufacturing practice today. Other antioxidants, such as sodium erythrobate, also inhibit synthesis of nitrosamines.

Much nitrite and nitrate in the U.S. food supply occurs naturally in foods, primarily in vegetables and baked goods. About one third to two thirds of nitrites and one seventh of nitrates in our food supply are added in manufacturing.

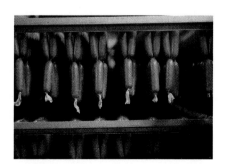

Figure 19-5 Cured meats derive their pink color from nitrates. The National Cancer Institute advises moderation in use with these foods, as the nitrates/nitrites pose some cancer risk.

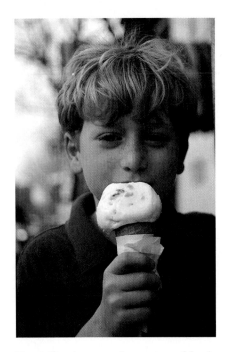

Emulsifiers improve the texture of foods such as ice cream, baked goods, and candies.

- - - - - - - - - - - - - -

Infants are more sensitive to MSG than adults, in part because infants have not yet developed a complete blood-brain barrier. This means they cannot fully exclude such substances as MSG from the brain.

- - - - - - - - - - - - - -

You might wonder why, if nitrates and nitrites form chemical substances that can cause cancer, they aren't banned by the Delaney Clause? In the U.S., USDA regulates the use of chemicals in meats. The laws that govern USDA functions are separate from the 1983 Federal Food, Drug, and Cosmetics Act. Because of this, the Delaney Clause, an amendment to the 1938 law, does not apply to USDA actions. Currently, USDA sees no clear threat to public safety from the regulated use of nitrates and nitrites in meats, so no action has been taken.

Emulsifiers. These products, by distributing and suspending fat in water, improve the uniformity, smoothness, and body of foods, such as bakery goods, ice cream, and candies. In mayonnaise, for example, egg yolks act as emulsifiers in holding together the oil and the acids, such as vinegar or lemon juice. Lecithins, derived from soybeans, act as emulsifiers in chocolate and margarine. Monoglycerides and diglycerides, found also as by-products of fat digestion in the intestinal tract, are used as emulsifiers in cake mixes.

Extenders. Extenders are used to add texture and bulk to a product. Hydrolyzed protein (HP), hydrolyzed vegetable protein (HVP), hydrolyzed plant protein (HPP), textured protein (TP), texturized vegetable protein (TVP), and texturized plant protein (TPP) are often used in this manner.

Fat Replacements. Fat replacements, such as Paselli SA2, Dur-Low, Oatrim, and Sta-Slim 143, are being produced for commercial use to provide body to products like fat-free mayonnaise. They do so primarily by binding water. These carbohydrate-based products join the fat replacement Simplesse, a protein-based compound we discussed in Chapter 4.

Flavors and Flavoring Agents. Naturally occurring and artificial agents can impart flavor to foods. These agents include extracts from spices and herbs, as well as man-made agents. You probably recognize flavors of some spices and of liquid derivatives of onion, garlic, cloves, and peppermint in foods. To meet the demands of industry, manufacturers have developed synthetic flavors that taste like natural flavors but also have the advantage of stability. Often artificial flavors, such as butter or banana, have the same chemical composition that makes up part of the natural flavor.

Flavor Enhancers. These substances—monosodium glutamate (MSG), for example—help bring out the natural flavors of foods. Glutamate is an amino acid present in protein. When in the free form—not attached to a protein—it enhances flavor. Some people are sensitive to MSG and experience flushing, chest pain, facial pressure, dizziness, sweating, rapid heart rate, nausea, vomiting, headaches, and high blood pressure after exposure, especially when taken on an empty stomach. Because MSG is often used in Chinese food, reactions have been called the *Chinese restaurant syndrome*. Symptoms typically occur about 10 to 20 minutes after ingestion and may last from 2 to 3 hours or more. For most people, typical use of MSG poses no health risk. Some people, however, may feel that they are sensitive to MSG. If so, they should read labels to help avoid significant sources. It may be present alone (look for the word glutamate), as well as in any isolated protein source (caseinate, texturized vegetable protein, etc.), yeast extract, bouillon, soup stock, and seasonings. Tomatoes, mushrooms, and parmesan cheese are also sources of free glutamate.

Humectants. These chemicals, such as glycerol, propylene glycol, and sorbitol, are added to foods to help retain proper moisture, fresh flavor, and texture. They are often used in candies, shredded coconut, and marshmallows.

Leavening Agents. Air and steam can be used to create a light texture in breads and cakes; however, carbon dioxide bubbles are much more reliable for this purpose. Common leavening agents that produce carbon dioxide gas include yeast, baking powder, and baking soda. Baking soda needs to react with acids to generate carbon dioxide. Baking powder can be used in either acid or alkaline conditions.

Maturing and Bleaching Agents. Compounds such as bromates, peroxides, and ammonium chloride hasten the natural aging and whitening processes of milled flour. Freshly milled flour lacks the qualities necessary to make a stable, elastic dough and otherwise requires several months of aging to be useful in baking.

Nutrient Supplements. Vitamin and mineral supplements are added to foods to improve their nutritional quality. Sometimes they replace nutrients lost in processing, as is the intent of enriching flour. Vitamin A is added to margarine and to some forms of milk. Vitamin D is added to some dairy products. Potassium iodide is added to salt, and calcium to some flours, fruit juices, and other products. Breakfast cereals often contain a variety of added nutrients.

Stabilizers and Thickeners. These additives impart a smooth texture and uniform color and flavor to candies, ice cream and other frozen desserts, chocolate milk, and artificially sweetened beverages. Commonly used substances are pectins, vegetable gums (such as guar gum and carrageenan), gelatins, and agars. They work by absorbing water. Without stabilizers and thickeners, ice crystals form in ice cream and other frozen desserts, and particles of chocolate separate from chocolate milk. Stabilizers are also used to prevent evaporation and deterioration of flavorings used in cakes, puddings, and gelatin mixes.

Sequestrants. These compounds include EDTA and citric acid. They bind many free chemical ions, and by doing so, help preserve food quality by reducing the ability of ions to cause rancidity in products containing fat.

• • •

In general, if you consume a variety of foods in moderation, the chances of food additives jeopardizing your health are minimal. Pay attention to your body. If you suspect an intolerance or sensitivity, consult your physician for further evaluation. Remember that, in the short run, you are more likely to suffer either from hazardous food-handling practices that allow bacteria and other microbes to grow in food or from consuming raw animal foods than from eating additives.

Look at the ingredients listed on a typical box of flavored gelatin dessert. Besides the expected sugar and gelatin, there is a long list of vitamins and minerals, adipic acid, disodium phosphate, fumaric acid, artificial color, and artificial flavor. You may wonder whether this is a smart food choice. If you are bewildered or concerned about additives creeping into your diet, you can easily avoid most of them by emphasizing unprocessed whole foods. However, there is no evidence to show that this will make you healthier. It amounts to a personal decision. Do you have faith that FDA and food manufacturers are adequately protecting your health and welfare, or do you want to take more personal control by minimizing your intake of compounds not naturally found in foods (Figure 19-6)?

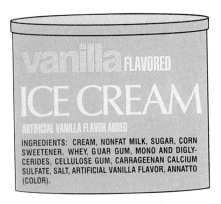

Figure 19-6 Depending on food choices, a diet can be either essentially devoid of or rich in food additives.

CONCEPT CHECK

Food additives are used to reduce spoilage from microbial growth, oxygen, metals, and other compounds. Additives are also used to adjust pH, improve flavor and color, leaven, provide nutritional fortification, thicken, and emulsify food components. Additives are classified as intentional (direct), which are those purposely added to foods, and incidental (indirect), which are those that turn up in foods due to environmental contamination or various manufacturing practices. The amount of an additive allowed in a food is limited to $\frac{1}{100}$ of the highest amount that has no observable effect when fed to animals. In most cases, the Delaney Clause further limits intentional addition of cancer-causing compounds to food in the United States. Carcinogens that incidentally enter foods have maximum amounts set for their presence in foods.

Substances That Occur Naturally in Foods and Can Cause Illness

Foods contain a variety of naturally occurring substances that can cause illness. Following are some of the more important examples[13]:

Safrole—found in sassafras, mace, and nutmeg; causes cancer.

Solanine—found in potato shoots and green spots on potato skins; inhibits the action of neurotransmitters.

Mushroom toxins—found in some species of mushrooms and can cause stomach upset, dizziness, hallucinations, and other neurological symptoms. The more lethal varieties can cause liver and kidney failure, coma, and even death. FDA regulates commercially grown and harvested mushrooms. These are cultivated in concrete buildings or caves. However, there are no systematic controls on individual gatherers harvesting wild species, except in Michigan and Illinois.[27]

Avidin—found in raw egg whites; binds biotin in a way that prevents its absorption.

Thiaminase—found in raw clams and mussels; destroys the vitamin thiamin.

Glycyrrhizic acid—found in pure licorice extracts; causes hypertension.

Tetrodotoxin—found in puffer fish; causes respiratory paralysis.

Protease inhibitor—found in raw soybeans; inhibits digestive enzymes.

Saponins—found in alfalfa sprouts; can destroy red blood cell membranes.

Oxalic acid—found in spinach; binds calcium and iron.

Herbal teas—containing senna or comfrey; can cause diarrhea and liver damage.

Nitrates—found in spinach, lettuce, and beets; can be converted to the carcinogen nitrosamine.

Browning products—found in toasted grains; can cause DNA mutations.

People have coexisted for centuries with these naturally occurring substances and have learned to avoid some of them and limit intake in other cases. Today they pose little health risk. Farmers know potatoes must be stored in the dark so that solanine won't be synthesized. And we have developed cooking and food preparation methods to limit the potency of other substances. Nevertheless, it is important to understand that some potentially harmful chemicals in foods occur naturally.

Environmental Contaminants in Food

A variety of environmental contaminants may be found in foods. Aside from pesticide residues and products of fungal growth, other important contaminants deserve attention.

LEAD

Ingesting lead can cause anemia, kidney disease, and damage to the nervous system and can interfere with nerve impulse conduction. Because it has a high atomic weight, it is a "heavy" metal. Many heavy metals are toxic at low doses.

Lead toxicity is especially a problem for children because it is associated with IQ deficits, behavior disorders, slowed growth, and impaired hearing.[1] Exposed children who eat a high-fat diet low in calcium and low in iron absorb more lead. In 1991 the Centers for Disease Control and Prevention (CDC) changed its guidelines for acceptable concentration of lead in the blood. Responding to mounting evidence of lead toxicity at lower blood concentrations, CDC set 10 µg/100 ml as a dangerous amount.

Despite the reduction of lead exposure in children over the last 20 years, associated with the decline in leaded gasoline and lead solder used in homes and in the canning industry, approximately 1.7 million children age 1 to 5 years still have elevated blood lead. Medical costs for a child with lead intoxication average $2,500 per treatment, and most children require two or more treatments.[1]

Poor, African-American children, who reside disproportionately in inner cities, are at increased risk for harmful lead exposure because of the lead-based paint present on the interiors and exteriors of the surrounding buildings. As this paint flakes off of walls or is abraded from window trim as windows are opened and closed, lead paint chips enter the environment and may be ingested.

Other sources of lead in general include brass fittings on water pumps used in wells and imported wine from areas where leaded gasoline is still used (especially Eastern Europe). It is important also not to store food in a can with a lead solder joint after the can has been opened. Contact with air speeds degradation of the solder joint and the release of lead into the food product. This is especially important for acidic food products, such as tomatoes. Because most domestic can manufacturers and food processors no longer make or use lead-soldered cans, the primary risk is from canned goods imported to the United States. In addition, never store acidic products such as fruit juice, sauerkraut, or pickled vegetables in galvanized, tin, or other metal containers, except stainless steel. Acid can dissolve the metal, and lead leaches into the food product.

Lead can also leach out of solder joints in copper pipes, so let tap water run a minute or so before drinking it or cooking with it, especially first thing in the morning or when the water has been off for a few hours. Use only cold water for drinking, cooking, and preparing infant formula. Lead in drinking water makes up about 20% of the average person's total lead exposure. Drinking water can be tested for lead content for about $20 to $50 by laboratories certified by the Environmental Protection Agency (EPA). Avoid softening drinking water because soft water can leach lead from pipes.

Finally, lead can enter the food supply via leaded crystal and pottery glazes. Lead is no longer used in glazes on commercially produced dishes in the United States because of this hazard. However, there is no way to ensure the safety of homemade or imported pottery items. It is important not to use antiques or collectibles, including any leaded glass, for food or beverage storage because of potential lead contamination.

DIOXIN

Dioxin is a chemical containing chlorine and benzene. It can be created by incineration of chlorine-based material like plastics together with hydrocarbon-based material, such as paper. Dioxin causes cancer and other harmful effects in animals, even in small doses, and likely does so in humans as well. Besides exposure from trash-burning incinerators, other sources of dioxin are bottom-feeding fish from the Great Lakes—an area with a great deal of industrial activity and chemical production.

or process and whether cancellation would decrease productivity.[30] After determining the dollar cost to the farmer, EPA then looks at costs to processors and consumers as well.

Once a pesticide is approved for use, at least a 100-fold margin of safety is a standard requirement for contamination in food to minimize health effects other than cancer (such as kidney damage or birth defects). In other words, the tolerances (limits) used for foods set the safety standard at 100 times less than the highest dose at which the pesticide causes no ill effects in animals—or lower. If the pesticide causes cancer, its use must not cause more than one cancer case in 1 million people. And if the pesticide causes cancer and its concentration in finished foods is much greater than that allowed for use on crops, generally its use is banned by the Delaney Clause. We noted earlier that there are proposals to stop the use of the Delaney Clause for pesticides and replace it with a simple standard, such as a risk of "no more than one cancer case in the lifetime of one million people" as a guideline for use. This proposal is currently under debate. FDA is responsible for enforcing pesticide tolerances on all foods except meat, poultry, and certain egg products, which are monitored by USDA.

How Safe Are Pesticides?

Dangers from exposure to pesticides through food depend on how potent the chemical toxin is, how concentrated it is in the food, how much and how frequently it's eaten, and the consumer's resistance or susceptibility to the substance. Pesticide use is clearly associated with declining water quality. Accumulating information also links pesticide use to increased cancer rates in farm communities. For rural counties in the U.S. the incidence of lymph, genital, brain, and digestive tract cancers increases with higher-than-average herbicide use.[3] Respiratory cancer cases increase with greater insecticide use. In tests using laboratory animals, scientists have found that some of the chemicals present in pesticide residues cause birth defects, sterility, tumors, organ damage, and injury to the central nervous system. Some pesticides persist in the environment for years.

Still, some researchers argue that the cancer risk from pesticide residues is hundreds of times less than the risk from eating such common foods as peanut butter, brown mustard, and basil. Plants manufacture their own toxic substances to defend themselves against insects, birds, and grazing animals (including humans). When plants are stressed or damaged, they produce even more of these toxins. Because of this, many foods contain naturally occurring chemicals considered toxic, even carcinogenic. Other scientists argue that if natural carcinogens are already in the food supply, then we should reduce the number of added carcinogens whenever possible. In other words, we should do what we can to decrease the problem.

The mere presence of a pesticide in food or water at any concentration frightens some people. But the concentrations of pesticide residues found in foods are almost always well below the tolerances that have been set to meet safety concerns. High and obviously hazardous concentrations are very rare and are usually the result of spills or improper uses. But the major challenge for scientists and regulators goes beyond detecting and measuring pesticide residues; it is rather a question of what, if any, biological significance they have.[30]

The Risks of Pesticides to Children

Any discussions of pesticides and associated health risks need to focus attention on children. They are not simply small adults in a biological sense. Children face a higher risk from pesticide exposure than adults do for several reasons[3]:

1. Their exposure is greater; children eat more food in proportion to their body weight than do adults.
2. Children consume more foods that are potential sources of pesticide residues than do adults. They eat more fruit, for example.
3. Exposure at an early age carries a greater risk than does exposure later in life; residues can accumulate to toxic amounts over a longer period. Also, cancer has more time to develop.

4. Physiological susceptibility to the effects of carcinogens and neurotoxins in pesticides may be greater; the cells in children are dividing rapidly, and the enzyme systems that detoxify chemicals are not fully developed.

Until recent years, EPA did not consider these factors in risk calculations. EPA now looks at age-related consumption data for approval of new pesticides. Although children are at greater risk from pesticides, the magnitude of that risk and how best to calculate it are open to debate. A recent report by the National Academy of Sciences advocates changes to the current pesticide regulatory system to ensure the safety of foods eaten by children. In addition, its authors stress the value of including fruits and vegetables in children's diets and caution parents not to change their children's diets to avoid certain foods.[4] Carefully washing fruits and vegetables and consuming a wide variety are sufficient recommendations. Peeling fruits and vegetables is another option. A final general precaution is to keep children away from lawns, gardens, and flower beds that have recently been treated with pesticides and herbicides.

Testing Amounts of Pesticides in Foods

FDA tests thousands of raw products each year for pesticide residues. (A pesticide is considered illegal in this case if it is not approved for use on the crop in question or if the amount used exceeds the allowed tolerance.) A 1993 FDA study showed no residues in 64% of domestic samples and 69% of imported samples. Less than 1% of domestic and imported samples had residues that were over tolerance, and 1% of domestic and 3% of import samples had residues for which there was no tolerance.[9] The findings for 1993 continue to demonstrate that pesticide residues in foods are generally well below EPA tolerances, and they confirm the safety of the food supply relative to pesticide residues.

Residues sometimes appear on the wrong crops or in excessive amounts because of contamination from nearby farms via wind or water. When a problem is identified, FDA takes steps to make sure it's corrected and that the tainted food in question never reaches the consumer. However, of 600 pesticides available on international markets, many are not even detected by any of FDA's multiresidue tests.[3] This has raised concern by pesticide critics with regard to imported foods. Better tests that detect single residues are less frequently used because of cost.

Personal Action

We often take risks in our own lives, but we prefer to have a choice in the matter after weighing the pros and cons. For instance, we can choose not to immunize a child, but we do so with the understanding that the child might get sick. Or we can drive recklessly. These are personal risks that we choose to take. We can also choose to risk cancer from smoking or to avoid that risk. But in regard to pesticides in food, someone else is deciding what is acceptable and what is not.[30] Our only choice is whether to buy or avoid pesticide-containing foods. And in reality it is almost impossible to avoid pesticides entirely because even "organic" produce often contains traces of pesticides, probably because of cross-contamination from nearby farms.

Short-term studies of the effects of pesticides on laboratory animals cannot pinpoint long-term cancer risks precisely. But it should be clearly understood that the presence of minute traces of an environmental chemical in a food does not mean that any adverse effect will result from eating that food.

FDA feels that the hazards are comparatively low and, in the short run, are less than the hazards of food-borne illness created in our own kitchens. We can't avoid pesticide risks entirely, but we can limit exposure by following the advice previously given in this chapter.

In the future, we can also encourage farmers to use fewer pesticides to reduce exposure to our foods and water supplies, but we will have to settle for produce that isn't perfect in appearance. Are you concerned enough about pesticides on food to change your shopping habits or take more political action?

CHAPTER TWENTY

Under-nutrition throughout the World

T he images are both vivid and heartrending: emaciated children with enormous eyes and stomachs, staring at us from news photos and television. Each year, more than 15 million children worldwide die of undernutrition and related diseases.

Today, nearly one in five people in the developing world is chronically undernourished—too hungry to lead a productive, active life.[3] The incidence of undernourishment has approximately doubled in the past decade, testament to the widespread and growing problems of poverty and undernutrition. Although about two thirds of undernourished people live in Asia, the incidence of undernutrition is increasing most rapidly among the peoples of eastern Africa, particularly in Ethiopia, Sudan, Rwanda, Burundi, Eritrea, Kenya, Somalia, and Tanzania. Theirs are the eyes that haunt us.[31]

In this chapter we examine various concepts related to undernutrition, its frequency and consequences, and the many conditions that contribute to its existence. Finally we discuss some approaches for reducing undernutrition based on its underlying causes.

NUTRITION AWARENESS

NUTRITION AWARENESS INVENTORY

Answer these 15 statements about under-nutrition worldwide to test your current knowledge. If you think the answer is true or mostly true, circle T. If you think the answer is false or mostly false, circle F. Use the scoring key at the end of the book to compute your total score. Repeat this test after you have read this chapter, and compare your results.

1. **T F** Hunger is partly the psychological state resulting when not enough food is eaten.
2. **T F** The primary cause of undernutrition is poverty.
3. **T F** Diabetes is more common when food supplies are low.
4. **T F** Undernutrition is the most common form of malnutrition among the poor.
5. **T F** The risk of dying from pregnancy-related causes highlights the gap between developing and industrialized countries.
6. **T F** The greatest risk from undernutrition during pregnancy is borne by the fetus (infant).
7. **T F** A 9-year-old child suffering from undernutrition can look like a 4-year-old.
8. **T F** Marginal deficiencies of iron affect few people worldwide.
9. **T F** The effects of years of undernutrition can be overcome in several weeks on a high-protein, high-carbohydrate diet.
10. **T F** Compared with other industrialized countries, the United States has one of the lowest infant mortality rates in the world.
11. **T F** Homelessness in the United States is much more evident today than in the early 1980s.
12. **T F** World population is rapidly outstripping the global food supply.
13. **T F** Traditionally, poorer people bear more children.
14. **T F** In Third World countries, the urban population consists mostly of the poor.
15. **T F** Wherever they live, a key factor for the health of people is a safe water supply.

World Hunger: A Continuing Plague

In November 1974, the United Nations World Food Conference proclaimed the bold objective "that within a decade no child will go to bed hungry, that no family will fear for its next day's bread, and that no human being's future and capacities will be stunted by malnutrition." Not only does this promise remain unfulfilled, but in the mid-1990s hunger is a daily experience for one in five people in the developing world and one in eight people in the United States. Currently a third of Africa's population eats less than what is considered necessary for healthy life, which in turn impairs physical and mental health.[3]

The famines that occurred in Ethiopa in the 1980s called special attention to the problem of undernutrition in the developing world. The plight of millions of starving people consolidated widespread public support for immediate aid for the victims of famine. Still, hunger has not abated. Quite the opposite, as frequent news stories remind us. Continuing civil wars in Africa and the former Yugoslavia in Eastern Europe, coupled with drought in many parts of the world, have brought an additional 30 million people to the brink of starvation in recent years, about two thirds of whom live in Africa.[3] Relief aid has been arriving, but often too little and too late. The deadly combination of war and poor weather has also recently led to increasing hunger in Bangladesh, Afghanistan, the Philippines, and Cambodia. As you might surmise, undernutrition in developing nations is an ongoing threat that requires political and technological solutions.

We begin our look at these problems by first defining some key terms. **Hunger** is the physiological state that results when not enough food is eaten to meet energy needs. It also describes an uneasiness, discomfort, weakness, or pain caused by lack of food. If hunger is not alleviated, the resulting medical and social costs from undernutrition are high: premature births, mental retardation beginning in infancy, inadequate growth and development in childhood, poor school performance, de-

TABLE 20-I

The realities of undernutrition

- Nearly one in five people in the developing world is chronically undernourished—too hungry to lead a productive, active life.
- About 60,000 people die of hunger each day—two thirds of them children.
- Approximately half of all children who die each year in developing countries do so from causes that could be prevented at low cost.
- At least 250,000 children are permanently blinded each year simply through a lack of vitamin A.
- Women in poor countries average up to four times more births than women in the United States.
- Every day, the world produces about 2400 kcal for each person, meeting average energy needs for many adults.
- Poor women in Third World countries face a 300-fold increased risk of death in pregnancy compared with women in the United States.
- In many developing countries, life expectancy of the population is one half to two thirds of that in the United States.
- Almost half of the world's people earn less than $200 a year—many use 80% to 90% of that income to obtain food. About $2000 to $3000 each year per person is needed if life expectancy is to reach that seen the United States.
- Of the nearly 5.7 billion people on earth, more than 1 billion drink contaminated water.
- About 2 billion people in the world are without proper sanitation facilities.
- Developing countries have two thirds of the 15 million AIDS cases worldwide.

creased work output in adulthood, and chronic disease (Table 20-1).[16] Symptoms of chronic hunger are found not only in the developing world, but also among many people living at or below the poverty level in the United States.[3]

The primary cause of chronic hunger is poverty. Unemployment and underemployment, homelessness, drug addiction, functional illiteracy, single-parent families (often headed by a woman who has limited earning potential), wage discrimination, poor health, inadequate governmental programs, and war and civil strife all contribute to this poverty. In developing nations, civil strife (frequently arising from ethnic and religious fighting), a lack of resources, and inadequate governmental programs combine to intensify the problem of hunger.[3]

Malnutrition is a condition of impaired development or function caused by a long-term deficiency, excess, or imbalance in energy and/or nutrient intake. The occurrence of specific diseases of malnutrition depends mostly on the food-population ratio. When food supplies are low and the population is large, undernutrition leading to nutritional deficiency diseases, such as goiter (enlarged thyroid gland) and xerophthalmia (dryness and keratinization of the epithelium in the eye from a vitamin A deficiency), is common.[9,16,29] However, when the food supply is ample or overabundant, poor food choices coupled with an excessive intake can lead to nutrition-related chronic diseases, such as certain forms of diabetes.[20] Note, however, that pockets of undernutrition among the poor may still be found in food-abundant areas, such as the United States.[4]

Genetic background contributes to both forms of malnutrition. Not every child in Thailand who eats mainly rice develops **protein-energy malnutrition (PEM);** similarly, not every adult in New York City who consumes a high-fat, energy-rich diet suffers a heart attack. Genetics influences the development of these diseases.[19]

Undernutrition, referred to many times in this book, is the malnutrition that results from an inadequate intake, absorption, or use of the nutrients or energy needed for optimal growth, development, and body function. The earliest response

malnutrition Failing health that results from longstanding faulty nutrition that either fails to meet or greatly exceeds nutritional needs.

protein-energy malnutrition (PEM) A condition associated with body wasting and increased susceptibility to infections that results from prolonged consumption of insufficient amounts of food energy and protein.

undernutrition Failing health that results from a longstanding dietary intake that does not meet nutritional needs.

to undernutrition is reduced physical activity, allowing the individual to preserve energy for growth and other vital functions.[30] With persistent undernutrition, the second response is a reduced rate of weight gain or poor weight maintenance. In addition, in children the rate of growth in height is reduced.[32]

Undernutrition is the most common form of malnutrition among the poor in both developing and developed countries. Currently about half of the 4 million African children who die annually before the age of 5 are undernourished. This condition is also the primary cause of specific nutrient deficiencies that in turn can result in muscle wasting, blindness (from xerophthalmia), scurvy, pellagra, beriberi, anemia, rickets, goiter, and a host of other effects (Table 20-2).[16] For example, more than 250,000 children develop blindness from xerophthalmia each year.[18] The deficiency of vitamin A that causes this disease also increases the risk for other diseases, such as measles. The United Nations International Children's Fund reports that the lives of 1 to 3 million children could be saved annually in the developing world if vitamin A supplements were provided a few times a year. The annual cost per child would be about 6 cents. About 30% to 60% of all women in the Third World suffer from iron-deficiency and related anemias. Of the 5.7 billion people in the world, at least 800 million exhibit some form of undernutrition.[3] Death and disease from infections, particularly those causing acute and prolonged diarrhea or acute respiratory disease, are dramatically increased when the infections are superimposed on a state of chronic undernutrition.[5]

Protein-energy malnutrition (PEM) is a form of undernutrition caused by an extremely deficient intake of energy and protein, which is generally exacerbated by an accompanying illness. The typically dramatic results of protein-energy malnutrition—kwashiorkor and marasmus—were covered in Chapter 5. We will concentrate in this chapter on the more subtle effects of a chronic lack of food.

Famine is the extreme shortage of food affecting many people. Although famines often are initiated by poor harvests caused by unfavorable weather, they are characterized by large-scale loss of life, social disruption, and economic chaos, which further decrease food production. As a result of these extremes, there is a downward spiral of events: human distress; sales of land, livestock, and other important farm assets; migration; division and impoverishment of the poorest families; crime; and the weakening of customary moral codes, as seen recently in Sudan and Rwanda. Antisocial behavior, such as hoarding and crime, increases. In the midst of all this, undernutrition rates soar, infectious diseases such as cholera spread, and people die in greater numbers.[3] Successfully halting this spiral requires more than just feeding those in need. Special efforts are needed to eradicate the fundamental causes.

Causes of famine vary by region and decade, but the most common underlying cause is crop failure. The most obvious causes of crop failure are bad weather, war and civil strife, or both. War deserves a special focus: it contributes to food crisis by drawing labor from food production, disrupting the marketing of crops, destroying fields, creating refugees, and hindering relief efforts. In this situation food relief can even become a weapon.[3] War is linked to many famines in recent years.[22] In fact, these types of man-made disasters absorb more than three quarters of the disaster assistance channeled through the World Food Program.

famine An extreme shortage of food that leads to massive starvation in a population; often associated with crop failure, war, and political strife.

- - - - - - - - - - - - - - -

More than 3 million people may have perished in the great Bengal, India, famine of 1943. In 1974 in the new country of Bangladesh, another 1.5 million starved. China suffered an almost unbelievable famine from 1959 to 1961—estimates of mortality range from 16 to 64 million.

- - - - - - - - - - - - - - -

Critical Life Stages for Undernutrition

Prolonged undernutrition is detrimental to health at any time throughout life. But the likelihood of undernutrition's developing is greater and its effects are more critical during pregnancy, growth periods of childhood, and throughout the early years (Figure 20-1).

PREGNANCY

The heavy nutrient needs of the developing fetus place both a pregnant woman and her fetus at risk of undernutrition, with potential serious consequences for each. Indeed pregnancy is the life stage posing the greatest risk for undernutrition and its associated health effects.

TABLE 20-2

Effects of nutrient-deficiency diseases that commonly accompany undernutrition

Disease and key nutrient involved	Typical effects	Foods rich in deficient nutrient	Where the problem still exists
Xerophthalmia Vitamin A	Blindness from chronic eye infections, poor growth, dryness and keratinization of epithelial tissues	Liver, fortified milk, sweet potatoes, spinach, greens, carrots, cantaloupe, apricots	Asia, Africa
Rickets (and osteomalacia) Vitamin D	Weakened bones, bowed legs, other bone deformities	Fortified milk, fish oils, sun exposure	Asia and Africa where religious practices encourage avoidance of sun exposure for women and children; elderly in developed nations
Beriberi Thiamin	Nerve degeneration, altered muscle coordination, cardiovascular problems	Sunflower seeds, pork, whole and enriched grains, dry beans	Famines, such as in Africa and Asia
Ariboflavinosis Riboflavin	Inflammation of face and oral cavity	Milk, mushrooms, spinach, liver, enriched grains	Famines, such as in Africa
Pellagra Niacin	Diarrhea, skin inflammation, dementia	Mushrooms, bran, tuna, chicken, beef, peanuts, whole and enriched grains	Famines, such as in Africa
Scurvy Vitamin C	Delayed wound healing, internal bleeding, abnormal formation of bones and teeth	Citrus fruits, strawberries, broccoli	Famines, such as in Africa
Iron-deficiency anemia Iron	Reduced work output, reduced growth, increased health risk in pregnancy, impaired learning capacity	Meats, spinach, seafood, broccoli, peas, bran, whole-grain and enriched breads	Worldwide
Goiter Iodide	Enlarged thyroid gland, poor growth in infancy and childhood, possible mental retardation, cretinism	Iodized salt, saltwater fish	South America, Eastern Europe, Africa

Note that often two or more nutrient-deficiency diseases are found in an undernourished person in the Third World. This separate discussion of nutrients just makes it easier to see the important role of each nutrient.

Maternal Risks

As we saw in Chapter 16, a pregnant woman needs to consume extra nutrients to meet her own needs, as well as those of her developing fetus. If the mother's nutrient intake is inadequate during pregnancy, her own health can be seriously jeopardized as stores of maternal nutrients are depleted to help provide for the fetus. Ma-

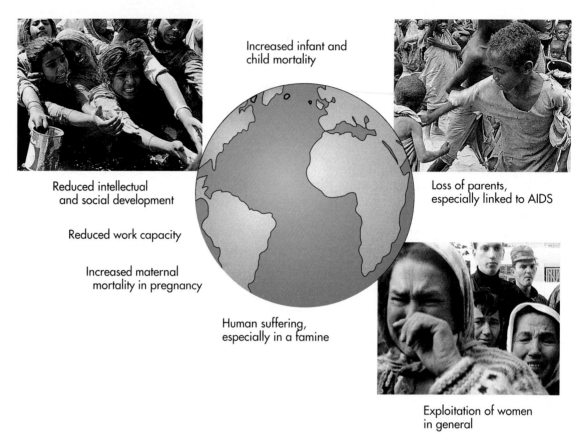

Figure 20-1 Undernutrition affects many aspects of human health and much of humanity.

ternal iron-deficiency anemia is one possible consequence. Pregnancy-induced hypertension (preeclampsia), a life-threatening condition involving rapid weight gain (from fluid retention) and a sharp increase in blood pressure, is also likely influenced by inadequate prenatal nutrition.

In Africa, women give birth, on average, to more than six live babies. Coupled with chronic undernutrition, these high birth rates create a 1 in 20 lifetime risk of dying from pregnancy-related causes for the mother. In contrast, American women, who on average have about two children, face a risk of 1 death per 6000 births from pregnancy-related causes. No other social indicator, whether literacy, life expectancy, or infant mortality, shows a wider gap between the developing world and the industrialized world.

Fetal and Newborn Risks

A great risk from undernutrition during gestation is also borne by the fetus. A growing fetus requires a diet rich in protein, vitamins, and minerals to support growth and development of the brain and other body tissues. When these needs are not met, birth often occurs prematurely, before the full term of gestation, which normally is about 40 weeks. An infant born earlier than 37 weeks' gestation (i.e., preterm) is most likely to have diminished lung function and a weakened immune system, conditions that compromise health and contribute to the death of newborns. Long-term impediments to growth and development may occur even if a preterm infant survives the first year.

Infants born preterm and weighing 2500 g (5.5 pounds) or less are 5 to 10 times more likely to die during the first year than full-term, normal-weight infants, primarily because of their poor lung development. When low birthweight is accompanied by other physical abnormalities, medical intervention can cost $100,000 or more. If severe retardation occurs, the lifetime cost of care can be over $2 million.

In the United States, low birthweight accounts for more than half of all infant deaths and for 75% of deaths of babies under 1 month of age. Currently about 7% of infants born in the United States have low birthweight. Worldwide, more than half of infant deaths stem from low birthweight.[3]

Childhood

The rapid growth years of early childhood compose another period of high risk from undernutrition. Because the human brain grows most rapidly from conception through early childhood, the brain and central nervous system are particularly vulnerable. After the preschool years, brain growth and development slow dramatically until maturity, when they cease. Nutritional deprivation, especially in early infancy, can lead to permanent brain impairment.[30] Beyond early childhood, learning may be jeopardized by a deprived environment, but the basic size and structure of the brain are set.

In general, poor children experience more nutritional deprivation and overall illness and are more severely affected than other children. For example, iron-deficiency anemia, indicated by the presence of an abnormally low concentration of hemoglobin in the blood, is much more common among poor children than nonpoor children. This deficiency can lead to reduced stamina, stunting, and learning problems.[1] Undernutrition in childhood can also weaken resistance to infection because immune function decreases when such nutrients as protein, vitamin A, and zinc are very low in a diet.[5] Poorly nourished youngsters are then at risk for more frequent colds, ear infections, and other infectious diseases.

When adequate nutrients are restored to the diet of children, improvements in health can be obvious. For example, in recent years the height of several groups of growth-retarded children in the United States, including Hispanic children in Colorado, has been shown to increase after zinc supplementation.

Elderly Years

A final group at risk for undernutrition comprises elderly persons, as well as those who are chronically ill.[3] Often advancing age and chronic illness coexist in the same individuals. These people generally require nutrient-dense foods, the amount depending on each person's state of health and degree of physical activity. Because many have fixed incomes and significant medical costs, food can end up as a low-priority item. In addition, elderly and chronically ill people are often unable to take care of all their own needs, are sometimes isolated, and are more apt to be depressed—all important factors that can influence food intake (see Chapter 18).

General Effects of Semistarvation

The results of undernutrition from semistarvation in the initial stages are often so mild that physical signs and symptoms are absent and blood tests typically do not detect the slight changes in metabolism. Even in the absence of clinical evidence, however, undernourishment may affect reproductive capacity, resistance to or recovery from disease, physical activity and work output, and attitudes and behavior.[16] Recall from Chapter 2 that as tissues continue to be depleted of nutrients, blood tests eventually detect biochemical changes, such as a drop in blood hemoglobin concentration. Physical symptoms, such as body weakness, become apparent with further depletion. Finally, the signs and symptoms of a full-blown deficiency disease become obvious enough to be recognized, such as **edema** associated with a protein deficiency.[20]

In general, the occurrence of severe deficiency in a few people in a population represents the tip of the iceberg. Typically a much greater number will have milder degrees of undernutrition. And, under certain circumstances even these mild nutrient deficiencies can cause real difficulties in maintaining health, as well as for life in general. These problems are especially important in the developing world. For example, combined deficiencies of certain vitamins and the minerals iron and zinc—

Growth failure in children is a common result of undernutrition and a warning sign that more extreme effects may follow. In a recent survey of 76 developing countries, stunting was seen in more than one third of children ages 2 to 5 years.

edema The build-up of excess fluid in extracellular spaces.

EXPERT OPINION

THE HUMAN SIDE OF HUNGER AND POVERTY IN AMERICA

SUSAN M. KRUEGER, M.S., R.D.

As a registered dietitian and college instructor of human nutrition, hunger is a very important issue to me. Good nutrition is vital to the health of our country. Yet, with 1 in 5 children living in poverty, up to 30 million Americans experiencing some degree of hunger on a regular basis, 1 in 10 Americans using food stamps, and 37 million people without health insurance, we obviously have problems with the health and well-being of many. All of the nutrition knowledge in the world will not help people if they lack the funds and assistance to purchase healthy foods.

Beginning in 1993, I have traveled each summer with my husband and four children, who now range in age from 8 to 15 years, to southern Appalachia to do volunteer work with poor residents in this region of our country. The first summer I departed from home equipped with many ideas, pamphlets, food guide displays, coloring books with nutrition themes, and other aids for teaching people how to improve their diets and thereby the quality of their lives. To my surprise, I did not use any of the items I had so carefully packed during that summer visit!

THE PEOPLE OF SOUTHERN APPALACHIA

I quickly realized that my teaching tools and nutrition expertise were largely superfluous in southern Appalachia. In the area where we worked, many people had greater, or at least more immediate, needs than nutrition education.

We found people living in tar paper shacks, in structures with large holes in the roofs, and in trailers with missing windows and doors. Some people had no running water or indoor plumbing facilities. We found children who owned no shoes. We met lonely elderly people in nursing homes who rarely had visitors, and others alone in their own homes, which were often in great need of repair.

We also found children craving the attention of adults, many of whom were performing adult responsibilities, especially in regards to child care, as well as household duties. We saw evidence of "silent undernutrition"—adults who looked old beyond their years and children who were very small and thin for their ages.

We came across a food pantry with no food. Food arrived while we were there, but the shelves were emptied soon after that. When food was available, recipients could get food only once a month simply because the amount of donated food was not enough for more frequent distribution to the many people requesting it. In contrast, at the pantry at home in Eau Claire, Wisconsin, where I have been volunteering weekly for the last five years, recipients can come weekly. This pantry receives surplus meats and high-protein foods, soups, vegetables, and potatoes from the dietary department of a local hospital. Foods such as canned beans and vegetables, cereal, soup, pasta, fresh produce, and bread are also distributed. This pantry receives generous support from individuals, churches, businesses, and grocery stores in the local area.

In our work with the poor in southern Appalachia we also found people who had a strong sense of pride, of wanting to make it on their own without "government handouts." We met others who were in desperate need of assistance but had no idea that they qualified for aid or were unaware of how to obtain it. In many people we also found a great love of family.

Southern Appalachia has an undeniably beautiful landscape. But this region is unattractive to industry because of its mountainous terrain and many hazardous two-lane highways that often have no shoulders—just mountains or rivers—on the sides. And many residents lack the education and training needed by modern industries.

HOW WE HELPED

During our time in southern Appalachia, my family and I have performed home repairs, from fixing roofs to painting, visited isolated elderly individuals, and conducted play activities with local children. One of my favorite job sites was a very depressed, tiny village where we would play with the local children three afternoons a week. On some days, 35 or more kids between the ages of 6 months and 15 years would show up! The homes in the area where these children lived were for the most part in extremely poor condition, and many did not have running water.

Overall, the children who attended these play groups were eager and trusting. I could not believe the enjoyment displayed by some of the older children, even teens, with some of the simple craft activities, such as making necklaces from beads and string or designing and coloring paper headbands. Some of my own young children were bored with the same activities!

We also worked with many adults. One of the jobs I was involved with during my first summer was building a storage shed to hold firewood next to a tar paper shack. The woman who lived there had been born with a disfiguring skin condition. When she was an infant the condition had caused her so much pain that her parents had to carry her on a pillow. When she was a child, her parents tried to send her to school, but she did not attend long because the other children were frightened of her appearance. She now lives alone, cannot read, does not know how old she is, uses an outhouse even in the cold winter months because she has no indoor plumbing, and heats her two-room home with a stove. She does have electricity and owns a black and white television, which is her major source of entertainment and companionship.

WHAT I HAVE LEARNED

My experiences in southern Appalachia have taught me much. They confirmed my belief that poor people are not really any different from those who have more. We all have the same basic needs and experience the same basic feelings that are all part of being human.

I also learned that people are poor and often hungry for many different reasons. Some of the people I have worked with are poor because they have lost their jobs and have not been able to find new ones. Many of the people who need assistance work! Some are working part-time jobs, but many are working full-time jobs that pay minimum wage, which keeps them below poverty level. According to the 1990 census, over 18 million people were working full-time, year-round jobs paying such low wages that they were living in poverty despite their efforts. Some of the people requiring assistance have problems with alcohol or drug abuse. Others have physical, and many have mental, disabilities that greatly diminish their ability to provide for themselves.

Many of the people whom I have encountered have not had the educational opportunities that could help break the cycle of poverty. Some of the people come from families with no academic tradition, and lack knowledge about how to find, finance, and make use of such opportunities.

Many people who seek assistance are the heads of single-parent families, who frequently experience difficulty in making ends meet and/or obtaining an education, especially when finding and paying for child care is involved. Finally, many people are poor because of continuing discrimination and economic problems faced by members of ethnic minority groups.

WHAT YOU CAN DO

Many students have asked how they can get involved in hunger issues. I recommend donating time, money, or food to local food banks and pantries. Even a couple boxes of macaroni and cheese can make a difference and help a family or individual stretch their food supply to the end of the week.

Keeping an open mind is also important. There are so many damaging myths that abound in our society concerning the poor, such as that people on welfare are lazy and do not want to work and that food stamp and welfare fraud is common. Problems of deceit in our society are not found predominantly among the less privileged, as a quick review of recent government and business scandals will reveal. Most of the poor whom I have encountered do not enjoy relying on government or private assistance and would rather be working a job that did not necessitate standing in line for food to get them through the week.

Finally, I would recommend becoming aware of poverty and hunger issues in our country, examining the potential solutions that are being offered, exercising your right to vote, and expressing your opinions to your representatives in government. These are all ways to be involved in the eradication of hunger while solutions for the more complex problem of poverty are being sought.

Susan M. Krueger is a senior lecturer in the Biology Department at the University of Wisconsin–Eau Claire. She is a member of the board of the St. Francis Food Pantry and has been involved with the Community Table soup kitchen in Eau Claire, Wisconsin. She and her family have been Passionist volunteers in Preston County, West Virginia, for the past three summers.

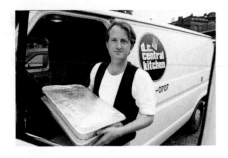

This Washington, D.C., operation collects leftover food from hotels, restaurants, and catering firms for delivery to homeless shelters, soup kitchens, and churches.

Undernutrition especially is a condition that need not exist. Nutrition programs and community intervention, if employed fully and effectively, could go a long way toward meeting the food needs of those at highest risk.[13] More training and employment opportunities could then help solidify the improvements. The near-elimination of wide-scale undernutrition in the United States in the 1970s demonstrates that a federal food safety net can help avert the problem.

Private emergency food network systems are also important, as we noted earlier, but are not sufficient to meet all food needs in the United States. Private donations often taper off during economic hardship in a given geographical area.[4] In addition, much of what is donated is limited in nutritional value. Of necessity, processed and canned grocery items predominate, rather than protein-rich foods or perishable items, such as fresh produce and milk.

Overall, the long-term solution to the problem of hunger in the United States is only partly governmental in nature. Education, training, housing, and food assistance when needed provide only part of the answer. An additional important part involves a cultural shift that emphasizes the responsibility of all citizens to provide as best they can for themselves, their families, and the less fortunate around them. Many Americans see more individual responsibility as a critical goal for our society at this time. Poverty and resulting hunger that stem from irresponsible individual behavior really cannot be "fixed" by government programs. Government programs, however, can be helpful in reducing or preventing poverty that results largely from lack of opportunity.

Clearly it is not fair to solely blame the victims of poverty. The difficulties faced by poorer Americans are substantial: substandard education and training, poor communication skills, lack of reliable and safe child care, inability to relocate, little employment experience, and no economic reserves to fall back on during crises.[3] Even when the desire for a better life is strong, people may get discouraged and then apathetic in the face of apparently insurmountable obstacles. Moreover, many poor Americans are ill equipped for the demands of a modern, dynamic society—in particular, elderly, sick, and handicapped persons and young single mothers and their children. Thus, regardless of how repugnant government assistance appears to some people, there likely will always be some need for it.

Since long-term undernutrition, especially among children, has both individual and societal consequences, all Americans, either directly or indirectly, are affected by this problem. The next few years are likely to bring changes in both government and private assistance programs, demanding new initiatives from all Americans. Your contribution to this process as an informed voter and, it's hoped, an active participant, is an important part of the process.

CONCEPT CHECK

Federal programs aimed at reducing hunger and malnutrition began during the Depression of the 1930s. In response to reports of widespread poverty and hunger during the early 1960s, Congress established several new federal food assistance programs and substantially increased funding for already existing programs. Largely as a result of these federal programs, undernutrition had decreased substantially by the mid-1970s. The improvement was short-lived, with the number of Americans experiencing poverty, homelessness, and undernutrition climbing during the 1980s and 1990s. The incidence of these three interrelated problems is influenced by economic, cultural, and individual factors, as well as government policies. The large, continuing federal budget deficits and serious questions about the long-term effectiveness of many government assistance programs may stimulate significant changes in their future administration, funding mechanisms, and program design. All citizens can help to reduce this problem.

Undernutrition in the Third World: Underlying Causes

Undernutrition in the Third World is also tied to poverty, so any true solution must address this problem. However, the countries that are considered to be Third World nations—those that have neither a productive free market economy nor a planned economy similar to that of the former Soviet Union—have a multitude of problems so complex and interrelated that they cannot be treated separately. Programs that have proved immensely helpful in the United States would be only a starting point in the Third World. All approaches to reducing undernutrition in these countries face major obstacles[3]:

- Extreme imbalances in the food/population ratio in different regions of a country
- War and political or civil unrest
- Rapid depletion of natural resources
- Cultural attitudes toward certain foods
- Poor **infrastructure,** especially poor housing, sanitation and storage facilities, education, communications, and transportation systems
- High external debt

Let's examine each of these problems and its relationship to poverty and undernutrition. Figure 20-2 depicts key factors that influence how much food is available for consumption by household members.

infrastructure The basic framework of a system of organization. The infrastructure of a society includes roads, bridges, telephones, and other basic technologies.

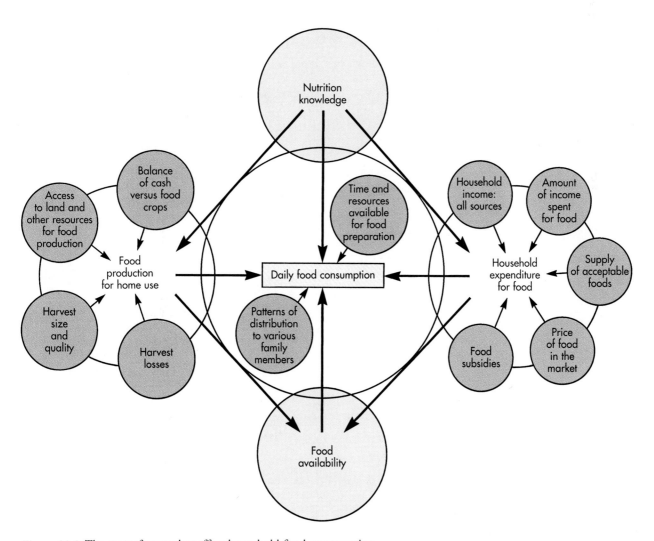

Figure 20-2 The many factors that affect household food consumption.

geometric progression A series of numbers in which the division of each number by the next smaller one yields the same value (in this case 2).

arithmetic progression A series of numbers in which the difference between each successive number is the same.

FOOD/POPULATION RATIO

Whether the earth can yield enough food for all people has been a longstanding question. As early as 1798, an English clergyman and political economist, Thomas Malthus, proposed a rather pessimistic view of the prospects for humans.[2] He said that given the passion between the genders (which he felt was something to be counseled against), the population would always increase in a **geometric progression**: 2, 4, 8, 16, 32, and so on. Meanwhile, at best, the food supply would increase in only an **arithmetic progression**: 2, 4, 6, 8, 10, and so on. As you can see from these progressions, Malthus's prediction was that by the time the population increased to "32" the food supply would have risen to only "10."

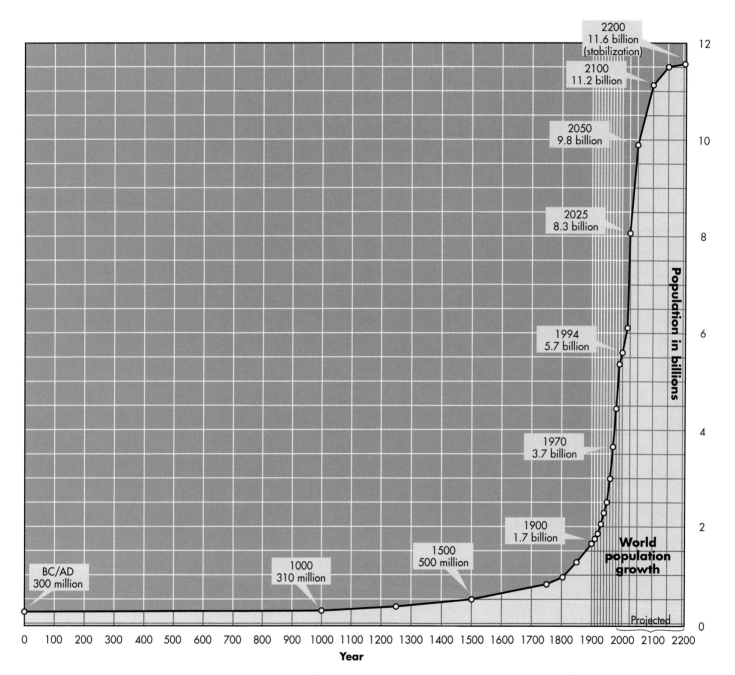

Figure 20-3 World population trends. Population growth is stabilizing in the industrialized countries of the world but continues to skyrocket in the developing countries. The current world population is 5.7 billion. These long-range projections show expected population values assuming continued decline in birth rates. Without this decline, population growth in the first half of the next century will likely be much more rapid than shown here. (From Overseas Development Council, United Nations Population Fund.)

Malthus felt that in the likely absence of sexual restraint, the growing population would be subject to recurring checks imposed by widespread starvation, war, or natural catastrophe brought on by disease. His proposals became the object of intense controversy in England and elsewhere, often meeting vigorous opposition. Eminent scientists in Britain pointed out that scientific advances in agriculture would greatly increase food production. In fact, that has been true. Nevertheless, the population explosion is just that. Malthus was correct in his prediction of geometric growth in the world population. So far this growth has not slowed significantly through natural checks, disease, or recent human interventions, such as birth control (Figure 20-3).[2]

No one can say what the earth's carrying capacity for humans may be, since it depends on unknown potential changes in technology and on the ability of economies to substitute new resources for ones that are running out. Some experts argue that the real threat is not that the earth will run out of land, topsoil, or water, but that nations will fail to pursue the economic, trade, and research policies that can increase the production of food, limit environmental damage, and ensure that resources reach the people who need them. In a free society, people are an asset, not a liability. Significant poverty and undernutrition persist mainly in those areas in the Third World where totalitarian governments dominate and suffocate economic activity. Still, ingenuity of this sort does not materialize automatically. And even if new solutions can be devised, some countries likely will lack the social and political inventiveness to take timely advantage of them.[3]

Currently, population growth does in fact exceed economic growth in many countries, and poverty is soaring.[2] Since efforts to speed up economic development have failed, the only way left to improve the situation may be to slow the growth of the population, as Malthus recommended. If we want to preserve a decent life for a widening share of humanity, then the growth in the earth's population should slow. According to the World Bank, 1 billion people are added to the world's population every 12 years, mostly in cities and in seacoast and river-basin areas, where the environment is very fragile. By 2030, the world thus will have nearly 3 billion more people than today—2 billion of them in countries where the average person earns less than $2 a day. Unless there is a catastrophe, more than 9 of 10 infants in the next generation will be born in the poorest parts of the world.

As one brake on population expansion, birth control programs have been effective in developed countries but have been relatively ineffective in developing countries that could really profit from them.[2] Whereas women in the United States average 2.1 live births each, women in some East African countries average 8.5 live births

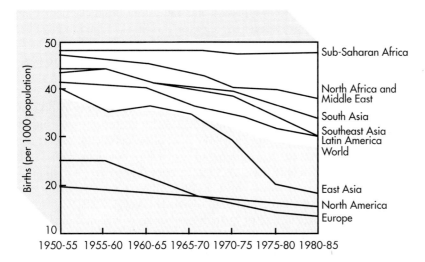

Figure 20-4 Birth rates in regions throughout the world. Rates have generally declined since the end of World War II. The only exception to this trend is in sub-Saharan Africa. As a result, Africa may account for nearly one fourth of the world's population by the late twenty-first century.

each, and for the world as a whole, women average 4 live births (Figure 20-4). At this time, there are about 5.7 billion people in the world. More than three quarters live in developing Third World countries, and more than half in Asia. Many experts believe that the global supply of food could provide adequate nutrition on average for all 5.7 billion, about 2400 kcal/per day, but food supplies are not distributed equally among consumers.[3] Gross disparities exist between developed and developing countries, among the rich and poor within countries, and even within families. In some instances, women and children get less to eat than do men, and sometimes among children, girls get less than boys.[14]

As well, food supply and population trends within the developing world itself clearly differ. Latin America and Russia have both had declining population growth rates since 1970, and their share of the world population will have risen only marginally between 1950 and 2025, given current trends. On the other hand, the population in Africa is projected to more than double to 19% of the world population over the same 75-year period.[2] The population of Africa likely will rise from 650 million in 1992 to 900 million by the year 2000.

Economists estimate that world food production will in fact continue to increase more rapidly than the world population in the near future, allowing the food/population ratio to increase through the year 2000. In the short run, then, the primary problem appears not to be food production, but distribution and use, especially in poverty-stricken areas of the developing nations.

Eventually, though, it is likely that food production will begin to lag behind population growth.[2] Most good farmland in the world is already in use, and because of inefficient farming practices or competing land-use demands, the number of farmable acres worldwide decreases annually. For many reasons, sustainable world food output—that which does not deplete the earth's resources—is now running well behind food consumption. This suggests that food production in less-developed countries will barely keep up with population growth and will soon lag behind. That in turn will reduce the reserves needed to both combat and help stave off undernutrition, particularly widespread starvation, in developing countries.[2]

Renewed Focus on Population Control

While efforts on the supply side of the food/population ratio are essential, many scientists in this area of research still feel there is no substitute for reducing the demand side.[2] They argue that the survival of our civilization depends on limiting reproduction.

For millions of years, maximizing reproduction has been a measure of biological success. Because disease and difficult living conditions often claimed young lives, producing many offspring was one strategy for carrying on the family. These conditions still hold in Third World countries and constitute as well a key method for providing support in old age. More children also means more helpers to farm, hunt, and prepare food.[2] Traditionally, poorer people bear more children, contrary to what you might predict.

Now, in the evolutionary blink of an eye—mere decades—poor people in developing nations are being asked to change their entire attitude toward having children. It is a difficult undertaking. In 1888, 1.5 billion people inhabited the earth. Now the population exceeds 5.7 billion and is growing fast. Currently the population increases by three people every second, or about a quarter of a million people every day. In essence, the world must accommodate a new population roughly equivalent to that of the United States and Canada every 3 years!

Even though the overall rate of growth has begun to decline, most population experts believe population size will still pass 8.3 billion by the year 2025. The poorest countries are increasing the most and will have an overall population of 7 billion, further straining their ability to cope. The world population likely will pass 9.8 billion in 2050 and 11 billion in 2100, before stability finally sets in at about 11.6 billion between 2150 and 2200. If population growth continues as these predictions indicate, governments will be forced to confront economic problems that they could more easily finesse in less crowded times. Overall, an increasing population stresses existing resources in developing countries such that many people's needs are not met, social unrest is intensified, and significant environmental devastation is more likely.[3]

Keys to Successful Family-Planning Programs

Attempts to implement family-planning programs in Third World nations have met only partial success. Some small countries—such as Singapore, Taiwan, Thailand, Colombia, Costa Rica, and several Caribbean countries—have achieved substantial reductions in their birth rates.[2] Larger countries, including India and Mexico, are struggling.

China, with its nearly 1.2 billion people, has explicitly recognized that it is already overpopulated—22% of the world's population is living on 7% of the world's arable land.[6] It has the world's most stringent family-planning program: the government allows only one child per urban couple—two at most in rural areas if the first child is a girl. The birth rate is now 1.8 children per couple. Penalties for having extra children include restricted housing and employment opportunities. Abortion is very common and is sometimes forced on unwilling women, as is sterilization. These policies have lowered China's population growth rate from 27.6 per thousand in 1964 to 11.5 per thousand in 1993. Despite its numerical success, China's program has encountered domestic opposition, and its coercive aspects have been criticized as human rights abuses by some.

Experience with family-planning programs in Third World countries and the historical changes in birth rates in many industrialized countries suggest an important conclusion: only when people have enough to eat and are financially secure do they feel safe having fewer children.[2] Based on this principle, many experts predict that more couples in Third World countries would choose to have fewer children if their income increased enough so they had access to food, shelter, and health care, and sufficient resources to provide for themselves in old age. Thus raising per capita income and education, especially for women in developing countries, is currently viewed as the most effective long-term approach to curbing excessive population growth.[3]

The experience of South Korea illustrates this approach. In 1960, South Korean families averaged six children each. Economic policies, coupled with a strong family-planning program, transformed South Korea from a struggling country to an economic success. Today, South Korean families average slightly fewer than two children each, and the population will soon stabilize. However, nations do not have to wait to become industrialized before launching population control programs. Indonesia, South Korea, and Thailand made great economic strides and at the same time controlled population growth.[2] Still, to date, population stabilization—as in Western countries—has mainly been accompanied by relative wealth and security. Note that currently the government in some parts of Germany has proposed paying couples to have children, as the birth rate has fallen since reunification of the country. People there realize it is hard to maintain an acceptable standard of living as the number of children in a household increases.

In addition to economics, another unavoidable roadblock to family-planning programs in the developing world lies with ancient cultural, religious, and traditional beliefs. In sub-Saharan Africa, being childless not only carries an aura of evil for the woman, but also marks the end of a line of descent. The Yoruba believe, for example, that a childless woman has made a pact with evil spirits before her own birth to kill her children and, devoid of descendants, will return to join these evil spirits in some other-worldly sphere. These women are almost as afraid of being rendered functionally infertile by the deaths of all their children as they are of bearing none. Thus female sterilization and even contraception are widely feared. Even women with four or five children fear, not unreasonably, that all the children may suddenly die.

- - - - - - - - - - - - - - -
Breastfeeding is important to family health and is also a valuable adjunct to family-planning programs because it helps naturally space births further apart. When an infant is nourished solely by breastfeeding, ovulation and hence the possibility of conception in the mother is prevented for an average of about 6 months (although this natural form of birth control is not completely reliable). In contrast, women who do not breast-feed generally begin to ovulate within a month or so after giving birth. When childbirths are more widely spaced, the health of mother and infant is aided, and fewer total births occur.
- - - - - - - - - - - - - - -

In India, a rigid class structure that leaves those in the lower classes destitute encourages these families to have more children for many of the economic reasons discussed previously. Also, Moslem and other religious groups typically promote large families.

Only by taking on the twin challenges of food insecurity and population growth can the developed world hope to escape the expensive trap of humanitarian intervention and crisis management for peoples in need.[3] Today it is likely that Malthus's gloomy mathematical prediction may soon become fact. If we cannot find ways of humanely controlling population growth, nature may solve the problem by killing off large portions of humanity in the ways Malthus predicted. Only the future will tell.

Concept Check

Although world food production is currently sufficient to meet the energy needs of the world's population, undernutrition exists because of poverty, politics, and unequal distribution of food resources. Projected population growth, however, may soon overwhelm food production. Limiting population growth, especially in Third World countries where birth rates are high, is a challenging priority encouraged by most scientists and world leaders.

WAR AND POLITICAL/CIVIL UNREST

The president of Mali recently stated, "Only by translating our sense of common destiny into action will we be able to resolve the paradox of currently spending $1000 billion each year in the production of lethal weapons, while only a fraction of that sum would make our planet a land of prosperity for millions of people who today suffer from illness, hunger, thirst, and ignorance."

Worldwide, military spending has doubled over the past 20 years to about $1.5 million per minute. The amount of money spent on weapons every minute could feed 2000 undernourished children for a year. Although Africa has been ravaged by economic decay and famines for years, military spending in Africa more than doubled in the 1970s and held firm through the early 1990s. Presently, less than one half of 1% of the total world yearly production of goods and services is devoted to economic development assistance, while approximately 6% goes to military expenditures.[3]

In the worst cases, civil disruptions and war contribute in large measure to massive undernutrition. War-related famine affects at least 20 million people in southern and northeastern Africa. In southern Sudan, 3 to 4 million men, women, and children were starving in 1991 because civil war prevented them from planting their fields and restocking their herds. Two other African countries, Rwanda and Somalia, once had productive economies but are now struggling with mass starvation resulting from ethnic and politically motivated fighting. These bloody civil wars have devastated these countries' infrastructures, creating millions of refugees in their wake. Most of these people are without shelter, clothing, or food, and lack any means of obtaining them.

Such civil strife is not limited to Africa. Following the break-up of the former Yugoslavia, warring ethnic and religious groups have conducted Europe's worst war since 1945. The destruction and disruption of daily life have brought manufacturing, commerce, and food production to a near standstill throughout Bosnia and in parts of Croatia and Serbia.[3]

Even when food is available in such situations, political divisions often impede its distribution so much that undernutrition continues to plague the affected people for years. In addition, many food aid programs aimed at the poor, especially during emergencies, have been undermined by poor administration, corruption, and political influence.[3]

During the 1960s and 1970s, undernutrition in less-developed countries was viewed primarily as a technical problem, requiring a technical solution: how to produce enough food for the growing world population. And as indicated already, impressive gains in agricultural productivity and world food production have occurred in the past three decades. Now, most undernutrition is seen as stemming from political causes, requiring a political solution: how to achieve cooperation among and within nations such that gains in food production and infrastructure are not wiped out by war. Note that when U.S. troops ended their mission in Somalia in the early 1990s, they left knowing they had helped end a famine, but could not pacify a hostile country. Today in Africa, war is destroying what the last 30 years of aid helped to build.

Only a combination of approaches—finding technical solutions that help reduce chronic hunger and poverty while solving political crises that otherwise lead to chaos, anarchy, and disrupted economies—will help.[3]

RAPID DEPLETION OF NATURAL RESOURCES

Population control has become more critical lately as we quickly deplete the earth's resources. The productive capacity of agriculture is approaching its limits worldwide. Food production—especially in parts of the Third World—is being undermined by environmentally unsustainable farming methods.

The **green revolution** refers to the dramatic rise in crop yields, beginning in the 1960s, in countries such as the Philippines, India, and Mexico. These gains resulted from use of more fertilizers, improved cultivation practices, and superior strains of key crops developed by extensive plant-breeding programs.[6] Most of the potential benefits of the green revolution technologies have now been realized. For example, rice yields have not increased significantly since the release of superior varieties in 1966. Wheat is another example. India more than tripled its wheat harvest between 1965 and 1983, a period when various high-yielding wheat strains were introduced. Since then, India's grain output has not increased.

Future gains in productivity may be much harder to accomplish because of the need to farm less productive soils. Until the introduction of additional superior wheat and rice strains, developing countries will not benefit greatly from the recent, more modest breakthroughs in biotechnology discussed in the Nutrition Perspective. Actually, the green revolution was never intended to solve the world's food problems, according to Dr. Norman Borlaug, its chief architect. It was just a stopgap measure until world leaders could control population growth.

Areas of the world that remain uncultivated or ungrazed are mostly of poor quality for farming: rocky, steep, infertile, too dry, too wet, or inaccessible. Much of this land is invaluable for providing crucial **ecosystem** benefits. This is particularly true for humid tropical areas, such as the Amazon basin rain forests, which significantly influence the earth's climate, notably through oxygen production. Some nations, such as Brazil, still have additional land that can sustain cultivation, but such countries are in the distinct minority. And even then, expansion of the cultivated area in Brazil would cause further rain forest devastation. The overwhelming experience over the past few decades has been overextension of agriculture onto erodible land, followed by predictable degradation, erosion, and abandonment.[3]

In Africa, an area of land twice the size of New Jersey is turned into unproductive desert each year because of soil erosion (Figure 20-5). The erosion results from overgrazing by livestock, destructive farming techniques, and destruction of mature rain forests. Also, cultivation of many **cash crops** in African countries damages the land, draining the soil of vital nutrients. Then, when the land has been used up, farmers move on to other areas, leaving behind desolated land ripe for soil erosion. In the short run, farmers can overplow and overpump with impressive results, but in doing so they use up natural resources on which long-term productivity depends. Soil erosion is also a problem in the United States. Currently farmland equivalent to the size of Ireland is lost here to erosion every year. New farming techniques, such as "no till" planting, are helping to reverse this trend.

green revolution Increases in crop yields arising from introduction of new agricultural technologies in less developed countries beginning in the 1960s. The key technologies were high-yielding, disease-resistant strains of rice, wheat, and corn, greater use of fertilizer, and improved cultivation practices.

ecosystem A community in nature that includes plants and animals and the environment associated with them.

cash crop A crop grown with the intent to export it, so that a country can obtain money to purchase goods from other countries. Cultivation of cash crops diverts needed agricultural resources from production of crops necessary to feed a country's own citizens. Examples of cash crops are coffee, tea, cocoa, and bananas.

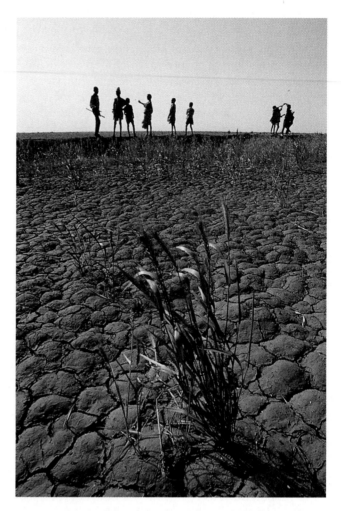

Figure 20-5 In Africa, land twice the size of New Jersey is turned into unproductive desert each year by overgrazing of livestock, destructive farming techniques, and harvesting of mature rain forests.

Nearly all irrigation water available worldwide is currently used, and groundwater supplies are becoming depleted at rapid rates in many regions. China, which has more than 20% of the world's irrigated land, is plagued with a growing scarcity of fresh water. In Third World countries, poultry, swine, and milk production is often concentrated around metropolitan areas, in turn polluting and drawing down the ground water excessively.[3]

The prospect of obtaining substantially more food from the oceans is also poor. In recent years the world fish catch has leveled off at about 100 million tons a year.

Clearly, we can exploit the earth's resources only so far without potentially invoking serious famine and death. The principle followed by the Food and Agricultural Organization (FAO) of the United Nations emphasizes this point: "The fight to ensure that all people have enough nutritious food to eat is worthy of our greatest efforts, but it must be fought with the full recognition that it cannot be won unless agricultural, fishery, and forestry production returns to the earth as much—or more—than it takes." This statement highlights the need for immediate steps to protect the earth's already deteriorated environment from further destruction if food production is to keep up with expanding population.[21]

CULTURAL ATTITUDES TOWARD CERTAIN FOODS

Culture affects food use just as it does family size. In India, for example, the Hindu reverence for cattle has multiplied some already significant nutrition problems.

These sacred cows consume food rather than provide it; the wandering cows also considerably damage vegetation that could otherwise feed humans. Although the cows provide milk, there is no effort to improve milk production through selective breeding practices. In certain areas of India, a child may not be fed milk curds because of a superstitious belief that these inhibit growth; some Indians avoid bananas because they supposedly cause convulsions.

In nearly all countries some potential foods are not commonly eaten for a variety of reasons. In the United States, for example, many people shun horse meat, insects, algae, and even soy products, all of which are consumed by many people in other countries. Such cultural attitudes are obstacles, but not roadblocks, to good nutrition. Given adequate food resources, a healthful diet that allows for individual food taboos and prejudices is possible.

INADEQUATE SHELTER AND SANITATION

In Third World countries the deaths of undernourished people are rarely caused simply by inadequate food intake. Rather, poor shelter and sanitation—two essential components of a country's infrastructure—almost always contribute to the human toll exacted by undernutrition. Poor sanitation and undernutrition individually increase the risk for infection; the combination is often fatal.[24]

Potentially dangerous sanitation conditions are commonly associated with inadequate shelter. Worldwide, more than 1 billion people currently live in inadequate and deteriorating shelter. The future looks even worse. By the year 2000, Mexico City will house more than 26 million people, with São Paulo, Calcutta, and Bombay not far behind. Many of the 15 million child deaths each year, half of them in children under 5 years old, could be prevented if standards of environmental hygiene were improved.

Urban populations in some developing countries are currently growing at an annual rate of 5% to 7%. This urban explosion is the result of both high birth rates and migration of people to the cities from the countryside.[24] People come to the cities to find employment and resources that the countryside can no longer provide (Figure 20-6). It is estimated that by the year 2000 about half the world's population will live in cities and towns. Such a skewed population distribution will result in further impoverishment.

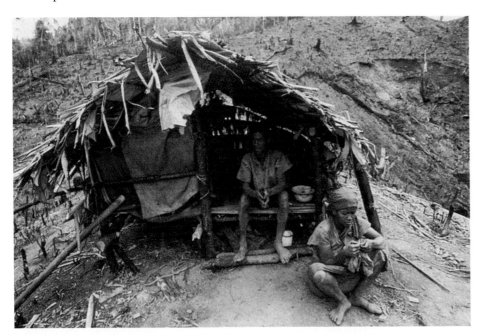

Figure 20-6 Losing ground in their effort to grow rice, farmers in Madagascar survey erosion on hills cleared of rain forest. Farming further depletes the soil, and in turn new land must be cleared. Slash-and-burn farming destroys 50 acres of rainforest an hour worldwide.

- - - - - - - - - - - - - -

Rural people displaced by multinational land developers in the north and northeast parts of Brazil have flooded into Rio de Janeiro and São Paulo, attracted by the prospect of jobs. These migrants have built shanty towns next to apartment towers and affluent suburbs, a common sight in Third World cities. Frequently, no jobs are available in the cities, so desperate urban poverty simply replaces rural impoverishment.

- - - - - - - - - - - - - -

In Third World countries, urban residents are poor and their needs for housing and community services often outstrip available governmental resources. These urban poor often live in overcrowded, self-made shelters that are only partially served by public utilities and lack a safe and adequate water supply. The general conditions in the shanty towns and ghettos of the Third World are typically worse than those in the rural areas the people left behind. And because the people now need cash to purchase food, they often find themselves with diets that are even more meager than the homegrown rural fare.[24] To make matters worse, makeshift shelters often lack facilities to protect food from spoilage caused by insects and rodents. In some developing countries, food losses can amount to as much as 30% to 40% of the perishable foods.

The shift from rural to urban life is hardest on infants and children. Infants tend to be weaned earlier from the breast in cities than in rural communities: their mothers may seek employment in cities or try to mimic the sophisticated, formula-using woman promoted in advertisements. Because infant formulas are relatively expensive, poor parents may provide too little to meet the baby's needs, or they may overdilute the mixture. In addition, many urban water supplies are unsafe, so prepared formula is likely to be contaminated with bacteria. In many nations, bottle-fed infants contract far more illnesses and are as much as 25 times more likely to die in childhood than those who are exclusively breastfed for the first 6 months of life. Human milk is generally much more hygienic, readily available, and nutritionally sound than formula and also provides infants with some immune protection.[28] In spite of the grim statistics, major corporations continue to market infant formulas in these regions.

Overall, provision of a safe and convenient water supply is the single most effective measure for improving and maintaining public health in any country. The World Health Organization (WHO) estimates that 1.2 billion people, about one fifth of all people, have an unsafe and inadequate water supply.[3]

Besides unsafe water, poor sanitation worsens critical public health problems in many places. It is common to see human feces, rotting garbage, and associated insect and rodent infestations in Third World cities. Human urine and feces are breeding grounds for many disease organisms, and thus are two of the most dangerous substances people encounter in routine daily living.[24] The inability to dispose of massive numbers of dead people resulting from recent civil wars has contributed further to the sanitation problem in some countries. In some developing countries, diarrheal diseases account for as many as one third of all deaths in children under 5 years of age. WHO estimates that even with progress in housing, 1.8 billion people in the world are still without proper sanitation.

To the usual public health problems widespread in Third World countries can be added the mounting devastation caused by infection with human immunodeficiency virus (HIV) and its associated disease, acquired immunodeficiency syndrome (AIDS).[27] Because impoverished individuals often have weakened immune systems, they tend to develop the symptoms of AIDS more quickly after HIV infection than do healthier people (see the Nutrition Focus). About two thirds of the world's estimated 19 million HIV-infected people live in developing countries, and their numbers are increasing rapidly. In already poor and undernourished populations, the long-term economic and social effects of the AIDS epidemic may rival those of a prolonged war.

HIGH EXTERNAL DEBT

Individuals sometimes take out high-interest loans from the neighborhood finance company to pay for necessary items of daily living—food, rent, medical care. If they can't keep up with the loan payments, they may be able to get another loan to pay off the first. But eventually, unless their income increases, they will be forced to sell off assets or perhaps declare bankruptcy. During the 1970s and 1980s many developing countries became trapped in the same cycle, borrowing repeatedly from foreign countries. Servicing these external debts, which now total about $1.3 trillion, has brought several countries to the verge of economic collapse.[20] Even the United States is not immune to such national financial problems. As the result of large annual federal deficits, our national debt is now so large that the yearly interest payments account for about 15% of all federal spending. This debt limits the ability of our country to help less developed countries, as well as disadvantaged Americans.

The external debt of Latin American countries represents 45% of the region's gross regional output of goods and services. Nearly 40% of total export earnings are spent paying off this debt. One approach pursued by Latin American nations to relieve the effects of this debt burden is to renegotiate their external loans on more favorable terms. Many African nations also carry large external debts. Low prices for the raw commodities they export, high prices for the oil they must import, and embezzlement of public funds by political officials are at the root of their financial problems.[3] As a result, African nations have had to curtail their domestic programs, further aggravating the problem of undernutrition in many countries.[20]

CONCEPT CHECK

Depletion of natural resources and the turmoil due to war and civil strife have decreased food production and seriously hampered efforts to end undernutrition in many Third World countries. In addition, the inadequate housing, impure water supplies, and poor sanitation prevalent in urban areas of less developed countries increase the risk for infection and disease. Infection then combines with undernutrition to further compromise the health status of impoverished people. Finally, many Third World countries are burdened by very high external debts, which severely limit their ability to mount programs aimed at reducing undernutrition.

Reducing Third World Undernutrition

As you have probably guessed, greatly reducing undernutrition in the Third World will be complicated. In the 1980s it was a common practice for the more affluent nations of the world to supply famished areas with direct food aid. Though highly publicized and praised at the time, direct food aid is not a long-term solution. While reducing the number of deaths from famine, such aid can also reduce incentives for local production by driving down local prices.[23] In addition, the affected countries may have little or no means of transporting the food to those who need it most. Furthermore, the donated foods may meet with little cultural acceptance.

In the short run, there appears to be no choice—aid must be given because people are starving. Still, improving the infrastructure available to poor people, especially rural people, is a better long-term focus. This is because the most significant factor contributing to undernutrition of people in impoverished areas of the world is their reliance on outside sources for basic needs. This dependence makes them constantly vulnerable.[3]

One American federal program that has helped improve the infrastructure of developing nations is the Peace Corps, which provides such services as assisting with education, distributing food and medical supplies, and building structures for local use. The aim of the Peace Corps is to provide infrastructure and education to help create independent, self-sustaining economies around the world.

TAILORING DEVELOPMENT TO LOCAL CONDITIONS

Recall that in the last 30 years world food supplies have grown faster than the population. Thus the increase in undernutrition during this period is caused by an increase in the number of people cut off from their fair share of this supply. Millions of farmers are losing access to resources they need to be self-reliant. And the num-

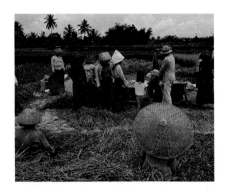

Labor-intensive agriculture, which is needed in these rice fields, may be the best choice for some less developed countries.

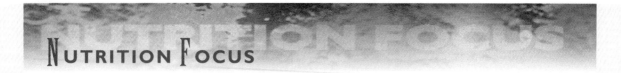

NUTRITION FOCUS

THE HUMAN IMPACT OF AIDS WORLDWIDE

The Black Plague, which left its grim mark on human civilization, took the lives of approximately 25 million people in the fourteenth century. By the year 2000, an estimated 30 to 120 million people around the world will be infected with the human immunodeficiency virus (HIV), and possibly 25 million people will have developed the symptoms of acquired immunodeficiency syndrome (AIDS). *Currently about 1 million Americans are infected with HIV;* of these people, 140,000 have full-blown AIDS. About 40,000 new HIV infections are detected each year in this country.[7]

AIDS is now the leading cause of death among men age 25 to 44 in the United States, and the fourth-leading cause of death among women in this age range. A disease with currently no known cure, AIDS represents certain death for the vast majority of people infected with HIV—the twentieth-century plague. Since the first cases of AIDS were diagnosed in the early 1980s, a total of about 240,000 Americans have died from it.

The devastating impact of AIDS on human civilization has been very rapid when measured on earth's scale of time, and the true costs to societies—other than the cost in human lives—have yet to be borne. Though AIDS has not replaced heart disease and stroke as the primary cause of death in America, the very nature of the disease is likely to wreak significant human devastation here and worldwide, partly because its primary route of transmission is a basic human behavior—sexual activity.

HOW HIV INFECTION SPREADS

The vectors, or vehicles of transmission, for HIV are blood and body fluids, including sexual secretions. Most cases have been transmitted through homosexual or heterosexual contact or by injection of intravenous drugs (generally illegal drugs) with contaminated needles that have been used by infected persons.[27] Among high-risk groups—sexually promiscuous people and intravenous drug abusers—following safe-sex practices and using clean needles have been shown to reduce spread of HIV infection and are keys to conquering AIDS.

After initial infection by HIV, a person may exhibit no obvious signs and symptoms for as long as 5 to 10 years, and so may be an unsuspecting carrier. During this period,

however, the virus gradually weakens the immune system. Eventually, the immune system is so debilitated that the person develops one or more opportunistic infections, such as tuberculosis and a rare type of pneumonia (see the Nutrition Perspective in Chapter 15). By this time, the downward course of AIDS is well on its way, and death typically can only be delayed, not averted.

WHO IS AT RISK FOR AIDS?

The belief that AIDS is a novel disease affecting a limited population of homosexual males on the East and West Coasts in the United States is dangerously inaccurate. Though homosexual people currently account for more than half the cases here, the number of AIDS cases in heterosexual people—especially women and the children that HIV-infected women bear—is rapidly increasing. This is evidenced by recent studies showing that about 20% of people in some South Florida towns have HIV infections, with heterosexual contact being the main method of contracting the virus.[27]

AIDS needs no passport. Heterosexually transmitted HIV flows freely in Thai sex parlors, along the truck routes of India, around Dominican Republic sugar cane plantations, and in the copper mines of Zambia. It is likely that one fourth of all adults in Zambia are infected with HIV. Heterosexual contact accounts for the majority of cases. A recent study warns that 57 countries risk major HIV outbreaks. Reported HIV cases are increasing rapidly in Africa, Asia, and Russia, with 2 million men, women, and children becoming infected yearly worldwide. The World Health Organization estimates that 70% of the world's 15 million people infected with the HIV virus are in Africa, with civil war refugees and migration contributing to its spread. The AIDS epicenter, however, is now shifting to Asia.

WHAT ARE THE COSTS OF AIDS?

Although a price can't be assigned to the human lives lost to AIDS, other costs linked to the AIDS epidemic can be calculated: the direct costs of AIDS research and medical care for AIDS patients; the lost contribution to a nation's economy that AIDS patients and victims, who mostly are young adults in their most productive years, would normally have made; and the economic hardship borne by families of patients and victims. By the year 2000 the AIDS plague could siphon off an estimated $81 to $107 billion from the U.S. economy and may drain $356 to $514 billion from the global economy. This is money that could be spent on goods and services to help maintain stable economies around the world.

The economic impact of AIDS will hit developing countries worst, because their economies are already small and their living standards low. Brazil, for example, would need to spend $600 million to adequately help its AIDS victims today. Such an economic burden would certainly mean rising budget deficits and expanding debt, especially for a country that is still struggling with a foreign debt load of more than $100 billion. Such situations may well be the plight of other developing nations.

Besides the mind-reeling direct public costs entailed in responding to AIDS, there are less obvious costs imposed on businesses, families, and society in general. In India and Thailand, for example, a significant proportion of the adult male populations will be forfeited to AIDS. Worker productivity will plummet because AIDS patients produce less and demand more, especially as they wither and waste away in the latter stages of the disease. Business productivity drops even further when relatives take time away from work or school to care for family members afflicted with AIDS. And AIDS demands a considerable amount of family income. Hard-pressed families that have to devote much of their income to doctors and medicines have little left for living expenses. Other family members must strain to keep up with daily duties because they must care for orphans left behind in the disease's wake. The number of youngsters orphaned by AIDS could more than double in the next 3 years to 3.7 million worldwide.

HAS THE RESPONSE TO AIDS WORLDWIDE BEEN ADEQUATE?

Governments in many countries have come under fire for their slow response in fighting AIDS. At present, neither the government nor the medical profession in developing countries has acted aggressively to stem the AIDS tide. In India, for example, Bombay's first AIDS clinic was opened in January 1993 by a private interest group. And governments of developing nations frequently can't afford to supply AIDS counseling or treatment. Even worse, they continue to act as if their countries remain immune to the scourge. Such a weak response on the part of government leaders, coupled with the resigned attitudes of citizens, will undoubtedly lead to a greater degree of poverty and illness worldwide.

On the individual level, behavioral changes that reduce the risk of being infected by HIV are required. Since there is no known cure for AIDS, prevention is the only completely effective way to avoid death from AIDS. Moreover, many scientists believe that even if AIDS vaccines were developed, they alone would not be able to eradicate the disease, further emphasizing the importance of behavior that reduces infection risk. Those who avoid sex with HIV-infected persons and contact with infected blood, blood products, and other body fluids will not become infected. The risk of infection can be reduced by so-called safe-sex practices and various other precautions.[27] For example, health-care workers, who often don't know whether a particular person is HIV infected or not, commonly use a variety of practices intended to reduce their chances of being infected by patients.

The role of nutrition in responding to AIDS is limited. Eating a balanced diet does not prevent HIV infection, does not cure AIDS, and does not permanently stave off death from it. What proper nutrition can do is help lessen the impact of the various infections that AIDS patients typically get. A poor nutritional status, in contrast, contributes to the more rapid onset of body wasting and other symptoms, leading to a quicker demise.[10]

Clearly, both public and private responses are needed to stop the spread of HIV. If the epidemic is not brought under control, the task of combating undernutrition throughout the world will become even more difficult. The medical ramifications of caring for those already infected with HIV will be troubling enough, especially in Third World countries. But if the AIDS epidemic continues to spread at the current rate, the resulting social and economic burdens could well spark crises that spread beyond national borders.

ber of households with insufficient means to support themselves is growing. In response, small-scale regional development is one option. There is a growing realization that the rural landless will flock to the overcrowded cities unless economic opportunities can be created for them.[24]

Small-scale rural enterprises and off-farm activities would ensure that poor people in rural areas who now have no access to land or other reliable means of support could acquire resources to obtain food. Such enterprises could be run by the people who stand to benefit, either as individuals or as members of small groups, using very limited capital. A prerequisite would be access to credit, appropriate technologies, a market, and the ability to transport the product to that market.[3] Households that presently have land could be helped in different ways, such as making credit available, so that they would be able to feed themselves.

For the most part, the most effective approach is teaching people to provide for themselves, rather than simply giving them the resources: that is, helping them meet most of their own needs and directing them to employment opportunities. Experience has shown that credit—along with training, food storage facilities, and marketing—allows rural people to participate in development to their benefit and the benefit of their families and communities.[24]

Suitable technologies for processing, preserving, marketing, and distributing nutritious local staples need to be encouraged so small farmers, both men and women, can flourish. Nutrition education on how to use these foods to create healthful diets, such as for vitamin A–rich vegetables (carotenoid-rich, to be specific), adds further benefit. Supplementing indigenous foods with nutrients in short supply, such as iron or iodide, also deserves consideration.[26]

Extensive land ownership, a key part of any solution, brings many advantages, particularly widespread and more equitable availability of food.[24,29] If food resources are instead concentrated in the hands of a few, as often results when relatively few people own most of the productive land, efficient transportation systems are needed to distribute the food. Inadequate and inequitable food distribution then becomes one more hindrance to reducing undernutrition.

Raising the economic status of impoverished people by employing them turns out then to be as important as expanding the food supply. If an increase in the food supply is achieved without an accompanying rise in employment, there may be no long-term change in the number of undernourished people. It is possible to see food prices fall with increased mechanization, use of fertilizers, and other modern technologies. But these very same advances can also displace people from jobs. When this happens, those who need the food most will be unable to afford it.

A shipment of high-technology tractors, for example, might put local farm laborers out of work. Rice might be planted more efficiently using farm machinery, but using human power eventually leaves more people with the resources to buy food. Success in reducing undernutrition in the Third World depends on employing more poor people more productively on available land or providing other jobs. From a Third World point of view, it is of little consequence that these jobs are technologically primitive by Western standards. As we mentioned before, an effort to increase both per capita income and education is needed. Employment must be part of that effort.[3]

It is also prudent to assume that developing countries will have to rely largely on their own resources to finance development. For decades, countries in Africa could count on the Cold War as an economic resource. The United States and the former Soviet Union opposed each other through African proxies, pouring in money to prop up pro-Western or pro-Communist governments. Now the big powers' priorities have turned inward. It is even more essential, then, to make full use of human resources available in the developing world itself. The optimal approach ends up depending on the relative need to employ people and the number of people available to do the work.

Overemphasizing cash crops, such as coffee, tea, rubber, and cocoa, as some developing countries, especially Latin American countries, have done is not likely to solve the nutritional problems of poor people. Cash crops are usually grown at the expense of food crops, on the assumption that money earned from the cash crops will be used to purchase enough food for the families of the workers. However, this is not always the case. Food can be bought, but it may not be enough and is generally not affordable. In such a situation poor families are at greater risk than others because the money earned from cash crops is often not sufficient to meet other basic family needs, let alone food needs. As with poor families in the United States, buying quality foods often takes second priority, resulting in nutritional deprivation.

Also detrimental are the economics of drug crops, such as cocaine, marijuana, or opium poppy seeds. Frequently viewing drugs as valuable cash crops, workers often believe that the large sums of money netted from these crops—which are often more easily grown than food crops—can meet family needs and increase the standard of living. The unfortunate reality is that many workers see little or no cash earnings and so become victims of their trade. Cash from drug crops often lines the pockets of criminals and corrupt government officials. It also reduces incentives to initiate production of subsistence-level food crops, which could provide employment and nourishment for many.

PREVENTING FAMINE

Policies to prevent famine focus on reducing war and civil strife. Increasing the productivity of rural people is also important, as we've just discussed. Then, as agricultural surpluses grow, producers can sell some, rather than consume all of their harvest. Livestock numbers will grow, absorbing surplus grain and providing animal protein. As rural wealth grows, food becomes a smaller portion of the household budget. If disaster strikes, food stocks will be adequate, livestock can be slaughtered, and price swings will be more tolerable. The conditions of scarcity that characterize famine then cease to arise.

In the end, positive government action is required to strengthen rural economies in Third World countries, thus ending the kind of desperate poverty that links natural or man-made disasters to famine and ultimately to widespread death.[3] However, little such preparedness for famine exists in Africa today. Famine-prone African countries are unusually dependent on international sources of supply for food, medicine, transport, and famine management. But international relief is likely to arrive on the scene after the famine has already peaked. Local remedies, such as food reserves, can be put into action much sooner.

Currently, world leaders are concerned about the "marginalization" of Third World problems, fearing that rich nations may dismiss war, disease, and famine as a way of life for the poorer nations who continue to struggle with life and death circumstances. In a recent survey, Americans listed world famine well after their concern about violence, drugs, and inflation. Ultimately, though, depletion of world resources, the massive debt incurred by poorer countries, the threat of danger to more prosperous countries nearby, and the toll taken in human lives affect the world economy and the well-being of all.

• • •

The battle against worldwide undernutrition, then, is twofold: to support systems intended to supply nutrients to the undernourished and to reduce the number of people in danger of undernutrition. The second part of this battle is critical for long-term improvement. The FAO stresses the need for strategies that supply food to vulnerable households, subsidize basic commodities purchased by the poor, and raise the levels of education, employment, and income-generating capacity of the poor.

Today, one third of the earth's population does not receive enough food to maintain an active working life, though enough food is produced to supply 2400

CRITICAL **T**HINKING

Stan has read about various relief efforts to help undernourished people in developing countries, especially the emergency food aid programs for famine-ravaged areas. Many of these efforts appear to be only temporary, and he wonders what long-range approaches might help solve the problem of undernutrition permanently. What suggestions would you give Stan about possible long-term solutions for undernutrition in Third World countries?

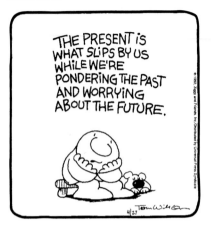

Figure 20-7 Ziggy.

kcal daily for every man, woman, and child on the planet.[3] And more than half of it is grown in the Third World. The economic loss from undernutrition is staggering, and the amount of human pain and suffering is incalculable. With all the international relief efforts, government assistance, and private organizations combined, we remain in the "dark ages" in our battle against this undernutrition (Figure 20-7). Life is not necessarily fair, but civilization should try to make it fairer.[3]

CONCEPT CHECK

Overall, the one important approach to reducing undernutrition in Third World countries lies in increasing farmers' access to land and other resources needed for food production and developing off-farm employment opportunities so people can purchase food for their families. Development programs must be sensitive to regional conditions to ensure that new technologies introduced don't intensify existing problems for the poorest people. Simple approaches are appropriate if people using them are left with the resources needed to feed their families. To prevent famine, more attention needs to be paid to the prevention and quick resolution of war and civil strife and to the strengthening of rural economies.

Summary

1. Poverty is a common thread wherever people suffer from undernutrition. Malnutrition can occur when the food supply is either scarce or abundant. The resulting deficiency conditions or degenerative diseases are influenced by genetic makeup.

2. Undernutrition is the most common form of malnutrition in developing countries. It results from inadequate intake, absorption, or use of nutrients or food energy. Many deficiency conditions appear, and infectious diseases thrive because the immune system cannot function properly.

3. The greatest risk of undernutrition occurs during critical periods of growth and development: gestation, infancy, and childhood. Low birthweight is a leading cause of infant deaths worldwide. Many developmental problems are caused by nutritional deprivation during critical periods of brain growth.

4. Undernutrition diminishes both physical and mental capabilities. In poor countries this is worsened by recurrent infections, poor sanitary conditions, extreme weather, inadequate shelter, and exposure to diseases.

5. In the United States, famine has been nonexistent since the 1930s, but undernutrition is present. Soup kitchens, food stamps, school lunch and breakfast programs, and the Supplemental Feeding Program for Women, Infants, and Children (WIC) have focused on improving the nutritional health of poor and at-risk people. These programs have proved effective in reducing undernutrition when adequately funded. The need to reduce out-of-

wedlock pregnancies remains a national priority, as single parents and their children are likely to live in poverty.

6. Multiple factors contribute to the problem of undernutrition in Third World countries. In densely populated countries, food resources may be inadequate, as well as the means for distributing food. Farming methods often encourage erosion, which deprives the soil of valuable nutrients, thus defeating future efforts to grow food. Limited water supplies hamper food production. Naturally occurring devastation from droughts, excessive rainfall, fire, and crop infestation, as well as urbanization, war and civil unrest, debt, and poor sanitation, all contribute to widespread undernutrition.

7. Any proposals to reduce undernutrition in Third World countries must consider the interaction of multiple factors, many of which are thoroughly embedded in cultural traditions. Family-planning programs, for example, may not succeed until life expectancy can be raised. Through education, efforts could be made to improve farming methods, encourage breastfeeding, and improve sanitation and hygiene. Direct food aid is only a short-term solution. In what may appear to be a step backward, a focus on subsistence-level farming, and away from the specialization of cash crops, is needed to increase the economic status of poor people. This and small-scale industrial development are ways to gain meaningful employment and purchasing power for vast numbers of the rural poor.

Study Questions

1. Briefly describe any evidence of undernutrition you have seen in the community where you grew up. What are or were the roots of these problems?

2. What do you believe primarily contributes to undernutrition in wealthy nations, such as the United States? What are some solutions to this problem?

3. What three points would you make to a group of seventh grade girls concerning the economic perils of teenage pregnancy and subsequent parenting?

4. How does the concept of personal responsibility relate to the problem of undernutrition in the United States? Does it apply to all causes of the problem?

5. A person you recently met asks you where to find food and shelter. Where would you first direct this person in your community for help? If you are unsure, find out by contacting a local shelter or county social services office.

6. Why is solving the problem of undernutrition a key factor in development of the full potential of Third World countries? What basic nutrients are keys to the health of these people?

7. Choose one problem that contributes to the complex picture of famine. In two paragraphs, describe the problem and discuss possible solutions.

8. Outline how war and civil unrest have intensified problems of chronic hunger in developing countries over the last few years.

9. How important is population control in solving the problem of world hunger? Support your answer with three main points.

10. Discuss how infrastructure could influence the causes and solutions of chronic hunger in a developing nation.

REFERENCES

1. Anageles IT and others: Decreased rate of stunting among anemic Indonesian preschool children through iron supplementation, *American Journal of Clinical Nutrition* 53:339, 1993.

2. Bongaarts J: Population policy options in the developing world, *Science* 263:771, 1994.

3. Bread for the World Institute: *Hunger 1995: causes of hunger,* Silver Spring, Md, 1994, Bread for the World Institute.

4. Brown JL, Allen D: Hunger in America, *Annual Review of Public Health* 9:503, 1988.

5. Chandra RK: Protein-energy malnutrition and immunological responses, *Journal of Nutrition* 122:597, 1992.

6. Clausi AS: The power of food, *Food Technology,* p 129, May 1995.

7. DesJarlais DC: Targeted HIV-prevention programs, *New England Journal of Medicine* 311:1451, 1994.

8. Etherton TD: The impact of biotechnology on animal agriculture and the consumer, *Nutrition Today* 29:12, 1994.

9. Fawzi WW and others: Vitamin A supplementation and child mortality, *Journal of the American Medical Association* 269:898, 1993.

10. Gorbach SL and others: Interactions between nutrition and infection with human immunodeficiency virus, *Nutrition Reviews* 51:226, 1993.

11. Henkel J: Genetic engineering: Fast forwarding to future foods, *FDA Consumer,* p 6, April 1995.

12. IUNS Declaration: Nutritional goals for the nineties: a call for advocacy and action, *Nutrition Today* 29:5, 1994.

13. Joy AB and others: Hunger in California: what interventions are needed? *Journal of the American Dietetic Association* 94:749, 1994.

14. Lewis S: Food security, environment, poverty, and the world's children, *Journal of Nutrition Education* 24:3S, 1992.

15. Li R and others: Functional consequences of iron supplementation in iron-deficient cotton mill workers in Beijing, China, *American Journal of Clinical Nutrition* 59:908, 1994.

16. Maberly GF and others: Programs against micronutrient malnutrition: ending hidden hunger, *Annual Review of Public Health,* 15:277, 1994.

17. Mayer J: Nutritional problems in the United States: then and now two decades later, *Nutrition Today,* Jan/Feb 1990, p 15.

18. Nestel P and others: Risk factors associated with xerophthalmia in Northern Sudan, *Journal of Nutrition* 123:2115, 1993.

19. Olson RE: World food production and problems in human nutrition, *Nutrition Today,* Jan/Feb 1989, p 18.

20. Pearce D and others: Debt and the environment, *Scientific American,* June 1995, p 51.

21. Plunknett DL, Winkelmann DL: Technology for sustainable agriculture, *Scientific American,* Sept 1995, p 182.

22. Ropp KL: New animal drug increases milk production, *FDA Consumer,* May 1994, p 24.

23. Singer HW: The African food crisis and the role of food aid, *Food Policy,* Aug 1989, p 196.

24. Solomons NW, Gross R: Urban nutrition in developing countries, *Nutrition Reviews* 53:90, 1995.

25. Splett PL: Federal food assistance programs, *Nutrition Today,* March/April 1994, p 6.

26. Stephenson LS: Possible new developments in community control of iron-deficiency anemia, *Nutrition Reviews* 53:23, 1995.

27. Stryker J and others: Prevention of HIV infection, *Journal of the American Medical Association* 273:1143, 1995.

28. Taren D, Chen J: A positive association between extended breast-feeding and nutritional status in rural Hubei Province, People's Republic of China, *American Journal of Clinical Nutrition* 58:862, 1993.

29. Tebeb HN: Goiter problems in Ethiopia, *American Journal of Clinical Nutrition* 57:315S, 1993.

30. Trowbridge FL and others: Coordinated strategies for controlling micronutrient malnutrition: a technical workshop, *Journal of Nutrition* 123:775, 1993.

31. Uvin P: The state of world hunger, *Nutrition Reviews* 52:151, 1994.

32. Waterlow JC: Childhood malnutrition in developing nations: looking back and looking forward, *Annual Review of Nutrition* 14:1, 1994.

TAKE ACTION

Addressing hunger on a personal level

The following are suggested activities for doing something about hunger and undernutrition in your own community. We encourage you to try to make a difference, even if it represents just one small step. Like any change in behavior, don't try to do too many things at once. Try one or two of them, representing your personal stand against this gigantic problem.

1. Fast for 1 or 2 days. Keep a diary of how you feel physically and emotionally during the day. At the end of the fasting period record what you learned about being without food. Note: If you have a medical problem such as diabetes that demands regular consumption of food or if you are pregnant, do not choose this activity.
2. Fast one meal per day for a month (e.g., lunch). Save an amount of money equivalent to the amount you would spend eating this meal out (e.g., $4.00). Donate the money to a voluntary agency in your community that works to reduce hunger.
3. Write a letter to a senator or member of congress asking what he or she is doing about ending domestic and world undernutrition.
4. Volunteer at a local soup kitchen or homeless shelter for a time-limited period (1 month).
5. Contribute to World Food Day activities each October 16th.
6. Organize students on your campus. At Miami University in Oxford, Ohio, two students initiated a year-long successful campaign to provide food for the homeless in the suburban Cincinnati area by distributing excess food from the university's dining halls. Let us know about your efforts!

Biotechnology: An Answer to Food Shortages?

The human ability to manipulate nature has enabled us to improve the production and yield of many important foods. Traditional **biotechnology** is almost as old as agriculture. The first farmer to selectively improve his stock by breeding the best bull with the best cows was implementing biotechnology in a simple sense. The first baker who used yeast to make bread rise likewise used biotechnology to produce an improved product.

By the 1930s, biotechnology had made it possible to selectively breed better plant hybrids; as a result, corn production in the United States quickly doubled. Through similar methods, strains of wheat used for centuries were crossed with wild grasses to acquire more desirable properties, such as greater yield, increased resistance to mildew and bacterial diseases, and tolerance to salt or adverse climatic conditions.[11]

Another type of biotechnology uses hormones rather than breeding. In the last decade, Canadian salmon have been treated with a hormone that allows them to mature three times faster than normal—without changing the fish in any other way. Overall, then, biotechnology involves the use of various techniques to manipulate the characteristics of plants, animals, and bacteria or to manufacture products.[8]

biotechnology A collection of processes that involve the use of biological systems for altering and, ideally, improving the characteristics of plants, animals, and other forms of life.

Genetic Engineering

During the 1970s scientists developed new techniques, collectively called **genetic engineering,** that differed from traditional biotechnology methods by directly changing some of the genetic material (DNA) in a living organism. No longer is cross-breeding the only tool for improving the characteristics of plants and animals. The new biotechnology includes a wide range of cell and subcell techniques for synthesizing and then placing specific pieces of DNA into organisms (Figure 20-8).[11]

Genetic engineering has numerous benefits for development of improved strains. It allows access to a wider gene pool, thus permitting faster and more precise production of new and more useful strains of bacteria, plants, and animals. Traditional breeding proceeds in a hit-or-miss fashion, whereas genetic engineering permits a planned, deliberate approach. Scientists select a desirable trait in one species and then introduce the gene controlling that trait into other species. However, it is important to note that genetic engineering does not replace conventional breeding practices; they work together.

Already genetic engineering has yielded numerous products and processes useful to farmers: new drought-tolerant crop varieties and disease-resistant varieties that can be grown without pesticides; microbial inoculants to stop pest and frost damage to plants; methods to better detect *Listeria* and other microbes that cause food-borne illness; and new varieties of potatoes resistant to spoilage that in turn reduce the need for preservatives.[11] There is even interest in putting certain animal genes into plants to improve various plant characteristics. To our eyes and palates the initial genetically engineered food products will seem only subtly different from traditional products because application of the new biotechnology is being introduced cautiously. But the ultimate benefits could be substantial.[8]

Questions surround the use of the new biotechnology. Take, for instance, research that has yielded the new Flavr Savr tomato, which is genetically engineered to allow it to stay firm longer. Is it still a tomato? It looks the same, feels the same, tastes the same, and even has the identical nutritional value as that of the original product. The only change researchers have made is to counteract the action of a single gene in the DNA that makes tomatoes rot rapidly (Figure 20-8). The reversal of just one gene out of 10,000 is the only change needed to make the biotech tomato significantly different from the standard garden variety.[11]

Still, the question remains—how many and which properties can be changed in a plant, animal, or bacterium before it becomes something else? A tomato altered in only one specific way still seems to be a tomato, but does it remain one if it is changed in 10 or 20 ways? When traditional methods crossed a tangerine with a grapefruit, the new genetic structure was clearly something else, now commonly known as a tangelo.

genetic engineering Alteration of genetic material in plants or animals with the intent of improving growth, disease resistance, or other characteristics.

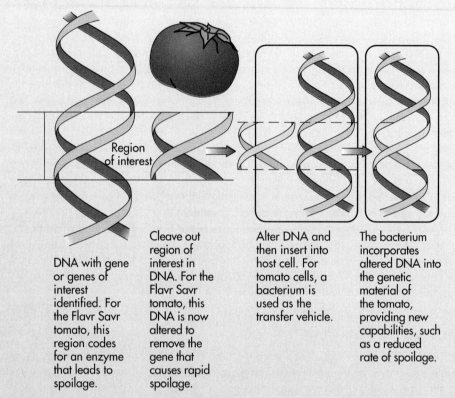

DNA with gene or genes of interest identified. For the Flavr Savr tomato, this region codes for an enzyme that leads to spoilage.

Cleave out region of interest in DNA. For the Flavr Savr tomato, this DNA is now altered to remove the gene that causes rapid spoilage.

Alter DNA and then insert into host cell. For tomato cells, a bacterium is used as the transfer vehicle.

The bacterium incorporates altered DNA into the genetic material of the tomato, providing new capabilities, such as a reduced rate of spoilage.

Figure 20-8 The new biotechnology involves various techniques for transferring foreign DNA into an organism. In this diagram, a sample of DNA is cleaved out of a larger DNA fragment and inserted into the DNA of a host cell. Thus the host cell contains new genetic information, with the potential of providing the cell with new capabilities. For the Flavr Savr tomato this means a reduced rate of spoilage. In other applications, bacteria can be engineered to produce the human form of the hormone insulin.

Controversy about the New Biotechnology

Public response to use of the new biotechnology in food production has been mixed. Use of genetically modified organisms may lead to reduction of environmentally detrimental activities, such as use of pesticides. But critics point out that past releases of foreign agents (e.g., insects and plants) into areas with no natural predators have sometimes had disastrous consequences. Although such risks associated with use of genetically engineered organisms may appear to be momentarily negligible, these risks may be cumulative and thus dangerous in the long run. Another potential problem is that genetic engineering may inadvertently introduce allergens—such as those naturally present in peanuts, milk, and shellfish—into foods that currently don't contain any. To reduce this risk, FDA carefully scrutinizes all biotech food products for allergens and will require labels that would list any potential allergens introduced into these foods.[11]

The alleged benefits of using biotechnology to boost agricultural production have been questioned in some countries (e.g., the United States, Canada, and Europe) that have large food reserves. Some people also object to use of biotech products because they are "unnatural" and may pose risks to the environment or consumers. Such concerns underlie the legal ban on the use of growth hormone produced using genetic engineering technology in beef production that has been enacted by Western European countries. The citizens in these countries felt that the increase in the meat supply resulting from use of growth hormone was not worth the perceived risks posed by the product. In the United States, FDA recently approved the first genetically engineered food product for humans, a substitute for the enzyme renin, which is traditionally used in making cheese. Will a protest arise over use of this biotech product, called cymasin, by cheesemakers?[11]

Other potentially beneficial applications of the new biotechnology are currently being studied by both scientists and concerned consumer groups. Bovine somatotropin (BST), a hormone produced by cattle, has been known since the 1930s to increase milk production when injected into dairy cattle. In the past the supply of BST was so limited that its routine use to boost milk yields was not feasible. But today BST can be produced using genetic engineering techniques; the biotech product, called Posilac, is structurally identical to naturally produced BST. Since large supplies of biotech BST are available, farmers now have the option of using it to greatly increase milk yield. Currently about 10% of dairy farmers in the U.S. do so. Because cows produce BST naturally, it has always been present in their milk. The amount of hormone in milk from treated and untreated cows is not different, nor is the milk's nutrient composition.[8] Moreover, because BST is a protein, any present in consumed milk is digested and, therefore, inactivated in the intestine.

FDA has determined that milk from BST-treated cows is safe for humans, but the agency is still evaluating its effects on animals and the environment.[22] One question is whether the increased milk production of treated cows will stress the health of the animals themselves, leading farmers to use more antibiotics, which can show up in milk. Some Americans are already opposed to use of BST in milk production, and the European Economic Community has banned this practice. Again, because of the current milk surpluses in the United States and Europe and the relatively low price of milk, consumers have little economic incentive to support this technology. Furthermore, dairy farmers in Wisconsin—as well as in other dairy-producing regions—are generally opposed to the introduction of the hormone because they fear negative consumer reaction will lower milk consumption. The industry is also concerned that a sharp increase in milk output would adversely affect prices and, in turn, harm thousands of small dairy farms facing an already precarious economic situation.

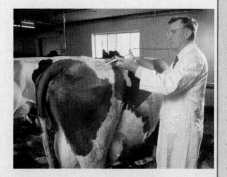

Milk yields can be increased using genetically engineered bovine somatotropin.

Role of Biotechnology in the Third World

Whether potential improvements in food production resulting from genetic engineering will help reduce Third World undernutrition remains to be seen. Unless food prices decrease as food production improves, landowners and suppliers of biotech products will capture the benefits of biotechnology and it will have little impact on undernutrition overall. The principle is simple: a poor person who couldn't afford food yesterday probably won't be able to afford biotech-produced food tomorrow unless it is also cheaper or he is richer.

In addition, the more successful farmers, often those with larger farms, will adopt the new biotechnology first, a common phenomenon with most innovations. Because of this, the present trend toward fewer, larger farms will continue in the Third World, a trend that is counterproductive in addressing the most pressing undernutrition issues there.[3] Furthermore, biotechnology does not promise a dramatically increased yield of most grains, the primary food resource in the world.

For the Third World, the primary focus should be on providing people with the resources to produce and/or purchase their own food, rather than on simply growing more food. Biotechnology is one useful tool, but not a panacea, for combating the complex scourge of world undernutrition. Improved crops yielded by this technology will aid in the battle, adding to needed political and other efforts.

Appendixes Contents

Food Composition Table

This food composition table, developed by Positive Input Corp., lists most of the foods in Mosby's NutriTrac software, which is available as a supplement to this text. As we go to press with this textbook, we are still adding foods to Mosby's NutriTrac so that it will be as complete as possible. For this reason, you will sometimes be able to find foods in Mosby's NutriTrac that are not listed in this food composition table.

The quickest way to find a food is to use the "Search For" feature in Mosby's NutriTrac software. However, if you do not have access to a computer or your computer time is limited, you can easily find a food using this food composition table. The foods in the table are arranged alphabetically. Note, however, that in some cases foods are arranged alphabetically within groups, such as Babyfood, Beef, and Bread, rather than by name alone.

Food from restaurants, including fast food (quick service), is cataloged separately, starting on p. A-62. These foods are listed alphabetically by restaurant name. If the fast-food/quick-service restaurant you are looking for is not listed, use the generic "Fast Food" category within the "Restaurant" section.

The code number in the left-hand column corresponds to the food data bank in Mosby's NutriTrac software. When you enter your intake into the software program, you may choose to use code numbers. Alternatively, you may choose to enter your intake into Mosby's NutriTrac by typing a food's name or partial name and selecting the "Search For" option.

Food Composition Table

Code	Name	Amount	Unit	Grams	Kilocalories	Carbohydrates (g)	Protein (g)	Fat (g)
11001	ALFALFA SEEDS, SPROUTED, FRESH	½	CUP	16.5	5	1	1	0
19065	ALMOND JOY CANDY BAR	1	BAR	50.0	232	29	2	14
12067	ALMONDS, TOASTED, UNBLANCHED	½	CUP	71.0	418	16	14	36
19066	ALPINE WHITE BAR W/ ALMONDS	1	BAR	35.0	197	18	4	13
15002	ANCHOVY, EUROPEAN, CND IN OIL	3	OUNCE	85.1	179	0	25	8
55188	ANGEL HAIR PASTA, LEAN CUISINE-STOUFFER'S	1	EACH	283.5	240	38	10	5
18150	ANIMAL CRACKERS	1	EACH	2.5	11	2	0	0
19294	APPLE BUTTER	1	TBSP.	18.0	33	9	0	0
19186	APPLE CRISP	1	CUP	282.0	460	91	5	10
9400	APPLE JUICE, UNSWEETENED	¾	CUP	185.8	87	22	0	0
18302	APPLE PIE	1	SLICE	155.0	411	58	4	19
9007	APPLES, CND, SWEETENED	½	CUP	102.0	68	17	0	0
9009	APPLES, DEHYDRATED, SULFURED	¼	CUP	15.0	52	14	0	0
9003	APPLES, FRESH, W/ SKIN	1	MEDIUM	138.0	81	21	0	0
9004	APPLES, FRESH, W/O SKIN	1	MEDIUM	128.0	73	19	0	0
9020	APPLESAUCE, SWEETENED	½	CUP	127.5	97	25	0	0
9019	APPLESAUCE, UNSWEETENED	½	CUP	122.0	52	14	0	0
9403	APRICOT NECTAR, CND, W/ ADDED VIT C	¾	CUP	188.2	105	27	1	0
9036	APRICOT NECTAR, CND, W/O ADDED VIT C	¾	CUP	188.2	105	27	1	0
9028	APRICOTS, CND, HEAVY SYRUP PACK	½	CUP	129.0	107	28	1	0
9024	APRICOTS, CND, JUICE PACK	½	CUP	124.0	60	15	1	0
9026	APRICOTS, CND, LIGHT SYRUP PACK	½	CUP	126.5	80	21	1	0
9022	APRICOTS, CND, WATER PACK	½	CUP	121.5	33	8	1	0
9030	APRICOTS, DEHYDRATED, SULFURED	¼	CUP	29.8	95	25	1	0
9032	APRICOTS, DRIED, SULFURED	¼	CUP	32.5	77	20	1	0
9021	APRICOTS, FRESH	3	MEDIUM	106.0	51	12	1	0
9035	APRICOTS, FROZEN, SWEETENED	½	CUP	121.0	119	30	1	0
11705	ASPARAGUS, CKD	½	CUP	90.0	23	4	2	0
11015	ASPARAGUS, CND	½	CUP	121.0	23	3	3	1
11011	ASPARAGUS, FRESH	½	CUP	67.0	15	3	2	0
11019	ASPARAGUS, FRZ, CKD	½	CUP	100.0	28	5	3	0
9037	AVOCADOS, FRESH	1	MEDIUM	201.0	324	15	4	31
3117	BABYFOOD, APPLESAUCE	1	OUNCE	28.4	10	3	0	0
3280	BABYFOOD, BANANAS W/ TAPIOCA	1	OUNCE	28.4	19	5	0	0
3681	BABYFOOD, BARLEY, PPD W/ WHOLE MILK	1	OUNCE	28.4	31	5	1	1
3003	BABYFOOD, BEEF	1	OUNCE	28.4	30	0	4	1
3049	BABYFOOD, BEEF AND RICE	1	OUNCE	28.4	23	2	1	1
3043	BABYFOOD, BEEF LASAGNA	1	OUNCE	28.4	22	3	1	1
3287	BABYFOOD, BEEF NOODLE	1	OUNCE	28.4	16	2	1	1
3052	BABYFOOD, BEEF STEW	1	OUNCE	28.4	14	2	1	0
3098	BABYFOOD, BEETS	1	OUNCE	28.4	10	2	0	0
3100	BABYFOOD, CARROTS	1	OUNCE	28.4	9	2	0	0
3013	BABYFOOD, CHICKEN	1	OUNCE	28.4	42	0	4	3
3069	BABYFOOD, CHICKEN NOODLE	1	OUNCE	28.4	14	2	1	0
3070	BABYFOOD, CHICKEN SOUP	1	OUNCE	28.4	14	2	0	0
3014	BABYFOOD, CHICKEN STICKS	1	STICK	10.0	19	0	1	1
3214	BABYFOOD, COOKIES, ARROWROOT	1	OUNCE	28.4	125	20	2	4
3120	BABYFOOD, CORN, CREAMED	1	OUNCE	28.4	18	5	0	0
3028	BABYFOOD, COTTAGE CHEESE W/ FRUIT	1	OUNCE	28.4	22	5	1	0
3018	BABYFOOD, EGG YOLKS	1	OUNCE	28.4	58	0	3	5
3201	BABYFOOD, EGG YOLKS AND BACON	1	OUNCE	28.4	22	2	1	1
3236	BABYFOOD, FRUIT DESSERT	1	OUNCE	28.4	18	5	0	0
3092	BABYFOOD, GREEN BEANS	1	OUNCE	28.4	7	2	0	0
3009	BABYFOOD, HAM	1	OUNCE	28.4	35	0	4	2
3166	BABYFOOD, JUICE, APPLE	¾	CUP	185.8	87	22	0	0
3179	BABYFOOD, JUICE, MIXED FRUIT	¾	CUP	185.8	87	22	0	0
3172	BABYFOOD, JUICE, ORANGE	¾	CUP	185.8	82	19	1	1
3090	BABYFOOD, MACARONI AND CHEESE	1	OUNCE	28.4	17	2	1	1
3045	BABYFOOD, MACARONI AND TOMATO AND BEEF	1	OUNCE	28.4	17	3	1	0
3021	BABYFOOD, MEAT STICKS	1	STICK	10.0	18	0	1	1
3279	BABYFOOD, MIXED VEGETABLES	1	OUNCE	28.4	9	2	0	0

Saturated fat (g)	Monounsaturated fat (g)	Polyunsaturated fat (g)	Fiber (g)	Cholesterol (g)	Folate (g)	Vitamin A (RE)	Vitamin B-6 (mg)	Vitamin B-12 (µg)	Vitamin C (mg)	Vitamin E (mg)	Riboflavin (mg)	Thiamin (mg)	Calcium (mg)	Iron (mg)	Magnesium (mg)	Niacin (mg)	Phosphorus (mg)	Potassium (mg)	Sodium (mg)	Zinc (mg)
0	0	0	0	0	6	3	0	0	1	-	0	0	5	.2	4	.1	12	13	1	.2
8	3	1	-	1	4	2	0	.1	0	-	.1	0	40	.6	33	.2	70	186	67	.4
3	23	8	8	0	45	0	.1	0	0	-	.4	.1	201	3.5	216	2	390	549	8	3.5
7	5	1	2	4	5	9	0	.3	0	-	.1	0	81	.2	13	0	82	146	26	.4
2	3	2	0	72	11	18	.2	.7	0	-	.3	.1	197	3.9	59	16.9	214	463	3120	2.1
1	-	1	-	10	-	250	-	-	6	-	.3	.3	80	1.5	-	2.9	-	500	410	-
0	0	0	-	0	0	0	0	0	0	-	0	0	1	.1	0	.1	3	3	10	0
-	-	-	0	0	0	0	0	0	0	-	0	0	1	0	1	0	1	16	0	0
2	4	3	-	0	14	87	.1	-	6	-	.2	.2	79	2.1	20	2.2	71	274	513	.5
0	0	0	-	0	0	0	.1	0	77	0	0	0	13	.7	6	-	13	221	6	.1
5	8	5	-	0	6	19	0	0	3	-	.2	.2	11	1.7	11	1.9	43	122	327	.3
0	0	0	2	0	0	5	0	0	0	-	0	0	4	.2	2	.1	5	69	3	0
0	0	0	2	0	0	1	0	0	0	-	0	0	3	.3	3	.1	8	96	19	0
0	0	0	4	0	4	7	.1	0	8	.8	0	0	10	.2	7	.1	10	159	0	.1
0	0	0	2	0	1	5	.1	0	5	.3	0	0	5	.1	4	.1	9	145	0	.1
0	0	0	2	0	1	1	0	0	2	-	0	0	5	.4	4	.2	9	78	4	.1
0	0	0	1	0	1	4	0	0	1	-	0	0	4	.1	4	.2	9	92	2	0
0	0	0	-	0	2	248	0	0	102	-	0	0	13	.7	9	.5	17	215	6	.2
0	0	0	1	0	2	248	0	0	1	-	0	0	13	.7	9	.5	17	215	6	.2
0	0	0	-	0	2	160	.1	0	4	-	0	0	12	.6	10	.5	17	173	14	.1
0	0	0	2	0	2	210	.1	0	6	-	0	0	15	.4	12	.4	25	205	5	.1
0	0	0	2	0	2	167	.1	0	3	-	0	0	14	.5	10	.4	16	175	5	.1
0	0	0	2	0	1	157	.1	0	4	-	0	0	10	.4	9	.5	16	233	4	.1
0	0	0	-	0	1	377	.2	0	3	-	0	0	18	1.9	19	1.1	47	550	4	.3
0	0	0	3	0	3	235	.1	0	1	-	0	0	15	1.5	15	1	38	448	3	.2
0	0	0	3	0	9	277	.1	0	11	-	0	0	15	.6	8	.6	20	314	1	.3
0	0	0	2	0	2	203	.1	0	11	-	0	0	12	1.1	11	1	23	277	5	.1
0	0	0	-	0	88	75	.1	0	24	-	.1	.1	22	.6	17	.9	55	279	216	.4
0	0	0	2	0	116	64	.1	0	22	-	.1	.1	19	2.2	12	1.2	52	208	472	.5
0	0	1	0	86	39	.1	0	9	-	26	.1	.1	14	.6	12	.8	38	183	.1	3
0	0	0	-	0	135	82	0	0	24	-	.1	.1	23	.6	13	1	55	218	4	.6
5	19	4	12	0	124	123	.6	0	16	-	.2	.2	22	2.1	78	3.9	82	1204	20	.8
-	-	-	0	-	0	0	0	0	11	-	0	0	1	.1	1	0	2	22	1	0
-	-	-	0	-	2	1	0	0	7	-	0	0	2	.1	3	.1	3	31	3	0
-	-	-	-	-	3	-	0	.1	-	-	.2	.1	65	3.5	9	1.7	43	54	14	.2
1	1	0	0	-	2	9	0	.4	1	-	0	0	2	.5	3	.9	20	54	19	.6
-	-	-	-	-	2	22	0	.1	1	-	0	0	3	.2	2	.4	10	34	101	.3
-	-	-	0	-	2	44	0	.1	1	-	0	0	5	.2	3	.4	11	35	129	.2
-	-	-	-	-	2	25	0	0	0	-	0	0	2	.1	2	.2	9	13	5	.1
0	0	0	0	4	2	65	0	.1	1	-	0	0	3	.2	3	.4	12	40	98	.2
-	-	-	1	-	9	1	0	0	1	-	0	0	4	.1	4	0	4	52	24	0
-	-	-	0	-	5	335	0	0	2	-	0	0	7	.1	3	.1	6	57	14	0
1	1	1	0	-	3	16	.1	.1	0	-	0	0	16	.3	3	1	26	35	14	.3
-	-	-	0	-	2	30	0	0	0	-	0	0	5	.1	3	.1	7	10	5	.1
-	-	-	0	-	1	63	0	0	0	-	0	0	10	.1	1	.1	7	19	5	.1
-	-	-	0	-	1	95	0	0	0	-	0	0	7	.2	1	.2	12	11	48	.1
1	3	0	0	0	3	-	0	0	2	-	.1	.1	9	.9	6	1.6	33	44	105	.2
-	-	-	1	-	4	2	0	0	1	-	0	0	5	.1	2	.1	9	23	15	.1
-	-	-	0	-	1	1	0	0	7	-	0	0	9	0	1	0	11	12	14	0
1	2	1	0	208	26	107	0	.4	0	-	.1	0	22	.8	2	0	81	22	11	.5
-	-	-	0	-	1	8	0	0	0	-	0	0	8	.1	1	.1	14	10	14	.1
-	-	-	0	-	1	7	0	0	1	-	0	0	3	.1	1	0	2	27	4	0
-	-	-	1	-	9	12	0	0	2	-	0	0	18	.3	6	.1	5	36	1	.1
1	1	0	0	-	1	3	.1	0	1	-	.1	0	1	.3	3	.8	25	60	19	.5
-	-	-	0	-	0	4	.1	0	108	-	0	0	7	1.1	6	.2	9	169	6	.1
-	-	-	0	-	12	7	.1	0	118	-	0	0	15	.6	9	.2	9	188	7	.1
-	-	-	0	-	49	11	.1	0	116	-	.1	.1	22	.3	17	.4	20	342	2	.1
-	-	-	0	-	0	1	0	0	0	-	0	0	14	.1	2	.2	17	12	22	.1
-	-	-	0	-	2	31	0	.1	0	-	0	0	4	.1	2	.2	12	20	5	.1
1	1	0	0	-	1	2	0	0	1	-	0	0	3	.1	1	.1	10	11	55	.2
-	-	-	-	-	2	69	0	0	1	-	0	0	5	.1	3	.1	6	32	3	.1

Food Composition Table—cont'd

Code	Name	Amount	Unit	Grams	Kilocalories	Carbohydrates (g)	Protein (g)	Fat (g)
3076	BABYFOOD, NOODLES AND CHICKEN	1	OUNCE	28.4	18	3	0	1
3228	BABYFOOD, PEACH COBBLER	1	OUNCE	28.4	19	5	0	0
3230	BABYFOOD, PEACH MELBA	1	OUNCE	28.4	17	5	0	0
3131	BABYFOOD, PEACHES W/SUGAR	1	OUNCE	28.4	20	5	0	0
3133	BABYFOOD, PEARS	1	OUNCE	28.4	12	3	0	0
3124	BABYFOOD, PEAS, BUTTERED	1	OUNCE	28.4	17	3	1	0
3135	BABYFOOD, PLUMS W/ TAPIOCA	1	OUNCE	28.4	21	6	0	0
3694	BABYFOOD, RICE, PPD W/ WHOLE MILK	1	OUNCE	28.4	33	5	1	1
3210	BABYFOOD, RICE, W/ MIXED FRUIT	1	OUNCE	28.4	24	5	0	0
3050	BABYFOOD, SPAGHETTI AND TOMATO AND MEAT	1	OUNCE	28.4	18	3	1	0
3103	BABYFOOD, SPINACH, CREAMED	1	OUNCE	28.4	12	2	1	0
3058	BABYFOOD, SPLIT PEA AND HAM	1	OUNCE	28.4	20	3	1	0
3105	BABYFOOD, SQUASH	1	OUNCE	28.4	7	2	0	0
3109	BABYFOOD, SWEETPOTATOES	1	OUNCE	28.4	17	4	0	0
3216	BABYFOOD, TEETHING BISCUITS	1	BISCUIT	11.0	43	8	1	0
3238	BABYFOOD, TROPICAL FRUIT	1	OUNCE	28.4	17	5	0	0
3016	BABYFOOD, TURKEY	1	OUNCE	28.4	37	0	4	2
3083	BABYFOOD, TURKEY AND RICE	1	OUNCE	28.4	14	2	1	0
3017	BABYFOOD, TURKEY STICKS	1	STICK	10.0	18	0	1	1
10124	BACON	1	SLICE	6.0	35	0	2	3
10131	BACON, CANADIAN-STYLE BACON, GRILLED	1	SLICE	21.0	39	0	5	2
62528	BACON, TURKEY	1	SLICE	14.0	25	0	3	2
18005	BAGELS, CINNAMON-RAISIN	1	3½ IN.	71.0	195	39	7	1
18006	BAGELS, CINNAMON-RAISIN, TOASTED	1	3½ IN.	66.0	194	39	7	1
18003	BAGELS, EGG	1	3½ IN.	71.0	197	38	8	1
18004	BAGELS, EGG, TOASTED	1	3½ IN.	66.0	197	38	8	1
18007	BAGELS, OAT BRAN	1	3½ IN.	71.0	181	38	8	1
18008	BAGELS, OAT BRAN, TOASTED	1	3½ IN.	66.0	181	38	8	1
18001	BAGELS, PLAIN	1	3½ IN.	71.0	195	38	7	1
18409	BAGELS, PLAIN, TOASTED	1	3½ IN.	66.0	195	38	7	1
55189	BAKED CHEESE RAVIOLI, LEAN CUISINE-STOUFFER'S	1	EACH	241.0	240	30	13	8
41297	BAKED CHEESE RAVIOLI-HEALTHY CHOICE	1	EACH	255.1	250	44	14	2
55190	BAKED POTATO W/ SOUR CREAM, LEAN CUISINE-STOUFFER'S	1	EACH	294.1	230	38	9	5
11028	BAMBOO SHOOTS, CND	½	CUP	65.5	12	2	1	0
11026	BAMBOO SHOOTS, FRESH	½	CUP	75.5	20	4	2	0
19400	BANANA CHIPS	1	OUNCE	28.4	147	17	1	10
18304	BANANA CREAM PIE	1	SLICE	148.0	398	49	7	20
41240	BANANA NUT MUFFIN-HEALTHY CHOICE	1	EACH	70.9	180	32	3	6
19311	BANANA PUDDING	1	CUP	298.1	379	63	7	11
9040	BANANAS, FRESH	1	MEDIUM	114.0	105	27	1	1
6150	BARBECUE SAUCE	½	CUP	125.0	94	16	2	2
7001	BARBEQUE LOAF, LUNCH MEAT	1	SLICE	23.0	40	1	4	2
15187	BASS, FRESHWATER, CKD, DRY HEAT	3	OUNCE	85.1	124	0	21	4
15188	BASS, STRIPED, CKD, DRY HEAT	3	OUNCE	85.1	105	0	19	3
41276	BEAN AND HAM SOUP-HEALTHY CHOICE	1	EACH	212.6	220	35	12	4
16006	BEANS, BAKED, CND, VEGETARIAN	½	CUP	127.0	118	26	6	1
16007	BEANS, BAKED, CND, W/ BEEF	½	CUP	133.0	161	22	8	5
16008	BEANS, BAKED, CND, W/ FRANKS	½	CUP	128.5	182	20	9	8
16009	BEANS, BAKED, CND, W/ PORK	½	CUP	126.5	134	25	7	2
16005	BEANS, BAKED, HOME PREPARED	½	CUP	126.5	191	27	7	7
16315	BEANS, BLACK, CKD	½	CUP	86.0	114	20	8	0
11056	BEANS, GREEN, CND	½	CUP	68.0	14	3	1	0
11052	BEANS, GREEN, FRESH	½	CUP	55.0	17	4	1	0
11061	BEANS, GREEN, FZN	½	CUP	67.5	18	4	1	0
16029	BEANS, KIDNEY, CND	½	CUP	128.0	104	19	7	0
16073	BEANS, LIMA, CND	½	CUP	120.5	95	18	6	0
11040	BEANS, LIMA, FZN	½	CUP	90.0	95	18	6	0
16039	BEANS, NAVY, CND	½	CUP	131.0	148	27	10	1
16044	BEANS, PINTO, CND	½	CUP	120.0	94	17	5	0
16103	BEANS, REFRIED, CND	½	CUP	126.5	135	23	8	1
11932	BEANS, YELLOW, CND	½	CUP	68.0	14	3	1	0

Saturated fat (g)	Monounsaturated fat (g)	Polyunsaturated fat (g)	Fiber (g)	Cholesterol (g)	Folate (g)	Vitamin A (RE)	Vitamin B-6 (mg)	Vitamin B-12 (µg)	Vitamin C (mg)	Vitamin E (mg)	Riboflavin (mg)	Thiamin (mg)	Calcium (mg)	Iron (mg)	Magnesium (mg)	Niacin (mg)	Phosphorus (mg)	Potassium (mg)	Sodium (mg)	Zinc (mg)
-	-	-	0	-	1	37	0	0	0	-	0	0	7	.1	3	.2	9	17	7	.1
-	-	-	0	-	0	4	0	0	6	-	0	0	1	0	1	.1	2	16	3	0
-	-	-	-	-	1	6	0	0	7	-	0	0	3	.1	1	.1	1	26	3	.1
-	-	-	0	-	1	5	0	0	5	-	0	0	1	.1	1	.2	3	44	1	0
-	-	-	1	-	1	1	0	0	6	-	0	0	2	.1	3	.1	3	33	1	0
-	-	-	-	-	10	12	-	-	4	-	0	0	13	.3	-	.4	-	33	1	-
-	-	-	0	-	0	3	0	0	0	-	0	0	2	.1	1	.1	2	24	2	0
-	-	-	-	-	2	-	0	.1	-	-	.1	.1	68	3.5	13	1.5	50	54	13	.2
-	-	-	0	-	1	1	.1	0	6	-	.2	.1	6	1.3	1	.8	7	9	3	.1
-	-	-	0	-	2	38	0	0	1	-	0	0	5	.2	2	.3	10	31	6	.1
-	-	-	1	-	20	104	0	0	1	-	0	0	32	.4	18	.1	14	63	16	.1
-	-	-	0	-	4	23	0	0	1	-	0	0	7	.1	-	.1	14	39	4	.2
-	-	-	1	-	4	57	0	0	2	-	0	0	7	.1	3	.1	5	52	0	0
-	-	-	0	-	3	188	0	0	3	-	0	0	5	.1	3	.1	7	69	6	0
-	-	-	0	-	2	1	0	0	1	-	.1	0	29	.4	4	.5	18	36	40	.1
1	1	0	0	-	3	48	0	.3	1	-	.1	0	8	.4	3	1	27	51	20	.5
0	0	0	0	-	1	42	0	0	0	-	0	0	7	.1	2	.1	5	10	4	.1
-	-	-	0	-	1	7	0	.1	0	-	0	0	7	.1	2	.2	10	9	48	.2
1	1	0	0	5	0	0	0	.1	2	-	0	0	1	.1	1	.4	20	29	96	.2
1	1	0	0	12	1	0	.1	.2	5	-	0	.2	2	.2	4	1.5	62	82	325	.4
1	-	-	-	10	-	0	-	-	0	-	-	-	0	0	-	-	-	-	170	-
0	0	0	-	0	15	6	0	0	0	-	.2	.3	13	2.7	15	2.2	55	108	229	.5
0	0	0	-	0	11	5	0	0	0	-	.2	.2	13	2.7	15	2	55	108	228	.5
0	0	0	-	17	16	23	.1	.1	0	-	.2	.4	9	2.8	18	2.4	60	48	359	.5
0	0	0	-	17	11	21	.1	.1	0	-	.1	.3	9	2.8	18	2.2	59	48	358	.5
0	0	0	-	0	33	0	.1	0	0	-	.2	.2	9	2.2	40	2.1	117	145	360	1.5
0	0	0	-	0	23	0	.1	0	0	-	.2	.2	9	2.2	41	1.9	117	145	360	1.5
0	0	0	1	0	16	0	0	0	0	-	.2	.4	53	2.5	21	3.2	68	72	379	.6
0	0	0	-	0	11	0	0	0	0	-	.2	.3	13	2.5	20	2.9	68	72	379	.6
3	-	-	-	55	-	60	-	-	36	-	.3	.1	160	.8	-	1.1	-	380	590	-
1	-	-	-	20	-	500	-	-	5	-	.3	.3	200	1.5	-	1.9	240	590	420	-
2	-	-	-	15	-	350	-	-	30	-	.3	.2	160	.6	-	1.1	-	900	570	-
0	0	0	2	0	2	1	.1	0	1	-	0	0	5	.2	3	.1	16	52	5	.4
0	0	0	2	0	5	2	.2	0	3	-	.1	.1	10	.4	2	.5	45	402	3	.8
8	1	0	2	0	4	2	.1	0	2	-	0	0	5	.4	22	.2	16	152	2	.2
6	8	5	-	75	16	104	.2	.4	2	-	.3	.2	111	1.5	24	1.6	136	244	355	.7
-	-	3	-	0	-	-	-	-	-	-	.1	.2	80	1	-	.8	160	250	80	-
2	5	4	-	0	6	89	.1	.5	1	-	.4	.1	253	.4	24	.5	206	328	584	.8
0	0	0	3	0	22	9	.7	0	10	.3	.1	.1	7	.4	33	.6	23	451	1	.2
0	1	1	1	0	5	109	.1	0	9	-	0	0	24	1.1	22	1.1	25	217	1019	.2
1	1	0	0	9	2	2	.1	.4	4	-	.1	.1	13	.3	4	.5	30	76	307	.6
1	2	1	0	74	14	30	.1	2	2	-	.1	.1	88	1.6	32	1.3	218	388	77	.7
1	1	1	0	88	9	26	.3	3.8	0	-	0	.1	16	.9	43	2.2	216	279	75	.4
1	-	1	-	5	-	60	-	-	2	-	.2	.2	48	1	-	1.1	220	630	480	-
0	0	0	6	0	30	22	.2	0	4	-	.1	.2	64	.4	41	.5	132	376	504	1.8
2	2	0	-	29	58	28	.1	0	2	-	.1	.1	60	2.1	33	1.3	108	426	632	1.6
3	4	1	9	8	39	19	.1	0	3	-	.1	.1	62	2.2	36	1.2	134	302	553	2.4
1	1	0	7	9	46	23	.1	0	3	-	0	.1	67	2.2	43	.6	137	391	524	1.8
2	3	1	7	6	61	0	.1	0	1	-	.1	.2	77	2.5	54	.5	138	453	534	.9
0	0	0	-	0	128	1	.1	0	0	-	.1	.2	23	1.8	60	.4	120	305	204	1
0	0	0	1	0	22	24	0	0	3	-	0	0	18	.6	9	.1	13	74	171	.2
0	0	0	2	0	20	37	0	0	9	-	.1	0	20	.6	14	.4	21	115	3	.1
0	0	0	2	0	6	36	0	0	6	-	0	0	30	.6	14	.3	16	76	9	.4
0	0	0	-	0	63	0	.1	0	2	-	.1	.1	35	1.6	40	.6	134	329	444	.7
0	0	0	6	0	61	0	.1	0	1	-	0	.1	25	2.2	47	.3	89	265	405	.8
0	0	0	-	0	14	15	.1	0	5	-	0	.1	25	1.8	50	.7	101	370	26	.5
0	0	0	7	0	82	0	.1	0	1	-	.1	.2	62	2.4	62	.6	176	377	587	1
0	0	0	4	0	72	0	.1	0	1	-	.1	.1	44	1.9	32	.4	110	361	499	.8
1	1	0	7	0	106	0	.1	0	-	-	.1	.1	58	2.2	49	.6	106	497	536	1.7
0	0	0	1	0	22	7	0	0	3	-	0	0	18	.6	9	.1	13	74	171	.2

Food Composition Table—cont'd

Code	Name	Amount	Unit	Grams	Kilocalories	Carbohydrates (g)	Protein (g)	Fat (g)
11722	BEANS, YELLOW, FRESH	½	CUP	55.0	17	4	1	0
41335	BEEF AND BEAN BURRITOS (MEDIUM)-HEALTHY CHOICE	1	EACH	148.8	270	42	12	7
41334	BEEF AND BEAN BURRITOS (MILD)-HEALTHY CHOICE	1	EACH	148.8	250	45	11	5
55191	BEEF AND BEAN ENCHILADAS, LEAN CUISINE-STOUFFER'S	1	EACH	262.2	240	32	15	6
41270	BEEF AND POTATO SOUP-HEALTHY CHOICE	1	EACH	212.6	110	17	9	1
14114	BEEF BROTH AND TOMATO JUICE, CND	¾	CUP	183.0	68	16	1	0
55192	BEEF CANNELLONI W/ SAUCE, LEAN CUISINE-STOUFFER'S	1	EACH	272.9	200	28	14	3
41249	BEEF ENCHILADA-HEALTHY CHOICE	1	EACH	379.2	370	66	15	5
19002	BEEF JERKY, CHOPPED AND FORMED	3	OUNCE	85.1	287	12	34	11
55149	BEEF PIE-STOUFFER'S	1	EACH	283.5	460	37	18	27
57806	BEEF POT PIE-SWANSON	1	PIE	198.5	370	36	12	19
43405	BEEF RAVIOLI, MICRO CUP-HORMEL	1	EACH	212.6	270	34	9	11
41251	BEEF SIRLOIN TIPS-HEALTHY CHOICE	1	EACH	318.9	270	29	22	7
43413	BEEF STEW, MICRO CUP-HORMEL	1	EACH	212.6	230	11	13	15
55158	BEEF STROGANOFF W/ PARSLEY NOODLES-STOUFFER'S	1	EACH	276.4	390	28	24	20
13347	BEEF, CORNED, BRISKET, CKD	3	OUNCE	85.1	213	0	15	16
13353	BEEF, CURED, LUNCH MEAT, JELLIED	3	OUNCE	85.1	94	0	16	3
13355	BEEF, CURED, PASTRAMI	3	OUNCE	85.1	297	3	15	25
13357	BEEF, CURED, SAUSAGE, SMOKED	3	OUNCE	85.1	265	2	12	23
13358	BEEF, CURED, SMOKED, CHOPPED BEEF	3	OUNCE	85.1	105	2	17	4
13360	BEEF, CURED, THIN-SLICED BEEF	3	OUNCE	85.1	151	5	24	3
13298	BEEF, GROUND, EXTRA LEAN, BROILED	3	OUNCE	85.1	218	0	22	14
13300	BEEF, GROUND, EXTRA LEAN, PAN-FRIED	3	OUNCE	85.1	217	0	21	14
13305	BEEF, GROUND, LEAN, BROILED	3	OUNCE	85.1	231	0	21	16
13307	BEEF, GROUND, LEAN, PAN-FRIED	3	OUNCE	85.1	234	0	21	16
13312	BEEF, GROUND, REGULAR, BROILED	3	OUNCE	85.1	246	0	20	18
13314	BEEF, GROUND, REGULAR, PAN-FRIED	3	OUNCE	85.1	260	0	20	19
13326	BEEF, LIVER, CKD, BRAISED	3	OUNCE	85.1	137	3	21	4
13327	BEEF, LIVER, CKD, PAN-FRIED	3	OUNCE	85.1	185	7	23	7
7042	BEEF, LOAVED, LUNCH MEAT	1	SLICE	28.4	87	1	4	7
13504	BEEF, STEAKS AND ROASTS, CKD, ½ IN. FAT	3	OUNCE	85.1	297	0	21	23
13361	BEEF, STEAKS AND ROASTS, CKD, FAT TRIMMED	3	OUNCE	85.1	232	0	23	15
13004	BEEF, STEAKS AND ROASTS, CKD., ¼ IN. FAT	3	OUNCE	85.1	259	0	22	18
7043	BEEF, THIN SLICED	1	SLICE	4.2	7	0	1	0
14006	BEER, LIGHT	12	FL OZ	354.0	99	5	1	0
14003	BEER, REGULAR	12	FL OZ	356.4	146	13	1	0
11081	BEETS, CKD	½	CUP	85.0	37	8	1	0
18009	BISCUITS, PLAIN OR BUTTERMILK	1	EACH	35.0	127	17	2	6
14008	BLOODY MARY	1	FL OZ	29.7	23	1	0	0
9052	BLUEBERRIES, CND, HEAVY SYRUP	½	CUP	128.0	113	28	1	0
9050	BLUEBERRIES, FRESH	½	CUP	72.5	41	10	0	0
9055	BLUEBERRIES, FROZEN, SWEETENED	½	CUP	115.0	93	25	0	0
9054	BLUEBERRIES, FROZEN, UNSWEETENED	½	CUP	77.5	40	9	0	0
41241	BLUEBERRY MUFFIN-HEALTHY CHOICE	1	EACH	70.9	190	39	3	4
18305	BLUEBERRY PIE	1	SLICE	125.0	290	44	2	13
15189	BLUEFISH, CKD, DRY HEAT	3	OUNCE	85.1	135	0	22	5
10126	BOLOGNA	1	SLICE	23.0	57	0	4	5
7007	BOLOGNA, BEEF	1	SLICE	28.4	88	0	3	8
41286	BONELESS BEEF RIBS W/ BARBECUE SAUCE-HEALTHY CHOICE	1	EACH	311.8	330	40	28	6
14413	BOURBON AND SODA	1	FL OZ	29.0	26	0	0	0
12078	BRAZILNUTS, DRIED, UNBLANCHED	½	CUP	70.0	459	9	10	46
19167	BREAD PUDDING	1	CUP	252.0	423	62	13	15
18080	BREAD STICKS, PLAIN	1	STICK	10.0	41	7	1	1
18083	BREAD STUFFING, PLAIN	1	CUP	232.0	390	52	9	17
18020	BREAD, BANANA	1	SLICE	60.0	203	33	3	7
18024	BREAD, CORNBREAD	1	PIECE	65.0	173	28	4	5
18025	BREAD, CRACKED-WHEAT	1	SLICE	25.0	65	12	2	1
18026	BREAD, CRACKED-WHEAT, TOASTED	1	SLICE	23.0	65	12	2	1
18344	BREAD, DINNER ROLL, EGG	1	EACH	35.0	107	18	3	2
18349	BREAD, DINNER ROLL, FRENCH	1	EACH	38.0	105	19	3	2
18345	BREAD, DINNER ROLL, OAT BRAN	1	EACH	33.0	78	13	3	2

Saturated fat (g)	Monounsaturated fat (g)	Polyunsaturated fat (g)	Fiber (g)	Cholesterol (g)	Folate (g)	Vitamin A (RE)	Vitamin B-6 (mg)	Vitamin B-12 (μg)	Vitamin C (mg)	Vitamin E (mg)	Riboflavin (mg)	Thiamin (mg)	Calcium (mg)	Iron (mg)	Magnesium (mg)	Niacin (mg)	Phosphorus (mg)	Potassium (mg)	Sodium (mg)	Zinc (mg)
0	0	0	1	0	20	6	0	0	9	-	.1	0	20	.6	14	.4	21	115	3	.1
3	0	3	-	15	-	20	-	-	4	-	.2	.4	48	1.5	-	1.9	180	270	520	-
1	-	2	-	10	-	20	-	-	1	-	.2	.4	32	2	-	2.9	130	330	450	-
3	-	1	-	45	-	80	-	-	6	-	.3	.2	80	1	-	1.9	-	470	480	-
-	-	-	-	-	20	-	-	-	2	-	-	0	-	.2	-	.4	-	100	550	-
0	0	0	-	0	8	24	0	.1	2	-	.1	0	20	1.1	5	.3	24	176	240	0
1	-	-	-	25	-	350	-	-	6	-	.2	.1	120	1.5	-	2.9	-	800	490	-
2	-	2	-	30	-	250	-	-	24	-	.3	.3	120	1	-	1.9	260	600	450	-
5	5	0	0	96	14	0	.4	3.4	0	-	.8	.1	9	4.7	43	7.8	323	508	2445	6.9
-	-	-	-	-	-	700	-	-	2	-	.4	.3	32	1.5	-	3.8	-	300	1130	-
-	-	-	-	-	-	250	-	-	-	-	.2	.2	16	1.5	-	2.9	-	-	730	-
4	5	1	-	20	-	100	-	-	11	-	.3	.2	48	.9	28	2.5	-	359	920	1.1
3	-	2	-	65	-	700	-	-	42	-	.2	.2	16	1	-	2.9	190	520	360	-
5	4	-	-	45	-	320	-	-	2	-	.1	0	16	.9	21	2.3	-	487	1140	2.4
-	-	-	-	-	-	40	-	-	1	-	.3	.1	48	1.5	-	2.9	-	300	1090	-
5	8	1	0	83	5	0	.2	1.4	14	-	.1	0	7	1.6	10	2.6	106	123	964	3.9
1	1	0	0	29	6	0	.2	4.4	15	-	.2	.1	9	2.9	15	4.1	118	342	1124	3
9	12	1	0	79	6	0	.2	1.5	3	-	.1	.1	8	1.6	15	4.3	128	194	1044	3.6
10	11	1	0	57	3	0	.1	1.6	10	-	.1	0	6	1.5	11	2.7	89	150	962	2.4
2	2	0	0	39	7	0	.3	1.5	18	-	.1	.1	7	2.4	18	3.9	154	321	1070	3.3
1	1	0	0	35	9	0	.3	2.2	12	-	.2	.1	9	2.3	16	4.5	143	365	1224	3.4
5	6	1	0	71	8	0	.2	1.8	0	-	.2	.1	6	2	18	4.2	137	266	60	4.6
5	6	1	0	69	8	0	.2	1.7	0	-	.2	.1	6	2	18	4	136	265	60	4.6
6	7	1	0	74	8	0	.2	2	0	-	.2	0	9	1.8	18	4.4	134	256	65	4.6
6	7	1	0	71	8	0	.2	1.9	0	-	.2	0	9	1.9	17	4.1	135	254	65	4.4
7	8	1	0	77	8	0	.2	2.5	0	-	.2	0	9	2.1	17	4.9	145	248	71	4.4
8	8	1	0	76	8	0	.2	2.3	0	-	.2	0	9	2.1	17	5	145	255	71	4.3
2	1	1	0	331	185	9017	.8	60.4	20	-	3.5	.2	6	5.8	17	9.1	344	200	60	5.2
2	1	1	0	410	187	9125	1.2	95.1	20	-	3.5	.2	9	5.3	20	12.3	392	310	90	4.6
3	3	0	0	18	1	0	.1	1.1	4	-	.1	0	3	.7	4	1	34	59	377	.7
9	10	1	0	77	6	0	.3	2	0	-	.2	.1	9	2.2	18	2.9	164	244	50	4.7
6	6	1	0	74	6	0	.3	2.1	0	-	.2	.1	8	2.3	20	3.1	179	275	53	5.2
7	8	1	0	75	6	0	.3	2.1	0	-	.2	.1	9	2.2	19	3.1	173	266	53	5
0	0	0	0	2	0	0	0	.1	1	-	0	0	0	.1	1	.2	7	18	60	.2
0	0	0	0	0	15	0	.1	0	0	-	.1	0	18	.1	18	1.4	42	64	11	.1
0	0	0	1	0	21	0	.2	.1	0	-	.1	0	18	.1	21	1.6	43	89	18	.1
0	0	0	1	0	68	3	.1	0	3	-	0	0	14	.7	20	.3	32	259	65	.3
1	2	2	-	2	0	0	0	0	0	-	.1	.1	17	1.2	6	1.2	151	78	368	.2
0	0	0	0	0	4	10	0	0	4	-	0	0	2	.1	2	.1	4	43	67	0
-	-	-	2	0	2	8	0	0	1	-	.1	0	6	.4	5	.1	13	51	4	.1
-	-	-	2	0	5	7	0	0	9	-	0	0	4	.1	4	.3	7	65	4	.1
-	-	-	2	0	8	5	.1	0	1	-	.1	0	7	.4	2	.3	8	69	1	.1
-	-	-	2	0	5	6	0	0	2	-	0	0	6	.1	4	.4	9	42	1	.1
-	-	2	-	0	-	-	-	-	4	-	.2	.2	80	.8	-	.8	160	200	110	-
2	7	2	-	0	5	43	0	0	3	-	0	0	10	.4	6	.4	26	63	406	.2
1	2	1	0	65	2	117	.4	5.3	0	-	.1	.1	8	.5	36	6.2	247	406	65	.9
2	2	0	0	14	1	0	.1	.2	8	-	0	.1	3	.2	3	.9	32	65	272	.5
3	4	0	0	16	1	0	0	.4	6	-	0	0	3	.5	3	.7	25	45	278	.6
2	-	2	-	70	-	60	-	-	5	-	.3	.2	48	1	-	2.9	220	670	530	-
0	0	0	-	0	0	0	0	0	0	-	0	0	1	0	0	0	1	1	4	0
11	16	17	4	0	3	0	.2	0	0	-	.1	.7	123	2.4	158	1.1	420	420	1	3.2
6	5	2	-	166	33	164	.2	-	2	-	.6	.2	287	2.8	48	1.6	275	564	582	1.3
0	0	0	-	0	3	0	0	0	0	-	.1	.1	2	.4	3	.5	12	12	66	.1
3	7	5	-	0	39	160	.1	0	4	-	.3	.4	148	3.8	35	3.7	114	304	1070	.7
2	3	2	-	26	7	14	.1	.1	1	-	.1	.1	11	.8	8	.9	34	79	119	.2
1	1	2	-	26	12	35	.1	.1	0	-	.2	.2	162	1.6	16	1.5	110	96	428	.4
0	0	0	1	0	10	0	.1	0	0	-	.1	.1	11	.7	13	.9	38	44	135	.3
0	0	0	-	0	7	0	.1	0	0	-	.1	.1	11	.7	13	.8	38	44	135	.3
1	1	0	1	18	19	8	0	.1	0	-	.2	.2	21	1.2	9	1.2	35	37	191	.3
0	1	0	-	0	13	0	0	0	0	-	.1	.2	35	1	8	1.7	32	43	231	.3
0	0	1	1	0	10	0	0	0	0	-	.1	.1	28	1.4	10	1.6	34	36	136	.3

Food Composition Table—cont'd

Code	Name	Amount	Unit	Grams	Kilocalories	Carbohydrates (g)	Protein (g)	Fat (g)
18342	BREAD, DINNER ROLL, PLAIN	1	EACH	35.0	105	18	3	3
18346	BREAD, DINNER ROLL, RYE	1	EACH	35.0	100	19	4	1
18347	BREAD, DINNER ROLL, WHEAT	1	EACH	33.0	90	15	3	2
18348	BREAD, DINNER ROLL, WHOLE-WHEAT	1	EACH	33.0	88	17	3	2
18027	BREAD, EGG	1	SLICE	40.0	115	19	4	2
18028	BREAD, EGG, TOASTED	1	SLICE	37.0	117	19	4	2
18029	BREAD, FRENCH OR VIENNA	1	SLICE	25.0	69	13	2	1
18030	BREAD, FRENCH OR VIENNA, TOASTED	1	SLICE	23.0	69	13	2	1
18033	BREAD, ITALIAN	1	SLICE	30.0	81	15	3	1
18034	BREAD, ITALIAN, TOASTED	1	SLICE	27.0	80	15	3	1
18049	BREAD, LO CAL, OAT BRAN	1	SLICE	23.0	46	9	2	1
18050	BREAD, LO CAL, OAT BRAN, TOASTED	1	SLICE	19.0	45	9	2	1
18051	BREAD, LO CAL, OATMEAL	1	SLICE	23.0	48	10	2	1
18052	BREAD, LO CAL, OATMEAL, TOASTED	1	SLICE	19.0	48	10	2	1
18053	BREAD, LO CAL, RYE	1	SLICE	23.0	47	9	2	1
18054	BREAD, LO CAL, RYE, TOASTED	1	SLICE	19.0	46	9	2	1
18055	BREAD, LO CAL, WHEAT	1	SLICE	23.0	46	10	2	1
18056	BREAD, LO CAL, WHEAT, TOASTED	1	SLICE	19.0	45	10	2	1
18057	BREAD, LO CAL, WHITE	1	SLICE	23.0	48	10	2	1
18058	BREAD, LO CAL, WHITE, TOASTED	1	SLICE	19.0	47	10	2	1
18035	BREAD, MIXED-GRAIN	1	SLICE	26.0	65	12	3	1
18036	BREAD, MIXED-GRAIN, TOASTED	1	SLICE	24.0	65	12	3	1
18037	BREAD, OAT BRAN	1	SLICE	30.0	71	12	3	1
18038	BREAD, OAT BRAN, TOASTED	1	SLICE	27.0	70	12	3	1
18039	BREAD, OATMEAL	1	SLICE	27.0	73	13	2	1
18040	BREAD, OATMEAL, TOASTED	1	SLICE	25.0	73	13	2	1
18041	BREAD, PITA, WHITE, ENRICHED	1	PITA	60.0	165	33	5	1
18042	BREAD, PITA, WHOLE-WHEAT	1	PITA	64.0	170	35	6	2
18044	BREAD, PUMPERNICKEL	1	SLICE	32.0	80	15	3	1
18045	BREAD, PUMPERNICKEL, TOASTED	1	SLICE	29.0	80	15	3	1
18046	BREAD, PUMPKIN	1	SLICE	60.0	199	31	2	8
18047	BREAD, RAISIN	1	SLICE	26.0	71	14	2	1
18048	BREAD, RAISIN, TOASTED	1	SLICE	24.0	71	14	2	1
18059	BREAD, RICE BRAN	1	SLICE	27.0	66	12	2	1
18384	BREAD, RICE BRAN, TOASTED	1	SLICE	25.0	66	12	2	1
18353	BREAD, ROLLS, HARD (INCLUDES KAISER)	1	EACH	57.0	167	30	6	2
18060	BREAD, RYE	1	SLICE	32.0	83	15	3	1
18061	BREAD, RYE, TOASTED	1	SLICE	29.0	82	15	3	1
18064	BREAD, WHEAT (INCLUDES WHEAT BERRY)	1	SLICE	25.0	65	12	2	1
18066	BREAD, WHEAT BRAN	1	SLICE	36.0	89	17	3	1
18067	BREAD, WHEAT BRAN, TOASTED	1	SLICE	33.0	90	17	3	1
18065	BREAD, WHEAT, TOASTED	1	SLICE	23.0	65	12	2	1
18069	BREAD, WHITE	1	SLICE	25.0	67	12	2	1
18070	BREAD, WHITE, TOASTED	1	SLICE	23.0	67	13	2	1
41348	BREADED FISH-HEALTHY CHOICE	1	STICK	9.8	15	2	1	1
43400	BREAST OF CHICKEN W/ SPANISH RICE, TOP SHELF-HORMEL	1	EACH	283.5	400	38	27	15
41252	BREAST OF TURKEY-HEALTHY CHOICE	1	EACH	297.7	290	39	21	5
62616	BROCCOLI AND CHEESE BAKED POTATO-WEIGHT WATCHERS	1	EACH	283.5	230	34	12	7
11091	BROCCOLI, CKD	½	CUP	78.0	22	4	2	0
11740	BROCCOLI, FLOWER CLUSTERS, FRESH	½	CUP	44.0	12	2	1	0
11093	BROCCOLI, FRZ, CHOPPED, CKD	½	CUP	92.0	26	5	3	0
18151	BROWNIES	1	EACH	56.0	227	36	3	9
11099	BRUSSELS SPROUTS, CKD	½	CUP	78.0	30	7	2	0
62601	BUFFALO (CHICKEN) WINGS	4	EACH	91.0	190	2	18	12
18351	BUNS, HAMBURGER OR HOT DOG, MIXED-GRAIN	1	EACH	43.0	113	19	4	3
18350	BUNS, HAMBURGER OR HOT DOG, PLAIN	1	EACH	43.0	123	22	4	2
18155	BUTTER COOKIES, ENRICHED	1	EACH	5.0	23	3	0	1
4136	BUTTER, W/ SALT	1	PAT	5.0	36	0	0	4
1145	BUTTER, W/O SALT	1	PAT	5.0	36	0	0	4
1002	BUTTER, WHIPPED	1	TBSP.	11.0	79	0	0	9

Saturated fat (g)	Monounsaturated fat (g)	Polyunsaturated fat (g)	Fiber (g)	Cholesterol (g)	Folate (g)	Vitamin A (RE)	Vitamin B-6 (mg)	Vitamin B-12 (µg)	Vitamin C (mg)	Vitamin E (mg)	Riboflavin (mg)	Thiamin (mg)	Calcium (mg)	Iron (mg)	Magnesium (mg)	Niacin (mg)	Phosphorus (mg)	Potassium (mg)	Sodium (mg)	Zinc (mg)
1	1	0	1	0	11	0	0	0	0	-	.1	.2	42	1.1	8	1.4	41	47	182	.3
0	0	0	-	0	8	0	0	0	0	-	.1	.1	11	.9	19	1.4	56	63	312	.4
1	1	0	-	0	5	0	0	0	0	-	.1	.1	58	1.2	14	1.3	39	44	112	.3
0	0	1	-	0	10	0	.1	0	0	-	.1	.1	35	.8	28	1.2	74	90	158	.7
1	1	0	-	20	28	9	0	0	0	-	.2	.2	37	1.2	8	1.9	42	46	197	.3
1	1	0	-	21	20	9	0	0	0	-	.2	.1	38	1.2	8	1.8	43	47	200	.3
0	0	0	1	0	8	0	0	0	0	-	.1	.1	19	.6	7	1.2	26	28	152	.2
0	0	0	-	0	6	0	0	0	0	-	.1	.1	19	.6	7	1.1	26	28	152	.2
0	0	0	1	0	9	0	0	0	0	-	.1	.1	23	.9	8	1.3	31	33	175	.3
0	0	0	-	0	6	0	0	0	0	-	.1	.1	23	.9	8	1.2	31	33	173	.3
0	0	0	-	0	8	0	0	0	0	-	0	.1	13	.7	11	.9	28	23	81	.2
0	0	0	-	0	5	0	0	0	0	-	0	.1	13	.7	10	.8	27	23	79	.2
0	0	0	-	0	8	0	0	-	0	-	.1	.1	26	.5	7	.7	27	35	89	.2
0	0	0	-	0	5	0	0	0	0	-	.1	.1	26	.5	6	.6	27	35	88	.2
0	0	0	-	0	5	0	0	0	0	-	.1	.1	17	.7	4	.6	19	23	93	.2
0	0	0	-	0	4	0	0	0	0	-	0	.1	17	.7	4	.5	19	22	92	.2
0	0	0	3	0	6	-	0	0	0	-	.1	.1	18	.7	6	.9	-	29	118	.2
0	0	0	-	0	4	0	0	0	0	-	.1	.1	18	.7	6	.8	21	28	116	.2
0	0	0	2	0	8	-	0	.1	0	-	.1	.1	22	.7	6	.8	31	17	104	.3
0	0	0	-	0	6	0	0	.1	0	-	.1	.1	21	.7	6	.7	30	17	102	.3
0	0	0	2	0	12	0	.1	0	0	-	.1	.1	24	.9	14	1.1	46	53	127	.3
0	0	0	-	0	9	0	.1	0	0	-	.1	.1	24	.9	14	1	46	53	127	.3
0	0	1	1	0	8	0	0	0	0	-	.1	.2	20	.9	9	1.4	32	34	122	.3
0	0	1	-	0	5	-	0	0	0	-	.1	.1	19	.9	9	1.3	31	33	121	.3
0	0	0	1	0	7	1	0	-	0	-	.1	.1	18	.7	10	.8	34	38	162	.3
0	0	0	-	0	5	1	0	0	0	-	.1	.1	18	.7	10	.8	34	39	163	.3
0	0	0	1	0	14	0	0	0	0	-	.2	.4	52	1.6	16	2.8	58	72	322	.5
0	0	1	5	0	22	0	.1	0	0	-	.1	.2	10	1.8	44	1.8	115	109	340	1
0	0	0	2	0	11	0	0	0	0	-	.1	.1	22	.9	17	1	57	67	215	.5
0	0	0	-	0	8	0	0	0	0	-	.1	.1	21	.9	17	.9	57	66	214	.5
1	2	4	-	26	7	334	0	0	1	-	.1	.1	11	1	8	.8	32	55	188	.2
0	1	0	1	0	9	0	0	0	0	-	.1	.1	17	.8	7	.9	28	59	101	.2
0	1	0	-	0	6	0	0	0	0	-	.1	.1	17	.8	7	.8	28	59	102	.2
0	0	0	-	0	8	-	.1	0	0	-	.1	.2	19	1	19	1.8	43	53	119	.3
0	0	0	-	0	6	0	.1	0	0	-	.1	.1	19	1	19	1.7	44	53	120	.3
0	1	1	-	0	9	0	0	0	0	-	.2	.3	54	1.9	15	2.4	57	62	310	.5
0	0	0	2	0	16	0	0	0	-	-	.1	.1	23	.9	13	1.2	40	53	211	.4
0	0	0	-	0	11	-	0	0	0	-	.1	.1	23	.9	12	1.1	40	53	210	.4
0	0	0	1	0	10	0	0	0	0	-	.1	.1	26	.8	12	1	38	50	133	.3
0	1	0	3	0	9	0	.1	0	0	-	.1	.1	27	1.1	29	1.6	67	82	175	.5
0	1	0	-	0	7	0	.1	0	0	-	.1	.1	27	1.1	29	1.4	67	82	176	.5
0	0	0	-	0	7	0	0	0	0	-	.1	.1	26	.8	12	.9	37	50	132	.3
0	0	0	1	0	9	0	0	0	-	-	.1	.1	27	.8	6	1	24	30	135	.2
0	0	0	-	0	6	0	0	0	0	-	.1	.1	27	.8	6	.9	24	30	136	.2
-	-	0	-	3	-	-	-	-	-	-	0	0	-	.1	-	.1	-	20	31	-
7	4	3	-	75	-	100	-	-	4	-	.3	.1	80	.4	35	7.6	-	584	810	1.7
-	-	-	-	45	-	40	-	-	48	-	.3	.5	32	1	-	5.7	270	540	420	-
-	-	6	10	-	200	-	-	9	-	-	-	-	300	.8	-	-	-	830	510	-
0	0	0	2	0	39	108	.1	0	58	-	.1	0	36	.7	19	.4	46	228	20	.3
0	0	0	-	0	31	132	.1	0	41	-	.1	0	21	.4	11	.3	29	143	12	.2
0	0	0	3	0	52	174	.1	0	37	-	.1	.1	47	.6	18	.4	51	166	22	.3
2	5	1	1	10	7	11	0	.1	0	-	.1	.1	16	1.3	17	1	57	83	175	.4
0	0	0	3	0	47	56	.1	0	48	-	.1	.1	28	.9	16	.5	44	247	16	.3
-	-	-	100	-	60	-	-	1	-	-	-	-	24	.4	-	-	-	-	900	-
	1	0	2	0	12	0	0	0	0	-	.1	.2	41	1.7	21	1.9	52	65	197	.5
	1	0	-	0	12	0	0	0	0	-	.1	.2	60	1.4	9	1.7	38	61	241	.3
1	0	0	0	4	0	8	0	0	0	-	0	0	1	.1	1	.2	5	6	18	0
3	1	0	0	11	0	38	0	0	0	-	.1	0	0	1	0	0	0	1	41	0
3	1	0	0	11	0	38	0	0	0	-	.1	0	0	1	0	0	0	1	1	0
6	3	0	0	24	0	83	0	0	0	-	0		3	0	0	0	3	3	91	0

Food Composition Table—cont'd

Code	Name	Amount	Unit	Grams	Kilocalories	Carbohydrates (g)	Protein (g)	Fat (g)
19069	BUTTERFINGER BAR	1	BAR	61.0	267	41	5	11
19070	BUTTERSCOTCH CANDY	1	PIECE	6.0	24	6	0	0
18307	BUTTERSCOTCH PUDDING PIE	1	SLICE	127.0	354	42	6	18
11110	CABBAGE, CKD	½	CUP	75.0	17	3	1	0
11749	CABBAGE, FRESH	1	CUP	70.0	17	4	1	0
18086	CAKE, ANGELFOOD	1	SLICE	28.4	73	16	2	0
18090	CAKE, BOSTON CREAM PIE	1	SLICE	92.0	232	39	2	8
8094	CAKE, CARROT, W/ CREAM CHEESE FROSTING	1	SLICE	111.0	484	52	5	29
18096	CAKE, CHOCOLATE, W/ CHOCOLATE FROSTING	1	SLICE	64.0	235	35	3	10
18110	CAKE, FRUITCAKE	1	PIECE	43.0	139	26	1	4
18113	CAKE, GERMAN CHOCOLATE, W/ FROSTING	1	SLICE	111.0	404	55	4	21
18115	CAKE, GINGERBREAD	1	SLICE	67.0	207	34	3	7
18119	CAKE, PINEAPPLE UPSIDE-DOWN	1	SLICE	115.0	367	58	4	14
18120	CAKE, POUND	1	SLICE	28.4	110	14	2	6
18133	CAKE, SPONGE	1	SLICE	38.0	110	23	2	1
18102	CAKE, WHITE, W/ COCONUT FROSTING	1	SLICE	112.0	399	71	5	12
18139	CAKE, WHITE, W/ FROSTING	1	SLICE	74.0	264	42	4	9
18140	CAKE, YELLOW, W/ CHOCOLATE FROSTING	1	SLICE	64.0	243	35	2	11
18141	CAKE, YELLOW, W/ VANILLA FROSTING	1	SLICE	64.0	239	38	2	9
55177	CANADIAN STYLE BACON, FRENCH BREAD PIZZAS-STOUFFER'S	1	EACH	163.0	370	40	18	15
19074	CARAMELS	1	PIECE	8.0	31	6	0	1
11655	CARROT JUICE, CND	¾	CUP	184.5	74	17	2	0
11960	CARROTS, BABY, FRESH	1	MEDIUM	10.0	4	1	0	0
11125	CARROTS, CKD	½	CUP	78.0	35	8	1	0
11128	CARROTS, CND, REG PK	½	CUP	73.0	17	4	0	0
11124	CARROTS, FRESH	1	MEDIUM	60.0	26	6	1	0
11131	CARROTS, FRZ, CKD	½	CUP	73.0	26	6	1	0
12585	CASHEW, DRY ROASTED	½	CUP	68.5	393	22	10	32
12586	CASHEW, OIL ROASTED	½	CUP	65.0	374	19	10	31
15235	CATFISH, CHANNEL, FARMED, CKD, DRY HEAT	3	OUNCE	85.1	129	0	16	7
15233	CATFISH, CHANNEL, WILD, CKD, DRY HEAT	3	OUNCE	85.1	89	0	16	2
15011	CATFISH, FRIED	3	OUNCE	85.1	195	7	15	11
11935	CATSUP	1	TBSP.	15.0	16	4	0	0
11949	CATSUP, LOW SODIUM	1	TBSP.	15.0	16	4	0	0
11136	CAULIFLOWER, CKD, BOILED	½	CUP	62.0	14	3	1	0
11135	CAULIFLOWER, FRESH	½	CUP	50.0	13	3	1	0
11138	CAULIFLOWER, FRZ, CKD	½	CUP	90.0	17	3	1	0
15012	CAVIAR, BLACK AND RED, GRANULAR	1	TBSP.	16.0	40	1	4	3
11144	CELERY, CKD	½	CUP	75.0	14	3	1	0
11143	CELERY, FRESH	½	CUP	60.0	10	2	0	0
8053	CEREALS, 100% BRAN	1	CUP	66.0	178	48	8	3
8054	CEREALS, 100% NATURAL CEREAL, PLAIN	1	CUP	104.0	489	65	12	22
8055	CEREALS, 100% NATURAL CEREAL, W/ APPLE AND CINN.	1	CUP	104.0	477	70	11	20
8056	CEREALS, 100% NATURAL CEREAL, W/ RAISINS AND DATES	1	CUP	110.0	496	72	11	20
8028	CEREALS, 40% BRAN FLAKES, KELLOGG'S	1	CUP	39.0	127	31	5	1
8029	CEREALS, 40% BRAN FLAKES, POST	1	CUP	47.0	152	37	5	1
8153	CEREALS, 40% BRAN FLAKES, RALSTON PURINA	1	CUP	49.0	159	39	6	1
8001	CEREALS, ALL-BRAN	1	CUP	85.2	212	63	12	2
8006	CEREALS, BRAN CHEX	1	CUP	49.0	156	39	5	1
8008	CEREALS, C.W. POST, PLAIN	1	CUP	97.0	432	69	9	15
8009	CEREALS, C.W. POST, W/ RAISINS	1	CUP	103.0	446	74	9	15
8010	CEREALS, CAP'N CRUNCH	1	CUP	37.0	156	30	2	3
8011	CEREALS, CAP'N CRUNCH'S CRUNCHBERRIES	1	CUP	35.0	146	29	2	3
8012	CEREALS, CAP'N CRUNCH'S PEANUT BUTTER	1	CUP	35.0	154	26	3	5
8013	CEREALS, CHEERIOS	1	CUP	22.7	89	16	3	1
8014	CEREALS, COCOA KRISPIES	1	CUP	36.0	139	32	2	1
8017	CEREALS, COOKIE-CRISP, CHOC CHIP AND VANILLA	1	CUP	30.0	120	26	2	1
8018	CEREALS, CORN BRAN	1	CUP	36.0	125	30	2	1
8019	CEREALS, CORN CHEX	1	CUP	28.4	111	25	2	0
8020	CEREALS, CORN FLAKES, KELLOGG'S	1	CUP	22.7	88	20	2	0

Saturated fat (g)	Monounsaturated fat (g)	Polyunsaturated fat (g)	Fiber (g)	Cholesterol (g)	Folate (g)	Vitamin A (RE)	Vitamin B-6 (mg)	Vitamin B-12 (µg)	Vitamin C (mg)	Vitamin E (mg)	Riboflavin (mg)	Thiamin (mg)	Calcium (mg)	Iron (mg)	Magnesium (mg)	Niacin (mg)	Phosphorus (mg)	Potassium (mg)	Sodium (mg)	Zinc (mg)
5	4	2	2	1	19	12	0	.1	2	-	0	.1	15	.6	27	2	58	129	83	.4
0	0	0	0	1	0	2	0	0	0	-	0	0	0	0	0	0	0	0	3	0
5	8	4	-	77	14	107	.1	.4	1	-	.3	.2	128	1.6	22	1.3	135	221	335	.7
0	0	0	2	0	15	10	.1	0	15	-	0	0	23	.1	6	.2	11	73	6	.1
0	0	0	-	0	40	9	.1	0	36	-	0	0	33	.4	11	.2	16	172	13	.1
0	0	0	0	0	1	0	0	-	0	-	.1	0	40	.1	3	.3	66	26	212	0
2	4	1	1	34	7	21	0	.1	0	-	.2	.4	21	.3	6	.2	45	36	132	.1
5	7	15	-	60	13	426	.1	.1	1	-	.2	.2	28	1.4	20	1.1	79	124	273	.5
3	6	1	2	29	5	18	-	.1	0	-	.1	0	28	1.4	22	.4	78	128	214	.4
0	2	1	2	2	1	8	0	.1	0	-	0	0	14	.9	7	.3	22	66	116	.1
5	9	5	-	53	4	23	0	.1	0	-	.1	.1	53	1.2	19	1.1	173	151	369	.5
2	4	1	2	23	7	11	0	0	0	-	.1	.1	46	2.2	11	1	113	161	307	.3
3	6	4	-	25	8	75	0	.1	1	-	.2	.2	138	1.7	15	1.4	94	129	367	.4
3	2	0	-	63	3	44	0	.1	0	-	.1	0	10	.4	3	.4	39	34	113	.1
0	0	0	-	39	5	17	0	.1	0	-	.1	1	27	1	4	.7	52	38	93	.2
4	4	2	-	1	6	12	0	.1	0	-	.2	.1	101	1.3	13	1.2	78	111	318	.4
2	4	2	-	1	5	12	0	.1	0	-	.2	.1	96	1.1	9	1.1	69	70	242	.2
3	6	1	1	35	5	17	0	.1	0	-	.1	.1	24	1.3	19	.8	103	114	216	.4
2	4	3	-	36	6	12	0	.1	0	-	0	.1	40	.7	4	.3	92	34	220	.2
-	-	-	-	-	80	-	-	-	6	-	.4	.6	160	1	-	3.8	-	300	1070	-
1	0	0	0	1	0	1	0	0	0	-	0	0	11	0	1	0	9	17	20	0
0	0	0	1	0	7	4751	.4	0	16	-	.1	.2	44	.8	26	.7	77	539	54	.3
0	0	0	-	0	3	20	0	0	1	-	0	0	2	.1	1	.1	4	28	4	0
0	0	0	3	0	11	1915	.2	0	2	-	0	0	24	.5	10	.4	23	177	51	.2
0	0	0	1	0	7	1005	.1	0	2	-	0	0	18	.5	6	.4	18	131	176	.2
0	0	0	2	0	8	1688	.1	0	6	-	0	.1	16	.3	9	.6	26	194	21	.1
0	0	0	3	0	8	1292	.1	0	2	-	0	0	20	.3	7	.3	19	115	43	.2
6	19	5	2	0	47	0	.2	0	0	-	.1	.1	31	4.1	178	1	336	387	438	3.8
6	18	5	2	0	44	0	.2	0	0	-	.1	.3	27	2.7	166	1.2	277	345	407	3.1
2	4	1	0	54	6	13	.1	2.4	1	-	.1	.4	8	.7	22	2.1	208	273	68	.9
1	1	1	0	61	9	13	.1	2.5	1	-	.1	.2	9	.3	24	2	259	356	43	.5
3	5	3	-	69	14	7	.2	1.6	0	-	.1	.1	37	1.2	23	1.9	184	289	238	.7
0	0	0	0	0	2	15	0	0	2	-	0	0	3	.1	3	.2	6	72	178	0
0	0	0	0	0	2	15	0	0	2	-	0	0	3	.1	3	.2	6	72	3	0
0	0	0	2	0	27	1	.1	0	27	-	0	0	10	.2	6	.3	20	88	9	.1
0	0	0	1	0	29	1	.1	0	23	-	0	0	11	.2	8	.3	22	152	15	.1
0	0	0	2	0	37	2	.1	0	28	-	0	0	15	.4	8	.3	22	125	16	.1
1	1	1	0	94	8	90	.1	3.2	0	-	.1	0	44	1.9	48	0	57	29	240	.2
0	0	0	1	0	17	10	.1	0	5	-	0	0	32	.3	9	.2	19	213	68	.1
0	0	0	1	0	17	8	.1	0	4	-	0	0	24	.2	7	.2	15	172	52	.1
1	1	2	20	0	47	0	2.1	6.3	63	-	1.8	1.6	46	8.1	312	20.9	801	824	457	5.7
15	4	2	9	1	31	-	.2	.1	0	-	.6	.3	181	3.1	125	2.4	383	514	45	2.4
15	2	1	7	1	17	-	.1	.3	1	-	.6	.3	157	2.9	72	1.9	350	514	52	2
14	4	2	7	1	45	-	.2	.1	0	-	.6	.3	160	3.1	124	2.1	348	538	47	2.1
-	-	-	5	0	138	516	.7	2.1	0	-	.6	.5	19	24.8	71	6.9	192	248	303	5.1
-	-	-	9	0	166	622	.8	2.5	0	-	.7	.6	21	7.5	102	8.3	296	251	431	2.5
-	-	-	7	0	173	649	.9	2.6	26	-	.7	.6	23	7.8	118	8.6	273	286	456	2
-	-	-	30	0	301	1128	1.5	0	45	-	1.3	1.1	69	13.5	318	15	794	1051	961	11.2
-	-	-	8	0	173	11	.9	2.6	26	-	.3	.6	29	7.8	126	8.6	327	394	455	2.1
11	2	1	7	0	342	1284	1.7	5.1	0	-	1.5	1.3	47	15.4	67	17.1	224	198	167	1.6
11	2	1	14	0	364	1364	1.9	5.5	0	-	1.5	1.3	50	16.4	74	18.1	232	261	161	1.6
2	0	1	1	0	238	5	1	2.3	0	-	.7	.7	6	9.8	15	8.6	47	48	278	4
2	0	0	1	0	128	5	.9	2.5	0	-	.7	.6	11	9	14	8.1	47	49	244	3.6
2	1	1	0	0	244	6	1	2.3	0	-	.7	.6	7	9.1	19	9	49	57	268	3.8
0	1	1	2	0	5	301	.4	1.2	12	-	.3	.3	39	3.6	31	4	107	81	246	.6
-	-	-	0	0	127	477	.6	0	19	-	.5	.5	6	2.3	12	6.3	47	53	275	1.9
-	-	-	0	0	3	397	.5	1.6	16	-	.4	.4	6	4.8	8	5.3	24	29	207	.3
-	-	-	7	0	232	8	.9	1.4	0	-	.7	.4	41	12.2	18	10.9	52	70	310	4
-	-	-	1	0	100	14	.5	1.5	15	-	.1	.4	3	1.8	4	5	11	23	272	.1.3
-	-	-	1	0	80	301	.4	0	12	-	.3	.3	1	1.4	3	4	14	21	232	.1

Food Composition Table—cont'd

Code	Name	Amount	Unit	Grams	Kilocalories	Carbohydrates (g)	Protein (g)	Fat (g)
8022	CEREALS, CORN FLAKES, LOW SODIUM	1	CUP	25.0	100	22	2	0
8021	CEREALS, CORN FLAKES, RALSTON PURINA	1	CUP	25.0	98	22	2	0
8023	CEREALS, CRACKLIN' BRAN	1	CUP	60.0	229	41	6	9
8168	CEREALS, CREAM OF RICE, CKD	1	CUP	244.0	127	28	2	0
8171	CEREALS, CREAM OF WHEAT, INSTANT	1	CUP	241.0	154	32	4	0
8170	CEREALS, CREAM OF WHEAT, QUICK	1	CUP	239.0	129	27	4	0
8169	CEREALS, CREAM OF WHEAT, REGULAR	1	CUP	251.0	133	28	4	1
8024	CEREALS, CRISP RICE, LOW SODIUM	1	CUP	26.0	105	24	1	0
8025	CEREALS, CRISPY RICE	1	CUP	28.0	111	25	2	0
8026	CEREALS, CRISPY WHEATS 'N RAISINS	1	CUP	43.0	150	35	3	1
8027	CEREALS, FORTIFIED OAT FLAKES	1	CUP	48.0	177	35	9	1
8030	CEREALS, FRUIT LOOPS	1	CUP	28.4	111	25	2	1
8035	CEREALS, GOLDEN GRAHAMS	1	CUP	39.0	150	33	2	1
8036	CEREALS, GRAHAM CRACKOS	1	CUP	30.0	108	26	2	0
8037	CEREALS, GRANOLA, HOMEMADE	1	CUP	122.0	594	67	15	33
8038	CEREALS, GRAPE-NUTS	1	CUP	113.6	406	93	13	0
8039	CEREALS, GRAPE-NUTS FLAKES	1	CUP	32.5	116	27	3	0
8040	CEREALS, HEARTLAND NATURAL CEREAL, PLAIN	1	CUP	115.0	499	79	12	18
8041	CEREALS, HEARTLAND NATURAL CEREAL, W/ COCNT	1	CUP	105.0	463	71	11	17
8042	CEREALS, HEARTLAND NATURAL CEREAL, W/ RAISINS	1	CUP	110.0	468	76	11	16
8043	CEREALS, HONEY AND NUT CORN FLAKES	1	CUP	37.9	151	31	2	2
8045	CEREALS, HONEY NUT CHEERIOS	1	CUP	33.0	125	26	4	1
8044	CEREALS, HONEYBRAN	1	CUP	35.0	119	29	3	1
8046	CEREALS, HONEYCOMB	1	CUP	22.0	86	20	1	0
8048	CEREALS, KIX	1	CUP	18.9	74	16	2	0
8049	CEREALS, LIFE, PLAIN AND CINN PRODUCTS	1	CUP	44.0	162	32	8	1
8050	CEREALS, LUCKY CHARMS	1	CUP	32.0	125	26	3	1
8178	CEREALS, MALT-O-MEAL, PLAIN AND CHOC	1	CUP	240.0	122	26	4	0
8179	CEREALS, MAYPO, CKD W/ WATER, W/ SALT	1	CUP	240.0	170	32	6	2
8119	CEREALS, MAYPO, CKD W/ WATER, W/O SALT	1	CUP	240.0	170	32	6	2
8051	CEREALS, MOST BRAND	1	CUP	52.0	175	40	7	1
8052	CEREALS, NATURE VALLEY GRANOLA	1	CUP	113.0	503	75	12	20
8149	CEREALS, NUTRI-GRAIN, BARLEY	1	CUP	41.0	153	34	4	0
8150	CEREALS, NUTRI-GRAIN, CORN	1	CUP	42.0	160	35	3	1
8151	CEREALS, NUTRI-GRAIN, RYE	1	CUP	40.0	144	34	3	0
8152	CEREALS, NUTRI-GRAIN, WHEAT	1	CUP	44.0	158	37	4	0
8123	CEREALS, OATS, INSTANT, PLAIN	1	PKT.	177.0	104	18	4	2
8125	CEREALS, OATS, INSTANT, W/ APPLES AND CINN	1	PKT.	149.0	136	26	4	2
8127	CEREALS, OATS, INSTANT, W/ BRAN&RSNS	1	PKT.	195.0	158	30	5	2
8129	CEREALS, OATS, INSTANT, W/ CINN AND SPICE	1	PKT.	161.0	177	35	5	2
8131	CEREALS, OATS, INSTANT, W/ MAPL&BRN SUG FLAV	1	PKT.	155.0	163	32	5	2
8133	CEREALS, OATS, INSTANT, W/ RAISINS AND SPICE	1	PKT.	158.0	161	32	4	2
8180	CEREALS, OATS, REG AND QUICK AND INSTANT	1	CUP	234.0	145	25	6	2
8058	CEREALS, PRODUCT 19	1	CUP	33.0	126	27	3	0
8059	CEREALS, QUISP	1	CUP	30.0	124	25	2	2
8060	CEREALS, RAISIN BRAN, KELLOGG'S	1	CUP	49.2	154	37	5	1
8061	CEREALS, RAISIN BRAN, POST	1	CUP	56.8	174	43	5	1
8062	CEREALS, RAISIN BRAN, RALSTON PURINA	1	CUP	56.0	178	46	4	0
8063	CEREALS, RAISINS, RICE AND RYE	1	CUP	46.0	155	39	3	0
8064	CEREALS, RICE CHEX	1	CUP	25.2	100	23	1	0
8065	CEREALS, RICE KRISPIES	1	CUP	28.4	112	25	2	0
8156	CEREALS, RICE, PUFFED	1	CUP	14.0	56	13	1	0
8067	CEREALS, SPECIAL K	1	CUP	21.3	83	16	4	0
8068	CEREALS, SUGAR CORN POPS	1	CUP	28.4	108	26	1	0
8069	CEREALS, SUGAR FROSTED FLAKES	1	CUP	35.0	133	32	2	0
8074	CEREALS, TASTEEOS	1	CUP	24.0	94	19	3	1
8075	CEREALS, TEAM	1	CUP	42.0	164	36	3	1
8077	CEREALS, TOTAL	1	CUP	33.0	116	26	3	1
8078	CEREALS, TRIX	1	CUP	28.0	108	25	2	0
8080	CEREALS, WHEAT 'N RAISIN CHEX	1	CUP	54.0	185	43	5	0

Saturated fat (g)	Monounsaturated fat (g)	Polyunsaturated fat (g)	Fiber (g)	Cholesterol (g)	Folate (g)	Vitamin A (RE)	Vitamin B-6 (mg)	Vitamin B-12 (µg)	Vitamin C (mg)	Vitamin E (mg)	Riboflavin (mg)	Thiamin (mg)	Calcium (mg)	Iron (mg)	Magnesium (mg)	Niacin (mg)	Phosphorus (mg)	Potassium (mg)	Sodium (mg)	Zinc (mg)
-	-	-	0	0	2	10	0	0	0	-	0	0	11	.6	3	.1	12	18	3	.1
-	-	-	0	0	2	10	0	0	0	-	0	.1	2	.6	3	1.1	10	22	239	.1
-	-	-	10	0	212	794	1.1	0	32	-	.9	.8	40	3.8	116	10.6	241	355	487	3.2
-	-	-	-	0	7	0	.1	0	0	-	0	0	7	.5	7	1	41	49	422	.4
-	-	-	-	0	10	0	0	0	0	-	0	.2	60	12.1	14	1.7	43	48	364	.4
-	-	-	-	0	10	0	0	0	0	-	0	.2	50	10.3	12	1.4	100	45	464	.3
-	-	-	-	0	10	0	0	0	0	-	0	.3	50	10.3	10	1.5	43	43	336	.3
-	-	-	-	0	3	0	0	0	0	-	0	0	17	.8	10	.4	27	20	3	.4
-	-	-	0	0	3	0	0	.1	1	-	0	.1	5	.7	12	2	31	27	206	.5
-	-	-	3	0	15	569	.8	2.3	0	-	.6	.6	71	6.8	34	7.6	117	174	204	.5
-	-	-	1	0	169	636	.9	2.5	0	-	.7	.6	68	13.7	58	8.4	176	343	429	1.5
-	-	-	1	0	100	376	.5	0	15	-	.4	.4	3	4.5	7	5	24	26	145	3.7
1	0	0	1	0	6	516	.7	2.1	21	-	.6	.5	24	6.2	16	6.9	56	86	385	.3
-	-	-	2	0	106	397	.5	0	16	-	.4	.4	14	1.9	25	5.3	66	108	196	1.6
6	9	17	13	0	99	-	.4	0	1	-	.3	.7	76	4.8	142	2.1	494	612	12	4.5
-	-	-	11	0	401	1504	2	6	0	-	1.7	1.5	11	4.9	76	20	285	379	790	2.5
-	-	-	3	0	115	430	.6	1.7	0	-	.5	.4	13	9.3	36	5.7	97	113	183	.6
-	-	-	7	0	64	-	.2	0	1	-	.2	.4	75	4.3	147	1.6	416	385	293	3
-	-	-	7	0	57	-	.2	0	1	-	.1	.3	66	5.4	138	1.8	380	384	213	2.7
-	-	-	6	0	44	-	.2	0	1	-	.1	.3	66	4	141	1.5	376	415	226	2.8
-	-	-	0	0	134	501	.7	0	20	-	.6	.5	5	2.4	8	6.7	17	48	301	.1
0	0	0	1	0	21	437	.6	1.7	17	-	.5	.4	23	5.2	39	5.8	122	115	299	.9
-	-	-	4	0	23	463	.6	1.9	19	-	.5	.5	16	5.6	46	6.2	132	151	202	.9
-	-	-	1	0	78	291	.4	1.2	0	-	.3	.3	4	2.1	7	3.9	22	70	124	1.2
0	0	0	0	0	67	251	.3	1	10	-	.3	.2	24	5.4	8	3.3	26	30	194	.2
-	-	-	3	0	37	-	.1	0	-	-	1	1	154	11.6	14	11.6	238	197	229	1.5
0	0	0	1	0	6	424	.6	1.7	17	-	.5	.4	36	5.1	27	5.6	89	66	227	.6
-	-	-	-	0	5	0	0	0	0	-	.2	.5	5	9.6	5	5.8	24	31	324	.2
-	-	-	-	0	10	703	1	2.9	29	-	.7	.7	125	8.4	50	9.4	247	211	259	1.5
-	-	-	6	0	10	703	1	2.9	29	-	.7	.7	125	8.4	50	9.4	247	211	10	1.5
-	-	-	7	0	734	2754	3.7	11	110	-	3.1	2.8	79	33	103	36.7	361	340	276	2.8
13	3	3	6	0	85	-	.1	0	0	-	.2	.4	71	3.8	115	.8	354	389	233	2.2
-	-	-	2	0	145	543	.7	2.2	22	-	.6	.5	11	1.4	32	7.2	126	108	277	5.4
-	-	-	3	0	148	556	.8	2.2	22	-	.6	.5	1	.9	27	7.4	121	98	276	5.5
-	-	-	3	0	141	530	.7	2.1	21	-	.6	.5	8	1.1	30	7	104	72	272	5.3
-	-	-	3	0	155	583	.8	2.3	23	-	.7	.6	12	1.2	34	7.7	165	120	299	5.8
-	-	-	3	0	150	453	.7	0	0	-	.3	.5	163	6.3	42	5.5	133	99	285	.9
-	-	-	-	0	137	435	.7	0	0	-	.3	.5	158	6.1	34	5.1	118	107	222	.7
-	-	-	-	0	156	480	.8	0	0	-	.6	.6	174	7.6	57	8.1	207	236	248	1.3
-	-	-	3	0	153	473	.8	0	0	-	.3	.6	172	6.6	52	5.7	145	105	280	1
-	-	-	-	0	146	451	.7	0	0	-	.3	.5	161	6.4	42	5.3	143	102	279	.9
-	-	-	2	0	150	441	.7	0	0	-	.4	.5	166	6.6	36	5.5	133	150	226	.7
0	1	1	-	0	9	-	0	0	0	-	0	.3	19	1.6	56	.3	178	131	374	1.1
-	-	-	1	0	466	1748	2.3	7	70	-	2	1.7	4	21	12	23.3	47	51	378	.5
1	0	0	1	0	8	5	.9	2.6	0	-	.8	.5	9	6.3	12	5.8	25	45	241	.2
-	-	-	5	0	133	500	.7	2	0	-	.6	.5	17	22.3	63	6.7	183	256	273	5
-	-	-	8	0	201	752	1	3	0	-	.9	.7	27	9	97	10	238	350	370	3
-	-	-	8	0	148	556	.7	2.2	2	-	.6	.6	27	27.3	85	7.4	248	287	486	1.7
-	-	-	3	0	125	468	.6	1.9	0	-	.6	.5	10	5.6	20	6.3	50	144	350	4.7
-	-	-	0	0	89	2	.5	1.3	13	-	0	.4	4	1.6	6	4.4	25	29	211	.3
-	-	-	0	0	100	376	.5	0	15	-	.4	.4	4	1.8	10	5	34	30	341	.5
-	-	-	-	0	3	0	0	0	0	-	.3	.4	1	4.4	4	4.9	14	16	0	.1
-	-	-	1	0	75	282	.4	0	11	-	.3	.3	6	3.4	12	3.7	41	37	199	2.8
-	-	-	0	0	100	376	.5	0	15	-	.4	.4	1	1.8	2	5	28	17	104	1.5
-	-	-	1	0	124	463	.6	0	19	-	.5	.5	1	2.2	3	6.2	26	22	284	0
-	-	-	3	0	9	318	.4	1.3	13	-	.4	.3	11	3.8	26	4.2	96	71	183	.7
-	-	-	1	0	7	556	.8	2.2	22	-	.6	.5	6	2.6	18	7.4	65	71	260	1
0	0	0	4	0	466	1748	2.3	7	70	-	2	1.7	282	21	37	23.3	137	123	326	.8
-	-	-	0	0	3	371	.5	1.5	15	-	.4	.4	6	4.5	6	4.9	19	26	179	.1
-	-	-	4	0	143	0	.7	2.2	2	-	.6	.5	24	7.7	53	7.1	163	227	306	1.2

Food Composition Table—cont'd

Code	Name	Amount	Unit	Grams	Kilocalories	Carbohydrates (g)	Protein (g)	Fat (g)
8082	CEREALS, WHEAT CHEX	1	CUP	46.0	169	38	5	1
8147	CEREALS, WHEAT, SHREDDED, LARGE BISCUIT	1	BISCUIT	23.6	83	19	3	0
8148	CEREALS, WHEAT, SHREDDED, SMALL BISCUIT	1	CUP	33.1	119	26	4	1
8143	CEREALS, WHEATENA, CKD W/ WATER	1	CUP	243.0	136	29	5	1
8182	CEREALS, WHEATENA, CKD W/ WATER, W/ SALT	1	CUP	243.0	136	29	5	1
8089	CEREALS, WHEATIES	1	CUP	29.0	101	23	3	0
8183	CEREALS, WHOLE WHEAT HOT NATURAL CEREAL	1	CUP	242.0	150	33	5	1
55832	CHEDDAR CHEESE SAUCE-STOUFFER'S	1	CUP	283.9	731	22	26	60
55764	CHEDDAR CHEESE SOUP-STOUFFER'S	1	CUP	283.9	441	18	21	31
55772	CHEDDAR CHEESE, HEAT'N SERVE SOUP -STOUFFER'S	1	CUP	307.6	488	22	22	36
55196	CHEESE CANNELLONI, LEAN CUISINE-STOUFFER'S	1	EACH	258.7	270	27	23	8
55108	CHEESE ENCHILADAS-STOUFFER'S	1	EACH	276.4	490	33	23	29
41331	CHEESE FRENCH BREAD PIZZA-HEALTHY CHOICE	1	EACH	159.5	290	46	19	4
41300	CHEESE MANICOTTI-HEALTHY CHOICE	1	EACH	262.2	220	34	15	3
55796	CHEESE MANICOTTI-STOUFFER'S	1	OUNCE	28.4	29	3	2	1
55822	CHEESE RAVIOLI-STOUFFER'S	1	OUNCE	28.4	54	6	3	2
1150	CHEESE SPREAD, PAST. PROCESSED, AMERICAN	2	OUNCE	56.7	165	5	9	12
55808	CHEESE STUFFED SHELLS-STOUFFER'S	1	OUNCE	28.4	28	3	2	1
55819	CHEESE TORTELLINI W/ EGG PASTA-STOUFFER'S	1	EACH	145.3	212	22	11	8
55821	CHEESE TORTELLINI W/ SPINACH PASTA-STOUFFER'S	1	OUNCE	28.4	56	6	3	2
1147	CHEESE, AMERICAN, PASTUERIZED PROCESSED	2	OUNCE	56.7	213	1	13	18
1004	CHEESE, BLUE	1½	OUNCE	42.5	150	1	9	12
1005	CHEESE, BRICK	1½	OUNCE	42.5	158	1	10	13
1006	CHEESE, BRIE	1½	OUNCE	42.5	142	0	9	12
1008	CHEESE, CARAWAY	1½	OUNCE	42.5	160	1	11	12
1009	CHEESE, CHEDDAR, AMERICAN DOMESTIC	1½	OUNCE	42.5	171	1	11	14
62577	CHEESE, CHEDDAR, REDUCED FAT	1½	OUNCE	42.5	120	2	12	8
1011	CHEESE, COLBY	1½	OUNCE	42.5	167	1	10	14
1012	CHEESE, COTTAGE, CREAMED	1½	OUNCE	42.5	44	1	5	2
1013	CHEESE, COTTAGE, CREAMED, W/ FRUIT	1½	OUNCE	42.5	53	6	4	1
1016	CHEESE, COTTAGE, LOWFAT, 1% FAT	1½	OUNCE	42.5	31	1	5	0
1015	CHEESE, COTTAGE, LOWFAT, 2% FAT	1½	OUNCE	42.5	38	2	6	1
1014	CHEESE, COTTAGE, UNCREAMED, DRY	1½	OUNCE	42.5	36	1	7	0
1017	CHEESE, CREAM	1½	OUNCE	42.5	148	1	3	15
62554	CHEESE, CREAM, FAT FREE	2	TBSP.	35.0	35	2	5	0
62553	CHEESE, CREAM, LIGHT	2	TBSP.	32.0	70	2	3	5
1018	CHEESE, EDAM	1½	OUNCE	42.5	152	1	11	12
62579	CHEESE, FAT FREE SLICES, WHITE	1	SLICE	21.3	30	2	5	0
62578	CHEESE, FAT FREE SLICES, YELLOW	1	SLICE	21.3	30	2	5	0
1019	CHEESE, FETA	1½	OUNCE	42.5	112	2	6	9
1020	CHEESE, FONTINA	1½	OUNCE	42.5	165	1	11	13
1156	CHEESE, GOAT, HARD TYPE	1½	OUNCE	42.5	192	1	13	15
1157	CHEESE, GOAT, SEMISOFT TYPE	1½	OUNCE	42.5	155	1	9	13
1159	CHEESE, GOAT, SOFT TYPE	1½	OUNCE	42.5	114	0	8	9
1022	CHEESE, GOUDA	1½	OUNCE	42.5	152	1	11	12
1023	CHEESE, GRUYERE	1½	OUNCE	42.5	176	0	13	14
1024	CHEESE, LIMBURGER	1½	OUNCE	42.5	139	0	9	12
1025	CHEESE, MONTEREY	1½	OUNCE	42.5	159	0	10	13
62576	CHEESE, MONTEREY, REDUCED FAT	1½	OUNCE	42.5	120	2	12	8
1028	CHEESE, MOZZARELLA, PART SKIM MILK	1½	OUNCE	42.5	108	1	10	7
1029	CHEESE, MOZZARELLA, PART SKIM MILK, LOW MOISTURE	1½	OUNCE	42.5	119	1	12	7
1026	CHEESE, MOZZARELLA, WHOLE MILK	1½	OUNCE	42.5	120	1	8	9
1027	CHEESE, MOZZARELLA, WHOLE MILK, LOW MOISTURE	1½	OUNCE	42.5	135	1	9	10
1161	CHEESE, MOZZERELLA, SUBSTITUTE	1½	OUNCE	42.5	105	10	5	5
1030	CHEESE, MUENSTER	1½	OUNCE	42.5	157	0	10	13
1032	CHEESE, PARMESAN, GRATED	1	TBSP.	5.0	23	0	2	2
62608	CHEESE, PARMESAN, GRATED, FAT FREE	1	TBSP.	5.0	5	1	1	0
1033	CHEESE, PARMESAN, PIECE	1½	OUNCE	42.5	167	1	15	11
1146	CHEESE, PARMESAN, SHREDDED	1½	OUNCE	42.5	176	1	16	12
1035	CHEESE, PROVOLONE	1½	OUNCE	42.5	149	1	11	11

Saturated fat (g)	Monounsaturated fat (g)	Polyunsaturated fat (g)	Fiber (g)	Cholesterol (g)	Folate (g)	Vitamin A (RE)	Vitamin B-6 (mg)	Vitamin B-12 (µg)	Vitamin C (mg)	Vitamin E (mg)	Riboflavin (mg)	Thiamin (mg)	Calcium (mg)	Iron (mg)	Magnesium (mg)	Niacin (mg)	Phosphorus (mg)	Potassium (mg)	Sodium (mg)	Zinc (mg)
-	-	-	4	0	162	0	.8	2.4	24	-	.2	.6	18	7.3	58	8.1	182	173	308	1.2
-	-	-	2	0	12	0	.1	0	0	-	.1	.1	10	.7	40	1.1	86	77	0	.6
-	-	-	3	0	17	0	.1	0	0	-	.1	.1	13	1.4	44	1.7	117	120	3	1.1
-	-	-	7	0	17	0	0	0	0	-	0	0	10	1.4	49	1.3	146	187	5	1.7
-	-	-	-	0	17	0	0	0	0	-	0	0	10	1.4	49	1.3	146	187	578	1.7
0	0	0	3	0	102	384	.5	1.5	15	-	.4	.4	44	4.6	32	5.1	100	108	276	.6
-	-	-	-	0	27	0	.2	0	0	-	.1	.2	17	1.5	53	2.2	167	172	564	1.2
-	-	-	-	130	-	-	-	-	-	0	0	0	6329	.1	-	0	-	341	1392	-
-	-	-	-	70	-	-	-	-	-	0	0	0	4967	0	-	.2	-	511	681	-
-	-	-	-	98	-	-	-	-	-	0	0	0	4947	.1	-	.2	-	553	770	-
4	-	-	-	25	-	60	-	-	21	-	.3	.1	240	.4	-	1.5	-	400	590	-
-	-	-	-	-	-	150	-	-	6	-	.3	.1	480	.8	-	1.5	-	400	550	-
2	-	1	-	15	-	20	-	-	0	-	.3	.5	240	2	-	2.9	240	310	390	-
2	-	-	-	30	-	250	-	-	6	-	.3	.3	120	1.5	-	1.9	210	590	310	-
-	-	-	-	4	-	-	-	-	2	-	0	0	296	0	-	0	-	45	108	-
-	-	-	-	14	-	-	-	-	0	-	0	0	336	0	-	0	-	16	52	-
8	4	0	0	31	4	107	.1	.2	0	-	.2	0	319	.2	16	.1	496	137	921	1.5
-	-	-	-	3	-	-	-	-	1	-	0	0	248	0	-	.1	-	53	59	-
-	-	-	-	63	-	-	-	-	0	-	0	0	1524	.1	-	.2	-	71	272	-
-	-	-	-	19	-	-	-	-	0	-	0	0	456	0	-	.1	-	26	79	-
11	5	1	0	54	4	164	0	.4	0	-	.2	0	349	.2	13	.1	252	92	369	1.7
8	3	0	0	32	15	97	.1	.5	0	-	.2	0	224	.1	10	.4	165	109	593	1.1
8	4	0	0	40	9	128	0	.5	0	-	.1	0	286	.2	10	.1	192	58	238	1.1
7	3	0	0	43	28	77	.1	.7	0	-	.2	0	78	.2	9	.2	80	65	268	1
8	4	0	0	40	8	123	0	.1	0	-	.2	0	286	.3	9	.1	208	40	293	1.3
9	4	0	0	45	8	129	0	.4	0	-	.2	0	307	.3	12	0	218	42	264	1.3
5	-	-	0	23	-	90	-	-	0	-	-	-	360	0	-	-	-	35	270	-
9	4	0	0	40	8	117	0	.4	0	-	.2	0	291	.3	11	0	194	54	257	1.3
1	1	0	0	6	5	20	0	.3	0	-	.1	0	26	.1	2	.1	56	36	172	.2
1	0	0	0	5	4	15	0	.2	0	-	.1	0	20	0	2	0	44	28	172	.1
0	0	0	0	2	5	5	0	.3	0	-	.1	0	26	.1	2	.1	57	36	173	.2
1	0	0	0	4	6	9	0	.3	0	-	.1	0	29	.1	3	.1	64	41	173	.2
0	0	0	0	3	6	3	0	.4	0	-	.1	0	13	.1	2	.1	44	14	5	.2
9	4	1	0	47	6	186	0	.2	0	-	.1	0	34	.5	3	0	44	51	126	.2
0	-	-	-	5	-	100	-	-	0	-	-	-	120	0	-	-	-	-	180	-
4	-	-	-	15	-	80	-	-	0	-	-	-	48	0	-	-	-	-	150	-
7	3	0	0	38	7	108	0	.7	0	-	.2	0	311	.2	13	0	228	80	410	1.6
0	-	-	0	0	-	40	-	-	0	-	-	-	120	0	-	-	-	18	310	-
0	-	-	0	0	-	40	-	-	0	-	-	-	120	0	-	-	-	18	310	-
6	2	0	0	38	14	54	.2	.7	0	-	.4	.1	209	.3	8	.4	143	26	475	1.2
8	4	1	0	49	3	123	0	.7	0	-	.1	0	234	.1	6	.1	147	27	340	1.5
10	3	0	-	45	2	663	0	.1	0	-	.5	.1	381	.8	23	1	310	20	147	.7
9	3	0	0	34	1	702	0	.1	0	-	.3	0	127	.7	12	.5	159	67	219	.3
6	2	0	0	20	5	578	.1	.1	0	-	.2	0	60	.8	7	.2	109	11	156	.4
7	3	0	0	48	9	74	0	.7	0	-	.1	0	298	.1	12	0	232	51	348	1.7
8	4	1	0	47	4	128	0	.7	0	-	.1	0	430	.1	15	0	257	34	143	1.7
7	4	0	0	38	24	134	0	.4	0	-	.2	0	211	.1	9	.1	167	54	340	.9
8	4	0	0	38	8	108	0	.4	0	-	.2	0	317	.3	11	0	189	34	228	1.3
5	-	-	0	23	-	90	-	-	0	-	-	-	360	0	-	-	-	27	270	-
4	2	0	0	25	4	75	0	.3	0	-	.1	0	275	.1	10	0	197	36	198	1.2
5	2	0	0	23	4	81	0	.4	0	-	.1	0	311	.1	11	.1	223	40	224	1.3
6	3	0	0	33	3	102	0	.3	0	-	.1	0	220	.1	8	0	158	29	159	.9
7	3	0	0	38	3	117	0	.3	0	-	.1	0	244	.1	9	0	175	32	176	1
2	3	1	0	0	5	186	0	.3	0	-	.2	0	259	.2	17	.1	248	193	291	.8
8	4	0	0	41	5	134	0	.6	0	-	.1	0	305	.2	12	0	199	57	267	1.2
1	0	0	0	4	0	9	0	.1	0	-	0	0	69	0	3	0	40	5	93	.2
0	0	0	0	2	-	0	-	-	0	-	-	-	16	0	-	-	-	10	15	-
7	3	0	0	29	3	63	0	.5	0	-	.1	0	503	.3	19	.1	295	39	681	1.2
7	4	0	0	31	3	74	0	.6	0	-	.1	0	533	.4	22	.1	313	41	721	1.4
7	3	0	0	29	4	112	0	.6	0	-	.1	0	321	.2	12	.1	211	59	372	1.4

Food Composition Table—cont'd

Code	Name	Amount	Unit	Grams	Kilocalories	Carbohydrates (g)	Protein (g)	Fat (g)
1037	CHEESE, RICOTTA, PART SKIM MILK	1½	OUNCE	42.5	59	2	5	3
1036	CHEESE, RICOTTA, WHOLE MILK	1½	OUNCE	42.5	74	1	5	6
1038	CHEESE, ROMANO	1½	OUNCE	42.5	164	2	14	11
1039	CHEESE, ROQUEFORT	1½	OUNCE	42.5	157	1	9	13
1040	CHEESE, SWISS, DOMESTIC	1½	OUNCE	42.5	160	1	12	12
1044	CHEESE, SWISS, PASTEURIZED PROCESSED	2	OUNCE	56.7	189	1	14	14
18147	CHEESECAKE, COMMERCIALLY PREPARED	1	SLICE	85.0	273	22	5	19
18149	CHEESECAKE, HOMEMADE	1	SLICE	85.0	303	21	6	22
18148	CHEESECAKE, NO-BAKE TYPE	1	SLICE	80.0	219	28	4	10
18382	CHEESECAKE, PLAIN, W/ CHERRY TOPPING	1	SLICE	90.0	258	24	5	17
9066	CHERRIES, SOUR, RED, CND, HEAVY SYRUP PACK	½	CUP	128.0	116	30	1	0
9065	CHERRIES, SOUR, RED, CND, LIGHT SYRUP PACK	½	CUP	126.0	95	24	1	0
9064	CHERRIES, SOUR, RED, CND, WATER PACK	½	CUP	122.0	44	11	1	0
9067	CHERRIES, SOUR, RED, CND, X-HEAVY SYRUP PACK	½	CUP	130.5	149	38	1	0
9063	CHERRIES, SOUR, RED, FRESH	½	CUP	51.5	26	6	1	0
9074	CHERRIES, SWEET, CND, HEAVY SYRUP PACK	½	CUP	128.5	107	27	1	0
9072	CHERRIES, SWEET, CND, JUICE PACK	½	CUP	125.0	67	17	1	0
9073	CHERRIES, SWEET, CND, LIGHT SYRUP PACK	½	CUP	126.0	84	22	1	0
9071	CHERRIES, SWEET, CND, WATER PACK	½	CUP	124.0	57	15	1	0
9075	CHERRIES, SWEET, CND, X-HEAVY SYRUP PACK	½	CUP	130.5	133	34	1	0
9070	CHERRIES, SWEET, FRESH	½	CUP	72.5	52	12	1	1
9076	CHERRIES, SWEET, FROZEN, SWEETENED	½	CUP	129.5	115	29	1	0
18308	CHERRY PIE	1	SLICE	125.0	325	50	3	14
18444	CHERRY PIE, FRIED	1	PIE	128.0	404	55	4	21
19163	CHEWING GUM	1	STICK	3.0	10	3	0	0
19033	CHEX MIX	1	CUP	42.5	181	28	5	7
55109	CHICKEN A LA KING W/ RICE-STOUFFER'S	1	EACH	269.3	270	38	18	5
43397	CHICKEN A LA KING, TOP SHELF-HORMEL	1	EACH	283.5	360	49	18	10
57799	CHICKEN A LA KING-SWANSON	1	EACH	250.0	319	15	17	20
55197	CHICKEN A LA ORANGE, LEAN CUISINE-STOUFFER'S	1	EACH	226.8	280	33	27	4
41301	CHICKEN A LA ORANGE-HEALTHY CHOICE	1	EACH	255.1	240	36	20	2
55792	CHICKEN AND DUMPLINGS-STOUFFER'S	1	EACH	220.0	303	24	15	16
57801	CHICKEN AND DUMPLINGS-SWANSON	1	EACH	200.0	207	18	10	10
41253	CHICKEN AND PASTA DIVAN-HEALTHY CHOICE	1	EACH	340.2	300	41	25	4
55794	CHICKEN AND VEG. ORIENTAL-STOUFFER'S	1	EACH	220.0	186	14	12	9
55198	CHICKEN AND VEG. W/ VERMICELLI, LEAN CUISINE-STOUFFER'S	1	EACH	333.1	240	30	18	5
41302	CHICKEN AND VEGETABLES-HEALTHY CHOICE	1	EACH	326.0	210	31	20	1
55199	CHICKEN CACCIATORE, LEAN CUISINE-STOUFFER'S	1	EACH	308.3	280	31	22	7
43398	CHICKEN CACCIATORE, TOP SHELF-HORMEL	1	EACH	283.5	210	25	21	3
55200	CHICKEN CHOW MEIN W/ RICE, LEAN CUISINE-STOUFFER'S	1	EACH	255.1	240	34	14	5
55110	CHICKEN CHOW MEIN W/ RICE-STOUFFER'S	1	EACH	304.8	250	39	13	5
41303	CHICKEN CHOW MEIN-HEALTHY CHOICE	1	EACH	241.0	220	31	18	3
62611	CHICKEN CHOW MEIN-WEIGHT WATCHERS	1	EACH	255.2	200	34	12	2
55807	CHICKEN CLASSICA -STOUFFER'S	1	OUNCE	28.4	22	2	2	1
41336	CHICKEN CON QUESO BURRITOS (MILD)-HEALTHY CHOICE	1	EACH	148.8	280	40	15	8
41254	CHICKEN DIJON-HEALTHY CHOICE	1	EACH	311.8	250	40	21	3
55111	CHICKEN DIVAN-STOUFFER'S	1	EACH	226.8	220	11	24	10
62618	CHICKEN ENCHILADAS SUIZA-WEIGHT WATCHERS	1	EACH	255.2	250	28	15	8
55201	CHICKEN ENCHILADAS, LEAN CUISINE-STOUFFER'S	1	EACH	280.0	290	34	17	9
41304	CHICKEN ENCHILADAS-HEALTHY CHOICE	1	EACH	269.3	310	44	14	9
55112	CHICKEN ENCHILADAS-STOUFFER'S	1	EACH	283.5	490	31	21	31
41305	CHICKEN FAJITAS-HEALTHY CHOICE	1	EACH	198.5	200	25	17	3
55203	CHICKEN FETTUCINI, LEAN CUISINE-STOUFFER'S	1	EACH	255.1	280	33	23	6
41306	CHICKEN FETTUCINI-HEALTHY CHOICE	1	EACH	241.0	240	29	22	4
62620	CHICKEN FETTUCINI-WEIGHT WATCHERS	1	EACH	233.9	280	25	22	9
55763	CHICKEN GUMBO SOUP-STOUFFER'S	1	CUP	283.9	110	9	7	5
55202	CHICKEN IN BBQ SAUCE, LEAN CUISINE-STOUFFER'S	1	EACH	248.1	260	32	20	6
55204	CHICKEN ITALIANO, LEAN CUISINE-STOUFFER'S	1	EACH	255.1	270	33	22	6
55789	CHICKEN ITALIENNE-STOUFFER'S	1	OUNCE	28.4	22	1	2	1
55755	CHICKEN NOODLE SOUP-STOUFFER'S	1	CUP	283.9	130	10	7	7

Saturated fat (g)	Monounsaturated fat (g)	Polyunsaturated fat (g)	Fiber (g)	Cholesterol (g)	Folate (g)	Vitamin A (RE)	Vitamin B-6 (mg)	Vitamin B-12 (μg)	Vitamin C (mg)	Vitamin E (mg)	Riboflavin (mg)	Thiamin (mg)	Calcium (mg)	Iron (mg)	Magnesium (mg)	Niacin (mg)	Phosphorus (mg)	Potassium (mg)	Sodium (mg)	Zinc (mg)
2	1	0	0	13	6	48	0	.1	0	-	.1	0	116	.2	6	0	78	53	53	.6
4	2	0	0	22	5	57	0	.1	0	-	.1	0	88	.2	5	0	67	44	36	.5
7	3	0	0	44	3	60	0	.5	0	-	.2	0	452	.3	17	0	323	37	510	1.1
8	4	1	0	38	21	127	.1	.3	0	-	.2	0	281	.2	13	.3	167	39	769	.9
8	3	0	0	39	3	108	0	.7	0	-	.2	0	409	.1	15	0	257	47	111	1.7
9	4	0	0	48	3	130	0	.7	0	-	.2	0	438	.3	17	0	432	122	777	2
10	7	1	2	47	13	137	0	.1	1	-	.2	0	43	.5	9	.2	79	77	176	.4
12	7	2	-	103	10	273	0	.2	0	-	.2	0	49	1.1	7	.3	82	87	241	.5
6	3	1	2	34	14	79	0	.2	0	-	.2	.1	138	.4	15	.4	187	169	304	.4
9	5	1	-	77	9	217	0	.2	1	-	.1	0	39	1.1	6	.3	64	84	183	.4
0	0	0	1	0	10	91	.1	0	3	-	0	0	13	1.7	8	.2	13	119	9	.1
0	0	0	-	0	10	92	.1	0	3	-	0	0	13	1.7	8	.2	13	120	9	.1
0	0	0	1	0	10	92	.1	0	3	-	.1	0	13	1.7	7	.2	12	120	9	.1
0	0	0	-	0	10	91	.1	0	2	-	0	0	13	1.6	7	.2	12	119	9	.1
0	0	0	1	0	4	66	0	0	5	.1	0	0	8	.2	5	.2	8	89	2	.1
0	0	0	1	0	5	19	0	0	5	-	.1	0	12	.4	12	.5	23	186	4	.1
0	0	0	1	0	5	16	0	0	3	-	0	0	17	.7	15	.5	27	164	4	.1
0	0	0	1	0	5	20	0	0	5	-	.1	0	11	.5	11	.5	23	186	4	.1
0	0	0	1	0	5	20	0	0	3	-	.1	0	14	.4	11	.5	19	162	1	.1
0	0	0	-	0	5	20	0	0	5	-	.1	0	12	.5	10	.5	22	185	4	.1
0	0	0	2	0	3	15	0	0	5	-	0	0	11	.3	8	.3	14	162	0	0
0	0	0	1	0	5	25	0	0	1	-	.1	0	16	.5	13	.2	21	258	1	.1
3	7	3	1	0	10	-	.1	0	1	-	0	0	15	.6	10	.3	36	101	308	.2
3	10	7	-	-	4	22	0	.1	2	-	.1	.2	28	1.6	13	1.8	55	83	479	.3
-	-	-	0	0	0	0	0	0	0	-	0	0	0	0	0	0	0	0	0	0
-	-	-	-	0	0	6	.7	5.3	20	-	.2	.7	15	10.5	27	7.2	80	114	432	.9
-	-	-	-	-	-	20	-	-	1	-	.2	.1	160	.8	-	2.9	32	260	800	-
4	4	2	-	37	-	250	-	-	1	-	.2	.1	48	.2	28	8.6	-	476	890	1.2
-	-	-	-	-	-	-	-	-	-	-	.2	.1	54	.3	-	3.2	-	-	1159	-
1	-	-	-	55	-	80	-	-	12	-	.2	.2	32	.4	-	9.5	-	490	290	-
2	-	-	-	45	-	150	-	-	27	-	.1	.2	16	.8	-	5.7	230	430	220	-
-	-	-	-	70	-	-	-	-	0	-	0	0	1055	.2	-	.4	-	248	660	-
-	-	-	-	-	-	75	-	-	-	-	.1	0	15	.4	-	1.8	-	-	922	-
2	-	1	-	50	-	800	-	-	72	-	.3	.4	120	1	-	4.8	270	500	520	-
-	-	-	-	31	-	-	-	-	5	-	0	0	372	.1	-	.6	-	349	1079	-
1	-	1	-	30	-	150	-	-	6	-	.3	.3	64	1	-	5.7	-	500	500	-
-	-	-	-	35	-	150	-	-	9	-	.2	.3	32	1.5	-	3.8	190	390	490	-
2	-	1	-	45	-	100	-	-	9	-	.2	.2	32	.8	-	5.7	-	560	570	-
-	-	-	-	50	-	100	-	-	2	-	.3	.2	80	1	-	6.7	-	-	810	-
1	-	1	-	30	-	60	-	-	6	-	.2	.2	32	.6	-	4.8	-	350	530	-
-	-	-	-	-	-	80	-	-	12	-	.2	0	16	.4	-	1.9	-	340	720	-
1	-	1	-	45	-	80	-	-	4	-	.1	.2	16	.8	-	3.8	290	290	440	-
1	-	-	3	25	-	300	-	-	36	-	-	-	48	.4	-	-	-	360	430	-
1	-	-	-	5	-	-	-	-	1	-	0	0	112	0	-	.1	-	50	83	-
2	-	3	-	20	-	20	-	-	6	-	.3	.5	80	1.5	-	2.9	170	260	500	-
1	-	-	-	40	-	100	-	-	9	-	.1	.2	16	1	-	9.5	300	350	470	-
-	-	-	-	-	-	60	-	-	4	-	.2	.5	200	2	-	3.8	32	490	610	-
3	-	-	4	25	-	40	-	-	1	-	-	-	360	.8	-	-	-	470	570	-
3	-	2	-	55	-	250	-	-	6	-	.3	.2	120	1.5	-	2.9	-	450	500	-
3	-	1	-	35	-	80	-	-	21	-	.2	.2	80	.8	-	4.8	160	380	480	-
-	-	-	-	-	-	60	-	-	2	-	.3	.1	240	.6	-	2.9	-	420	860	-
1	-	1	-	35	-	150	-	-	9	-	.2	.2	64	1.5	-	3.8	210	360	310	-
3	-	-	-	35	-	-	-	-	-	-	.4	.3	120	.8	-	5.7	-	420	500	-
2	-	2	-	45	-	-	-	-	-	-	.2	.2	64	1	-	2.9	210	190	370	-
3	-	-	2	40	-	40	-	-	0	-	-	-	240	1	-	-	-	730	590	-
-	-	-	-	20	-	-	-	-	0	-	0	0	160	.1	-	.2	-	180	1422	-
1	-	2	-	50	-	250	-	-	18	-	.2	.2	48	.8	-	5.7	-	650	500	-
1	-	2	-	40	-	100	-	-	24	-	.3	.3	80	.8	-	5.7	-	600	590	-
-	-	-	-	7	-	-	-	-	1	-	0	0	48	0	-	.1	-	57	128	-
-	-	-	-	20	-	-	-	-	0	-	0	0	80	.1	-	.2	-	140	1282	-

Food Composition Table—cont'd

Code	Name	Amount	Unit	Grams	Kilocalories	Carbohydrates (g)	Protein (g)	Fat (g)
55768	CHICKEN NOODLE, HEAT'N SERVE SOUP-STOUFFER'S	1	CUP	283.9	320	28	13	17
55205	CHICKEN ORIENTAL, LEAN CUISINE-STOUFFER'S	1	EACH	255.1	280	31	22	7
41256	CHICKEN ORIENTAL-HEALTHY CHOICE	1	EACH	318.9	200	32	19	1
41257	CHICKEN PARMIGIANA-HEALTHY CHOICE	1	EACH	326.0	280	45	22	4
41271	CHICKEN PASTA SOUP-HEALTHY CHOICE	1	EACH	212.6	100	13	7	2
55113	CHICKEN PIE-STOUFFER'S	1	EACH	283.5	440	32	16	27
57807	CHICKEN POT PIE-SWANSON	1	EACH	198.5	380	35	11	22
55790	CHICKEN PRIMAVERA-STOUFFER'S	1	OUNCE	28.4	17	1	2	1
5280	CHICKEN ROLL, LIGHT MEAT	3	OUNCE	85.1	135	2	17	6
5283	CHICKEN SALAD SANDWICH SPREAD	3	OUNCE	85.1	170	6	10	11
5281	CHICKEN SPREAD, CND	3	OUNCE	85.1	163	5	13	10
41295	CHICKEN STIR FRY W/ BROCCOLI-HEALTHY CHOICE	1	EACH	340.2	280	35	21	6
55206	CHICKEN TENDERLOINS, LEAN CUISINE-STOUFFER'S	1	EACH	269.3	240	19	29	5
55820	CHICKEN TORTELLINI W/ EGG PASTA-STOUFFER'S	1	OUNCE	28.4	51	6	3	2
41248	CHICKEN W/ BARBEQUE SAUCE-HEALTHY CHOICE	1	EACH	361.5	410	65	24	6
41277	CHICKEN W/ RICE SOUP-HEALTHY CHOICE	1	EACH	212.6	90	14	5	1
5054	CHICKEN, BACK, MEAT ONLY, CKD, FRIED	3	OUNCE	85.1	245	5	26	13
5055	CHICKEN, BACK, MEAT ONLY, CKD, ROASTED	3	OUNCE	85.1	203	0	24	11
5056	CHICKEN, BACK, MEAT ONLY, CKD, STEWED	3	OUNCE	85.1	178	0	22	10
5049	CHICKEN, BACK, MEAT&SKIN, CKD, FRIED, BATTER	3	OUNCE	85.1	282	9	19	19
5050	CHICKEN, BACK, MEAT&SKIN, CKD, FRIED, FLR	3	OUNCE	85.1	282	6	24	18
5051	CHICKEN, BACK, MEAT&SKIN, CKD, ROASTED	3	OUNCE	85.1	255	0	22	18
5052	CHICKEN, BACK, MEAT&SKIN, CKD, STEWED	3	OUNCE	85.1	219	0	19	15
5063	CHICKEN, BREAST, MEAT ONLY, CKD, FRIED	3	OUNCE	85.1	159	0	28	4
5064	CHICKEN, BREAST, MEAT ONLY, CKD, ROASTED	3	OUNCE	85.1	140	0	26	3
5065	CHICKEN, BREAST, MEAT ONLY, CKD, STEWED	3	OUNCE	85.1	128	0	25	3
5058	CHICKEN, BREAST, MEAT&SKIN, CKD, FRIED, BATTER	3	OUNCE	85.1	221	8	21	11
5059	CHICKEN, BREAST, MEAT&SKIN, CKD, FRIED, FLR	3	OUNCE	85.1	189	1	27	8
5060	CHICKEN, BREAST, MEAT&SKIN, CKD, ROASTED	3	OUNCE	85.1	168	0	25	7
5061	CHICKEN, BREAST, MEAT&SKIN, CKD, STEWED	3	OUNCE	85.1	156	0	23	6
5044	CHICKEN, DARK MEAT, MEAT ONLY, CKD, FRIED	3	OUNCE	85.1	203	2	25	10
5045	CHICKEN, DARK MEAT, MEAT ONLY, CKD, ROASTED	3	OUNCE	85.1	174	0	23	8
5046	CHICKEN, DARK MEAT, MEAT ONLY, CKD, STEWED	3	OUNCE	85.1	163	0	22	8
5035	CHICKEN, DARK MEAT, MEAT&SKIN, CKD, FRIED, BATTER	3	OUNCE	85.1	253	8	19	16
5036	CHICKEN, DARK MEAT, MEAT&SKIN, CKD, FRIED, FLR	3	OUNCE	85.1	242	3	23	14
5037	CHICKEN, DARK MEAT, MEAT&SKIN, CKD, ROASTED	3	OUNCE	85.1	215	0	22	13
5038	CHICKEN, DARK MEAT, MEAT&SKIN, CKD, STEWED	3	OUNCE	85.1	198	0	20	12
5072	CHICKEN, DRUMSTICK, MEAT ONLY, CKD, FRIED	3	OUNCE	85.1	166	0	24	7
5073	CHICKEN, DRUMSTICK, MEAT ONLY, CKD, ROASTED	3	OUNCE	85.1	146	0	24	5
5074	CHICKEN, DRUMSTICK, MEAT ONLY, CKD, STEWED	3	OUNCE	85.1	144	0	23	5
5067	CHICKEN, DRUMSTICK, MEAT&SKIN, CKD, FRIED, BATTER	3	OUNCE	85.1	228	7	19	13
5068	CHICKEN, DRUMSTICK, MEAT&SKIN, CKD, FRIED, FLR	3	OUNCE	85.1	208	1	23	12
5069	CHICKEN, DRUMSTICK, MEAT&SKIN, CKD, ROASTED	3	OUNCE	85.1	184	0	23	9
5070	CHICKEN, DRUMSTICK, MEAT&SKIN, CKD, STEWED	3	OUNCE	85.1	174	0	22	9
5021	CHICKEN, GIBLETS, CKD, FRIED	3	OUNCE	85.1	236	4	28	11
5022	CHICKEN, GIBLETS, CKD, SIMMERED	3	OUNCE	85.1	134	1	22	4
5026	CHICKEN, HEART, CKD, SIMMERED	3	OUNCE	85.1	157	0	22	7
5081	CHICKEN, LEG, MEAT ONLY, CKD, FRIED	3	OUNCE	85.1	177	1	24	8
5082	CHICKEN, LEG, MEAT ONLY, CKD, ROASTED	3	OUNCE	85.1	162	0	23	7
5083	CHICKEN, LEG, MEAT ONLY, CKD, STEWED	3	OUNCE	85.1	157	0	22	7
5076	CHICKEN, LEG, MEAT&SKIN, CKD, FRIED, BATTER	3	OUNCE	85.1	232	7	19	14
5077	CHICKEN, LEG, MEAT&SKIN, CKD, FRIED, FLOUR	3	OUNCE	85.1	216	2	23	12
5078	CHICKEN, LEG, MEAT&SKIN, CKD, ROASTED	3	OUNCE	85.1	197	0	22	11
5079	CHICKEN, LEG, MEAT&SKIN, CKD, STEWED	3	OUNCE	85.1	187	0	21	11
5028	CHICKEN, LIVER, CKD, SIMMERED	3	OUNCE	85.1	134	1	21	5
5012	CHICKEN, MEAT ONLY, CKD, FRIED	3	OUNCE	85.1	186	1	26	8
5013	CHICKEN, MEAT ONLY, ROASTED	3	OUNCE	85.1	162	0	25	6
5014	CHICKEN, MEAT ONLY, STEWED	3	OUNCE	85.1	151	0	23	6
5097	CHICKEN, THIGH, MEAT ONLY, CKD, FRIED	3	OUNCE	85.1	185	1	24	9
5098	CHICKEN, THIGH, MEAT ONLY, CKD, ROASTED	3	OUNCE	85.1	178	0	22	9

Saturated fat (g)	Monounsaturated fat (g)	Polyunsaturated fat (g)	Fiber (g)	Cholesterol (g)	Folate (g)	Vitamin A (RE)	Vitamin B-6 (mg)	Vitamin B-12 (µg)	Vitamin C (mg)	Vitamin E (mg)	Riboflavin (mg)	Thiamin (mg)	Calcium (mg)	Iron (mg)	Magnesium (mg)	Niacin (mg)	Phosphorus (mg)	Potassium (mg)	Sodium (mg)	Zinc (mg)
-	-	-	-	60	-	-	-	-	6	-	0	0	240	.2	-	.6	-	310	1793	-
2	-	2	-	35	-	40	-	-	6	-	.2	.2	32	1	-	6.7	-	470	480	-
-	-	-	-	35	-	250	-	36	-	.1	.2	32	.8	-	7.6	200	400	440	-	
2	-	-	-	45	-	900	-	12	-	.2	.2	80	1	-	9.5	260	500	370	-	
-	-	-	-	15	-	60	-	-	-	-	-	0	-	-	-	.4	-	70	560	-
-	-	-	-	-	-	500	-	-	1	-	.4	.3	80	1	-	4.8	-	320	750	-
-	-	-	-	-	-	400	-	-	-	-	.2	.2	16	1	-	2.9	-	-	760	-
-	-	-	-	5	-	-	-	-	1	-	0	0	48	0	-	.1	-	40	119	-
2	3	1	0	43	2	20	.2	.1	0	-	.1	.1	37	.8	16	4.5	134	194	497	.6
3	3	5	0	26	4	36	.1	.3	1	-	.1	0	9	.5	9	1.4	28	156	321	.9
3	4	2	0	44	3	21	.1	.1	0	-	.1	0	106	2	10	2.3	76	90	328	1
3	-	-	-	55	-	20	-	-	-	-	.3	.2	48	1.5	-	2.9	260	630	500	-
2	-	1	-	60	-	200	-	-	5	-	.3	.2	120	.4	-	7.6	-	750	490	-
-	-	-	-	20	-	-	-	-	0	-	0	0	72	0	-	.1	-	31	57	-
2	-	2	-	55	-	100	-	-	12	-	.1	.1	48	1.5	-	8.6	250	670	550	-
-	-	-	-	10	-	80	-	-	6	-	.1	0	16	.2	-	1.9	70	140	510	-
4	5	3	0	79	8	25	.3	.3	0	-	.2	.1	22	1.4	21	6.5	150	213	84	2.4
3	4	3	0	77	6	24	.3	.3	0	-	.2	.1	20	1.2	19	6	140	202	82	2.3
3	3	2	0	72	6	23	.2	.2	0	-	.1	0	18	1.1	14	3.9	111	134	57	2
5	8	4	-	75	8	31	.2	.2	0	-	.2	.1	22	1.3	16	5	117	153	270	1.7
5	7	4	-	76	7	31	.3	.2	0	-	.2	.1	20	1.4	20	6.2	141	192	77	2.1
5	7	4	0	75	5	84	.2	.2	0	-	.2	.1	18	1.2	17	5.7	131	179	74	1.9
4	6	3	0	66	4	75	.1	.2	0	-	.1	0	15	1	14	3.7	102	123	54	1.6
1	1	1	0	77	3	6	.5	.3	0	-	.1	.1	14	1	26	12.6	209	235	67	.9
1	1	1	0	72	3	5	.5	.3	0	-	.1	.1	13	.9	25	11.7	194	218	63	.9
1	1	1	0	65	3	5	.3	.2	0	-	.1	0	11	.7	20	7.2	140	159	54	.8
3	5	3	0	72	5	17	.4	.3	0	-	.1	.1	17	1.1	20	8.9	157	171	234	.8
2	3	2	-	76	3	13	.5	.3	0	-	.1	.1	14	1	26	11.7	198	220	65	.9
2	3	1	0	71	3	23	.5	.3	0	-	.1	.1	12	.9	23	10.8	182	208	60	.9
2	2	1	0	64	3	20	.2	.2	0	-	.1	0	11	.8	19	6.6	133	151	53	.8
3	4	2	0	82	8	20	.3	.3	0	-	.2	.1	15	1.3	21	6	159	215	82	2.5
2	3	2	0	79	7	19	.3	.3	0	-	.2	.1	13	1.1	20	5.6	152	204	79	2.4
2	3	2	0	75	6	18	.2	.2	0	-	.2	0	12	1.2	17	4	122	154	63	2.3
4	6	4	-	76	8	26	.2	.2	0	-	.2	.1	18	1.2	17	4.8	123	157	251	1.8
4	6	3	-	78	7	26	.3	.3	0	-	.2	.1	14	1.3	20	5.8	150	196	76	2.2
4	5	3	0	77	6	49	.3	.2	0	-	.2	.1	13	1.2	19	5.4	143	187	74	2.1
3	5	3	0	70	5	46	.1	.2	0	-	.2	0	12	1.1	15	3.8	113	141	60	1.9
2	3	2	0	80	8	15	.3	.3	0	-	.2	.1	10	1.1	20	5.2	158	212	82	2.7
1	2	1	0	79	8	15	.3	.3	0	-	.2	.1	10	1.1	20	5.2	156	209	81	2.7
1	2	1	0	75	7	14	.2	.2	0	-	.2	0	9	1.2	18	3.7	128	169	68	2.6
4	5	3	-	73	8	22	.2	.2	0	-	.2	.1	14	1.1	17	4.3	125	158	229	2
3	5	3	-	77	7	21	.3	.3	0	-	.2	.1	10	1.1	20	5.1	150	195	76	2.5
3	4	2	0	77	6	26	.3	.3	0	-	.2	.1	10	1.1	20	5.1	149	195	77	2.4
2	3	2	0	71	6	23	.2	.2	0	-	.2	0	9	1.1	17	3.6	120	156	65	2.3
3	4	3	0	379	322	3044	.5	11.3	7	-	1.3	.1	15	8.8	21	9.3	243	281	96	5.3
1	1	1	0	334	320	1896	.3	8.6	7	-	.8	.1	10	5.5	17	3.5	195	134	49	3.9
2	2	2	0	206	68	8	.3	6.2	2	-	.6	.1	16	7.7	17	2.4	169	112	41	6.2
2	3	2	0	84	8	17	.3	.3	0	-	.2	.1	11	1.2	21	5.7	164	216	82	2.5
2	3	2	0	80	7	16	.3	.3	0	-	.2	.1	10	1.1	20	5.4	156	206	77	2.4
2	2	2	0	76	7	15	.2	.2	0	-	.2	.1	9	1.2	18	4.1	127	162	66	2.4
4	6	3	-	77	8	23	.2	.2	0	-	.2	.1	15	1.2	17	4.6	129	161	237	1.8
3	5	3	-	80	7	24	.2	.3	0	-	.2	.1	11	1.2	20	5.6	155	198	75	2.2
3	4	3	0	78	6	33	.3	.3	0	-	.2	.1	10	1.1	20	5.3	148	191	74	2.2
3	4	2	0	71	5	31	.2	.2	0	-	.2	0	9	1.1	17	3.9	118	150	62	2.1
2	1	1	0	537	655	4179	.5	16.5	13	-	1.5	.1	12	7.2	18	3.8	265	119	43	3.7
2	3	2	0	80	6	15	.4	.3	0	-	.2	.1	14	1.1	23	8.2	174	219	77	1.9
2	2	1	0	76	5	14	.4	.3	0	-	.2	.1	13	1	21	7.8	166	207	73	1.8
2		1	0	71	5	13	.2	.2	0	-	.1	0	12	1	18	5.2	128	153	60	1.7
2	3	2	0	87	8	18	.3	.3	0	-	.2	.1	11	1.2	22	6.1	169	220	81	2.4
3	4	2	0	81	7	17	.3	.3	0	-	.2	.1	10	1.1	20	5.5	156	202	75	2.2

Food Composition Table—cont'd

Code	Name	Amount	Unit	Grams	Kilocalories	Carbohydrates (g)	Protein (g)	Fat (g)
5099	CHICKEN, THIGH, MEAT ONLY, CKD, STEWED	3	OUNCE	85.1	166	0	21	8
5092	CHICKEN, THIGH, MEAT&SKIN, CKD, FRIED, BATTER	3	OUNCE	85.1	236	8	18	14
5093	CHICKEN, THIGH, MEAT&SKIN, CKD, FRIED, FLR	3	OUNCE	85.1	223	3	23	13
5094	CHICKEN, THIGH, MEAT&SKIN, CKD, ROASTED	3	OUNCE	85.1	210	0	21	13
5095	CHICKEN, THIGH, MEAT&SKIN, CKD, STEWED	3	OUNCE	85.1	197	0	20	13
5106	CHICKEN, WING, MEAT ONLY, CKD, FRIED	3	OUNCE	85.1	179	0	26	8
5107	CHICKEN, WING, MEAT ONLY, CKD, ROASTED	3	OUNCE	85.1	173	0	26	7
5108	CHICKEN, WING, MEAT ONLY, CKD, STEWED	3	OUNCE	85.1	154	0	23	6
5101	CHICKEN, WING, MEAT&SKIN, CKD, FRIED, BATTER	3	OUNCE	85.1	276	9	17	19
5102	CHICKEN, WING, MEAT&SKIN, CKD, FRIED, FLR	3	OUNCE	85.1	273	2	22	19
5103	CHICKEN, WING, MEAT&SKIN, CKD, ROASTED	3	OUNCE	85.1	247	0	23	17
5104	CHICKEN, WING, MEAT&SKIN, CKD, STEWED	3	OUNCE	85.1	212	0	19	14
16058	CHICKPEAS, CND	½	CUP	120.0	143	27	6	1
41272	CHILI BEEF SOUP-HEALTHY CHOICE	1	EACH	212.6	150	22	11	1
55114	CHILI CON CARNE W/ BEANS-STOUFFER'S	1	EACH	248.1	280	28	20	10
43411	CHILI MAC, MICRO CUP-HORMEL	1	EACH	212.6	192	18	10	9
43408	CHILI NO BEANS, MICRO CUP-HORMEL	1	EACH	209.1	290	15	18	17
55767	CHILI W/ BEANS SOUP-STOUFFER'S	1	CUP	283.9	240	25	14	9
16059	CHILI W/ BEANS, CND	½	CUP	127.5	143	15	7	7
43409	CHILI W/ BEANS, MICRO CUP-HORMEL	1	EACH	209.1	250	23	15	11
43369	CHILI W/ BEANS-HORMEL	1	CUP	253.2	357	32	18	18
43368	CHILI W/O BEANS-HORMEL	1	CUP	253.2	429	17	19	32
18198	CHOCOLATE CHIP COOKIES, DIETARY	1	EACH	7.0	32	5	0	1
18159	CHOCOLATE CHIP COOKIES, HIGHER FAT, ENR	1	EACH	10.0	48	7	1	2
18158	CHOCOLATE CHIP COOKIES, LOWER FAT	1	EACH	10.0	45	7	1	2
18160	CHOCOLATE CHIP COOKIES, SOFT-TYPE	1	EACH	15.0	69	9	1	4
18310	CHOCOLATE CREME PIE	1	SLICE	113.0	344	38	3	22
18312	CHOCOLATE MOUSSE PIE	1	SLICE	95.0	247	28	3	15
19183	CHOCOLATE PUDDING	1	CUP	298.1	396	68	8	12
18157	CHOCOLATE WAFERS	1	EACH	6.0	26	4	0	1
19119	CHUNKY BAR	1	BAR	35.0	173	20	3	10
43370	CHUNKY CHILI W/ BEANS-HORMEL	1	CUP	253.2	345	30	18	17
14187	CLAM AND TOMATO JUICE, CND	¾	CUP	181.1	83	20	1	0
15158	CLAM, CKD, BREADED AND FRIED	3	OUNCE	85.1	172	9	12	9
15159	CLAM, CKD, MOIST HEAT	3	OUNCE	85.1	126	4	22	2
15160	CLAM, CND, DRAINED SOLIDS	3	OUNCE	85.1	126	4	22	2
15162	CLAM, CND, SOLIDS AND LIQUIDS	3	OUNCE	85.1	2	0	0	0
14121	CLUB SODA	12	FL OZ	355.2	0	0	0	0
19219	COCONUT CREAM PUDDING	1	CUP	280.0	291	50	9	7
18313	COCONUT CREME PIE	1	SLICE	64.0	191	24	1	11
18316	COCONUT CUSTARD PIE	1	SLICE	104.0	270	31	6	14
15016	COD, ATLANTIC, CKD, DRY HEAT	3	OUNCE	85.1	89	0	19	1
15017	COD, ATLANTIC, CND	3	OUNCE	85.1	89	0	19	1
14209	COFFEE, BREWED	6	FL OZ	177.6	4	1	0	0
14219	COFFEE, INSTANT, DECAFFEINATED	6	FL OZ	179.2	4	1	0	0
14215	COFFEE, INSTANT, REGULAR	6	FL OZ	179.2	4	1	0	0
18104	COFFEECAKE	1	SLICE	63.0	263	29	4	15
18103	COFFEECAKE, CHEESE	1	SLICE	76.0	258	34	5	12
18106	COFFEECAKE, FRUIT	1	SLICE	50.0	156	26	3	5
14400	COLA	12	FL OZ	369.6	152	38	0	0
62530	COLA, DIET	12	FL OZ	355.2	0	0	0	0
11159	COLESLAW	½	CUP	64.0	44	8	1	2
11162	COLLARDS, CKD	½	CUP	64.0	17	4	1	0
11161	COLLARDS, FRESH	1	CUP	36.0	11	3	1	0
11164	COLLARDS, FRZ, CHOPPED, CKD	½	CUP	85.0	31	6	3	0
19049	COMBOS SNACKS CHEDDAR PRETZEL	1	OUNCE	28.4	136	18	3	6
55799	CONFETTI RICE-STOUFFER'S	1	OUNCE	28.4	24	5	1	0
55824	CORN PUDDING-STOUFFER'S	1	OUNCE	28.4	38	5	1	2
55168	CORN SOUFFLE-STOUFFER'S	1	EACH	170.1	240	27	7	11
20092	CORN, CKD	½	CUP	70.0	88	20	2	1

Saturated fat (g)	Monounsaturated fat (g)	Polyunsaturated fat (g)	Fiber (g)	Cholesterol (g)	Folate (g)	Vitamin A (RE)	Vitamin B-6 (mg)	Vitamin B-12 (µg)	Vitamin C (mg)	Vitamin E (mg)	Riboflavin (mg)	Thiamin (mg)	Calcium (mg)	Iron (mg)	Magnesium (mg)	Niacin (mg)	Phosphorus (mg)	Potassium (mg)	Sodium (mg)	Zinc (mg)
2	3	2	0	77	6	16	.2	.2	0	-	.2	.1	9	1.2	18	4.4	127	156	64	2.2
4	6	3	-	79	8	25	.2	.2	0	-	.2	.1	15	1.2	18	4.9	132	163	245	1.7
3	5	3	-	82	7	25	.3	.3	0	-	.2	.1	12	1.3	21	5.9	159	202	75	2.1
4	5	3	0	79	6	41	.3	.2	0	-	.2	.1	10	1.1	19	5.4	148	189	71	2
3	5	3	0	71	5	37	.1	.2	0	-	.2	0	9	1.2	16	4.2	118	145	60	1.9
2	3	2	0	71	3	15	.5	.3	0	-	.1	0	13	1	18	6.2	139	177	77	1.8
2	2	2	0	72	3	15	.5	.3	0	-	.1	0	14	1	18	6.2	141	179	78	1.8
2	2	1	0	63	3	14	.3	.2	0	-	.1	0	11	1	15	4.4	114	130	62	1.7
5	8	4	-	67	5	29	.3	.2	0	-	.1	.1	17	1.1	14	4.5	103	117	272	1.2
5	8	4	-	69	3	32	.3	.2	0	-	.1	0	13	1.1	16	5.7	128	151	65	1.5
5	6	4	0	71	3	40	.4	.2	0	-	.1	0	13	1.1	16	5.7	128	156	70	1.5
4	6	3	0	60	3	34	.2	.2	0	-	.1	0	10	1	14	3.9	103	118	57	1.4
0	0	1	5	0	80	2	.6	0	5	-	0	0	38	1.6	35	.2	108	206	359	1.3
-	-	-	-	15	-	20	-	-	6	-	0	.1	16	.6	-	.4	-	290	560	-
-	-	-	-	-	-	200	-	-	15	-	.3	.2	64	2	-	2.9	-	700	910	-
4	4	-	-	22	-	210	-	-	-	-	.2	.1	-	1.5	35	2.1	-	443	977	2.1
8	8	1	-	60	-	400	-	-	-	-	.2	.1	48	1.6	35	2.5	-	507	830	3.9
-	-	-	-	30	-	-	-	-	0	-	0	0	721	.3	-	.6	-	711	991	-
3	3	0	6	22	29	43	.2	0	2	-	.1	.1	60	4.4	57	.5	196	465	666	2.6
4	4	-	-	49	-	190	-	-	-	-	.2	.1	48	1.9	46	1.7	-	677	977	2.7
6	7	1	-	65	-	250	-	-	-	-	.2	.1	57	1.9	58	2	-	913	1226	2.5
13	15	1	-	71	-	786	-	-	-	-	.3	.1	48	1.7	42	2.9	-	592	1024	3.2
1	0	0	0	0	0	0	0	0	0	-	0	0	2	.2	2	.2	6	14	1	0
1	1	0	0	0	1	0	0	0	0	-	0	0	3	.3	3	.3	11	14	32	.1
0	1	0	-	0	1	0	0	0	0	-	0	0	2	.3	3	.3	8	12	38	.1
1	2	0	0	0	1	0	0	0	0	-	0	0	2	.4	5	.2	8	14	49	.1
6	12	3	2	6	8	-	0	0	0	-	.1	0	41	1.2	24	.8	77	144	154	.3
8	5	1	-	21	3	96	0	.2	0	-	.1	0	73	1	30	.6	219	271	437	.6
2	5	4	3	9	9	33	.1	0	5	-	.5	.1	268	1.5	63	1	238	537	385	1.3
0	0	0	-	0	1	0	0	0	0	-	0	0	2	.2	3	.2	8	13	35	.1
8	0	2	2	4	8	4	0	.1	0	-	.1	0	50	.4	26	.7	73	187	19	.6
-	-	-	-	60	-	-	-	-	-	-	-	-	-	-	-	-	-	-	929	-
0	0	0	-	0	29	40	.2	55.4	7	-	.1	.1	22	1.1	40	.3	141	163	724	2
2	4	2	-	52	15	77	.1	34.2	9	-	.2	.1	54	11.8	12	1.8	160	277	310	1.2
0	0	0	0	57	24	145	.1	84.1	19	-	.4	.1	78	23.8	15	2.9	287	534	95	2.3
0	0	0	0	57	24	145	.1	84.1	19	-	.4	.1	78	23.8	15	2.9	287	534	95	2.3
0	0	0	0	3	2	8	0	4.3	1	-	0	0	11	.3	9	.2	97	127	183	.1
0	0	0	0	0	0	0	0	0	0	-	0	0	18	0	4	0	0	7	75	.4
5	1	0	-	20	11	140	.4	.7	2	-	.4	.1	316	.6	45	.3	249	445	456	1
5	4	1	-	0	3	13	0	-	0	-	.1	0	19	.5	13	.1	54	42	163	.4
6	6	1	2	36	4	28	0	.1	0	-	.2	.1	84	.8	19	.4	127	182	348	.7
0	0	0	0	47	7	12	.2	.9	1	-	.1	.1	12	.4	36	2.1	117	208	66	.5
0	0	0	0	47	7	12	.2	.9	1	-	.1	.1	18	.4	35	2.1	221	449	185	.5
0	0	0	0	0	0	0	0	0	0	-	0	0	4	.1	9	.4	2	96	4	0
0	0	0	-	0	0	0	0	0	0	-	0	0	5	.1	7	.5	5	63	5	.1
0	0	0	-	0	0	0	0	0	0	-	0	0	5	.1	7	.5	5	64	5	.1
4	8	2	2	20	20	18	0	.1	0	-	.1	.1	34	1.2	14	1.1	68	77	221	.5
4	6	1	1	26	44	54	0	.1	0	-	.1	.1	45	.5	11	.5	75	220	258	.4
1	3	1	1	11	10	10	0	0	0	-	.1	0	23	1.2	9	1.3	59	45	193	.3
0	-	-	0	0	0	0	0	0	0	-	0	0	11	.1	4	0	44	4	15	0
-	-	-	0	-	-	-	-	-	-	-	-	-	-	-	-	-	-	-	30	-
0	0	1	-	5	17	52	.1	0	21	-	0	0	29	.4	6	.2	20	116	15	.1
-	-	-	1	0	4	175	0	0	8	-	0	0	15	.1	4	.2	5	84	10	.1
-	-	-	1	0	4	120	0	0	8	-	0	0	10	.1	3	.1	4	61	7	0
-	-	-	0	65	508	.1	0	22	-	.1	0	179	1	26	.5	23	213	43	.2
-	-	-	-	3	2	2	0	0	0	-	.2	0	54	.9	6	.9	41	37	317	.2
-	-	-	-	1	-	-	-	-	0	-	0	0	24	0	-	0	-	14	136	-
-	-	-	-	15	-	-	-	-	1	-	0	0	88	0	-	.1	-	51	125	-
-	-	-	-	-	60	-	-	-	-	-	.3	.2	48	.4	-	1.1	-	200	760	-
0	0	0	3	0	4	4	0	0	0	-	0	0	1	.2	25	.4	53	22	0	.4

Food Composition Table—cont'd

Code	Name	Amount	Unit	Grams	Kilocalories	Carbohydrates (g)	Protein (g)	Fat (g)
11901	CORN, SWEET, WHITE, CKD	½	CUP	82.0	89	21	3	1
11905	CORN, SWEET, WHITE, CND	½	CUP	82.0	66	15	2	1
11906	CORN, SWEET, WHITE, CND, CREAM STYLE	½	CUP	128.0	92	23	2	1
11900	CORN, SWEET, WHITE, FRESH	½	CUP	77.0	66	15	2	1
11168	CORN, SWEET, YELLOW, CKD	½	CUP	82.0	89	21	3	1
11172	CORN, SWEET, YELLOW, CND, BRINE PK	½	CUP	82.0	66	15	2	1
11174	CORN, SWEET, YELLOW, CND, CREAM STYLE	½	CUP	128.0	92	23	2	1
11167	CORN, SWEET, YELLOW, FRESH	½	CUP	77.0	66	15	2	1
43366	CORNED BEEF HASH-HORMEL	1	CUP	253.2	420	18	27	27
7020	CORNED BEEF LOAF, JELLIED	1	SLICE	28.4	43	0	6	2
19401	CORNNUTS, BARBECUE-FLAVOR	1	OUNCE	28.4	124	20	3	4
19402	CORNNUTS, NACHO-FLAVOR	1	OUNCE	28.4	124	20	3	4
19009	CORNNUTS, PLAIN	1	OUNCE	28.4	124	21	2	4
41278	COUNTRY VEGETABLE SOUP-HEALTHY CHOICE	1	EACH	212.6	120	23	3	1
15137	CRAB, ALASKA KING, CKD, MOIST HEAT	3	OUNCE	85.1	82	0	16	1
15138	CRAB, ALASKA KING, IMITATION	3	OUNCE	85.1	87	9	10	1
15140	CRAB, BLUE, CKD, MOIST HEAT	3	OUNCE	85.1	87	0	17	2
15141	CRAB, BLUE, CND	3	OUNCE	85.1	84	0	17	1
15142	CRAB, BLUE, CRAB CAKES	3	OUNCE	85.1	132	0	17	6
15226	CRAB, DUNGENESS, CKD, MOIST HEAT	3	OUNCE	85.1	94	1	19	1
15227	CRAB, QUEEN, CKD, MOIST HEAT	3	OUNCE	85.1	98	0	20	1
9077	CRABAPPLES, FRESH	½	CUP	55.0	42	11	0	0
18214	CRACKERS, CHEESE, REGULAR	1	EACH	1.0	5	1	0	0
18215	CRACKERS, CHEESE, W/ PEANUT BUTTER FILLING	1	EACH	7.0	34	4	1	2
18216	CRACKERS, CRISPBREAD, RYE	1	EACH	10.0	37	8	1	0
18218	CRACKERS, MATZO, EGG	1	EACH	28.4	111	22	3	1
18400	CRACKERS, MATZO, EGG AND ONION	1	EACH	28.4	111	22	3	1
18217	CRACKERS, MATZO, PLAIN	1	EACH	28.4	112	24	3	0
18219	CRACKERS, MATZO, WHOLE-WHEAT	1	EACH	28.4	100	22	4	0
18220	CRACKERS, MELBA TOAST, PLAIN	1	EACH	5.0	20	4	1	0
18424	CRACKERS, MELBA TOAST, PLAIN, W/O SALT	1	EACH	5.0	20	4	1	0
18221	CRACKERS, MELBA TOAST, RYE	1	EACH	5.0	19	4	1	0
18222	CRACKERS, MELBA TOAST, WHEAT	1	EACH	5.0	19	4	1	0
18229	CRACKERS, RITZ	1	EACH	3.0	15	2	0	1
18427	CRACKERS, RITZ, LOW SODIUM	1	EACH	3.0	15	2	0	1
18225	CRACKERS, RYE, W/ CHEESE FILLING	1	EACH	7.0	34	4	1	2
18226	CRACKERS, RYE, WAFERS, PLAIN	1	EACH	25.0	84	20	2	0
18227	CRACKERS, RYE, WAFERS, SEASONED	1	EACH	22.0	84	16	2	2
18228	CRACKERS, SALTINES	1	EACH	3.0	13	2	0	0
18425	CRACKERS, SALTINES, LOW SALT	1	EACH	3.0	13	2	0	0
18230	CRACKERS, SNACK-TYPE, W/ CHEESE FILLING	1	EACH	7.0	33	4	1	1
18231	CRACKERS, SNACK-TYPE, W/ PEANUT BUTTER FILLING	1	EACH	7.0	34	4	1	2
18428	CRACKERS, WHEAT, LOW SALT	1	EACH	2.0	9	1	0	0
18232	CRACKERS, WHEAT, REGULAR	1	EACH	2.0	9	1	0	0
18233	CRACKERS, WHEAT, W/ CHEESE FILLING	1	EACH	7.0	35	4	1	2
18234	CRACKERS, WHEAT, W/ PEANUT BUTTER FILLING	1	EACH	7.0	35	4	1	2
18235	CRACKERS, WHOLE-WHEAT	1	EACH	4.0	18	3	0	1
18429	CRACKERS, WHOLE-WHEAT, LOW SALT	1	EACH	4.0	18	3	0	1
9078	CRANBERRIES, FRESH	½	CUP	47.5	23	6	0	0
9080	CRANBERRY JUICE BOTTLED	¾	CUP	189.4	108	27	0	0
9081	CRANBERRY SAUCE, CND, SWEETENED	½	CUP	138.5	209	54	0	0
14238	CRANBERRY-APPLE JUICE DRINK, BOTTLED	¾	CUP	183.4	123	31	0	0
14240	CRANBERRY-APRICOT JUICE DRINK, BOTTLED	¾	CUP	183.4	117	30	0	0
14241	CRANBERRY-GRAPE JUICE DRINK, BOTTLED	¾	CUP	183.4	103	26	0	0
9082	CRANBERRY-ORANGE RELISH, CND	½	CUP	137.5	245	64	0	0
15243	CRAYFISH, FARMED, CKD, MOIST HEAT	3	OUNCE	85.1	74	0	15	1
15146	CRAYFISH, WILD, CKD, MOIST HEAT	3	OUNCE	85.1	75	0	14	1
55762	CREAM OF BROCCOLI SOUP-STOUFFER'S	1	CUP	283.9	300	16	12	21
55765	CREAM OF POTATO SOUP-STOUFFER'S	1	CUP	283.9	300	34	11	13
18238	CREAM PUFFS, SHELL, W/ CUSTARD FILLING	1	EACH	130.0	335	30	9	20

Saturated fat (g)	Monounsaturated fat (g)	Polyunsaturated fat (g)	Fiber (g)	Cholesterol (g)	Folate (g)	Vitamin A (RE)	Vitamin B-6 (mg)	Vitamin B-12 (µg)	Vitamin C (mg)	Vitamin E (mg)	Riboflavin (mg)	Thiamin (mg)	Calcium (mg)	Iron (mg)	Magnesium (mg)	Niacin (mg)	Phosphorus (mg)	Potassium (mg)	Sodium (mg)	Zinc (mg)
0	0	0	5	0	38	0	0	0	5	-	.1	.2	2	.5	26	1.3	84	204	14	.4
0	0	0	1	0	40	0	0	0	7	-	.1	0	4	.7	16	1	53	160	265	.3
0	0	0	2	0	57	0	.1	0	6	-	.1	0	4	.5	22	1.2	65	172	365	.7
0	0	0	2	0	35	0	0	0	5	-	0	.2	2	.4	28	1.3	69	208	12	.3
0	0	0	2	0	38	18	0	0	5	-	.1	.2	2	.5	26	1.3	84	204	14	.4
0	0	0	2	0	40	13	0	0	7	-	.1	0	4	.7	16	1	53	160	265	.3
0	0	0	2	0	57	13	.1	0	6	-	.1	0	4	.5	22	1.2	65	172	365	.7
0	0	0	2	0	35	22	0	0	5	-	0	.2	2	.4	28	1.3	69	208	12	.3
9	18	-	0	80	-	-	-	-	-	-	.2	-	71	1.8	31	3.4	-	625	991	4
1	1	0	0	13	2	0	0	.4	2	-	0	0	3	.6	3	.5	21	29	270	1.2
1	2	1	2	0	0	10	.1	0	0	-	0	.1	5	.5	31	.4	80	81	277	.5
1	2	1	2	1	4	1	.1	0	4	-	0	.1	10	.5	31	.3	88	88	180	.5
1	2	1	2	0	0	0	.1	0	0	-	0	0	3	.5	32	.5	78	79	156	.5
-	-	-	-	0	-	200	-	-	6	-	.1	.1	32	.4	-	1.5	100	380	540	-
0	0	0	0	45	43	8	.2	9.8	6	-	0	0	50	.6	54	1.1	238	223	912	6.5
0	0	1	0	17	1	17	0	1.4	0	-	0	0	11	.3	37	.2	240	77	715	.3
0	0	1	0	85	43	2	.2	6.2	3	-	0	.1	88	.8	28	2.8	175	276	237	3.6
0	0	0	0	76	36	2	.1	.4	2	-	.1	.1	86	.7	33	1.2	221	318	283	3.4
1	2	2	0	128	35	69	.1	5	2	-	.1	.1	89	.9	28	2.5	181	276	281	3.5
0	0	0	0	65	36	26	.1	8.8	3	-	.2	0	50	.4	49	3.1	149	347	321	4.7
0	0	0	0	60	36	44	.1	8.8	6	-	.2	.1	28	2.4	54	2.5	109	170	588	3.1
0	0	0	-	0	-	2	-	0	4	-	0	0	10	.2	4	.1	8	107	1	-
0	0	0	0	0	0	0	0	0	0	-	0	0	2	0	0	0	2	1	10	0
0	1	0	0	0	2	-	.1	0	0	-	0	0	6	.2	4	.5	23	17	69	.1
0	0	0	2	0	2	0	0	0	0	-	0	0	3	.2	8	.1	27	32	26	.2
0	0	0	-	25	8	4	0	.1	0	-	.2	.2	11	.8	7	1.4	45	43	6	.2
0	0	0	1	15	3	5	0	.1	0	-	.1	.2	10	1.2	9	1.4	25	24	81	.2
0	0	0	1	0	4	0	0	0	0	-	.1	.1	4	.9	7	1.1	25	32	1	.2
0	0	0	3	0	10	0	0	0	0	-	.1	.1	7	1.3	38	1.5	86	90	1	.7
0	0	0	0	0	1	0	0	0	0	-	0	0	5	.2	3	.2	10	10	41	.1
0	0	0	-	0	1	0	0	0	0	-	0	0	5	.2	3	.2	10	10	1	.1
0	0	0	0	0	1	-	0	0	0	-	0	0	4	.2	2	.2	9	10	45	.1
0	0	0	0	0	1	0	0	0	0	-	0	0	2	.2	3	.3	8	7	42	.1
0	0	0	0	0	0	0	0	0	0	-	0	0	4	.1	1	.1	7	4	25	0
0	0	0	-	0	0	0	0	0	0	-	0	0	4	.1	1	.1	7	11	11	0
0	1	0	-	1	1	0	0	0	0	-	0	0	16	.2	3	.2	24	24	73	0
0	0	0	-	0	11	1	.1	0	0	-	.1	.1	10	1.5	30	.4	84	124	199	.7
0	1	0	-	0	11	-	0	0	0	-	0	.1	10	.7	23	.5	68	100	195	.6
0	0	0	0	0	1	0	0	0	0	-	0	0	4	.2	1	.2	3	4	39	0
0	0	0	-	0	1	0	0	0	0	-	0	0	4	.2	1	.2	3	22	19	0
0	1	0	-	0	1	0	0	0	0	-	0	0	18	.2	3	.3	28	30	98	0
0	1	0	-	0	2	0	0	0	0	-	0	0	7	.2	4	.4	17	16	66	.1
0	0	0	-	0	0	0	0	0	0	-	0	0	1	.1	1	.1	4	4	6	0
0	0	0	-	0	0	0	0	0	0	-	0	0	1	.1	1	.1	4	4	16	0
0	1	0	-	0	1	1	0	0	0	-	0	0	14	.2	4	.2	27	21	64	.1
0	1	0	-	0	3	0	0	0	0	-	0	0	12	.2	3	.4	24	21	56	.1
0	0	0	0	0	1	0	0	0	0	-	0	0	2	.1	4	.2	12	12	26	.1
0	0	0	-	0	1	0	0	0	0	-	0	0	2	.1	4	.2	12	12	10	.1
-	-	-	2	0	1	2	0	0	6	-	0	0	3	.1	2	0	4	34	0	.1
-	-	-	-	0	0	0	0	0	67	-	0	0	6	.3	4	.1	4	34	4	.1
-	-	-	1	0	-	3	0	0	3	-	0	0	6	.3	4	.1	8	36	40	.1
0	-	-	0	0	0	0	0	0	59	-	0	0	13	.1	4	.1	6	50	4	.1
0	-	-	0	0	1	84	0	0	0	-	0	0	17	.3	6	.2	9	112	4	.1
0	-	-	0	0	1	0	.1	0	59	-	0	0	15	0	6	.2	7	44	6	.1
-	-	-	-	0	-	10	-	0	25	-	0	0	15	.3	5	.1	11	52	44	-
0	0	0	0	117	9	13	.1	2.6	0	-	.1	0	43	.9	28	1.4	205	202	82	1.3
0	0	0	0	113	37	13	.1	1.8	1	-	.1	0	51	.7	28	1.9	230	252	80	1.5
-	-	-	-	60	-	-	-	-	0	-	0	0	2484	0	-	0	-	431	791	-
-	-	-	-	30	-	-	-	-	0	-	0	0	2083	.1	-	.2	-	791	1422	-
5	8	5	-	174	20	259	.1	.5	0	-	.4	.2	86	1.5	16	1.1	142	150	443	.8

Food Composition Table—cont'd

Code	Name	Amount	Unit	Grams	Kilocalories	Carbohydrates (g)	Protein (g)	Fat (g)
14130	CREAM SODA	12	FL OZ	370.8	189	49	0	0
1067	CREAM SUBSTITUTE, NONDAIRY, LIQUID	1	TBSP.	15.0	20	2	0	1
1069	CREAM SUBSTITUTE, NONDAIRY, POWDERED	1	TSP.	2.0	11	1	0	1
1049	CREAM, HALF AND HALF, CREAM AND MILK	1	TBSP.	15.0	20	1	0	2
1053	CREAM, HEAVY WHIPPING	1	TBSP.	15.0	52	0	0	6
1052	CREAM, LIGHT WHIPPING	1	TBSP.	15.0	44	0	0	5
1050	CREAM, LIGHT, COFFEE OR TABLE	1	TBSP.	15.0	29	1	0	3
1051	CREAM, MEDIUM, 25% FAT	1	TBSP.	15.0	37	1	0	4
1054	CREAM, WHIPPED, PRESSURIZED	1	TBSP.	3.0	8	0	0	1
55788	CREAMED CHICKEN-STOUFFER'S	1	OUNCE	28.4	48	1	3	4
55777	CREAMED CHIPPED BEEF-STOUFFER'S	1	OUNCE	28.4	45	2	2	3
55169	CREAMED SPINACH-STOUFFER'S	1	EACH	127.6	190	8	4	16
55756	CREAMY CHICKEN SOUP-STOUFFER'S	1	CUP	283.9	240	25	17	8
14034	CREME DE MENTHE, 72 PROOF	1	FL OZ	33.6	125	14	0	0
18240	CROISSANTS, APPLE	1	MEDIUM	57.0	145	21	4	5
18239	CROISSANTS, BUTTER	1	MEDIUM	57.0	231	26	5	12
18241	CROISSANTS, CHEESE	1	MEDIUM	57.0	236	27	5	12
18242	CROUTONS, PLAIN	1	CUP	30.0	122	22	4	2
18243	CROUTONS, SEASONED	1	CUP	40.0	186	25	4	7
11205	CUCUMBER, FRESH	½	CUP	52.0	7	1	0	0
14010	DAIQUIRI	1	FL OZ	30.2	56	2	0	0
14009	DAIQUIRI, CND	1	FL OZ	30.5	38	5	0	0
18245	DANISH PASTRY, CHEESE	1	EACH	71.0	266	26	6	16
18244	DANISH PASTRY, CINNAMON	1	EACH	65.0	262	29	5	15
18246	DANISH PASTRY, FRUIT	1	EACH	71.0	263	34	4	13
18433	DANISH PASTRY, LEMON	1	EACH	71.0	263	34	4	13
18247	DANISH PASTRY, NUT	1	EACH	65.0	280	30	5	16
18435	DANISH PASTRY, RASPBERRY	1	EACH	71.0	263	34	4	13
9087	DATES, DOMESTIC, NATURAL AND DRY	½	CUP	89.0	245	65	2	0
17165	DEER, CKD, ROASTED	3	OUNCE	85.1	134	0	26	3
1073	DESSERT TOPPING, NONDAIRY	1	TBSP.	4.0	13	1	0	1
43375	DINTY MOORE BEEF STEW-HORMEL	1	CUP	253.2	246	18	12	15
43376	DINTY MOORE CHICKEN STEW-HORMEL	1	CUP	253.2	310	18	13	21
43377	DINTY MOORE MEATBALL STEW-HORMEL	1	CUP	253.2	268	16	12	18
43378	DINTY MOORE VEGETABLE STEW-HORMEL	1	CUP	253.2	173	22	6	7
19032	DOO DADS SNACK MIX, ORIGINAL FLAVOR	1	CUP	56.7	259	36	6	10
18251	DOUGHNUTS, CHOCOLATE, SUGARED OR GLAZED	1	EACH	42.0	175	24	2	8
18253	DOUGHNUTS, FRENCH CRULLERS, GLAZED	1	EACH	41.0	169	24	1	8
18255	DOUGHNUTS, GLAZED	1	EACH	60.0	242	27	4	14
18248	DOUGHNUTS, PLAIN	1	EACH	47.0	198	23	2	11
18249	DOUGHNUTS, PLAIN, CHOCOLATE-COATED OR FROSTED	1	EACH	43.0	204	21	2	13
18250	DOUGHNUTS, PLAIN, SUGARED OR GLAZED	1	EACH	45.0	192	23	2	10
18254	DOUGHNUTS, W/ CREME FILLING	1	EACH	85.0	307	26	5	21
18256	DOUGHNUTS, W/ JELLY FILLING	1	EACH	85.0	289	33	5	16
18252	DOUGHNUTS, WHEAT, SUGARED OR GLAZED	1	EACH	45.0	162	19	3	9
14153	DR. PEPPER	12	FL OZ	368.4	151	38	0	0
5142	DUCK, DOMESTICATED, MEAT ONLY, ROASTED	3	OUNCE	85.1	171	0	20	10
5140	DUCK, DOMESTICATED, MEAT&SKIN, ROASTED	3	OUNCE	85.1	287	0	16	24
7021	DUTCH BRAND LOAF, LUNCH MEAT	1	SLICE	28.4	68	2	4	5
18257	ECLAIRS, CUSTARD-FILLED W/ CHOCOLATE GLAZE	1	EACH	62.0	162	15	4	10
18317	EGG CUSTARD PIE	1	SLICE	105.0	221	22	6	12
19168	EGG CUSTARDS	1	CUP	282.0	296	30	14	13
1142	EGG SUBSTITUTE, FROZEN	1	CUP	240.0	384	8	27	27
1143	EGG SUBSTITUTE, LIQUID	1	CUP	251.0	211	2	30	8
1057	EGGNOG	1	CUP	254.0	342	34	10	19
11210	EGGPLANT, CKD	½	CUP	48.0	13	3	0	0
11209	EGGPLANT, FRESH	½	CUP	41.0	11	2	0	0
1128	EGGS, CHICKEN, WHOLE, CKD, FRIED	1	LARGE	46.0	92	1	6	7
1129	EGGS, CHICKEN, WHOLE, CKD, HARD-BOILED	1	LARGE	50.0	78	1	6	5
1130	EGGS, CHICKEN, WHOLE, CKD, OMELET	1	LARGE	59.0	90	1	6	7

Saturated fat (g)	Monounsaturated fat (g)	Polyunsaturated fat (g)	Fiber (g)	Cholesterol (g)	Folate (g)	Vitamin A (RE)	Vitamin B-6 (mg)	Vitamin B-12 (µg)	Vitamin C (mg)	Vitamin E (mg)	Riboflavin (mg)	Thiamin (mg)	Calcium (mg)	Iron (mg)	Magnesium (mg)	Niacin (mg)	Phosphorus (mg)	Potassium (mg)	Sodium (mg)	Zinc (mg)
0	0	0	0	0	0	0	0	0	0	-	0	0	19	.2	4	0	0	4	44	.3
0	1	0	0	0	0	1	0	0	0	-	0	0	1	0	0	0	10	29	12	0
1	0	0	0	0	0	0	0	0	0	-	0	0	0	0	0	0	8	16	4	0
1	0	0	0	6	0	16	0	0	0	-	0	0	16	0	2	0	14	19	6	.1
3	2	0	0	21	1	63	0	0	0	-	0	0	10	0	1	0	9	11	6	0
3	1	0	0	17	1	44	0	0	0	-	0	0	10	0	1	0	9	15	5	0
2	1	0	0	10	0	27	0	0	0	-	0	0	14	0	1	0	12	18	6	0
2	1	0	0	13	0	35	0	0	0	-	0	0	14	0	1	0	11	17	6	0
0	0	0	0	2	0	6	0	0	0	-	0	0	3	0	0	0	3	4	4	0
-	-	-	-	14	-	-	-	-	0	-	0	0	352	0	-	.1	-	37	119	-
-	-	-	-	13	-	-	-	-	0	-	0	0	184	0	-	.2	-	57	176	-
-	-	-	-	-	-	400	-	-	6	-	.2	0	80	.4	-	-	-	400	400	-
-	-	-	-	20	-	-	-	-	0	-	0	0	2484	0	-	.2	-	511	1282	-
0	0	0	0	0	0	0	0	0	0	-	0	0	0	0	0	0	0	0	2	0
3	1	0	1	29	7	42	0	0	0	-	.1	.1	17	.6	7	.9	33	51	156	.6
7	3	1	2	43	16	78	0	.2	0	-	.1	.2	21	1.2	9	1.2	60	67	424	.4
5	4	2	2	36	19	89	0	.2	0	-	.2	.3	30	1.2	14	1.2	74	75	316	.5
0	1	0	2	0	7	0	0	0	0	-	.1	.2	23	1.2	9	1.6	34	37	209	.3
2	4	1	2	1	16	2	0	0	0	-	.2	.2	38	1.1	17	1.9	56	72	495	.4
0	0	0	0	0	7	11	0	0	3	-	0	0	7	.1	6	.1	10	75	1	.1
0	0	0	0	0	1	0	0	0	0	-	0	0	1	0	1	0	2	6	2	0
0	-	-	0	0	0	0	0	0	0	-	0	0	0	0	0	0	1	3	12	0
5	8	2	-	32	18	44	0	.2	0	-	.2	.1	25	1.1	11	1.4	77	70	320	.6
4	8	2	1	20	21	7	0	.1	0	-	.2	.2	46	1.3	12	1.9	70	81	241	.5
3	7	2	1	15	11	11	-	.1	3	-	.2	.2	33	1.3	11	1.4	63	59	251	.4
3	7	2	-	-	11	38	-	-	3	-	.1	0	33	.5	11	.5	63	59	251	.4
4	8	4	1	30	18	9	.1	.1	1	-	.2	.1	61	1.2	21	1.5	72	62	236	.6
3	7	2	-	-	11	43	-	-	3	-	.1	0	33	.5	11	.5	63	59	251	.4
-	-	-	7	0	11	4	.2	0	0	-	.1	.1	28	1	31	2	36	580	3	.3
1	1	1	0	95	-	0	-	-	0	-	.5	.2	6	3.8	20	5.7	192	285	46	2.3
1	0	0	0	0	0	3	0	0	0	-	0	0	0	0	0	0	0	1	1	0
7	6	1	-	33	-	815	-	-	3	-	.1	0	27	1	23	2.5	-	588	971	2.8
5	7	8	-	95	-	476	-	-	2	-	.3	.1	38	.7	25	3.6	-	610	1012	1.3
8	8	1	-	33	-	279	-	-	1	-	.2	.1	27	1.2	27	3.2	-	586	1094	2.7
2	1	2	-	16	-	714	-	-	2	-	.1	.1	36	.7	31	1.7	-	509	949	.8
-	-	-	4	1	23	24	.1	0	0	-	.1	.2	42	1.4	34	3	168	157	721	1.3
2	5	1	1	24	7	11	0	.1	0	-	0	0	89	1	14	.2	68	50	143	.2
2	4	1	-	5	3	-	0	0	0	-	.1	.1	11	.6	5	.6	50	32	141	.1
3	8	2	1	4	13	-	0	.1	0	-	.1	.2	26	1.2	13	1.7	56	65	205	.5
2	5	4	1	17	4	8	0	.1	0	-	.1	.1	21	.9	9	.9	126	60	257	.3
4	7	2	1	25	7	13	0	.2	0	-	0	.1	15	1.1	17	.6	87	49	184	.3
2	5	1	-	14	5	1	0	.1	0	-	.1	.1	27	.5	8	.7	53	46	181	.2
6	11	3	-	20	12	7	0	.1	0	-	.1	.3	21	1.6	17	1.9	65	68	263	.7
4	9	2	-	22	14	7	0	.1	1	-	.1	.3	21	1.5	17	1.8	72	67	249	.6
1	4	3	-	9	7	9	0	.1	0	-	.1	.1	22	.5	10	.8	47	67	160	.3
0	-	-	0	0	0	0	0	0	0	-	0	0	11	.1	0	0	41	4	37	.1
4	3	1	0	76	9	20	.2	.3	0	-	.4	.2	10	2.3	17	4.3	173	214	55	2.2
8	11	3	0	71	5	54	.2	.3	0	-	.2	.1	9	2.3	14	4.1	133	174	50	1.6
2	2	1	0	13	1	0	.1	.4	5	-	.1	.1	24	.4	6	.7	46	107	354	.5
3	4	2	-	79	9	118	0	.2	0	-	.2	.1	39	.7	9	.5	66	73	209	.4
3	6	2	1	35	21	53	.1	.5	0	-	.2	0	84	.6	12	.3	118	111	252	.5
7	4	1	-	245	28	169	.1	.9	1	-	.6	.1	316	.8	39	.2	319	431	217	1.5
5	6	15	0	5	39	324	.3	.8	1	-	.9	.3	175	4.8	36	.3	172	512	479	2.4
2	2	4	0	3	37	542	0	.7	0	-	.8	.3	133	5.3	22	.3	304	828	444	3.3
11	6	1	0	149	2	203	.1	1.1	4	-	.5	.1	330	.5	47	.3	278	420	138	1.2
0	0	0	1	0	7	3	0	0	1	-	0	0	3	.2	6	.3	11	119	1	.1
0	0	0	1	0	8	3	0	0	1	-	0	0	3	.1	6	.2	9	89	1	.1
2	3	1	0	211	17	114	.1	.4	0	-	.2	0	25	.7	5	.2	89	61	162	.5
2	2	1	0	212	22	84	.1	.6	0	-	.3	0	25	.6	5	0	86	63	62	.5
2	3	1	0	207	17	110	.1	.4	0	-	.2	0	25	.7	5	0	87	60	159	.5

Food Composition Table—cont'd

Code	Name	Amount	Unit	Grams	Kilocalories	Carbohydrates (g)	Protein (g)	Fat (g)
1131	EGGS, CHICKEN, WHOLE, CKD, POACHED	1	LARGE	50.0	75	1	6	5
1132	EGGS, CHICKEN, WHOLE, CKD, SCRAMBLED	½	CUP	110.0	183	2	12	13
1123	EGGS, CHICKEN, WHOLE, FRESH, AND FROZEN	1	LARGE	50.0	75	1	6	5
41242	ENGLISH MUFFIN SANDWICH-HEALTHY CHOICE	1	EACH	120.5	200	30	16	3
18260	ENGLISH MUFFINS, MIXED-GRAIN (INCLUDES GRANOLA)	1	EACH	66.0	155	31	6	1
18261	ENGLISH MUFFINS, MIXED-GRAIN, TOASTED	1	EACH	61.0	156	31	6	1
18258	ENGLISH MUFFINS, PLAIN	1	EACH	57.0	134	26	4	1
18259	ENGLISH MUFFINS, PLAIN, TOASTED	1	EACH	52.0	133	26	4	1
18262	ENGLISH MUFFINS, RAISIN-CINNAMON	1	EACH	57.0	139	28	4	2
18263	ENGLISH MUFFINS, RAISIN-CINNAMON, TOASTED	1	EACH	52.0	137	28	4	2
18264	ENGLISH MUFFINS, WHEAT	1	EACH	57.0	127	26	5	1
18265	ENGLISH MUFFINS, WHEAT, TOASTED	1	EACH	52.0	126	25	5	1
18266	ENGLISH MUFFINS, WHOLE-WHEAT	1	EACH	66.0	134	27	6	1
18267	ENGLISH MUFFINS, WHOLE-WHEAT, TOASTED	1	EACH	61.0	135	27	6	1
55170	ESCALLOPED APPLES-STOUFFER'S	1	EACH	170.1	200	41	0	4
55117	ESCALLOPED CHICKEN AND NOODLES-STOUFFER'S	1	EACH	283.5	420	30	21	24
62592	FAT FREE CINNAMON GRAHAM SNACKS-SNACKWELL	20	EACH	13.4	49	12	1	0
62606	FAT FREE CRACKED PEPPER CRACKERS-SNACKWELL	7	EACH	15.0	60	13	2	0
62589	FAT FREE DEVILS FOOD COOKIE CAKES-SNACKWELL	1	EACH	16.0	50	13	1	0
62591	FAT FREE DOUBLE FUDGE COOKIE CAKES-SNACKWELL	1	EACH	16.0	50	12	1	0
62590	FAT FREE WHEAT CRACKERS-SNACKWELL	5	EACH	15.0	60	12	2	0
62621	FETTUCINI ALFREDO WITH BROCCOLI-WEIGHT WATCHERS	1	EACH	241.0	220	24	15	6
55208	FETTUCINI ALFREDO, LEAN CUISINE-STOUFFER'S	1	EACH	255.1	280	41	14	7
55171	FETTUCINI ALFREDO-STOUFFER'S	1	EACH	141.8	245	22	8	14
55209	FETTUCINI PRIMAVERA, LEAN CUISINE-STOUFFER'S	1	EACH	283.5	260	32	14	8
55831	FETTUCINI SAUCE (ALFREDO STYLE)-STOUFFER'S	1	CUP	283.9	701	11	14	67
41288	FETTUCINI W/ TURKEY AND VEGETABLES-HEALTHY CHOICE	1	EACH	354.4	350	45	29	6
62612	FIESTA CHICKEN-WEIGHT WATCHERS	1	EACH	241.0	220	38	12	2
55773	FIESTA MEXICALI HEAT'N SERVE SOUP -STOUFFER'S	1	CUP	283.9	110	18	3	3
19098	FIFTH AVENUE BAR	1	BAR	60.0	280	41	5	13
18170	FIG BARS	1	EACH	16.0	56	11	1	1
55210	FILET OF FISH DIVAN, LEAN CUISINE-STOUFFER'S	1	EACH	294.1	210	13	27	5
55211	FILET OF FISH FLORENTINE, LEAN CUISINE-STOUFFER'S	1	EACH	272.9	220	13	26	7
15027	FISH FILLETS AND STICKS, FRIED	3	OUNCE	85.1	231	20	13	10
15029	FLOUNDER, CKD, DRY HEAT	3	OUNCE	85.1	100	0	21	1
55178	FRENCH BREAD PIZZA, CHEESE-STOUFFER'S	1	EACH	145.3	350	40	16	14
41332	FRENCH BREAD PIZZA, DELUXE-HEALTHY CHOICE	1	EACH	180.7	330	41	23	7
55181	FRENCH BREAD PIZZA, DELUXE-STOUFFER'S	1	EACH	173.6	420	40	21	19
55180	FRENCH BREAD PIZZA, DOUBLE CHEESE-STOUFFER'S	1	EACH	166.6	420	43	22	18
55182	FRENCH BREAD PIZZA, HAMBURGER-STOUFFER'S	1	EACH	173.6	410	39	23	18
55183	FRENCH BREAD PIZZA, PEPPERONI-STOUFFER'S	1	EACH	159.5	400	39	19	19
55185	FRENCH BREAD PIZZA, SAUSAGE-STOUFFER'S	1	EACH	170.1	430	40	20	21
55187	FRENCH BREAD PIZZA, VEGETABLE DELUXE-STOUFFER'S	1	EACH	180.7	420	41	18	20
55761	FRENCH ONION SOUP-STOUFFER'S	1	CUP	283.9	100	10	4	4
18268	FRENCH TOAST, FROZEN, READY-TO-HEAT	1	SLICE	59.0	126	19	4	4
18269	FRENCH TOAST, MADE W/ LOWFAT (2%) MILK	1	SLICE	65.0	149	16	5	7
18381	FRENCH TOAST, MADE W/ WHOLE MILK	1	SLICE	65.0	151	16	5	7
19226	FROSTINGS, CHOCOLATE, CREAMY	1	OUNCE	28.4	113	18	0	5
19713	FROSTINGS, CREAM CHEESE-FLAVOR	1	OUNCE	28.4	117	19	0	5
19229	FROSTINGS, SOUR CREAM-FLAVOR	1	OUNCE	28.4	117	19	0	5
19230	FROSTINGS, VANILLA, CREAMY	1	OUNCE	28.4	119	20	0	5
41319	FROZEN DESSERT, BORDEAUX CHERRY-HEALTHY CHOICE	1	CUP	133.0	240	46	6	4
41320	FROZEN DESSERT, BUTTER PECAN CRUNCH-HEALTHY CHOICE	1	CUP	133.0	280	52	6	4
41321	FROZEN DESSERT, CHOCOLATE CHIP-HEALTHY CHOICE	1	CUP	133.0	260	48	6	4
41322	FROZEN DESSERT, COFFEE TOFFEE-HEALTHY CHOICE	1	CUP	133.0	260	50	6	4
41323	FROZEN DESSERT, COOKIES 'N CREAM-HEALTHY CHOICE	1	CUP	133.0	260	48	8	4
41324	FROZEN DESSERT, DOUBLE FUDGE SWIRL-HEALTHY CHOICE	1	CUP	133.0	260	48	6	4
41325	FROZEN DESSERT, FUDGE BROWNIE-HEALTHY CHOICE	1	CUP	133.0	280	54	6	4
41326	FROZEN DESSERT, MINT CHOCOLATE CHIP-HEALTHY CHOICE	1	CUP	133.0	280	50	6	4
41327	FROZEN DESSERT, NEAPOLITAN-HEALTHY CHOICE	1	CUP	133.0	240	44	6	4

Saturated fat (g)	Monounsaturated fat (g)	Polyunsaturated fat (g)	Fiber (g)	Cholesterol (g)	Folate (g)	Vitamin A (RE)	Vitamin B-6 (mg)	Vitamin B-12 (µg)	Vitamin C (mg)	Vitamin E (mg)	Riboflavin (mg)	Thiamin (mg)	Calcium (mg)	Iron (mg)	Magnesium (mg)	Niacin (mg)	Phosphorus (mg)	Potassium (mg)	Sodium (mg)	Zinc (mg)
2	2	1	0	212	18	95	.1	.4	0	-	.2	0	25	.7	5	0	89	60	140	.6
4	5	2	0	387	33	215	.1	.8	0	-	.5	.1	78	1.3	13	.1	187	152	308	1.1
2	2	1	0	213	24	96	.1	.5	0	-	.3	0	25	.7	5	0	89	61	63	.6
1	-	1	-	20	-	60	-	-	4	-	.4	.5	120	2	-	2.9	220	200	510	-
0	1	0	-	0	23	1	.1	0	0	-	.2	.3	129	2	29	2.4	98	103	275	.6
0	1	0	-	0	16	1	.1	0	0	-	.2	.2	130	2	29	2.1	99	103	276	.6
0	0	1	-	0	21	0	0	0	0	-	.2	.3	99	1.4	12	2.2	76	75	264	.4
0	0	1	-	0	15	0	0	0	0	-	.1	.2	98	1.4	11	2	75	74	262	.4
0	0	1	-	0	18	0	0	0	0	-	.2	.2	84	1.4	9	2	44	119	255	.6
0	0	1	-	0	13	0	0	0	0	-	.1	.2	83	1.4	9	1.8	44	118	253	.6
0	0	0	-	0	22	0	.1	0	0	-	.2	.2	101	1.6	22	1.9	66	106	218	.6
0	0	0	-	0	16	0	0	0	0	-	.1	.2	100	1.6	22	1.7	64	105	216	.6
0	0	1	4	0	32	0	.1	0	0	-	.1	.2	175	1.6	47	2.3	186	139	420	1.1
0	0	1	-	0	23	0	.1	0	0	-	.1	.2	176	1.6	47	2	187	139	422	1.1
-	-	-	-	-	-	-	-	-	30	-	-	0	-	-	-	-	-	90	15	-
0	0	0	0	0	-	0	-	-	0	-	-	-	0	.3	-	-	-	-	40	-
0	0	0	0	0	-	0	-	-	0	-	-	-	24	.4	-	-	-	-	150	-
0	0	0	1	0	-	0	-	-	0	-	-	-	0	0	-	-	-	-	25	-
0	0	0	1	0	-	0	-	-	0	-	-	-	0	.2	-	-	-	-	70	-
0	0	0	1	0	-	0	-	-	0	-	-	-	24	.4	-	-	-	45	170	-
3	-	-	6	15	-	60	-	-	1	-	-	-	300	1.5	-	-	-	510	540	-
3	-	-	-	15	-	-	-	-	-	-	.4	.3	200	.8	-	1.5	-	270	570	-
-	-	-	-	-	-	-	-	-	-	-	.3	.2	120	.4	-	1	-	100	400	-
3	-	-	-	45	-	400	-	-	18	-	.4	.3	240	.8	-	1.5	-	400	510	-
-	-	-	-	180	-	-	-	-	0	-	0	0	2724	0	-	0	-	341	1813	-
3	-	2	-	60	-	150	-	-	-	-	.5	.5	120	1.5	-	3.8	310	450	480	-
1	-	-	5	25	-	450	-	-	42	-	-	-	72	1.5	-	-	-	490	480	-
-	-	-	-	10	-	-	-	-	6	-	0	0	2404	1	-	.2	-	431	711	-
-	-	-	-	-	2	33	5	.1	.1	0	-	.1	0	42	.6	38	2	90	197	112	.6
0	1	0	1	0	2	1	0	0	0	-	0	0	10	.5	4	.3	10	33	56	.1
2	-	1	-	65	-	20	-	-	27	-	.3	.2	120	.4	-	1.9	-	800	490	-
3	-	2	-	65	-	500	-	-	1	-	.3	.2	120	.4	-	1.9	-	780	590	-
3	4	3	0	95	15	26	.1	1.5	0	-	.2	.1	17	.6	21	1.8	154	222	495	.6
0	0	0	0	58	8	9	.2	2.1	0	-	.1	.1	15	.3	49	1.9	246	293	89	.5
-	-	-	-	-	-	60	-	-	4	-	.3	.5	200	1.5	-	2.9	-	300	630	-
3	-	1	-	35	-	80	-	-	-	-	.3	.5	200	2.5	-	3.8	280	350	500	-
-	-	-	-	-	-	100	-	-	6	-	.4	.5	160	1.5	-	3.8	-	350	950	-
-	-	-	-	-	-	40	-	-	6	-	.5	.5	360	1.5	-	3.8	-	320	850	-
-	-	-	-	-	-	60	-	-	6	-	.3	.4	160	1.5	-	3.8	-	340	650	-
-	-	-	-	-	-	100	-	-	6	-	.4	.5	160	1.5	-	3.8	-	300	880	-
-	-	-	-	-	-	80	-	-	6	-	.4	.6	160	1.5	-	3.8	-	340	840	-
-	-	-	-	-	-	250	-	-	4	-	.4	.5	280	1.5	-	3.8	-	230	830	-
-	-	-	0	-	-	-	-	-	0	-	0	0	240	0	-	0	-	170	2073	-
1	1	1	2	48	14	32	.3	1	0	-	.2	.2	63	1.3	10	1.6	82	79	292	.5
2	3	2	-	75	15	86	0	.2	0	-	.2	.1	65	1.1	11	1.1	76	87	311	.4
2	3	2	-	76	15	81	0	.2	0	-	.2	.1	64	1.1	11	1.1	76	86	311	.4
2	3	1	-	0	0	56	0	0	0	-	0	0	2	.4	6	0	22	56	52	.1
1	3	1	-	0	0	0	0	0	0	-	0	0	1	0	1	0	1	10	11	0
1	3	1	-	0	0	35	0	0	0	-	0	0	1	0	1	.2	1	55	58	0
1	2	1	-	0	0	64	0	0	0	-	0	0	1	0	0	0	11	10	26	0
0	-	2	-	10	-	-	-	-	-	-	.3	.1	160	-	-	-	200	300	100	-
-	-	2	-	10	-	-	-	-	2	-	.3	.1	160	-	-	-	160	300	160	-
0	-	2	-	10	-	-	-	-	2	-	.3	.1	160	.4	-	-	160	320	140	-
-	-	2	-	10	-	-	-	-	2	-	.3	.1	160	-	-	-	160	320	160	-
0	-	2	-	10	-	-	-	-	-	-	.3	.1	240	-	-	-	200	360	160	-
-	-	2	-	10	-	-	-	-	-	-	.3	.1	160	.8	-	-	200	420	140	-
0	-	2	-	10	-	-	-	-	-	-	.3	.1	160	.4	-	-	160	380	140	-
0	-	4	-	10	-	-	-	-	-	-	.3	.1	160	.4	-	-	-	340	160	-
0	-	2	-	10	-	-	-	-	-	-	.3	.1	160	-	-	-	200	320	120	-

Food Composition Table—cont'd

Code	Name	Amount	Unit	Grams	Kilocalories	Carbohydrates (g)	Protein (g)	Fat (g)
41328	FROZEN DESSERT, PRALINE AND CARAMEL-HEALTHY CHOICE	1	CUP	133.0	260	52	6	4
41329	FROZEN DESSERT, ROCKY ROAD-HEALTHY CHOICE	1	CUP	133.0	320	64	6	4
41330	FROZEN DESSERT, VANILLA-HEALTHY CHOICE	1	CUP	133.0	240	42	8	4
19263	FRUIT AND JUICE BARS	1	BAR	77.0	63	16	1	0
9100	FRUIT HVY SYRUP	½	CUP	127.5	93	24	0	0
9097	FRUIT JUICE PACK	½	CUP	124.0	57	15	1	0
9099	FRUIT LT SYRUP	½	CUP	126.0	72	19	1	0
18319	FRUIT PIE, FRIED	1	PIE	128.0	404	55	4	21
14267	FRUIT PUNCH DRINK, CND	¾	CUP	185.8	87	22	0	0
9105	FRUIT SALAD, HVY SYRUP	½	CUP	127.5	93	24	0	0
9103	FRUIT SALAD, JUICE PACK	½	CUP	124.5	62	16	1	0
9104	FRUIT SALAD, LT SYRUP	½	CUP	126.0	73	19	0	0
9102	FRUIT SALAD, WATER PACK	½	CUP	122.5	37	10	0	0
9096	FRUIT WATER PACK	½	CUP	122.5	39	10	1	0
9188	FRUIT, MIXED, DRIED	¼	CUP	37.5	91	24	1	0
9189	FRUIT, MIXED, FRZN, SWTND, THAWD	½	CUP	125.0	123	30	2	0
9187	FRUIT, MIXED, HVY SYRUP	½	CUP	127.5	92	24	0	0
19381	FUDGE, BROWN SUGAR W/ NUTS	1	PIECE	14.0	55	11	0	1
19100	FUDGE, CHOCOLATE	1	PIECE	17.0	65	14	0	1
19101	FUDGE, CHOCOLATE W/ NUTS	1	PIECE	19.0	81	14	1	3
19102	FUDGE, PEANUT BUTTER	1	PIECE	16.0	59	13	1	1
19103	FUDGE, VANILLA	1	PIECE	16.0	59	13	0	1
19104	FUDGE, VANILLA W/ NUTS	1	PIECE	15.0	62	11	0	2
41337	GARDEN POTATO CASSEROLE-HEALTHY CHOICE	1	EACH	262.2	180	23	12	4
55774	GARDEN TOMATO HEAT'N SERVE SOUP-STOUFFER'S	1	CUP	283.9	110	16	4	3
41273	GARDEN VEGETABLE SOUP-HEALTHY CHOICE	1	EACH	212.6	100	18	3	1
19215	GELATIN POPS	1	EACH	44.0	31	7	1	0
14011	GIN AND TONIC	1	FL OZ	30.0	23	2	0	0
14136	GINGER ALE	12	FL OZ	366.0	124	32	0	0
62532	GINGER ALE, DIET	12	FL OZ	355.2	0	0	0	0
18172	GINGERSNAPS	1	EACH	7.0	29	5	0	1
43399	GLAZED BREAST OF CHICKEN, TOP SHELF-HORMEL	1	EACH	283.5	170	19	19	2
55212	GLAZED CHICKEN W/ VEG. LEAN CUISINE-STOUFFER'S	1	EACH	241.0	250	24	21	7
41307	GLAZED CHICKEN-HEALTHY CHOICE	1	EACH	241.0	220	27	21	3
55784	GLAZED CHICKEN-STOUFFER'S	1	OUNCE	28.4	26	1	3	1
19105	GOOBERS	1	PIECE	1.0	5	0	0	0
18173	GRAHAM CRACKERS, PLAIN OR HONEY	1	EACH	7.0	30	5	0	1
19016	GRANOLA BARS, HARD, ALMOND	1	EACH	28.4	140	18	2	7
19017	GRANOLA BARS, HARD, CHOCOLATE CHIP	1	EACH	28.4	124	20	2	5
19019	GRANOLA BARS, HARD, PEANUT	1	EACH	28.4	136	18	3	6
19420	GRANOLA BARS, HARD, PEANUT BUTTER	1	EACH	28.4	137	18	3	7
19015	GRANOLA BARS, HARD, PLAIN	1	EACH	28.4	134	18	3	6
19404	GRANOLA BARS, SOFT, CHOCOLATE CHIP	1	EACH	28.4	119	20	2	5
19406	GRANOLA BARS, SOFT, NUT AND RAISIN	1	EACH	28.4	129	18	2	6
19021	GRANOLA BARS, SOFT, PEANUT BUTTER	1	EACH	28.4	121	18	3	4
19027	GRANOLA BARS, SOFT, PEANUT BUTTER AND CHOC CHIP	1	EACH	28.4	122	18	3	6
19020	GRANOLA BARS, SOFT, PLAIN	1	EACH	28.4	126	19	2	5
19022	GRANOLA BARS, SOFT, RAISIN	1	EACH	28.4	127	19	2	5
14277	GRAPE DRINK, CND	¾	CUP	187.6	84	22	0	0
14282	GRAPE JUICE DRINK, CND	¾	CUP	187.6	94	24	0	0
9135	GRAPE JUICE, CND OR BOTTLED, UNSWEETENED	¾	CUP	189.4	116	28	1	0
14142	GRAPE SODA	12	FL OZ	372.0	160	42	0	0
9124	GRAPEFRUIT JUICE, CND, SWEETENED	¾	CUP	187.0	86	21	1	0
9123	GRAPEFRUIT JUICE, CND, UNSWEETENED	¾	CUP	185.2	70	17	1	0
9404	GRAPEFRUIT JUICE, PINK, FRESH	¾	CUP	185.3	72	17	1	0
9128	GRAPEFRUIT JUICE, WHITE, FRESH	¾	CUP	185.3	72	17	1	0
9112	GRAPEFRUIT, FRESH, PINK & RED	1	MEDIUM	146.0	44	11	1	0
9116	GRAPEFRUIT, FRESH, WHITE	1	MEDIUM	136.0	45	11	1	0
9120	GRAPEFRUIT, SECTIONS, CND, JUICE PACK	½	CUP	124.5	46	11	1	0
9121	GRAPEFRUIT, SECTIONS, CND, LIGHT SYRUP PACK	½	CUP	127.0	76	20	1	0

Saturated fat (g)	Monounsaturated fat (g)	Polyunsaturated fat (g)	Fiber (g)	Cholesterol (g)	Folate (g)	Vitamin A (RE)	Vitamin B-6 (mg)	Vitamin B-12 (µg)	Vitamin C (mg)	Vitamin E (mg)	Riboflavin (mg)	Thiamin (mg)	Calcium (mg)	Iron (mg)	Magnesium (mg)	Niacin (mg)	Phosphorus (mg)	Potassium (mg)	Sodium (mg)	Zinc (mg)
0	-	2	-	10	-	-	-	-	-	-	.3	.1	160	-	-	-	200	320	140	-
0	-	2	-	10	-	-	-	-	-	-	.3	.1	160	-	-	-	200	380	140	-
0	-	2	-	10	-	-	-	-	-	-	.5	.1	240	-	-	-	200	360	120	-
-	-	-	-	0	5	2	0	0	7	-	0	0	4	.1	3	.1	5	41	3	0
0	0	0	1	0	3	26	.1	0	2	-	0	0	8	.4	6	.5	14	112	8	.1
0	0	0	1	0	3	38	.1	0	3	-	0	0	10	.3	9	.5	17	118	5	.1
0	0	0	1	0	3	26	.1	0	2	-	0	0	8	.4	6	.5	14	112	8	.1
3	10	7	3	0	4	4	0	.1	2	-	.1	.2	28	1.6	13	1.8	55	83	479	.3
0	0	0	0	0	2	2	0	0	55	-	0	0	15	.4	4	0	2	46	41	.2
0	0	0	1	0	3	64	0	0	3	-	0	0	8	.4	6	.4	11	102	8	.1
0	0	0	-	0	3	75	0	0	4	-	0	0	14	.3	10	.4	17	144	6	.2
0	0	0	-	0	3	54	0	0	3	-	0	0	9	.4	6	.5	11	103	8	.1
0	0	0	-	0	3	54	0	0	2	-	0	0	9	.4	6	.5	11	96	4	.1
0	0	0	1	0	3	31	.1	0	3	-	0	0	6	.3	9	.4	13	115	5	.1
0	0	0	-	0	1	92	.1	0	1	-	.1	0	14	1	15	.7	29	299	7	.2
0	0	0	2	0	9	40	0	0	94	-	0	0	9	.3	7	.5	15	164	4	.1
0	0	0	-	0	4	24	0	0	88	-	.1	0	1	.5	6	.8	13	107	5	.1
0	0	1	-	1	2	2	0	0	0	-	0	0	16	.3	7	0	12	52	14	.1
1	0	0	0	2	0	8	0	0	0	-	0	0	7	.1	4	0	10	18	11	.1
1	1	1	0	3	2	9	0	0	0	-	0	0	10	.1	9	0	18	30	11	.1
0	0	0	-	1	2	2	0	0	0	-	0	0	7	0	4	.2	10	21	12	.1
1	0	0	0	3	0	8	0	0	0	-	0	0	6	0	1	0	5	8	11	0
1	0	1	0	2	2	7	0	0	0	-	0	0	7	.1	4	0	11	17	9	.1
2	-	-	-	20	-	-	-	-	-	-	-	-	-	-	-	-	-	600	360	-
-	-	-	-	10	-	-	-	-	0	-	0	0	240	.3	-	.2	-	431	1052	-
-	-	-	-	0	-	350	-	-	9	-	.1	.1	16	.4	-	.8	-	230	560	-
-	-	-	0	0	0	0	0	0	0	-	0	0	1	0	0	0	0	1	20	0
0	0	0	-	0	0	0	0	0	0	-	0	0	1	0	0	0	0	2	1	0
0	-	-	0	0	0	0	0	0	0	-	0	0	11	.7	4	0	0	4	26	.2
-	-	-	-	0	-	-	-	-	-	-	-	-	-	-	-	-	-	-	30	-
0	0	0	0	0	0	0	0	0	0	-	0	0	5	.4	3	.2	6	24	46	0
1	1	1	-	35	-	400	-	-	4	-	.2	.1	32	.4	35	7.6	-	804	780	1.1
2	-	4	-	50	-	20	-	-	4	-	.2	.2	16	.2	-	7.6	-	580	590	-
1	-	1	-	45	-	-	-	-	1	-	.1	.2	-	.6	-	6.7	240	370	510	-
-	-	-	-	9	-	-	-	-	0	-	0	0	24	0	-	.2	-	45	105	-
0	0	0	-	0	0	0	0	0	0	-	0	0	1	0	1	.1	3	5	0	0
0	0	0	0	0	1	0	0	0	0	-	0	0	2	.3	2	.3	7	9	42	.1
4	2	1	-	0	3	1	0	0	0	-	0	.1	9	.7	23	.2	65	77	73	.4
3	1	0	1	0	4	1	0	0	0	-	0	.1	22	.9	20	.2	58	71	98	.5
1	2	3	-	0	7	1	0	0	0	-	0	.1	11	.7	31	.4	85	86	79	.6
1	2	3	-	0	5	1	0	0	0	-	0	.1	12	.7	16	.6	39	82	80	.4
1	1	3	2	0	7	4	0	0	0	-	0	.1	17	.8	27	.4	79	95	83	.6
3	1	1	1	0	6	1	0	0	0	-	0	.1	26	.7	22	.3	65	96	77	.4
3	1	2	2	0	9	1	0	.1	0	-	.1	.1	24	.6	26	.7	68	111	72	.5
1	2	1	1	0	9	1	0	.1	0	-	0	.1	26	.6	24	.9	71	82	116	.5
2	2	1	1	0	9	1	0	.1	0	-	0	0	23	.5	25	.9	74	107	93	.5
2	1	2	1	0	7	0	0	.1	0	-	0	.1	30	.7	21	.1	65	92	79	.4
3	1	1	1	0	6	0	0	.1	0	-	0	.1	29	.7	20	.3	62	103	80	.4
0	0	0	0	0	1	0	0	0	64	-	0	0	6	.3	4	0	2	9	11	.2
0	0	0	0	0	2	0	0	0	30	-	0	0	6	.2	8	.2	8	66	2	.1
0	0	0	0	0	5	2	.1	0	0	-	.1	0	17	.5	19	.5	21	250	6	.1
0	0	0	0	0	0	0	0	0	0	-	0	0	11	.3	4	0	0	4	56	.3
0	0	0	0	0	19	0	0	0	50	-	0	.1	15	.7	19	.6	21	303	4	.1
0	0	0	0	0	19	2	0	0	54	.1	0	.1	13	.4	19	.4	20	283	2	.2
0	0	0	-	0	19	82	.1	0	70	-	0	.1	17	.4	22	.4	28	300	2	.1
0	0	0	0	0	19	2	.1	0	70	-	0	.1	17	.4	22	.4	28	300	2	.1
0	0	0	-	0	18	38	.1	0	56	-	0	0	16	.2	12	.3	13	188	2	.1
0	0	0	1	0	14	1	.1	0	45	-	0	.1	16	.1	12	.4	11	201	0	.1
0	0	0	0	0	11	0	0	0	42	-	0	0	19	.3	14	.3	15	210	9	.1
0	0	0	1	0	11	0	0	0	27	-	0	0	18	.5	13	.3	13	164	3	.1

Food Composition Table—cont'd

Code	Name	Amount	Unit	Grams	Kilocalories	Carbohydrates (g)	Protein (g)	Fat (g)
9119	GRAPEFRUIT, SECTIONS, CND, WATER PACK	½	CUP	122.0	44	11	1	0
9131	GRAPES, AMERICAN TYPE, FRESH	½	CUP	46.0	29	8	0	0
6114	GRAVY, AU JUS, CND	¼	CUP	59.6	10	1	1	0
6116	GRAVY, BEEF, CND	¼	CUP	58.3	31	3	2	1
6119	GRAVY, CHICKEN, CND	¼	CUP	59.6	47	3	1	3
6121	GRAVY, MUSHROOM, CND	¼	CUP	59.6	30	3	1	2
6125	GRAVY, TURKEY, CND	¼	CUP	59.6	30	3	2	1
6527	GRAVY, UNSPECIFIED TYPE	¼	CUP	65.4	22	4	1	0
55172	GREEN BEAN MUSHROOM CASSEROLE-STOUFFER'S	1	EACH	134.7	160	13	5	10
55118	GREEN PEPPER STEAK W/ RICE-STOUFFER'S	1	EACH	297.7	310	35	20	10
55780	GREEN PEPPER STEAK-STOUFFER'S	1	OUNCE	28.4	28	1	3	1
62617	GRILLED SALISBURY STEAK-WEIGHT WATCHERS	1	EACH	241.0	250	24	19	9
15032	GROUPER, CKD, DRY HEAT	3	OUNCE	85.1	100	0	21	1
62534	GUAVA JUICE	¾	CUP	179.9	66	16	-	0
19106	GUMDROPS	1	EACH	3.5	14	3	0	0
15034	HADDOCK, CKD, DRY HEAT	3	OUNCE	85.1	95	0	21	1
15035	HADDOCK, SMOKED	3	OUNCE	85.1	99	0	21	1
15037	HALIBUT, CKD, DRY HEAT	3	OUNCE	85.1	119	0	23	3
15196	HALIBUT, GREENLAND, CKD, DRY HEAT	3	OUNCE	85.1	203	0	16	15
55159	HAM AND ASPARAGUS BAKE-STOUFFER'S	1	EACH	269.3	520	32	18	35
7032	HAM AND CHEESE LOAF(OR ROLL), LUNCH MEAT	1	SLICE	28.4	73	0	5	6
7033	HAM AND CHEESE SPREAD, LUNCH MEAT	1	TBSP.	15.0	37	0	2	3
7031	HAM SALAD SPREAD	1	TBSP.	15.0	32	2	1	2
7029	HAM, APPROX 11% FAT, SLICED	1	SLICE	28.4	52	1	5	3
7027	HAM, CHOPPED, NOT CND	3	OUNCE	85.1	195	0	15	15
7026	HAM, CHOPPED, SPICED, CND	3	OUNCE	85.1	203	0	14	16
7028	HAM, EXTRA LEAN, APPX 5% FAT	1	SLICE	28.4	37	0	5	1
7030	HAM, MINCED	3	OUNCE	85.1	224	2	14	18
62626	HAMBURGER PATTY, MEATLESS	1	EACH	90.0	140	8	18	4
55809	HEARTLAND MEDLEY-STOUFFER'S	1	OUNCE	28.4	17	2	1	0
41279	HEARTY BEEF SOUP-HEALTHY CHOICE	1	EACH	212.6	120	17	9	1
41280	HEARTY CHICKEN SOUP-HEALTHY CHOICE	1	EACH	212.6	110	17	7	2
41258	HERB ROASTED CHICKEN-HEALTHY CHOICE	1	EACH	347.3	300	50	22	5
15040	HERRING, CKD, DRY HEAT	3	OUNCE	85.1	173	0	20	10
15042	HERRING, KIPPERED	3	OUNCE	85.1	185	0	21	11
15197	HERRING, PACIFIC, CKD, DRY HEAT	3	OUNCE	85.1	213	0	18	15
15041	HERRING, PICKLED	3	OUNCE	85.1	223	8	12	15
41311	HOMESTYLE TURKEY W/ VEGETABLES-HEALTHY CHOICE	1	EACH	269.3	260	34	26	2
20030	HOMINY, CND, WHITE	½	CUP	80.0	58	11	1	1
20330	HOMINY, CND, YELLOW	½	CUP	80.0	58	11	1	1
19296	HONEY	1	TBSP.	21.0	64	17	0	0
7035	HONEY LOAF, LUNCH MEAT	1	SLICE	28.4	36	2	4	1
55214	HONEY MUSTARD CHICKEN, LEAN CUISINE-STOUFFER'S	1	EACH	212.6	230	30	18	4
41312	HONEY MUSTARD CHICKEN-HEALTHY CHOICE	1	EACH	269.3	310	41	26	4
43371	HOT CHILI NO BEANS-HORMEL	1	EACH	212.6	360	14	16	27
43410	HOT CHILI W/ BEANS, MICRO CUP-HORMEL	1	EACH	209.1	250	24	15	11
43372	HOT CHILI W/ BEANS-HORMEL	1	EACH	212.6	300	27	15	15
7022	HOT DOG, BEEF	1	EACH	57.0	180	1	7	16
7024	HOT DOG, CHICKEN	1	EACH	45.0	116	3	6	9
62605	HOT DOG, FAT FREE	1	EACH	50.0	40	2	7	0
7025	HOT DOG, TURKEY	1	EACH	45.0	102	1	6	8
16137	HUMMUS, FRESH	½	CUP	123.0	210	25	6	10
18270	HUSH PUPPIES	1	EACH	22.0	74	10	2	3
18271	ICE CREAM CONES, CAKE OR WAFER-TYPE	1	EACH	4.0	17	3	0	0
18272	ICE CREAM CONES, SUGAR, ROLLED-TYPE	1	EACH	10.0	40	8	1	0
19270	ICE CREAM, CHOCOLATE	½	CUP	66.0	143	19	3	7
19090	ICE CREAM, FRENCH VANILLA, SOFT-SERVE	½	CUP	66.5	143	15	3	9
19271	ICE CREAM, STRAWBERRY	½	CUP	66.0	127	18	2	6
19095	ICE CREAM, VANILLA	½	CUP	66.0	133	16	2	7
19089	ICE CREAM, VANILLA, RICH	½	CUP	66.5	160	15	2	11

Saturated fat (g)	Monounsaturated fat (g)	Polyunsaturated fat (g)	Fiber (g)	Cholesterol (g)	Folate (g)	Vitamin A (RE)	Vitamin B-6 (mg)	Vitamin B-12 (µg)	Vitamin C (mg)	Vitamin E (mg)	Riboflavin (mg)	Thiamin (mg)	Calcium (mg)	Iron (mg)	Magnesium (mg)	Niacin (mg)	Phosphorus (mg)	Potassium (mg)	Sodium (mg)	Zinc (mg)
0	0	0	0	0	11	0	0	0	27	-	0	0	18	.5	12	.3	12	161	2	.1
0	0	0	1	0	2	5	.1	0	2	-	0	0	6	.1	2	.1	5	88	1	0
0	0	0	-	0	1	0	0	.1	1	-	0	0	2	.4	1	.5	18	48	30	.6
1	1	0	0	2	1	0	0	.1	0	-	0	0	3	.4	1	.4	17	47	326	.6
1	2	1	0	1	1	66	0	.1	0	-	0	0	12	.3	1	.3	17	65	344	.5
0	1	1	0	0	7	0	0	0	0	-	0	0	4	.4	1	.4	9	63	340	.4
0	1	0	0	1	1	0	0	.1	0	-	0	0	2	.4	1	.8	17	65	344	.5
0	0	0	-	0	1	0	0	0	0	-	0	0	9	.1	3	.2	12	16	356	.1
-	-	-	-	-	-	40	-	-	2	-	.2	.1	64	.2	-	.4	-	200	550	-
-	-	-	-	-	-	40	-	-	6	-	.2	.2	16	1	-	3.8	-	410	700	-
-	-	-	7	-	-	-	-	-	4	-	0	0	48	0	-	.1	-	51	164	-
3	-	-	4	30	-	60	-	-	0	-	-	-	120	1.5	-	-	-	450	590	-
0	0	0	0	40	9	43	.3	.6	0	-	0	.1	18	1	31	.3	122	404	45	.4
-	-	-	0	-	-	0	-	-	30	-	-	-	0	0	-	-	-	-	18	-
0	0	0	0	0	0	0	0	0	0	-	0	0	0	0	0	0	0	0	2	0
0	0	0	0	63	11	16	.3	1.2	0	-	0	0	36	1.1	43	3.9	205	339	74	.4
0	0	0	0	65	13	19	.3	1.4	0	-	0	0	42	1.2	46	4.3	213	353	649	.4
0	1	1	0	35	12	46	.3	1.2	0	-	.1	.1	51	.9	91	6.1	242	490	59	.5
3	9	1	0	50	1	15	.4	.8	0	-	.1	.1	3	.7	28	1.6	179	293	88	.4
-	-	-	-	-	-	60	-	-	36	-	.5	.5	160	.8	-	2.9	-	360	1100	-
2	3	1	0	16	1	7	.1	.2	7	-	.1	.2	16	.3	5	1	72	83	381	.6
1	1	0	0	9	0	14	0	.1	1	-	0	0	33	.1	3	.3	74	24	180	.3
1	1	0	0	6	0	0	0	.1	1	-	0	.1	1	.1	2	.3	18	22	137	.2
1	1	0	0	16	1	0	.1	.2	8	-	.1	.2	2	.3	5	1.5	70	94	373	.6
5	7	2	0	43	1	0	.3	.8	17	-	.2	.5	6	.7	14	3.3	132	271	1166	1.6
5	8	2	0	42	1	0	.3	.6	2	-	.1	.5	6	.8	11	2.7	118	242	1161	1.6
0	1	0	0	13	1	0	.1	.2	7	-	.1	.3	2	.2	5	1.4	62	99	405	.5
6	8	2	0	60	1	0	.2	.8	26	-	.2	.6	9	.7	14	3.5	134	265	1059	1.6
2	-	1	5	0	-	0	-	-	0	-	-	.3	96	1.5	-	4	-	-	380	7.5
-	-	-	3	-	-	-	-	-	1	-	0	0	40	0	-	.1	-	60	85	-
-	-	-	-	20	-	150	-	-	9	-	.1	.1	32	.4	-	1.9	90	280	540	-
-	-	-	-	25	-	200	-	-	2	-	.2	.1	32	.4	-	1.9	90	190	520	-
2	-	1	-	40	-	250	-	-	24	-	.1	.2	32	.8	-	7.6	280	370	560	-
2	4	2	0	65	10	26	.3	11.2	1	-	.3	.1	63	1.2	35	3.5	258	356	98	1.1
2	4	2	0	70	12	33	.4	15.9	1	-	.3	.1	71	1.3	39	3.7	276	380	781	1.2
4	7	3	0	84	5	30	.4	8.2	0	-	.2	.1	90	1.2	35	2.4	248	461	81	.6
2	10	1	0	11	2	219	.1	3.6	0	-	.1	0	65	1	7	2.8	76	59	740	.5
-	-	-	-	30	-	100	-	-	5	-	.1	0	32	-	-	-	-	100	550	-
0	0	0	2	0	1	0	0	0	0	-	0	0	8	.5	13	0	28	7	168	.8
0	0	0	-	0	1	9	0	0	0	-	0	0	8	.5	13	0	28	7	168	.8
-	-	0	0	0	0	0	0	0	0	-	0	0	1	.1	0	0	1	11	1	0
0	1	0	0	10	2	0	.1	.3	6	-	.1	.1	5	.4	5	.9	41	97	374	.7
1	-	1	-	40	-	200	-	-	2	-	.2	.2	16	.4	-	3.8	-	340	540	-
1	-	-	-	45	-	100	-	-	4	-	.2	.2	16	.8	-	1.5	-	110	520	-
11	13	1	-	60	-	330	-	-	-	-	.2	.2	40	1.4	35	2.5	-	497	860	2.7
4	4	-	-	49	-	190	-	-	-	-	.2	.1	48	1.9	46	1.7	-	677	977	2.7
5	6	1	-	55	-	210	-	-	-	-	.2	.1	48	1.8	49	1.7	-	777	1030	2.3
7	8	1	0	35	2	0	.1	.9	14	-	.1	0	11	.8	2	1.4	50	95	585	1.2
2	4	2	0	45	2	17	.1	.1	0	-	.1	0	43	.9	5	1.4	48	38	617	.5
0	0	0	0	15	-	0	-	-	0	-	-	-	0	.2	-	-	-	-	460	-
3	3	2	0	48	4	0	.1	.1	0	-	.1	.1	48	.8	6	1.9	60	81	642	1.4
2	4	4	6	0	73	2	.5	0	10	-	.1	.1	61	1.9	36	.5	138	214	300	1.4
0	1	2	1	10	4	9	0	0	0	-	.1	.1	61	.7	5	.6	42	32	147	.1
0	0	0	0	0	0	0	0	0	0	-	0	0	1	.1	1	.2	4	4	6	0
0	0	0	0	0	1	0	0	0	0	-	0	.1	4	.4	3	.5	10	15	32	.1
4	2	0	-	22	11	79	0	.2	0	-	.1	0	72	.6	19	.1	71	164	50	.4
5	2	0	-	61	6	102	0	.3	1	-	.1	0	87	.1	8	.1	77	118	41	.3
-	-	-	-	19	8	51	0	.2	5	-	.2	0	79	.1	9	.1	66	124	40	.2
4	2	0	0	29	3	77	0	.3	0	-	.2	0	84	.1	9	.1	69	131	53	.5
7	3	0	0	41	3	122	0	.2	0	-	.1	0	78	Trace	7	.1	63	106	37	.3

Food Composition Table—cont'd

Code	Name	Amount	Unit	Grams	Kilocalories	Carbohydrates (g)	Protein (g)	Fat (g)
19088	ICE MILK, VANILLA	½	CUP	66.5	92	15	3	3
19096	ICE MILK, VANILLA, SOFT SERVE	½	CUP	66.5	84	14	3	2
19283	ICE POPS	1	BAR	52.0	37	10	0	0
19717	ICE POPS, W/ ADDED ASCORBIC ACID	1	BAR	52.0	37	10	0	0
62547	ICED TEA, BOTTLED, ALL FLAVORS	1	CUP	236.6	118	29	0	0
62548	ICED TEA, BOTTLED, ALL FLAVORS, DIET	1	CUP	236.6	0	1	0	0
62622	ITALIAN CHEESE LASAGNA-WEIGHT WATCHERS	1	EACH	311.9	300	28	29	8
43395	ITALIAN LASAGNA, TOP SHELF-HORMEL	1	EACH	283.5	350	30	23	16
55798	ITALIAN STYLE VEGETABLES-STOUFFER'S	1	OUNCE	28.4	10	2	0	0
19297	JAMS AND PRESERVES	1	TBSP.	20.0	48	13	0	0
19300	JELLIES	1	TBSP.	19.0	51	13	0	0
19108	JELLYBEANS	1	EACH	1.1	4	1	0	0
19109	KIT KAT WAFER BAR	1	BAR	46.0	235	28	3	13
9148	KIWIFRUIT, FRESH	1	MEDIUM	76.0	46	11	1	0
19110	KRACKEL CHOCOLATE BAR	1	BAR	47.0	236	29	3	13
17225	LAMB, GROUND, CKD, BROILED	3	OUNCE	85.1	241	0	21	17
17016	LAMB, LEG, SHANK, MEAT AND FAT, CKD, RSTD	3	OUNCE	85.1	191	0	22	11
17018	LAMB, LEG, SHANK, MEAT ONLY, CKD, RSTD	3	OUNCE	85.1	153	0	24	6
17020	LAMB, LEG, SIRLOIN, MEAT AND FAT, CKD, RSTD	3	OUNCE	85.1	248	0	21	18
17022	LAMB, LEG, SIRLOIN, MEAT ONLY, CKD, RSTD	3	OUNCE	85.1	174	0	24	8
17012	LAMB, LEG, WHOLE, MEAT AND FAT, CKD, RSTD	3	OUNCE	85.1	219	0	22	14
17014	LAMB, LEG, WHOLE, MEAT ONLY, CKD, RSTD	3	OUNCE	85.1	162	0	24	7
17024	LAMB, LOIN, MEAT AND FAT, CKD, BROILED	3	OUNCE	85.1	269	0	21	20
17025	LAMB, LOIN, MEAT AND FAT, CKD, ROASTED	3	OUNCE	85.1	263	0	19	20
17027	LAMB, LOIN, MEAT ONLY, CKD, BROILED	3	OUNCE	85.1	184	0	26	8
17028	LAMB, LOIN, MEAT ONLY, CKD, ROASTED	3	OUNCE	85.1	172	0	23	8
17002	LAMB, MEAT AND FAT, CKD	3	OUNCE	85.1	250	0	21	18
17004	LAMB, MEAT ONLY, CKD	3	OUNCE	85.1	175	0	24	8
17030	LAMB, RIB, MEAT AND FAT, CKD, BROILED	3	OUNCE	85.1	307	0	19	25
17031	LAMB, RIB, MEAT AND FAT, CKD, ROASTED	3	OUNCE	85.1	305	0	18	25
17033	LAMB, RIB, MEAT ONLY, CKD, BROILED	3	OUNCE	85.1	200	0	24	11
17034	LAMB, RIB, MEAT ONLY, CKD, ROASTED	3	OUNCE	85.1	197	0	22	11
4002	LARD	¼	CUP	51.3	462	0	0	51
62613	LASAGNA FLORENTINE-WEIGHT WATCHERS	1	EACH	283.5	210	37	13	2
55215	LASAGNA W/ MEAT SAUCE, LEAN CUISINE-STOUFFER'S	1	EACH	290.6	280	36	20	6
41308	LASAGNA W/ MEAT SAUCE-HEALTHY CHOICE	1	EACH	283.5	260	37	18	5
62623	LASAGNA WITH MEAT SAUCE-WEIGHT WATCHERS	1	EACH	290.6	290	34	24	7
43403	LASAGNA, MICRO CUP-HORMEL	1	EACH	212.6	250	25	8	13
55134	LASAGNA-STOUFFER'S	1	EACH	283.5	340	40	18	12
11247	LEEKS, CKD	½	CUP	52.0	16	4	0	0
11246	LEEKS, FRESH	½	CUP	52.0	32	7	1	0
18320	LEMON MERINGUE PIE	1	SLICE	113.0	303	53	2	10
41259	LEMON PEPPER FISH-HEALTHY CHOICE	1	EACH	304.8	300	52	13	5
18445	LEMON PIE, FRIED	1	PIE	128.0	404	55	4	21
19380	LEMON PUDDING	1	CUP	298.1	373	75	0	9
14145	LEMON-LIME SODA	12	FL OZ	368.4	147	38	0	0
62529	LEMON-LIME SODA, DIET	12	FL OZ	355.2	0	0	0	0
14297	LEMONADE FLAVOR DRINK	1	CUP	266.0	112	29	0	0
14543	LEMONADE, PINK	1	CUP	247.8	99	26	0	0
14290	LEMONADE, LOW CALORIE	1	CUP	243.7	5	1	0	0
14293	LEMONADE, WHITE	1	CUP	247.8	99	26	0	0
9150	LEMONS, FRESH, W/O PEEL	1	MEDIUM	58.0	17	5	1	0
41274	LENTIL SOUP-HEALTHY CHOICE	1	EACH	212.6	140	23	8	1
11250	LETTUCE, BUTTERHEAD, FRESH	1	CUP	56.0	7	1	1	0
11252	LETTUCE, ICEBERG, FRESH	1	CUP	56.0	7	1	1	0
11253	LETTUCE, LOOSELEAF, FRESH	1	CUP	56.0	10	2	1	0
11251	LETTUCE, ROMAINE, FRESH	1	CUP	56.0	9	1	1	0
55216	LINGUINI W/ CLAM SAUCE, LEAN CUISINE-STOUFFER'S	1	EACH	272.9	280	36	17	8
14415	LIQUEUR, COFFEE W/ CREAM, 34 PROOF	1	FL OZ	31.1	102	6	1	5
14414	LIQUEUR, COFFEE, 53 PROOF	1	FL OZ	34.8	117	16	0	0

Saturated fat (g)	Monounsaturated fat (g)	Polyunsaturated fat (g)	Fiber (g)	Cholesterol (g)	Folate (g)	Vitamin A (RE)	Vitamin B-6 (mg)	Vitamin B-12 (µg)	Vitamin C (mg)	Vitamin E (mg)	Riboflavin (mg)	Thiamin (mg)	Calcium (mg)	Iron (mg)	Magnesium (mg)	Niacin (mg)	Phosphorus (mg)	Potassium (mg)	Sodium (mg)	Zinc (mg)
2	1	0	0	9	4	31	0	.4	1	-	.2	0	92	.1	10	.1	72	140	57	.3
1	1	0	0	8	4	19	0	.3	1	-	.1	0	104	0	9	.1	80	147	47	.4
-	-	-	0	0	0	0	0	0	0	-	0	0	0	0	1	0	0	2	6	0
-	-	-	0	0	0	0	0	0	6	-	0	0	0	0	1	0	0	2	6	0
0	-	-	0	0	-	0	-	-	0	-	-	-	0	0	-	-	-	-	10	-
0	-	-	0	0	-	0	-	-	0	-	-	-	0	0	-	-	-	-	0	-
3	-	-	7	25	-	350	-	-	15	-	-	-	780	1.5	-	-	-	720	560	-
8	5	1	-	60	-	100	-	-	2	-	.5	.3	240	1.5	49	3.8	-	728	840	3.2
-	-	-	-	0	-	-	-	-	2	-	0	0	72	0	-	0	-	62	147	-
0	0	0	0	0	7	0	0	0	2	-	0	0	4	.1	1	0	2	15	8	0
-	-	-	0	0	0	0	0	0	0	-	0	0	2	0	1	0	1	12	7	0
-	-	-	0	0	0	0	0	0	0	-	0	0	0	0	0	0	0	0	0	0
8	4	0	0	12	0	14	0	.3	1	-	.1	0	83	.4	20	.2	80	142	46	.5
-	-	-	3	0	-	14	-	0	74	-	0	0	20	.3	23	.4	30	252	4	-
6	3	3	-	9	4	6	0	.3	0	-	.1	0	84	.4	26	.2	104	161	64	.6
7	7	1	0	82	16	0	.1	2.2	-	.1	.2	.1	19	1.5	20	5.7	171	288	69	4
4	4	1	0	77	19	0	.1	2.3	0	.1	.2	.1	9	1.7	21	5.6	168	277	55	4
2	2	0	0	74	20	0	.1	2.3	0	.2	.2	.1	7	1.8	22	5.4	177	291	56	4.3
7	7	1	0	82	14	0	.1	2.2	0	.1	.2	1	9	1.7	19	5.6	156	256	58	3.5
3	3	1	0	78	18	0	.1	2.2	0	.1	.3	.1	7	1.9	21	5.3	173	283	60	4.1
6	6	1	0	79	17	0	.1	2.2	0	.1	.2	.1	9	1.7	20	5.6	162	266	56	3.7
2	3	0	0	76	20	0	.1	2.2	0	.2	.2	.1	7	1.8	22	5.4	175	287	58	4.2
8	8	1	0	85	15	0	.1	2.1	0	.1	.2	.1	17	1.5	20	6	167	278	65	3
9	8	2	0	81	16	0	.1	1.9	0	.1	.2	.1	15	1.8	20	6	153	209	54	2.9
3	4	1	0	81	20	0	.1	2.1	0	.1	.2	.1	16	1.7	24	5.8	192	320	71	3.5
3	3	1	0	74	21	0	.1	1.8	0	.1	.2	.1	14	2.1	23	5.8	175	227	56	3.5
8	8	1	0	82	15	0	.1	2.2	0	-	.2	.1	14	1.6	20	5.7	160	264	61	3.8
3	4	1	0	78	20	0	.1	2.2	0	.2	.2	.1	13	1.7	22	5.4	179	293	65	4.5
11	10	2	0	84	12	0	.1	2.2	0	.1	.2	.1	16	1.6	20	6	151	230	65	3.4
11	11	2	0	82	13	0	.1	1.9	0	.1	.2	.1	19	1.4	17	5.7	141	230	62	3
4	4	1	0	77	18	0	.1	2.2	0	.2	.2	.1	14	1.9	25	5.6	181	266	72	4.5
4	5	1	0	75	19	0	.1	1.8	0	.1	.2	.1	18	1.5	20	5.2	166	268	69	3.8
20	23	6	0	49	0	0	0	0	0	.6	0	0	0	0	0	0	0	0	0	.1
1	-	-	5	10	-	300	-	-	15	-	-	-	300	1.5	-	-	-	440	420	-
3	-	-	-	25	-	100	-	-	6	-	.3	.2	120	1	-	2.9	-	700	560	-
2	-	1	-	20	-	150	-	-	2	-	.3	.3	80	1.5	-	1.9	210	500	420	-
3	-	-	7	15	-	250	-	-	12	-	-	-	480	1.5	-	-	-	720	580	-
6	4	2	-	23	-	100	-	-	2	-	.2	.1	40	.8	25	1.9	-	331	949	1.1
-	-	-	-	-	-	150	-	-	6	-	.3	.2	200	1	-	6.7	-	570	840	-
0	0	0	-	0	13	3	.1	0	2	-	0	0	16	.6	7	.1	9	45	5	0
0	0	0	1	0	33	5	.1	0	6	-	0	0	31	1.1	15	.2	18	94	10	.1
2	4	3	1	51	9	59	0	.2	4	-	.2	.1	63	.7	17	.7	119	101	165	.6
1	-	2	-	40	-	80	-	-	48	-	.1	.2	32	.6	-	1.1	180	410	370	-
3	10	7	-	4	4	0	.1	0	-	.1	.2	28	1.6	13	1.8	55	83	479	.3	
1	4	3	-	0	0	0	0	0	0	-	0	0	6	.2	3	0	15	3	417	.1
0	0	0	0	0	0	0	0	0	0	-	0	0	7	.3	4	.1	0	4	41	.2
-	-	-	0	-	-	-	-	-	-	-	-	-	-	-	-	-	-	-	30	-
0	0	0	-	0	0	0	0	0	34	-	0	0	29	.1	3	0	3	3	19	.1
0	0	0	-	0	5	0	0	0	10	-	.1	0	7	.4	5	0	5	37	7	.1
0	-	-	0	0	0	0	0	0	6	-	0	0	51	.1	2	0	24	0	7	.1
0	0	0	-	0	5	5	0	0	10	-	.1	0	7	.4	5	0	5	37	7	.1
0	0	0	2	0	6	2	0	0	31	-	0	0	15	.3	5	.1	9	80	1	0
-	-	-	-	0	-	60	-	-	2	-	0	.1	-	.6	-	.4	-	160	480	-
0	0	0	1	0	41	54	0	0	4	-	0	0	18	.2	7	.2	13	144	3	.1
0	0	0	1	0	31	18	0	0	2	-	0	0	11	.3	5	.1	11	88	5	.1
0	0	0	1	0	28	106	0	0	10	-	0	0	38	.8	6	.2	14	148	5	.2
0	0	0	1	0	76	146	0	0	13	-	.1	.1	20	.6	3	.3	25	162	4	.1
2	-	2	-	30	-	-	-	-	-	-	.2	.3	32	1.5	-	1.9	-	90	560	-
3	1	0	0	5	0	13	0	0	0	-	0	0	5	0	1	0	16	10	29	0
0	0	0	0	0	0	0	0	0	0	-	0	0	0	0	1	.1	2	10	3	0

Food Composition Table—cont'd

Code	Name	Amount	Unit	Grams	Kilocalories	Carbohydrates (g)	Protein (g)	Fat (g)
14534	LIQUEUR, COFFEE, 63 PROOF	1	FL OZ	34.8	107	11	0	0
14533	LIQUOR, DISTILLED, ALL 100 PROOF	1	FL OZ	27.8	82	0	0	0
14037	LIQUOR, DISTILLED, ALL 80 PROOF	1	FL OZ	27.8	64	0	0	0
14550	LIQUOR, DISTILLED, ALL 86 PROOF	1	FL OZ	27.8	70	0	0	0
14551	LIQUOR, DISTILLED, ALL 90 PROOF	1	FL OZ	27.8	73	0	0	0
14532	LIQUOR, DISTILLED, ALL 94 PROOF	1	FL OZ	27.8	76	0	0	0
15148	LOBSTER, NORTHERN, CKD, MOIST HEAT	3	OUNCE	85.1	83	1	17	1
15228	LOBSTER, SPINY, CKD, MOIST HEAT	3	OUNCE	85.1	122	3	22	2
19107	LOLLIPOP	1	EACH	6.0	22	6	0	0
19140	M&M'S PEANUT	1	PKG	49.0	243	29	5	13
19141	M&M'S PLAIN	1	PKG	48.0	228	33	3	11
12131	MACADAMIA DRIED	½	CUP	67.0	470	9	6	49
12633	MACADAMIA OIL ROASTED	½	CUP	67.0	481	9	5	51
55217	MACARONI AND BEEF IN SAUCE, LEAN CUISINE-STOUFFER'S	1	EACH	283.5	250	35	14	6
55137	MACARONI AND BEEF W/ TOMATOES-STOUFFER'S	1	EACH	326.0	340	38	21	12
41338	MACARONI AND BEEF-HEALTHY CHOICE	1	EACH	241.0	200	32	12	3
62533	MACARONI AND CHEESE	1	CUP	111.9	360	44	1	13
57808	MACARONI AND CHEESE POT PIE-SWANSON	1	EACH	198.5	200	24	7	8
55218	MACARONI AND CHEESE, LEAN CUISINE-STOUFFER'S	1	EACH	255.1	290	37	15	9
43406	MACARONI AND CHEESE, MICRO CUP-HORMEL	1	EACH	212.6	260	28	12	11
41339	MACARONI AND CHEESE-HEALTHY CHOICE	1	EACH	255.1	280	45	12	6
55155	MACARONI AND CHEESE-STOUFFER'S	1	EACH	170.1	250	23	11	13
62624	MACARONI AND CHEESE-WEIGHT WATCHERS	1	EACH	255.2	260	43	15	6
20100	MACARONI, CKD, ENRICHED	1	CUP	140.0	197	40	7	1
20400	MACARONI, CKD, UNENRICHED	1	CUP	140.0	197	40	7	1
20106	MACARONI, VEGETABLE, CKD, ENRICHED	1	CUP	134.0	172	36	6	0
20108	MACARONI, WHOLE-WHEAT, CKD	1	CUP	140.0	174	37	7	1
41309	MANDARIN CHICKEN-HEALTHY CHOICE	1	EACH	311.8	260	39	23	2
62535	MANGO JUICE	¾	CUP	179.9	66	16	-	0
9176	MANGOS, FRESH	½	CUP	82.5	54	14	0	0
14012	MANHATTAN	1	FL OZ	28.5	64	1	0	0
4067	MARGARINE, HARD, CORN&SYBN	1	TSP.	4.7	34	0	0	4
4071	MARGARINE, HARD, CORN(HYDR)	1	TSP.	4.7	34	0	0	4
4128	MARGARINE, IMITATION (APPX 40% FAT)	1	TSP.	4.8	17	0	0	2
4132	MARGARINE, REGULAR, W/ SALT ADDED	1	TSP.	4.7	34	0	0	4
4131	MARGARINE, REGULAR, W/O ADDED SALT	1	TSP.	4.7	34	0	0	4
4130	MARGARINE, SOFT, W/ SALT ADDED	1	TSP.	4.7	34	0	0	4
4129	MARGARINE, SOFT, W/O ADDED SALT	1	TSP.	4.7	34	0	0	4
11256	MARINARA SAUCE	½	CUP	125.0	85	13	2	4
55830	MARINARA SAUCE-STOUFFER'S	1	CUP	283.9	180	18	3	11
19303	MARMALADE, ORANGE	1	TBSP.	20.0	49	13	0	0
19116	MARSHMALLOWS	1	CUP	46.0	146	37	1	0
14014	MARTINI	1	FL OZ	28.2	63	0	0	0
4018	MAYONNAISE	1	TBSP.	14.7	57	4	0	5
62610	MAYONNAISE, FAT FREE	1	TBSP.	15.0	10	3	0	0
62609	MAYONNAISE, LIGHT	1	TBSP.	15.0	25	1	0	2
55219	MEATLOAF W/ MAC. AND CHEESE, LEAN CUISINE-STOUFFER'S	1	EACH	265.8	280	26	26	8
41260	MEATLOAF-HEALTHY CHOICE	1	EACH	340.2	340	48	17	8
55779	MEATLOAF-STOUFFER'S	1	OUNCE	28.4	57	2	4	3
9185	MELON BALLS, FROZEN, UNTHAWED	½	CUP	86.5	29	7	1	0
9181	MELONS, CANTALOUP, FRESH	1	WEDGE	80.0	28	7	1	0
9183	MELONS, CASABA, FRESH	1	WEDGE	164.0	43	10	1	0
9184	MELONS, HONEYDEW, FRESH	1	WEDGE	129.0	45	12	1	0
55812	MEXICALI CHICKEN-STOUFFER'S	1	OUNCE	28.4	20	2	1	1
19120	MILK CHOCOLATE	1	BAR	44.0	226	26	3	13
19126	MILK CHOCOLATE COATED PEANUTS	1	OUNCE	28.4	147	14	4	9
19127	MILK CHOCOLATE COATED RAISINS	1	OUNCE	28.4	111	19	1	4
19132	MILK CHOCOLATE W/ ALMONDS	1	BAR	41.0	216	22	4	14
1110	MILK SHAKES, THICK CHOCOLATE	1	CUP	345.4	410	73	11	9
1111	MILK SHAKES, THICK VANILLA	1	CUP	345.4	386	61	13	10

Saturated fat (g)	Monounsaturated fat (g)	Polyunsaturated fat (g)	Fiber (g)	Cholesterol (g)	Folate (g)	Vitamin A (RE)	Vitamin B-6 (mg)	Vitamin B-12 (µg)	Vitamin C (mg)	Vitamin E (mg)	Riboflavin (mg)	Thiamin (mg)	Calcium (mg)	Iron (mg)	Magnesium (mg)	Niacin (mg)	Phosphorus (mg)	Potassium (mg)	Sodium (mg)	Zinc (mg)
0	0	0	-	0	0	0	0	0	0	-	0	0	0	0	1	.1	2	10	3	0
0	0	0	-	0	0	0	0	0	0	-	0	0	0	0	0	0	1	1	0	0
0	0	0	0	0	0	0	0	0	0	-	0	0	0	0	0	0	1	1	0	0
0	0	0	0	0	0	0	0	0	0	-	0	0	0	0	0	0	1	1	0	0
0	0	0	0	0	0	0	0	0	0	-	0	0	0	0	0	0	1	1	0	0
0	0	0	-	0	0	0	0	0	0	-	0	0	0	0	0	0	1	1	0	0
0	0	0	0	61	9	22	.1	2.6	0	-	.1	0	52	.3	30	.9	157	299	323	2.5
0	0	1	0	77	1	5	.1	3.4	2	-	0	0	54	1.2	43	4.2	195	177	193	6.2
-	-	-	0	0	0	0	0	0	0	-	0	0	0	0	0	0	0	0	2	0
-	-	-	2	6	27	4	.1	.2	0	-	.1	0	65	.7	40	1.6	134	191	46	.7
-	-	-	1	7	4	12	0	.2	0	-	.1	0	81	.7	32	.3	94	188	49	.6
7	39	1	6	0	11	0	.1	0	0	-	.1	.2	47	1.6	78	1.4	91	247	3	1.1
8	40	1	6	0	11	1	.1	0	0	-	.1	.1	30	1.2	78	1.4	134	220	174	.7
1	-	1	-	25	-	100	-	-	4	-	.2	.2	48	1.5	-	2.9	-	450	540	-
-	-	-	-	-	-	60	-	-	6	-	.1	.1	32	.8	-	1.9	-	300	1440	-
1	-	-	-	15	-	200	-	-	15	-	.3	.3	32	1	-	0	-	530	420	-
8	-	-	16	40	-	100	-	-	0	-	-	-	240	1.5	-	-	-	-	1029	-
-	-	-	-	-	-	80	-	-	-	-	.2	.1	120	.6	-	.8	-	-	740	-
4	-	-	-	30	-	-	-	-	-	-	.4	.3	200	.8	-	1.5	-	160	550	-
6	3	1	-	45	-	80	-	-	6	-	.3	.1	80	.6	25	1.1	-	209	650	1.1
3	-	1	-	20	-	-	-	-	-	-	.3	.3	120	1	-	1.1	230	220	520	-
-	-	-	-	-	-	20	-	-	-	-	.3	.2	160	.4	-	.4	-	140	640	-
2	-	-	7	20	-	100	-	-	0	-	-	-	300	1	-	-	-	410	550	-
0	0	0	2	0	10	0	0	0	0	-	.1	.3	10	2	25	2.3	76	43	1	.7
0	0	0	2	0	10	-	0	0	0	-	0	0	10	.7	25	.6	76	43	1	.7
0	0	0	6	0	8	7	0	0	0	-	.1	.2	15	.7	25	1.4	67	42	8	.6
0	0	0	6	0	7	0	.1	0	0	-	.1	.2	21	1.5	42	1	125	62	4	1.1
-	-	-	-	50	-	250	-	-	9	-	.2	.2	16	1	-	4.8	200	400	400	-
-	-	-	-	-	0	-	-	-	30	-	-	-	0	0	-	-	-	-	18	-
0	0	0	1	0	-	321	.1	0	23	.9	0	0	8	.1	7	.5	9	129	2	0
0	0	0	-	0	0	0	0	0	0	-	0	0	1	0	1	0	2	7	1	0
1	2	1	0	0	0	47	0	0	0	.5	0	0	1	0	0	0	1	2	44	0
1	2	1	0	0	0	47	0	0	0	.5	0	0	1	0	0	0	1	2	44	-
0	1	1	0	0	0	48	0	0	0	.2	0	0	1	0	0	0	1	1	46	0
1	2	1	0	0	0	47	0	0	0	.4	0	0	1	0	0	0	1	2	44	0
1	2	1	0	0	0	47	0	0	0	.4	0	0	1	0	0	0	1	1	0	0
1	1	2	0	0	0	47	0	0	0	.3	0	0	1	0	0	0	1	2	51	0
1	2	1	0	0	0	47	0	0	0	.3	0	0	1	0	0	0	1	2	1	0
1	2	1	-	0	17	120	.3	0	16	-	.1	.1	22	1	30	2	44	530	786	.3
-	-	-	-	0	-	-	-	-	66	-	0	0	721	.2	-	.4	-	681	1222	-
-	-	-	0	0	7	1	0	0	1	-	0	0	8	0	0	0	1	7	11	0
-	-	-	0	0	0	0	0	0	0	-	0	0	1	0	.1	1	0	4	2	22	0
0	0	0	-	0	0	0	0	0	0	-	0	0	1	0	1	0	1	5	1	0
1	1	3	0	4	1	12	0	0	0	.6	0	0	2	0	0	0	4	1	104	0
0	-	-	0	0	-	0	-	-	0	-	-	-	0	0	-	-	-	10	105	-
0	-	-	-	5	-	0	-	-	0	-	-	-	0	0	-	-	-	5	130	-
3	-	1	-	55	-	60	-	-	9	-	.4	.2	120	2	-	3.8	-	550	540	-
3	-	1	-	40	-	-	-	-	-	-	-	-	-	-	-	-	240	690	560	-
-	-	-	-	15	-	-	-	-	0	-	0	0	48	.1	-	.1	-	4	193	-
-	-	-	1	0	22	153	.1	0	5	-	0	.1	9	.3	12	.6	10	242	27	.1
-	-	-	1	0	14	258	.1	0	34	.1	0	0	9	.2	9	.5	14	247	7	.1
-	-	-	1	0	-	5	-	0	26	-	0	.1	8	.7	13	.7	11	344	20	-
-	-	-	1	0	-	5	.1	0	32	-	0	.1	8	.1	9	.8	13	350	13	-
-	-	-	5	-	-	-	-	-	4	-	0	0	88	0	-	.1	-	68	48	-
8	4	0	2	10	3	21	0	.2	0	-	.1	0	84	.6	26	.1	95	169	36	.6
4	4	1	1	3	2	0	.1	.1	0	-	0	0	29	.4	26	1.2	60	142	12	.5
2	1	0	1	1	1	2	0	.1	0	-	0	0	24	.5	13	.1	41	146	10	.2
7	6	1	3	8	5	6	0	.2	0	-	.2	0	92	.7	37	.3	108	182	30	.5
6	3	0	1	36	17	73	.1	1.1	0	-	.8	.2	456	1.1	55	.4	435	774	383	1.7
7	3	0	0	41	23	97	.1	1.8	0	-	.7	.1	505	.3	41	.5	398	631	330	1.3

Food Composition Table—cont'd

Code	Name	Amount	Unit	Grams	Kilocalories	Carbohydrates (g)	Protein (g)	Fat (g)
1075	MILK SUBSTITUTES, FLUID W/ HYDR VEGETABLE OILS	1	CUP	244.0	150	15	4	8
1076	MILK SUBSTITUTES, FLUID, W/ LAURIC ACID OIL	1	CUP	244.0	150	15	4	8
1088	MILK, BUTTERMILK	1	CUP	245.0	99	12	8	2
1104	MILK, CHOCOLATE DRINK, LOWFAT, 1% FAT	1	CUP	250.0	158	26	8	2
1103	MILK, CHOCOLATE DRINK, LOWFAT, 2% FAT	1	CUP	250.0	179	26	8	5
1102	MILK, CHOCOLATE DRINK, WHOLE	1	CUP	250.0	208	26	8	8
1105	MILK, CHOCOLATE HOMEMADE HOT COCOA	1	CUP	250.0	218	26	9	9
1095	MILK, CND, CONDENSED, SWEETENED	¼	CUP	76.3	245	42	6	7
1153	MILK, CND, EVAPORATED	¼	CUP	63.0	85	6	4	5
1097	MILK, CND, EVAPORATED, SKIM	¼	CUP	63.8	50	7	5	0
1082	MILK, LOWFAT, 1% FAT	1	CUP	244.0	102	12	8	3
1079	MILK, LOWFAT, 2% FAT	1	CUP	244.0	121	12	8	5
1099	MILK, MALTED, BEVERAGE	1	CUP	265.0	236	27	10	10
1101	MILK, MALTED, CHOCOLATE FLAVOR, BEVERAGE	1	CUP	265.0	228	30	9	9
1085	MILK, SKIM	1	CUP	245.0	86	12	8	0
1077	MILK, WHOLE, 3.3% FAT	1	CUP	244.0	150	11	8	8
1078	MILK, WHOLE, 3.7% FAT	1	CUP	244.0	157	11	8	9
19135	MILKY WAY BAR	1	BAR	60.0	251	44	3	9
18322	MINCE MEAT PIE	1	SLICE	165.0	477	79	4	18
55770	MINESTRONE HEAT'N SERVE SOUP-STOUFFER'S	1	CUP	283.9	130	18	5	4
41281	MINESTRONE SOUP-HEALTHY CHOICE	1	EACH	212.6	160	30	6	1
55760	MINESTRONE SOUP-STOUFFER'S	1	CUP	283.9	140	20	6	3
12635	MIXED NUTS W/ PEANUTS, DRY ROASTED	½	CUP	68.5	407	17	12	35
12637	MIXED NUTS W/ PEANUTS, OIL ROASTED	½	CUP	71.0	438	15	12	40
12638	MIXED NUTS W/O PEANUTS, OIL ROASTED	½	CUP	72.0	443	16	11	40
18177	MOLASSES COOKIES	1	EACH	15.0	65	11	1	2
19142	MOUNDS CANDY BAR	1	BAR	20.0	72	12	1	4
19143	MR. GOODBAR CHOCOLATE BAR	1	BAR	50.0	257	26	6	16
18274	MUFFINS, BLUEBERRY	1	LARGE	65.0	180	31	4	4
18279	MUFFINS, CORN	1	LARGE	65.0	198	33	4	5
18283	MUFFINS, OAT BRAN	1	LARGE	65.0	176	31	5	5
18273	MUFFINS, PLAIN	1	LARGE	65.0	192	27	4	7
18287	MUFFINS, WHEAT BRAN	1	LARGE	65.0	184	27	5	8
15056	MULLET, STRIPED, CKD, DRY HEAT	3	OUNCE	85.1	128	0	21	4
41313	MUSHROOM GRAVY OVER BEEF SIRLOIN TIPS-HEALTHY CHOICE	1	EACH	269.3	310	43	22	5
11261	MUSHROOMS, CKD	½	CUP	78.0	21	4	2	0
11264	MUSHROOMS, CND, DRAINED SOLIDS	½	CUP	78.0	19	4	1	0
11950	MUSHROOMS, ENOKI, FRESH	1	MEDIUM	3.0	1	0	0	0
11260	MUSHROOMS, FRESH	½	CUP	35.0	9	2	1	0
11269	MUSHROOMS, SHIITAKE, CKD	½	CUP	72.5	40	10	1	0
11268	MUSHROOMS, SHIITAKE, DRIED	1	MEDIUM	3.6	11	3	0	0
15165	MUSSELS, BLUE, CKD, MOIST HEAT	3	OUNCE	85.1	146	6	20	4
62619	NACHO GRANDE CHICKEN ENCHILADAS-WEIGHT WATCHERS	1	EACH	255.2	290	42	15	8
41340	NACHO MACARONI AND CHEESE-HEALTHY CHOICE	1	EACH	255.1	280	44	13	5
55754	NAVY BEAN W/ HAM SOUP-STOUFFER'S	1	CUP	283.9	240	31	11	8
19145	NESTLE CRUNCH	1	BAR	40.0	198	26	2	10
55757	NEW ENGLAND CLAM CHOWDER SOUP-STOUFFER'S	1	CUP	283.9	341	21	14	23
55829	NEWBURG SAUCE SUPREME-STOUFFER'S	1	CUP	283.9	481	20	7	41
43407	NOODLES AND CHICKEN, MICRO CUP-HORMEL	1	EACH	212.6	174	19	7	7
55804	NOODLES ROMANOFF-STOUFFER'S	1	CUP	283.9	441	36	17	25
20113	NOODLES, CHINESE, CHOW MEIN	½	CUP	22.5	119	13	2	7
20310	NOODLES, EGG, CKD, ENRICHED	½	CUP	80.0	106	20	4	1
20510	NOODLES, EGG, CKD, UNENRICHED	½	CUP	80.0	106	20	4	1
20112	NOODLES, EGG, SPINACH, CKD, ENRICHED	½	CUP	80.0	106	19	4	1
20115	NOODLES, JAPANESE, SOBA, CKD	½	CUP	57.0	56	12	3	0
18200	OATMEAL COOKIES, DIETARY	1	EACH	7.0	31	5	0	1
18178	OATMEAL COOKIES, REGULAR	1	EACH	18.0	81	12	1	3
18179	OATMEAL COOKIES, SOFT-TYPE	1	EACH	15.0	61	10	1	2
15058	OCEAN PERCH, ATLANTIC, CKD, DRY HEAT	3	OUNCE	85.1	103	0	20	2
4053	OIL, OLIVE	1	TBSP.	13.5	119	0	0	14

Saturated fat (g)	Monounsaturated fat (g)	Polyunsaturated fat (g)	Fiber (g)	Cholesterol (g)	Folate (g)	Vitamin A (RE)	Vitamin B-6 (mg)	Vitamin B-12 (μg)	Vitamin C (mg)	Vitamin E (mg)	Riboflavin (mg)	Thiamin (mg)	Calcium (mg)	Iron (mg)	Magnesium (mg)	Niacin (mg)	Phosphorus (mg)	Potassium (mg)	Sodium (mg)	Zinc (mg)
2	5	1	0	0	0	0	0	0	0	-	.2	0	79	1	16	0	181	279	191	2.9
7	0	0	0	0	0	0	0	0	0	-	.2	0	79	1	16	0	181	279	191	2.9
1	1	0	0	9	12	20	.1	.5	2	-	.4	.1	285	.1	27	.1	219	371	257	1
2	1	0	0	7	12	147	.1	.9	2	-	.4	.1	287	.6	33	.3	256	425	152	1
3	1	0	4	17	12	142	.1	.8	2	-	.4	.1	284	.6	33	.3	254	422	150	1
5	2	0	4	30	12	72	.1	.8	2	-	.4	.1	280	.6	33	.3	251	417	149	1
6	3	0	4	33	12	85	.1	.9	2	-	.4	.1	298	.8	55	.4	270	480	123	1.2
4	2	0	0	26	9	62	0	.3	2	-	.3	.1	216	.1	20	.2	193	284	97	.7
3	1	0	0	19	5	34	0	.1	1	-	.2	0	164	.1	15	.1	127	191	67	.5
0	0	0	0	2	5	75	0	.2	1	-	.2	0	185	.2	17	.1	124	211	73	.6
2	1	0	0	10	12	144	.1	.9	2	-	.4	.1	300	.1	34	.2	235	381	123	1
3	1	0	0	18	12	139	.1	.9	2	-	.4	.1	297	.1	33	.2	232	377	122	1
6	3	1	0	37	22	95	.2	1	3	-	.6	.2	355	.3	53	1.3	302	530	223	1.1
6	3	0	0	34	16	80	.1	.9	3	-	.4	.1	305	.6	48	.6	265	498	172	1.1
0	0	0		4	13	149	.1	.9	2	-	.3	.1	302	.1	28	.2	247	406	126	1
5	2	0	0	33	12	76	.1	.9	2	-	.4	.1	291	.1	33	.2	228	370	120	.9
6	3	0	0	35	12	83	.1	.9	4	-	.4	.1	290	.1	33	.2	227	368	119	.9
5	3	0	1	12	5	28	0	.3	1	-	.1	0	78	.5	20	.2	98	145	144	.4
4	8	5	-	0	8	3	.1	0	10	-	.2	.2	36	2.5	23	2	69	335	419	.4
-	-	-	-	0	-	-	-	-	0	-	0	0	481	.2	-	0	-	310	1192	-
-	-	-	-	0	-	60	-	-	15	-	.1	.1	32	.6	-	1.5	130	440	520	-
-	-	-	-	10	-	-	-	-	0	-	0	0	721	.2	-	.2	-	371	1282	-
5	22	7	6	0	35	1	.2	0	0	-	.1	.1	48	2.5	154	3.2	298	409	458	2.6
6	23	9	6	0	59	1	.2	0	0	-	.2	.4	77	2.3	167	3.6	329	413	463	3.6
7	24	8	4	0	41	1	.1	0	0	-	.3	.4	76	1.9	181	1.4	323	392	504	3.4
0	1	0	-	0	1	0	0	0	0	-	0	.1	11	1	8	.5	14	52	69	.1
2	1	0	1	0	1	0	0	0	0	-	0	0	5	.8	14	0	24	42	25	.2
9	6	1	2	10	36	5	.1	.2	0	-	.1	0	56	.6	48	2.4	140	225	17	.9
1	2	1	2	20	10	-	0	.4	1	-	.1	.1	37	1	10	.7	128	80	291	.3
1	2	2	-	33	22	23	.1	.1	0	-	.2	.2	48	1.8	24	1.3	185	45	339	.5
1	1	3	5	0	12	-	.1	0	0	-	.1	.2	41	2.7	102	.3	244	330	255	1.2
1	2	4	2	25	8	26	0	.1	0	-	.2	.2	130	1.6	11	1.5	99	79	304	.4
1	2	4	-	21	34	163	.2	.1	5	-	.3	.2	122	2.7	51	2.6	185	207	382	1.8
1	1	1	0	54	8	36	.4	.2	1	-	.1	.1	26	1.2	28	5.4	208	390	60	.7
2	-	-	-	35	-	60	-	-	2	-	0	-	-	.2	-	.4	-	80	500	-
0	0	0	2	0	14	0	.1	0	3	-	.2	.1	5	1.4	9	3.5	68	278	2	.7
0	0	0	2	0	10	0	0	0	0	-	.1	0	9	.6	12	1.2	51	101	332	.6
0	0	0	-	0	1	0	0	0	0	-	0	0	0	0	0	.1	3	11	0	0
0	0	0	0	0	7	0	0	0	1	-	.2	0	2	.4	4	1.4	36	130	1	.3
0	0	0	2	0	15	0	.1	0	0	-	.1	0	2	.3	10	1.1	21	85	3	1
0	0	0	0	0	6	0	0	0	0	-	0	0	0	.1	5	.5	11	55	0	.3
1	1	1	0	48	64	77	.1	20.4	12	-	.4	.3	28	5.7	31	2.6	242	228	314	2.3
3	-	-	4	20	-	300	-	-	12	-	-	-	360	.6	-	-	-	600	560	-
3	-	-	-	20	-	0	-	-	0	-	.5	.6	160	.8	-	0	-	420	560	-
-	-	-	-	20	-	-	-	-	0	-	0	0	70	3	-	.2	-	571	1252	-
6	4	0	1	8	4	6	0	.2	0	-	.1	0	68	.3	18	.2	71	138	59	.4
-	-	-	-	40	-	-	-	-	0	-	0	0	2484	.1	-	.2	-	571	961	-
-	-	-	-	120	-	-	-	-	0	-	0	0	1843	0	-	0	-	371	1052	-
2	3	2	-	29	-	270	-	-	8	-	.1	.1	32	.7	21	1.7	-	254	1009	.8
-	-	-	-	40	-	-	-	-	0	-	0	0	1602	.2	-	.2	-	260	1993	-
1	2	4	1	0	5	2	0	0	0	-	.1	.1	5	1.1	12	1.3	36	27	99	.3
0	0	0	-	26	6	5	0	.1	0	-	.1	.1	10	1.3	15	1.2	55	22	132	.5
0	0	0	-	26	6	5	0	.1	0	-	0	0	10	.5	15	.3	55	22	132	.5
0	0	0	2	26	17	11	.1	.1	0	-	.1	.2	15	.9	19	1.2	46	30	10	.5
0	0	0	0	0	4	0	0	0	0	-	0	.1	2	.3	5	.3	14	20	34	.1
1	1	0	-	0	1	0	0	0	0	-	0	0	3	.2	2	.1	10	12	1	0
1	2	0	1	0	1	0	0	0	0	-	0	0	7	.5	6	.4	25	26	69	.1
0	1	0	0	1	1	1	0	0	0	-	0	0	14	.4	5	.3	31	20	52	.1
0	1	0	0	46	9	12	.2	1	1	-	.1	.1	117	1	33	2.1	236	298	82	.5
2	10	1	0	0	0	0	0	0	0	1.6	0	0	0	.1	0	0	0	0	0	0

Food Composition Table—cont'd

Code	Name	Amount	Unit	Grams	Kilocalories	Carbohydrates (g)	Protein (g)	Fat (g)
4042	OIL, PEANUT	1	TBSP.	13.5	119	0	0	14
4058	OIL, SESAME	1	TBSP.	13.6	121	0	0	14
4044	OIL, SOYBEAN	1	TBSP.	13.6	121	0	0	14
4034	OIL, SOYBEAN, (HYDR)	1	TBSP.	13.6	121	0	0	14
4543	OIL, SOYBEAN, (HYDR)&CTTNSD	1	TBSP.	13.6	121	0	0	14
4518	OIL, VEGETABLE, CORN	1	TBSP.	13.6	121	0	0	14
4582	OIL, VEGETABLE, CANOLA	1	TBSP.	13.6	121	0	0	14
4501	OIL, VEGETABLE, COCOA BUTTER	1	TBSP.	13.6	121	0	0	14
4502	OIL, VEGETABLE, COTTONSEED	1	TBSP.	13.6	121	0	0	14
4055	OIL, VEGETABLE, PALM	1	TBSP.	13.6	121	0	0	14
4513	OIL, VEGETABLE, PALM KERNEL	1	TBSP.	13.6	118	0	0	14
4510	OIL, VEGETABLE, SAFFLOWER, LINOLEIC	1	TBSP.	13.6	121	0	0	14
4511	OIL, VEGETABLE, SAFFLOWER, OLEIC	1	TBSP.	13.6	121	0	0	14
4584	OIL, VEGETABLE, SUNFLOWER	1	TBSP.	13.6	121	0	0	14
11279	OKRA, CKD	½	CUP	80.0	26	6	1	0
11278	OKRA, FRESH	½	CUP	50.0	19	4	1	0
11281	OKRA, FRZ, CKD	½	CUP	92.0	34	8	2	0
11280	OKRA, FRZ, UNPREPARED	½	CUP	71.3	21	5	1	0
41282	OLD FASHIONED CHICKEN NOODLE SOUP-HEALTHY CHOICE	1	EACH	212.6	90	11	5	2
55806	OLD-FASHION STUFF'N-STOUFFER'S	½	CUP	142.0	310	31	6	19
10161	OLIVE LOAF, LUNCH MEAT	1	SLICE	28.4	67	3	3	5
7051	OLIVE LOAF, PORK, LUNCH MEAT	1	SLICE	28.4	67	3	3	5
9194	OLIVES, RIPE, CANNED (JUMBO-SUPER COLOSSAL)	1	JUMBO	8.3	7	0	0	1
9193	OLIVES, RIPE, CANNED (SMALL-EXTRA LARGE)	1	SMALL	3.2	4	0	0	0
11283	ONIONS, CKD	½	CUP	119.9	53	12	2	0
11285	ONIONS, CND, SOL&LIQ	½	CUP	112.0	21	4	1	0
11282	ONIONS, FRESH	½	CUP	79.9	30	7	1	0
14327	ORANGE AND APRICOT JUICE DRINK, CND	¾	CUP	187.0	95	24	1	0
14323	ORANGE DRINK, CND	¾	CUP	185.8	95	24	0	0
9206	ORANGE JUICE, FRESH	¾	CUP	186.0	84	19	1	0
9215	ORANGE JUICE, FROM CONCENTRATE	¾	CUP	186.4	84	20	1	0
62558	ORANGE JUICE, W/ ADDED CALCIUM	¾	CUP	186.4	84	20	1	0
9200	ORANGES, FRESH	1	MEDIUM	131.0	62	15	1	0
9205	ORANGES, FRESH, W/ PEEL	1	MEDIUM	159.0	64	25	2	0
18199	OREOS, DIETARY	1	EACH	10.0	46	7	0	2
18166	OREOS, REGULAR	1	EACH	10.0	47	7	0	2
18168	OREOS, W/ EXTRA CREME FILLING	1	EACH	13.0	65	9	0	3
55220	ORIENTAL BEEF W/ VEG., LEAN CUISINE-STOUFFER'S	1	EACH	244.5	290	31	20	9
41314	ORIENTAL CHICKEN W/ SPICY PEANUT SAUCE-HEALTHY CHOICE	1	EACH	269.3	340	40	33	5
19031	ORIENTAL MIX, RICE-BASED	1	OUNCE	28.4	155	9	6	12
55221	OVEN BAKED CHICKEN, LEAN CUISINE-STOUFFER'S	1	EACH	226.8	200	21	17	5
15168	OYSTER, EASTERN, BREADED AND FRIED	3	OUNCE	85.1	168	10	7	11
15170	OYSTER, EASTERN, CND	3	OUNCE	85.1	59	3	6	2
18288	PANCAKES PLAIN, FROZEN	1	4 IN.	9.0	21	4	0	0
18294	PANCAKES, BLUEBERRY	1	4 IN.	9.5	21	3	1	1
18390	PANCAKES, BUTTERMILK	1	4 IN.	9.5	22	3	1	1
18298	PANCAKES, DIETARY	1	3 IN.	22.0	44	9	1	0
18293	PANCAKES, PLAIN	1	4 IN.	9.5	22	3	1	1
18300	PANCAKES, WHOLE-WHEAT	1	4 IN.	44.0	92	13	4	3
9229	PAPAYA NECTAR, CND	¾	CUP	187.0	107	27	0	0
9226	PAPAYAS, FRESH	1	MEDIUM	304.0	119	30	2	0
11808	PARSNIPS, CKD, W/ SALT	½	CUP	78.0	63	15	1	0
11299	PARSNIPS, CKD, W/O SALT	½	CUP	78.0	63	15	1	0
11298	PARSNIPS, FRESH	½	CUP	66.5	50	12	1	0
9232	PASSION-FRUIT JUICE, PURPLE, FRESH	¾	CUP	185.2	94	25	1	0
9233	PASSION-FRUIT JUICE, YELLOW, FRESH	¾	CUP	185.2	111	27	1	0
55800	PASTA FLORENTINE-STOUFFER'S	½	CUP	142.0	190	16	8	11
41294	PASTA ITALIANO-HEALTHY CHOICE	1	EACH	340.2	350	59	16	5
55810	PASTA ROMA-STOUFFER'S	½	CUP	142.0	130	16	8	4
41292	PASTA SHELLS W/ TOMATO SAUCE-HEALTHY CHOICE	1	EACH	340.2	330	53	24	3

Saturated fat (g)	Monounsaturated fat (g)	Polyunsaturated fat (g)	Fiber (g)	Cholesterol (g)	Folate (g)	Vitamin A (RE)	Vitamin B-6 (mg)	Vitamin B-12 (µg)	Vitamin C (mg)	Vitamin E (mg)	Riboflavin (mg)	Thiamin (mg)	Calcium (mg)	Iron (mg)	Magnesium (mg)	Niacin (mg)	Phosphorus (mg)	Potassium (mg)	Sodium (mg)	Zinc (mg)
2	6	4	0	0	0	0	0	0	0	1.6	0	0	0	0	0	0	0	0	0	0
2	5	6	0	0	0	0	0	0	0	.2	0	0	0	0	0	0	0	0	0	0
2	3	8	0	0	0	0	0	0	0	1.5	0	0	0	0	0	0	0	0	0	0
2	6	5	0	0	0	0	0	0	0	1.1	0	0	0	0	0	0	0	0	0	0
2	4	7	0	0	0	0	0	0	0	1.7	0	0	0	0	0	0	0	0	0	0
2	3	8	0	0	0	0	0	0	0	2	0	0	0	0	0	0	0	0	0	0
1	8	4	0	-	0	0	0	0	0	-	0	0	0	0	0	0	0	0	0	0
8	4	0	0	0	0	0	0	0	0	.2	0	0	0	0	0	0	0	0	0	0
4	2	7	0	0	0	0	0	0	0	4.8	-	0	0	0	0	0	0	0	0	0
7	5	1	0	0	0	0	0	0	0	2.6	0	0	0	0	0	0	0	0	0	-
11	2	0	0	0	0	0	0	0	0	-	0	0	0	0	0	0	0	0	0	0
1	2	10	0	0	0	0	0	0	0	4.7	0	0	0	0	0	0	0	0	0	0
1	10	2	0	0	0	0	0	0	0	4.7	0	0	0	0	0	0	0	0	0	0
1	11	1	0	-	0	0	0	0	0	-	0	0	0	0	0	0	0	0	0	0
0	0	0	2	0	37	46	.1	0	13	-	0	.1	50	.4	46	.7	45	258	4	.4
0	0	0	1	0	44	33	.1	0	11	-	0	.1	41	.4	29	.5	32	152	4	.3
0	0	0	3	0	134	47	0	0	11	-	.1	.1	88	.6	47	.7	42	215	3	.6
0	0	0	2	0	105	33	0	0	9	-	.1	.1	58	.4	31	.5	30	150	2	.4
-	-	-	-	20	-	80	-	-	12	-	.1	0	16	.2	-	1.9	60	130	540	-
-	-	-	-	5	-	-	-	-	0	-	0	0	361	.2	-	.4	-	100	561	-
2	2	1	0	11	1	6	.1	.4	2	-	.1	.1	31	.2	5	.5	36	84	421	.4
2	2	1	0	11	1	0	.1	.4	3	-	.1	.1	31	.2	5	.5	36	84	421	.4
0	0	0	-	0	0	3	0	0	0	-	0	0	8	.3	0	0	0	1	75	0
0	0	0	-	0	0	1	0	0	0	-	0	0	3	.1	0	0	0	0	28	0
0	0	0	2	0	18	0	.2	0	6	-	0	.1	26	.3	13	.2	42	199	4	.3
0	0	0	1	0	11	0	.2	0	5	-	0	0	50	.1	7	.1	31	124	416	.3
0	0	0	1	0	15	0	.1	0	5	.2	0	0	16	.2	8	.1	26	125	2	.2
0	0	0	0	0	11	108	.1	0	37	-	0	0	9	.2	7	.4	15	150	4	.1
0	0	0	0	0	4	4	0	0	63	-	0	0	11	.5	4	.1	2	33	30	.2
0	0	0	0	0	56	37	.1	0	93	.1	.1	.2	20	.4	20	.7	32	372	2	.1
0	0	0	0	0	82	15	.1	0	73	-	0	.1	17	.2	19	.4	30	354	2	.1
0	0	0	0	0	82	15	.1	0	73	-	0	.1	224	.2	19	.4	30	354	2	.1
0	0	0	3	0	40	28	.1	0	70	.3	.1	.1	52	.1	13	.4	18	237	0	.1
0	0	0	4	0	-	40	.1	0	113	-	.1	.2	111	1.3	22	.8	35	312	3	-
1	1	0	-	0	1	0	0	0	0	-	0	0	6	.5	7	.3	18	30	24	.1
0	1	0	0	0	1	0	0	0	0	-	0	0	3	.4	5	.2	10	18	60	.1
1	2	0	-	0	1	0	0	0	0	-	0	0	3	.4	4	.2	12	16	64	.1
2	-	-	-	40	-	150	-	-	1	-	.2	.1	16	1	-	2.9	-	400	590	-
1	-	1	-	45	-	-	-	-	2	-	-	-	-	.2	-	.4	-	50	470	-
5	3	3	4	0	25	1	.1	0	0	-	0	.1	22	.8	40	3	112	147	235	1.3
2	-	-	-	35	-	350	-	-	6	-	.2	.2	16	.8	-	7.6	-	550	480	-
3	4	3	-	69	12	77	.1	13.3	3	-	.2	.1	53	5.9	49	1.4	135	208	355	74.1
1	0	1	0	47	8	77	.1	16.3	4	-	.1	.1	38	5.7	46	1.1	118	195	95	77.4
0	0	0	-	1	1	3	0	0	0	-	0	0	6	.3	1	.4	33	7	46	.1
0	0	0	-	5	1	5	0	0	0	-	0	0	20	.2	2	.1	14	13	39	.1
0	0	0	-	6	1	3	0	0	0	-	0	0	15	.2	1	.1	13	14	50	.1
0	0	0	-	0	1	2	0	0	0	-	0	0	13	.4	6	.4	75	85	58	.2
0	0	0	-	6	1	5	0	0	0	-	0	0	21	.2	2	.1	15	13	42	.1
1	1	1	-	27	9	28	0	.1	0	-	.2	.1	110	1.4	20	1	164	123	252	.5
0	0	0	1	0	4	21	0	0	6	-	0	0	19	.6	6	.3	0	58	9	.3
0	0	0	5	0	116	85	.1	0	188	-	.1	.1	73	.3	30	1	15	781	9	.2
0	0	0	-	0	45	0	.1	0	10	-	0	.1	29	.5	23	.6	54	286	192	.2
0	0	0	3	0	45	0	.1	0	10	-	0	.1	29	.5	23	.6	54	286	8	.2
0	0	0	3	0	44	0	.1	0	11	-	0	.1	24	.4	19	.5	47	249	7	.4
-	-	-	0	0	-	133	-	0	55	-	.2	0	7	.4	31	2.7	24	515	11	-
-	-	-	0	0	-	446	-	0	34	-	.2	-	7	.7	31	4.1	46	515	11	-
-	-	-	-	25	-	-	-	-	0	-	0	0	1723	.1	-	.1	-	200	446	-
2	-	3	-	30	-	60	-	-	-	-	.5	.5	48	2	-	2.9	180	540	530	-
-	-	-	-	15	-	-	-	-	3	-	0	.1	521	.2	-	.5	-	300	391	-
2	-	-	-	35	-	100	-	-	21	-	.4	.5	320	1.5	-	2.9	240	640	470	-

Food Composition Table—cont'd

Code	Name	Amount	Unit	Grams	Kilocalories	Carbohydrates (g)	Protein (g)	Fat (g)
55142	PASTA SHELLS, CHEESE W/ SAUCE-STOUFFER'S	1	EACH	262.2	300	28	17	13
41287	PASTA W/ CACCIATORE CHICKEN-HEALTHY CHOICE	1	EACH	354.4	310	47	26	3
41293	PASTA W/ TERIYAKI CHICKEN-HEALTHY CHOICE	1	EACH	357.9	350	58	24	3
20321	PASTA, CKD, ENRICHED, W/ ADDED SALT	½	CUP	70.0	99	20	3	0
20121	PASTA, CKD, ENRICHED, W/O ADDED SALT	½	CUP	70.0	99	20	3	0
20094	PASTA, FRESH-REFRIGERATED, PLAIN, CKD	½	CUP	73.0	96	18	4	1
20096	PASTA, FRESH-REFRIGERATED, SPINACH, CKD	½	CUP	73.0	95	18	4	1
20097	PASTA, HOMEMADE, MADE W/ EGG, CKD	½	CUP	73.6	96	17	4	1
20098	PASTA, HOMEMADE, MADE W/O EGG, CKD	½	CUP	73.6	91	18	3	1
20127	PASTA, SPINACH, CKD	½	CUP	70.0	91	18	3	0
20125	PASTA, WHOLE-WHEAT, CKD	½	CUP	70.0	87	19	4	0
9251	PEACH NECTAR, CND, W/O ADDED VIT C	¾	CUP	186.4	101	26	1	0
9241	PEACHES, CND, HEAVY SYRUP PACK	½	CUP	128.0	95	26	1	0
9238	PEACHES, CND, JUICE PACK	½	CUP	124.0	55	14	1	0
9240	PEACHES, CND, LIGHT SYRUP PACK	½	CUP	125.5	68	18	1	0
9237	PEACHES, CND, WATER PACK	½	CUP	122.0	29	7	1	0
9242	PEACHES, CND, X-HEAVY SYRUP PACK	½	CUP	131.0	126	34	1	0
9239	PEACHES, CND, X-LIGHT SYRUP	½	CUP	123.5	52	14	0	0
9244	PEACHES, DEHYDRATED, SULFURED	¼	CUP	29.0	94	24	1	0
9246	PEACHES, DRIED, SULFURED	¼	CUP	40.0	96	25	1	0
9236	PEACHES, FRESH	1	MEDIUM	87.0	37	10	1	0
9250	PEACHES, FROZEN, SLICED, SWEETENED	½	CUP	125.0	118	30	1	0
19147	PEANUT BAR	1	BAR	40.0	209	19	6	13
19148	PEANUT BRITTLE	1	OUNCE	28.4	128	20	2	5
18185	PEANUT BUTTER COOKIES, REGULAR	1	EACH	15.0	72	9	1	4
18186	PEANUT BUTTER COOKIES, SOFT-TYPE	1	EACH	15.0	69	9	1	4
18201	PEANUT BUTTER SANDWICH COOKIES, DIETARY	1	EACH	10.0	54	5	1	3
18190	PEANUT BUTTER SANDWICH COOKIES, REGULAR	1	EACH	14.0	67	9	1	3
16097	PEANUT BUTTER, CHUNK STYLE, W/ SALT	2	TBSP.	32.3	190	7	8	16
16397	PEANUT BUTTER, CHUNK STYLE, W/O SALT	2	TBSP.	32.3	190	7	8	16
16098	PEANUT BUTTER, SMOOTH STYLE, W/ SALT	2	TBSP.	32.3	190	7	8	16
16398	PEANUT BUTTER, SMOOTH STYLE, W/O SALT	2	TBSP.	32.3	190	7	8	16
12681	PEANUT KERNELS, OIL ROASTED	½	CUP	72.0	418	14	19	35
16088	PEANUTS, ALL TYPES, CKD, BOILED, W/ SALT	½	CUP	31.5	100	7	4	7
16090	PEANUTS, ALL TYPES, DRY-ROASTED, W/ SALT	½	CUP	73.0	427	16	17	36
16390	PEANUTS, ALL TYPES, DRY-ROASTED, W/O SALT	½	CUP	73.0	427	16	17	36
16087	PEANUTS, ALL TYPES, FRESH	½	CUP	73.0	414	12	19	36
16089	PEANUTS, ALL TYPES, OIL-ROASTED, W/ SALT	½	CUP	72.0	418	14	19	35
16389	PEANUTS, ALL TYPES, OIL-ROASTED, W/O SALT	½	CUP	72.0	418	14	19	35
16091	PEANUTS, SPANISH, FRESH	½	CUP	73.0	416	12	19	36
16092	PEANUTS, SPANISH, OIL-ROASTED, W/ SALT	½	CUP	73.5	426	13	21	36
16392	PEANUTS, SPANISH, OIL-ROASTED, W/O SALT	½	CUP	73.5	426	13	21	36
16093	PEANUTS, VALENCIA, FRESH	½	CUP	73.0	416	15	18	35
16094	PEANUTS, VALENCIA, OIL-ROASTED, W/ SALT	½	CUP	72.0	424	12	19	37
16394	PEANUTS, VALENCIA, OIL-ROASTED, W/O SALT	½	CUP	72.0	424	12	19	37
16095	PEANUTS, VIRGINIA, FRESH	½	CUP	73.0	411	12	18	36
16096	PEANUTS, VIRGINIA, OIL-ROASTED, W/ SALT	½	CUP	71.5	413	14	18	35
16396	PEANUTS, VIRGINIA, OIL-ROASTED, W/O SALT	½	CUP	71.5	413	14	18	35
9340	PEARS, ASIAN, FRESH	1	MEDIUM	122.0	51	13	1	0
9257	PEARS, CND, HEAVY SYRUP PACK	½	CUP	127.5	94	24	0	0
9254	PEARS, CND, JUICE PACK	½	CUP	124.0	62	16	0	0
9256	PEARS, CND, LIGHT SYRUP PACK	½	CUP	125.5	72	19	0	0
9253	PEARS, CND, WATER PACK	½	CUP	122.0	35	10	0	0
9258	PEARS, CND, X-HEAVY SYRUP PACK	½	CUP	130.5	127	33	0	0
9255	PEARS, CND, X-LIGHT SYRUP PACK	½	CUP	123.5	58	15	0	0
9252	PEARS, FRESH	1	MEDIUM	166.0	98	25	1	1
11318	PEAS AND CARROTS, CND	½	CUP	76.0	29	6	2	0
11323	PEAS AND CARROTS, FRZ, CKD	½	CUP	80.0	38	8	2	0
11324	PEAS AND ONIONS, CND	½	CUP	60.0	31	5	2	0
11327	PEAS AND ONIONS, FRZ, CKD	½	CUP	90.0	41	8	2	0

Saturated fat (g)	Monounsaturated fat (g)	Polyunsaturated fat (g)	Fiber (g)	Cholesterol (g)	Folate (g)	Vitamin A (RE)	Vitamin B-6 (mg)	Vitamin B-12 (μg)	Vitamin C (mg)	Vitamin E (mg)	Riboflavin (mg)	Thiamin (mg)	Calcium (mg)	Iron (mg)	Magnesium (mg)	Niacin (mg)	Phosphorus (mg)	Potassium (mg)	Sodium (mg)	Zinc (mg)
-	-	-	-	-	-	150	-	-	9	-	.3	.1	280	1	-	1.9	-	480	820	-
-	-	1	-	35	-	100	-	-	6	-	.4	.5	32	1.5	-	6.7	250	660	430	-
1	-	2	-	45	-	100	-	-	6	-	.3	.3	48	1.5	-	3.8	200	390	370	-
0	0	0	-	0	5	-	0	0	0	-	.1	.1	5	1	13	1.2	38	22	70	.4
0	0	0	1	0	5	-	0	0	0	-	.1	.1	5	1	13	1.2	38	22	1	.4
0	0	0	-	24	5	4	0	.1	0	-	.1	.2	4	.8	13	.7	46	18	4	.4
0	0	0	-	24	13	10	.1	.1	0	-	.1	.1	13	.8	18	.7	42	27	4	.5
0	0	0	-	30	14	13	0	.1	0	-	.1	.1	7	.9	10	.9	38	15	61	.3
0	0	0	-	0	13	0	0	0	0	-	.1	.1	4	.8	10	1	29	14	54	.3
0	0	0	-	0	8	11	.1	0	0	-	.1	.1	21	.7	43	1.1	76	41	10	.8
0	0	0	3	0	4	0	.1	0	0	-	0	.1	11	.7	21	.5	62	31	2	.6
0	0	0	1	0	3	48	0	0	10	-	0	0	9	.4	7	.5	11	75	13	.1
0	0	0	1	0	4	42	0	0	4	-	0	0	4	.3	6	.8	14	118	8	.1
0	0	0	1	0	4	47	0	0	4	-	0	0	7	.3	9	.7	21	159	5	.1
0	0	0	1	0	4	44	0	0	3	-	0	0	4	.5	6	.7	14	122	6	.1
0	0	0	1	0	4	65	0	0	4	-	0	0	2	.4	6	.6	12	121	4	.1
0	0	0	-	0	4	17	0	0	2	-	0	0	4	.4	7	.7	14	109	10	.1
0	0	0	-	0	4	33	0	0	4	-	0	0	6	.4	6	1	14	91	6	.1
0	0	0	-	0	2	41	0	0	3	-	0	0	11	1.6	17	1.4	47	392	3	.2
0	0	0	3	0	0	86	0	0	2	-	.1	0	11	1.6	17	1.8	48	398	3	.2
0	0	0	2	0	3	47	0	0	6	-	0	0	4	.1	6	.9	10	171	0	.1
0	0	0	2	0	4	35	0	0	118	-	0	0	4	.5	6	.8	14	162	7	.1
2	7	4	1	3	24	20	0	0	0	-	.1	0	31	.4	30	3.2	61	163	96	.5
1	2	1	1	4	20	13	0	0	0	-	0	.1	9	.4	14	1	31	59	128	.3
1	1	1	-	0	5	1	0	0	0	-	0	0	5	.4	7	.6	13	25	62	.1
1	2	1	0	0	1	0	0	0	0	-	0	0	2	.1	5	.3	13	16	50	.1
1	2	1	-	0	3	0	0	0	0	-	0	0	5	.2	5	.5	19	29	41	.2
1	2	1	-	0	2	0	0	0	0	-	0	0	7	.4	7	.5	26	27	52	.1
3	8	5	2	0	30	0	.1	0	0	-	0	0	13	.6	51	4.4	102	241	157	.9
3	8	5	2	0	30	0	.1	0	0	-	0	0	13	.6	51	4.4	102	241	5	.9
3	8	5	2	0	25	0	.1	0	0	-	0	0	11	.5	51	4.2	104	233	154	.8
3	8	5	-	0	25	0	.1	0	0	-	0	0	11	.5	51	4.2	104	233	5	.8
5	18	11	6	0	91	0	.2	0	0	-	.1	.2	63	1.3	133	10.3	372	491	312	4.8
1	3	2	3	0	23	0	0	0	0	-	0	.1	17	.3	32	1.7	62	57	237	.6
5	18	11	6	0	106	0	.2	0	0	5.7	.1	.3	39	1.6	128	9.9	261	480	593	2.4
5	18	11	6	0	106	0	.2	0	0	-	.1	.3	39	1.6	128	9.9	261	480	4	2.4
5	18	11	6	0	175	0	.3	0	0	6.1	.1	.5	67	3.3	123	8.8	274	515	13	2.4
5	18	11	7	0	91	0	.2	0	0	5	.1	.2	63	1.3	133	10.3	372	491	312	4.8
5	18	11	7	0	91	0	.2	0	0	-	.1	.2	63	1.3	133	10.3	372	491	4	4.8
6	16	13	7	0	175	0	.3	0	0	-	.1	.5	77	2.9	137	11.6	283	543	16	1.5
6	16	13	-	0	93	0	.2	0	0	-	.1	.2	74	1.7	123	11	284	570	318	1.5
6	16	13	-	0	93	0	.2	0	0	-	.1	.2	74	1.7	123	11	284	570	4	1.5
5	16	12	-	0	179	0	.2	0	0	-	.2	.5	45	1.5	134	9.4	245	242	1	2.4
6	17	13	-	0	90	0	.2	0	0	-	.1	.1	39	1.2	115	10.3	230	441	556	2.2
6	17	13	-	0	90	0	.2	0	0	-	.1	.1	39	1.2	115	10.3	230	441	4	2.2
5	18	11	-	0	174	0	.3	0	0	-	.1	.5	65	1.9	125	9	277	504	7	3.2
5	18	10	-	0	90	0	.2	0	0	-	.1	.2	61	1.2	134	10.5	362	466	310	4.7
5	18	10	-	0	90	0	.2	0	0	-	.1	.2	61	1.2	134	10.5	362	466	4	4.7
0	0	0	4	0	10	0	0	0	5	-	0	0	5	0	10	.3	13	148	0	0
0	0	0	3	0	2	0	0	0	1	-	0	0	6	.3	5	.3	9	83	6	.1
0	0	0	2	0	1	1	0	0	2	-	0	0	11	.4	9	.2	15	119	5	.1
0	0	0	3	0	2	0	0	0	1	-	0	0	6	.4	5	.2	9	83	6	.1
0	0	0	2	0	1	0	0	0	1	-	0	0	5	.3	5	.1	9	65	2	.1
0	0	0	-	0	2	0	0	0	1	-	0	0	7	.3	5	.3	9	84	7	.1
0	0	0	-	0	1	0	0	0	2	-	0	0	9	.2	6	.5	9	56	2	.1
0	0	0	4	0	12	3	0	0	7	-	0	.1	18	.4	10	.2	18	208	0	.2
0	0	0	3	0	14	438	.1	0	5	-	0	.1	17	.6	11	.4	35	76	197	.4
0	0	0	3	0	21	621	.1	0	6	-	.1	.2	18	.8	13	.9	39	126	54	.4
0	0	0	-	0	16	10	.1	0	2	-	0	.1	10	.5	10	.8	31	58	265	.3
0	0	0	3	0	18	32	.1	0	6	-	.1	.1	13	.8	12	.9	31	105	33	.3

Food Composition Table—cont'd

Code	Name	Amount	Unit	Grams	Kilocalories	Carbohydrates (g)	Protein (g)	Fat (g)
11300	PEAS, EDIBLE-PODDED, FRESH	½	CUP	72.5	30	5	2	0
11305	PEAS, GREEN, CKD	½	CUP	80.0	67	13	4	0
11308	PEAS, GREEN, CND	½	CUP	85.0	59	11	4	0
11310	PEAS, GREEN, CND, SEASONED	½	CUP	85.0	43	8	3	0
11304	PEAS, GREEN, FRESH	½	CUP	72.5	59	10	4	0
11313	PEAS, GREEN, FRZ, CKD	½	CUP	80.0	62	11	4	0
18324	PECAN PIE	1	SLICE	113.0	452	65	5	21
12142	PECANS, DRIED	½	CUP	54.0	360	10	4	37
41333	PEPPERONI FRENCH BREAD PIZZA-HEALTHY CHOICE	1	EACH	170.1	310	38	20	7
62625	PEPPERONI PIZZA-WEIGHT WATCHERS	1	EACH	157.6	390	46	23	12
11329	PEPPERS, HOT CHILI, GREEN, CND	1	EACH	73.0	18	4	1	0
11670	PEPPERS, HOT CHILI, GREEN, FRESH	1	EACH	45.0	18	4	1	0
11820	PEPPERS, HOT CHILI, RED, CND	1	EACH	73.0	18	4	1	0
11819	PEPPERS, HOT CHILI, RED, FRESH	1	EACH	45.0	18	4	1	0
11632	PEPPERS, JALAPEÑO, CND	¼	CUP	34.0	8	2	0	0
11333	PEPPERS, SWEET, GREEN, FRESH	1	MEDIUM	74.0	20	5	1	0
11821	PEPPERS, SWEET, RED, FRESH	1	MEDIUM	74.0	20	5	1	0
11951	PEPPERS, SWEET, YELLOW, FRESH	1	MEDIUM	74.0	20	5	1	0
15061	PERCH, CKD, DRY HEAT	3	OUNCE	85.1	100	0	21	1
55827	PESTO SAUCE-STOUFFER'S	¼	CUP	71.0	193	5	9	15
10162	PICKLE AND PIMENTO LOAF, LUNCH MEAT	1	SLICE	28.4	74	2	3	6
7058	PICKLE AND PIMENTO LOAF, PORK, LUNCH MEAT	1	SLICE	28.4	74	2	3	6
11958	PICKLE RELISH, HAMBURGER	1	TBSP.	15.0	19	5	0	0
11944	PICKLE RELISH, HOT DOG	1	TBSP.	15.0	14	4	0	0
11945	PICKLE RELISH, SWEET	1	TBSP.	15.0	19	5	0	0
11941	PICKLE, CUCUMBER, SOUR	1	SLICE	7.0	1	0	0	0
11937	PICKLE, CUCUMBER, DILL	1	SLICE	6.0	1	0	0	0
11947	PICKLE, CUCUMBER, DILL, LOW SODIUM	1	SLICE	6.0	1	0	0	0
11946	PICKLE, CUCUMBER, SOUR, LOW SODIUM	1	SLICE	7.0	1	0	0	0
11940	PICKLE, CUCUMBER, SWEET	1	SLICE	6.0	7	2	0	0
11948	PICKLE, CUCUMBER, SWEET, LOW SODIUM	1	SLICE	6.0	7	2	0	0
7062	PICNIC LOAF, LUNCH MEAT	1	SLICE	28.4	66	1	4	5
15063	PIKE, NORTHERN, CKD, DRY HEAT	3	OUNCE	85.1	96	0	21	1
15204	PIKE, WALLEYE, CKD, DRY HEAT	3	OUNCE	85.1	101	0	21	1
14017	PINA COLADA	1	FL OZ	31.4	58	9	0	1
12147	PINE NUTS	1	TBSP.	10.0	52	1	2	5
14334	PINEAPPLE AND GRAPEFRUIT JUICE DRINK, CND	¾	CUP	187.6	88	22	0	0
14341	PINEAPPLE AND ORANGE JUICE DRINK, CND	¾	CUP	187.6	94	22	2	0
9273	PINEAPPLE JUICE, CND	¾	CUP	187.6	105	26	1	0
9270	PINEAPPLE, CND, HEAVY SYRUP PACK	½	CUP	127.5	99	26	0	0
9268	PINEAPPLE, CND, JUICE PACK	½	CUP	125.0	75	20	1	0
9269	PINEAPPLE, CND, LIGHT SYRUP PACK	½	CUP	126.0	66	17	0	0
9267	PINEAPPLE, CND, WATER PACK	½	CUP	123.0	39	10	1	0
9271	PINEAPPLE, CND, X-HEAVY SYRUP PACK	½	CUP	130.0	108	28	0	0
9266	PINEAPPLE, FRESH	1	SLICE	84.0	41	10	0	0
12151	PISTACHIO, DRIED	½	CUP	64.0	369	16	13	31
12652	PISTACHIO, DRY ROASTED	½	CUP	64.0	388	18	10	34
9284	PLUMS, CND, PURPLE, HEAVY SYRUP PACK	½	CUP	129.0	115	30	0	0
9282	PLUMS, CND, PURPLE, JUICE PACK	½	CUP	126.0	73	19	1	0
9283	PLUMS, CND, PURPLE, LIGHT SYRUP PACK	½	CUP	126.0	79	21	0	0
9281	PLUMS, CND, PURPLE, WATER PACK	½	CUP	124.5	51	14	0	0
9285	PLUMS, CND, PURPLE, X-HEAVY SYRUP PACK	½	CUP	130.5	132	34	0	0
9279	PLUMS, FRESH	1	MEDIUM	66.0	36	9	1	0
15205	POLLOCK, ATLANTIC, CKD, DRY HEAT	3	OUNCE	85.1	100	0	21	1
15069	POMPANO, FLORIDA, CKD, DRY HEAT	3	OUNCE	85.1	179	0	20	10
19034	POPCORN, AIR-POPPED	1	CUP	8.0	31	6	1	0
19806	POPCORN, AIR-POPPED, WHITE POPCORN	1	CUP	8.0	31	6	1	0
19036	POPCORN, CAKES	1	CAKE	10.0	38	8	1	0
19038	POPCORN, CARAMEL-COATED, W/ PEANUTS	1	CUP	35.2	141	28	2	3
19039	POPCORN, CARAMEL-COATED, W/O PEANUTS	1	CUP	35.2	152	28	1	5

Saturated fat (g)	Monounsaturated fat (g)	Polyunsaturated fat (g)	Fiber (g)	Cholesterol (g)	Folate (g)	Vitamin A (RE)	Vitamin B-6 (mg)	Vitamin B-12 (µg)	Vitamin C (mg)	Vitamin E (mg)	Riboflavin (mg)	Thiamin (mg)	Calcium (mg)	Iron (mg)	Magnesium (mg)	Niacin (mg)	Phosphorus (mg)	Potassium (mg)	Sodium (mg)	Zinc (mg)
0	0	0	2	0	30	10	.1	0	44	-	.1	.1	31	1.5	17	.4	38	145	3	.2
0	0	0	4	0	51	48	.2	0	11	-	.1	.2	22	1.2	31	1.6	94	217	2	1
0	0	0	3	0	38	65	.1	0	8	-	.1	.1	17	.8	14	.6	57	147	186	.6
0	0	0	-	0	24	37	.1	0	10	-	.1	.1	13	1	13	.6	46	104	216	.6
0	0	0	4	0	47	46	.1	0	29	.1	.1	.2	18	1.1	24	1.5	78	177	4	.9
0	0	0	4	0	47	54	.1	0	8	-	.1	.2	19	1.3	23	1.2	72	134	70	.8
4	12	3	4	36	7	53	0	.1	1	-	.1	.1	19	1.2	20	.3	87	84	479	.6
3	23	9	4	0	21	7	.1	0	1	-	.1	.5	19	1.2	69	.5	157	212	1	3
3	-	1	-	30	-	150	-	-	-	-	.3	.5	160	2.5	-	3.8	240	350	470	-
4	-	-	4	45	-	80	-	-	5	-	-	-	540	1	-	-	-	320	650	-
0	0	0	1	0	7	45	.1	0	50	-	0	0	5	.4	10	.6	12	137	856	.1
0	0	0	1	0	11	35	.1	0	109	-	0	0	8	.5	11	.4	21	153	3	.1
0	0	0	1	0	7	868	.1	0	50	-	0	0	5	.4	10	.6	12	137	856	.1
0	0	0	1	0	11	484	.1	0	109	-	0	0	8	.5	11	.4	21	153	3	.1
0	0	0	1	0	5	58	.1	0	4	-	0	0	9	1	4	.2	6	46	497	.1
0	0	0	1	0	16	47	.2	0	66	.5	0	0	7	.3	7	.4	14	131	1	.1
0	0	0	2	0	16	422	.2	0	141	.5	0	0	7	.3	7	.4	14	131	1	.1
-	-	-	-	0	19	18	.1	0	136	-	0	0	8	.3	9	.7	18	157	1	.1
0	0	0	0	98	5	9	.1	1.9	1	-	.1	.1	87	1	32	1.6	219	293	67	1.2
-	-	-	-	18	-	-	-	-	3	-	0	0	1422	.1	-	.1	-	155	341	-
2	3	1	0	10	1	2	.1	.3	4	-	.1	.1	27	.3	5	.6	40	96	394	.4
2	3	1	0	10	1	2	.1	.3	4	-	.1	.1	27	.3	5	.6	40	96	394	.4
0	0	0	0	0	0	4	0	0	0	-	0	0	1	.2	1	.1	3	11	164	0
0	0	0	-	0	0	3	0	0	0	-	0	0	1	.2	3	.1	6	12	164	0
0	0	0	-	0	0	2	0	0	0	-	0	0	0	.1	1	0	2	4	122	0
0	0	0	0	0	0	1	0	0	0	-	0	0	0	0	0	0	1	2	85	0
0	0	0	0	0	0	2	0	0	0	-	0	0	1	0	1	0	1	7	77	0
0	0	0	-	0	0	2	0	0	0	-	0	0	1	0	1	0	1	7	1	0
0	0	0	0	0	-	1	-	0	0	-	0	0	0	0	0	0	1	2	1	0
0	0	0	0	0	0	1	0	0	0	-	0	0	0	0	0	0	1	2	56	0
0	0	0	0	0	0	1	0	0	0	-	0	0	0	0	0	0	1	2	1	0
2	2	1	0	11	1	0	.1	.4	5	-	.1	.1	13	.3	4	.7	35	76	330	.6
0	0	0	0	43	15	20	.1	2	3	-	.1	.1	62	.6	34	2.4	240	282	42	.7
0	0	0	0	94	14	20	.1	2	0	-	.2	.3	120	1.4	32	2.4	229	424	55	.7
0	0	0	-	0	3	0	0	0	1	-	0	0	3	.1	3	0	2	22	2	0
1	2	2	0	6	0	0	0	0	0	-	0	.1	3	.9	23	.4	51	60	0	.4
0	0	0	0	0	20	8	.1	0	86	-	0	.1	13	.6	11	.5	11	114	26	.1
0	0	0	0	0	20	99	.1	0	42	-	0	.1	9	.5	11	.4	8	86	6	.1
0	0	0	0	0	43	0	.2	0	20	-	0	.1	32	.5	24	.5	15	251	2	.2
0	0	0	1	0	6	1	.1	0	9	-	0	.1	18	.5	20	.4	9	133	1	.2
0	0	0	1	0	6	5	.1	0	12	-	0	.1	17	.3	17	.4	7	152	1	.1
0	0	0	1	0	6	1	.1	0	9	-	0	.1	18	.5	20	.4	9	132	1	.2
0	0	0	1	0	6	2	.1	0	9	-	0	.1	18	.5	22	.4	5	156	1	.1
0	0	0	-	0	6	1	.1	0	9	-	0	.1	18	.5	20	.4	9	133	1	.1
0	0	0	1	0	9	2	.1	0	13	.1	0	.1	6	.3	12	.4	6	95	1	.1
4	21	5	7	0	37	15	.2	0	5	-	.1	.5	86	4.3	101	.7	322	700	4	.9
4	23	5	7	0	38	15	.2	0	5	-	.2	.3	45	2	83	.9	305	621	499	.9
0	0	0	1	0	3	34	0	0	1	-	0	0	12	1.1	6	.4	17	117	25	.1
0	0	0	1	0	3	127	0	0	4	-	.1	0	13	.4	10	.6	19	194	1	.1
0	0	0	1	0	3	33	0	0	1	-	0	0	11	1.1	6	.4	16	117	25	.1
0	0	0	1	0	3	113	0	0	3	-	.1	0	9	.2	6	.5	16	157	1	.1
0	0	0	-	0	3	33	0	0	1	-	0	0	12	1.1	7	.4	16	116	25	.1
0	0	0	1	0	1	21	.1	0	6	-	.1	0	3	.1	5	.3	7	114	0	.1
0	0	1	0	77	3	10	.3	3.1	0	-	.2	0	65	.5	73	3.4	241	388	94	.5
4	3	1	0	54	15	31	.2	1	0	-	.1	.6	37	.6	26	3.2	290	541	65	.6
0	0	0	-	0	2	2	0	0	0	-	0	0	1	.2	10	.2	24	24	0	.3
0	0	0	-	0	2	0	0	0	0	-	0	0	1	.2	10	.2	24	24	0	.3
0	0	0	0	0	2	1	0	0	0	-	0	0	1	.2	16	.6	28	33	29	.4
0	1	1	1	0	6	2	.1	0	0	-	0	0	23	1.4	28	.7	45	125	104	.4
1	1	2	2	2	1	4	0	0	0	-	0	0	15	.6	12	.8	29	38	73	.2

Food Composition Table—cont'd

Code	Name	Amount	Unit	Grams	Kilocalories	Carbohydrates (g)	Protein (g)	Fat (g)
19040	POPCORN, CHEESE-FLAVOR	1	CUP	11.0	58	6	1	4
19035	POPCORN, OIL-POPPED	1	CUP	11.0	55	6	1	3
19807	POPCORN, OIL-POPPED, WHITE POPCORN	1	CUP	11.0	55	6	1	3
62602	POPSICLES	1	EACH	56.0	40	11	0	0
19408	PORK SKINS, BARBECUE-FLAVOR	1	OUNCE	28.4	153	0	16	9
19041	PORK SKINS, PLAIN	1	OUNCE	28.4	155	0	17	9
10193	PORK, BACKRIBS	3	OUNCE	85.1	315	0	21	25
10127	PORK, BRAUNSCHWEIGER	3	OUNCE	85.1	305	3	11	27
7045	PORK, CND, LUNCH MEAT	1	SLICE	21.0	70	0	3	6
10220	PORK, GROUND, CKD	3	OUNCE	85.1	253	0	22	18
10154	PORK, HAM AND CHEESE LOAF OR ROLL	3	OUNCE	85.1	220	1	14	17
10147	PORK, HAM PATTIES, GRILLED	3	OUNCE	85.1	291	1	11	26
10148	PORK, HAM SALAD SPREAD	3	OUNCE	85.1	184	9	7	13
10143	PORK, HAM, CHOPPED, CND	3	OUNCE	85.1	203	0	14	16
10138	PORK, HAM, CND, EXTRA LEAN (APPX 4% FAT), ROASTED	3	OUNCE	85.1	116	0	18	4
10185	PORK, HAM, CND, EXTRA LEAN AND REG, ROASTED	3	OUNCE	85.1	142	0	18	7
10184	PORK, HAM, CND, EXTRA LEAN AND REG, UNHEATED	3	OUNCE	85.1	122	0	15	6
10140	PORK, HAM, CND, REGULAR (APPROX 13% FAT), ROASTED	3	OUNCE	85.1	192	0	17	13
10134	PORK, HAM, EXTRA LEAN (5% FAT), ROASTED	3	OUNCE	85.1	123	1	18	5
10133	PORK, HAM, EXTRA LEAN (5% FAT), UNHEATED	3	OUNCE	85.1	111	1	16	4
10183	PORK, HAM, EXTRA LEAN AND REG, ROASTED	3	OUNCE	85.1	140	0	19	7
10182	PORK, HAM, EXTRA LEAN AND REG, UNHEATED	3	OUNCE	85.1	138	2	16	7
10151	PORK, HAM, MEAT AND FAT, ROASTED	3	OUNCE	85.1	207	0	18	14
10153	PORK, HAM, MEAT ONLY, ROASTED	3	OUNCE	85.1	134	0	21	5
10136	PORK, HAM, REGULAR (11% FAT), ROASTED	3	OUNCE	85.1	151	0	19	8
10135	PORK, HAM, REGULAR (11% FAT), UNHEATED	3	OUNCE	85.1	155	3	15	9
10172	PORK, SMOKED LINK SAUSAGE, GRILLED	3	OUNCE	85.1	331	2	19	27
10089	PORK, SPARERIBS, MEAT AND FAT, CKD, BRAISED	3	OUNCE	85.1	338	0	25	26
10221	PORK, TENDERLOIN, MEAT AND FAT, CKD, BROILED	3	OUNCE	85.1	171	0	25	7
10223	PORK, TENDERLOIN, MEAT ONLY, CKD, BROILED	3	OUNCE	85.1	159	0	26	5
19042	POTATO CHIPS, BARBECUE-FLAVOR	1	OUNCE	28.4	139	15	2	9
19421	POTATO CHIPS, CHEESE-FLAVOR	1	OUNCE	28.4	141	16	2	8
19422	POTATO CHIPS, LIGHT	1	OUNCE	28.4	134	19	2	6
19411	POTATO CHIPS, PLAIN, SALTED	1	OUNCE	28.4	152	15	2	10
19811	POTATO CHIPS, PLAIN, UNSALTED	1	OUNCE	28.4	152	15	2	10
19412	POTATO CHIPS, PRINGLES, CHEESE-FLAVOR	1	OUNCE	28.4	156	14	2	10
19045	POTATO CHIPS, PRINGLES, LIGHT	1	OUNCE	28.4	142	18	2	7
19410	POTATO CHIPS, PRINGLES, PLAIN	1	OUNCE	28.4	158	14	2	11
19046	POTATO CHIPS, PRINGLES, SOUR-CREAM&ONION-FLAVOR	1	OUNCE	28.4	155	15	2	10
19043	POTATO CHIPS, SOUR-CREAM-AND-ONION-FLAVOR	1	OUNCE	28.4	151	15	2	10
11920	POTATO CHIPS, W/O SALT ADDED	1	OUNCE	28.4	148	15	2	10
11672	POTATO PANCAKES, HOME-PREPARED	1	OUNCE	28.4	77	8	2	4
11399	POTATO PUFFS, FRZ, PREPARED	1	EACH	7.0	16	2	0	1
11414	POTATO SALAD	½	CUP	125.0	179	14	3	10
19415	POTATO STICKS	1	OUNCE	28.4	148	15	2	10
55174	POTATOES, AU GRATIN-STOUFFER'S	1	EACH	163.0	170	17	5	9
11843	POTATOES, AU GRATIN, HOME-PREPARED	½	CUP	122.5	162	14	6	9
11363	POTATOES, BAKED, W/O SKIN	1	MEDIUM	202.0	188	44	4	0
11364	POTATOES, BAKED, SKIN ONLY	1	EACH	58.0	115	27	2	0
11674	POTATOES, BAKED, W/ SKIN	1	MEDIUM	202.0	220	51	5	0
11365	POTATOES, BOILED, CKD IN SKIN, W/O SKIN	1	MEDIUM	202.0	176	41	4	0
11367	POTATOES, BOILED, CKD, W/O SKIN	1	MEDIUM	202.0	174	40	3	0
11366	POTATOES, BOILED, SKIN ONLY	1	EACH	34.0	27	6	1	0
11376	POTATOES, CND, DRAINED SOLIDS	½	CUP	90.0	54	12	1	0
11374	POTATOES, CND, SOLIDS AND LIQUIDS	½	CUP	150.0	60	13	2	0
11370	POTATOES, HASHED BROWN	½	CUP	78.0	119	6	2	11
11657	POTATOES, MASHED, HOME-PREPARED	½	CUP	105.0	81	18	2	1
11930	POTATOES, MASHED, PREPARED FROM FLAKES	½	CUP	105.0	119	16	2	6
11368	POTATOES, MICROWAVED, W/O SKIN	½	CUP	78.0	78	18	2	0
11369	POTATOES, MICROWAVED, SKIN ONLY	1	EACH	58.0	77	17	3	0

Saturated fat (g)	Monounsaturated fat (g)	Polyunsaturated fat (g)	Fiber (g)	Cholesterol (g)	Folate (g)	Vitamin A (RE)	Vitamin B-6 (mg)	Vitamin B-12 (μg)	Vitamin C (mg)	Vitamin E (mg)	Riboflavin (mg)	Thiamin (mg)	Calcium (mg)	Iron (mg)	Magnesium (mg)	Niacin (mg)	Phosphorus (mg)	Potassium (mg)	Sodium (mg)	Zinc (mg)
1	1	2	1	1	1	5	0	.1	0	-	0	0	12	.2	10	.2	40	29	98	.2
1	1	1	1	0	2	2	0	0	0	-	0	0	1	.3	12	.2	27	25	97	.3
1	1	1	-	0	2	0	0	0	0	-	0	0	1	.3	12	.2	27	25	97	.3
0	0	0	0	0	-	0	-	-	1	-	-	-	0	0	-	-	-	-	10	-
3	4	1	-	33	9	52	0	0	0	-	.1	0	12	.3	0	1	62	51	756	.2
3	4	1	-	27	0	11	0	.2	0	-	.1	0	9	.2	3	.4	24	36	521	.2
9	11	2	-	100	3	3	.3	.5	0	-	.2	.4	38	1.2	18	3	166	268	86	2.9
9	13	3	0	133	37	3589	.3	17.1	8	-	1.3	.2	8	8	9	7.1	143	169	972	2.4
2	3	1	0	13	1	0	0	.2	0	-	0	.1	1	.2	2	.7	17	45	271	.3
7	8	2	0	80	5	2	.3	.5	1	-	.2	.6	19	1.1	20	3.6	192	308	62	2.7
6	8	2	0	48	3	20	.2	.7	21	-	.2	.5	49	.8	14	2.9	215	250	1142	1.7
9	12	3	0	61	3	0	.1	.6	0	-	.2	.3	8	1.4	9	2.8	86	208	904	1.6
4	6	2	0	31	1	0	.1	.6	5	-	.1	.4	7	.5	9	1.8	102	128	776	.9
5	8	2	0	42	1	0	.3	.6	2	-	.1	.5	6	.8	11	2.7	118	242	1161	1.6
1	2	0	0	26	4	0	.4	.6	23	-	.2	.9	5	.8	18	4.2	178	296	965	1.9
2	3	1	0	35	4	0	.3	.7	19	-	.2	.8	6	.9	17	4.3	188	299	908	2
2	3	1	0	32	5	0	.4	.7	21	-	.2	.7	5	.8	14	3.9	176	284	1085	1.6
4	6	2	0	53	4	0	.3	.9	12	-	.2	.7	7	1.2	14	4.5	207	304	800	2.1
2	2	0	0	45	3	0	.3	.6	18	-	.2	.6	7	1.3	12	3.4	167	244	1023	2.4
1	2	0	0	40	3	0	.4	.6	22	-	.2	.8	6	.6	14	4.1	185	298	1215	1.6
2	3	1	0	48	3	0	.3	.6	19	-	.2	.6	7	1.2	16	4.5	211	308	1178	2.2
2	3	1	0	45	3	0	.3	.7	23	-	.2	.8	6	.8	15	4.3	201	253	1087	1.7
5	7	2	0	53	3	0	.3	.5	-	-	.2	.5	6	.7	16	3.8	182	243	1010	2
2	2	1	0	47	3	0	.4	.6	-	-	.2	.6	6	.8	19	4.3	193	269	1129	2.2
3	4	1	0	50	3	0	.3	.6	19	-	.3	.6	7	1.1	19	5.2	239	348	1276	2.1
3	4	1	0	48	3	0	.3	.7	24	-	.2	.7	6	.8	16	4.5	210	282	1120	1.8
10	12	3	0	58	4	0	.3	1.4	2	-	.2	.6	26	1	16	3.9	138	286	1276	2.4
9	11	2	0	103	3	3	.3	.9	-	-	.3	.3	40	1.6	20	4.7	222	272	79	3.9
2	3	1	-	80	5	2	.4	.8	1	-	.3	.8	4	1.2	30	4.3	247	378	54	2.5
2	2	0	-	80	5	2	.4	.9	1	-	.3	.8	4	1.2	31	4.4	251	384	55	2.5
2	2	5	1	0	24	6	.2	0	10	-	.1	.1	14	.5	21	1.3	53	357	213	.3
2	2	3	-	1	0	2	.1	0	15	-	0	0	20	.5	21	1.4	85	433	225	.3
1	1	3	-	0	8	0	.2	0	7	-	.1	.1	6	.4	25	2	55	494	139	0
3	3	3	1	0	13	0	.2	0	9	-	.1	0	7	.5	19	1.1	47	361	168	.3
3	3	3	-	0	13	0	.2	0	9	-	.1	0	7	.5	19	1.1	47	361		.3
3	2	5	-	1	5	0	.1	0	2	-	0	.1	31	.5	15	.7	46	108	214	.2
1	2	4	1	0	7	0	.2	0	3	-	0	.1	10	.4	18	1.2	44	285	121	.2
3	2	6	1	0	2	0	0	0	2	-	0	.1	7	.4	16	.9	45	286	186	.2
3	2	5	-	1	7	28	.1	0	3	-	0	.1	18	.4	16	.7	48	141	204	.2
3	2	5	1	2	18	6	.2	.3	11	-	.1	.1	20	.5	21	1.1	50	377	177	.3
3	2	5	1	0	13	0	.1	0	12	-	0	0	7	.3	17	1.2	43	368	2	.3
1	1	2	1	27	7	4	.1	.1	6	-	0	0	7	.4	9	.6	31	223	144	.2
0	0	0	0	0	1	0	0	0	0	-	0	0	2	.1	1	.2	3	27	52	0
2	3	5	-	85	8	41	.2	0	12	-	.1	.1	24	.8	19	1.1	65	317	661	.4
3	2	5	1	0	11	0	.1	0	13	-	0	0	5	.6	18	1.4	49	351	71	.3
-	-	-	-	-	20	-	-	-	4	-	.1	0	5	.6	18	1.4	49	351	71	.3
4	3	1	-	18	10	47	.2	0	12	-	.1	.1	146	.8	24	1.2	138	485	530	.8
0	0	0	3	0	18	0	.6	0	26	-	0	.2	10	.7	51	2.8	101	790	10	.6
0	0	0	2	0	13	0	.4	0	8	-	.1	.1	20	4.1	25	1.8	59	332	12	.3
0	0	0	5	0	22	0	.7	0	26	-	.1	.2	20	2.7	55	3.3	115	844	16	.6
0	0	0	4	0	20	0	.6	0	26	-	0	.2	10	.6	44	2.9	89	766	8	.6
0	0	0	4	0	18	0	.5	0	15	-	0	.2	16	.6	40	2.7	81	663	10	.5
0	0	0	-	0	3	0	.1	0	2	-	0	0	15	2.1	10	.4	18	138	5	.1
0	0	0	-	0	6	0	.2	0	5	-	0	.1	4	1.1	13	.8	25	206	234	.3
0	0	0	2	0	7	0	.2	0	19	-	0	.1	45	1.5	21	1.3	33	364	451	.6
4	5	1	2	-	6	0	.2	0	4	-	0	0	6	.6	16	1.6	33	250	19	.3
0	0	0	2	2	9	20	.2	0	7	-	0	.1	27	.3	19	1.2	50	314	318	.3
2	2	2	-	4	8	22	0	0	10	-	.1	.1	51	.2	19	.7	59	245	349	.2
0	0	0	-	0	10	0	.2	0	12	-	0	.1	4	.3	20	1.3	85	321	5	.3
0	0	0	-	0	10	0	.3	0		-	0	0	27	3.4	21	1.3	48	377	9	.3

Food Composition Table—cont'd

Code	Name	Amount	Unit	Grams	Kilocalories	Carbohydrates (g)	Protein (g)	Fat (g)
11675	POTATOES, MICROWAVED, W/ SKIN	1	MEDIUM	202.0	212	49	5	0
11671	POTATOES, O'BRIEN, HOME-PREPARED	½	CUP	97.0	79	15	2	1
11844	POTATOES, SCALLOPED	½	CUP	122.5	105	13	4	5
19216	PRALINE	1	PIECE	39.0	177	24	1	9
19047	PRETZELS, HARD, PLAIN, SALTED	1	OUNCE	28.4	108	22	3	1
19814	PRETZELS, HARD, PLAIN, UNSALTED	1	OUNCE	28.4	108	22	3	1
19050	PRETZELS, HARD, WHOLE-WHEAT	1	OUNCE	28.4	103	23	3	1
9294	PRUNE JUICE, CND	¾	CUP	191.8	136	33	1	0
9289	PRUNES, DEHYDRATED	¼	CUP	33.0	112	29	1	0
9293	PRUNES, DRIED, STEWED, W/ ADDED SUGAR	¼	CUP	59.5	74	20	1	0
9292	PRUNES, DRIED, STEWED, W/O ADDED SUGAR	¼	CUP	53.0	57	15	1	0
9291	PRUNES, DRIED, UNCOOKED	¼	CUP	40.3	96	25	1	0
19072	PUDDING POPS, CHOCOLATE	1	EACH	47.0	72	12	2	2
19073	PUDDING POPS, VANILLA	1	EACH	47.0	75	13	2	2
18326	PUMPKIN PIE	1	SLICE	109.0	229	30	4	10
11423	PUMPKIN, CKD	½	CUP	122.5	24	6	1	0
11424	PUMPKIN, CND, W/O SALT	½	CUP	122.5	42	10	1	0
11429	RADISHES, FRESH	½	CUP	58.0	10	2	0	0
11431	RADISHES, ORIENTAL, CKD	½	CUP	73.5	12	3	0	0
11432	RADISHES, ORIENTAL, DRIED	½	CUP	58.0	157	37	5	0
11430	RADISHES, ORIENTAL, FRESH	½	CUP	44.0	8	2	0	0
11637	RADISHES, WHITE ICICLE, FRESH	½	CUP	50.0	7	1	1	0
18191	RAISIN COOKIES, SOFT-TYPE	1	EACH	15.0	60	10	1	2
19149	RAISINETS	10	PIECE	10.0	41	7	0	2
9297	RAISINS, GOLDEN SEEDLESS	½	CUP	72.5	219	58	2	0
9299	RAISINS, SEEDED	½	CUP	72.5	215	57	2	0
9298	RAISINS, SEEDLESS	½	CUP	72.5	218	57	2	0
9304	RASPBERRIES, CND, RED, HEAVY SYRUP PACK	½	CUP	128.0	116	30	1	0
9302	RASPBERRIES, FRESH	½	CUP	61.5	30	7	1	0
9306	RASPBERRIES, FROZEN, RED, SWEETENED	½	CUP	125.0	129	33	1	0
62536	RAVIOLI, BEEF	1	CUP	243.9	230	36	9	5
62537	RAVIOLI, CHEESE	1	CUP	243.9	220	38	9	3
62557	RED BEANS AND RICE	2	OUNCE	56.7	189	40	8	1
62607	REDUCED FAT CHOCOLATE CHIP COOKIES	13	EACH	5.8	26	4	0	1
62595	REDUCED FAT CHOCOLATE SANDWICH COOKIES-SNACKWELL	2	EACH	25.0	100	–	1	3
62593	REDUCED FAT CLASSIC GOLDEN CRACKERS-SNACKWELL	6	EACH	14.0	60	11	1	1
62594	REDUCED FAT CREME SANDWICH COOKIES-SNACKWELL	2	EACH	26.0	110	21	1	3
62597	REDUCED FAT FRENCH ONION SNACK CRACKERS-SNACKWELL	32	EACH	30.0	120	23	2	2
62598	REDUCED FAT OATMEAL RAISIN COOKIES-SNACKWELL	2	EACH	27.0	110	20	2	3
62525	REDUCED FAT ZESTY CHEESE SNACK CRACKERS-SNACKWELL	32	EACH	30.0	120	23	3	2
19150	REESE'S PEANUT BUTTER CUPS	1	EACH	7.0	34	3	1	2
19151	REESE'S PIECES CANDY	1	PKG	55.0	258	34	7	11
19052	RICE CAKES, BROWN RICE, BUCKWHEAT	1	CAKE	9.0	34	7	1	0
19817	RICE CAKES, BROWN RICE, BUCKWHEAT, UNSALTED	1	CAKE	9.0	34	7	1	0
19413	RICE CAKES, BROWN RICE, CORN	1	CAKE	9.0	35	7	1	0
19414	RICE CAKES, BROWN RICE, MULTIGRAIN	1	CAKE	9.0	35	7	1	0
19818	RICE CAKES, BROWN RICE, MULTIGRAIN, UNSALTED	1	CAKE	9.0	35	7	1	0
19051	RICE CAKES, BROWN RICE, PLAIN	1	CAKE	9.0	35	7	1	0
19816	RICE CAKES, BROWN RICE, PLAIN, UNSALTED	1	CAKE	9.0	35	7	1	0
19416	RICE CAKES, BROWN RICE, RYE	1	CAKE	9.0	35	7	1	0
19193	RICE PUDDING	1	CUP	298.1	486	66	6	22
20037	RICE, BROWN, LONG-GRAIN, CKD	½	CUP	97.5	108	22	3	1
20041	RICE, BROWN, MEDIUM-GRAIN, CKD	½	CUP	97.5	109	23	2	1
20045	RICE, WHITE, LONG-GRAIN, CKD	½	CUP	79.0	103	22	2	0
20049	RICE, WHITE, LONG-GRAIN, INSTANT, ENRICHED	½	CUP	82.5	81	18	2	0
20051	RICE, WHITE, MEDIUM-GRAIN, CKD	½	CUP	93.0	121	27	2	0
20053	RICE, WHITE, SHORT-GRAIN, CKD	½	CUP	93.0	121	27	2	0
20057	RICE, WHITE, W/ PASTA, CKD	½	CUP	101.0	123	22	3	3
55222	RIGATONI BAKE, LEAN CUISINE-STOUFFER'S	1	EACH	276.4	250	27	18	8
41341	RIGATONI IN MEAT SAUCE-HEALTHY CHOICE	1	EACH	269.3	260	34	16	6

Saturated fat (g)	Monounsaturated fat (g)	Polyunsaturated fat (g)	Fiber (g)	Cholesterol (g)	Folate (g)	Vitamin A (RE)	Vitamin B-6 (mg)	Vitamin B-12 (μg)	Vitamin C (mg)	Vitamin E (mg)	Riboflavin (mg)	Thiamin (mg)	Calcium (mg)	Iron (mg)	Magnesium (mg)	Niacin (mg)	Phosphorus (mg)	Potassium (mg)	Sodium (mg)	Zinc (mg)
0	0	0	-	0	24	0	.7	0	31	-	.1	.2	22	2.5	55	3.5	212	903	16	.7
1	0	0	-	4	8	55	.2	0	16	-	.1	.1	35	.5	17	1	49	258	210	.3
2	2	1	-	7	11	23	.2	0	13	-	.1	.1	70	.7	23	1.3	77	463	410	.5
1	6	2	-	0	5	2	0	0	0	-	0	.1	12	.5	20	.1	43	82	24	.8
0	0	0	1	0	24	0	0	0	0	-	.2	.1	10	1.2	10	1.5	32	41	486	.2
0	0	0	1	0	24	0	0	0	0	-	.2	.1	10	1.2	10	1.5	32	41	82	.2
0	0	0	-	0	15	0	.1	0	0	-	.1	.1	8	.8	9	1.9	35	122	58	.2
0	0	0	2	0	1	0	.4	0	8	-	.1	0	23	2.3	27	1.5	48	529	8	.4
0	0	0	-	0	1	58	.2	0	0	-	.1	0	24	1.2	21	1	37	349	2	.1
0	0	0	2	0	0	17	.1	0	2	-	.1	0	12	.6	11	.4	20	186	1	.1
0	0	0	3	0	0	16	.1	0	2	-	.1	0	12	.6	11	.4	19	177	1	.1
0	0	0	3	0	1	80	.1	0	1	-	.1	0	21	1	18	.8	32	300	2	.2
-	-	-	0	1	1	16	0	.3	0	-	.1	0	66	.2	10	.1	53	105	78	.2
-	-	-	0	1	2	24	0	.2	0	-	.1	0	61	0	5	0	47	65	50	.2
2	5	2	3	22	16	523	.1	.4	2	-	.2	.1	65	.9	16	.2	77	168	307	.5
0	0	0	-	0	10	132	.1	0	6	-	.1	0	18	.7	11	.5	37	282	1	.3
0	0	0	3	0	15	2702	.1	0	5	-	.1	0	32	1.7	28	.4	43	252	6	.2
0	0	0	1	0	16	1	0	0	13	-	0	0	12	.2	5	.2	10	135	14	.2
0	0	0	1	0	13	0	0	0	11	-	0	0	12	.1	7	.1	18	209	10	.1
0	0	0	-	0	171	0	.4	0	0	-	.4	.2	365	3.9	99	2	118	2027	161	1.2
0	0	0	1	0	12	0	0	0	10	-	0	0	12	.2	7	.1	10	100	9	.1
0	0	0	-	0	7	0	0	0	15	-	0	0	14	.4	5	.2	14	140	8	.1
1	1	0	-	0	1	2	0	0	0	-	0	0	7	.3	3	.3	12	21	51	0
1	1	0	-	0	1	1	0	0	0	-	0	0	11	.1	5	0	14	51	4	.1
0	0	0	3	0	2	3	.2	0	2	-	.1	0	38	1.3	25	.8	83	541	9	.2
0	0	0	5	0	2	0	.1	0	4	-	.1	.1	20	1.9	22	.8	54	598	20	.1
0	0	0	3	0	2	1	.2	0	2	-	.1	.1	36	1.5	24	.6	70	544	9	.2
0	0	0	4	0	13	4	.1	0	11	-	0	0	14	.5	15	.6	12	120	4	.2
0	0	0	4	0	16	8	0	0	15	.2	.1	0	14	.4	11	.6	7	93	0	.3
0	0	0	5	0	32	7	0	0	21	-	.1	0	19	.8	16	.3	21	142	1	.2
2	-	-	4	20	-	150	-	-	2	-	-	-	0	1.5	-	-	-	-	1150	-
1	-	-	4	15	-	60	-	-	1	-	-	-	24	1.5	-	-	-	-	1280	-
0	-	-	7	0	-	99	-	-	6	-	-	.2	48	1.5	-	2.8	-	-	786	-
0	0	0	0	0	-	0	-	-	0	-	-	-	0	.1	-	-	-	-	34	-
1	1	0	1	0	-	0	-	-	0	-	-	-	0	.4	-	-	-	-	190	-
0	0	0	0	0	-	0	-	-	0	-	-	-	24	.4	-	-	-	-	140	-
1	1	0	1	0	-	0	-	-	0	-	-	-	24	.2	-	-	-	-	95	-
0	1	-	1	23	-	0	-	-	0	-	-	-	48	.6	-	-	-	-	290	-
0	1	1	1	0	-	0	-	-	0	-	-	-	24	.4	-	-	-	-	135	-
1	1	0	1	5	0	0	0	0	0	0	0	0	48	.6	0	0	0	0	350	0
2	0	0	0	1	2	1	0	0	0	-	0	0	5	.1	6	.3	17	28	20	.1
-	-	-	2	2	31	2	.1	.2	0	-	.1	0	73	.8	45	3.1	127	242	83	.6
0	0	0	0	0	2	0	0	0	0	-	0	0	1	.1	14	.7	34	27	10	.2
0	0	0	-	0	2	0	0	0	0	-	0	0	1	.1	14	.7	34	27	0	.2
0	0	0	0	0	2	0	0	0	0	-	0	0	1	.1	10	.6	29	25	26	.2
0	0	0	0	0	2	0	0	0	0	-	0	0	2	.2	12	.6	33	26	23	.2
0	0	0	-	0	2	0	0	0	0	-	0	0	2	.2	12	.6	33	26	0	.2
0	0	0	0	0	2	0	0	0	0	-	0	0	1	.1	12	.7	32	26	29	.3
0	0	0	0	0	2	0	0	0	0	-	0	0	1	.1	12	.7	32	26	2	.3
0	0	0	0	0	0	0	0	0	0	-	0	0	2	.2	13	.6	34	28	10	.3
3	10	8	-	3	9	104	.1	.6	1	-	.2	.1	155	.9	24	.5	203	179	253	1.5
0	0	0	2	0	4	0	.1	0	0	-	0	.1	10	.4	42	1.5	81	42	5	.6
0	0	0	-	0	4	0	.1	0	0	-	0	.1	10	.5	43	1.3	75	77	1	.6
0	0	0	0	0	2	0	.1	0	0	-	0	.1	8	.9	9	1.2	34	28	1	.4
0	0	0	0	0	3	0	0	0	0	-	0	.1	7	.5	4	.7	12	3	2	.2
0	0	0	0	0	2	0	0	0	0	-	0	.2	3	1.4	12	1.7	34	27	0	.4
0	0	0	-	0	2	0	.1	0	0	-	0	.2	1	1.4	7	1.4	31	24	0	.4
1	1	1	4	1	7	0	.1	.1	0	-	.1	.1	8	.9	12	1.8	37	42	574	.3
3	-	1	-	25	-	200	-	-	6	-	.3	.2	160	1.5	-	3.8	-	620	430	-
2	-	-	-	30	-	200	-	-	2	-	.3	.3	120	1.5	-	2.9	200	700	540	-

Food Composition Table—cont'd

Code	Name	Amount	Unit	Grams	Kilocalories	Carbohydrates (g)	Protein (g)	Fat (g)
55782	RIGATONI W/ MEAT SAUCE-STOUFFER'S	½	CUP	142.0	145	16	8	6
62614	ROAST TURKEY MEDALLIONS-WEIGHT WATCHERS	1	EACH	241.0	190	34	10	2
41310	ROASTED TURKEY AND MUSHROOMS IN GRAVY-HEALTHY CHOICE	1	EACH	241.0	200	26	18	3
15071	ROCKFISH, PACIFIC, CKD, DRY HEAT	3	OUNCE	85.1	103	0	20	2
15207	ROE, CKD, DRY HEAT	3	OUNCE	85.1	174	2	24	7
14157	ROOT BEER	12	FL OZ	369.6	152	39	0	0
62531	ROOT BEER, DIET	12	FL OZ	355.2	0	0	0	0
15232	ROUGHY, ORANGE, CKD, DRY HEAT	3	OUNCE	85.1	76	0	16	1
62541	SALAD DRESSING, BLUE CHEESE	2	TBSP.	32.0	90	5	1	7
62542	SALAD DRESSING, BLUE CHEESE, FAT FREE	2	TBSP.	35.0	50	12	1	0
4120	SALAD DRESSING, FRENCH	2	TBSP.	31.3	134	5	0	13
62545	SALAD DRESSING, FRENCH, FAT FREE	2	TBSP.	35.0	50	12	0	0
4020	SALAD DRESSING, FRENCH, LO FAT	2	TBSP.	32.5	44	7	0	2
4114	SALAD DRESSING, ITALIAN	2	TBSP.	29.4	137	3	0	14
62543	SALAD DRESSING, ITALIAN, FAT FREE	2	TBSP.	31.0	10	2	0	0
4021	SALAD DRESSING, ITALIAN, LO CAL	2	TBSP.	30.0	32	1	0	3
62539	SALAD DRESSING, RANCH	2	TBSP.	29.0	170	2	0	18
62540	SALAD DRESSING, RANCH, FAT FREE	2	TBSP.	35.0	50	11	0	0
4015	SALAD DRESSING, RUSSIAN	2	TBSP.	30.7	151	3	0	16
4022	SALAD DRESSING, RUSSIAN, LOW CAL	2	TBSP.	32.5	46	9	0	1
4016	SALAD DRESSING, SESAME SEED	2	TBSP.	30.7	136	3	1	14
4017	SALAD DRESSING, THOUSAND ISLAND	2	TBSP.	31.3	118	5	0	11
4023	SALAD DRESSING, THOUSAND ISLAND, LO CAL	2	TBSP.	30.7	49	5	0	3
62544	SALAD DRESSING, THOUSAND ISLAND, FAT FREE	2	TBSP.	35.0	45	11	0	0
4135	SALAD DRESSING, VINEGAR AND OIL	2	TBSP.	31.3	140	1	0	16
41290	SALISBURY STEAK W/ MUSHROOM GRAVY-HEALTHY CHOICE	1	EACH	311.8	280	35	21	6
43402	SALISBURY STEAK, TOP SHELF-HORMEL	1	EACH	283.5	320	22	25	15
15209	SALMON, ATLANTIC, WILD, CKD, DRY HEAT	3	OUNCE	85.1	155	0	22	7
15210	SALMON, CHINOOK, CKD, DRY HEAT	3	OUNCE	85.1	196	0	22	11
15211	SALMON, CHUM, CKD, DRY HEAT	3	OUNCE	85.1	131	0	22	4
15239	SALMON, COHO, FARMED, CKD, DRY HEAT	3	OUNCE	85.1	151	0	21	7
15247	SALMON, COHO, WILD, CKD, DRY HEAT	3	OUNCE	85.1	118	0	20	4
15082	SALMON, COHO, WILD, CKD, MOIST HEAT	3	OUNCE	85.1	156	0	23	6
15212	SALMON, PINK, CKD, DRY HEAT	3	OUNCE	85.1	127	0	22	4
62546	SALSA	2	TBSP.	33.0	20	5	0	0
41262	SALSA CHICKEN-HEALTHY CHOICE	1	EACH	318.9	240	36	20	2
2047	SALT, TABLE	1	TSP.	6.0	0	0	0	0
15088	SARDINE, ATLANTIC, CND IN OIL	3	OUNCE	85.1	177	0	21	10
6313	SAUCE, WHITE	½	CUP	131.9	120	11	5	7
11439	SAUERKRAUT, CND, SOL&LIQ	½	CUP	118.0	22	5	1	0
7003	SAUSAGE, BEERWURST, PORK	1	SLICE	23.0	55	0	3	4
7006	SAUSAGE, BOCKWURST	1	LINK	65.0	200	0	9	18
7013	SAUSAGE, BRATWURST	1	LINK	85.0	256	2	12	22
7089	SAUSAGE, ITALIAN, CKD	1	LINK	83.0	268	1	17	21
7037	SAUSAGE, KIELBASA, KOLBASSY	1	LINK	85.0	264	2	11	23
7038	SAUSAGE, KNOCKWURST	1	LINK	68.0	209	1	8	19
7075	SAUSAGE, LINK, PORK AND BEEF	1	LINK	68.0	228	1	9	21
16107	SAUSAGE, MEATLESS	1	LINK	25.0	64	2	5	5
7057	SAUSAGE, PEPPERONI	1	SLICE	5.5	27	0	1	2
7059	SAUSAGE, POLISH-STYLE	1	EACH	227.0	740	4	32	65
7064	SAUSAGE, PORK, LINKS OR BULK, CKD	1	LINK	13.0	48	0	3	4
7072	SAUSAGE, SALAMI, BEEF AND PORK, DRY	1	SLICE	10.0	42	0	2	3
7068	SAUSAGE, SALAMI, BEEF, CKD	1	SLICE	23.0	60	1	3	5
7074	SAUSAGE, SMOKED LINK, PORK	1	LINK	68.0	265	1	15	22
15173	SCALLOP, BREADED AND FRIED	3	OUNCE	85.1	183	9	15	9
15174	SCALLOP, IMITATION	3	OUNCE	85.1	84	9	11	0
43412	SCALLOPED POTATOES AND HAM, MICRO CUP-HORMEL	1	EACH	212.6	260	21	8	16
55175	SCALLOPED POTATOES-STOUFFER'S	1	EACH	163.0	130	16	4	6
14018	SCREWDRIVER	1	FL OZ	30.4	25	3	0	0
15092	SEA BASS, CKD, DRY HEAT	3	OUNCE	85.1	105	0	20	2

Saturated fat (g)	Monounsaturated fat (g)	Polyunsaturated fat (g)	Fiber (g)	Cholesterol (g)	Folate (g)	Vitamin A (RE)	Vitamin B-6 (mg)	Vitamin B-12 (µg)	Vitamin C (mg)	Vitamin E (mg)	Riboflavin (mg)	Thiamin (mg)	Calcium (mg)	Iron (mg)	Magnesium (mg)	Niacin (mg)	Phosphorus (mg)	Potassium (mg)	Sodium (mg)	Zinc (mg)
-	-	-	-	15	-	-	-	-	24	-	0	0	1042	.2	-	.4	-	310	426	-
1	-	-	4	20	-	100	-	-	5	-	-	-	24	1	-	-	-	220	530	-
1	-	1	-	40	-	200	-	-	-	-	.1	.1	16	.8	-	2.9	150	260	380	-
0	0	1	0	37	9	56	.2	1	0	-	.1	0	10	.5	29	3.3	194	442	65	.5
2	2	3	0	407	78	77	.2	9.8	14	-	.8	.2	24	.7	22	1.9	438	241	100	1.1
0	0	0	0	0	0	0	0	0	0	-	0	0	18	.2	4	0	0	4	48	.3
-	-	-	0	-	-	-	-	-	-	-	-	-	-	-	-	-	-	-	30	-
0	1	0	0	22	7	20	.3	2	0	-	.2	.1	32	.2	32	3.1	218	327	69	.8
4	-	-	0	10	-	0	-	-	0	-	-	-	24	0	-	-	-	-	470	-
0	-	-	0	0	-	0	-	-	0	.4	-	-	0	0	-	-	-	-	340	-
3	3	7	0	18	1	6	0	0	0	1.6	0	0	3	.1	0	0	4	25	428	0
0	-	-	0	0	-	100	-	-	0	-	-	-	0	0	-	-	-	-	300	-
0	0	1	0	2	0	0	0	0	0	.3	0	0	4	.1	0	0	5	26	256	.1
2	3	8	0	0	1	7	0	0	0	1.5	0	0	3	.1	0	0	1	4	231	0
0	-	-	0	0	-	0	-	-	0	-	-	-	0	0	-	-	-	-	290	-
0	1	2	0	2	0	0	0	0	0	.3	0	0	1	.1	0	0	2	5	236	0
3	-	-	0	5	-	0	-	-	0	-	-	-	0	0	-	-	-	-	270	-
0	-	-	0	0	-	0	-	-	0	.6	-	-	0	0	-	-	-	-	310	-
2	4	9	0	6	3	63	0	.1	2	1.8	0	0	6	.2	0	.2	11	48	266	.1
0	0	1	0	2	1	5	0	0	2	.1	0	0	6	.2	0	0	12	51	282	0
2	4	8	-	0	0	63	0	0	0	1.5	0	0	6	.2	0	0	11	48	307	0
2	3	6	1	8	2	30	0	.1	0	1.3	0	0	3	.2	1	0	5	35	219	0
0	1	2	0	5	2	29	0	.1	0	.3	0	0	3	.2	0	0	5	35	307	0
0	-	-	0	0	-	0	-	-	0	-	-	-	0	0	-	-	-	-	300	-
3	5	8	0	0	0	0	0	0	0	1.3	0	0	0	0	0	0	0	2	0	0
3	-	-	-	55	-	-	-	-	-	-	-	-	-	-	-	-	260	630	500	-
7	8	1	-	70	-	0	-	-	4	-	.3	0	16	1.5	35	4.8	-	801	910	5.7
1	2	3	0	60	25	11	.8	2.6	0	-	.4	.2	13	.9	31	8.6	218	534	48	.7
3	5	2	0	72	30	127	.4	2.4	3	-	.1	0	24	.8	104	8.5	316	430	51	.5
1	2	1	0	81	4	29	.4	2.9	0	-	.2	.1	12	.6	24	7.3	309	468	54	.5
2	3	2	0	54	12	50	.5	2.7	1	-	.1	.1	10	.3	29	6.3	282	391	44	.4
1	1	1	0	47	11	33	.5	4.3	1	-	.1	.1	-	.5	28	6.8	274	369	49	.5
1	2	2	0	48	8	27	.5	3.8	1	-	.1	.1	39	.6	30	6.6	253	387	45	.4
1	1	1	0	57	4	35	.2	2.9	0	-	.1	.2	14	.8	28	7.3	251	352	73	.6
0	-	-	0	0	-	80	-	-	4	-	-	-	0	0	-	-	-	-	240	-
1	-	-	-	50	-	200	-	-	66	-	.2	.2	64	.6	-	3.8	200	540	450	-
0	0	0	0	0	0	0	0	0	0	-	0	0	3	0	0	0	0	0	2325	0
1	3	4	0	121	10	57	.1	7.6	0	-	.2	.1	325	2.5	33	4.5	417	338	430	1.1
3	2	1	-	17	8	46	0	.5	1	-	.2	0	212	.1	132	.3	128	222	398	.3
0	0	0	3	0	28	2	.2	0	17	-	0	0	35	1.7	15	.2	24	201	780	.2
1	2	1	0	14	1	0	.1	.2	7	-	0	.1	2	.2	3	.7	24	58	285	.4
7	8	2	0	38	4	4	.1	.5	0	-	.1	.3	10	.4	12	2.7	95	176	718	1
8	10	2	0	51	2	0	.2	.8	1	-	.2	.4	37	1.1	13	2.7	127	180	473	2
8	10	3	0	65	4	0	.3	1.1	2	-	.2	.5	20	1.2	15	3.5	141	252	765	2
8	11	3	0	57	4	0	.2	1.4	18	-	.2	.2	37	1.2	14	2.4	126	230	915	1.7
7	9	2	0	39	1	0	.1	.8	18	-	.1	.2	7	.6	7	1.9	67	135	687	1.1
7	10	2	0	48	1	0	.1	1	13	-	.1	.2	7	1	8	2.2	73	129	643	1.4
1	1	2	1	0	7	16	.2	0	0	-	.1	.6	16	.9	9	2.8	56	58	222	.4
1	1	0	0	4	0	0	0	.1	0	-	0	0	1	.1	1	.3	7	19	112	.1
23	31	7	0	159	5	0	.4	2.2	2	-	.3	1.1	27	3.3	32	7.8	309	538	1989	4.4
1	2	0	0	11	0	0	0	.2	0	-	0	.1	4	.2	2	.6	24	47	168	.3
1	2	0	0	8	0	0	.1	.2	3	-	0	.1	1	.2	2	.5	14	38	186	.3
2	2	0	0	15	0	0	0	.7	4	-	0	0	2	.5	3	.7	26	52	270	.5
8	10	3	0	46	3	0	.2	1.1	1	-	.2	.5	20	.8	13	3.1	110	228	1020	1.9
2	4	2	-	52	15	19	.1	1.1	2	-	.1	0	36	.7	50	1.3	201	283	395	.9
0	0	0	0	19	1	17	0	1.4	0	-	0	0	7	.3	37	.3	240	88	676	.3
6	8	2	-	33	-	-	-	-	11	-	.1	.1	32	.4	21	2.1	-	425	768	.9
-	-	-	-	-	-	-	-	-	2	-	.1	.1	80	.2	-	.8	-	375	610	-
0	0	0	-	0	11	2	0	0	9	-	0	0	2	0	2	0	4	47	0	0
1	0	1	0	45	5	54	.4	.3	0	-	.1	.1	11	.3	45	1.6	211	279	74	.4

Food Composition Table—cont'd

Code	Name	Amount	Unit	Grams	Kilocalories	Carbohydrates (g)	Protein (g)	Fat (g)
12036	SEEDS, SUNFLOWER, DRIED	½	CUP	72.0	410	14	16	36
12537	SEEDS, SUNFLOWER, DRY ROASTED, W/ SALT ADDED	½	CUP	64.0	372	15	12	32
12037	SEEDS, SUNFLOWER, DRY ROASTED, W/O SALT	½	CUP	64.0	372	15	12	32
12538	SEEDS, SUNFLOWER, OIL ROASTED, W/ SALT ADDED	½	CUP	67.5	415	10	14	39
12038	SEEDS, SUNFLOWER, OIL ROASTED, W/O SALT	½	CUP	67.5	415	10	14	39
12539	SEEDS, SUNFLOWER, TOASTED, W/ SALT ADDED	½	CUP	67.0	415	14	12	38
12039	SEEDS, SUNFLOWER, TOASTED, W/O SALT	½	CUP	67.0	415	14	12	38
19418	SESAME STICKS, WHEAT-BASED, SALTED	1	OUNCE	28.4	153	13	3	10
19820	SESAME STICKS, WHEAT-BASED, UNSALTED	1	OUNCE	28.4	153	13	3	10
14346	SHAKE, CHOCOLATE	1	CUP	226.4	288	46	8	8
14428	SHAKE, STRAWBERRY	1	CUP	226.4	256	43	8	6
14347	SHAKE, VANILLA	1	CUP	226.4	251	41	8	7
11640	SHALLOTS, FREEZE-DRIED	½	CUP	7.2	25	6	1	0
11677	SHALLOTS, FRESH	½	CUP	79.9	58	13	2	0
15096	SHARK, CKD, BATTER-DIPPED AND FRIED	3	OUNCE	85.1	194	5	16	12
19097	SHERBET, ALL FLAVORS	1	CUP	192.0	265	58	2	4
18193	SHORTBREAD COOKIES, PECAN	1	EACH	14.0	76	8	1	5
18192	SHORTBREAD COOKIES, PLAIN	1	EACH	8.0	40	5	0	2
41263	SHRIMP MARINARA-HEALTHY CHOICE	1	EACH	297.7	260	51	10	1
62615	SHRIMP MARINARA-WEIGHT WATCHERS	1	EACH	255.2	190	35	9	2
15150	SHRIMP, CKD, BREADED AND FRIED	3	OUNCE	85.1	206	10	18	10
15151	SHRIMP, CKD, MOIST HEAT	3	OUNCE	85.1	84	0	18	1
15152	SHRIMP, CND	3	OUNCE	85.1	102	1	20	2
15149	SHRIMP, FRESH	3	OUNCE	85.1	90	1	17	1
15153	SHRIMP, IMITATION	3	OUNCE	85.1	86	8	11	1
55143	SINGLE SERVING STUFFED PEPPER-STOUFFER'S	1	EACH	283.5	220	28	10	8
41264	SIRLOIN BEEF W/ BARBECUE SAUCE-HEALTHY CHOICE	1	EACH	311.8	280	44	17	4
19370	SKITTLES BITE SIZE CANDIES	1	PKG	65.0	255	62	0	2
41291	SLICED TURKEY BREAST W/ GRAVY AND DRESSING-HEALTHY CHOICE	1	EACH	283.5	270	30	27	4
41296	SLICED TURKEY BREAST W/ GRAVY-HEALTHY CHOICE	1	EACH	340.2	290	46	19	3
55225	SLICED TURKEY W/ DRESSING, LEAN CUISINE-STOUFFER'S	1	EACH	223.3	200	23	16	5
19407	SLIM JIMS, SMOKED	1	OUNCE	28.4	156	2	6	14
15100	SMELT, RAINBOW, CKD, DRY HEAT	3	OUNCE	85.1	105	0	19	3
15102	SNAPPER, CKD, DRY HEAT	3	OUNCE	85.1	109	0	22	1
19155	SNICKERS BAR	1	BAR	61.0	278	37	6	14
62599	SORBET, ALL FLAVORS	½	CUP	90.0	100	25	0	0
6474	SOUP, BEAN W/ BACON	1	CUP	264.9	106	16	5	2
6007	SOUP, BEAN W/ HAM	1	CUP	243.0	231	27	13	9
6406	SOUP, BEAN W/ HOT DOGS	1	CUP	250.0	187	22	10	7
6404	SOUP, BEAN W/ PORK	1	CUP	253.0	172	23	8	6
6008	SOUP, BEEF BROTH OR BOUILLON	1	CUP	240.0	17	0	3	1
6547	SOUP, BEEF MUSHROOM	1	CUP	244.0	73	6	5	3
6409	SOUP, BEEF NOODLE	1	CUP	244.0	83	9	5	3
6070	SOUP, BEEF, CHUNKY	1	CUP	240.0	170	20	12	5
6402	SOUP, BLACK BEAN	1	CUP	247.0	116	20	6	2
6478	SOUP, CAULIFLOWER	1	CUP	256.1	69	11	3	2
6411	SOUP, CHEESE	1	CUP	247.0	156	11	5	10
6480	SOUP, CHICKEN BROTH OR BOUILLON	1	CUP	244.0	22	1	1	1
6417	SOUP, CHICKEN GUMBO	1	CUP	244.0	56	8	3	1
6549	SOUP, CHICKEN MUSHROOM	1	CUP	244.0	132	9	4	9
6419	SOUP, CHICKEN NOODLE	1	CUP	241.0	75	9	4	2
6018	SOUP, CHICKEN NOODLE, CHUNKY	1	CUP	240.0	175	17	13	6
6485	SOUP, CHICKEN RICE	1	CUP	252.8	61	9	2	1
6022	SOUP, CHICKEN RICE, CHUNKY	1	CUP	240.0	127	13	12	3
6425	SOUP, CHICKEN VEGETABLE	1	CUP	241.0	75	9	4	3
6024	SOUP, CHICKEN VEGETABLE, CHUNKY	1	CUP	240.0	166	19	12	5
6412	SOUP, CHICKEN W/ DUMPLINGS	1	CUP	241.0	96	6	6	6
6423	SOUP, CHICKEN W/ RICE	1	CUP	241.0	60	7	4	2
6015	SOUP, CHICKEN, CHUNKY	1	CUP	251.0	178	17	13	7
6426	SOUP, CHILI BEEF	1	CUP	250.0	170	21	7	7

Saturated fat (g)	Monounsaturated fat (g)	Polyunsaturated fat (g)	Fiber (g)	Cholesterol (g)	Folate (g)	Vitamin A (RE)	Vitamin B-6 (mg)	Vitamin B-12 (µg)	Vitamin C (mg)	Vitamin E (mg)	Riboflavin (mg)	Thiamin (mg)	Calcium (mg)	Iron (mg)	Magnesium (mg)	Niacin (mg)	Phosphorus (mg)	Potassium (mg)	Sodium (mg)	Zinc (mg)
4	7	24	8	0	164	4	.6	0	1	-	.2	1.6	84	4.9	255	3.2	508	496	2	3.6
3	6	21	4	0	152	0	.5	0	1	-	.2	.1	45	2.4	83	4.5	739	544	499	3.4
3	6	21	6	0	152	0	.5	0	1	-	.2	.1	45	2.4	83	4.5	739	544	2	3.4
4	7	26	5	0	158	3	.5	0	1	-	.2	.2	38	4.5	86	2.8	769	326	407	3.5
4	7	26	5	0	158	3	.5	0	1	-	.2	.2	38	4.5	86	2.8	769	326	2	3.5
4	7	25	-	0	159	0	.5	0	1	-	.2	.2	38	4.6	86	2.8	776	329	411	3.6
4	7	25	-	0	159	0	.5	0	1	-	.2	.2	38	4.6	86	2.8	776	329	2	3.6
2	3	5	1	0	6	3	0	0	0	-	0	0	48	.2	13	.4	39	50	422	.3
2	3	5	-	0	6	3	0	0	0	-	0	0	48	.2	13	.4	39	50	8	.3
5	2	0	-	29	8	52	.1	.8	1	-	.6	.1	256	.7	38	.4	231	453	220	.9
4	-	-	-	25	7	66	.1	.7	2	-	.4	.1	256	.2	29	.4	226	412	188	.8
4	2	0	-	25	7	72	.1	.8	2	-	.4	.1	276	.2	27	.4	231	394	186	.8
0	0	0	-	0	8	404	.1	0	3	-	0	0	13	.4	7	.1	21	119	4	.1
0	0	0	-	0	27	998	.3	0	6	-	0	0	30	1	17	.2	48	267	10	.3
3	5	3	0	50	4	46	.3	1	0	-	.1	.1	43	.9	37	2.4	165	132	104	.4
2	1	0	-	10	8	27	.1	.2	8	-	.1	0	104	.3	15	.2	77	184	88	.9
1	3	1	0	5	1	0	0	0	0	-	0	0	4	.3	3	.3	12	10	39	.1
0	1	0	-	2	1	1	0	0	0	-	0	0	3	.2	1	.3	9	8	36	0
-	-	-	-	60	-	100	-	-	114	-	.1	.2	48	1.5	-	1.1	130	390	320	-
1	-	-	4	40	-	150	-	-	6	-	-	-	120	1	-	-	-	440	400	-
2	3	4	-	151	7	48	.1	1.6	1	-	.1	.1	57	1.1	34	2.6	185	191	293	1.2
0	0	0	0	166	3	56	.1	1.3	2	-	0	0	33	2.6	29	2.2	117	155	191	1.3
0	0	1	0	147	2	15	.1	1	2	-	0	0	50	2.3	35	2.3	198	179	144	1.1
0	0	1	0	129	3	46	.1	1	2	-	0	0	44	2	31	2.2	174	157	126	.9
0	0	1	0	31	1	17	0	1.4	0	-	0	0	16	.5	37	.1	240	76	600	.3
-	-	-	-	-	-	20	-	-	6	-	.2	.2	32	1	-	2.9	-	400	1010	-
2	-	1	-	25	-	-	-	-	-	-	-	-	-	-	-	-	190	630	240	-
-	-	-	0	0	0	0	0	0	0	-	0	0	2	.1	1	0	2	15	30	0
2	-	1	-	50	-	150	-	-	-	-	.3	.3	48	1	-	7.6	310	590	530	-
1	-	1	-	20	-	150	-	-	27	-	.1	.2	16	.6	-	1.5	-	360	520	-
1	-	2	-	25	-	500	-	-	6	-	.3	.2	32	.8	-	4.8	-	400	590	-
6	6	1	-	38	0	48	.1	.3	2	-	.1	0	19	1	6	1.3	51	73	420	.7
0	1	1	0	77	4	14	.1	3.4	0	-	.1	0	65	1	32	1.5	251	316	65	1.8
0	0	1	0	40	5	30	.4	3	1	-	0	0	34	.2	31	.3	171	444	48	.4
7	4	1	2	7	24	19	.1	.3	0	-	.1	0	70	.5	37	1.8	129	199	163	.7
0	-	-	1	0	-	0	-	-	12	-	-	-	0	0	-	-	-	-	10	-
1	1	0	9	3	8	5	0	0	1	-	.3	.1	56	1.3	29	.4	90	326	927	.7
3	4	1	11	22	29	396	.1	.1	4	-	.1	.1	78	3.2	46	1.7	143	425	972	1.1
2	3	2	-	12	30	87	.1	.1	1	-	.1	.1	87	2.3	47	1	165	477	1092	1.2
2	2	2	9	3	32	89	0	.1	2	-	0	.1	81	2	46	.6	132	402	951	1
0	0	0	0	0	5	0	0	.2	0	-	.1	0	14	.4	5	1.9	31	130	782	0
1	1	0	-	7	10	0	0	.2	5	-	.1	0	5	.9	10	1	34	154	942	1.5
1	1	0	1	5	4	63	0	.2	0	-	.1	.1	15	1.1	5	1.1	46	100	952	1.5
3	2	0	1	14	13	262	.1	.6	7	-	.2	.1	31	2.3	5	2.7	120	336	866	2.6
0	1	0	4	0	25	49	.1	0	1	-	.1	.1	44	2.1	42	.5	106	274	1198	1.4
0	1	1	-	0	3	0	0	.2	3	-	.1	.1	10	.5	3	.5	51	105	843	.3
7	3	0	-	30	5	109	0	0	0	-	.1	0	141	.7	5	.4	136	153	958	.6
0	0	0	0	0	2	12	0	0	0	-	0	0	15	.1	5	.2	12	24	1484	0
0	1	0	2	5	5	15	.1	0	5	-	0	0	24	.9	5	.7	24	76	954	.4
2	4	2	-	10	0	112	0	0	0	-	.1	0	29	.9	10	1.6	27	154	942	1
1	1	1	1	7	2	72	0	.1	0	-	.1	.1	17	.8	5	1.4	36	55	1106	.4
1	3	2	4	19	5	122	0	.3	0	-	.2	.1	24	1.4	10	4.3	72	108	850	1
0	1	0	1	3	1	0	0	.1	0	-	0	0	8	0	0	.4	10	10	981	.1
1	1	1	1	12	4	586	0	.3	4	-	.1	0	34	1.9	10	4.1	72	108	888	1
1	1	1	1	10	5	265	0	.1	1	-	.1	0	17	.9	7	1.2	41	154	945	.4
1	2	1	-	17	12	600	.1	.2	6	-	.2	0	26	1.5	10	3.3	106	367	1068	2.2
1	3	1	1	34	2	53	0	.2	0	-	.1	0	14	.6	5	1.8	60	116	860	.4
0	1	0	1	7	1	65	0	.1	0	-	0	0	17	.7	0	1.1	22	101	815	.3
2	3	1	2	30	5	131	.1	.3	1	-	.2	.1	25	1.7	8	4.4	113	176	889	1
3	3	0	9	12	17	150	.2	.3	4	-	.1	.1	42	2.1	30	1.1	147	525	1035	1.4

Food Composition Table—cont'd

Code	Name	Amount	Unit	Grams	Kilocalories	Carbohydrates (g)	Protein (g)	Fat (g)
6027	SOUP, CLAM CHOWDER, MANHATTAN STYLE	1	CUP	240.0	134	19	7	3
6230	SOUP, CLAM CHOWDER, NEW ENGLAND	1	CUP	248.0	164	17	9	7
6034	SOUP, CRAB	1	CUP	244.0	76	10	5	2
6201	SOUP, CREAM OF ASPARAGUS	1	CUP	248.0	161	16	6	8
6210	SOUP, CREAM OF CELERY	1	CUP	248.0	164	15	6	10
6216	SOUP, CREAM OF CHICKEN	1	CUP	248.0	191	15	7	11
6243	SOUP, CREAM OF MUSHROOM	1	CUP	248.0	203	15	6	14
6246	SOUP, CREAM OF ONION	1	CUP	248.0	186	18	7	9
6253	SOUP, CREAM OF POTATO	1	CUP	248.0	149	17	6	6
6256	SOUP, CREAM OF SHRIMP	1	CUP	248.0	164	14	7	9
6501	SOUP, CREAM OF VEGETABLE	1	CUP	260.1	107	12	2	6
6036	SOUP, GAZPACHO	1	CUP	244.0	56	1	9	2
6037	SOUP, LENTIL W/ HAM	1	CUP	248.0	139	20	9	3
6440	SOUP, MINESTRONE	1	CUP	241.0	82	11	4	3
6039	SOUP, MINESTRONE, CHUNKY	1	CUP	240.0	127	21	5	3
6493	SOUP, MUSHROOM	1	CUP	253.0	96	11	2	5
6445	SOUP, ONION	1	CUP	241.0	58	8	4	2
6249	SOUP, PEA, GREEN	1	CUP	254.0	239	32	13	7
6451	SOUP, PEA, SPLIT W/ HAM	1	CUP	253.0	190	28	10	4
6050	SOUP, PEA, SPLIT W/ HAM, CHUNKY	1	CUP	240.0	185	27	11	4
6359	SOUP, TOMATO	1	CUP	248.0	161	22	6	6
6461	SOUP, TOMATO BEEF W/ NOODLE	1	CUP	244.0	139	21	4	4
6463	SOUP, TOMATO RICE	1	CUP	247.0	119	22	2	3
6499	SOUP, TOMATO VEGETABLE	1	CUP	253.0	56	10	2	1
6465	SOUP, TURKEY NOODLE	1	CUP	244.0	68	9	4	2
6466	SOUP, TURKEY VEGETABLE	1	CUP	241.0	72	9	3	3
6064	SOUP, TURKEY, CHUNKY	1	CUP	236.0	135	14	10	4
6500	SOUP, VEGETABLE BEEF	1	CUP	253.1	53	8	3	1
6067	SOUP, VEGETABLE, CHUNKY	1	CUP	240.0	122	19	4	4
6468	SOUP, VEGETARIAN VEGETABLE	1	CUP	241.0	72	12	2	2
1056	SOUR CREAM	1	TBSP.	12.0	26	1	0	3
62556	SOUR CREAM, FAT FREE	1	TBSP.	16.0	13	3	1	0
1055	SOUR CREAM, HALF AND HALF, CULTURED	1	TBSP.	15.0	20	1	0	2
1074	SOUR CREAM, IMITATION, NONDAIRY, CULTURED	1	TBSP.	14.4	30	1	0	3
62555	SOUR CREAM, LIGHT	1	TBSP.	16.0	16	1	1	1
41265	SOUTHWESTERN STYLE CHICKEN-HEALTHY CHOICE	1	EACH	354.4	340	51	25	5
6134	SOY SAUCE	1	TBSP.	18.0	10	2	1	0
16109	SOYBEANS, BOILED	½	CUP	86.0	149	9	14	8
16111	SOYBEANS, DRY ROASTED	½	CUP	86.0	387	28	34	19
43404	SPAGHETTI AND MEATBALLS, MICRO CUP-HORMEL	1	EACH	212.6	210	27	10	7
11455	SPAGHETTI SAUCE	½	CUP	124.5	136	20	2	6
55226	SPAGHETTI W/ MEAT SAUCE, LEAN CUISINE-STOUFFER'S	1	EACH	326.0	290	45	15	6
43396	SPAGHETTI W/ MEAT SAUCE, TOP SHELF-HORMEL	1	EACH	283.5	260	37	14	6
41342	SPAGHETTI W/ MEAT SAUCE-HEALTHY CHOICE	1	EACH	283.5	280	42	14	6
55247	SPAGHETTI W/ MEAT SAUCE-STOUFFER'S	1	EACH	365.0	320	38	16	12
55150	SPAGHETTI W/ MEATBALLS-STOUFFER'S	1	EACH	276.4	290	37	14	9
19164	SPECIAL DARK SWEET CHOCOLATE BAR	1	BAR	79.0	376	49	4	24
55176	SPINACH SOUFFLE-STOUFFER'S	1	EACH	170.1	220	11	9	15
11458	SPINACH, CKD	½	CUP	90.0	21	3	3	0
11461	SPINACH, CND, DRAINED SOLIDS	½	CUP	107.0	25	4	3	1
11459	SPINACH, CND, REG PK, SOL&LIQ	½	CUP	117.0	22	3	2	0
11457	SPINACH, FRESH	1	CUP	56.0	12	2	2	0
11464	SPINACH, FRZ, CKD	½	CUP	95.0	27	5	3	0
11463	SPINACH, FRZ, UNPREPARED	½	CUP	78.0	19	3	2	0
41283	SPLIT PEA AND HAM SOUP-HEALTHY CHOICE	1	EACH	212.6	170	25	10	3
55766	SPLIT PEA SOUP W/ HAM-STOUFFER'S	1	CUP	283.9	220	35	15	3
11642	SQUASH, SUMMER, CKD	½	CUP	90.0	18	4	1	0
11641	SQUASH, SUMMER, FRESH	½	CUP	65.0	13	3	1	0
11644	SQUASH, WINTER, BAKED	½	CUP	102.5	40	9	1	1
11643	SQUASH, WINTER, FRESH	½	CUP	58.0	21	5	1	0

Saturated fat (g)	Monounsaturated fat (g)	Polyunsaturated fat (g)	Fiber (g)	Cholesterol (g)	Folate (g)	Vitamin A (RE)	Vitamin B-6 (mg)	Vitamin B-12 (μg)	Vitamin C (mg)	Vitamin E (mg)	Riboflavin (mg)	Thiamin (mg)	Calcium (mg)	Iron (mg)	Magnesium (mg)	Niacin (mg)	Phosphorus (mg)	Potassium (mg)	Sodium (mg)	Zinc (mg)
2	1	0	3	14	9	329	.3	7.9	12	-	.1	.1	67	2.6	19	1.8	84	384	1001	1.7
3	2	1	1	22	10	40	.1	10.2	3	-	.2	.1	186	1.5	22	1	156	300	992	.8
0	1	0	1	10	15	51	.1	.2	0	-	.1	.2	66	1.2	15	1.3	88	327	1235	1.5
3	2	2	1	22	30	84	.1	.5	4	-	.3	.1	174	.9	20	.9	154	360	1042	.9
4	2	3	1	32	8	67	.1	.5	1	-	.2	.1	186	.7	22	.4	151	310	1009	.2
5	4	2	0	27	8	94	.1	.5	1	-	.3	.1	181	.7	17	.9	151	273	1047	.7
5	3	5	0	20	10	37	.1	.5	2	-	.3	.1	179	.6	20	.9	156	270	1076	.6
4	3	2	1	32	12	67	.1	.5	2	-	.3	.1	179	.7	22	.6	154	310	1004	.6
4	2	1	0	22	9	67	.1	.5	1	-	.2	.1	166	.5	17	.6	161	322	1061	.7
6	3	0	0	35	10	55	.4	1	1	-	.2	.1	164	.6	22	.5	146	248	1037	.8
1	3	1	1	0	8	3	0	.1	4	-	.1	1.2	31	.5	10	.5	55	96	1170	.3
0	1	1	4	0	10	20	.1	0	3	-	0	0	24	1	7	.9	37	224	1183	.2
1	1	0	-	7	50	35	.2	.3	4	-	.1	.2	42	2.7	22	1.4	184	357	1319	.7
1	1	1	1	2	16	234	.1	0	1	-	0	.1	34	.9	7	.9	55	313	911	.7
1	1	0	2	5	31	434	.2	0	5	-	.1	.1	60	1.8	14	1.2	110	612	864	1.4
1	2	2	1	0	5	0	0	.3	1	-	.1	.3	66	.5	5	.5	76	200	1020	.1
0	1	1	1	0	15	0	0	0	1	-	0	0	27	.7	2	.6	12	67	1053	.6
4	2	1	3	18	8	58	.1	.4	3	-	.3	.2	173	2	56	1.3	239	376	1046	1.8
2	2	1	-	8	3	46	.1	.3	2	-	.1	.1	23	2.3	48	1.5	213	400	1007	1.3
2	2	1	4	7	5	487	.2	.2	7	-	.1	.1	34	2.1	38	2.5	178	305	965	3.1
3	2	1	0	17	21	109	.2	.4	68	-	.2	.1	159	1.8	22	1.5	149	449	932	.3
2	2	1	1	5	7	54	.1	.2	0	-	.1	.1	17	1.1	7	1.9	56	220	917	.8
1	1	1	1	2	14	77	.1	0	15	-	0	.1	22	.8	5	1.1	35	331	815	.5
0	0	0	1	0	10	20	.1	0	6	-	0	.1	8	.6	20	.8	30	104	1146	.2
1	1	0	1	5	2	29	0	.1	0	-	.1	.1	12	1	5	1.4	49	76	815	.6
1	1	1	0	2	5	243	0	.2	0	-	0	0	17	.8	5	1	41	176	906	.6
1	2	1	-	9	11	715	.3	2.1	6	-	.1	0	50	1.9	24	3.6	104	361	923	2.1
1	0	0	1	0	8	23	.1	.3	1	-	0	0	13	.9	23	.5	35	76	1002	.3
1	2	1	1	0	17	588	.2	0	6	-	.1	.1	55	1.6	7	1.2	72	396	1010	3.1
0	1	1	0	0	11	301	.1	0	1	-	0	.1	22	1.1	7	.9	34	210	822	.5
2	1	0	0	5	1	23	0	0	0	-	0	0	14	1	0	1	10	17	6	0
0	-	-	-	3	-	30	-	-	0	-	-	-	36	0	-	-	-	-	18	-
1	1	0	0	6	2	17	0	0	0	-	0	0	16	0	2	0	14	19	6	.1
3	0	0	0	0	0	0	0	0	0	-	0	0	0	.1	1	0	6	23	15	.2
1	-	-	-	5	-	18	-	-	0	-	-	-	22	0	-	-	-	27	9	-
2	-	2	-	60	-	-	-	-	-	-	-	-	-	-	-	-	260	560	550	-
0	0	0	0	0	3	0	0	0	0	-	0	0	3	.4	6	.6	20	32	1029	.1
1	2	4	5	0	46	1	.2	0	1	-	.2	.1	88	4.4	74	.3	211	443	1	1
3	4	10	7	0	176	2	.2	0	4	-	.6	.4	232	3.4	196	.9	558	1173	2	4.1
3	3	1	-	20	-	140	-	-	4	-	.3	.1	32	1.1	25	2.3	-	341	930	1.1
1	3	2	4	0	27	153	.4	0	14	-	.1	.1	35	.8	30	1.9	45	478	618	.3
2	-	2	-	20	-	100	-	-	6	-	.3	.3	48	2	-	3.8	-	500	500	-
2	2	1	-	20	-	100	-	-	2	-	.3	.2	48	1.5	46	3.8	-	879	980	2.4
2	-	2	-	20	-	250	-	-	5	-	.3	.4	48	2	-	1.9	160	540	480	-
-	-	12	-	-	-	150	-	-	6	-	.2	.2	80	1.5	-	3.8	-	800	560	-
-	-	-	-	-	-	100	-	-	6	-	.3	.3	64	1.5	-	3.8	-	550	790	-
-	-	-	4	0	3	2	0	0	0	-	.2	0	15	1.7	91	.5	126	269	8	1.2
-	-	-	-	-	-	200	-	-	6	-	.3	.1	120	.4	-	.4	-	345	820	-
0	0	0	2	0	131	737	.2	0	9	-	.2	.1	122	3.2	78	.4	50	419	63	.7
0	0	0	-	0	105	939	.1	0	15	-	.1	0	136	2.5	81	.4	47	370	29	.5
0	0	0	3	0	68	752	.1	0	16	-	.1	0	97	1.8	66	.3	37	269	373	.5
0	0	0	2	0	109	376	.1	0	16	-	.1	0	55	1.5	44	.4	27	312	44	.3
0	0	0	3	0	102	739	.1	0	12	-	.2	.1	139	1.4	66	.4	46	283	82	.7
0	0	0	2	0	93	605	.1	0	19	-	.1	.1	87	1.6	45	.3	32	252	58	.3
1	-	-	-	10	-	100	-	-	6	-	.1	.2	16	.6	-	1.9	190	450	460	-
-	-	-	-	10	-	-	-	-	0	-	0	0	240	.2	-	.4	-	571	1192	-
0	0	0	1	0	18	26	.1	0	5	-	0	0	24	.3	22	.5	35	173	1	.4
0	0	0	1	0	17	13	.1	0	10	-	0	0	13	.3	15	.4	23	127	1	.2
0	0	0	3	0	29	365	.1	0	10	-	0	.1	14	.3	8	.7	21	448	1	.3
0	0	0	1	0	13	235	0	0	7	-	0	.1	18	.3	12	.5	19	203	2	.1

Food Composition Table—cont'd

Code	Name	Amount	Unit	Grams	Kilocalories	Carbohydrates (g)	Protein (g)	Fat (g)
11953	SQUASH, ZUCCHINI, BABY, FRESH	1	MEDIUM	11.0	2	0	0	0
15176	SQUID, FRIED	3	OUNCE	85.1	149	7	15	6
9316	STRAWBERRIES, FRESH	½	CUP	74.5	22	5	0	0
9320	STRAWBERRIES, FROZEN, SWEETENED	½	CUP	127.5	122	33	1	0
9318	STRAWBERRIES, FROZEN, UNSWEETENED	½	CUP	74.5	26	7	0	0
14351	STRAWBERRY FLAVOR BEVERAGE	1	CUP	266.0	234	33	8	8
18354	STRUDEL, APPLE	1	EACH	71.0	195	29	2	8
55781	STUFFED CABBAGE NO SAUCE-STOUFFER'S	1	OUNCE	28.4	39	3	2	2
55228	STUFFED CABBAGE W/ MEAT, LEAN CUISINE-STOUFFER'S	1	EACH	269.3	210	26	13	6
55778	STUFFED CABBAGE-STOUFFER'S	1	OUNCE	28.4	29	3	1	1
55157	STUFFED GREEN PEPPERS-STOUFFER'S	1	EACH	219.7	200	22	9	8
18203	SUGAR COOKIES, DIETARY	1	EACH	7.0	30	5	1	1
18204	SUGAR COOKIES, REGULAR (INCLUDES VANILLA)	1	EACH	15.0	72	10	1	3
15218	SUNFISH, CKD, DRY HEAT	3	OUNCE	85.1	97	0	21	1
55229	SWEDISH MEATBALLS W/ PASTA, LEAN CUISINE-STOUFFER'S	1	EACH	258.7	290	31	23	8
55148	SWEDISH MEATBALLS W/ PASTA-STOUFFER'S	1	EACH	262.2	420	32	24	21
41266	SWEET AND SOUR CHICKEN-HEALTHY CHOICE	1	EACH	326.0	280	52	20	2
18359	SWEET ROLLS W/ RAISINS AND NUTS	1	EACH	57.0	196	30	4	7
18355	SWEET ROLLS, CHEESE	1	EACH	66.0	238	29	5	12
18356	SWEET ROLLS, CINNAMON W/ RAISINS	1	EACH	60.0	223	31	4	10
11508	SWEET POTATOES, BAKED IN SKIN	½	CUP	100.0	103	24	2	0
11510	SWEET POTATOES, BOILED, W/O SKIN	½	CUP	164.0	172	40	3	0
11659	SWEET POTATOES, CANDIED	½	CUP	113.4	155	32	1	4
11514	SWEET POTATOES, MASHED	½	CUP	127.5	129	30	3	0
11647	SWEET POTATOES, SYRUP PACK, DRAINED SOLIDS	½	CUP	98.0	106	25	1	0
15111	SWORDFISH, CKD, DRY HEAT	3	OUNCE	85.1	132	0	22	4
19093	SYMPHONY MILK CHOCOLATE BAR	1	BAR	68.0	355	39	5	22
19348	SYRUP, CHOCOLATE, FUDGE-TYPE	1	TBSP.	21.0	73	12	1	3
19349	SYRUP, CORN, DARK	1	TBSP.	20.0	56	15	0	0
19351	SYRUP, CORN, HIGH-FRUCTOSE	1	TBSP.	19.0	53	14	0	0
19350	SYRUP, CORN, LIGHT	1	TBSP.	20.0	56	15	0	0
19352	SYRUP, MALT	1	TBSP.	24.0	76	17	1	0
19353	SYRUP, MAPLE	1	TBSP.	20.0	52	13	0	0
19128	SYRUP, PANCAKE, LO CAL	1	TBSP.	20.0	33	9	0	0
19360	SYRUP, PANCAKE, W/ 2% MAPLE	1	TBSP.	20.0	53	14	0	0
19113	SYRUP, PANCAKE, W/ BUTTER	1	TBSP.	20.0	59	15	0	0
18360	TACO SHELLS, BAKED	1	MEDIUM	13.0	61	8	1	3
18448	TACO SHELLS, BAKED, W/O ADDED SALT	1	MEDIUM	13.0	61	8	1	3
43438	TACO SHELLS, CHI-CHI'S-HORMEL	1	EACH	20.0	99	12	1	5
19382	TAFFY	1	PIECE	15.0	56	14	0	0
9223	TANGERINE JUICE, CND, SWEETENED	¾	CUP	186.4	93	22	1	0
9221	TANGERINE JUICE, FRESH	¾	CUP	185.2	80	19	1	0
9219	TANGERINES, CND, JUICE PACK	½	CUP	124.5	46	12	1	0
9220	TANGERINES, CND, LIGHT SYRUP PACK	½	CUP	126.0	77	20	1	0
9218	TANGERINES, FRESH	1	MEDIUM	84.0	37	9	1	0
19218	TAPIOCA PUDDING	1	CUP	298.1	355	58	6	11
19524	TARO CHIPS	1	OUNCE	28.4	141	19	1	7
14355	TEA, BREWED	8	FL OZ	236.8	2	1	0	0
14381	TEA, HERB, BREWED	8	FL OZ	236.8	2	0	0	0
14371	TEA, INSTANT, SWEETENED	8	FL OZ	259.0	88	22	0	0
14367	TEA, INSTANT, UNSWEETENED	8	FL OZ	236.8	2	0	0	0
43401	TENDER BEEF ROAST, TOP SHELF-HORMEL	1	EACH	283.5	240	19	28	6
14020	TEQUILA SUNRISE	1	FL OZ	31.2	34	3	0	0
41267	TERIYAKI CHICKEN-HEALTHY CHOICE	1	EACH	347.3	290	39	24	4
6112	TERIYAKI SAUCE	1	TBSP.	18.0	15	3	1	0
55811	THREE BEAN CHILI-STOUFFER'S	1	CUP	283.9	210	32	10	5
19159	THREE MUSKETEERS BAR	1	BAR	60.0	250	46	2	8
14382	THIRST QUENCHER DRINK, BOTTLED	12	FL OZ	361.2	90	23	0	0
18361	TOASTER PASTRIES, BROWN-SUGAR-CINN.	1	EACH	52.0	214	35	3	7
18362	TOASTER PASTRIES, FRUIT	1	EACH	52.0	204	37	2	5

Saturated fat (g)	Monounsaturated fat (g)	Polyunsaturated fat (g)	Fiber (g)	Cholesterol (g)	Folate (g)	Vitamin A (RE)	Vitamin B-6 (mg)	Vitamin B-12 (µg)	Vitamin C (mg)	Vitamin E (mg)	Riboflavin (mg)	Thiamin (mg)	Calcium (mg)	Iron (mg)	Magnesium (mg)	Niacin (mg)	Phosphorus (mg)	Potassium (mg)	Sodium (mg)	Zinc (mg)
0	0	0	-	0	2	5	0	0	4	-	0	0	2	.1	4	.1	10	50	0	.1
2	2	2	0	221	5	9	0	1	4	-	.4	0	33	.9	32	2.2	213	237	260	1.5
0	0	0	2	0	13	2	0	0	42	.1	0	0	10	.3	7	.2	14	124	1	.1
0	0	0	2	0	19	3	0	0	53	-	.1	0	14	.8	9	.5	17	125	4	.1
0	0	0	2	0	13	3	0	0	31	.2	0	0	12	.6	8	.3	10	110	1	.1
5	2	0	-	32	12	74	.1	.9	2	-	.4	.1	293	.2	32	.2	229	370	128	.9
2	4	1	2	20	4	6	0	.1	1	-	0	0	11	.3	6	.2	23	69	191	.1
-	-	-	-	5	-	-	-	-	1	-	0	0	72	0	-	.1	-	48	150	-
2	-	1	-	30	-	80	-	-	6	-	.2	.1	64	1.5	-	3.8	-	600	560	-
-	-	-	-	4	-	-	-	-	3	-	0	0	48	0	-	.1	-	51	145	-
-	-	-	-	-	-	60	-	-	6	-	.1	.1	32	.8	-	2.9	-	380	650	-
0	1	0	-	0	0	0	0	0	0	-	0	0	2	.3	1	.2	6	7	0	0
1	2	0	-	8	2	4	0	0	0	-	0	0	3	.3	2	.4	12	9	54	.1
0	0	0	0	73	14	14	.1	2	1	-	.1	.1	88	1.3	32	1.2	196	382	88	1.7
3	-	1	-	55	-	20	-	-	-	-	.3	.2	48	1.5	-	3.8	-	450	550	-
-	-	-	-	-	-	20	-	-	1	-	.3	.2	48	1.5	-	2.9	-	350	740	-
-	-	-	-	35	-	250	-	-	30	-	.2	.2	32	1	-	8.6	220	480	320	-
1	3	3	-	13	18	60	.1	.1	0	-	.2	.2	36	1.5	16	1.3	63	123	185	.4
4	6	1	-	37	20	41	0	.1	0	-	.1	.1	78	.5	13	.5	65	87	236	.4
3	5	1	1	40	14	38	.1	.1	1	-	.2	.2	43	1	10	1.4	46	67	230	.4
0	0	0	3	0	23	2182	.2	0	25	-	.1	.1	28	.4	20	.6	55	348	10	.3
0	0	0	4	0	18	2796	.4	0	28	-	.2	.1	34	.9	16	1	44	302	21	.4
2	1	0	-	9	13	475	0	0	8	-	0	0	29	1.3	12	.4	29	214	79	.2
0	0	0	-	0	14	1929	.3	0	7	-	.1	0	38	1.7	31	1.2	66	268	96	.3
0	0	0	-	0	8	702	.1	0	11	-	0	0	17	.9	12	.3	25	189	38	.2
1	2	1	0	43	2	35	.3	1.7	1	-	.1	0	5	.9	29	10	287	314	98	1.3
-	-	-	-	19	5	9	0	.3	0	-	.3	.1	160	.7	37	.2	170	262	58	.8
1	1	1	0	3	1	5	0	.1	0	-	0	0	21	.3	10	0	36	45	27	.2
-	-	-	0	0	0	0	0	0	0	-	0	0	4	.1	2	0	2	9	31	0
-	-	-	0	0	0	0	0	0	0	-	0	0	0	0	0	0	0	0	0	0
-	-	-	-	0	0	0	0	0	0	-	0	0	1	0	0	0	0	1	24	0
-	-	-	-	0	3	0	.1	0	0	-	.1	0	15	.2	17	1.9	57	77	8	0
-	-	-	0	0	0	0	0	0	0	-	0	0	13	.2	3	0	0	41	2	.8
-	-	-	0	0	0	0	0	0	0	-	0	0	0	0	0	0	9	1	40	0
-	-	-	0	0	0	0	0	0	0	-	0	0	1	0	0	0	2	1	12	0
0	0	0	-	1	0	3	0	0	0	-	0	0	0	0	0	0	2	1	20	0
0	1	1	1	0	1	5	0	0	0	-	0	0	21	.3	14	.2	32	23	48	.2
0	1	1	-	0	1	-	-	0	0	-	0	0	21	.3	14	.2	32	23	2	.2
-	-	-	-	0	-	-	-	-	-	-	.1	.1	-	.1	-	.5	-	-	4	-
0	0	0	-	1	0	5	0	0	0	-	0	0	0	0	0	0	0	1	13	0
0	0	0	0	0	9	78	.1	0	41	-	0	.1	34	.4	15	.2	26	332	2	.1
0	0	0	0	0	9	78	.1	0	57	-	0	.1	33	.4	15	.2	26	330	2	.1
0	0	0	1	0	6	106	.1	0	43	-	0	.1	14	.3	14	.6	12	166	6	.6
0	0	0	1	0	6	106	.1	0	25	-	.1	.1	9	.5	10	.6	13	98	8	.3
0	0	0	2	0	17	77	.1	0	26	-	0	.1	12	.1	10	.1	8	132	1	.2
2	5	4	0	3	12	0	.3	.3	2	-	.3	.1	250	.7	24	.9	236	310	352	.8
2	1	4	2	0	6	0	.1	0	1	-	0	0	17	.3	24	.1	37	214	97	.1
0	0	0	0	0	12	0	0	0	0	-	0	0	0	0	7	0	2	88	7	0
0	0	0	0	0	1	0	0	0	0	-	0	0	5	.2	2	0	0	21	2	.1
0	0	0	0	0	10	0	0	0	0	-	0	0	5	.1	5	.1	3	49	8	.1
0	0	0	0	0	1	0	0	0	0	-	0	0	5	0	5	.1	2	47	7	.1
2	2	1	-	60	-	400	-	-	2	-	.4	.8	16	1.5	42	5.7	-	933	880	4.5
0	0	0	-	0	3	3	0	0	6	-	0	0	2	.1	2	.1	3	32	1	0
1	-	2	-	55	-	20	-	-	6	-	.1	.1	32	.8	-	7.6	250	520	560	-
0	0	0	0	0	4	0	0	0	0	-	0	0	5	.3	11	.2	28	41	690	0
-	-	-	-	20	-	-	-	-	6	-	0	0	1202	.4	-	.6	-	891	861	-
4	3	0	1	7	0	16	0	.1	0	-	.1	0	50	.4	17	.1	55	80	116	.3
0	0	0	0	0	0	0	0	0	0	-	0	0	0	.2	4	0	33	40	144	.1
2	4	1	-	0	42	116	.2	.1	0	-	.3	.2	18	2.1	12	2.4	69	59	220	.3
1	2	2	-	0	42	55	.2	0	0	-	.2	.2	14	1.8	9	2	58	58	218	.3

Food Composition Table—cont'd

Code	Name	Amount	Unit	Grams	Kilocalories	Carbohydrates (g)	Protein (g)	Fat (g)
19383	TOFFEE	1	PIECE	12.0	65	8	0	4
16126	TOFU, FRESH, FIRM	1	OUNCE	28.4	41	1	4	2
16127	TOFU, FRESH, REGULAR	1	OUNCE	28.4	22	1	2	1
16129	TOFU, FRIED	1	OUNCE	28.4	77	3	5	6
16429	TOFU, FRIED, PREPARED W/ CALCIUM SULFATE	1	OUNCE	28.4	77	3	5	6
16130	TOFU, OKARA	1	OUNCE	28.4	22	4	1	0
16132	TOFU, SALTED AND FERMENTED (FUYU)	1	OUNCE	28.4	33	1	2	2
14023	TOM COLLINS	1	FL OZ	29.6	16	0	0	0
11954	TOMATILLOS, FRESH	1	MEDIUM	34.0	11	2	0	0
41284	TOMATO GARDEN SOUP-HEALTHY CHOICE	1	EACH	212.6	130	22	4	3
11540	TOMATO JUICE, CND, W/ SALT	¾	CUP	183.0	31	8	1	0
11886	TOMATO JUICE, CND, W/O SALT	¾	CUP	183.0	31	8	1	0
11530	TOMATOES, CKD, BOILED	½	CUP	120.0	32	7	1	0
11660	TOMATOES, CKD, STEWED	½	CUP	50.5	40	7	1	1
11533	TOMATOES, CND, STEWED	½	CUP	127.5	33	8	1	0
11537	TOMATOES, CND, W/ GREEN CHILIES	½	CUP	120.5	18	4	1	0
11535	TOMATOES, CND, WEDGES IN TOMATO JUICE	½	CUP	130.5	34	8	1	0
11531	TOMATOES, CND, WHOLE, REG PK	½	CUP	120.0	24	5	1	0
11529	TOMATOES, FRESH	1	MEDIUM	123.0	26	6	1	0
11527	TOMATOES, GREEN, FRESH	1	MEDIUM	123.0	30	6	1	0
11955	TOMATOES, SUN-DRIED	¼	CUP	13.5	35	8	2	0
11956	TOMATOES, SUN-DRIED, PACKED IN OIL	¼	CUP	27.5	59	6	1	4
14155	TONIC WATER	12	FL OZ	366.0	124	32	0	0
19364	TOPPINGS, BUTTERSCOTCH	1	TBSP.	20.5	52	14	0	0
62550	TOPPINGS, CARAMEL	1	TBSP.	16.7	52	13	0	-
62549	TOPPINGS, HOT FUDGE	1	TBSP.	19.0	70	11	1	2
19365	TOPPINGS, MARSHMALLOW CREAM	1	TBSP.	20.5	64	16	0	0
19367	TOPPINGS, NUTS IN SYRUP	1	TBSP.	20.5	84	11	1	5
19366	TOPPINGS, PINEAPPLE	1	TBSP.	21.3	54	14	0	0
19137	TOPPINGS, STRAWBERRY	1	TBSP.	21.3	54	14	0	0
62538	TORTELLINI, BEEF	1	CUP	257.9	230	46	5	1
55160	TORTELLINI-CHEESE IN ALFREDO SAUCE-STOUFFER'S	1	EACH	251.6	580	35	26	37
55161	TORTELLINI-CHEESE W/ TOMATO SAUCE-STOUFFER'S	1	EACH	262.2	360	39	18	15
19057	TORTILLA CHIPS, NACHO-FLAVOR	1	OUNCE	28.4	141	18	2	7
19424	TORTILLA CHIPS, NACHO-FLAVOR, LIGHT	1	OUNCE	28.4	126	20	2	4
19056	TORTILLA CHIPS, PLAIN	1	OUNCE	28.4	142	18	2	7
19058	TORTILLA CHIPS, RANCH-FLAVOR	1	OUNCE	28.4	139	18	2	7
19063	TORTILLA CHIPS, TACO-FLAVOR	1	OUNCE	28.4	136	18	2	7
18363	TORTILLAS, CORN	1	MEDIUM	25.0	56	12	1	1
18449	TORTILLAS, CORN, W/O ADDED SALT	1	MEDIUM	25.0	56	12	1	1
18364	TORTILLAS, FLOUR	1	MEDIUM	35.0	114	19	3	2
18450	TORTILLAS, FLOUR, W/O ADDED SALT	1	MEDIUM	35.0	114	19	3	2
19059	TRAIL MIX, REGULAR	1	CUP	150.0	693	67	21	44
19821	TRAIL MIX, REGULAR, UNSALTED	1	CUP	150.0	693	67	21	44
19062	TRAIL MIX, REGULAR, W/ CHOCOLATE CHIPS	1	CUP	146.0	707	66	21	47
19061	TRAIL MIX, TROPICAL	1	CUP	140.0	570	92	9	24
14269	TROPICAL FRUIT JUICE, BLEND	¾	CUP	185.2	85	22	0	0
15219	TROUT, CKD, DRY HEAT	3	OUNCE	85.1	162	0	23	7
15241	TROUT, RAINBOW, FARMED, CKD, DRY HEAT	3	OUNCE	85.1	144	0	21	6
15116	TROUT, RAINBOW, WILD, CKD, DRY HEAT	3	OUNCE	85.1	128	0	19	5
19138	TRUFFLES	1	PIECE	12.0	59	5	1	4
55162	TUNA NOODLE CASSEROLE-STOUFFER'S	1	EACH	283.5	280	33	17	15
15128	TUNA SALAD	3	OUNCE	85.1	159	8	14	8
15183	TUNA, LIGHT MEAT, CND IN OIL	3	OUNCE	85.1	168	0	25	7
15184	TUNA, LIGHT MEAT, CND IN WATER	3	OUNCE	85.1	111	0	25	0
15121	TUNA, LIGHT, CND IN WATER	3	OUNCE	85.1	99	0	22	1
15220	TUNA, SKIPJACK, CKD, DRY HEAT	3	OUNCE	85.1	112	0	24	1
15185	TUNA, WHITE MEAT, CND IN OIL	3	OUNCE	85.1	158	0	23	7
15186	TUNA, WHITE MEAT, CND IN WATER	3	OUNCE	85.1	116	0	23	2
15221	TUNA, YELLOWFIN, CKD, DRY HEAT	3	OUNCE	85.1	118	0	25	1

Saturated fat (g)	Monounsaturated fat (g)	Polyunsaturated fat (g)	Fiber (g)	Cholesterol (g)	Folate (g)	Vitamin A (RE)	Vitamin B-6 (mg)	Vitamin B-12 (µg)	Vitamin C (mg)	Vitamin E (mg)	Riboflavin (mg)	Thiamin (mg)	Calcium (mg)	Iron (mg)	Magnesium (mg)	Niacin (mg)	Phosphorus (mg)	Potassium (mg)	Sodium (mg)	Zinc (mg)
2	1	0	-	13	0	38	0	0	0	-	0	0	4	0	0	0	4	6	22	0
0	1	1	1	0	8	5	0	0	0	-	0	0	58	3	27	.1	54	67	4	.4
0	0	1	0	0	4	3	0	0	0	-	0	0	30	1.5	29	.1	27	34	2	.2
1	1	3	1	0	8	0	0	0	0	-	0	0	105	1.4	17	0	81	41	5	.6
1	1	3	-	0	8	0	0	0	0	-	0	0	272	1.4	27	0	81	41	5	.6
0	0	0	-	0	7	0	0	0	0	-	0	0	23	.4	7	0	17	60	3	.2
0	1	1	-	0	8	5	0	0	0	-	0	0	13	.6	15	.1	21	21	814	.4
0	0	0	-	0	0	0	0	0	1	-	0	0	1	0	0	0	0	2	5	0
-	-	-	1	0	2	4	0	0	4	-	0	0	2	.2	7	.6	13	91	0	.1
1	-	-	-	5	-	100	-	-	6	-	.1	.1	32	.4	-	1.1	70	440	510	-
0	0	0	1	0	36	102	.2	0	33	-	.1	.1	16	1.1	20	1.2	35	403	661	.3
0	0	0	1	0	36	102	.2	0	33	-	.1	.1	16	1.1	20	1.2	35	403	18	.3
0	0	0	1	0	16	89	.1	0	27	-	.1	.1	7	.7	17	.9	37	335	13	.1
0	1	0	1	0	6	34	0	0	9	-	0	.1	13	.5	8	.6	19	125	230	.1
0	0	0	-	0	7	70	0	0	17	-	0	.1	42	.9	15	.9	26	305	324	.2
0	0	0	-	0	11	47	.1	0	7	-	0	0	24	.3	13	.8	17	129	483	.2
0	0	0	-	0	13	76	.2	0	19	-	0	.1	34	.6	14	.9	30	328	283	.2
0	0	0	1	0	9	72	.1	0	18	-	0	.1	31	.7	14	.9	23	265	196	.2
0	0	0	1	0	18	76	.1	0	23	.4	.1	.1	6	.6	14	.8	30	273	11	.1
0	0	0	2	0	11	79	.1	0	29	-	0	.1	16	.6	12	.6	34	251	16	.1
0	0	0	2	0	9	12	0	0	5	-	.1	.1	15	1.2	26	1.2	48	463	283	.3
1	2	1	-	0	6	35	.1	0	28	-	.1	.1	13	.7	22	1	38	430	73	.2
0	0	0	0	0	0	0	0	0	0	-	0	0	4	0	0	0	0	0	15	.4
0	0	0	-	0	0	6	0	0	0	-	0	0	11	0	1	0	10	17	72	0
-	-	-	-	-	-	-	0	0	0	-	0	0	9	-	-	-	5	6	11	0
1	-	-	-	0	-	0	-	-	0	-	-	-	36	.2	-	-	-	-	35	-
-	-	-	-	0	0	0	0	0	0	-	0	0	1	0	0	0	2	1	9	0
0	1	3	0	0	4	1	0	0	0	-	0	0	8	.2	13	.1	23	43	9	.2
-	-	-	-	0	0	1	0	0	12	-	0	0	5	.1	0	0	2	67	13	.1
-	-	-	-	0	0	0	0	0	5	-	0	0	5	.2	1	0	3	16	4	.1
0	-	-	9	15	-	150	-	-	4	-	-	-	96	1.5	-	-	-	-	770	-
-	-	-	-	-	-	40	-	-	4	-	.5	.3	320	.8	-	1.9	-	270	830	-
-	-	-	-	-	-	150	-	-	6	-	.3	.2	240	1	-	1.9	-	420	720	-
1	4	1	2	1	4	12	.1	0	1	-	.1	0	42	.4	23	.4	69	61	201	.3
1	3	1	-	1	7	12	.1	0	0	-	.1	.1	45	.5	27	.1	90	77	284	-
1	4	1	2	0	3	6	.1	0	0	-	.1	0	44	.4	25	.4	58	56	150	.4
1	4	1	-	0	5	8	.1	0	0	-	.1	0	40	.4	25	.4	68	69	174	.4
1	4	1	-	1	6	26	.1	0	0	-	.1	.1	44	.6	25	.6	68	62	223	.4
0	0	0	1	0	4	6	.1	0	0	-	0	0	44	.4	16	.4	79	39	40	.2
0	0	0	-	0	4	-	.1	0	0	-	0	0	44	.4	16	.4	79	39	3	.2
0	1	1	1	0	4	0	0	0	0	-	.1	.2	44	1.2	9	1.3	43	46	167	.2
0	1	1	-	0	4	0	0	0	0	-	.1	.2	14	1.2	9	1.3	43	46	167	.2
8	19	14	-	0	107	3	.4	0	2	-	.3	.7	117	4.6	237	7.1	518	1028	344	4.8
8	19	14	-	0	107	3	.4	0	2	-	.3	.7	117	4.6	237	7.1	518	1028	15	4.8
9	20	16	-	6	95	7	.4	0	2	-	.3	.6	159	4.9	235	6.4	565	946	177	4.6
12	3	7	-	0	59	7	.5	0	11	-	.2	.6	80	3.7	134	2.1	260	993	14	1.6
0	0	0	-	0	2	2	0	0	81	-	0	0	7	.2	4	0	2	24	7	.1
1	4	2	0	63	13	16	.2	6.4	0	-	.4	.4	47	1.6	24	4.9	267	394	57	.7
2	2	2	0	58	20	73	.3	4.2	3	-	.1	.2	-	.3	27	7.5	226	375	36	.4
1	1	2	0	59	13	13	.3	5.4	2	-	.1	.1	-	.3	26	4.9	229	381	48	.4
3	1	0	-	6	0	17	0	0	0	-	0	0	19	.1	6	0	21	37	9	.1
-	-	-	-	-	-	20	-	-	0	-	.3	.2	120	.6	-	3.8	-	380	1090	-
1	2	4	0	11	6	23	.1	1	2	-	.1	0	14	.9	16	5.7	151	151	342	.5
1	3	2	0	15	5	20	.1	1.9	0	-	.1	0	11	1.2	26	10.5	265	176	43	.8
0	0	0	0	15	4	20	.3	1.9	0	-	.1	0	10	2.7	25	10.5	158	267	43	.4
0	0	0	0	26	3	14	.3	2.5	0	-	.1	0	9	1.3	23	11.3	139	202	287	.7
0	0	0	0	51	9	15	.8	1.9	1	-	.1	0	31	1.4	37	16	242	444	40	.9
1	2	3	0	26	4	20	.4	1.9	0	-	.1	0	3	.6	29	9.9	227	283	43	.4
1	1	1	0	36	3	20	.4	1.9	0	-	0	0	3	.5	29	4.9	227	241	43	.4
0	0	0	0	49	2	17	.9	.5	1	-	0	.4	18	.8	54	10.2	208	484	40	.6

Food Composition Table—cont'd

Code	Name	Amount	Unit	Grams	Kilocalories	Carbohydrates (g)	Protein (g)	Fat (g)
55814	TURKEY AND GRAVY-STOUFFER'S	1	EACH	255.0	78	2	12	2
5297	TURKEY BOLOGNA	1	SLICE	21.0	42	0	3	3
7079	TURKEY BREAST MEAT	1	SLICE	21.0	23	0	5	0
55232	TURKEY DIJON, LEAN CUISINE-STOUFFER'S	1	EACH	269.3	210	20	20	6
55791	TURKEY DIJONNAISE-STOUFFER'S	1	EACH	260.0	113	7	8	5
5287	TURKEY LUNCH MEAT	1	SLICE	28.4	36	0	5	1
5289	TURKEY PASTRAMI	1	SLICE	28.4	40	0	5	2
5292	TURKEY PATTIES, BREADED, BATTERED, FRIED	3	OUNCE	85.1	241	13	12	15
55163	TURKEY PIE-STOUFFER'S	1	EACH	283.5	410	33	16	24
57809	TURKEY POT PIE-SWANSON	1	EACH	198.0	191	18	6	11
5296	TURKEY ROAST, ROASTED	3	OUNCE	85.1	132	3	18	5
5291	TURKEY ROLL, LIGHT AND DARK MEAT	3	OUNCE	85.1	127	2	15	6
5290	TURKEY ROLL, LIGHT MEAT	3	OUNCE	85.1	125	0	16	6
5299	TURKEY SALAMI	1	SLICE	28.4	56	0	5	4
41243	TURKEY SAUSAGE OMELET ON ENGLISH MUFFIN-HEALTHY CHOICE	1	EACH	134.7	210	30	16	4
5300	TURKEY STICKS, BREADED, BATTERED, FRIED	3	OUNCE	85.1	237	14	12	14
41268	TURKEY TETRAZZINI-HEALTHY CHOICE	1	EACH	357.9	340	49	23	6
55164	TURKEY TETRAZZINI-STOUFFER'S	1	EACH	283.5	400	26	22	23
5294	TURKEY THIGH, PREBASTED, MEAT&SKIN, CKD, ROASTED	3	OUNCE	85.1	134	0	16	7
41275	TURKEY VEGETABLE SOUP-HEALTHY CHOICE	1	EACH	212.6	110	17	4	3
5190	TURKEY, BACK, MEAT&SKIN, CKD, ROASTED	3	OUNCE	85.1	207	0	23	12
5192	TURKEY, BREAST, MEAT&SKIN, CKD, ROASTED	3	OUNCE	85.1	161	0	24	6
5164	TURKEY, CKD, ROASTED, MEAT&SKIN&GIBLETS&NECK	3	OUNCE	85.1	174	0	24	8
5188	TURKEY, DARK MEAT, CKD, ROASTED	3	OUNCE	85.1	159	0	24	6
5184	TURKEY, DARK MEAT, MEAT&SKIN, CKD, ROASTED	3	OUNCE	85.1	188	0	23	10
5172	TURKEY, GIBLETS, CKD, SIMMERED, SOME GIBLET FAT	3	OUNCE	85.1	142	2	23	4
5306	TURKEY, GROUND, CKD	3	OUNCE	85.1	200	0	23	11
5194	TURKEY, LEG, MEAT&SKIN, CKD, ROASTED	3	OUNCE	85.1	177	0	24	8
5186	TURKEY, LIGHT MEAT, CKD, ROASTED	3	OUNCE	85.1	134	0	25	3
5182	TURKEY, LIGHT MEAT, MEAT&SKIN, CKD, ROASTED	3	OUNCE	85.1	168	0	24	7
5168	TURKEY, MEAT ONLY, CKD, ROASTED	3	OUNCE	85.1	145	0	25	4
5166	TURKEY, MEAT&SKIN, CKD, ROASTED	3	OUNCE	85.1	177	0	24	8
5288	TURKEY, THIN SLICED	3	OUNCE	85.1	94	0	19	1
5196	TURKEY, WING, MEAT&SKIN, CKD, ROASTED	3	OUNCE	85.1	195	0	23	11
11565	TURNIPS, CKD	½	CUP	78.0	14	4	1	0
11564	TURNIPS, FRESH	½	CUP	65.0	18	4	1	0
19160	TWIX	1	EACH	57.0	272	37	3	13
19112	TWIZZLERS STRAWBERRY CANDY	1	PKG	71.0	263	66	2	1
18328	VANILLA CREAM PIE	1	SLICE	126.0	350	41	6	18
19201	VANILLA PUDDING	1	CUP	298.1	388	65	7	11
18210	VANILLA SANDWICH COOKIES W/ CREME FILLING	1	EACH	10.0	48	7	0	2
18213	VANILLA WAFERS, HIGHER FAT	1	EACH	6.0	28	4	0	1
18212	VANILLA WAFERS, LOWER FAT	1	EACH	4.0	18	3	0	1
17089	VEAL, MEAT AND FAT, CKD	3	OUNCE	85.1	196	0	26	10
17091	VEAL, MEAT ONLY, CKD	3	OUNCE	85.1	167	0	27	6
41285	VEGETABLE BEEF SOUP-HEALTHY CHOICE	1	EACH	212.6	130	21	8	1
55759	VEGETABLE BEEF W/ BARLEY SOUP-STOUFFER'S	1	CUP	283.9	190	15	4	13
55797	VEGETABLE CHOW MEIN-STOUFFER'S	1	OUNCE	28.4	14	2	0	1
11578	VEGETABLE JUICE CND	¾	CUP	181.5	34	8	1	0
55166	VEGETABLE LASAGNA-STOUFFER'S	1	EACH	274.0	400	33	23	20
41343	VEGETABLE PASTA ITALIANO-HEALTHY CHOICE	1	EACH	283.5	220	46	7	1
11581	VEGETABLES, MIXED, CND	½	CUP	81.5	38	8	2	0
11584	VEGETABLES, MIXED, FRZ	½	CUP	91.0	54	12	3	0
55758	VEGETARIAN VEGETABLE SOUP-STOUFFER'S	1	CUP	283.9	120	20	6	2
55828	VELOUTE SAUCE SUPREME-STOUFFER'S	1	CUP	307.6	564	21	9	50
62629	VITAMIN SUPPLEMENT, CENTRUM	1	EACH	1.0	-	-	-	-
62628	VITAMIN SUPPLEMENT, ONE-A-DAY	1	EACH	1.0	-	-	-	-
62630	VITAMIN SUPPLEMENT, STRESSTAB	1	EACH	1.0	-	-	-	-
18392	WAFFLES, BUTTERMILK	1	EACH	75.0	217	25	6	10
18367	WAFFLES, PLAIN	1	EACH	75.0	218	25	6	11

Saturated fat (g)	Monounsaturated fat (g)	Polyunsaturated fat (g)	Fiber (g)	Cholesterol (g)	Folate (g)	Vitamin A (RE)	Vitamin B-6 (mg)	Vitamin B-12 (μg)	Vitamin C (mg)	Vitamin E (mg)	Riboflavin (mg)	Thiamin (mg)	Calcium (mg)	Iron (mg)	Magnesium (mg)	Niacin (mg)	Phosphorus (mg)	Potassium (mg)	Sodium (mg)	Zinc (mg)
-	-	-	-	23	-	-	-	-	0	-	0	0	85	0	-	.9	-	406	296	-
1	1	1	0	21	1	0	0	.1	0	-	0	0	18	.3	3	.7	28	42	184	.4
0	0	0	0	9	1	0	.1	.4	0	-	0	0	1	.1	4	1.7	48	58	301	.2
2	-	-	-	45	-	400	-	-	2	-	.3	.2	120	.4	-	4.8	-	640	590	-
-	-	-	-	28	-	-	-	-	1	-	0	0	480	.1	-	.3	-	176	356	-
0	0	0	0	16	2	0	.1	.1	0	-	.1	0	3	.8	5	1	54	92	282	.8
1	1	0	0	15	1	0	.1	.1	0	-	.1	0	3	.5	4	1	57	74	296	.6
4	6	4	0	53	7	9	.2	.2	0	-	.2	.1	12	1.9	13	2	230	234	680	1.2
-	-	-	-	-	-	250	-	-	-	-	.4	.3	80	1	-	3.8	-	290	750	-
-	-	-	-	-	-	176	-	-	-	-	.1	.1	8	.5	-	1.4	-	-	363	-
2	1	1	0	45	4	0	.2	1.3	-	-	.1	0	4	1.4	19	5.3	208	253	578	2.2
2	2	2	0	47	4	0	.2	.2	0	-	.2	.1	27	1.1	15	4.1	143	230	498	1.7
2	2	1	0	37	3	0	.3	.2	0	-	.2	.1	34	1.1	14	6	156	213	416	1.3
1	1	1	0	23	1	0	.1	.1	0	-	0	0	6	.5	4	1	30	69	285	.5
2	-	1	-	20	-	60	-	-	-	-	.5	.4	160	2	-	2.9	250	590	470	-
4	6	4	-	54	8	10	.2	.2	0	-	.2	.1	12	1.9	13	1.8	199	221	713	1.2
3	-	2	-	40	-	-	-	-	72	-	.3	.2	80	1	-	3.8	250	510	490	-
-	-	-	-	-	-	20	-	-	-	-	.4	.2	80	.8	-	2.9	-	300	960	-
2	2	2	0	53	5	0	.2	.2	0	-	.2	.1	7	1.3	14	2	145	205	372	3.5
1	-	1	-	15	-	150	-	-	5	-	0	0	16	.2	-	.4	-	140	540	-
4	4	3	0	77	7	0	.3	.3	0	-	.2	0	28	1.9	19	2.9	161	221	62	3.3
2	2	2	0	63	5	0	.4	.3	0	-	.1	0	18	1.2	23	5.4	179	245	54	1.7
2	3	2	0	81	17	58	.3	1.1	0	-	.2	0	22	1.7	20	4.2	170	231	57	2.7
2	1	2	0	72	8	0	.3	.3	0	-	.2	.1	27	2	20	3.1	174	247	67	3.8
3	3	3	0	76	8	0	.3	.3	0	-	.2	0	28	1.9	20	3	167	233	65	3.5
1	1	1	0	356	293	1527	.3	20.4	1	-	.8	0	11	5.7	14	3.8	174	170	50	3.1
3	4	3	0	87	6	0	.3	.3	0	-	.1	0	21	1.6	20	4.1	167	230	91	2.4
3	2	2	0	72	8	0	.3	.3	0	-	.2	.1	27	2	20	3	169	238	65	3.6
1	0	1	0	59	5	0	.5	.3	0	-	.1	.1	16	1.1	24	5.8	186	259	54	1.7
2	2	2	0	65	5	0	.4	.3	0	-	.1	.1	16	1.1	24	5.8	186	259	54	1.7
1	1	1	0	65	6	0	.4	.3	0	-	.2	0	18	1.2	22	5.3	177	242	54	1.7
2	3	2	0	70	6	0	.3	.3	0	-	.2	.1	21	1.5	22	4.6	181	253	60	2.6
0	0	0	0	35	3	0	.3	1.7	0	-	.1	0	22	1.5	21	4.3	173	238	58	2.5
3	4	3	0	69	5	0	.4	.3	0	-	.1	0	6	.3	17	7.1	195	236	1217	1
0	0	0	2	0	7	0	.1	0	9	-	0	0	20	1.2	21	4.9	168	226	52	1.8
0	0	0	1	0	9	0	.1	0	14	-	0	0	17	.2	6	.2	15	105	39	.2
-	-	-	1	5	4	18	0	.2	0	-	.1	0	20	.2	7	.3	18	124	44	.2
-	-	-	-	0	0	0	0	0	0	-	0	0	67	.4	17	.2	76	117	115	.4
5	8	4	-	78	14	107	.1	.4	1	-	.3	0	25	.4	4	.1	220	45	197	.1
2	5	4	0	21	0	18	0	.3	0	-	.4	.2	113	1.3	16	1.2	131	159	328	.7
0	1	0	0	0	0	0	-	0	0	-	0	.1	262	.4	24	.8	203	337	402	.7
0	1	0	-	0	0	0	0	0	0	-	0	0	3	.2	1	.3	8	9	35	0
0	0	0	-	2	0	1	0	0	0	-	0	0	2	.1	1	.2	4	6	18	0
4	4	1	0	97	13	0	.3	1.3	0	.3	.3	.1	19	1	22	6.8	203	276	74	4
2	2	1	0	100	14	0	.3	1.4	0	.4	.3	.1	20	1	24	7.2	213	287	76	4.3
-	-	-	-	15	-	150	-	-	15	-	.1	.1	32	.4	-	1.9	120	360	530	-
-	-	-	-	10	-	-	-	-	0	-	0	0	240	.1	-	.2	-	341	1252	-
-	-	-	-	0	-	-	-	-	1	-	0	0	24	0	-	0	-	26	156	-
0	0	0	1	0	38	212	.3	0	50	-	.1	.1	20	.8	20	1.3	31	350	662	.4
-	-	-	-	-	-	250	-	-	-	-	.4	.1	160	.6	-	.8	-	350	760	-
-	-	-	-	0	-	250	-	-	0	-	.3	.5	32	2.5	-	1.5	-	380	330	-
0	0	0	-	0	19	949	.1	0	4	-	0	0	22	.9	13	.5	34	237	121	.3
0	0	0	5	0	17	389	.1	0	3	-	.1	.1	23	.7	20	.8	46	154	32	.4
-	-	-	-	0	-	-	-	-	0	-	0	0	401	.1	-	.2	-	401	911	-
-	-	-	-	98	-	-	-	-	0	-	0	0	2257	0	-	0	-	369	1410	-
-	-	-	-	-	400	1000	2	6	60	10	1.7	1.5	162	18	100	20	109	40	-	15
-	-	-	-	-	400	1000	2	6	60	10	1.7	1.5	-	-	-	20	-	-	-	-
-	-	-	-	-	400	-	-	5	12	500	10	-	10	-	18	-	100	-	-	-
2	3	5	-	50	11	26	0	.2	0	-	.3	.2	137	1.6	14	1.5	124	128	451	.6
2	3	5	-	52	11	49	0	.2	0	-	.3	.2	191	1.7	14	1.6	143	119	383	.5

Food Composition Table—cont'd

Code	Name	Amount	Unit	Grams	Kilocalories	Carbohydrates (g)	Protein (g)	Fat (g)
18403	WAFFLES, PLAIN, FROZEN, TOASTED	1	EACH	33.0	87	13	2	3
12154	WALNUTS, BLACK, DRIED	½	CUP	62.5	379	8	15	35
12155	WALNUTS, ENGLISH OR PERSIAN, DRIED	½	CUP	60.0	385	11	9	37
55167	WELSH RAREBIT-STOUFFER'S	1	EACH	141.8	270	9	13	20
41244	WESTERN STYLE OMELET ON ENGLISH MUFFIN-HEALTHY CHOICE	1	EACH	134.7	200	29	16	3
55826	WHIPPED SWEET POTATOES-STOUFFER'S	½	CUP	142.0	205	30	2	9
14032	WHISKEY SOUR	1	FL OZ	29.9	41	2	0	0
15223	WHITEFISH, CKD, DRY HEAT	3	OUNCE	85.1	146	0	21	6
15131	WHITEFISH, SMOKED	3	OUNCE	85.1	92	0	20	1
20089	WILD RICE, CKD	½	CUP	82.0	83	17	3	0
14536	WINE, DESSERT, DRY	3	FL OZ	90.0	113	4	0	0
14057	WINE, DESSERT, SWEET	3	FL OZ	90.0	138	11	0	0
14084	WINE, TABLE, ALL	3	FL OZ	88.5	62	1	0	0
14096	WINE, TABLE, RED	3	FL OZ	88.5	64	2	0	0
14104	WINE, TABLE, ROSE	3	FL OZ	88.5	63	1	0	0
14106	WINE, TABLE, WHITE	3	FL OZ	88.5	60	1	0	0
11602	YAM, BAKED	½	CUP	68.0	79	19	1	0
41269	YANKEE POT ROAST-HEALTHY CHOICE	1	EACH	311.8	260	36	19	4
15225	YELLOWTAIL, CKD, DRY HEAT	3	OUNCE	85.1	159	0	25	6
15135	YELLOWTAIL, FRESH	3	OUNCE	85.1	124	0	20	4
62552	YOGURT, FROZEN, FAT FREE	½	CUP	67.0	100	22	4	0
62604	YOGURT, FRUIT, FAT FREE	1	CUP	248.0	233	48	10	0
62627	YOGURT, FRUIT, FAT FREE, LIGHT	1	CUP	248.0	110	19	10	0
1121	YOGURT, FRUIT, LOWFAT, 10 G PROTEIN PER 8 OZ	1	CUP	227.0	231	43	10	2
1122	YOGURT, FRUIT, LOWFAT, 11 G PROTEIN PER 8 OZ	1	CUP	227.0	239	42	11	3
1120	YOGURT, FRUIT, LOWFAT, 9 G PROTEIN PER 8 OZ	1	CUP	227.0	225	42	9	3
62603	YOGURT, PLAIN, FAT FREE	1	CUP	248.0	120	17	13	0
1117	YOGURT, PLAIN, LOWFAT, 12 G PROTEIN PER 8 OZ	1	CUP	227.0	144	16	12	4
1118	YOGURT, PLAIN, SKIM MILK, 13 G PROTEIN PER 8 OZ	1	CUP	227.0	127	17	13	0
1116	YOGURT, PLAIN, WHOLE MILK, 8 G PROTEIN PER 8 OZ	1	CUP	227.0	139	11	8	7
19393	YOGURT, SOFT-SERVE, CHOCOLATE	1	CUP	144.1	231	36	6	9
19293	YOGURT, SOFT-SERVE, VANILLA	1	CUP	144.1	229	35	6	8
1119	YOGURT, VANILLA, LOWFAT, 11 G PROTEIN PER 8 OZ	1	CUP	227.0	194	31	11	3
19091	YORK PEPPERMINT PATTIE	1	SM PATTY	11.0	38	9	0	1
55233	ZUCCHINI LASAGNA, LEAN CUISINE-STOUFFER'S	1	EACH	311.8	260	34	17	6
41344	ZUCCHINI LASAGNA-HEALTHY CHOICE	1	EACH	326.0	250	41	14	3

Saturated fat (g)	Monounsaturated fat (g)	Polyunsaturated fat (g)	Fiber (g)	Cholesterol (g)	Folate (g)	Vitamin A (RE)	Vitamin B-6 (mg)	Vitamin B-12 (μg)	Vitamin C (mg)	Vitamin E (mg)	Riboflavin (mg)	Thiamin (mg)	Calcium (mg)	Iron (mg)	Magnesium (mg)	Niacin (mg)	Phosphorus (mg)	Potassium (mg)	Sodium (mg)	Zinc (mg)
0	1	1	-	8	12	120	.3	.8	0	-	.2	.1	77	1.5	7	1.5	139	42	260	.2
2	8	23	3	0	41	19	.3	0	2	-	.1	.1	36	1.9	126	.4	290	328	1	2.1
3	9	23	3	0	40	7	.3	0	2	-	.1	.2	56	1.5	101	.6	190	301	6	1.6
-	-	-	-	-	-	40	-	-	-	-	.3	0	280	.2	-	-	-	140	460	-
2	-	-	-	15	-	100	-	-	4	-	.5	.5	160	2	-	1.9	240	220	480	-
-	-	-	-	30	-	-	-	-	0	-	0	0	240	.1	-	.1	-	200	556	-
0	0	0	-	0	2	0	0	0	4	-	0	.1	2	0	1	0	2	16	3	0
1	2	2	0	65	14	33	.3	.8	0	-	.1	.1	28	.4	36	3.3	294	345	55	1.1
0	0	0	0	28	6	48	.3	2.8	0	-	.1	0	15	.4	20	2	112	360	867	.4
0	0	0	1	0	21	0	.1	0	0	-	.1	0	2	.5	26	1.1	67	83	2	1.1
0	0	0	0	0	0	0	0	0	0	-	0	0	7	.2	8	.2	8	83	8	.1
0	0	0	0	0	0	0	0	0	0	-	0	0	7	.2	8	.2	8	83	8	.1
0	0	0	0	0	1	0	0	0	0	-	0	0	7	.4	9	.1	12	79	7	.1
0	0	0	-	0	2	0	0	0	0	-	0	0	7	.4	12	.1	12	99	4	.1
0	0	0	-	0	1	0	0	0	0	-	0	0	7	.3	9	.1	13	88	4	.1
0	0	0	-	0	0	0	0	0	0	-	0	0	8	.3	9	.1	12	71	4	.1
0	0	0	3	0	11	0	.2	0	8	-	0	.1	10	.4	12	.4	33	456	5	.1
2	-	-	-	55	-	100	-	-	9	-	.2	.2	32	1	-	1.5	150	350	400	-
-	-	-	0	60	3	26	.2	1.1	2	-	0	.1	25	.5	32	7.4	171	458	43	.6
1	2	1	0	47	3	25	.1	1.1	2	-	0	.1	20	.4	26	5.8	134	357	33	.4
0	-	-	-	0	-	20	-	-	0	-	-	-	96	0	-	-	-	-	70	-
0	0	0	0	7	-	0	-	-	0	-	-	-	438	0	-	-	-	423	153	-
0	0	0	0	5	-	0	-	-	15	-	-	-	420	.2	-	-	-	510	160	-
2	1	0	0	10	21	25	.1	1.1	1	-	.4	.1	345	.2	33	.2	271	442	133	1.7
2	1	0	0	12	24	34	.1	1.2	2	-	.4	.1	383	.2	37	.2	301	491	147	1.9
2	1	0	0	10	19	27	.1	1	1	-	.4	.1	314	.1	30	.2	247	402	121	1.5
0	0	0	0	5	-	0	-	-	4	-	.2	-	480	0	-	-	0	600	170	-
2	1	0	0	14	25	36	.1	1.3	2	-	.5	.1	415	.2	40	.3	326	531	159	2
0	0	0	0	4	28	5	.1	1.4	2	-	.5	.1	452	.2	43	.3	355	579	174	2.2
5	2	0	0	29	17	68	.1	.8	1	-	.3	.1	274	.1	26	.2	215	351	105	1.3
5	3	0	0	7	16	62	.1	.4	0	-	.3	.1	212	1.8	39	.4	200	376	141	.7
5	2	0	0	3	9	82	.1	.4	1	-	.3	.1	206	.4	20	.4	186	304	125	.6
2	1	0	0	11	24	30	.1	1.2	2	-	.5	.1	389	.2	37	.2	306	498	149	1.9
-	-	-	-	0	0	0	0	0	0	-	0	0	2	.2	7	.1	10	13	4	.1
2	-	-	-	20	-	150	-	-	6	-	.3	.2	200	.8	-	1.9	-	650	520	-
2	-	-	-	15	-	350	-	-	6	-	.3	.4	200	1.5	-	1.9	250	830	400	-

Restaurants, Including Fast Food (Quick Service

Code	Name	Amount	Unit	Grams	Kilocalories	Carbohydrates (g)	Protein (g)	Fat (g)
32391	ARBY'S-BEEF'N CHEDDAR SANDWICH	1	EACH	194.0	443	30	35	20
32433	ARBY'S-BOSTON CLAM CHOWDER	1	EACH	226.8	207	18	10	11
32400	ARBY'S-CHICKEN BREAST FILLET SANDWICH	1	EACH	204.0	547	53	26	28
32434	ARBY'S-CREAM OF BROCCOLI SOUP	1	EACH	226.8	180	19	9	8
32413	ARBY'S-CURLY FRIES	1	EACH	99.2	337	43	4	18
32405	ARBY'S-FISH FILLET SANDWICH	1	EACH	221.0	526	50	23	27
32411	ARBY'S-FRENCH FRIES	1	EACH	70.9	246	30	2	13
32406	ARBY'S-HAM'N CHEESE SANDWICH	1	EACH	170.1	411	38	24	19
32390	ARBY'S-REGULAR ROAST BEEF	1	EACH	155.9	388	38	25	16
32393	ARBY'S-SUPER ROAST BEEF	1	EACH	241.0	516	51	26	23
32410	ARBY'S-TURKEY SUB	1	EACH	277.0	599	54	33	28
32438	ARBY'S-WISCONSIN CHEESE SOUP	1	EACH	226.8	287	19	9	19
34858	BURGER KING-BACON DOUBLE CHEESEBURGER	1	EACH	202.0	613	29	34	40
34856	BURGER KING-CHEESEBURGER	1	EACH	134.7	360	35	18	16
34857	BURGER KING-DOUBLE CHEESEBURGER	1	EACH	191.4	537	32	33	30
34855	BURGER KING-HAMBURGER	1	EACH	122.9	310	35	16	12
34843	BURGER KING-SALAD W/ 1000 ISLAND	1	EACH	176.0	145	9	2	12
34842	BURGER KING-SALAD W/ BLEU CHEESE	1	EACH	176.0	184	7	3	16
34844	BURGER KING-SALAD W/ FRENCH	1	EACH	176.0	152	13	2	11
34845	BURGER KING-SALAD W/ GOLDEN ITALIAN	1	EACH	176.0	162	7	2	14
34841	BURGER KING-SALAD W/ HOUSE DRESSING	1	EACH	176.0	159	8	3	13
34846	BURGER KING-SALAD W/ REDUCED-CALORIE ITALIAN	1	EACH	176.0	42	7	2	1
34859	BURGER KING-WHOPPER	1	EACH	283.5	684	54	28	39
37167	DUNKIN' DONUTS-ALMOND CROISSANT	1	EACH	105.0	420	38	8	27
37160	DUNKIN' DONUTS-APPLE 'N SPICE MUFFIN	1	EACH	100.0	300	52	6	8
37146	DUNKIN' DONUTS-APPLE FILLED W/ CINNAMON SUGAR	1	EACH	79.0	250	33	5	11
37159	DUNKIN' DONUTS-BANANA NUT MUFFIN	1	EACH	103.0	310	49	7	10
37147	DUNKIN' DONUTS-BAVARIAN FILLED /W CHOCOLATE	1	EACH	79.0	240	32	5	11
37149	DUNKIN' DONUTS-BLUEBERRY FILLED	1	EACH	67.0	210	29	4	8
37156	DUNKIN' DONUTS-BLUEBERRY MUFFIN	1	EACH	101.0	280	46	6	8
37157	DUNKIN' DONUTS-BRAN MUFFIN W/ RAISINS	1	EACH	104.0	310	51	6	9
37151	DUNKIN' DONUTS-CAKE RING, PLAIN	1	EACH	62.0	270	25	4	17
37163	DUNKIN' DONUTS-CHOCOLATE CHUNK COOKIE	1	EACH	43.0	200	25	3	10
37164	DUNKIN' DONUTS-CHOCOLATE CHUNK COOKIE W/ NUTS	1	EACH	43.0	210	23	3	11
37168	DUNKIN' DONUTS-CHOCOLATE CROISSANT	1	EACH	94.0	440	38	7	29
37145	DUNKIN' DONUTS-CHOCOLATE FROSTED YEAST RING	1	EACH	55.0	200	25	4	10
37158	DUNKIN' DONUTS-CORN MUFFIN	1	EACH	96.0	340	51	7	12
37161	DUNKIN' DONUTS-CRANBERRY NUT MUFFIN	1	EACH	98.0	290	44	6	9
37166	DUNKIN' DONUTS-CROISSANT, PLAIN	1	EACH	72.0	310	27	7	19
37153	DUNKIN' DONUTS-GLAZED BUTTERMILK RING	1	EACH	74.0	290	37	4	14
37152	DUNKIN' DONUTS-GLAZED CHOCOLATE RING	1	EACH	71.0	324	34	4	21
37144	DUNKIN' DONUTS-GLAZED COFFEE ROLL	1	EACH	81.0	280	37	5	12
37155	DUNKIN' DONUTS-GLAZED FRENCH CRULLER	1	EACH	38.0	140	16	2	8
37143	DUNKIN' DONUTS-GLAZED YEAST RING	1	EACH	55.0	200	26	4	9
37150	DUNKIN' DONUTS-JELLY FILLED	1	EACH	67.0	220	31	4	9
37148	DUNKIN' DONUTS-LEMON FILLED	1	EACH	79.0	260	33	4	12
37162	DUNKIN' DONUTS-OAT BRAN MUFFIN	1	EACH	100.0	330	50	7	11
37165	DUNKIN' DONUTS-OATMEAL PECAN RAISIN COOKIE	1	EACH	46.0	200	28	3	9
21002	FAST FOOD-BISCUIT W/ EGG	1	EACH	136.0	316	24	11	20
21003	FAST FOOD-BISCUIT W/ EGG AND BACON	1	EACH	150.0	458	29	17	31
21004	FAST FOOD-BISCUIT W/ EGG AND HAM	1	EACH	192.0	442	30	20	27
21005	FAST FOOD-BISCUIT W/ EGG AND SAUSAGE	1	EACH	180.0	581	41	19	39
21007	FAST FOOD-BISCUIT W/ EGG, CHEESE, AND BACON	1	EACH	144.0	477	33	16	31
21008	FAST FOOD-BISCUIT W/ HAM	1	EACH	113.0	386	44	13	18
21009	FAST FOOD-BISCUIT W/ SAUSAGE	1	EACH	124.0	485	40	12	32
21010	FAST FOOD-BISCUIT W/ STEAK	1	EACH	141.0	455	44	13	26
21001	FAST FOOD-BISCUIT, PLAIN	1	EACH	74.0	276	34	4	13
21027	FAST FOOD-BROWNIE	1	EACH	60.0	243	39	3	10
21060	FAST FOOD-BURRITO W/ BEANS	1	EACH	108.5	224	36	7	7
21061	FAST FOOD-BURRITO W/ BEANS AND CHEESE	1	EACH	93.0	189	27	8	6

Saturated fat (g)	Monounsaturated fat (g)	Polyunsaturated fat (g)	Fiber (g)	Cholesterol (g)	Folate (g)	Vitamin A (RE)	Vitamin B-6 (mg)	Vitamin B-12 (µg)	Vitamin C (mg)	Vitamin E (mg)	Riboflavin (mg)	Thiamin (mg)	Calcium (mg)	Iron (mg)	Magnesium (mg)	Niacin (mg)	Phosphorus (mg)	Potassium (mg)	Sodium (mg)	Zinc (mg)
10	4	4	1	85	45	64	.4	2.3	1	.4	.5	.4	202	5.6	44	6.5	442	380	1801	6
4	5	2	1	28	9	100	.1	9.4	4	.1	.2	.1	170	1.4	20	.9	143	319	1157	.7
6	11	11	2	101	35	17	.7	.4	0	2.9	.4	.5	123	3.9	51	16.4	322	366	1130	1.9
5	2	1	2	3	46	50	.2	.6	9	1.4	.4	.1	237	.8	55	.8	193	455	1113	.7
7	8	2	-	0	-	-	-	-	-	-	.1	.1	16	.8	-	1.9	-	724	167	-
7	9	11	-	44	-	-	-	-	1	-	.3	.3	72	2.1	-	5.3	-	450	872	-
3	6	5	-	0	-	-	-	-	4	-	-	.1	-	.6	-	1.9	-	240	114	-
7	8	2	1	68	83	112	.2	.6	3	1.3	.6	.4	151	3.8	19	3.1	177	338	899	1.6
4	8	2	1	58	45	71	.3	1.4	2	.2	.3	.4	61	4.7	35	6.6	268	354	888	3.8
9	8	6	2	41	42	0	.5	4.4	0	.4	.6	.6	118	6.6	60	9.7	414	518	822	11
6	7	8	-	82	-	-	-	-	-	-	.4	.5	94	3.2	-	9.4	-	-	1432	-
8	8	3	2	31	7	90	.1	0	2	.4	.2	0	252	1.3	7	.7	241	441	1129	1.1
17	15	6	1	115	32	74	.4	3.4	8	1.6	.4	.3	162	4.1	39	8.4	386	480	833	6.6
-	-	-	-	-	-	-	-	-	-	-	-	-	-	-	-	-	-	-	705	-
14	12	2	2	111	34	111	.3	2	7	2	.3	.2	210	3.3	34	5.5	339	383	947	4.5
-	-	-	-	-	-	-	-	-	-	-	-	-	-	-	-	-	-	-	560	-
-	-	-	-	17	-	-	-	-	26	-	0	0	336	.1	98	.2	528	405	251	.1
-	-	-	-	22	-	-	-	-	25	-	0	0	528	.1	102	.2	664	382	333	.1
-	-	-	-	0	-	-	-	-	26	-	0	0	320	.1	98	.2	480	410	330	.1
-	-	-	-	0	-	-	-	-	25	-	0	0	320	.1	98	.2	480	389	292	.1
-	-	-	-	11	-	-	-	-	25	-	0	0	352	.1	95	.2	592	402	293	.1
-	-	-	-	0	-	-	-	-	25	-	0	0	320	.1	105	.2	472	390	430	.1
18	15	2	3	113	34	209	.3	3.1	14	4.2	0	0	113	6.5	54	5.6	339	565	1075	5.8
-	-	-	3	0	-	-	-	-	-	-	-	-	-	-	-	-	-	-	280	-
-	-	-	2	25	-	-	-	-	-	-	-	-	-	-	-	-	-	-	360	-
-	-	-	1	0	-	-	-	-	-	-	-	-	-	-	-	-	-	-	280	-
-	-	-	3	30	-	-	-	-	-	-	-	-	-	-	-	-	-	-	410	-
-	-	-	2	0	-	-	-	-	-	-	-	-	-	-	-	-	-	-	260	-
-	-	-	2	0	-	-	-	-	-	-	-	-	-	-	-	-	-	-	240	-
-	-	-	2	30	-	-	-	-	-	-	-	-	-	-	-	-	-	-	340	-
-	-	-	4	15	-	-	-	-	-	-	-	-	-	-	-	-	-	-	560	-
-	-	-	1	0	-	-	-	-	-	-	-	-	-	-	-	-	-	-	330	-
-	-	-	1	30	-	-	-	-	-	-	-	-	-	-	-	-	-	-	110	-
-	-	-	2	30	-	-	-	-	-	-	-	-	-	-	-	-	-	-	100	-
-	-	-	3	0	-	-	-	-	-	-	-	-	-	-	-	-	-	-	220	-
-	-	-	1	0	-	-	-	-	-	-	-	-	-	-	-	-	-	-	190	-
-	-	-	1	40	-	-	-	-	-	-	-	-	-	-	-	-	-	-	560	-
-	-	-	2	25	-	-	-	-	-	-	-	-	-	-	-	-	-	-	360	-
-	-	-	2	0	-	-	-	-	-	-	-	-	-	-	-	-	-	-	240	-
-	-	-	1	10	-	-	-	-	-	-	-	-	-	-	-	-	-	-	370	-
-	-	-	2	0	-	-	-	-	-	-	-	-	-	-	-	-	-	-	383	-
-	-	-	2	0	-	-	-	-	-	-	-	-	-	-	-	-	-	-	310	-
-	-	-	0	30	-	-	-	-	-	-	-	-	-	-	-	-	-	-	130	-
-	-	-	1	0	-	-	-	-	-	-	-	-	-	-	-	-	-	-	230	-
-	-	-	1	0	-	-	-	-	-	-	-	-	-	-	-	-	-	-	230	-
-	-	-	1	0	-	-	-	-	-	-	-	-	-	-	-	-	-	-	280	-
-	-	-	3	0	-	-	-	-	-	-	-	-	-	-	-	-	-	-	450	-
-	-	-	1	25	-	-	-	-	-	-	-	-	-	-	-	-	-	-	100	-
6	8	4	-	233	30	178	.1	.7	0	-	.3	.3	154	3.1	20	.7	185	160	654	1.1
10	13	6	-	353	30	53	.1	1	3	-	.2	.1	189	3.7	24	2.4	239	251	999	1.6
8	11	5	-	300	33	240	.3	1.2	0	-	.6	.7	221	4.6	31	2	317	319	1382	2.2
15	16	4	-	302	40	164	.2	1.4	0	-	.5	.5	155	4	25	3.6	490	320	1141	2.2
11	14	3	-	261	37	166	.1	1.1	2	-	.4	.3	164	2.5	20	2.3	459	230	1260	1.5
11	5	1	-	25	8	34	.1	0	0	-	.3	.5	160	2.7	23	3.5	554	197	1433	1.6
14	13	3	1	35	9	14	.1	.5	0	-	.3	.4	128	2.6	20	3.3	446	198	1071	1.6
7	11	6	-	25	11	16	.2	.9	0	-	.4	.4	116	4.3	27	4.2	204	234	795	2.7
9	3	1	-	5	6	24	0	.1	0	-	.2	.3	90	1.6	9	1.6	260	87	584	.3
3	4	3	-	10	4	2	0	.2	3	-	.1	.1	25	1.3	16	.6	88	83	153	.6
3	2	1	-	2	59	16	.2	.5	1	-	.3	.3	56	2.3	43	2	49	327	493	.8
3	1	1	-	14	41	119	.1	.4	1	-	.4	.1	107	1.1	40	1.8	90	248	583	.8

Restaurants, Including Fast Food (Quick Service)—cont'd

Code	Name	Amount	Unit	Grams	Kilocalories	Carbohydrates (g)	Protein (g)	Fat (g)
21062	FAST FOOD-BURRITO W/ BEANS AND CHILI PEPPERS	1	EACH	102.0	206	29	8	7
21063	FAST FOOD-BURRITO W/ BEANS AND MEAT	1	EACH	115.5	254	33	11	9
21064	FAST FOOD-BURRITO W/ BEANS, CHEESE, AND BEEF	1	EACH	101.5	165	20	7	7
21065	FAST FOOD-BURRITO W/ BEANS, CHEESE, AND CHILI PEPPERS	1	EACH	167.0	329	42	17	11
21066	FAST FOOD-BURRITO W/ BEEF	1	EACH	110.0	262	29	13	10
21067	FAST FOOD-BURRITO W/ BEEF AND CHILI PEPPERS	1	EACH	100.5	213	25	11	8
21068	FAST FOOD-BURRITO W/ BEEF, CHEESE, AND CHILI PEPPERS	1	EACH	152.0	316	32	20	12
21069	FAST FOOD-BURRITO W/ FRUIT (APPLE OR CHERRY)	1	EACH	74.0	231	35	3	10
21100	FAST FOOD-CHEESEBURGER, LARGE, DOUBLE PATTY	1	EACH	258.0	704	40	38	44
21098	FAST FOOD-CHEESEBURGER, LARGE, SINGLE PATTY	1	EACH	219.0	563	38	28	33
21097	FAST FOOD-CHEESEBURGER, LARGE, SINGLE PATTY W/ BCN&COND	1	EACH	195.0	608	37	32	37
21096	FAST FOOD-CHEESEBURGER, LARGE, SINGLE PATTY, PLAIN	1	EACH	185.0	609	47	30	33
21095	FAST FOOD-CHEESEBURGER, REGULAR, DOUBLE PATTY	1	EACH	228.0	650	53	30	35
21091	FAST FOOD-CHEESEBURGER, REGULAR, SINGLE PATTY	1	EACH	154.0	359	28	18	20
21089	FAST FOOD-CHEESEBURGER, REGULAR, SINGLE PATTY, PLAIN	1	EACH	102.0	319	32	15	15
21101	FAST FOOD-CHEESEBURGER, TRIPLE PATTY, PLAIN	1	EACH	304.0	796	27	56	51
21103	FAST FOOD-CHICKEN FILLET SANDWICH W/ CHEESE	1	EACH	228.0	632	42	29	39
21102	FAST FOOD-CHICKEN FILLET SANDWICH, PLAIN	1	EACH	182.0	515	39	24	29
21037	FAST FOOD-CHICKEN NUGGETS, PLAIN	1	EACH	17.0	48	3	3	3
21038	FAST FOOD-CHICKEN NUGGETS, W/ BARB. SAUCE	1	EACH	17.0	43	3	2	2
21039	FAST FOOD-CHICKEN NUGGETS, W/ HONEY	1	EACH	17.0	49	4	2	3
21040	FAST FOOD-CHICKEN NUGGETS, W/ MUST. SAUCE	1	EACH	17.0	42	3	2	2
21041	FAST FOOD-CHICKEN NUGGETS, W/ SWEET AND SOUR	1	EACH	17.0	45	4	2	2
21042	FAST FOOD-CHILI CON CARNE	1	CUP	253.0	256	22	25	8
21070	FAST FOOD-CHIMICHANGA, W/ BEEF	1	EACH	174.0	425	43	20	20
21071	FAST FOOD-CHIMICHANGA, W/ BEEF AND CHEESE	1	EACH	183.0	443	39	20	23
21030	FAST FOOD-CHOCOLATE CHIP COOKIES	1	BOX	55.0	233	36	3	12
21043	FAST FOOD-CLAMS, BREADED AND FRIED	3	OUNCE	85.1	333	29	9	20
21128	FAST FOOD-CORN ON THE COB W/ BUTTER	1	EACH	146.0	155	32	4	3
21045	FAST FOOD-CRAB, SOFT-SHELL, FRIED	1	EACH	125.0	334	31	11	18
21011	FAST FOOD-CROISSANT W/ EGG AND CHEESE	1	EACH	127.0	368	24	13	25
21012	FAST FOOD-CROISSANT W/ EGG, CHEESE, AND BACON	1	EACH	129.0	413	24	16	28
21013	FAST FOOD-CROISSANT W/ EGG, CHEESE, AND HAM	1	EACH	152.0	474	24	19	34
21014	FAST FOOD-CROISSANT W/ EGG, CHEESE, AND SAUSAGE	1	EACH	160.0	523	25	20	38
21015	FAST FOOD-DANISH PASTRY, CHEESE	1	EACH	91.0	353	29	6	25
21016	FAST FOOD-DANISH PASTRY, CINNAMON	1	EACH	88.0	349	47	5	17
21017	FAST FOOD-DANISH PASTRY, FRUIT	1	EACH	94.0	335	45	5	16
21104	FAST FOOD-EGG AND CHEESE SANDWICH	1	EACH	146.0	340	26	16	19
21018	FAST FOOD-EGG, SCRAMBLED	2	EGGS	94.0	199	2	13	15
21074	FAST FOOD-ENCHILADA W/ CHEESE	1	EACH	163.0	319	29	10	19
21075	FAST FOOD-ENCHILADA W/ CHEESE AND BEEF	1	EACH	192.0	323	30	12	18
21076	FAST FOOD-ENCHIRITO W/ CHEESE, BEEF, AND BEANS	1	EACH	193.0	344	34	18	16
21019	FAST FOOD-ENG. MUFFIN W/ BUTTER	1	EACH	63.0	189	30	5	6
21020	FAST FOOD-ENG. MUFFIN W/ CHEESE AND SAUSAGE	1	EACH	115.0	393	29	15	24
21021	FAST FOOD-ENG. MUFFIN W/ EGG, CHEESE, AND CAN. BACON	1	EACH	146.0	383	31	20	20
21022	FAST FOOD-ENG. MUFFIN W/ EGG, CHEESE, AND SAUSAGE	1	EACH	165.0	487	31	22	31
21047	FAST FOOD-FISH FILLET, BATTERED AND FRIED	1	EACH	91.0	211	15	13	11
21105	FAST FOOD-FISH SANDWICH W/ TARTAR SAUCE	1	EACH	158.0	431	41	17	23
21106	FAST FOOD-FISH SANDWICH W/ TARTAR SAUCE AND CHEESE	1	EACH	183.0	523	48	21	29
21023	FAST FOOD-FRENCH TOAST W/ BUTTER	1	SLICE	67.5	178	18	5	9
21031	FAST FOOD-FRIED PIE, FRUIT (APPLE, CHERRY, OR LEMON)	1	EACH	85.0	266	33	2	14
21077	FAST FOOD-FRIJOLES W/ CHEESE	3	OUNCE	85.1	115	15	6	4
21116	FAST FOOD-HAM AND CHEESE SANDWICH	1	EACH	146.0	352	33	21	15
21117	FAST FOOD-HAM, EGG, AND CHEESE SANDWICH	1	EACH	143.0	347	31	19	16
21114	FAST FOOD-HAMBURGER, DOUBLE PATTY W/ COND AND VEG	1	EACH	226.0	540	40	34	27
21111	FAST FOOD-HAMBURGER, DOUBLE PATTY W/ CONDIMENTS	1	EACH	215.0	576	39	32	32
21110	FAST FOOD-HAMBURGER, DOUBLE PATTY, PLAIN	1	EACH	176.0	544	43	30	28
21113	FAST FOOD-HAMBURGER, LARGE, SINGLE PATTY W/ COND&VEG	1	EACH	218.0	512	40	26	27
21112	FAST FOOD-HAMBURGER, LARGE, SINGLE PATTY, PLAIN	1	EACH	137.0	426	32	23	23
21108	FAST FOOD-HAMBURGER, SINGLE PATTY W/ CONDIMENTS	1	EACH	107.0	275	33	14	10

Saturated fat (g)	Monounsaturated fat (g)	Polyunsaturated fat (g)	Fiber (g)	Cholesterol (g)	Folate (g)	Vitamin A (RE)	Vitamin B-6 (mg)	Vitamin B-12 (ug)	Vitamin C (mg)	Vitamin E (mg)	Riboflavin (mg)	Thiamin (mg)	Calcium (mg)	Iron (mg)	Magnesium (mg)	Niacin (mg)	Phosphorus (mg)	Potassium (mg)	Sodium (mg)	Zinc (mg)
4	3	0	-	16	59	10	.1	.6	1	-	.4	.2	50	2.3	36	2.2	57	290	522	1.7
4	4	1	-	24	37	32	.2	.9	1	-	.4	.3	53	2.4	42	2.7	70	328	668	1.9
4	2	1	-	62	30	75	.1	.5	3	-	.4	.2	65	1.9	25	1.9	70	205	495	1.2
6	4	1	-	78	72	190	.2	1	3	-	.6	.3	144	3.8	48	3.8	142	402	1024	3
5	4	0	-	32	20	14	.2	1	1	-	.5	.1	42	3	41	3.2	87	370	746	2.4
4	3	0	-	27	18	23	.2	.6	1	-	.4	.2	43	2.2	30	2.5	70	249	558	2.2
5	5	1	-	85	29	56	.2	1	2	-	.6	.3	111	3.9	35	4.2	158	333	1046	4
5	3	1	-	4	4	37	.1	.5	1	-	.2	.2	16	1.1	7	1.9	15	104	212	.4
18	17	5	-	142	49	54	.4	3.4	1	-	.5	.4	240	5.9	52	7.2	395	596	1148	6.7
15	13	2	-	88	28	129	.3	2.6	8	1.2	.5	.4	206	4.7	44	7.4	311	445	1108	4.6
16	14	3	-	111	33	80	.3	2.3	2	-	.4	.3	162	4.7	45	6.6	400	332	1043	6.8
15	13	2	-	96	39	148	.3	2.5	0	-	.6	.5	91	5.5	39	11.2	422	644	1589	5.6
13	13	6	-	93	34	84	.3	2.1	3	2	.4	.6	169	4.7	36	8.3	349	390	921	4.1
9	7	1	-	52	22	71	.2	1.2	2	-	.2	.3	182	2.6	26	6.4	216	229	976	2.6
6	6	2	-	50	27	37	.1	1	0	-	.4	.4	141	2.4	21	3.7	196	164	500	2.4
22	22	3	-	161	52	85	.6	5.9	3	-	.6	.6	283	8.3	61	11.5	541	821	1213	10.9
12	14	10	-	78	46	128	.4	.5	3	-	.5	.4	258	3.6	43	9.1	406	333	1238	2.9
9	10	8	-	60	29	31	.2	.4	9	-	.2	.3	60	4.7	35	6.8	233	353	957	1.9
1	1	0	0	10	2	5	.1	.1	0	-	0	0	3	.2	3	1.1	34	42	90	.2
1	1	0	-	8	4	6	0	0	0	-	0	0	3	.2	3	.9	28	42	108	.1
1	1	0	-	9	2	4	0	0	0	-	0	0	3	.2	3	1	30	38	79	.2
1	1	0	-	8	2	4	0	0	0	-	0	0	3	.2	3	.9	29	37	103	.1
1	1	0	-	8	2	10	0	0	0	-	0	0	3	.2	3	.9	28	36	89	.1
3	3	1	-	134	30	167	.3	1.1	2	-	1.1	.1	68	5.2	46	2.5	197	691	1007	3.6
9	8	1	-	9	31	16	.3	1.5	5	-	.6	.5	63	4.5	63	5.8	124	586	910	5
11	9	1	-	51	33	126	.2	1.3	3	-	.9	.4	238	3.8	60	4.7	187	203	957	3.4
5	5	1	-	12	16	15	0	.1	1	.4	.2	.1	20	1.5	17	1.4	52	82	188	.3
5	8	5	-	65	7	27	0	.8	0	-	.2	.2	15	2.3	23	2.1	176	196	617	1.2
2	1	1	-	6	44	96	.3	0	7	-	.1	.2	4	.9	41	2.2	108	359	29	.9
4	8	5	-	45	20	4	.2	4.5	1	-	.1	.1	55	1.8	25	1.8	131	163	1118	1.1
14	8	1	-	216	37	255	.1	.8	0	-	.4	.2	244	2.2	22	1.5	348	174	551	1.8
15	9	2	-	215	35	120	.1	.9	2	-	.3	.3	151	2.2	23	2.2	276	201	889	1.9
17	11	2	-	213	36	117	.2	1	11	-	.3	.5	144	2.1	26	3.2	336	272	1081	2.2
18	14	3	-	216	38	109	.1	.9	0	-	.3	1	144	3	24	4	290	283	1115	2.1
5	16	2	-	20	15	43	.1	.2	3	-	.2	.3	70	1.8	15	2.5	80	116	319	.6
3	11	2	-	27	14	5	.1	.2	3	-	.2	.3	37	1.8	14	2.2	74	96	326	.5
3	10	2	-	19	15	24	.1	.2	2	-	.2	.3	22	1.4	14	1.8	69	110	333	.5
7	8	3	-	291	37	181	.1	1.1	1	-	.6	.3	225	3	22	2.1	302	188	804	1.6
6	6	2	0	400	53	252	.2	.9	3	.9	.5	.1	54	2.4	13	.2	227	138	211	1.6
11	6	1	-	44	34	186	.4	.7	1	-	.4	.1	324	1.3	51	1.9	134	240	784	2.5
9	6	1	-	40	192	142	.3	1	1	-	.4	.1	228	3.1	83	2.5	167	574	1319	2.7
8	7	0	-	50	253	133	.2	1.6	5	-	.7	.2	218	2.4	71	3	224	560	1251	2.8
2	2	1	-	13	17	33	0	0	1	.1	.3	.3	103	1.6	13	2.6	85	69	386	.4
10	10	3	-	59	18	86	.1	.7	1	-	.3	.7	168	2.3	24	4.1	186	215	1036	1.7
9	7	2	-	234	44	158	.2	.8	1	.6	.5	.5	207	3.3	34	3.9	320	213	784	1.8
12	13	3	-	274	54	172	.2	1.4	1	-	.5	.8	196	3.5	30	4.5	287	294	1135	2.4
3	2	6	-	31	51	11	.1	1	0	-	.1	.1	16	1.9	22	1.9	156	291	484	.4
5	8	8	-	55	44	30	.1	1.1	3	.9	.2	.3	84	2.6	33	3.4	212	340	615	1
8	9	9	-	68	31	97	.1	1.1	3	1.8	.4	.5	185	3.5	37	4.2	311	353	939	1.2
-	-	-	-	58	15	73	0	.2	0	-	.2	.3	36	.9	8	2	73	88	257	.3
7	6	1	-	13	4	33	0	.1	1	.4	.1	.1	13	.9	8	1	37	51	325	.2
2	1	0	-	19	57	36	.1	.3	1	-	.2	.1	96	1.1	43	.8	89	308	449	.9
6	7	1	-	58	72	76	.2	.5	3	.3	.5	.3	130	3.2	16	2.7	152	291	771	1.4
7	6	2	-	246	43	149	.2	1.2	3	-	.6	.4	212	3.1	26	4.2	346	210	1005	2
11	10	3	-	122	27	11	.5	4.1	1	-	.4	.4	102	5.9	50	7.6	314	570	791	5.7
12	14	3	-	103	45	4	.4	3.3	1	-	.4	.3	92	5.5	45	6.7	284	527	742	5.8
10	12	2	-	99	37	0	.3	2.9	0	1.3	.4	.3	86	4.6	37	8.3	234	363	554	5.7
10	11	2	-	87	37	33	.3	2.4	3	-	.4	.4	96	4.9	44	7.3	233	480	824	4.9
8	10	2	-	71	32	0	.2	2.1	0	-	.3	.3	74	3.6	27	6.2	175	267	474	4.1
4	4	2	-	43	17	13	.1	.8	3	.4	.3	.3	51	2.5	22	4.7	110	215	564	2.1

Restaurants, Including Fast Food (Quick Service)—cont'd

Code	Name	Amount	Unit	Grams	Kilocalories	Carbohydrates (g)	Protein (g)	Fat (g)
21107	FAST FOOD-HAMBURGER, SINGLE PATTY, PLAIN	1	EACH	90.0	275	31	12	12
21115	FAST FOOD-HAMBURGER, TRIPLE PATTY W/ CONDIMENTS	1	EACH	259.0	692	29	50	41
21119	FAST FOOD-HOT DOG W/ CHILI	1	EACH	114.0	296	31	14	13
21120	FAST FOOD-HOT DOG W/ CORN FLOUR COATING (CORNDOG)	1	EACH	175.0	460	56	17	19
21118	FAST FOOD-HOT DOG, PLAIN	1	EACH	98.0	242	18	10	15
21028	FAST FOOD-ICE MILK, VANILLA, SOFT-SERVE W/ CONE	1	EACH	103.0	164	24	4	6
21078	FAST FOOD-NACHOS W/ CHEESE	3	OUNCE	85.1	260	27	7	14
21079	FAST FOOD-NACHOS W/ CHEESE AND JALAPENO PEPPERS	3	OUNCE	85.1	253	25	7	14
21080	FAST FOOD-NACHOS W/ CHEESE, BEANS, GROUND BEEF	3	OUNCE	85.1	190	19	7	10
21081	FAST FOOD-NACHOS W/ CINNAMON AND SUGAR	3	OUNCE	85.1	462	49	6	28
21130	FAST FOOD-ONION RINGS, BREADED AND FRIED	1	EACH	10.0	33	4	0	2
21048	FAST FOOD-OYSTERS, BATTERED OR BREADED, AND FRIED	3	OUNCE	85.1	225	24	8	11
21025	FAST FOOD-PANCAKES W/ BUTTER AND SYRUP	1	EACH	74.0	166	29	3	4
21049	FAST FOOD-PIZZA W/ CHEESE	1	SLICE	63.0	140	21	8	3
21050	FAST FOOD-PIZZA W/ CHEESE, SAUSAGE, AND VEGETABLES	1	SLICE	79.0	184	21	13	5
21051	FAST FOOD-PIZZA W/ PEPPERONI	1	SLICE	71.0	181	20	10	7
21131	FAST FOOD-POTATO, BAKED W/ CHEESE SAUCE	1	EACH	296.0	474	47	15	29
21132	FAST FOOD-POTATO, BAKED W/ CHEESE SAUCE AND BACON	1	EACH	299.0	451	44	18	26
21133	FAST FOOD-POTATO, BAKED W/ CHEESE SAUCE AND BROCCOLI	1	EACH	339.0	403	47	14	21
21134	FAST FOOD-POTATO, BAKED W/ CHEESE SAUCE AND CHILI	1	EACH	395.0	482	56	23	22
21135	FAST FOOD-POTATO, BAKED W/ SOUR CREAM AND CHIVES	1	EACH	302.0	393	50	7	22
21136	FAST FOOD-POTATO, FRENCH FRIED IN BEEF TALLOW	1	LARGE	115.0	359	44	5	19
21137	FAST FOOD-POTATO, FRENCH FRIED IN BEEF TALLOW AND VEG OIL	1	LARGE	115.0	358	44	5	19
21138	FAST FOOD-POTATO, FRENCH FRIED IN VEGETABLE OIL	1	LARGE	115.0	355	44	5	19
21139	FAST FOOD-POTATOES, MASHED	½	CUP	120.0	100	19	3	1
21026	FAST FOOD-POTATOES, HASHED BROWN	½	CUP	72.0	151	16	2	9
21122	FAST FOOD-ROAST BEEF SANDWICH W/ CHEESE	1	EACH	176.0	473	45	32	18
21121	FAST FOOD-ROAST BEEF SANDWICH, PLAIN	1	EACH	139.0	346	33	22	14
21052	FAST FOOD-SALAD, W/O DRESSING	½	CUP	69.3	11	2	1	0
21053	FAST FOOD-SALAD, W/O DRESSING, W/ CHEESE AND EGG	½	CUP	72.3	34	2	3	2
21054	FAST FOOD-SALAD, W/O DRESSING, W/ CHICKEN	½	CUP	72.7	35	1	6	1
21055	FAST FOOD-SALAD, W/O DRESSING, W/ PASTA AND SEAFOOD	½	CUP	139.0	126	11	5	7
21056	FAST FOOD-SALAD, W/O DRESSING, W/ SHRIMP	½	CUP	78.7	35	2	5	1
21058	FAST FOOD-SCALLOPS, BREADED AND FRIED	1	EACH	24.0	64	6	3	3
21059	FAST FOOD-SHRIMP, BREADED AND FRIED	1	OUNCE	28.4	79	7	3	4
21123	FAST FOOD-STEAK SANDWICH	1	EACH	140.0	315	36	21	10
21124	FAST FOOD-SUBMARINE SANDWICH W/ COLDCUTS	1	EACH	228.0	456	51	22	19
21125	FAST FOOD-SUBMARINE SANDWICH W/ ROAST BEEF	1	EACH	216.0	410	44	29	13
21126	FAST FOOD-SUBMARINE SANDWICH W/ TUNA SALAD	1	EACH	256.0	584	55	30	28
21032	FAST FOOD-SUNDAE, CARAMEL	1	EACH	155.0	304	49	7	9
21033	FAST FOOD-SUNDAE, HOT FUDGE	1	EACH	158.0	284	48	6	9
21034	FAST FOOD-SUNDAE, STRAWBERRY	1	EACH	153.0	268	45	6	8
21082	FAST FOOD-TACO	1	LARGE	263.0	568	41	32	32
21083	FAST FOOD-TACO SALAD	½	CUP	66.0	93	8	4	5
21084	FAST FOOD-TACO SALAD W/ CHILI CON CARNE	½	CUP	87.0	97	9	6	4
21088	FAST FOOD-TOSTADA W/ GUACAMOLE	1	OUNCE	28.4	39	3	1	3
21085	FAST FOOD-TOSTADA, W/ BEANS AND CHEESE	1	EACH	144.0	223	27	10	10
21086	FAST FOOD-TOSTADA, W/ BEANS, BEEF, AND CHEESE	1	EACH	225.0	333	30	16	17
21087	FAST FOOD-TOSTADA, W/ BEEF AND CHEESE	1	EACH	163.0	315	23	19	16
40349	HARDEE'S-BIG CHEESE	1	EACH	141.8	495	28	30	30
40350	HARDEE'S-BIG DELUXE	1	EACH	248.1	675	46	31	41
40356	HARDEE'S-BIG FISH SANDWICH	1	EACH	191.4	514	49	20	26
40353	HARDEE'S-BIG ROAST BEEF	1	EACH	163.0	365	39	22	13
40351	HARDEE'S-BIG TWIN	1	EACH	141.8	369	28	19	20
40358	HARDEE'S-BISCUIT	1	EACH	78.0	275	35	5	13
40348	HARDEE'S-CHEESEBURGER	1	EACH	100.6	335	29	17	17
40357	HARDEE'S-CHICKEN FILLET	1	EACH	191.4	510	42	27	26
40347	HARDEE'S-HAMBURGER	1	EACH	100.1	305	29	17	13
40354	HARDEE'S-HOT DOG	1	EACH	50.0	346	26	11	22
40355	HARDEE'S-HOT HAM & CHEESE	1	EACH	141.8	376	37	23	15

Saturated fat (g)	Monounsaturated fat (g)	Polyunsaturated fat (g)	Fiber (g)	Cholesterol (g)	Folate (g)	Vitamin A (RE)	Vitamin B-6 (mg)	Vitamin B-12 (ug)	Vitamin C (mg)	Vitamin E (mg)	Riboflavin (mg)	Thiamin (mg)	Calcium (mg)	Iron (mg)	Magnesium (mg)	Niacin (mg)	Phosphorus (mg)	Potassium (mg)	Sodium (mg)	Zinc (mg)
4	5	1	-	35	25	0	.1	.9	0	.5	.3	.3	63	2.4	19	3.7	103	145	387	2
16	18	3	-	142	31	16	.6	4.9	1	-	.5	.3	65	8.3	54	11	394	785	712	10.7
5	7	1	-	51	50	6	0	.3	3	-	.4	.2	19	3.3	10	3.7	192	166	480	.8
5	9	3	-	79	60	37	.1	.4	0	-	.7	.3	102	6.2	18	4.2	166	263	973	1.3
5	7	2	-	44	29	0	0	.5	0	-	.3	.2	24	2.3	13	3.6	97	143	670	2
4	2	0	-	28	5	52	.1	.2	1	.4	.3	.1	153	.2	15	.3	139	169	92	.6
6	6	2	-	14	8	69	.2	.6	1	-	.3	.1	205	1	42	1.2	208	129	614	1.3
6	6	2	-	35	8	196	.2	.4	0	-	.2	.1	259	1	45	1.2	164	122	724	1.2
4	4	2	-	7	13	156	.1	.3	2	-	.2	.1	128	.9	32	1.1	129	151	600	1.2
14	9	3	-	31	6	9	.1	1.3	6	-	.3	.1	66	2.3	15	3.1	26	61	343	.5
1	1	0	-	2	1	0	0	0	0	0	0	0	9	.1	2	.1	10	16	52	0
3	4	3	-	66	8	66	0	.6	3	-	.2	.2	17	2.7	14	2.7	120	111	414	9.6
2	2	1	-	19	11	22	0	.1	1	.4	.2	.1	41	.8	16	1.1	152	80	352	.3
2	1	0	-	9	59	74	0	.3	1	-	.2	.2	117	.6	16	2.5	113	110	336	.8
2	3	1	-	21	27	101	.1	.4	2	-	.2	.2	101	1.5	18	2	131	179	382	1.1
2	3	1	-	14	53	55	.1	.2	2	-	.2	.1	65	.9	9	3	75	153	267	.5
11	11	6	-	18	27	228	.7	.2	26	-	.2	.2	311	3	65	3.3	320	1166	382	1.9
10	10	5	-	30	30	173	.7	.3	29	-	.2	.3	308	3.1	69	4	347	1178	972	2.2
9	8	4	-	20	61	278	.8	.3	48	-	.3	.3	336	3.3	78	3.6	346	1441	485	2
13	7	1	-	32	51	174	.9	.2	32	-	.4	.3	411	6.1	111	4.2	498	1572	699	3.8
10	8	3	-	24	33	278	.8	.2	34	-	.2	.3	106	3.1	69	3.7	184	1383	181	.9
9	8	1	-	21	38	3	.3	.1	6	-	0	.2	18	1.6	38	2.6	153	819	187	.6
8	8	2	-	16	38	3	.3	.1	6	-	0	.2	18	1.6	38	2.6	153	819	187	.6
6	9	3	-	0	38	3	.3	.1	6	-	0	.2	18	1.6	38	2.6	153	819	187	.6
1	0	0	-	2	10	12	.3	.1	0	-	.1	.1	25	.6	22	1.4	66	353	272	.4
4	4	0	-	9	8	3	.2	0	5	.1	0	.1	7	.5	16	1.1	69	267	290	.2
9	4	4	-	77	40	46	.3	2.1	0	-	.5	.4	183	5.1	40	5.9	401	345	1633	5.4
4	7	2	-	51	40	21	.3	1.2	2	-	.3	.4	54	4.2	31	5.9	239	316	792	3.4
0	0	0	-	0	26	79	.1	0	16	-	0	0	9	.4	8	.4	27	119	18	.1
1	1	0	-	33	28	38	0	.1	3	-	.1	0	33	.2	8	.3	44	124	40	.3
0	0	0	-	24	23	32	.1	.1	6	-	0	0	12	.4	11	2	57	149	70	.3
1	2	3	-	17	33	213	.1	.6	13	-	.1	.1	24	1.1	17	1.2	68	200	524	.6
0	0	0	-	60	29	26	0	1.3	3	-	.1	0	20	.3	13	.4	53	135	163	.4
1	2	0	-	18	7	7	0	.1	0	-	.1	0	3	.3	5	0	49	49	153	.2
1	3	0	-	35	8	6	0	0	0	-	.2	0	14	.5	7	0	60	32	250	.2
3	4	2	-	50	62	31	.3	1.1	4	-	.3	.3	63	3.5	34	5	204	360	547	3.1
7	8	2	-	36	55	80	.1	1.1	12	-	.8	1	189	2.5	68	5.5	287	394	1651	2.6
7	2	3	-	73	45	50	.3	1.8	6	-	.4	.4	41	2.8	67	6	192	330	845	4.4
5	13	7	-	49	56	41	.2	1.6	4	-	.3	.5	74	2.6	79	11.3	220	335	1293	1.9
5	3	1	0	25	12	68	0	.6	3	.9	.3	.1	189	.2	28	.9	217	318	195	.8
5	2	1	0	21	9	57	.1	.6	2	.7	.3	.1	207	.6	33	1.1	228	395	182	.9
4	3	1	0	21	18	58	.1	.6	2	.8	.3	.1	161	.3	24	.9	155	271	92	.7
17	10	1	-	87	37	226	.4	1.6	3	-	.7	.2	339	3.7	108	4.9	313	729	1233	6
2	2	0	-	15	13	26	.1	.2	1	-	.1	0	64	.8	17	.8	48	139	254	.9
2	2	0	-	2	21	71	.2	.2	1	-	.2	.1	82	.9	17	.8	51	130	295	1.1
1	1	0	-	4	12	24	0	.1	0	-	.1	0	46	.2	8	.2	25	71	87	.4
5	3	1	-	30	75	85	.2	.7	1	-	.3	.1	210	1.9	59	1.3	117	403	543	1.9
11	4	1	-	74	97	173	.2	1.1	4	-	.5	.1	189	2.5	68	2.9	173	491	871	3.2
10	3	1	-	41	15	96	.2	1.2	3	-	.6	.1	217	2.9	64	3.1	179	572	897	3.7
-	-	-	-	-	-	-	-	-	-	-	-	-	-	-	-	-	-	-	1251	-
-	-	-	-	-	-	-	-	-	-	-	-	-	-	-	-	-	-	-	1063	-
-	-	-	-	-	-	-	-	-	-	-	-	-	-	-	-	-	-	-	314	-
6	6	2	1	55	29	0	.3	3	0	.2	.4	.4	80	4.5	40	6.6	280	389	1071	7.4
9	7	4	1	45	28	14	.2	1.9	2	.7	.3	.2	66	3.3	29	5.5	161	229	475	3.8
-	-	-	-	-	-	-	-	-	-	-	-	-	-	-	-	-	-	-	650	-
-	-	-	-	-	-	-	-	-	2	-	.3	.5	-	-	-	5.5	-	-	789	-
-	-	-	-	-	-	-	-	-	-	-	-	-	-	-	-	-	-	-	360	-
-	-	-	-	-	-	-	-	-	2	-	.6	.6	-	-	-	6.4	-	-	682	-
-	-	-	-	-	-	-	-	-	-	-	-	-	-	-	-	-	-	-	744	-
-	-	-	-	-	-	-	-	-	-	-	-	-	-	-	-	-	-	-	1067	-

Restaurants, Including Fast Food (Quick Service)—cont'd

Code	Name	Amount	Unit	Grams	Kilocalories	Carbohydrates (g)	Protein (g)	Fat (g)
40352	HARDEE'S-ROAST BEEF SANDWICH	1	EACH	141.8	323	39	19	11
44118	JACK IN THE BOX-BACON CHEESEBURGER	1	EACH	242.0	705	41	35	45
44101	JACK IN THE BOX-BREAKFAST JACK	1	EACH	126.0	313	29	19	14
44141	JACK IN THE BOX-CHEESECAKE	1	EACH	99.0	309	29	8	18
44115	JACK IN THE BOX-JUMBO JACK	1	EACH	222.0	497	41	25	26
44116	JACK IN THE BOX-JUMBO JACK W/ CHEESE	1	EACH	242.0	559	40	28	31
44136	JACK IN THE BOX-REGULAR FRENCH FRIES	1	EACH	109.0	351	45	4	17
44135	JACK IN THE BOX-SMALL FRENCH FRIES	1	EACH	68.0	219	28	3	11
47265	K.F.C.-COLONEL'S CHICKEN SANDWICH	1	EACH	166.0	482	39	21	27
47261	K.F.C.-FRENCH FRIES	1	EACH	77.0	244	31	3	12
47260	K.F.C.-MASHED POTATOES AND GRAVY	1	EACH	98.0	71	12	2	2
47239	K.F.C.-ORIGINAL RECIPE CENTER BREAST	1	EACH	103.0	261	9	25	15
47240	K.F.C.-ORIGINAL RECIPE DRUMSTICK	1	EACH	57.0	169	5	12	12
47241	K.F.C.-ORIGINAL RECIPE THIGH	1	EACH	95.0	324	11	16	24
47237	K.F.C.-ORIGINAL RECIPE WING	1	EACH	53.0	172	5	12	11
48215	MCDONALD'S-APPLE DANISH	1	EACH	115.0	390	51	6	17
48204	MCDONALD'S-BACON, EGG AND CHEESE BISCUIT	1	EACH	153.0	432	32	18	26
48174	MCDONALD'S-BIG MAC	1	EACH	215.0	560	43	25	32
48205	MCDONALD'S-BISCUIT W/ SPREAD	1	EACH	75.0	260	32	5	13
48170	MCDONALD'S-CHEESEBURGER	1	EACH	116.0	310	30	15	13
48187	MCDONALD'S-CHEF SALAD	1	EACH	265.0	215	7	20	12
48181	MCDONALD'S-CHICKEN MCNUGGETS	1	EACH	18.5	45	3	3	3
48226	MCDONALD'S-CHOCOLATE LOWFAT MILK SHAKE	1	EACH	294.1	321	66	11	2
48189	MCDONALD'S-CHUNKY CHICKEN SALAD	1	EACH	255.0	143	5	23	3
48217	MCDONALD'S-CINNAMON RAISIN DANISH	1	EACH	110.0	440	58	6	21
48198	MCDONALD'S-EGG MCMUFFIN	1	EACH	135.0	284	27	18	11
48201	MCDONALD'S-ENGLISH MUFFIN W/ SPREAD	1	EACH	58.0	170	26	5	4
48175	MCDONALD'S-FILET O' FISH	1	EACH	141.0	437	38	14	26
48188	MCDONALD'S-GARDEN SALAD	1	EACH	189.0	50	6	4	2
48169	MCDONALD'S-HAMBURGER	1	EACH	102.0	255	30	12	9
48209	MCDONALD'S-HASH BROWN POTATOES	1	EACH	53.0	130	15	1	7
48210	MCDONALD'S-HOTCAKES W/ MARGARINE AND SYRUP	1	EACH	174.0	440	74	8	12
48216	MCDONALD'S-ICED CHEESE DANISH	1	EACH	110.0	390	42	7	21
48180	MCDONALD'S-LARGE FRENCH FRIES	1	EACH	122.0	400	46	6	22
48176	MCDONALD'S-MCCHICKEN	1	EACH	187.0	415	39	19	20
48223	MCDONALD'S-MCDONALDLAND COOKIES	1	EACH	56.7	290	47	4	9
48172	MCDONALD'S-MCLEAN DELUXE	1	EACH	206.0	320	35	22	10
48179	MCDONALD'S-MEDIUM FRENCH FRIES	1	EACH	97.0	320	36	4	17
48171	MCDONALD'S-QUARTER POUNDER	1	EACH	166.0	410	34	23	20
48218	MCDONALD'S-RASPBERRY DANISH	1	EACH	117.0	410	62	6	16
48207	MCDONALD'S-SAUSAGE BISCUIT	1	EACH	118.0	420	32	12	28
48203	MCDONALD'S-SAUSAGE BISCUIT W/ EGG	1	EACH	175.0	505	33	19	33
48199	MCDONALD'S-SAUSAGE MCMUFFIN	1	EACH	135.0	345	27	15	20
48200	MCDONALD'S-SAUSAGE MCMUFFIN W/ EGG	1	EACH	159.0	430	27	21	25
48208	MCDONALD'S-SCRAMBLED EGGS	1	EACH	100.0	140	1	12	10
48190	MCDONALD'S-SIDE SALAD	1	EACH	106.0	30	4	2	1
48178	MCDONALD'S-SMALL FRENCH FRIES	1	EACH	68.0	220	26	3	12
48227	MCDONALD'S-STRAWBERRY LOWFAT MILK SHAKE	1	EACH	294.1	320	67	11	1
48225	MCDONALD'S-VANILLA LOWFAT MILK SHAKE	1	EACH	294.1	290	60	11	1
52366	PIZZA HUT-CHEESE PIZZA, HAND TOSSED	1	SLICE	70.0	259	28	17	10
52359	PIZZA HUT-CHEESE PIZZA, PAN	1	SLICE	70.0	246	29	15	9
53322	PIZZA HUT-CHEESE PIZZA, THIN'N CRISPY	1	SLICE	70.0	199	19	14	9
52363	PIZZA HUT-PEPPERONI PIZZA, THIN'N CRISPY	1	SLICE	70.0	207	18	13	10
52370	PIZZA HUT-PEPPERONI PERSONAL PAN PIZZA	1	EACH	250.0	675	76	37	29
52367	PIZZA HUT-PEPPERONI PIZZA, HAND TOSSED	1	SLICE	70.0	250	25	14	12
52360	PIZZA HUT-PEPPERONI PIZZA, PAN	1	SLICE	70.0	270	31	15	11
52365	PIZZA HUT-SUPER SPRM PIZZA, THIN'N CRISPY	1	SLICE	70.0	232	22	15	11
52362	PIZZA HUT-SUPER SUPREME PIZZA, PAN	1	SLICE	70.0	282	27	17	13
52369	PIZZA HUT-SUPER SUPREME, HAND TOSSED	1	SLICE	70.0	278	27	17	13
52371	PIZZA HUT-SUPREME PERSONAL PAN PIZZA	1	EACH	250.0	647	76	33	28

Saturated fat (g)	Monounsaturated fat (g)	Polyunsaturated fat (g)	Fiber (g)	Cholesterol (g)	Folate (g)	Vitamin A (RE)	Vitamin B-6 (mg)	Vitamin B-12 (µg)	Vitamin C (mg)	Vitamin E (mg)	Riboflavin (mg)	Thiamin (mg)	Calcium (mg)	Iron (mg)	Magnesium (mg)	Niacin (mg)	Phosphorus (mg)	Potassium (mg)	Sodium (mg)	Zinc (mg)
5	5	2	1	44	25	0	.3	2.6	0	.2	.4	.3	70	3.9	35	5.7	244	323	908	6.5
15	16	9	-	113	-	70	-	-	8	-	.5	.2	200	2.8	-	8.4	-	-	1240	-
5	5	3	-	190	-	138	.1	1.1	3	-	.5	.4	184	2.6	25	5.3	323	198	1080	1.9
9	7	2	-	63	-	-	-	-	-	-	.2	0	88	.3	-	1.9	-	-	208	-
10	11	2	-	72	-	67	.3	2.4	4	-	.3	.4	121	4.1	40	10.5	236	444	1023	3.8
13	11	2	-	98	-	196	.3	2.7	4	-	.3	.5	243	4.1	44	10.1	366	444	1482	4.3
4	7	-	-	0	-	-	-	-	26	-	0	.2	-	.7	-	3.6	-	-	194	-
3	7	-	-	0	-	-	-	-	16	-	-	.1	-	.4	-	2.3	-	-	121	-
6	4	9	1	47	29	14	.6	.3	0	2.3	.3	.4	100	3.1	41	10.6	261	297	1060	1.5
3	7	1	-	2	-	-	-	-	16	-	.1	.2	-	.3	-	1.9	-	-	139	-
1	0	0	-	-	-	-	-	-	-	-	0	-	16	.2	-	1.1	-	-	339	-
4	4	2	0	87	4	15	.6	.4	0	.5	.1	.1	16	1.2	31	14	238	265	603	1.1
2	3	2	-	59	5	14	.2	.2	0	.4	.1	0	7	.7	13	3.4	99	130	268	1.7
6	6	3	0	103	8	28	.3	.3	0	.5	.2	.1	13	1.4	23	6.5	176	224	549	2.4
3	6	2	-	59	-	-	-	-	-	-	.1	0	24	.3	-	2.9	-	-	383	-
4	11	2	2	25	3	35	0	0	15	3.8	.2	.3	14	1.4	8	2.2	31	69	370	.2
8	16	2	1	248	18	157	.2	.6	0	1.5	.3	.4	181	2.6	30	2.5	442	232	1206	1.7
10	20	2	-	103	21	106	.3	1.8	2	-	.4	.5	256	4	38	6.8	314	237	950	4.7
3	9	1	1	1	6	0	0	.1	0	1.8	.1	.2	75	1.3	14	1.5	168	100	730	.7
5	8	1	-	50	18	118	.1	.9	2	.5	.2	.3	199	2.3	21	3.9	177	223	750	2.1
6	6	1	-	120	-	385	-	-	13	-	.3	.3	240	1.4	-	3.4	-	-	459	-
1	2	0	-	9	-	-	-	-	0	-	0	0	-	.1	-	1.3	-	-	97	-
1	1	0	-	10	-	92	-	-	0	-	.5	.1	333	.8	-	.4	-	-	241	-
1	2	1	1	80	28	373	.6	.6	20	11	.2	.2	35	1	38	8.7	262	445	235	3
5	13	2	-	34	-	33	-	-	4	-	.3	.3	32	1	-	2.9	-	-	430	-
4	6	1	1	221	43	147	.2	.8	1	1.8	.3	.5	250	2.7	32	3.6	312	208	724	1.8
2	2	1	2	9	51	37	.1	-	0	.1	.1	.3	151	1.6	12	2.5	60	74	285	.4
5	10	11	1	50	20	44	.1	.8	-	-	.1	.3	164	1.8	27	2.7	227	149	1023	.9
1	1	0	-	65	-	900	-	-	21	-	.1	.1	32	.8	-	.4	-	-	70	-
3	5	1	-	37	-	40	-	-	2	-	.2	.3	80	1.5	-	3.8	-	-	490	-
1	4	2	-	0	-	-	-	-	1	-	-	.1	-	-	-	.8	-	-	330	-
2	5	5	-	8	-	40	-	-	-	-	.3	.3	80	1	-	2.9	-	-	685	-
6	13	2	-	47	-	40	-	-	-	-	.3	.3	32	.8	-	1.9	-	-	420	-
5	15	2	-	0	-	-	-	-	15	-	-	.2	-	.6	-	2.9	-	-	20	-
4	9	7	-	50	-	20	-	-	2	-	.2	.9	120	1.5	-	8.6	-	-	830	-
1	7	1	-	0	-	-	-	-	-	-	.2	.2	-	1	-	1.9	-	-	300	-
4	5	1	-	60	-	100	-	-	6	-	.3	.4	120	2	-	6.7	-	-	670	-
4	12	2	-	0	-	-	-	-	12	-	-	.2	-	.4	-	2.9	-	-	150	-
8	11	1	-	85	-	40	-	-	4	-	.3	.4	120	2	-	6.7	-	-	645	-
3	11	2	-	26	-	-	-	-	4	-	.2	.3	-	.8	-	1.9	-	-	310	-
8	17	3	-	44	-	-	-	-	-	-	.2	.5	64	1	-	3.8	-	-	1040	-
10	20	3	-	260	-	60	-	-	-	-	.3	.5	80	2	-	3.8	-	-	1210	-
7	11	2	-	57	-	40	-	-	-	-	.3	.5	160	1.5	-	4.8	-	-	770	-
8	14	3	-	270	-	100	-	-	-	-	.4	.5	200	2	-	4.8	-	-	920	-
3	5	2	-	425	-	100	-	-	-	-	.3	.1	48	1	-	-	-	-	290	-
0	1	0	-	33	-	800	-	-	12	-	.1	.1	16	.4	-	-	-	-	35	-
3	8	1	-	0	-	-	-	-	9	-	-	.2	-	.2	-	1.9	-	-	110	-
1	1	0	-	10	-	60	-	-	-	-	.5	.1	280	-	-	.4	-	-	170	-
1	1	0	-	10	-	60	-	-	-	-	.5	.1	280	-	-	-	-	-	170	-
7	3	-	-	28	-	50	-	.3	5	-	.2	.2	300	1.5	32	2.6	220	198	638	2.3
5	5	-	-	17	-	45	-	.3	4	-	.3	.3	252	1.5	26	2.5	188	160	470	2
5	3	-	-	17	-	35	-	.3	2	-	.2	.2	264	.9	21	2.3	188	131	434	1.8
5	5	-	-	23	-	35	-	.3	3	-	.2	.2	180	.9	19	2.5	148	144	493	1.7
13	17	-	-	53	-	120	-	.4	10	-	.7	.6	584	3.2	53	7.8	360	408	1335	3.8
6	5	-	-	25	-	50	-	.3	4	-	.3	.3	176	1.4	26	2.7	156	208	634	1.9
5	7	-	-	21	-	50	-	.3	4	-	.2	.3	208	1.8	25	2.6	176	203	564	2.1
5	5	-	-	28	-	50	-	.4	4	-	.2	.3	184	1.4	26	2.6	168	232	668	2.3
6	7	-	-	28	-	60	-	.4	5	-	.3	.4	216	1.9	32	3	188	266	724	2.7
7	6	-	-	27	-	55	-	.4	6	-	.3	.4	176	1.9	33	3.5	168	258	824	2.4
11	17	-	-	49	-	120	-	.5	11	-	.7	.6	416	3.7	53	7.6	320	487	1313	3.8

Restaurants, Including Fast Food (Quick Service)—cont'd

Code	Name	Amount	Unit	Grams	Kilocalories	Carbohydrates (g)	Protein (g)	Fat (g)
52368	PIZZA HUT-SUPREME PIZZA, HAND TOSSED	1	SLICE	70.0	270	25	16	13
52361	PIZZA HUT-SUPREME PIZZA, PAN	1	SLICE	70.0	295	27	16	15
52364	PIZZA HUT-SUPREME PIZZA, THIN'N CRISPY	1	SLICE	70.0	230	21	14	11
54494	RED LOBSTER-ATLANTIC OCEAN PERCH, LUNCH	1	EACH	141.8	130	1	24	4
54506	RED LOBSTER-CALAMARI, BRDED AND FRIED, LUNCH	1	EACH	141.8	360	30	13	21
54486	RED LOBSTER-CATFISH, LUNCH PORTION	1	EACH	141.8	170	0	20	10
54514	RED LOBSTER-CHICKEN BREAST, SKINLESS, LUNCH	1	EACH	113.4	140	0	26	3
54487	RED LOBSTER-COD, ATLANTIC, LUNCH PORTION	1	EACH	141.8	100	0	23	1
54510	RED LOBSTER-DEEP SEA SCALLOPS, LNCH PORTION	1	EACH	141.8	130	2	26	2
54488	RED LOBSTER-FLOUNDER, LUNCH PORTION	1	EACH	141.8	100	1	21	1
54489	RED LOBSTER-GROUPER, LUNCH PORTION	1	EACH	141.8	110	0	26	1
54490	RED LOBSTER-HADDOCK, LUNCH PORTION	1	EACH	141.8	110	2	24	1
54491	RED LOBSTER-HALIBUT, LUNCH PORTION	1	EACH	141.8	110	1	25	1
54513	RED LOBSTER-HAMBURGER, LUNCH PORTION	1	EACH	151.2	410	0	37	28
54504	RED LOBSTER-KING CRAB LEGS, LUNCH PORTION	1	EACH	453.6	170	6	32	2
54507	RED LOBSTER-LANGOSTINO, LUNCH PORTION	1	EACH	141.8	120	2	26	1
54500	RED LOBSTER-LEMON SOLE, LUNCH PORTION	1	EACH	141.8	120	1	27	1
54524	RED LOBSTER-LIVE MAINE LOBSTER	1	EACH	510.3	240	5	36	8
54492	RED LOBSTER-MACKEREL, LUNCH PORTION	1	EACH	141.8	190	1	20	12
54493	RED LOBSTER-MONKFISH, LUNCH PORTION	1	EACH	141.8	110	0	24	1
54498	RED LOBSTER-NORWEGIAN SALMON, LUNCH	1	EACH	141.8	230	3	27	12
54495	RED LOBSTER-POLLOCK, LUNCH PORTION	1	EACH	141.8	120	1	28	1
54502	RED LOBSTER-RAINBOW TROUT, LUNCH PORTION	1	EACH	141.8	170	0	23	9
54496	RED LOBSTER-RED ROCKFISH, LUNCH PORTION	1	EACH	141.8	90	0	21	1
54497	RED LOBSTER-RED SNAPPER, LUNCH PORTION	1	EACH	141.8	110	0	25	1
54509	RED LOBSTER-ROCK LOBSTER, LUNCH PORTION	1	EACH	368.5	230	2	49	3
54511	RED LOBSTER-SHRIMP, LUNCH PORTION	1	EACH	198.5	120	0	25	2
54505	RED LOBSTER-SNOW CRAB LEGS, LUNCH PORTION	1	EACH	453.6	150	1	33	2
54499	RED LOBSTER-SOCKEYE SALMON, LUNCH PORTION	1	EACH	141.8	160	3	28	4
54512	RED LOBSTER-STRIP STEAK, LUNCH PORTION	1	EACH	255.1	560	0	47	40
54501	RED LOBSTER-SWORDFISH, LUNCH PORTION	1	EACH	141.8	100	0	17	4
54503	RED LOBSTER-YELLOW FIN TUNA, LUNCH PORTION	1	EACH	141.8	180	6	32	2
62527	SUBWAY-BMT, ON HONEY WHEAT BREAD	1	12 IN.	220.0	1011	88	45	57
62559	SUBWAY-BMT, ON ITALIAN ROLL	1	12 IN.	213.0	982	83	44	55
62560	SUBWAY-CLUB SANDWICH, ON HONEY WHEAT ROLL	1	12 IN.	220.0	722	89	47	23
62561	SUBWAY-CLUB SANDWICH, ON ITALIAN ROLL	1	12 IN.	213.0	693	83	46	22
62562	SUBWAY-COLD CUT COMBO, ON ITALIAN ROLL	1	12 IN.	184.0	853	83	46	40
62563	SUBWAY-COLD CUT COMBO, ON WHEAT ROLL	1	12 IN.	184.0	853	88	48	41
62564	SUBWAY-HAM AND CHEESE, ON ITALIAN ROLL	1	12 IN.	184.0	643	81	38	18
62526	SUBWAY-HAM AND CHEESE, ON WHEAT	1	12 IN.	194.0	673	86	39	22
62565	SUBWAY-MEAT BALL SANDWICH, ON ITALIAN ROLL	1	12 IN.	215.0	918	96	42	44
62566	SUBWAY-MEAT BALL SANDWICH, ON WHEAT ROLL	1	12 IN.	224.0	947	101	44	45
62567	SUBWAY-ROAST BEEF, ON ITALIAN ROLL	1	12 IN.	184.0	689	84	42	23
62568	SUBWAY-ROAST BEEF, ON WHEAT ROLL	1	12 IN.	189.0	717	89	41	24
62569	SUBWAY-SEAFOOD, ON ITALIAN ROLL	1	12 IN.	210.0	986	94	29	57
62570	SUBWAY-SEAFOOD, ON WHEAT ROLL	1	12 IN.	219.0	1015	100	31	58
62571	SUBWAY-SPICY ITALIAN, ON ITALIAN ROLL	1	12 IN.	213.0	1043	83	42	63
62572	SUBWAY-STEAK AND CHEESE, ON ITALIAN ROLL	1	12 IN.	213.0	765	83	43	32
62573	SUBWAY-TURKEY BREAST, ON WHEAT ROLL	1	12 IN.	192.0	674	88	42	20
58318	TACO BELL-BEAN BURRITO	1	EACH	206.0	387	63	15	14
58319	TACO BELL-BEEF BURRITO	1	EACH	206.0	431	48	25	21
58321	TACO BELL-BURRITO SUPREME	1	EACH	198.0	440	55	20	22
62585	TACO BELL-LIGHT 7-LAYER BURRITO	1	EACH	276.0	440	67	19	9
62583	TACO BELL-LIGHT BEAN BURRITO	1	EACH	198.0	330	55	14	6
62586	TACO BELL-LIGHT BURRITO SUPREME	1	EACH	248.0	350	50	20	8
62584	TACO BELL-LIGHT CHICKEN BURRITO	1	EACH	170.0	290	45	12	6
62587	TACO BELL-LIGHT CHICKEN BURRITO SUPREME	1	EACH	248.0	410	62	18	10
62582	TACO BELL-LIGHT CHICKEN SOFT TACO	1	EACH	120.0	180	26	9	5
62575	TACO BELL-LIGHT SOFT TACO	1	EACH	99.0	180	19	13	5
62581	TACO BELL-LIGHT SOFT TACO SUPREME	1	EACH	128.0	200	23	14	5

Saturated fat (g)	Monounsaturated fat (g)	Polyunsaturated fat (g)	Fiber (g)	Cholesterol (g)	Folate (g)	Vitamin A (RE)	Vitamin B-6 (mg)	Vitamin B-12 (µg)	Vitamin C (mg)	Vitamin E (mg)	Riboflavin (mg)	Thiamin (mg)	Calcium (mg)	Iron (mg)	Magnesium (mg)	Niacin (mg)	Phosphorus (mg)	Potassium (mg)	Sodium (mg)	Zinc (mg)
6	7	-	-	28	-	55	-	.4	6	-	.3	.3	192	2.3	35	3.4	184	289	735	2.9
7	8	-	-	24	-	60	-	.4	5	-	.4	.4	200	1.4	33	2.9	184	290	832	2.8
6	6	-	-	21	-	50	-	.3	5	-	.2	.3	172	1.7	30	2.6	160	272	664	2.3
1	-	1	-	75	-	-	-	.3	-	-	.1	.1	-	-	21	1.5	160	-	190	.3
6	-	2	-	140	-	-	-	2	-	-	.1	.2	-	.6	21	1.5	360	-	1150	.9
3	-	2	-	85	-	-	-	0	-	-	.1	.3	-	-	21	1.9	160	-	50	.3
1	-	1	-	70	-	-	-	.1	-	-	.1	.1	-	.4	21	11.4	160	-	60	.9
0	-	1	-	70	-	-	-	.6	-	-	.1	0	-	-	28	.8	200	-	200	.3
0	-	2	-	50	-	-	-	.4	-	-	.1	-	-	-	53	1.9	240	-	260	1.5
0	-	1	-	70	-	-	-	.3	-	-	-	0	16	-	21	1.5	48	-	95	.3
0	-	1	-	65	-	-	-	.1	-	-	0	.1	32	-	28	1.5	200	-	70	.3
0	-	1	-	85	-	-	-	.2	-	-	.1	0	-	-	21	2.9	160	-	180	.3
0	-	1	-	60	-	-	-	.3	-	-	-	.2	-	-	28	2.9	240	-	105	-
11	-	1	-	130	-	-	-	1.2	-	-	.3	.1	-	1.5	28	7.6	200	-	115	7.5
1	-	2	-	100	-	-	-	1.6	-	-	.2	.1	48	-	70	1.9	320	-	900	6
0	-	1	-	210	-	-	-	2	-	-	-	.1	16	.8	35	1.1	160	-	410	1.5
0	-	0	-	65	-	-	-	.4	-	-	.1	.1	-	-	21	.4	64	-	90	.3
2	-	4	-	310	-	-	-	2	-	-	.2	.2	320	.8	53	2.9	320	-	550	6.8
4	-	5	-	100	-	-	-	.8	-	-	.4	.2	16	.8	21	5.7	200	-	250	1.2
0	-	1	-	80	-	40	-	.2	-	-	.1	.1	-	1	14	.8	64	-	95	.3
3	-	5	-	80	-	-	-	.2	-	-	.1	.2	16	-	35	6.7	240	-	60	.3
0	-	1	-	90	-	-	-	1	-	-	.2	.1	-	-	28	.4	160	-	90	.3
3	-	4	-	90	-	-	-	1	-	-	.2	.1	80	-	21	2.9	200	-	90	.9
0	-	1	-	85	-	-	-	.6	-	-	.1	.1	-	-	21	.8	120	-	95	.3
0	-	1	-	70	-	-	-	.3	-	-	0	.1	-	-	21	4.8	120	-	140	.3
1	-	1	-	200	-	-	-	.5	-	-	.1	-	48	-	88	3.8	400	-	1090	6
1	-	1	-	230	-	-	-	.5	-	-	0	-	32	-	35	1.9	120	-	110	1.5
1	-	2	-	130	-	-	-	1.6	-	-	.1	0	80	.2	70	1.9	200	-	1630	6
1	-	2	-	50	-	-	-	2	-	-	.1	.4	-	-	35	7.6	280	-	60	.3
17	-	2	-	150	-	-	-	1.2	-	-	.3	.2	-	2	35	7.6	280	-	115	9
1	-	1	-	100	-	20	-	.3	-	-	.1	.1	-	-	28	3.8	80	-	140	.6
1	-	2	-	70	-	-	-	1.6	-	-	0	.1	-	.6	35	13.3	240	-	70	.3
20	25	7	6	133	-	-	-	-	-	-	-	-	-	-	-	-	-	1002	3199	-
20	24	7	5	133	63	67	.5	2.3	5	5.1	.3	.3	64	4.3	66	5.1	308	917	3139	6.1
7	9	4	6	84	43	83	.5	.4	15	4.2	.4	.5	96	3.2	40	9.3	247	1055	2777	1.4
7	8	4	5	84	47	74	.6	1	20	1.3	.3	.5	58	3.1	66	12.5	384	971	2717	2.5
12	15	10	5	166	39	87	.2	1.2	17	.9	.3	.4	227	2.9	28	3.8	315	876	2218	2.7
12	15	10	6	166	41	90	.2	1.3	18	.9	.4	.4	235	3	29	3.9	327	1010	2278	2.8
7	8	4	5	73	45	174	.3	.8	17	3.8	.4	.5	304	2.2	50	3.6	527	834	1710	2.8
7	8	4	6	73	-	-	-	-	-	-	-	-	-	-	-	-	-	918	2508	-
17	17	4	3	88	35	72	.4	3.2	19	1	.4	.3	78	5	47	9.4	263	1210	2022	6.2
17	18	4	-	88	-	-	-	-	-	-	-	-	-	-	-	-	-	1498	2082	-
8	9	4	5	83	54	58	.4	2	5	4.4	.3	.2	55	3.7	57	4.4	266	910	2288	5.3
8	9	4	6	75	56	59	.4	2.1	5	4.5	.3	.2	56	3.8	59	4.5	273	994	2348	5.4
11	15	28	-	56	91	107	.3	6.5	5	2.5	.4	.5	230	4.4	32	7	336	641	2027	5.3
11	16	28	3	56	-	-	-	-	-	-	-	-	-	-	-	-	-	557	1967	-
23	28	7	5	137	-	-	-	-	-	-	-	-	-	-	-	-	-	880	2282	-
12	12	4	6	82	36	119	.4	2.5	6	.8	.5	.3	231	4.2	43	5.1	456	909	1556	6.8
6	7	7	7	67	-	-	-	-	-	-	-	-	-	-	-	-	-	605	2520	-
4	-	2	3	9	-	-	-	53	-	2	-	.4	190	4	-	2.8	-	495	1148	-
8	-	2	2	57	-	-	-	2	-	-	.3	.4	150	3	-	3.2	-	380	1311	-
8	-	2	3	33	-	-	-	26	-	2.1	-	.4	190	4	-	3.6	-	501	1181	-
-	-	-	-	5	-	350	-	-	5	-	-	-	300	2.5	-	-	-	-	1130	-
-	-	-	-	5	-	300	-	-	2	-	-	-	120	2	-	-	-	-	1340	-
-	-	-	-	25	-	600	-	-	9	-	-	-	96	1.5	-	-	-	-	1160	-
-	-	-	-	30	-	200	-	-	4	-	-	-	72	1.5	-	-	-	-	900	-
-	-	-	-	65	-	250	-	-	5	-	-	-	72	1.5	-	-	-	-	1190	-
-	-	-	-	30	-	150	-	-	5	-	-	-	48	.8	-	-	-	-	570	-
4	-	1	2	25	-	40	-	-	0	-	.2	.4	48	.6	-	2.8	-	196	554	-
-	-	-	-	25	-	100	-	-	2	-	-	-	48	.6	-	-	-	-	610	-

Restaurants, Including Fast Food (Quick Service)—cont'd

Code	Name	Amount	Unit	Grams	Kilocalories	Carbohydrates (g)	Protein (g)	Fat (g)
62574	TACO BELL-LIGHT TACO	1	EACH	78.0	140	11	11	5
62588	TACO BELL-LIGHT TACO SALAD	1	EACH	464.0	330	35	30	9
62580	TACO BELL-LIGHT TACO SUPREME	1	EACH	106.0	160	23	14	5
58328	TACO BELL-MEXICAN PIZZA	1	EACH	223.0	575	40	21	37
58325	TACO BELL-NACHOS	1	EACH	106.0	346	37	7	18
58323	TACO BELL-NACHOS BELL GRANDE	1	EACH	287.0	649	61	22	35
58329	TACO BELL-PINTOS 'N CHEESE	1	EACH	128.0	190	19	9	9
58337	TACO BELL-SALSA	1	EACH	10.0	18	4	1	0
58314	TACO BELL-SOFT TACO	1	EACH	92.0	225	18	12	12
58313	TACO BELL-TACO	1	EACH	78.0	183	11	10	11
58332	TACO BELL-TACO SALAD	1	EACH	575.0	905	55	34	61
58333	TACO BELL-TACO SALAD W/O SHELL	1	EACH	520.0	484	22	28	31
58316	TACO BELL-TOSTADA	1	EACH	156.0	243	27	9	11
61273	WENDY'S-BIG CLASSIC	1	EACH	251.0	480	44	27	23
62322	WENDY'S-BKD POTATO W/ BACON AND CHEESE	1	EACH	380.0	510	75	17	17
61287	WENDY'S-BKD POTATO W/ BROCCOLI AND CHEESE	1	EACH	411.0	450	77	9	14
62524	WENDY'S-BKD POTATO W/ CHEESE	1	EACH	383.0	550	74	14	24
61281	WENDY'S-CHICKEN CLUB SANDWICH	1	EACH	220.0	520	44	30	25
61292	WENDY'S-CHILI, LARGE	1	EACH	340.0	290	31	28	9
61291	WENDY'S-CHILI, SMALL	1	EACH	227.0	190	21	19	6
61285	WENDY'S-FRENCH FRIES, BIGGIE	1	EACH	170.0	450	62	6	22
61284	WENDY'S-FRENCH FRIES, MEDIUM	1	EACH	136.0	360	50	5	17
61283	WENDY'S-FRENCH FRIES, SMALL	1	EACH	91.0	240	33	3	12
61302	WENDY'S-FROSTY DAIRY DESSERT, LARGE	1	EACH	402.2	570	95	15	17
61301	WENDY'S-FROSTY DAIRY DESSERT, MEDIUM	1	EACH	321.8	460	76	12	13
61300	WENDY'S-FROSTY DAIRY DESSERT, SMALL	1	EACH	241.3	340	57	9	10
61271	WENDY'S-PLAIN SINGLE	1	EACH	133.0	350	31	25	15
61272	WENDY'S-SINGLE W/ EVERYTHING	1	EACH	219.0	440	36	26	23
62477	WHITE CASTLE-CHEESEBURGER SANDWICH	1	EACH	64.8	200	16	8	11
62481	WHITE CASTLE-CHICKEN SANDWICH	1	EACH	63.8	186	20	8	7
62478	WHITE CASTLE-FISH SANDWICH, W/O TARTAR	1	EACH	59.3	155	21	6	5
62483	WHITE CASTLE-FRENCH FRIES	1	EACH	96.9	301	38	2	15
62476	WHITE CASTLE-HAMBURGER SANDWICH	1	EACH	58.5	161	15	6	8
62485	WHITE CASTLE-ONION CHIPS	1	EACH	92.1	329	39	4	17
62484	WHITE CASTLE-ONION RINGS	1	EACH	60.2	245	27	3	13
62479	WHITE CASTLE-SAUSAGE AND EGG SANDWICH	1	EACH	96.3	322	16	13	22
62480	WHITE CASTLE-SAUSAGE SANDWICH	1	EACH	48.7	196	13	7	12

Saturated fat (g)	Monounsaturated fat (g)	Polyunsaturated fat (g)	Fiber (g)	Cholesterol (g)	Folate (g)	Vitamin A (RE)	Vitamin B-6 (mg)	Vitamin B-12 (μg)	Vitamin C (mg)	Vitamin E (mg)	Riboflavin (mg)	Thiamin (mg)	Calcium (mg)	Iron (mg)	Magnesium (mg)	Niacin (mg)	Phosphorus (mg)	Potassium (mg)	Sodium (mg)	Zinc (mg)
4	-	1	1	20	-	40	-	-	0	-	.1	.1	0	0	-	1.2	-	159	276	-
-	-	-	-	50	-	1200	-	-	27	-	-	-	120	1.5	-	-	-	-	1610	-
-	-	-	-	20	-	100	-	-	2	-	-	-	0	0	-	-	-	-	340	-
11	-	10	3	52	-	-	-	-	31	-	.3	.3	257	4	-	3	-	408	1031	-
6	-	2	1	9	-	-	-	-	2	-	.2	-	191	1	-	.6	-	159	399	-
12	-	3	4	36	-	-	-	-	58	-	.3	.1	297	3	-	2.2	-	674	997	-
4	-	1	2	16	-	-	-	-	52	-	.2	.1	156	1	-	.4	-	384	642	-
0	-	0	0	0	-	-	-	-	-	-	.1	-	36	1	-	-	-	376	376	-
5	-	1	2	32	-	-	-	-	1	-	.2	.4	116	2	-	2.8	-	196	554	-
5	-	1	1	32	-	-	-	-	1	-	.1	.1	84	1	-	1.2	-	159	276	-
19	-	12	4	80	-	-	-	-	75	-	.6	.5	320	6	-	4.8	-	673	910	-
14	-	2	3	80	-	-	-	-	74	-	.4	.2	290	4	-	3.2	-	612	680	-
4	-	1	2	16	-	-	-	-	45	-	.2	.1	180	2	-	.6	-	401	596	-
7	8	7	-	75	-	60	-	-	12	-	.3	.5	120	3.5	-	6.7	-	500	850	-
4	3	8	-	15	-	100	-	-	36	-	.2	.5	80	2.5	-	6.7	-	1370	1170	-
2	3	7	-	0	-	200	-	-	60	-	.1	.3	80	2.5	-	4.8	-	1310	450	-
8	6	7	-	30	-	150	-	-	36	-	.2	.3	240	2	-	3.8	-	1210	640	-
6	7	9	-	75	-	20	-	-	9	-	.4	.6	80	8	-	15.2	-	470	980	-
4	2	1	-	60	-	150	-	-	12	-	.2	.2	80	4.5	-	2.9	-	660	1000	-
2	1	1	-	40	-	100	-	-	6	-	.1	.1	64	3	-	1.9	-	440	670	-
5	15	1	-	0	-	-	-	-	12	-	.1	.3	16	.8	-	3.8	-	950	280	-
4	12	1	-	0	-	-	-	-	9	-	0	.2	16	.6	-	2.9	-	760	220	-
2	8	1	-	0	-	-	-	-	6	-	0	.2	-	.4	-	1.9	-	510	150	-
9	4	1	-	70	-	100	-	-	-	-	1.4	.2	400	1	-	.8	-	1040	330	-
7	3	1	-	55	-	100	-	-	-	-	1	.2	320	.8	-	.8	-	830	260	-
5	3	-	-	40	-	80	-	-	-	-	.8	.1	240	.6	-	.4	-	630	200	-
6	7	2	-	70	-	-	-	-	-	-	.2	.4	80	3	-	5.7	-	280	510	-
7	7	7	-	75	-	60	-	-	9	-	.2	.4	80	3	-	6.7	-	430	850	-
-	-	-	3	-	-	-	-	-	-	-	-	-	-	-	-	-	-	-	361	-
-	-	-	2	-	-	-	-	-	-	-	-	-	-	-	-	-	-	-	497	-
-	-	-	1	-	-	-	-	-	-	-	-	-	-	-	-	-	-	-	201	-
-	-	-	5	-	-	-	-	-	-	-	-	-	-	-	-	-	-	-	193	-
-	-	-	2	-	-	-	-	-	-	-	-	-	-	-	-	-	-	-	266	-
-	-	-	4	-	-	-	-	-	-	-	-	-	-	-	-	-	-	-	823	-
-	-	-	3	-	-	-	-	-	-	-	-	-	-	-	-	-	-	-	566	-
-	-	-	3	-	-	-	-	-	-	-	-	-	-	-	-	-	-	-	698	-
-	-	-	2	-	-	-	-	-	-	-	-	-	-	-	-	-	-	-	488	-

Chemistry: A Tool for Understanding Nutrition

An understanding of basic chemistry can make the study of nutrition easier and more interesting. It helps to connect nutrient characteristics with the structural and chemical characteristics of the individual compounds.

You have already taken at least one basic high school or college course in chemistry; consequently this appendix serves only to review key chemistry principles that arise in the study of nutrition. One concept to keep firmly in mind is that the physical and chemical properties of almost anything are intimately related to its structure. This is true of atoms, molecules, organisms—anything composed of matter. A basic knowledge of chemical structures can help you visualize important concepts in nutrition.

Let's briefly review those aspects of chemistry that are closely related to nutrition. We hope that this overview will make it easier to see what nutrition is all about.

Matter and Mass

All living and nonliving things are composed of matter. Two characteristics of matter are its mass and its volume. Mass is related to the amount of force it takes to move the object—it takes less force to move a paper clip than a car; therefore the clip has less mass. Volume is related to the amount of space an object occupies—a pint of water occupies less space than a gallon; therefore a pint has a smaller volume. Both of these properties depend on how much of the substance there is: a lake has a larger volume and a larger mass than a puddle of water.

A more fundamental property of matter is its density, which is defined as the mass of an object divided by its volume (d = mass/volume). Density is a more fundamental property than matter because it is independent of how much matter is available. The density of water in the lake and in the puddle is about 1 gram per milliliter (g/ml). The units of density are usually reported in units of g/ml (g ml^{-1}) for solids and liquids and g/L (g L^{-1}) for gases.

The density of pure water is 1 g/ml; lean body tissue has a density of about 1.1 g/ml; and the density of body fat is about 0.9 g/ml. Substances that are less dense than water are buoyant (they tend to float), while substances that are more dense than water tend to sink. The more fat a person has, the more buoyant he or she is when placed in water. This physical property—the tendency to float or sink in water—is used to determine the amount of body fat stored in a person (see Chapter 8).

Elements and Atoms

Most matter is composed of atoms (from Greek *atomos,* meaning "uncuttable"). Atoms cannot be broken down into simpler forms by ordinary chemical means. An element is composed of atoms of only one kind. For example, the element carbon is composed only of carbon atoms, and the element oxygen is composed only of oxygen atoms. There are more than 100 elements, such as hydrogen, oxygen, carbon, iron, and nitrogen. Many of these elements can be found in molecules found in foods. Over 99% of the mass of most cells is composed of a combination of carbon, hydrogen, oxygen, and nitrogen.

Atomic Structure

Atoms are composed of protons (possessing a unit positive charge), neutrons (zero charge), and electrons (unit negative charge). All atoms are spherically shaped. At the center of the sphere is the nucleus, which contains all the protons and neutrons. This nucleus then is surrounded by an electron cloud. The volume occupied by the electron cloud is about 10,000 times greater than the volume occupied by the nucleus. Consequently, the volume of the electron cloud defines the atomic volume.

Protons and neutrons have about the same mass, which is 2000 times greater than the mass of the electron. Essentially, all the mass of an atom is located within the nucleus. The structure of an atom can therefore be pictured as a very tiny, highly dense nuclear core surrounded by a cloud of electrons.

Electrons surrounding the nucleus have a somewhat peculiar nonintuitive behavior. For instance, it's impossible to know precisely where any given electron is located at any particular moment. It is possible only to define a volume of space where the electron is most likely to be found. This volume has a specific size and shape and is called an *orbital*. Any orbital can contain up to two electrons.

Different orbitals have different energies. Orbitals of similar energy are grouped together into electron shells. A shell can contain 1, 4, 9, or 16 different orbitals. Therefore shells can hold a maximum of 2, 8, 18, or 32 electrons, depending on the number of orbitals in the shell. Any shell can hold less than the maximum number of electrons. Most atoms have electrons occupying more than one shell. Carbon has two shells, the first holding two electrons (the maximum number) and the second holding four electrons (four less than the maximum number of eight). Shells themselves are always spherical, and this gives rise to the spherical shape of the atoms. The outermost shell in an atom is called the *valence shell*. The number of electrons in the valence shell and the energy of those electrons determine chemical behavior. Since these are unique for each element, each element has a unique chemistry.

Atoms that have not undergone chemical change are electrically neutral. This means that the number of protons equals the number of electrons in these atoms. Each element has a unique number of protons in its atoms. All neutral atoms of carbon, for example, contain six protons and six electrons, although the number of neutrons may vary (see the next section). The number of protons contained in the atom of an element is defined as the atomic number. Each element has a unique atomic number. The atomic number of each element and its symbol are given (among other things) in the periodic table (Table B-1).

Isotopes

In the previous section it was pointed out that all the atoms of a given element contain the same number of protons, but that the number of neutrons in the nuclei of elements such as carbon, nitrogen, or oxygen may vary. Carbon nuclei, for example can contain six, seven, or eight neutrons. Atoms with identical numbers of protons and different numbers of neutrons are called isotopes. Scientists distinguish between isotopes by adding the number of protons and neutrons together and writing the resultant sum as a superscript to the left of the elemental symbol. For example, consider carbon with its six protons. The predominant isotope of carbon contains six neutrons and is written as ^{12}C. The isotope containing seven neutrons is labeled ^{13}C, and the isotope containing eight neutrons is labeled ^{14}C. Note that because all these atoms have six protons, they are all carbon atoms, but because they possess different numbers of neutrons, they represent isotopes of carbon (see margin).

While the ordinary chemical behavior of different isotopes of the same element is virtually identical, the *radiochemical* behavior is sometimes different. These radioactive isotopes are frequently important in nutrition research. The element phosphorus has radioactive isotopes, such as ^{32}P. These isotopes emit radiation that can be detected and measured by instruments designed for that purpose. Other isotopes are not radioactive but still can be traced in body fluids or tissues, again using instruments designed for that purpose. Examples include ^{13}C and ^{15}N; these are called *stable isotopes.*

Carbon 14
6 Protons
8 Neutrons
6 Electrons

Carbon 12
6 Protons
6 Neutrons
6 Electrons

Carbon 13
6 Protons
7 Neutrons
6 Electrons

TABLE B-1

Periodic table of the elements

Main-group elements / Transitional metals / Inner-Transitional metals

Key: Atomic number / Symbol / Atomic weight — example: 1 / H / 1.00794

Period	1 IA	2 IIA	3 IIIB	4 IVB	5 VB	6 VIB	7 VIIB	8	9 VIIB	10	11 IB	12 IIB	13 IIIA	14 IVA	15 VA	16 VIA	17 VIIA	18 VIIIA
1	1 H 1.00794																	2 He 4.002602
2	3 Li 6.941	4 Be 9.012182											5 B 10.811	6 C 12.011	7 N 14.00674	8 O 15.9994	9 F 18.998403	10 Ne 20.1797
3	11 Na 22.989768	12 Mg 24.3050											13 Al 26.981539	14 Si 28.0855	15 P 30.973762	16 S 32.066	17 Cl 35.4527	18 Ar 39.948
4	19 K 39.0983	20 Ca 40.078	21 Sc 44.955910	22 Ti 47.88	23 V 50.9415	24 Cr 51.9961	25 Mn 54.93805	26 Fe 55.847	27 Co 58.93320	28 Ni 58.69	29 Cu 63.546	30 Zn 65.39	31 Ga 69.723	32 Ge 72.61	33 As 74.92159	34 Se 78.96	35 Br 79.904	36 Kr 83.80
5	37 Rb 85.4678	38 Sr 87.62	39 Y 88.90585	40 Zr 91.224	41 Nb 92.90638	42 Mo 95.94	43 Tc (98)	44 Ru 101.07	45 Rh 102.90550	46 Pd 106.42	47 Ag 107.8682	48 Cd 112.411	49 In 114.82	50 Sn 118.710	51 Sb 121.75	52 Te 127.60	53 I 126.90447	54 Xe 131.29
6	55 Cs 132.90543	56 Ba 137.327	57 La* 138.9055	72 Hf 178.49	73 Ta 180.9479	74 W 183.85	75 Re 186.207	76 Os 190.2	77 Ir 192.22	78 Pt 195.08	79 Au 196.96654	80 Hg 200.59	81 Tl 204.3833	82 Pb 207.2	83 Bi 208.98037	84 Po (209)	85 At (210)	86 Rn (222)
7	87 Fr (223)	88 Ra (226)	89 Ac** (227)	104 Unq (261)	105 Unp (262)	106 Unh (263)	107 Uns (262)	108 Uno (265)	109 Une (267)									

*Lanthanides

58 Ce 140.115	59 Pr 140.90765	60 Nd 144.24	61 Pm (145)	62 Sm 150.36	63 Eu 151.965	64 Gd 157.25	65 Tb 158.92534	66 Dy 162.50	67 Ho 164.93032	68 Er 167.266	69 Tm 168.93421	70 Yb 173.04	71 Lu 174.967

**Actinides

90 Th 232.0381	91 Pa (231)	92 U 238.0289	93 Np (237)	94 Pu (244)	95 Am (243)	96 Cm (247)	97 Bk (247)	98 Cf (251)	99 Es (252)	100 Fm (257)	101 Md (258)	102 No (259)	103 Lr (262)

Key to abbreviations

Name	Symbol	Name	Symbol	Name	Symbol	Name	Symbol
Actinium	Ac	Europium	Eu	Molybdenum	Mo	Samarium	Sm
Aluminum	Al	Fermium	Fm	Neodymium	Nd	Scandium	Sc
Americium	Am	Fluorine	F	Neon	Ne	Selenium	Se
Antimony	Sb	Francium	Fr	Neptunium	Np	Silicon	Si
Argon	Ar	Gadolinium	Gd	Nickel	Ni	Silver	Ag
Arsenic	As	Gallium	Ga	Niobium	Nb	Sodium	Na
Astatine	At	Germanium	Ge	Nitrogen	N	Strontium	Sr
Barium	Ba	Gold	Au	Nobelium	No	Sulfur	S
Berkelium	Bk	Hafnium	Hf	Osmium	Os	Tantalum	Ta
Beryllium	Be	Hahnium	Ha	Oxygen	O	Technetium	Tc
Bismuth	Bi	Helium	He	Palladium	Pd	Tellurium	Te
Boron	B	Holmium	Ho	Phosphorus	P	Terbium	Tb
Bromine	Br	Hydrogen	H	Platinum	Pt	Thallium	Tl
Cadmium	Cd	Indium	In	Plutonium	Pu	Thorium	Th
Calcium	Ca	Iodine	I	Polonium	Po	Thulium	Tm
Californium	Cf	Iridium	Ir	Potassium	K	Tin	Sn
Carbon	C	Iron	Fe	Praseodymium	Pr	Titanium	Ti
Cerium	Ce	Krypton	Kr	Promethium	Pm	Tungsten	W
Cesium	Cs	Lanthanum	La	Protactinium	Pa	Uranium	U
Chlorine	Cl	Lawrencium	Lw	Radium	Ra	Vanadium	V
Chromium	Cr	Lead	Pb	Radon	Rn	Xenon	Xe
Cobalt	Co	Lithium	Lui	Rhenium	Re	Ytterbium	Yb
Copper	Cu	Lutetium	Lu	Rhodium	Rh	Yttrium	Y
Curium	Cm	Magnesium	Lw	Rubidium	Rb	Zinc	Zn
Dysprosium	Dy	Manganese	Mg	Ruthenium	Ru	Zirconium	Zr
Einsteinium	Es	Mendelevium	Mm	Rutherfordium	Rf		
Erbium	Er	Mercury	Md				

Isotope "markers" such as ^{32}P and ^{13}C can be used to trace nutrients as they follow the chemical pathways in which they are metabolized. For example, researchers can "mark" a glucose molecule with a radioactive carbon atom (^{14}C). This allows them to see where the carbons of glucose end up in the body and also helps indicate what chemical transformations glucose undergoes when metabolized. Such studies have demonstrated that glucose can become part of the lipid stored in adipose cells or form CO_2 (detected as $^{14}CO_2$) that is exhaled in the breath. Isotope techniques are widely used in nutrition research.

Atomic and Molar Mass

The atomic masses that appear in the periodic table are obtained by measuring the mass of each element relative to the mass of the ^{12}C isotope. The units are called daltons (Da), and one ^{12}C atom has the arbitrarily assigned mass of 12.000 Da. One carbon atom also has a mass of 1.993×10^{-23} g (grams being a much more familiar unit than daltons).

In nature, however, not all the atoms of a given element have the same mass. For example, naturally occurring carbon is 98.90% ^{12}C and 1.10% ^{13}C. (The ^{14}C used in the experiments involving glucose described earlier is man made.) These masses are averaged ([12 Da $\times$ 0.989] + [13 Da $\times$ 0.110] = 12.011 Da) to give the average mass of the isotopes that occur in nature. It is the average masses that appear in the periodic table. So, for example, if you look up the mass of carbon in the periodic table you will find 12.011 and not 12.000.

A mole is defined to be the number of "things" equal to the number of atoms in 12 g of ^{12}C. The number of atoms in 12 g of ^{12}C is:

$$12 \text{g C} \times \frac{1 \text{ atom}}{1.993 \times 10^{-23} \text{g C}} = 6.023 \times 10^{23} \text{ atoms}$$

Therefore the number of "objects" in a mole is 6.02×10^{23}, which is frequently called Avogadro's number. This concept of grams per mole can be extended directly. For example, based on its atomic mass, one mole of naturally occurring hydrogen has a mass of 1.00795 g.

Ions

Atoms are electrically neutral because they have identical numbers of positively charged protons and negatively charged electrons. The electrons in metal atoms (those elements that have luster and conduct electricity) are not tightly bound to the nucleus, so when metals undergo chemical transformations they frequently lose one or more electrons. This results in a metallic species containing more protons than electrons, and therefore possessing a net positive charge. A species with a net positive charge is called a *cation*.

$$Na \rightarrow Na^+ + e^- \text{ (a sodium atom loses an electron, forming a cation)}$$

In nonmetallic elements, the electrons are very tightly held by the nucleus and cations are rarely formed, and then only under forcing conditions. Instead, nonmetallic elements generally accept additional electrons. This results in a species with a net negative charge, called an *anion*.

$$Cl + e^- \rightarrow Cl^- \text{ (a chlorine atom gains an electron to form an anion)}$$

These charged atoms—where electron(s) have been added or removed—are collectively known as *ions*. Sodium (Na^+), potassium (K^+), and calcium (Ca^{2+}) are found in the body as cations. Chloride (Cl^-) is a common anion in the body. Note that when an element gains an electron to become a negative ion, its name is modified by changing the suffix to *-ide*. In this example, chlor*ine* becomes chlor*ide*. A more complete list of common ions found in the body is given in Table B-2.

TABLE B-2

Important ions in the human body

Common ions	Symbol	Some functions
Calcium	Ca^{2+}	Component of bones and teeth, necessary for blood clotting, muscle contraction, and nerve transmission
Sodium	Na^+	Helps maintain membrane potentials (electrical charge differences across a membrane) and water balance
Potassium	K^+	Helps maintain membrane potentials
Hydrogen	H^+	Helps maintain acid-base balance
Hydroxide	OH^-	Helps maintain acid-base balance
Chloride	Cl^-	Helps maintain acid-base balance
Bicarbonate	HCO_3^-	Helps maintain acid-base balance
Ammonium	NH^{4+}	Helps maintain acid-base balance
Phosphate	PO_4^{3-}	Component of bone and teeth, involved in energy exchange and acid-base balance
Iron	Fe^{2+}	Necessary for red blood cell formation and function
Magnesium	Mg^{2+}	Necessary for enzyme function

Salts

Salts are substances composed of cations and anions. Table salt (Na^+ Cl^- or simply NaCl) is a good example. The oppositely charged sodium (Na^+) and chloride (Cl^-) ions are attracted to each other by electrostatic force, and the resulting ionic compound is known chemically as *sodium chloride*. Salts can be formed by interaction of acids and bases in a neutralization reaction; water is also formed in such reactions. In this type of reaction, hydrogen ions of an acid are replaced by the positive ions of a base, and a salt forms (see a later description of acids and bases if these are unfamiliar terms). For example, when hydrochloric acid reacts with sodium hydroxide (NaOH), table salt is produced.

$$HCl + NaOH \rightarrow NaCl + H_2O \text{ (neutralization reaction)}$$

The formula for salts can be misleading. For example, NaCl suggests that table salt exists as a discrete entity containing one sodium ion and one chloride ion. An inspection of the actual chemical structure of table salt, however, shows that table salt is actually a three-dimensional stack of layers—much like having a ream of paper with all the pages glued together. In each layer, the sodium ions are surrounded by four chloride ions and vice versa. The layers are stacked on top of one another so that a chloride ion is below a sodium ion on the layer above, and above the sodium ion on the layer beneath (Figure B-1). The point of all this is that no sodium ion is "attached" to a single chloride ion; it can be thought of as being associated with all the neighboring chloride ions. Distinct NaCl molecules are not observed except under special laboratory situations and in the gas phase.

Salts dissociate—separate—to form positively and negatively charged ions when dissolved in water. Substances that dissolve in water and conduct electricity are called *electrolytes*. Sodium, potassium, calcium, and chloride form various electrolytes in the body.

Molecules

Molecules form when atoms combine with each other in associated groups. You know many examples—H_2O, N_2, O_2, and H_2SO_4 are all molecules with which you are familiar. The term *compound* refers to molecules composed of more than one element, H_2O for example. Not all chemical compounds exist as molecules. Some

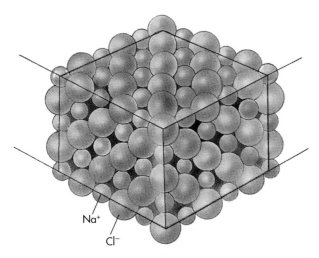

Figure B-1 Molecules of sodium chloride (table salt) in typical cube-shape formation.

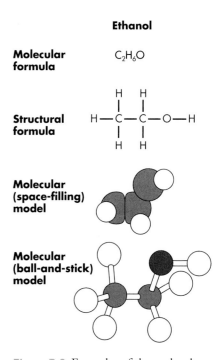

Glucose

Alanine

Butyric acid

Ethanol

Molecular formula C_2H_6O

Structural formula

Molecular (space-filling) model

Molecular (ball-and-stick) model

Figure B-2 Examples of the molecular and structural formulas and the molecular models of ethanol. The space-filling type of model gives a more realistic feeling of the space occupied by the atoms. On the other hand, the ball-and-stick type shows the bonds and bond angles more clearly.

compounds are made up of ions. Each molecule (or compound) possesses its own properties, such as color, taste, and density.

A molecular formula gives the elemental composition of a molecule or compound. This consists of the symbols of the atoms in the molecule plus a subscript denoting the number of each type of atom. If no subscript appears, then only one atom of that element is in the molecule. The molecular formula for ethanol (alcohol) is C_2H_6O, indicating that ethanol has two carbons, six hydrogens, and one oxygen atom in each molecule. A structural formula shows how the atoms are arranged with respect to each other. Molecular and ball-and-stick models approximate the shape of the molecule (Figure B-2). The structural formulas of several compounds important in nutrition are shown in the margin.

When molecules recombine with each other, atoms are conserved. This means that all the atoms present in the starting materials must be present in the products. For example, when glucose is combined with oxygen in the presence of a suitable catalyst, carbon dioxide (CO_2) and water (H_2O) are formed.

$$C_6H_{12}O_6 + 6\,O_2 \xrightarrow{\text{Catalyst}} 6\,CO_2 + 6\,H_2O$$
$$\text{Glucose}$$

Notice that all six carbons originally in glucose are present in carbon dioxide at the end of the transformation. Similar observations can be made about the total distribution of hydrogen and oxygen atoms between the molecules on both sides of the arrow. The products, then, are simply different combinations of the same atoms found in the original glucose and O_2. The overall process exhibits conservation of mass.

Chemical Bonding

Why do atoms combine to form molecules? The key lies in the structure of the atom. You know that the atom consists of a nucleus surrounded by a cloud of electrons. The nucleus is very dense and has a positive charge. The positive charge on the nucleus attracts the electrons in the atom, but it also attracts electrons in the valence shells of other atoms. When two atoms come in close proximity, each nucleus attracts the electrons in the valence shell of the other. This can result in each atom sharing electrons with the other atom. When this occurs, a covalent bond is formed. Specifically, when this type of bonding occurs, the atoms share valence electrons (up to six) with each other.

For example, consider a simple description of how methane (CH_4) is formed. Hydrogen has one electron in its valence shell, and that valence shell can hold a maximum of two electrons. Carbon has four electrons in its valence shell, and that

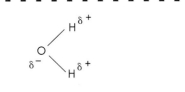

○ Hydrogen electrons
● Carbon electrons

shell can hold a maximum of eight electrons. Both carbon and hydrogen fill their valence shells to the maximum by sharing electrons with each other. This is illustrated in the margin at left. Notice that each hydrogen in methane contains two electrons and that the carbon atom has eight electrons in its valence shell. A good way to look at this is that the hydrogen atoms share one pair of electrons, while the carbon atom shares four pairs of electrons.

There are some guidelines that govern this behavior:

1. There must be room in the valence shell of each element to accommodate additional electrons.
2. Second-row nonmetallic elements of the periodic table (e.g., carbon, nitrogen, oxygen) and hydrogen typically fill their valence shells by sharing the necessary number of electrons with another element.
3. Third-row nonmetals and beyond the periodic table (e.g., phosphorus, sulfur, chloride) frequently make fewer covalent bonds than are necessary to fill the valence shell. Sulfur, for example, typically makes two bonds instead of the six that are possible. Phosphorus often forms five bonds.

A single bond exists when two atoms share one electron pair. A double bond forms when two atoms share two electron pairs. For example, fatty acids commonly have a few carbon-carbon double bonds (C=C), as shown below for oleic acid. This fatty acid is found in large amounts in olive oil and canola oil.

$$H-\overset{\overset{\displaystyle H}{|}}{\underset{\underset{\displaystyle H}{|}}{C}}-\overset{\overset{\displaystyle H}{|}}{\underset{\underset{\displaystyle H}{|}}{C}}-\overset{\overset{\displaystyle H}{|}}{\underset{\underset{\displaystyle H}{|}}{C}}-\overset{\overset{\displaystyle H}{|}}{\underset{\underset{\displaystyle H}{|}}{C}}-\overset{\overset{\displaystyle H}{|}}{\underset{\underset{\displaystyle H}{|}}{C}}-\overset{\overset{\displaystyle H}{|}}{\underset{\underset{\displaystyle H}{|}}{C}}-\overset{\overset{\displaystyle H}{|}}{\underset{\underset{\displaystyle H}{|}}{C}}-\overset{\overset{\displaystyle H}{|}}{C}=\overset{\overset{\displaystyle H}{|}}{C}-\overset{\overset{\displaystyle H}{|}}{\underset{\underset{\displaystyle H}{|}}{C}}-\overset{\overset{\displaystyle H}{|}}{\underset{\underset{\displaystyle H}{|}}{C}}-\overset{\overset{\displaystyle H}{|}}{\underset{\underset{\displaystyle H}{|}}{C}}-\overset{\overset{\displaystyle H}{|}}{\underset{\underset{\displaystyle H}{|}}{C}}-\overset{\overset{\displaystyle H}{|}}{\underset{\underset{\displaystyle H}{|}}{C}}-\overset{\overset{\displaystyle H}{|}}{\underset{\underset{\displaystyle H}{|}}{C}}-\overset{\overset{\displaystyle O}{||}}{C}-OH$$

The stability associated with completed electron shells for second-row elements and hydrogen is one reason why carbon is almost always found forming four bonds. For the same reason, nitrogen tends to make three bonds and oxygen two.

The backbone of large molecules found in biological systems consists of a chain of carbon atoms bound together (occasionally the chain contains a few atoms other than carbon). Variations in the length of the chains and their atomic combinations allow the formation of a wide variety of molecules. For example, some starches have thousands of carbons bound by covalent bonds to one another. Proteins typically contain many atoms, such as carbon, nitrogen, sulfur, hydrogen, and oxygen. Without the ability of atoms to form covalent bonds, the complex molecules that are common to living organisms could not exist.

When two different atoms form a covalent bond, the bonding electrons are never shared equally. Consider the H–O bond in water. It is unreasonable to expect that the hydrogen nucleus (containing one proton) and the oxygen nucleus (containing eight protons) have identical forces of attraction for the shared electron pair. In addition, other factors come into play—such as how many shells each atom has, how many electrons are in the shells, and the distance the shared electrons are from each nucleus. All of these lead to an unequal sharing of electrons in a covalent bond between different atoms.

The ability of an atom to attract electrons toward itself is called *electronegativity*. Elements toward the top right corner of the periodic table have the highest electronegativity, and those toward the bottom left have the lowest. Metals have low electronegativity, while nonmetals have relatively high electronegativity. Oxygen and nitrogen have the highest electronegativities of the elements typically found in compounds important to nutrition. The electronegativity values of atoms determine the type of chemical bond formed. If the electronegativity of two bonding atoms differs greatly, electron transfer occurs to yield an ionic bond, as in Na^+ Cl^-. If the electronegativity values are not very different, a covalent bond is formed.

In a water molecule, the electrons tend to be associated more closely with the more electronegative oxygen atom than with the hydrogen atoms. This unequal sharing of electrons can result in one end (an electrical pole) of the molecule having a charge opposite to that of the other end. The end containing the more elec-

O$^{\delta -}$ with H$^{\delta +}$ and H$^{\delta +}$

δ denotes partial charge

tronegative element is the negative end of the molecule. This results in a polar molecule, meaning that the molecule itself has a net polarity.

While all bonds formed between two different atoms are polar, not all molecules containing such bonds are polar. The distinction between bond polarity and molecular polarity is important. The figure in the margin shows that water, with two H–O bonds, is polar. However, CO_2, which contains two polar C–O bonds, is not polar, as shown below.

$$O=C=O$$

Although each C–O bond in carbon dioxide is polar, the molecule itself has zero polarity because the electrical vectors (to the left and right in the figure) are equal in magnitude and opposite in direction.

Polar molecules are weakly attracted both to ions and to other polar molecules. The positive end of the molecule can align itself with an anion or with the negative end of another molecule. These attractive forces, called respectively ion-dipole and dipole-dipole forces, are much weaker than covalent bonds individually, but when there are many of them, they make a significant contribution to the total energy of a collection of molecules. Water, for instance, has a much higher boiling point than expected because the molecules are "glued" together by such forces.

In fact, water and most other molecules containing an O–H or N–H bond exhibit a particularly strong interaction called *hydrogen bonding*. In this case, the hydrogen atom of one molecule is attracted to a nonbonded electron pair of a highly electronegative atom of a neighboring molecule, such as oxygen. Hydrogen bonds play an important role in determining the shape and stability of complex molecules, such as large proteins, because the hydrogen bonds between different parts of that molecule hold the molecule together.

Acids and Bases

Many molecules are classified as acids or bases. For most purposes, an acid is defined as a proton donor. Because a hydrogen atom without its electron is a proton (H^+), any substance that releases hydrogen ions when in water is an acid. For example, hydrogen chloride (HCl) forms hydrogen and chloride ions (H^+ and Cl^-) in solution and therefore is an acid.

$$HCl \rightarrow H^+ + Cl^-$$

A base is defined as a proton acceptor, so any substance that can accept hydrogen ions while in water is a base. Many bases can function as proton acceptors by releasing hydroxide ions (OH^-) when dissolved in water. For example, the base sodium hydroxide (NaOH) dissolves in water to form sodium and hydroxide ions:

$$NaOH \rightarrow Na^+ + OH^-$$

The hydroxide ions are proton acceptors as they go on to combine with hydrogen ions to form water:

$$OH^- + H^+ \rightarrow H_2O$$

Acids and bases are classified as strong or weak. Strong acids and strong bases dissociate completely when dissolved in water. Consequently, they release all of their hydrogen ions or hydroxide ions when dissolved. In general, the more completely an acid or base dissociates, the stronger it is. Hydrochloric acid, for example, is a strong acid because it completely dissociates in water.

Weak acids only partially dissociate in water. Consequently, they release only some of their acidic hydrogens. For example, when acetic acid ($CH_3\overset{O}{\overset{\|}{C}}$–OH, the principal component of vinegar) is dissolved in water, the acetic acid only partially dissociates.

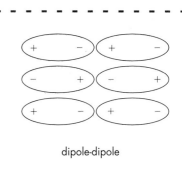

dipole-dipole

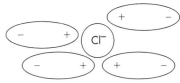

ion-dipole

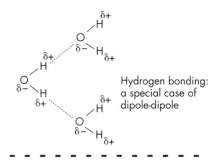

Hydrogen bonding: a special case of dipole-dipole

$$\underset{\textbf{Acetic acid}}{CH_3\overset{\displaystyle O}{\overset{\|}{C}}\!-\!OH} \;\rightleftharpoons\; \underset{\substack{\textbf{Acetate}\\\textbf{ion}}}{CH_3\overset{\displaystyle O}{\overset{\|}{C}}\!-\!O^-} + \underset{\textbf{Proton}}{H^+}$$

The equilibrium lies far to the left, so that only a small fraction of the acetic acid in a bottle of vinegar is dissociated into acetate ions and protons.

Most weak bases release hydroxide into solution by reacting with the water itself. For example, ammonia (NH_3) reacts with water to form NH^+_4 and OH^-.

$$NH_3 + H_2O \rightleftharpoons NH^+_4 + OH^-$$

pH

The term *pH* describes the hydrogen ion concentration (represented as $[H^+]$) of a solution. Specifically, a pH is equal to the negative logarithm of the hydrogen ion concentration ($pH = -\log_{10}[H^+]$). As the hydrogen ion concentration increases, the pH increases. Because of the exponential relationship, a one-unit change in pH represents a tenfold change in hydrogen ion concentration.

Keep in mind that a neutral pH is 7, an acid pH lies between 0 and 7, and alkaline or basic pH lies between 7 and 14.

The stomach has a pH of 1 to 2, and thus is very acidic. Since pH is based on an exponent, the stomach doesn't have merely seven times more hydrogen ions than the blood; it actually has one million times more hydrogen ions. Other common acidic solutions include coffee (pH 5), orange juice (pH 4), and vinegar (pH 3).

In a basic solution, hydroxide ions (OH^-) are present in greater amounts than hydrogen ions. Basic solutions include household ammonia (pH 12) and concentrated lye, or sodium hydroxide (pH 14). Figure B-3 shows the pH values of numerous familiar substances.

Free Radicals

We saw in a previous section that atoms tend to share electron pairs when forming chemical bonds, and there is a tendency to share enough electrons to completely fill the valence shell. A consequence is that atoms or elements are rarely found with an odd number of electrons. A molecule with an odd number of electrons is called a *free radical*. Free radicals are reactive, primarily because they contain an unpaired electron (shown as a dot). Free radicals seek an electron by attacking and removing electrons from other compounds, such as at the place where hydrogens are attached to carbon. This not only damages the molecule but transforms it into a free radical.

$$R\bullet + \!-\!CH_2 \longrightarrow RH + \!-\!\overset{\bullet}{C}H\!-$$

Free radicals are also formed when a covalent bond breaks and each atom or molecular fragment recovers the electron originally used to make the bond. In this case, energy—usually in the form of sunlight or heat—is needed to break the bond.

$$A\!-\!B + energy \rightarrow A\bullet + B\bullet$$

Because free radicals are so reactive, they can generate thousands of other free radicals within minutes in a chain-reaction process. The reactivity of free radicals sometimes produces detrimental effects in living systems. For instance, the development of some types of cancer, such as skin and lung cancer, is probably promoted by free radicals. However, some normal physiological functions in the body involve free-radical formation, such as respiration and killing of bacteria by various white blood cells.

Some substances are used extensively in the food industry to trap or prevent the formation of free radicals. This increases the storage time of food by decreasing

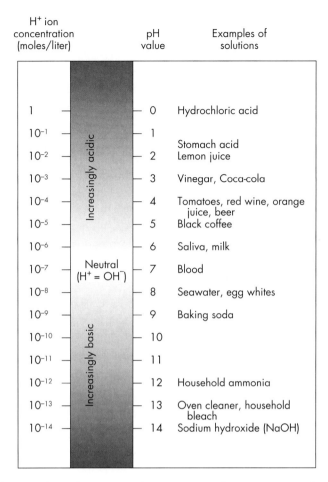

H⁺ ion concentration (moles/liter)	pH value	Examples of solutions

1	0	Hydrochloric acid
10^{-1}	1	
10^{-2}	2	Stomach acid Lemon juice
10^{-3}	3	Vinegar, Coca-cola
10^{-4}	4	Tomatoes, red wine, orange juice, beer
10^{-5}	5	Black coffee
10^{-6}	6	Saliva, milk
10^{-7}	7	Blood
10^{-8}	8	Seawater, egg whites
10^{-9}	9	Baking soda
10^{-10}	10	
10^{-11}	11	
10^{-12}	12	Household ammonia
10^{-13}	13	Oven cleaner, household bleach
10^{-14}	14	Sodium hydroxide (NaOH)

Increasingly acidic — Neutral ($H^+ = OH^-$) — Increasingly basic

Figure B-3 The pH values of common substances. Note that tomatoes aren't really that acidic.

chemical breakdown. These substances are part of the class of food additives called *preservatives* (see Chapter 19). Vitamin E in foods serves the same purpose; it can trap free radicals.

Isomerism

Molecules that have *identical* chemical formulas but *different* structures are called *isomers*. A simple example of this is two compounds with the formula C_2H_6O.

ethanol
CH_3CH_2OH

methyl ether
CH_3OCH_3

Ethanol is imbibed by millions of people daily; methyl ether is a foul-tasting poisonous substance that has little practical utility. This illustrates an important point about isomers: since they have different structures, they *must* have different properties.

The difference in properties between two isomers can be great (as in the example above) or very subtle, but the differences are there and are detectable. There are different types of isomerism, and we will briefly review two of the more common types.

STRUCTURAL ISOMERS

Isomers in which the number and kinds of bonds differ are called **structural isomers.** Look at ethanol and methyl ether, whose structures are shown in the margin. Ethanol has five C–H bonds, one O–H bond, and one C–C bond. Methyl ether has

Ethanol

Methyl ether

six C–H bonds and two C–O bonds. This analysis demonstrates that these two C_2H_6O molecules are structural isomers.

Molecules containing chains of carbon atoms typically have many structural isomers. Any variation in the way the chain is branched gives rise to a new isomer. For example, pentane C_5H_{12} has three isomers, as shown below:

Pentane $CH_3-CH_2-CH_2-CH_2-CH_3$

Neopentane $CH_3-CH_2-\underset{\underset{CH_3}{|}}{CH}-CH_3$

Isopentane $CH_3-\underset{\underset{CH_3}{|}}{\overset{\overset{CH_3}{|}}{C}}-CH_3$

STEREOISOMERS

Stereoisomers have the same number and types of bonds but different spatial arrangements (different configurations in space). The point is that the only difference between stereoisomers is the way the atoms are arranged in space.

A good way to illustrate this is to look at molecules containing double bonds. Because there is restricted rotation about a C=C bond, molecules containing double bonds frequently exhibit stereoisomerism. (C–C single bonds are easily rotated, like a pinwheel; if you put a second pin in the pinwheel, forming a "double bond," you wouldn't be able to spin it.) For example, in the relatively simple molecule 2-butene ($CH_3CH=CHCH_3$), the methyl groups ($-CH_3$) can be located on the same side of the double bond (*cis* isomer) or on opposite sides of the double bond (*trans* isomer). This is illustrated below.

$\underset{H}{\overset{H_3C}{>}}C=C\underset{H}{\overset{CH_3}{<}}$ *cis*-2-butene; the methyl groups are on the same side of the double bond

$\underset{H_3C}{\overset{H}{>}}C=C\underset{H}{\overset{CH_3}{<}}$ *trans*-2-butene; the methyl groups are on opposite sides of the double bond

Note that both isomers have one C=C bond, two C–C bonds, and eight C–H bonds. The only difference between the two isomers is the position of the methyl groups. Another example, involving a larger molecule, oleic acid and its isomer elaidic acid, is given in Figure B-4, *A*. Oleic acid is a *cis* isomer. In making margarine, some of the *trans* isomer forms, which is called *elaidic acid*. Collectively, these isomer types are sometimes called *geometric isomers*.

Another type of stereoisomerism occurs in molecules that cannot be superimposed on their mirror images—just like a right-hand glove cannot be superimposed on a left-hand glove. Isomers of this type occur very frequently in biological molecules; they are referred to as *optical isomers* because of their ability to rotate a beam of polarized light. In simple systems the isomers are distinguished by calling one isomer the D (or d) form and the other one the L (or l) form, as in D-alanine and L-alanine (Figure B-4, *B*). Just as the right-hand and left-hand gloves of a pair are nonsuperimposable mirror images of each other, D-alanine and L-alanine cannot be superimposed on each other. Nonsuperimposability of mirror images is the defining property of optical isomers.

The differences between D and L isomers are very subtle. For example, the chemistry of D-alanine is identical to the chemistry of L-alanine except when they react with other optical isomers, such as other amino acids; then the chemistry can be profoundly different. This is similar to trying to put a right-hand glove on the left hand—the glove doesn't interact as well with the wrong hand. Since most biological molecules are of one unique optical isomer form, this chemical difference that arises from isomerism can be very profound in biological systems. For example, L-alanine can be used by the body to make proteins, but the D form cannot.

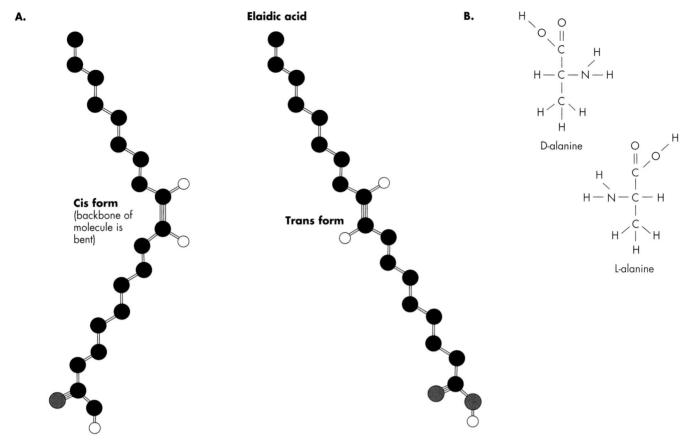

A. **Elaidic acid** **B.**

Cis form
(backbone of molecule is bent)

Trans form

D-alanine

L-alanine

Figure B-4 **A,** *Cis* and *trans* isomers of fatty acids. *Cis* forms are the most common forms in unprocessed foods. **B,** Optical isomers of alanine—an amino acid. The L isomer is the most commonly found amino acid in nature.

Chemical Reactions

One of the most important properties of chemical compounds is the reactions they undergo. It is chemical reactions that ultimately allow us to see, walk, and think.

In a chemical reaction, a compound or several compounds (the reactants) are converted into another compound or set of compounds (the products), accompanied by the absorption or release of energy (typically heat in biological processes). In effect, the reactants simply reshuffle their atoms to form products. Clearly, then, chemical reactions create and break down compounds. It is important to recognize that no atoms lose their identity during a chemical reaction, and no atoms are gained, lost, or converted to other atoms during the course of a normal chemical reaction.

Chemists have grouped reactions according to their similarities in chemical behavior. Some of these are performed over and over in body cells. What follows is a brief overview of some of these important reaction types.

CONDENSATION REACTIONS

A condensation reaction occurs when two molecules join together to form a larger molecule and a small molecule (usually water). The two reactant molecules each typically contain a hydroxyl group, meaning that there are two OH groups. A simple example is the condensation of ethanol to make ethyl ether and water:

$$CH_3CH_2OH + CH_3CH_2OH \rightarrow CH_3CH_2-O-CH_2CH_3 + H_2O$$
$$\text{ethanol} \qquad \text{ethanol} \qquad \text{ethyl ether}$$

While this reaction does not occur in the body, it illustrates the essential features of condensation reactions. One OH group gains a proton and forms a water molecule. The other OH group loses a proton and forms a bond with the other molecule—in exactly the same place that the water molecule leaves. Note that this is an overall description of what happens, not how it happens. The exact details of how some condensation reactions occur can be quite complex and are beyond the scope of this appendix. And while it is typical for both molecules to contain an OH group in a condensation reaction, it is not a requirement for the reaction. A condensation reaction can occur where only one of the reactants contains an OH group.

HYDROLYSIS REACTIONS

Hydrolysis reactions are reactions that occur when water is added to a compound. In biological systems, hydrolysis reactions are very frequently the reverse of condensation reactions. That is, water is added to a large molecule, which results in the formation of two smaller molecules. This can be illustrated by adding water to ethyl ether to form ethanol—the reverse of a reaction discussed earlier.

$$CH_3CH_2\text{--}O\text{--}CH_2CH_3 + H_2O \rightarrow 2\ CH_3CH_2OH$$

In fact, this reaction is reversible and can be run in either direction, depending on conditions.

Many important compounds in cells are formed using condensation reactions, and the breakdown of many compounds into smaller fragments occurs via hydrolysis reactions. For instance, hydrolysis of foodstuffs in the intestine yields smaller compounds that the body can absorb; breakdown of the lactose in milk into glucose and galactose illustrates this process. The converse occurs when the body makes protein for muscles, carbohydrates for storage in muscles, or fat to fuel muscles; all these synthetic processes use condensation reactions.

OXIDATION AND REDUCTION REACTIONS

The formal meaning of oxidation and reduction can be summarized as follows:

A species is oxidized when it loses one or more electrons.

A species is reduced when it gains one or more electrons.

Clearly, then, it is electron flow that governs oxidation-reduction processes. It is important to note that if one species loses electrons (is oxidized), another species *must* gain electrons (be reduced). The two processes go together; you cannot have one without the other. By way of illustration, consider the reaction between zinc and a Cu^{2+} ion.

$$Zn + Cu^{2+} \rightarrow Zn^{2+} + Cu$$

Here Zn is oxidized by losing two electrons ($Zn \rightarrow Zn^{2+} + 2e^-$), and copper is reduced by gaining two electrons ($Cu^{2+} + 2e^- \rightarrow Cu$).

Many oxidation-reduction reactions involving metallic atoms occur in the body. For example, the iron in hemoglobin is oxidized to Fe^{3+} and reduced to Fe^{2+} during the transport of oxygen to the body cells.

Oxidation-reduction reactions involving carbon-containing molecules are somewhat more difficult to visualize. A simple rule has been developed to determine oxidation-reduction in these cases:

If the molecule gains oxygen or loses hydrogen, it is oxidized; if it loses oxygen or gains hydrogen, the molecule is reduced.

The processes depicted below illustrate this definition:

This method of determining oxidation and reduction is extensively used in fields related to organic chemistry, namely biology and biochemistry. For example, pyruvic acid (made from glucose) is reduced to form lactic acid by gaining two hydrogens. This happens during intense exercise (see Chapter 10). Lactic acid is oxidized back to pyruvic acid by losing two hydrogens.

A compound that tends to remove electrons (hydrogens) from other compounds is called an **oxidizing agent.** In the body, strong oxidizing agents, including free radicals, can cause considerable damage by causing oxidation of important cellular constituents, especially DNA (the genetic material) and fatty acids in the cell membrane. Vitamin E and vitamin C in the body can donate electrons (hydrogens) to oxidizing agents, thereby preventing oxidative damage to critical molecules. Because of this property, these vitamins are called **antioxidants.**

Common Chemical Structures

As we saw earlier, carbon generally forms four bonds, nitrogen three, oxygen two, sulfur two, and hydrogen one. Most compounds in the body are composed of just carbon, hydrogen, and oxygen, with carbon often being the predominant element. Some commonly encountered combinations of atoms, called *functional groups,* have been given specific names because they appear in many molecules. You need to be familiar with them, for they are some of the most important features that differentiate molecules. These are summarized in the box on the next page. Study them because the names and structures of these groups appear frequently throughout the book.

Drawing Chemical Structures

Chemists have developed a short-hand notation for writing chemical formulas called *stick structures.* In stick structures neither carbon atoms nor the hydrogens bonded to the carbon atoms are expressly shown. What is shown is the bonds between the carbon atoms (the structure) and the position of all atoms other than carbon and hydrogen. The thing to keep in mind is that there are carbon atoms at the apices of every angle in the structure (with the appropriate number of hydrogens connected to the carbon) and at the terminal ends of the sticks. By way of illustration, look at a stick structure of propane ($CH_3CH_2CH_3$):

Propane   **Stick structure of propane**

In the margin, glucose, alanine, and butyric acid are depicted in stick structures. They appeared earlier in this appendix as chemical structures (p. B-7). The big advantage of using stick structures is that it allows for a clear representation of complex molecules without "cluttering up the picture." This notation will be used throughout the text, so you should become familiar with it. It becomes handy when large structures, such as those encountered in the body, have to be represented.

• • •

Glucose

Alanine

Butyric acid

Typical chemical groups found in nutrients

Functional group	Name	Typically found in	Example
$-OH$	hydroxide	alcohols	CH_3-OH
$-\overset{\displaystyle }{\underset{\displaystyle H}{C}}=O$	aldehyde	sugars	$CH_3\overset{\displaystyle }{\underset{\displaystyle H}{C}}=O$
$C-\overset{\displaystyle }{\underset{\displaystyle C}{C}}=O$	ketone	ketones	$CH_3\overset{\displaystyle }{\underset{\displaystyle CH_3}{C}}=O$
$-\overset{\displaystyle }{\underset{\displaystyle OH}{C}}=O$	carboxyl	acids	$CH_3\overset{\displaystyle }{\underset{\displaystyle OH}{C}}=O$
$-S-S-$	disulfide	proteins	$CH_3-S-S-CH_3$
$-\overset{\displaystyle }{\underset{\displaystyle |}{C}}=O$	carbonyl	aldehydes, ketones, carboxylic acids, amides	$(CH_3)_2C=O$
$-\overset{\displaystyle }{\underset{\displaystyle |}{C}}-NH_2$	amine	proteins	CH_3-NH_2
$-\overset{\displaystyle }{\underset{\displaystyle NH_2}{C}}=O$	amide	vitamins	$CH_3\overset{\displaystyle }{\underset{\displaystyle NH_2}{C}}=O$
$HO-\overset{\displaystyle OH}{\underset{\displaystyle OH}{P}}=O$	phosphate	high-energy compounds	$CH_2-O-\overset{\displaystyle OH}{\underset{\displaystyle O-CH_2-}{P}}=O$
$-\overset{\displaystyle }{\underset{\displaystyle O-C}{C}}=O$	ester	triglycerides	$CH_3-\overset{\displaystyle }{\underset{\displaystyle O-CH_2CH_3}{C}}=O$

This has been a brief overview of basic principles of chemistry. Ideally, it has reinforced earlier coursework. If these ideas are mostly new to you and you are confused, perhaps you have a classmate who can help you understand these key chemistry principles.

APPENDIX C Mathematical Tools for Use in Nutrition Study

The mathematical concepts you need for studying nutrition are few. Besides performing addition, subtraction, multiplication, and division, you need to calculate simple ratios and proportions (expressed as percentages) and convert English units of measurement to metric units. Note that Chapter 1 covered the conversion of kilocalories to kilojoules. This is important because many scientific journals today only use energy units of kilojoules (1 kcal = 4.18 kJ).

Percentages

The term *percent* (%) refers to a part of the total when the total represents 100 parts. For example, if you earn 80% on your first nutrition examination, you will have answered the equivalent of 80 out of 100 questions correctly. The best way to master this concept is to calculate some percentages. We have included some problems below.

Question	Answer
What is 6% of 45?	$0.06 \times 45 = 2.7$
What is 32% of 8?	$0.32 \times 8 = 2.6$
What percent of 16 is 6?	$6/16 = .375$ or 37.5%
What percent of 99 is 3?	$3/99 = 0.03$ or 3%

Joe ate 15% of the adult RDA for vitamin C at lunch. How many milligrams did he eat? (RDA = 60 mg)

$$0.15 \times 60 \text{ mg} = 9 \text{ mg}$$

Joe ate 200 g of carbohydrate, 100 g of fat, and 70 g of protein yesterday. Convert those values to percentages of total kilocalories:

$$\text{total kilocalories} = (200 \times 4) + (100 \times 9) + (70 \times 4) = 1980$$

$$\text{\% of kilocalories as carbohydrate} = (200 \times 4) \div 1980 = .404 \text{ or } 40.4\%$$

$$\text{\% of kilocalories as fat} = (100 \times 9) \div 1980 = .455 \text{ or } 45.5\%$$

$$\text{\% of kilocalories as protein} = (70 \times 4) \div 1980 = .141 \text{ or } 14.1\%$$

It is difficult to succeed in a nutrition course unless you know what a percentage is and how to calculate one. We use the concept of percentages frequently in referring to diets and nutrient composition.

The Metric System

The basic units of the metric system are the meter, for length; the gram, for weight; and the liter, for volume. The inside cover of this book contains factors for converting the English system units of pounds, feet, and cups to metric units. Here is a brief summary.

A meter is 39.4 inches long, or about 3 inches longer than 1 yard (3 feet). A meter can be divided into 100 units called *centimeters* or into 1000 units called *millimeters*. There are 2.54 centimeters in 1 inch, and about 30 centimeters in 1 foot. A 6-foot-tall person is 183 centimeters tall.

A gram is about $\frac{1}{28}$ of an ounce ($\frac{1}{28.3}$, to be exact). Thus an ounce equals about 28 g. Five grams of sugar or salt is about 1 teaspoon. A kilogram (kg) is 1000 g and is equivalent to 2.2 pounds. A 156-pound man weighs 71 kg. A gram is equal to 1000 milligrams (mg) or 1,000,000 micrograms.

Liters (L) can be divided into 1000 units called *milliliters* (ml). One teaspoon equals about 5 ml, 1 cup is about 240 ml, and 1 quart (4 cups) equals almost 1 L (0.946 L, to be exact).

If you plan to work in any realm of science, you should study the metric system until you become quite comfortable with it. For now, remember that a kilogram equals 2.2 pounds, 2.54 cm equals 1 inch, and a liter is almost the same as a quart. In addition, know what the prefixes *micro-, milli-, centi-,* and *kilo-* represent. With that knowledge you can convert any metric quantity to English units and convert English units to metric units.

U.S. Dietary Goals

U.S. dietary goals, 2nd edition, 1977

1. To avoid overweight, consume only as much energy (calories) as is expended; if overweight, decrease energy intake and increase energy expenditure.
2. Increase the consumption of complex carbohydrates and "naturally occurring" sugars from about 28% of energy intake to about 48% of energy intake.
3. Reduce the consumption of refined and processed sugars by about 45% to account for about 10% of total energy intake.
4. Reduce overall fat consumption from approximately 40% to about 30% of energy intake.
5. Reduce saturated fat consumption to account for about 10% of total energy intake, and balance that with polyunsaturated and monounsaturated fats, which should account for about 10% of energy intake each.
6. Reduce cholesterol consumption to about 300 mg a day.
7. Limit the intake of sodium by reducing the intake of salt to about 5 g a day.

The goals suggest the following changes in food selection and preparation:
1. Increase consumption of fruits and vegetables and whole grains.
2. Decrease consumption of refined and other processed sugars and foods high in such sugars.
3. Decrease consumption of foods high in total fat, and partially replace saturated fats, whether obtained from animal or vegetable sources, with polyunsaturated fats.
4. Decrease consumption of animal fat, and choose meats, poultry, and fish which will reduce saturated fat intake.
5. Except for young children, substitute low-fat and nonfat milk for whole milk, and low-fat dairy products for high-fat dairy products.
6. Decrease consumption of butterfat, eggs, and other high-cholesterol sources. Some consideration should be given to easing the cholesterol goal for premenopausal women, young children, and the elderly in order to obtain the nutritional benefits of eggs in the diet.
7. Decrease consumption of salt and foods high in salt content.

US Senate Select Committee on Nutrition and Human Needs: *Dietary goals for the United States,* ed 2, 1977.

Dietary Advice for Canadians

Canada has its own version of the RDAs, called Recommended Nutrient Intakes (RNIs), published by the Minister of National Health and Welfare.

Summary of examples of recommended nutrient intake based on energy expressed as daily rates

Age	Gender	Energy (kcal)	Thiamin (mg)	Riboflavin (mg)	Niacin (NE)*	ω-3 PUFA†(g)	ω-6 PUFA†(g)
Months							
0-4	Both	600	0.3	0.3	4	0.5	3
5-12	Both	900	0.4	0.5	7	0.5	3
Years							
1	Both	1100	0.5	0.6	8	0.6	4
2-3	Both	1300	0.6	0.7	9	0.7	4
4-6	Both	1800	0.7	0.9	13	1.0	6
7-9	M	2200	0.9	1.1	16	1.2	7
	F	1900	0.8	1.0	14	1.0	6
10-12	M	2500	1.0	1.3	18	1.4	8
	F	2200	0.9	1.1	16	1.2	7
13-15	M	2800	1.1	1.4	20	1.5	9
	F	2200	0.9	1.1	16	1.2	7
16-18	M	3200	1.3	1.6	23	1.8	11
	F	2100	0.8	1.1	15	1.2	7
19-24	M	3000	1.2	1.5	22	1.6	10
	F	2100	0.8	1.1	15	1.2	7
25-49	M	2700	1.1	1.4	19	1.5	9
	F	1900	0.8	1.0	14	1.1	7
50-74	M	2300	0.9	1.2	16	1.3	8
	F	1800	0.8‡	1.0‡	14‡	1.1‡	7‡
75+	M	2000	0.8	1.0	14	1.1	7
	F§	1700	0.8‡	1.0‡	14‡	1.1‡	7‡
Pregnancy (additional)							
1st trimester		100	0.1	0.1	1	0.05	0.3
2nd trimester		300	0.1	0.3	2	0.16	0.9
3rd trimester		300	0.1	0.3	2	0.16	0.9
Lactation		450	0.2	0.4	3	0.25	1.5

From Scientific Review Committee: *Nutrition recommendations,* Ottawa, Canada, 1990, Health and Welfare.
*Niacin equivalents.
†PUFA, polyunsaturated fatty acids.
‡Level below which intake should not fall.
§Assumes moderate physical activity.

| Summary of examples of recommended nutrient intake based on age and body weight expressed as daily rates |

Age	Gender	Weight (kg)	Pro-tein (g)	Vit. A (RE)*	Vit. D (μg)	Vit. E (mg)	Vit. C (mg)	Folate (μg)	Vit. B-12 (μg)	Cal-cium (mg)	Phos-phorus (mg)	Mag-nesium (mg)	Iron (mg)	Iodine (μg)	Zinc (mg)
Months															
0-4	Both	6	12†	400	10	3	20	25	0.3	250‡	150	20	0.3§	30	2
5-12	Both	9	12	400	10	3	20	40	0.4	400	200	32	7	40	3
Years															
1	Both	11	13	400	10	3	20	40	0.5	500	300	40	6	55	4
2-3	Both	14	16	400	5	4	20	50	0.6	550	350	50	6	65	4
4-6	Both	18	19	500	5	5	25	70	0.8	600	400	65	8	85	5
7-9	M	25	26	700	2.5	7	25	90	1.0	700	500	100	8	110	7
	F	25	26	700	2.5	6	25	90	1.0	700	500	100	8	95	7
10-12	M	34	34	800	2.5	8	25	120	1.0	900	700	130	8	125	9
	F	36	36	800	2.5	7	25	130	1.0	1100	800	135	8	110	9
13-15	M	50	49	900	2.5	9	30	175	1.0	1100	900	185	10	160	12
	F	48	46	800	2.5	7	30	170	1.0	1000	850	180	13	160	9
16-18	M	62	58	1000	2.5	10	40‖	220	1.0	900	1000	230	10	160	12
	F	53	47	800	2.5	7	30‖	190	1.0	700	850	200	12	160	9
19-24	M	71	61	1000	2.5	10	40‖	220	1.0	800	1000	240	9	160	12
	F	58	50	800	2.5	7	30‖	180	1.0	700	850	200	13	160	9
25-49	M	74	64	1000	2.5	9	40‖	230	1.0	800	1000	250	9	160	12
	F	59	51	800	2.5	6	30‖	185	1.0	700	850	200	13	160	9
50-74	M	73	63	1000	5	7	40‖	230	1.0	800	1000	250	9	160	12
	F	63	54	800	5	6	30‖	195	1.0	800	850	210	8	160	9
75+	M	69	59	1000	5	6	40‖	215	1.0	800	1000	230	9	160	12
	F	64	55	800	5	5	30‖	200	1.0	800	850	210	8	160	9
Pregnancy (additional)															
1st trimester			5	0	2.5	2	0	200	1.2	500	200	15	0	25	6
2nd trimester			20	0	2.5	2	10	200	1.2	500	200	45	5	25	6
3rd trimester			24	0	2.5	2	10	200	1.2	500	200	45	10	25	6
Lactation			20	400	2.5	3	25	100	0.2	500	200	65	0	50	6

From Scientific Review Committee: *Nutrition recommendations,* Ottawa, Canada, 1990, Health and Welfare.
*Retinol equivalents.
†Protein is assumed to be from breast milk and must be adjusted for infant formula.
‡Infant formula with high phosphorus should contain 375 mg calcium.
§Breast milk is assumed to be the source of the mineral.
‖Smokers should increase vitamin C values by 50%.

Summary of the Desired Characteristics of the Canadian Diet

1. **The Canadian diet should provide energy consistent with the maintenance of body weight within the recommended range.** Physical activity should be appropriate to circumstances and capabilities. While the importance of maintaining some activity throughout life can be stressed, it is not possible to specify a level of physical activity for the whole population. As a general guideline it is desirable that adults, for as long as possible, maintain an activity level that permits an energy intake of at least 1800 kcal while keeping weight within the recommended range.

2. **The Canadian diet should include essential nutrients in amounts recommended in this report.** While it is important that the diet provide the recommended amounts of nutrients, it should be understood that no evidence was found that intakes in excess of the RNI confer any health benefit. There is no general need for supplements except for vitamin D for infants and folate during pregnancy. Vitamin D supplementation might be required for elderly persons not exposed to the sun, and iron for pregnant women with low iron stores.

3. **The Canadian diet should include no more than 30% of energy as fat (33 g/1000 kcal) and no more than 10% as saturated fat (11 g/1000 kcal).** Dietary cholesterol, though not as influential in affecting levels of blood cholesterol, is not without importance. A reduction in cholesterol intake normally will accompany a reduction in total fat and saturated fat. The recommendation to reduce total fat intake does not apply to children under the age of 2 years.

4. **The Canadian diet should provide 55% of energy as carbohydrate (138 g/1000 kcal) from a variety of sources.** Sources should be selected that provide complex carbohydrates, a variety of dietary fiber, and beta-carotene.

5. **The sodium content of the Canadian diet should be reduced.** The present food supply provides sodium in an amount greatly exceeding requirements. While there is insufficient evidence to support a precise recommendation, potential benefit would be expected from a reduction in current sodium intake.

6. **The Canadian diet should include no more than 5% of total energy as alcohol, or two drinks daily, whichever is less.** The harmful influence of alcohol on blood pressure provides a more urgent reason for moderation. During pregnancy it is prudent to abstain from alcoholic beverages because a safe intake is not known with certainty.

7. **The Canadian diet should contain no more caffeine than the equivalent of four regular cups of coffee per day.** This is a prudent measure in view of the increased risk for cardiovascular disease associated with high intakes of caffeine.

8. **Community water supplies containing less fluoride than 1 mg/L should be fluoridated to that level.** Fluoridation of community water supplies has proven to be a safe, effective, and economical method of improving dental health.

In essence, suggested actions toward healthful eating as listed in Canada's *Guidelines for Healthy Eating* include the following:

- Enjoy a variety of foods.
- Emphasize cereals, breads, other grain products, vegetables, and fruits.
- Choose low-fat dairy products, lean meats, and foods prepared with little or no fat.
- Achieve and maintain a healthful body weight by enjoying regular physical activity and healthful eating.
- Limit salt, alcohol, and caffeine.

More details are available on RNI and diet recommendations in the 1990 publication *Nutrition Recommendations: The Report of the Scientific Review Committee.*

A separate Canadian food guide, illustrated on the following pages, provides a plan to meet these nutrient needs.

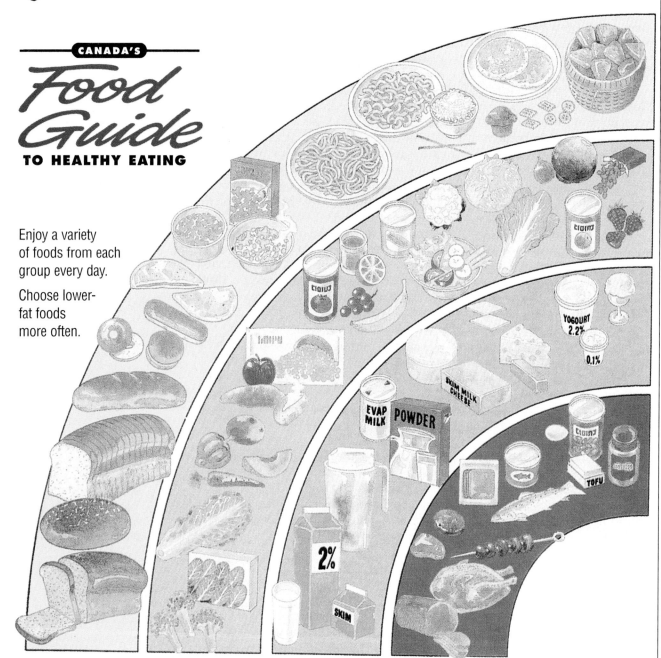

Healthy Canada

■✦■ Health and Welfare Canada   Santé et Bien-être social Canada

CANADA'S
Food Guide
TO HEALTHY EATING

Enjoy a variety of foods from each group every day.

Choose lower-fat foods more often.

Grain Products
Choose whole grain and enriched products more often.

Vegetables & Fruit
Choose dark green and orange vegetables and orange fruit more often.

Milk Products
Choose lower-fat milk products more often.

Meat & Alternatives
Choose leaner meats, poultry and fish, as well as dried peas, beans and lentils more often.

Canada ■✦■

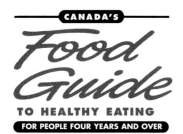

Different People Need Different Amounts of Food

The amount of food you need every day from the 4 food groups and other foods depends on your age, body size, activity level, whether you are male or female and if you are pregnant or breast-feeding. That's why the Food Guide gives a lower and higher number of servings for each food group. For example, young children can choose the lower number of servings, while male teenagers can go to the higher number. Most other people can choose servings somewhere in between.

Grain Products
5–12 SERVINGS PER DAY

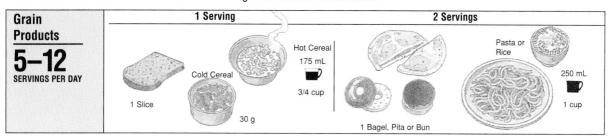

1 Serving
1 Slice
Cold Cereal — 30 g
Hot Cereal 175 mL — 3/4 cup

2 Servings
Pasta or Rice — 250 mL — 1 cup
1 Bagel, Pita or Bun

Vegetables & Fruit
5–10 SERVINGS PER DAY

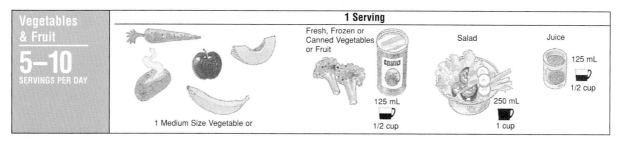

1 Serving
1 Medium Size Vegetable or
Fresh, Frozen or Canned Vegetables or Fruit — 125 mL — 1/2 cup
Salad — 250 mL — 1 cup
Juice — 125 mL — 1/2 cup

Milk Products

SERVINGS PER DAY
Children 4–9 years: 2–3
Youth 10–16 years: 3–4
Adults: 2–4
Pregnant & Breast-feeding Women: 3–4

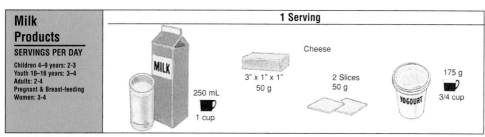

1 Serving
MILK — 250 mL — 1 cup
Cheese — 3" x 1" x 1" — 50 g
2 Slices — 50 g
YOGOURT — 175 g — 3/4 cup

Other Foods

Taste and enjoyment can also come from other foods and beverages that are not part of the 4 food groups. Some of these foods are higher in fat or Calories, so use these foods in moderation.

Meat & Alternatives
2–3 SERVINGS PER DAY

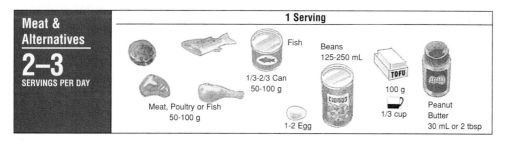

1 Serving
Meat, Poultry or Fish — 50–100 g
1-2 Egg
Fish — 1/3-2/3 Can — 50-100 g
Beans 125-250 mL
TOFU — 100 g — 1/3 cup
Peanut Butter — 30 mL or 2 tbsp

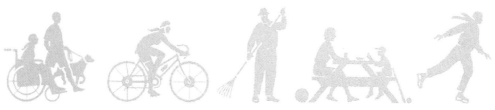

Enjoy eating well, being active and feeling good about yourself. That's VITALIT®

© Minister of Supply and Services Canada 1992   Cat. No. H39-252 / 1992E   No changes permitted. Reprint permission not required.
ISBN 0-662-19648-1

Exchange System Lists

Milk Exchange List

SKIM AND VERY-LOW-FAT MILK (12 g carbohydrate, 8 g protein, 0-3 g fat, 90 kcal)

1 cup	skim or nonfat milk (½% and 1%)
⅓ cup	powdered (nonfat dry, before adding liquid)
½ cup	canned, evaporated skim milk
1 cup	buttermilk made from nonfat or low-fat milk
¾ cup	yogurt made from nonfat milk (plain, unflavored)

LOW-FAT MILK (12 g carbohydrate, 8 g protein, 5 g fat, 120 kcal)

1 cup	2% milk
¾ cup	plain nonfat yogurt (added milk solids)
1 cup	sweet acidophilus milk

WHOLE MILK (12 g carbohydrate, 8 g protein, 8 g fat, 150 kcal)

1 cup	whole milk
½ cup	evaporated whole milk
1 cup	goat's milk
1 cup	kefir

Vegetable Exchange List

(5 g carbohydrate, 2 g protein, 0 g fat, 25 kcal)
1 vegetable exchange equals:
 ½ cup cooked vegetables or vegetable juice
 1 cup raw vegetables

artichoke	eggplant	peppers
artichoke hearts	green onions or scallions	radishes
asparagus	green pepper	salad greens
beans (green, wax, Italian)	greens (e.g., collard)	sauerkraut
bean sprouts	kohlrabi	spinach
beets	leeks	squash (summer)
broccoli	mixed vegetables (without	tomato (fresh, canned, sauce)
brussels sprouts	corn, peas, or pasta)	tomato/vegetable juice
cabbage	mushrooms, cooked	turnips
carrots	okra	waterchestnuts
cauliflower	onions	watercress
celery	pea pods	zucchini

Fruit Exchange List

FRUIT (15 g carbohydrate, 0 g protein, 0 g fat, 60 kcal)

1 fruit exchange equals:

1	apple (small)
4 rings	apple, dried
½ cup	applesauce (unsweetened)
4	apricots, fresh
8 halves	apricots, dried
1	banana (small)

¾ cup	blackberries
¾ cup	blueberries
⅓ melon	cantaloupe (small)
1 cup cubes	cantaloupe
12	cherries (3 oz)
½ cup	cherries, canned
3	dates
2	figs, fresh (3½ oz)
1½	figs, dried
½ cup	fruit cocktail
½	grapefruit
¾ cup	grapefruit sections
17	grapes (small)
1 slice	honeydew melon (or 1 cup cubes)
1	kiwi
¾ cup	mandarin orange sections
½	mango (or ½ cup cubes)
1	nectarine (small)
1	orange (small)
½	papaya (or 1 cup cubes)
1	peach, fresh (medium)
½ cup	peaches, canned
½	pear, fresh
½	pear, canned
¾ cup	pineapple, fresh
½ cup	pineapple, canned
2	plums (small)
½ cup	plums, canned
3	prunes, dried
2 tbsp	raisins
1 cup	raspberries
1¼ cup	strawberries (raw, whole)
2	tangerines
1 slice	watermelon (or 1¼ cups cubes)

FRUIT JUICE

½ cup	apple juice/cider
⅓ cup	cranberry juice cocktail
1 cup	cranberry juice cocktail, reduced-calorie
⅓ cup	fruit juice blends, 100% juice
⅓ cup	grape juice
½ cup	grapefruit juice
½ cup	orange juice
½ cup	pineapple juice
⅓ cup	prune juice

Starch Exchange List

(15 g carbohydrate, 3 g protein, 0-1 g fat, 80 kcal)
1 starch exchange equals:

BREAD

½ (1 oz)	bagel
2 slices (1½ oz)	bread, reduced-calorie
1 slice (1 oz)	bread, white, whole-wheat, pumpernickel, or rye
2 (⅔ oz)	bread sticks, crisp, 4 in. long × ½ in.
½	English muffin

½ (1 oz)	hot dog or hamburger bun
½	pita, 6 in. across
1 (1 oz)	roll, plain (small)
1 slice (1 oz)	raisin bread, unfrosted
1	tortilla, corn, 6 in. across
1	tortilla, flour, 7-8 in. across
1	waffle, 4½ in. square, reduced-fat

CEREALS AND GRAINS

½ cup	bran cereal
½ cup	bulgur
½ cup	cereal
¾ cup	cereal, unsweetened, read-to-eat
3 tbsp	cornmeal (dry)
⅓ cup	couscous
3 tbsp	flour (dry)
¼ cup	granola, low-fat
¼ cup	Grape-Nuts
½ cup	grits
½ cup	kasha
¼ cup	millet
¼ cup	muesli
½ cup	oats
½ cup	pasta
1½ cup	puffed cereal
½ cup	rice milk
⅓ cup	rice, white or brown
½ cup	Shredded Wheat
½ cup	sugar-frosted cereal
3 tbsp	wheat germ

STARCHY VEGETABLES

⅓ cup	baked beans
½ cup	corn
1 (5 oz)	corn on the cob (medium)
1 cup	mixed vegetables with corn, peas, or pasta
½ cup	peas, green
½ cup	plantain
1 (3 oz)	potato, baked or boiled (small)
½ cup	potato, mashed
1 cup	squash, winter (acorn, butternut)
½ cup	yam, sweet potato, plain

CRACKERS AND SNACKS

8	animal crackers
3	graham crackers, 2½ in. square
¾ oz	matzoh
4 slices	melba toast
24	oyster crackers
3 cups	popcorn (popped, no fat added or low-fat microwave)
¾ oz	pretzels
2	rice cakes, 4 in. across
6	saltine-type crackers
15-20 (¾ oz)	snack chips, fat-free (tortilla, potato)
2-5 (¾ oz)	whole-wheat crackers, no fat added

DRIED BEANS, PEAS, AND LENTILS

(counts as 1 starch exchange plus 1 very-lean-meat exchange)

½ cup	beans and peas (garbanzo, pinto, kidney, white, split, black-eyed).
⅔ cup	lima beans
½ cup	lentils
3 tbsp	miso

STARCHY FOODS PREPARED WITH FAT

(counts as 1 starch exchange plus 1 fat exchange)

1	biscuit, 2½ in. across
½ cup	chow mein noodles
1 (2 oz)	corn bread, 2 in. cube
6	crackers, round butter type
1 cup	croutons
16-25 (3 oz)	french-fried potatoes
¼ cup	granola
1 (1½ oz)	muffin (small)
2	pancakes, 4 in. across
3 cups	popcorn, microwave
3	sandwich crackers, cheese or peanut butter filling
⅓ cup	stuffing, bread (prepared)
2	taco shells, 6 in. across
1	waffle, 4½ in. square
4-6 (1 oz)	whole-wheat crackers, fat added

Other Carbohydrates Exchange List

One exchange equals 15 g carbohydrate, or 1 starch, or 1 fruit, or 1 milk

		Exchanges Per Serving
¹⁄₁₂th cake	angelfood cake, unfrosted	2 carbohydrates
2 in. square	brownie, unfrosted (small)	1 carbohydrate, 1 fat
2 in. square	cake, unfrosted	1 carbohydrate, 1 fat
2 in. square	cake, frosted	2 carbohydrates, 1 fat
2	cookies, fat-free (small)	1 carbohydrate
2	cookies or sandwich cookies with creme filling (small)	1 carbohydrate, 1 fat
1	cupcake, frosted (small)	2 carbohydrates, 1 fat
¼ cup	cranberry sauce, jellied	2 carbohydrates
1 (1½ oz)	doughnut, plain cake (medium)	1½ carbohydrates, 2 fats
3¾ in. across (2 oz)	doughnuts, glazed	2 carbohydrates, 2 fats
1 bar (3 oz)	fruit juice bars, frozen, 100% juice	1 carbohydrate
1 roll (¾ oz)	fruit snacks, chewy (puréed fruit concentrate)	1 carbohydrate
1 tbsp	fruit spread, 100% fruit	1 carbohydrate
½ cup	gelatin, regular	1 carbohydrate
3	gingersnaps	1 carbohydrate
1 bar	granola bar	1 carbohydrate, 1 fat
1 bar	granola bar, fat-free	2 carbohydrates
⅓ cup	hummus	1 carbohydrate, 1 fat
½ cup	ice cream	1 carbohydrate, 2 fats
½ cup	ice cream, light	1 carbohydrate, 1 fat
½ cup	ice cream, fat-free, no sugar added	1 carbohydrate
1 tbsp	jam or jelly, regular	1 carbohydrate
1 cup	milk, chocolate, whole	2 carbohydrates, 1 fat
⅙ pie	pie, fruit, 2 crusts	3 carbohydrates, 2 fats
⅛ pie	pie, pumpkin or custard	1 carbohydrate, 2 fats
12-18 (1 oz)	potato chips	1 carbohydrate, 2 fats

½ cup	pudding, regular (made with low-fat milk)	2 carbohydrates
½ cup	pudding, sugar-free (made with low-fat milk)	1 carbohydrate
¼ cup	salad dressing, fat-free	1 carbohydrate
½ cup	sherbet, sorbet	2 carbohydrates
½ cup	spaghetti or pasta sauce, canned	1 carbohydrate, 1 fat
1 (2½ oz)	sweet roll or Danish	2½ carbohydrates, 2 fats
2 tbsp	syrup, light	1 carbohydrate
1 tbsp	syrup, regular	1 carbohydrate
6-12 (1 oz)	tortilla chips	1 carbohydrate, 2 fats
⅓ cup	yogurt, frozen, low-fat or fat-free	1 carbohydrate, 0-1 fat
½ cup	yogurt, frozen, fat-free, no sugar added	1 carbohydrate
1 cup	yogurt, low-fat, with fruit	3 carbohydrates, 0-1 fat
5	vanilla wafers	1 carbohydrate, 1 fat

Meat and Meat Substitutes Exchange List

VERY-LEAN-MEAT AND SUBSTITUTES LIST (0 g carbohydrate, 7 g protein, 0-1 g fat, and 35 calories)

One very-lean-meat exchange equals:

Poultry:

1 oz chicken or turkey (white meat, no skin), Cornish hen (no skin)

Fish:

1 oz fresh or frozen cod, flounder, haddock, halibut, trout; tuna, fresh or canned in water

Shellfish:

1 oz clams, crab, lobster, scallops, shrimp, imitation shellfish

Game:

1 oz duck or pheasant (no skin), venison, buffalo, ostrich

Cheese with 1 g or less fat per ounce:

¼ cup nonfat or low-fat cottage cheese

1 oz fat-free cheese

Other:

1 oz processed sandwich meats with 1 g or less fat per ounce, such as deli thin, shaved meats, chipped beef, turkey ham

2 egg whites

¼ cup egg substitute, plain

1 oz hot dogs with 1 g or less fat per ounce

1 oz Kidney (high in cholesterol)

1 oz Sausage with 1 g or less fat per ounce

Counts as one very lean meat and one starch exchange:

½ cup dried beans, peas, lentils (cooked)

LEAN MEAT AND SUBSTITUTES LIST (0 g carbohydrate, 7 g protein, 3 g fat, and 55 calories)

One lean meat exchange equals:

Beef:

1 oz USDA Select or Choice grades of lean beef trimmed of fat, such as round, sirloin, and flank steak; tenderloin; roast (rib, chuck, rump); steak (T-bone, porterhouse, cubed), ground round

Pork:

1 oz lean pork, such as fresh ham; canned, cured, or boiled ham; Canadian bacon; tenderloin, center loin chop

Lamb:

1 oz roast, chop, leg

Veal:

1 oz lean chop, roast

	Poultry:
1 oz	chicken, turkey (dark meat, no skin), chicken white meat (with skin), domestic duck or goose (well-drained of fat, no skin)
	Fish:
1 oz	herring (uncreamed or smoked)
6	oysters (medium)
1 oz	salmon (fresh or canned), catfish
2	sardines (canned) (medium)
1 oz	tuna (canned in oil, drained)
	Game:
1 oz	goose (no skin), rabbit
	Cheese:
¼ cup	4.5%-fat cottage cheese
2 tbsp	grated Parmesan
1 oz	cheeses with 3 g or less fat per ounce
	Other:
1½ oz	hot dogs with 3 g or less fat per ounce
1 oz	processed sandwich meat with 3 g or less fat per ounce, such as turkey pastrami or kielbasa
1 oz	liver, heart (high in cholesterol)

MEDIUM-FAT MEAT AND SUBSTITUTES LIST (0 g carbohydrate, 7 g protein, 5 g fat, and 75 calories)

One medium-fat meat exchange equals:

	Beef:
1 oz	Most beef products fall into this category (ground beef, meatloaf, corned beef, short ribs, prime grades of meat trimmed of fat, such as prime rib)
	Pork:
1 oz	top loin, chop, Boston butt, cutlet
	Lamb:
1 oz	rib roast, ground
	Veal:
1 oz	cutlet (ground or cubed, unbreaded)
	Poultry:
1 oz	chicken dark meat (with skin), ground turkey or ground chicken, fried chicken (with skin)
	Fish:
1 oz	any fried fish product
	Cheese (with 5 g or less fat per ounce):
1 oz	feta
1 oz	mozzarella
¼ cup (2 oz)	ricotta
	Other:
1	egg (high in cholesterol, limit to 3 per week)
1 oz	sausage with 5 g or less fat per ounce
1 cup	soy milk
¼ cup	tempeh
4 oz or ½ cup	tofu

HIGH-FAT MEAT AND SUBSTITUTES LIST (0 g carbohydrate, 7 g protein, 8 g fat, and 100 calories)

One high-fat meat exchange equals:

	Pork:
1 oz	spareribs, ground pork, pork sausage
	Cheese:
1 oz	all regular cheeses, such as American cheddar, Monterey Jack, Swiss

Other:

1 oz	processed sandwich meats with 8 g or less fat per ounce, such as bologna, pimento loaf, salami
1 oz	sausage, such as bratwurst, Italian, knockwurst, Polish, snoked
1 (10/lb)	hot dog (turkey or chicken)
3 slices (20 slices/lb)	bacon

Counts as one high-fat meat plus one fat exchange:

1 (10/lb)	hot dog (beef, pork, or combination)
2 tbsp	peanut butter (contains unsaturated fat)

Fat Exchange List
MONOUNSATURATED FATS LIST (5 g fat and 45 calories)
One exchange equals:

⅛ (1 oz)	avocado (medium)
1 tsp	oil (canola, olive, peanut)
	olives:
8	ripe, black (large)
10	green, stuffed (large)
6 nuts	almonds, cashews
6 nuts	mixed (50% peanuts)
10 nuts	peanuts
4 halves	pecans
2 tsp	peanut butter, smooth or crunchy
1 tbsp	sesame seeds
2 tsp	tahini paste

POLYUNSATURATED FATS LIST (5 g fat and 45 calories)
One exchange equals:

	margarine:
1 tsp	stick, tub, or squeeze
1 tbsp	lower-fat (30% to 50% vegetable oil)
	mayonnaise:
1 tsp	regular
1 tbsp	reduced-fat
4 halves	nuts, walnuts, English
1 tsp	oil (corn, safflower, soybean)
	salad dressing:
1 tbsp	regular
2 tbsp	reduced-fat
	Miracle Whip Salad Dressing®:
2 tsp	regular
1 tbsp	reduced-fat
1 tbsp	seeds: pumpkin, sunflower

SATURATED FATS LIST (5 g fat and 45 calories)
One exchange equals:

1 slice (20 slices/lb)	bacon, cooked
1 tsp	bacon, grease
	butter:
1 tsp	stick
2 tsp	whipped
1 tbsp	reduced-fat
2 tbsp (½ oz)	chitterlings, boiled
2 tbsp	coconut, sweetened, shredded
2 tbsp	cream, half and half

	cream cheese:
1 tbsp (½ oz)	regular
2 tbsp (1 oz)	reduced-fat
	fatback or salt pork, see below†
1 tsp	shortening or lard
	sour cream:
2 tbsp	regular
3 tbsp	reduced-fat

†Use a piece 1 in. × 1 in. × ¼ in. if you plan to eat the fatback cooked with vegetables. Use a piece 2 in. × 1 in. × ½ in. when eating only the vegetables with the fatback removed.

Free Foods List

A *free food* is any food or drink that contains less than 20 calories or less than 5 g of carbohydrate per serving. Foods with a serving size listed should be limited to 3 servings per day. Foods listed without a serving size can be eaten as often as you like.

FAT-FREE OR REDUCED-FAT FOODS

1 tbsp	cream cheese, fat-free
1 tbsp	creamers, nondairy, liquid
2 tsp	creamers, nondairy, powdered
1 tbsp	mayonnaise, fat-free
1 tsp	mayonnaise, reduced-fat
4 tbsp	margarine, fat-free
1 tsp	margarine, reduced-fat
1 tbsp	Miracle Whip®, nonfat
1 tsp	Miracle Whip®, reduced-fat
	nonstick cooking spray
1 tbsp	salad dressing, fat-free
2 tbsp	salad dressing, fat-free, Italian
¼ cup	salsa
1 tbsp	sour cream, fat-free, reduced-fat
2 tbsp	whipped topping, regular or light

SUGAR-FREE OR LOW-SUGAR FOODS

1 candy	candy, hard, sugar-free
	gelatin dessert, sugar-free
	gelatin, unflavored
	gum, sugar-free
2 tsp	jam or jelly, low-sugar, or light
	sugar substitutes†
2 tbsp	syrup, sugar-free

†Sugar substitutes, alternatives, or replacements that are approved by the Food and Drug Administration (FDA) are safe to use. Common brand names include:
Equal® (aspartame)
Sprinkle Sweet® (saccharin)
Sweet One® (acesulfame K)
Sweet-10® (saccharin)
Sugar Twin® (saccharin)
Sweet `n Low® (saccharin)

DRINKS

	bouillon, broth, consommé
	bouillon or broth, low-sodium
	carbonated or mineral water
1 tbsp	cocoa powder, unsweetened
	coffee
	club soda
	diet soft drinks, sugar-free

	drink mixes, sugar-free
	tea
	tonic water, sugar-free

CONDIMENTS

1 tbsp	catsup
	horseradish
	lemon juice
	lime juice
	mustard
1½	pickles, dill (large)
	soy sauce, regular or light
1 tbsp	taco sauce
	vinegar

SEASONINGS

flavoring extracts
garlic
herbs, fresh or dried
pimento
spices
Tabasco® or hot pepper sauce
wine, used in cooking
worcestershire sauce

Combination Foods List

	Entrées:	**Exchanges Per Serving:**
1 cup (8 oz)	tuna noodle casserole, lasagna, spaghetti with meatballs, chili with beans, macaroni and cheese	2 carbohydrates, 2 medium-fat meats
2 cups (16 oz)	chow mein (without noodles or rice)	1 carbohydrate, 2 lean meats
¼ of 10 in. (5 oz)	pizza, cheese, thin crust	2 carbohydrates, 2 medium-fat meats, 1 fat
¼ of 10 in. (5 oz)	pizza, meat topping, thin crust	2 carbohydrates, 2 medium-fat meats, 2 fats
1 (7 oz)	pot pie	2 carbohydrates, 1 medium-fat meat, 4 fats
	Frozen entrées:	
1 (11 oz)	salisbury steak with gravy, mashed potato	2 carbohydrates, 3 medium-fat meats, 3-4 fats
1 (11 oz)	turkey with gravy, mashed potato, dressing	2 carbohydrates, 2 medium-fat meats, 2 fats
1 (8 oz)	entrée with less than 300 calories	2 carbohydrates, 3 lean meats
	Soups:	
1 cup	bean	1 carbohydrate, 1 very lean meat
1 cup (8 oz)	cream (made with water)	1 carbohydrate, 1 fat
½ cup (4 oz)	split pea (made with water)	1 carbohydrate
1 cup (8 oz)	tomato (made with water)	1 carbohydrate
1 cup (8 oz)	vegetable beef, chicken noodle, or other broth-type	1 carbohydrate

Fast (Quick-Service) Foods

		Exchanges Per Serving:
2	burritos with beef	4 carbohydrates, 2 medium-fat meats, 2 fats
6	chicken nuggets	1 carbohydrate, 2 medium-fat meats, 1 fat
1 each	chicken breast and wing, breaded and fried	1 carbohydrate, 4 medium-fat meats, 2 fats
1	fish sandwich/tartar sauce	3 carbohydrates, 1 medium-fat meat, 3 fats
20-25	french fries, thin	2 carbohydrates, 2 fats
1	hamburger (regular)	2 carbohydrates, 2 medium-fat meats
1	hamburger (large)	2 carbohydrates, 3 medium-fat meats, 1 fat
1	hot dog with bun	1 carbohydrate, 1 high-fat meat, 1 fat
1	individual pan pizza	5 carbohydrates, 3 medium-fat meats, 3 fats

Fast (Quick-Service) Foods—cont'd

		Exchanges Per Serving:
1	soft-serve cone (medium)	2 carbohydrates, 1 fat
1 sub (6 in.)	submarine sandwich	3 carbohydrates, 1 vegetable, 2 medium-fat meats, 1 fat
1 (6 oz)	taco, hard shell	2 carbohydrates, 2 medium-fat meats, 2 fats
1 (3 oz)	taco, soft shell	1 carbohydrate, 1 medium-fat meat, 1 fat

Dietary Intake and Energy Expenditure Assessment

Although it may seem overwhelming at first, it is actually very easy to track the foods you eat. One tip is to record foods and beverages consumed as soon as possible after the actual time of consumption.

I. Fill in the food record form that follows. We supply a blank copy (see the completed example on page G-3). Then, to estimate the nutrient values of the foods you are eating, consult food labels and the food composition table in Appendix A or use Mosby's NutriTrac nutrition software package. If these resources do not have the serving size you need, adjust the value. If you drink ½ cup of orange juice, for example, but a table has values only for 1 cup, halve all values before you record them. Then, consider pooling all the same food to save time; if you drink a cup of 1% milk three times throughout the day, enter your milk consumption only once as 3 cups. As you record your intake for use on the nutrient analysis form that follows, consider the following tips:

- Measure and record the amounts of foods eaten in portion sizes of cups, teaspoons, tablespoons, ounces, slices, or inches (or convert metric units to these units).
- Record brand names of all food products, such as "Quick Quaker Oats."
- Measure and record all those little extras, such as gravies, salad dressings, taco sauces, pickles, jelly, sugar, ketchup, and margarine.
- For beverages
  —List the type of milk, such as whole, skim, 2%, evaporated, chocolate, or reconstituted dry.
  —Indicate whether fruit juice is fresh, frozen, or canned.
  —Indicate type for other beverages, such as fruit drink, fruit-flavored drink, Kool-Aid, and hot chocolate made with water or milk.
- For fruits
  —Indicate whether fresh, frozen, dried, or canned.
  —If whole, record number eaten and size with approximate measurements (such as 1 apple—3 inches in diameter).
  —Indicate whether processed in water, light syrup, or heavy syrup.
- For vegetables
  —Indicate whether fresh, frozen, dried, or canned.
  —Record as portion of cup, teaspoon, or tablespoon, or as pieces (such as carrot sticks—4 inches long, ½ inch thick).
  —Record preparation method.
- For cereals
  —Record cooked cereals in portions of tablespoon or cup (a level measurement after cooking).
  —Record dry cereal in level portions of tablespoon or cup.
  —If margarine, milk, sugar, fruit, or something else is added, measure and record amount and type.
- For breads
  —Indicate whether whole wheat, rye, white, and so on.
  —Measure and record number and size of portion (biscuit—2 inches across, 1 inch thick; slice of homemade rye bread—3 inches by 4 inches, ¼ inch thick).
  —Sandwiches: list ALL ingredients (lettuce, mayonnaise, tomato, and so on).

- For meat, fish, poultry, and cheese
  —Give size (length, width, thickness) in inches or weight in ounces after cooking for meat, fish, and poultry (such as cooked hamburger patty—3 inches across, ½ inch thick).
  —Give size (length, width, thickness) in inches or weight in ounces for cheese.
  —Record measurements only for the cooked edible part—without bone or fat that is left on the plate.
  —Describe how meat, poultry, or fish was prepared.
- For eggs
  —Record as soft or hard cooked, fried, scrambled, poached, or omelet.
  —If milk, butter, or drippings are used, specify kinds and amount.
- For desserts
  —List commercial brand or "homemade" or "bakery" under brand.
  —Purchased candies, cookies, and cakes: specify kind and size.
  —Measure and record portion size of cakes, pies, and cookies by specifying thickness, diameter, and width or length, depending on the item.

Time	Minutes spent eating	M or S*	H† (0-3)	Activity while eating	Place of eating	Food and quantity	Others present	Reason for food choice

*M or S: Meal or snack
†Degree of hunger (0 = none; 3 = maximum).

TABLE G-1

One day's food record. This activity can help you understand more about your food habits.

Time	Minutes spent eating	M or S*	H†	Activity while eating	Place of eating	Food and quantity	Others present	Reason for choice
7:10 a.m.	15	M	2	standing, fixing lunch	kitchen	1 cup orange juice 1 cup raisin bran ½ cup 2% milk 2 tsp sugar Black coffee	—	health habit health taste habit
10:00 a.m.	4	S	1	sitting, taking notes	classroom	12 oz diet cola	class	weight control
12:15 p.m.	40	M	2	sitting, talking	student union	1 chicken sandwich with lettuce and mayonnaise 1 pear 1 cup 2% milk	friends	taste health health
2:30 p.m.	10	S	1	sitting, studying	library	12 oz regular cola	friend	hunger
6:30 p.m.	35	M	3	sitting, talking	kitchen	1 pork chop 1 baked potato 2 tbsp margarine Lettuce and tomato salad 2 tbsp ranch dressing ½ cup peas 1 cup whole milk 1 piece cherry pie	boyfriend	convenience health taste health taste health habit taste
9:10 p.m.	10	S	2	sitting, studying	living room	1 apple 1 glass mineral water	—	weight control weight control

*M or S: Meal or snack
†H: Degree of hunger (0 = none; 3 = maximum).

II. Now complete the nutrient analysis form as shown, using your food record. A blank copy of this form is printed at left for your use. Note that Mosby's NutriTrac software will create this table for you if you simply enter all food eaten.

Nutrient Analysis Form (Sample)

Name	Quantity	Kilocalories	Carbohydrates (g)	Protein (g)	Total fat (g)	Saturated fat (g)	Monounsaturated fat (g)	Polyunsaturated fat (g)	Dietary fiber (g)	Cholesterol (mg)	Folate (μg)	Vitamin A (RE)
Egg bagel, 3.5 inch diameter	1 ea.	180	34.7	7.45	1.00	0.171	0.286	0.400	0.748	44.0	16.3	7.00
Jelly	1 tbsp	49.0	12.7	0.018	0.018	0.005	0.005	0.005	—	—	2.00	0.200
Orange juice, prepared fresh or frozen	1½ cup	165	40.2	2.52	0.210	0.025	0.037	0.045	1.49	—	163	28.5
Cheeseburger, McDonald's	2 ea.	636	57.0	30.2	32.0	13.3	12.2	2.18	0.460	80.0	42.0	134
French fries, McDonald's	1 order	220	26.1	3.00	11.5	4.61	4.37	0.570	4.19	8.57	19.0	5.00
Cola beverage, regular	1½ cup	151	38.5	—	—	—	—	—	—	—	—	—
Pork loin chop, broiled, lean	4 oz.	261	—	36.2	11.9	4.09	5.35	1.43	—	112	6.77	3.15
Baked potato with skin	1 ea.	220	51.0	4.65	0.200	0.052	0.004	0.087	3.90	—	22.2	—
Peas, frozen, cooked	½ cup	63.0	11.4	4.12	0.220	0.039	0.019	0.103	3.61	—	46.9	53.4
Margarine, regular or soft, 80% fat	20 g	143	0.100	0.160	16.1	2.76	5.70	6.92	—	—	0.211	199
Iceberg lettuce, chopped	2 cup	14.6	2.34	1.13	0.212	0.028	0.008	0.112	1.68	—	62.8	37.0
French dressing	2 oz	300	3.63	0.318	32.0	4.94	14.2	12.4	0.431	—	—	0.023
2% low-fat milk	1 cup	121	11.7	8.12	4.78	2.92	1.35	0.170	—	22.0	12.0	140
Graham crackers	2 ea.	60.0	10.8	1.04	1.46	0.400	0.600	0.400	1.40	—	1.80	—
Totals		2584	300	99.0	112	33.4	44.1	24.8	17.9	266	395	607
RDA or minimal requirement*		2900		58						—	200	1000
% of RDA		89		170						—	198	61

*Values from inside cover. The values listed are for a male age 19 to 24 years. Note that number of kilocalories is just a rough estimate. It is better to base energy needs on actual energy output.

Vitamin B-6 (mg)	Vitamin B-12 (µg)	Vitamin C (mg)	Vitamin E (mg)	Riboflavin (mg)	Thiamin (mg)	Calcium (mg)	Iron (mg)	Magnesium (mg)	Niacin (mg)	Phosphorus (mg)	Potassium (mg)	Sodium (mg)	Zinc (mg)
0.030	0.065	—	1.80	0.197	2.58	20.0	2.10	18.0	2.40	61.0	65.0	300	0.612
0.005	—	0.710	0.016	0.005	0.002	2.00	0.120	0.720	0.036	1.00	16.0	4.00	—
0.165	—	145	0.714	0.060	0.300	33.0	0.411	36.0	0.750	60.0	711	3.00	0.192
0.230	1.82	4.10	0.560	0.480	0.600	338	5.68	45.8	8.66	410	314	1460	5.20
0.218	0.027	12.5	0.203	0.020	0.122	9.10	0.605	26.7	2.26	101	564	109	0.320
—	—	—	—	—	—	9.00	0.120	3.00	—	46.0	4.00	15.0	0.049
0.535	0.839	0.454	0.405	0.350	1.30	5.67	1.04	34.0	6.28	277	476	88.2	2.54
0.701	—	26.1	0.100	0.067	0.216	20.0	2.75	55.0	3.32	115	844	16.0	0.650
0.090	—	7.90	0.400	0.140	0.226	19.0	1.25	23.0	1.18	72.0	134	70.0	0.750
0.002	0.017	0.028	2.19	0.006	0.002	5.29	—	0.467	0.004	4.06	7.54	216	0.041
0.044	—	4.36	0.120	0.034	0.052	21.2	0.560	10.1	0.210	22.4	177	10.1	0.246
0.006	—		15.9	—	—	7.10	0.227	5.81	—	3.63	7.03	666	0.045
0.105	0.888	2.32	0.080	0.403	0.095	297	0.120	33.0	0.210	232	377	122	0.963
0.011	—	—		0.030	0.020	6.00	0.367	6.00	0.600	20.0	36.0	86.0	0.113
2.14	3.65	204	22.5	1.79	5.52	792	15.4	298	25.9	1425	3732	3165	11.7
2	2	60	10	1.7	1.5	1200	10	350	19	1200	2000	500	15
107	180	340	225	105	368	66	154	85	132	118	187	633	78

Nutrient Analysis Form (Sample)

Name	Quantity	Kilocalories	Carbohydrates (g)	Protein (g)	Total fat (g)	Saturated fat (g)	Monounsaturated fat (g)	Polyunsaturated fat (g)	Dietary fiber (g)	Cholesterol (mg)	Folate (μg)	Vitamin A (RE)
Totals												
RDA or minimal requirement*												
% of RDA												

*Values from inside cover. Note that number of kilocalories is just a rough estimate. It is better to base energy needs on actual energy output.

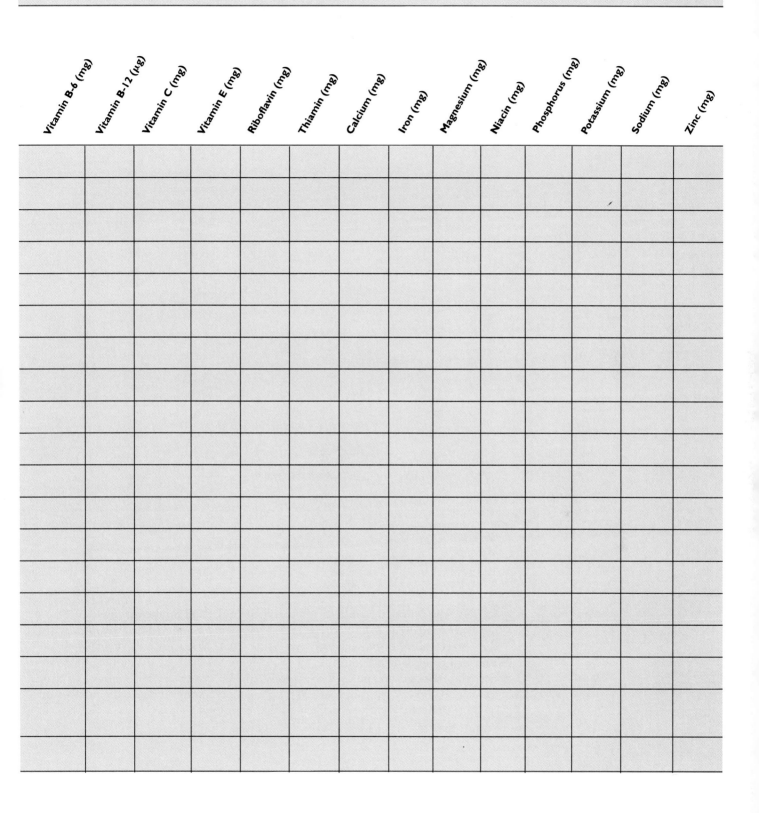

Vitamin B-6 (mg)	Vitamin B-12 (μg)	Vitamin C (mg)	Vitamin E (mg)	Riboflavin (mg)	Thiamin (mg)	Calcium (mg)	Iron (mg)	Magnesium (mg)	Niacin (mg)	Phosphorus (mg)	Potassium (mg)	Sodium (mg)	Zinc (mg)

III. Complete the following table as you summarize your dietary intake.

Percentage of kilocalories from protein, fat, carbohydrate, and alcohol

Intake
Protein (P):   _____ g/day × 4 kcal/g   =   (P)_____ kcal/day
Fat (F):   _____ g/day × 9 kcal/g   =   (F)_____ kcal/day
Carbohydrate (C):   _____ g/day × 4 kcal/g   =   (C)_____ kcal/day
Alcohol (A):   (A)_____ kcal/day*
                     Total kcal (T)/day   =   (T)_____ kcal/day

Percentage of kilocalories from protein:
$$\frac{(P)}{(T)} \times 100 = \underline{\quad} \% \text{ of total kilocalories}$$

Percentage of kilocalories from fat:
$$\frac{(F)}{(T)} \times 100 = \underline{\quad} \% \text{ of total kilocalories}$$

Percentage of kilocalories from carbohydrate:
$$\frac{(C)}{(T)} \times 100 = \underline{\quad} \% \text{ of total kilocalories}$$

Percentage of kilocalories from alcohol:
$$\frac{(A)}{(T)} \times 100 = \underline{\quad} \% \text{ of total kilocalories}$$

NOTE: The four percentages can total 99, 100, or 101, depending on the way in which figures were rounded off earlier.

*To calculate how many kilocalories in a beverage are from alcohol, look up the beverage in Appendix A. Determine how many kilocalories are from carbohydrate (multiply carbohydrate grams times 4), fat (fat grams times 9), and protein (protein grams times 4). The remaining kilocalories are from alcohol.

IV. Use the following table to again record your food intake for one day, placing each food item in the correct category of the Food Guide Pyramid, with the correct number of servings (see Table 2-1). Note that a food such as toast with margarine would contribute to two categories—namely, to the bread, cereal, rice, and pasta group and to the fats, oils, and sweets group. You can expect that many food choices will contribute to more than one group. Indicate the number of servings from the Food Guide Pyramid that each food yields.

Indicate the number of servings from the Food Guide Pyramid that each food yields

Food or beverage	Amount eaten	Milk, yogurt, and cheese	Meat, poultry, fish, dry beans, eggs, and nuts	Fruits	Vegetables	Bread, cereal, rice, and pasta	Fats, oils, and sweets
Group totals							
Recommended servings							in moderation
Shortages in numbers of servings							

V. Evaluation. Are there weaknesses suggested in your nutrient intake that correspond to missing servings in the Food Guide Pyramid? Consider replacing the missing servings to improve your nutrient intake.

VI. For the same day you keep your food record, also keep a 24-hour record of your activities. Include sleeping, sitting, and walking, as well as the obvious forms of exercise. Calculate your kilocalorie expenditure for these activities using Appendix K or Mosby's NutriTrac software. Try to substitute a similar activity if your particular activity is not listed. Calculate the total kilocalories you used for the day (total for column 3). Below is an example of an activity record. A blank form follows for your use. Ask your professor whether you are to turn in the form or the activity printout from the software.

Weight (lb or kg):

Energy Cost

Activity	Time (minutes); convert to hours	Column I kcal/hr (from App. K)	Column 2: time in hr	Column 3 (Column I × Column 2)
Example for a 150 lb man: Brisk walking	(30 min) 0.5 hr	299	0.5	150

Weight (lb or kg):

Energy Cost

Activity	Time (minutes); convert to hours	Column I kcal/hr (from table)	Column 2: time in hr	Column 3 (Column I × Column 2)
Total kilocalories expended (from adding all of column 3):				

Fatty Acids, Including Omega-3 Fatty Acids in Foods

Chain length, number, and site of double bonds for common fatty acids	
Common name of fatty acid	**Number of carbon atoms and number and site of double bond(s), counting from methyl end ($-CH_3$)**
Saturated fatty acids (no double bonds)	
Formic	1
Acetic	2
Propionic	3
Butyric	4
Valeric	5
Caproic	6
Caprylic	8
Capric	10
Lauric	12
Myristic	14
Palmitic	16
Stearic	18
Unsaturated fatty acids	
Oleic	18:1 (9-10) ω-9
Linoleic	18:2 (6-7, 9-10) ω-6
Alpha-linolenic	18:3 (3-4, 6-7, 9-10) ω-3
Arachidonic	20:4 (6-7, 9-10, 12-13, 15-16) ω-6
Eicosapentaenoic	20:5 (3-4, 6-7, 9-10, 12-13, 15-16) ω-3
Docosahexaenoic	22:6 (3-4, 6-7, 9-10, 12-13, 15-16, 18-19) ω-3

Fatty acid composition of selected foods*

Food item	<C12:0	Saturated C12:0	14:0	C16:0	C18:0	C18:1 ω-9	C18:2 ω-6	C18:3 ω-3	C20:5 ω-3	C22:6 ω-3
Fats and oils		Lauric acid	Myristic acid	Palmitic acid	Stearic acid	Oleic acid	Linoleic acid	Alpha-linolenic acid	EPA‡	DHA‡
Beef tallow	—	0.9	3.7	24.9	18.9	36.0	3.1	0.6	—	—
Butter	7.0	2.3	8.2	21.3	9.8	20.4	1.8	1.2	—	—
Cocoa butter	—	—	0.1	25.4	33.2	32.6	2.8	0.1	—	—
Corn oil	—	—	—	12.0	2.0	25.0	60.0	0.5	—	—
Cottonseed oil	—	—	0.8	22.7	2.3	17.0	51.5	0.2	—	—
Lard	0.1	0.2	1.3	23.8	13.5	41.2	10.2	1.0	—	—
Olive oil	—	—	—	13.0	2.5	74.0	9.0	0.5	—	—
Palm kernel oil	7.2	47.0	16.4	8.1	2.8	11.4	1.6	—	—	—
Palm oil	—	0.1	1.0	43.5	4.0	36.6	9.1	0.2	—	—
Safflower oil	—	—	—	6.5	2.5	11.5	79.0	0.5	—	—
Shortening§	0.2	0.4	0.4	19.3	9.9	50.6	13.5	0.6	—	—
Margarine, stick	2	1	10	23	9	31	7	1	—	—
Margarine, tub	1	1	1	12	8	22	52	1	—	—
Canola oil	—	—	—	5	1	62	22	9	—	—
Soybean oil	—	—	—	10	4	24	51	7	—	—
Coconut oil	14	45	17	8	3	6	2	—	—	—
Meat, fish, and poultry										
Beef, lean only, uncooked	—	—	0.17	1.4	0.74	2.4	0.2	0.01	—	—
Chicken, white meat, uncooked	—	—	0.01	0.3	0.1	0.3	0.2	0.01	0.01	0.02
Salmon, coho, raw	—	—	0.3	0.6	0.2	1.2	0.3	0.2	0.3	0.5
Tuna, light, canned in oil	—	—	0.03	1.4	0.1	2.8	2.7	0.07	0.03	0.1

*Only major fatty acids are presented.
†Values represent grams per 100 g edible portion.
‡EPA eicosapentaenoic acid ⎱ fish oil fatty acids
  DHA docosahexaenoic acid ⎰
§Soybean and palm oils, hydrogenated.
From USDA Agriculture Handbook No. 8-4.

Omega-3 fatty acids in foods

Food item	Edible portion, raw (grams/100 g)	Food item	Edible portion, raw (grams/100 g)
Fish oils		**Fats and oils—cont'd**	
Cod liver oil	19.2	Margarine, liquid, hydrogenated soybean oil, soybean oil, and cottonseed oil	2.4
Herring oil	12.0	Margarine, soft, hydrogenated soybean oil and cottonseed oil	1.6
Menhaden oil	21.7		
Salmon oil	20.9	Margarine, soft, hydrogenated soybean oil and palm oil	1.9
Finned fish		Margarine, soft, soybean oil, hydrogenated soybean oil, and hydrogenated cotton-seed oil	2.8
Anchovy, European	1.4		
Bluefish	1.2		
Dogfish, spiny	1.9	Rapeseed oil (canola)	11.1
Carp	0.6	Rice bran oil	1.6
Catfish	0.3	Salad dressing, commercial, blue cheese, regular	3.7
Cod	0.3		
Flounder	0.2	Salad dressing, commercial, Italian, regular	3.3
Halibut	0.9	Salad dressing, commercial, mayonnaise (imitation), soybean, without cholesterol	4.6
Herring, Atlantic	1.7		
Herring, Pacific	1.8	Salad dressing, commercial, mayonnaise, safflower and soybean	3.0
Mackerel, Atlantic	2.6		
Mackerel, king	2.2	Salad dressing, commercial, mayonnaise, soybean	4.2
Mullet, unspecified	1.1		
Perch	0.4	Salad dressing, commercial, mayonnaise-type	2.0
Sablefish	1.5		
Salmon, Atlantic	1.4	Salad dressing, commercial, Thousand Island, regular	2.5
Salmon, Chinook	1.5		
Scad, Muroaji	2.1	Salad dressing, home recipe, French	1.9
Shark	0.5	Salad dressing, home recipe, vinegar and soybean oil	1.4
Smelt	0.7		
Sprat	1.3	Shortening, special purpose, for bread, soybean (hydrogenated) and cottonseed	4.0
Sturgeon, Atlantic	1.5		
Swordfish	0.2	Shortening, special purpose, heavy-duty, frying, soybean (hydrogenated)	2.4
Trout, lake	2.0		
Tuna, albacore	1.5	Soybean lecithin	5.1
Tuna, bluefin	1.6	Soybean oil	6.8
Whitefish, lake	1.3	Walnut oil	10.4
Fats and oils		**Legumes**	
Butter	1.2	Soybeans, dry	1.6
Butter oil	1.5		
Chicken fat	1.0	**Nuts and seeds**	
Duck fat	1.0	Beechnuts, dried	1.7
Lard	1.0	Butternuts, fresh	1.7
Linseed oil	53.3	Butternuts, dried	8.7
Margarine, hard, soybean	1.5	Chia seeds, dried	3.9
Margarine, hard, soybean oil and hydro-genated soybean oil	1.9	Walnuts, black	3.3
		Walnuts, English/Persian	6.8
Margarine, hard, hydrogenated soybean oil and palm oil	2.3	**Vegetables**	
Margarine, hard, hydrogenated soybean oil and cottonseed oil	2.8	Soybeans, green, raw	3.2
		Soybeans, mature seeds, sprouted, cooked	2.1
Margarine, hard, hydrogenated palm oil	3.0		

From U.S. Department of Agriculture Human Nutrition Information Service: *Provisional tables on the content of omega-3 fatty acids and other fat components of selected foods,* HNIS/PT-103, 1988.

Metabolic Pathways—Glycolysis and the Citric Acid Cycle

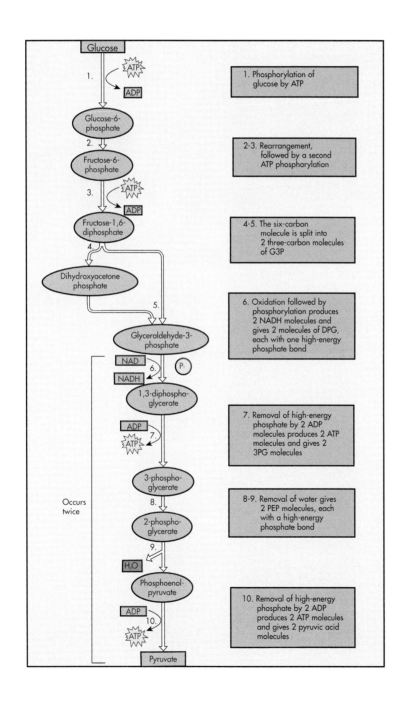

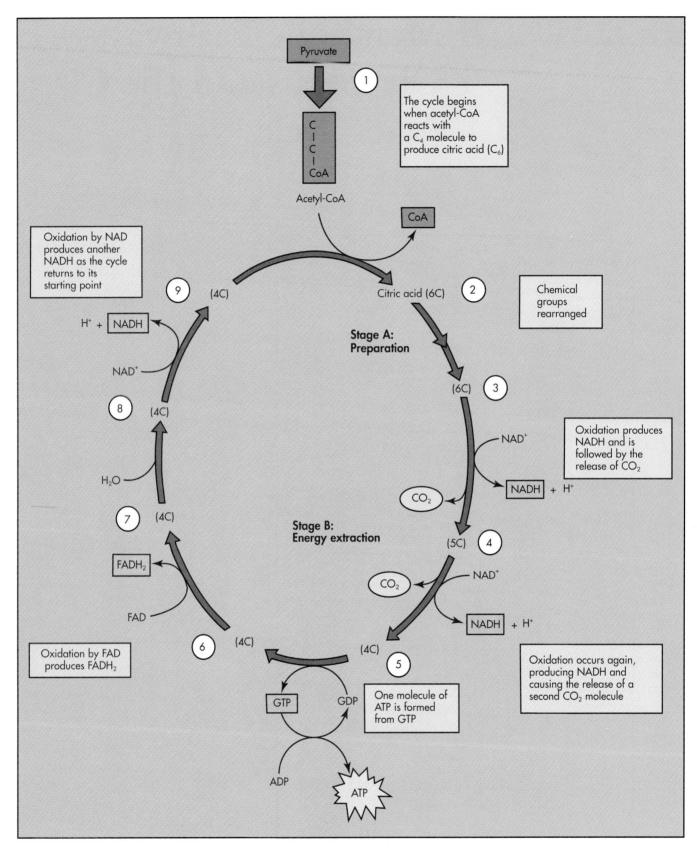

1. pyruvate
2. citrate
3. isocitrate
4. alpha-ketoglutarate
5. succinyl-CoA
6. succinate
7. fumarate
8. malate
9. oxaloacetate

Energy Cost of Various Activities

Activity	Body weight		
	120 pounds (54 kilograms) kcal/hour	150 pounds (68 kilograms) kcal/hour	180 pounds (82 kilograms) kcal/hour
Aerobics—heavy	435	544	653
Aerobics—medium	272	340	408
Aerobics—light	163	204	244
Backpacking	489	612	734
Badminton	277	346	416
Ballroom dancing	166	208	249
Basketball—vigorous	544	680	816
Bicycling (5.5 mph)	163	204	244
Bicycling (13 mph)	527	659	791
Billiards	108	136	163
Bowling	212	265	318
Calisthenics—heavy	435	544	653
Calisthenics—light	217	272	326
Canoeing (2.5 mph)	179	224	269
Carpentry—general	272	340	408
Circuit training	604	755	906
Cleaning (F)	202	253	303
Cleaning (M)	189	236	284
Climbing (100 ft/hr)	391	489	587
Cooking (F)	146	183	220
Cooking (M)	156	195	235
Disco dancing	326	408	489
Ditch digging—hand	315	394	473
Dressing/showering	85	106	128
Driving	93	117	140
Eating (sitting)	75	93	112
Fencing	239	299	359
Food shopping (F)	202	253	303
Food shopping (M)	189	236	284
Football—touch	380	476	571
Gardening	174	217	261
Gardening—digging	411	514	617
Gardening—raking	176	220	264
Golf	195	244	293
Horseback riding—trotting	277	346	416
Housework—cleaning	217	272	326
Ice skating (10 mph)	315	394	473
Jazzercize—heavy	435	544	653
Jazzercize—medium	272	340	408
Jazzercize—light	163	204	244
Jogging—medium	489	612	734

From *Nutritionist 3 software,* Salem, Ore, N-Squared Computing.   *Continued.*

Activity	Body weight		
	120 pounds (54 kilograms) kcal/hour	150 pounds (68 kilograms) kcal/hour	180 pounds (82 kilograms) kcal/hour
Jogging—slow	380	476	571
Judo	636	795	955
Lawn mowing (hand)	212	265	318
Lawn mowing (power)	195	244	293
Lying—at ease	71	89	107
Piano playing	130	163	195
Racquetball—social	435	544	653
Roller skating	277	346	416
Rowboating (2.5 mph)	239	299	359
Running or jogging (10 mph)	718	897	1077
Scull rowing (race)	669	836	1004
Sewing—hand	104	130	156
Shuffleboard/skeet	163	204	244
Sitting quietly	68	85	102
Skiing (10 mph)	478	598	718
Sleeping	64	80	97
Square dancing	277	346	416
Squash or handball	478	598	718
Swimming (.25 mph)	239	299	359
Table tennis	282	353	424
Tennis	331	414	497
Volleyball	277	346	416
Walking (2.5 mph)	163	204	244
Walking (3.75 mph)	239	299	359
Water skiing	380	476	571
Weightlifting—heavy	489	612	734
Weightlifting—light	217	272	326
Window cleaning (F)	192	240	288
Window cleaning (M)	189	236	284
Wood chopping/sawing	315	394	473
Writing (sitting)	94	118	142

Determination of Frame Size

METHOD 1

Height is recorded without shoes.

Wrist circumference is measured just beyond the bony (styloid) process at the wrist joint on the right arm, using a tape measure.

The following formula is used:

$$r = \frac{\text{height (cm)}}{\text{wrist circumference (cm)}}$$

Frame size can be determined as follows:

Males	Females
r > 10.4 small	r > 11 small
r = 9.6-10.4 medium	r = 10.1-11 medium
r < 9.6 large	r < 10.1 large

From Grant JP: *Handbook of Total Parenteral Nutrition*, Philadelphia, 1980, WB Saunders.

METHOD 2

The patient's right arm is extended forward perpendicular to the body, with the arm bent so the angle at the elbow forms 90 degrees, with the fingers pointing up and the palm turned away from the body. The greatest breadth across the elbow joint is measured with a sliding caliper along the axis of the upper arm, on the two prominent bones on either side of the elbow. This is recorded as the elbow breadth. The following tables give elbow breadth measurements for medium-framed men and women of various heights. Measurements lower than those listed indicate a small frame size; higher measurements indicate a large frame size.

Men		Women	
Height in 1″ heels	Elbow breadth	Height in 1″ heels	Elbow breadth
5′2″-5′3″	2½-2⅞	4′10″-4′11″	2¼-2½
5′4″-5′7″	2⅝-2⅞	5′0″-5′3″	2¼-2½
5′8″-5′11″	2¾-3	5′4″-5′7″	2⅜-2⅝
6′0″-6′3″	2¾-3⅛	5′8″-5′11″	2⅜-2⅝
6′4″ and over	2⅞-3¼	6′0″ and over	2½-2¾

From Metropolitan Life Insurance Co., 1983.

Caffeine Content of Foods

Beverages	mg
Carbonated beverages*	
Cherry Coke, Coca-Cola—12 fl oz (370 g)	46
cherry cola, Slice—12 fl oz (360 g)	48
Cherry RC—12 fl oz (360 g)	12
Coca-Cola—12 fl oz (370 g)	46
Coca-Cola Classic—12 fl oz (369 g)	46
Cola, RC—12 fl oz (360 g)	18
Mello Yello—12 fl oz (372 g)	52
Mr. Pibb—12 fl oz (369 g)	40
Mountain Dew—12 fl oz (360 g)	54
Dr. Pepper-type soda—12 fl oz (368 g)	37
Pepsi Cola—12 fl oz (360 g)	38
Carbonated beverages, low calorie*	
diet Cherry Coke, Coca-Cola—12 fl oz (354 g)	46
diet cherry cola, Slice—12 fl oz (360 g)	41
diet Coke, Coca-Cola—12 fl oz (354 g)	46
diet cola, aspartame-sweetened—12 fl oz (355 g)	50
diet Pepsi—12 fl oz (360 g)	36
diet RC—12 fl oz (360 g)	48
Pepsi Light—12 fl oz (360 g)	36
Tab—12 fl oz (354 g)	46
Coffee	
brewed—6 fl oz (177 g)	103
instant powder—1 tsp (1.8 g)	57
decaffeinated—1 rounded tsp (1.8 g)	2
with chicory—1 tsp (1.8 g)	37
prepared from instant powder—6 fl oz & 1 tsp powder (179 g)	57
amaretto, General Foods—6 fl oz & 11.5 g powder (189 g)	60
amaretto, sugar-free, General Foods—6 fl oz water & 7.7 g powder (185 g)	60
decaffeinated—6 fl oz water & 1 tsp powder (179 g)	2
Francais, General Foods—6 fl oz water & 11.5 g powder (189 g)	53
Francais, sugar-free, General Foods—6 fl oz water & 7.7 g powder (185 g)	59
Irish creme, General Foods—6 fl oz water & 12.8 g powder (190 g)	53
Irish creme, sugar free, General Foods—6 fl oz water & 7.1 g powder (185 g)	48
Irish mocha mint, General Foods—6 fl oz water & 11.5 g powder (189 g)	27
Irish mocha mint, sugar-free, General Foods—6 fl oz water & 6.4 g powder (189 g)	25

From Pennington JAT: *Bowes and Church's food values of portions commonly consumed,* ed 16, Philadelphia, 1993, JB Lippincott.

*Caffeine-free carbonated beverages and most noncola carbonated beverages contain no caffeine.

Continued.

Coffee—cont'd

orange cappuccino, General Foods—6 fl oz water & 14 g powder (191 g)	73
orange cappuccino, sugar-free, General Foods—6 fl oz water & 6.7 g powder (184 g)	71
Suisse mocha, General Foods—6 fl oz water & 11.5 g powder (189 g)	41
Suisse mocha, sugar-free, General Foods—6 fl oz water & 6.4 g powder (184 g)	40
Vienna, General Foods—6 fl oz water & 14 g powder (191 g)	56
Vienna, sugar-free, General Foods—6 fl oz water & 6.7 g powder (184 g)	55
with chicory—6 fl oz water & 1 tsp powder (179 g)	38

Tea, hot/iced

brewed 3 min—6 fl oz water (178 g)	36
instant powder—1 tsp (0.7 g)	31
with lemon flavor—1 rounded tsp (1.4 g)	25
with sugar & lemon flavor—3 tsp (23 g)	29
with sodium saccharin & lemon flavor—2 tsp (1.6 g)	36
prepared from instant powder	
1 tsp powder in 8 fl oz water (237 g)	31
Crystal Light—8 fl oz (238 g)	11
with lemon flavor—1 tsp powder in 8 fl oz water (238 g)	26
with sugar & lemon flavor—3 tsp powder in 8 fl oz water (259 g)	29
with sodium, saccharin & lemon flavor—2 tsp powder in 8 fl oz water (238 g)	36

Candy

chocolate	
German sweet, Bakers—1 oz square (28 g)	8
semi-sweet, Bakers—1 oz square (28 g)	13
chocolate chips	
Bakers—¼ cup (43 g)	12
German sweet, Bakers—¼ cup (43 g)	15
semi-sweet, Bakers—¼ cup (43 g)	14

Desserts
Frozen desserts

pudding pops, Jell-O	
chocolate—1 pop (47 g)	2
chocolate caramel swirl—1 pop (47 g)	1
chocolate fudge—1 pop (47 g)	3
chocolate vanilla swirl—1 pop (47 g)	2
chocolate with chocolate coating—1 pop (49 g)	3
double chocolate swirl—1 pop (47 g)	2
milk chocolate—1 pop (47 g)	2

Pies

chocolate mousse, from mix, Jell-O—⅛ pie (95 g)	6

Puddings, from instant mix

chocolate	
Jell-O—½ cup (150 g)	5
sugar-free, D-Zerta—½ cup (130 g)	4
sugar-free, Jell-O—½ cup (133 g)	4
chocolate fudge	
Jell-O—½ cup (150 g)	8
chocolate fudge mousse, Jell-O—½ cup (86 g)	12
chocolate mousse, Jell-O—½ cup (86 g)	9

Puddings, from instant mix—cont'd

chocolate tapioca, Jell-O—½ cup (147 g)	8
milk chocolate, Jell-O—½ cup (150 g)	5

Milk beverages

chocolate flavor mix in whole milk—2-3 tsp powder in 8 fl oz milk (266 g)	8
chocolate malted milk flavor powder	
in whole milk—3 tsp powder in 8 fl oz milk (265 g)	8
with added nutrients in whole milk—4-5 tsp powder in 8 fl oz milk (265 g)	5
chocolate syrup in whole milk—2 tbsp syrup in 8 fl oz milk (282 g)	6
cocoa/hot chocolate, prepared with water from mix—3-4 tsp powder in 6 fl oz water (206 g)	4

Milk beverage mixes

chocolate flavor mix, powder—2-3 tsp (22 g)	8
chocolate malted milk flavor mix, powder—¾ oz (3 tsp) (21 g)	8
chocolate malted milk flavor mix with added nutrients, powder—¾ oz (4-5 tsp) (21 g)	6
chocolate syrup—2 tbsp (1 fl oz) (38 g)	5
cocoa mix powder—1 oz pkt (3-4 tsp) (28 g)	5

Miscellaneous

baking chocolate, unsweetened, Bakers—1 oz (28 g)	25

Carotenoid Content of Selected Fruits and Vegetables

Fruit or vegetable (numbers apply to raw food unless otherwise indicated)	Total carotenoids* (μg)
Tomato juice, canned (1 cup)	23,546
Kale, cooked (⅔ cup)	22,610
Collard greens, cooked (⅔ cup)	18,445
Spinach, cooked, drained (½ cup)	15,385
Sweet potato, cooked (1)	12,848
Swiss chard, cooked (½ cup)	12,488
Watermelon (2 cups)	12,166
Spinach (1½ cups)	12,155
Pumpkin, canned (½ cup)	10,920
Mustard greens, cooked (⅔ cup)	10,710
Carrot (1)	9173
Beet greens, cooked (½ cup)	8724
Red pepper, raw or cooked (½)	7701
Apricots, dried (10 halves)	7386
Grapefruit, pink (½)	7195
Lettuce, romaine (1½ cups)	6460
Okra, cooked (½ cup)	5948
Celery, raw or cooked (2 stalks)	4741
Cantaloupe (¼)	4067
Peaches, dried (3 halves)	3878
Tomato, raw or cooked (½)	3162
Broccoli, cooked (½ cup)	2636
Lettuce, leaf (1½ cups)	2551
Ketchup (1 tbsp)	2267
Winter squash, cooked (½ cup)	2083
Green peas, cooked (½ cup)	1756
Lettuce, iceberg (1½ cups)	1601
Brussels sprouts, cooked (½ cup)	1518
Tomato sauce, canned (½ cup)	1488
Summer squash, cooked (½ cup)	1387
Green beans, cooked (⅔ cup)	1202
Asparagus (5 spears)	1021
Scallions (⅓ cup)	887
Plums (2)	884
Green pepper, raw or cooked (½)	800
Papaya (1 cup)	797
Yellow corn, cooked (1 ear)	793
Orange (1)	342
Kiwis (2)	330
Tangerines (2)	309

Continued.

Fruit or vegetable (numbers apply to raw food unless otherwise indicated)	Total carotenoids (µg)
Orange juice (1 cup)	276
Peaches (2)	271
Nectarine (1)	225
Pear (1)	211
Cucumber (⅓)	209
Cabbage, white, cooked (½ cup)	196
Grapes (1½ cups)	146
Raspberries (1 cup)	123
Prunes, dried (5)	116
Apple (1)	109
Avocado (⅙)	97
Strawberries (8)	62
Yellow onion (3 tbsp)	53
Blueberries (1 cup)	52
Grapefruit, white (½)	39
Cabbage, red (½ cup)	36
Cauliflower, cooked (⅔ cup)	35

*Note that fruits and vegetables contain various carotenoids. For example, alpha-carotene is abundant in orange vegetables. Beta-carotene is found widely in leafy vegetables, broccoli, carrots, and dried peaches and apricots. Lutein and zeaxanthin are found largely in green vegetables. Lycopene is especially plentiful in tomatoes, watermelon, and pink grapefruit.
From *Journal of the American Dietetic Association* 93:284, 1993.

Prenatal Weight Gain Chart

Prenatal Weight Gain Chart

Prepregnancy BMI <19.8 (·······). Prepregnancy BMI 19.8–26.0 (Normal Body Weight) (------), Prepregnancy BMI >26.0 (— — —)

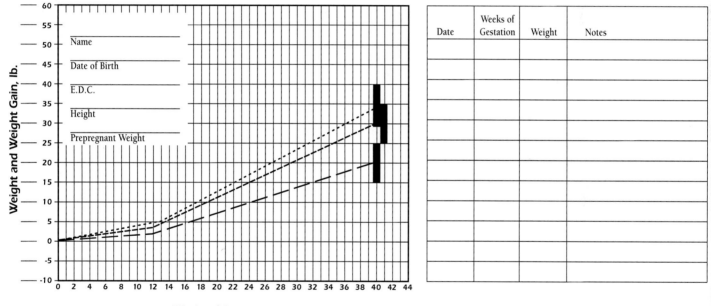

Date	Weeks of Gestation	Weight	Notes

Weeks of Pregnancy

From Institute of Medicine: *Nutrition during pregnancy and lactation: an implementation guide,* Washington, DC, 1992, National Academy Press. *E.D.C.,* Estimated date of conception.

Common Food Additives

Functions of some of the more than 2800 additives allowed in the U.S. food supply

Additive	Function	Additive	Function
A		**D**	
Acetic acid	pH control‡	Dehydrated beets	color
Acetone peroxide	mat-bleach-condit§	Dextrose	sweetener
Apidic acid	pH control‡	Diglycerides	emulsifier
Ammonium alginate	stabil-thick-tex*	Dioctyl sodium sulfosuccinate	emulsifier
Annatto extract	color	Disodium guanylate	flavor enhancer
Arabinogalactan	stabil-thick-tex*	Disodium inosinate	flavor enhancer
Ascorbic acid	nutrient	Dried algae meal	color
	preservative		
	antioxidant	**E**	
Azodicarbonamide	mat-bleach-condit§	EDTA (ethylenediamine tetraacetic acid)	antioxidant
B			
Benzoic acid	preservative	**F**	
Benzoyl peroxide	mat-bleach-condit§	FD&C Colors:	
Beta-apo-8′ carotenal	color	Blue No. 1	color
Beta carotene	nutrient	Red No. 3	color
	color	Red No. 40	color
BHA (butylated hydroxyanisole)	antioxidant	Yellow No. 5	color
BHT (butylated hydroxytoluene)	antioxidant	Fructose	sweetener
Butylparaben	preservative		
		G	
C		Gelatin	stabil-thick-tex*
Calcium alginate	stabil-thick-tex*	Glucose	sweetener
Calcium bromate	mat-bleach-condit§	Glycerine	humectant
Calcium lactate	preservative	Glycerol monostearate	humectant
Calcium phosphate	leavening†	Grape skin extract	color
Calcium silicate	anticaking‖	Guar gum	stabil-thick-tex*
Calcium sorbate	preservative	Gum arabic	stabil-thick-tex*
Canthaxanthin	color	Gum ghatti	stabil-thick-tex*
Caramel	color		
Carob bean gum	stabil-thick-tex*	**H**	
Carrageenan	emulsifier	Heptylparaben	preservative
	stabil-thick-tex*	Hydrogen peroxide	mat-bleach-condit§
Carrot oil	color	Hydrolyzed vegetable protein	flavor enhancer
Cellulose	stabil-thick-tex*		
Citric acid	preservative	**I**	
	antioxidant	Invert sugar	sweetener
	pH control‡	Iodine	nutrient
Citrus Red No. 2	color	Iron	nutrient
Cochineal extract	color	Iron-ammonium citrate	anticaking‖
Corn endosperm	color	Iron oxide	color
Corn syrup	sweetener		

From Lehmann P: *More than you ever thought you would know about food additives*, FDA Consumer reprint, Health and Human Services Publication No. (FDA) 79-2115, 1979.
Key to abbreviations: *stabil-thick-tex = stabilizers-thickeners-texturizers; †leavening = leavening agents; ‡pH control = pH control agents; §mat-bleach-condit = maturing and bleaching agents, dough conditioners; ‖anticaking = anticaking agents.

Additive	Function	Additive	Function
K		Sodium alginate	stabil-thick-tex*
Karaya gum	stabil-thick-tex*	Sodium aluminum sulfate	leavening†
		Sodium benzoate	preservative
L		Sodium bicarbonate	leavening†
Lactic acid	pH control‡	Sodium calcium alginate	stabil-thick-tex*
	preservative	Sodium citrate	pH control‡
Larch gum	stabil-thick-tex*	Sodium diacetate	preservative
Lecithin	emulsifier	Sodium erythrobate	preservative
Locust bean gum	stabil-thick-tex*	Sodium nitrate	preservative
		Sodium propionate	preservative
M		Sodium sorbate	preservative
Mannitol	sweetener	Sodium stearyl fumarate	mat-bleach-condit§
	anticaking‖	Sorbic acid	preservative
	stabil-thick-tex*	Sorbitan monostearate	emulsifier
Methylparaben	preservative	Sorbital	humectant
Modified food starch	stabil-thick-tex*		sweetener
Monoglycerides	emulsifier	Spices	flavor
MSG (monosodium glutamate)	flavor enhancer	Sucrose (table sugar)	sweetener
N		**T**	
Niacinamide (niacin)	nutrient	Tagetes (Aztec Marigold)	color
		Tartaric acid	pH control‡
P		TBHQ (tertiary butyl hydro-quinone)	antioxidant
Paprika (and oleoresin)	flavor		
	color	Thiamin	nutrient
Pectin	stabil-thick-tex*	Titanium dioxide	color
Phosphates	pH control‡	Toasted, partially defatted cooked cottonseed flour	color
Phosphoric acid	pH control‡		
Polysorbates	emulsifiers	Tocopherols (vitamin E)	nutrient
Potassium alginate	stabil-thick-tex*		antioxidant
Potassium bromate	mat-bleach-condit†	Tragacanth gum	stabil-thick-tex*
Potassium iodide	nutrient	Turmeric (oleoresin)	flavor
Potassium propionate	preservative		color
Potassium sorbate	preservative		
Propionic acid	preservative	**U**	
Propyl gallate	antioxidant	Ultramarine blue	color
Propylene glycol	stabil-thick-tex*	**V**	
	humectant		
Propylparaben	preservative	Vanilla, vanillin	flavor
		Vitamin A	nutrient
R		Vitamin C (ascorbic acid)	nutrient
Riboflavin	nutrient		preservative
	color		antioxidant
		Vitamin D (D-2, D-3)	nutrient
S		Vitamin E (tocopherols)	nutrient
Saccharin	sweetener	**Y**	
Saffron	color		
Silicon dioxide	anticaking‖	Yeast-malt sprout extract	flavor enhancer
Sodium acetate	pH control‡	Yellow prussiate of soda	anticaking‖

APPENDIX Q Sources of Nutrition Information

Consider the following reliable sources of food and nutrition information:

Journals that regularly cover nutrition topics:

American Family Physician*
American Journal of Clinical Nutrition
American Journal of Epidemiology
American Journal of Medicine
American Journal of Nursing
American Journal of Obstetrics and
    Gynecology
American Journal of Physiology
American Journal of Public Health
American Scientist
Annals of Internal Medicine
Annual Reviews of Medicine
Annual Reviews of Nutrition
Archives of Disease in Childhood
Archives of Internal Medicine
British Journal of Nutrition
BMJ (British Medical Journal)
Cancer
Cancer Research
Circulation
Diabetes
Diabetes Care
Disease-a-Month
FASEB Journal
FDA Consumer*
Food Chemical Toxicology
Food Engineering
Gastroenterology
Geriatrics
Gut
Human Nutrition: Applied Nutrition
Human Nutrition: Clinical Nutrition
Journal of the American College of
    Nutrition*

Journal of The American Dietetic Associa-
    tion*
Journal of The American Geriatric Society
JAMA (Journal of the American Medical
    Association)
Journal of Applied Physiology
Journal of Canadian Dietetic Association*
Journal of Clinical Investigation
Journal of Food Service
Journal of Food Technology
JNCI (Journal of the National Cancer In-
    stitute)
Journal of Nutrition
Journal of Nutritional Education*
Journal of Nutrition for the Elderly
Journal of Nutrition Research
Journal of Pediatrics
Lancet
Mayo Clinic Proceedings
Medicine and Science in Sports and
    Exercise
Nature
New England Journal of Medicine
Nutrition
Nutrition Reviews
Nutrition Today*
Pediatrics
The Physician and Sports Medicine
Postgraduate Medicine*
Proceedings of the Nutrition Society
Science
Science News*
Scientific American*

The majority of these journals are available in college or university libraries or in a specialty library on campus, such as one designated for health services or home economics. As indicated, a few journals will be filed under their abbreviations, rather than the first word in their full name. A reference librarian can help you locate any of these sources. The asterisked (*) journals are ones we think you will find especially interesting and useful because of the number of nutrition articles presented each month or the less technical nature of the presentation.

Magazines for the consumer that cover nutrition topics:

Better Homes and Gardens
Consumer Reports
Good Housekeeping

Health
Parents
Self

Textbooks and other sources for advanced study of nutrition topics:

Brody T: *Nutritional biochemistry,* San Diego, 1994, Academic Press.

Food and Nutrition Board: *Recommended dietary allowances,* ed 10, Washington, DC, 1989, National Academy of Sciences.

Groff JL, Gropper SS, Hunt SM: *Advanced human nutrition and metabolism,* St Paul, Minn, 1995, West.

International Life Sciences Institute: *Present knowledge in nutrition,* ed 6, 1990, The Nutrition Foundation.

Linder MC: *Nutritional biochemistry and metabolism with clinical applications,* New York, 1991, Elsevier Science Publishing.

Mahan LK, Arlin MT: *Krause's food, nutrition, and diet therapy,* Philadelphia, 1992, WB Saunders.

Murray RK and others: *Harper's biochemistry,* ed 21, Norwalk, Conn, 1993, Appleton & Lange.

Schils ME, Olson JA, Shike M: *Modern nutrition in health and disease,* ed 8, Philadelphia, 1994, Lea & Febiger.

Woteki CE, Thomas PR: *Eat for life,* Washington, DC, 1992, National Academy Press.

Newsletters that cover nutrition issues on a regular basis:

CNI Nutrition Week
Community Nutrition Institute
910 17th St. N.W., Suite 413
Washington, DC 20006

Dairy Council Digest
National Dairy Council
10255 West Higgins Road, Suite 900
Rosemont, IL 60018
(inexpensive)

Dietetic Currents
Ross Laboratories
Director of Professional Services
625 Cleveland Ave.
Columbus, OH 43216
(free)

Egg Nutrition Center
1819 H St. N.W., No. 510
Washington, DC 20009
(free)

Environmental Nutrition
52 Riverside Dr.
New York, NY 10024

Food and Nutrition News
National Livestock and Meat Board
444 Michigan Ave.
Chicago, IL 60611
(free)

Harvard Medical School Health Letter
Department of Continuing Education
25 Shattuck St.
Boston, MA 02115

Healthline
830 Menlo Ave. #100
Menlo Park, CA 94025

National Council Against Health Fraud
Newsletter (NCAHF)
P.O. Box 1276
Loma Linda, CA 92354

Nutrition Forum
George Stickley Co.
210 Washington Square
Philadelphia, PA 19106

Nutrition & the M.D.
Raven Press
1185 Avenue of the Americas
New York, NY 10036

Nutrition Research Newsletter
P.O. Box 700
Pallisades, NY 10964

Tufts University Diet & Nutrition Letter
P.O. Box 10948
Des Moines, IA 50940

University of California at Berkeley
Wellness Letter
P.O. Box 420148
Palm Coast, FL 32142

Professional organizations with a commitment to nutrition issues:

American Academy of Pediatrics
P.O. Box 1034
Evanston, IL 60204

American Cancer Society
90 Park Ave.
New York, NY 10016

American College of Sports Medicine
P.O. Box 1440
Indianapolis, IN 46204

American Dental Association
211 E. Chicago Ave.
Chicago, IL 60611

American Diabetes Association
2 Park Ave.
New York, NY 10016

American Dietetic Association
216 W. Jackson Blvd.
Suite 800
Chicago, IL 60606

American Geriatrics Society
770 Lexington Ave.
Suite 400
New York, NY 10021

American Heart Association
7272 Greenville Ave.
Dallas, TX 75231

American Home Economics Association
2010 Massachusetts Ave. N.W.
Washington, DC 20036

American Institute for Cancer Research
1759 R St. N.W.
Washington, DC 20009

American Institute of Nutrition
9650 Rockville Pike
Bethesda, MD 20014

American Medical Association
Nutrition Information Section
535 N. Dearborn St.
Chicago, IL 60610

American Public Health Association
1015 Fifteenth St. N.W.
Washington, DC 20005

American Society for Clinical Nutrition
9650 Rockville Pike
Bethesda, MD 20014

The Canadian Diabetes Association
123 Edwards St.
Suite 601
Toronto, Ontario M5G 1E2 Canada

The Canadian Dietetic Association
480 University Ave.
Suite 601
Toronto, Ontario M5G 1V2 Canada

The Canadian Society for Nutritional
  Sciences
Department of Foods and Nutrition
University of Manitoba
Winnipeg, Manitoba, R3T 2N2 Canada

Food and Nutrition Board
National Research Council
National Academy of Sciences
2101 Constitution Ave. N.W.
Washington, DC 20418

Institute of Food Technologies
221 N. LaSalle St.
Chicago, IL 60601

National Council on the Aging
1828 L St. N.W.
Washington, DC 20036

National Institute of Nutrition
1335 Carling Ave.
Suite 210
Ottawa, Ontario K1Z OL2 Canada

National Osteoporosis Foundation
1150 Seventeenth St. N.W., Suite 500
Washington, DC 20036

Nutrition Foundation, Inc.
1126 Sixteenth St. N.W.
Suite 111
Washington, DC 20036

Nutrition Today Society
428 E. Preston St.
Baltimore, MD 21202

Society for Nutrition Education
2001 Killebrew Dr., Suite 340
Minneapolis, MN 55425

Professional or lay organizations concerned with nutrition issues:

Bread for the World Institute
1100 Wayne Ave.
Silver Springs, MO 20910

California Council Against Health
  Fraud, Inc.
P.O. Box 1276
Loma Linda, CA 92354

Center for Science in the Public
  Interest (CSPI)
1875 Connecticut Ave. N.W.
Suite 100
Washington, DC 20009

Children's Foundation
1420 New York Ave. N.W.
Suite 800
Washington, DC 20005

Food Research and Action Center
  (FRAC)
1875 Connecticut Ave. N.W. #540
Washington, DC 20009

Institute for Food and Development
  Policy
1885 Mission St.
San Francisco, CA 94103

La Leche League International, Inc.
9616 Minneapolis Ave.
Franklin Park, IL 60131

March of Dimes Birth Defects Foundation
(National Headquarters)
1275 Mamaroneck Ave.
White Plains, NY 10605

Overeaters Anonymous (OA)
2190 190th St.
Torrance, CA 90504

Oxfam America
115 Broadway
Boston, MA 02116

Local resources for advice on nutrition issues:

Cooperative extension agents in county extension offices
Dietitians (Contact the state or local Dietetics Association.)
Nutrition faculty affiliated with departments of food and nutrition, home economics,
  and dietetics
Registered Dietitians (RDs) in city, county, or state agencies

**Government agencies that are concerned with nutrition issues
or that distribute nutrition information:**

United States
The Consumer Information Center
Department 609K
Pueblo, CO 81009

Food and Drug Administration (FDA)
5600 Fishers Lane
Rockville, MD 20852

Food and Nutrition Information and
  Education Resources Center
National Library of Congress
Beltsville, MD 20705

Human Nutrition Research Division
Agricultural Research Center
Beltsville, MD 20705

National Center for Health Statistics
3700 East-West
Hyattsville, MD 20782

National Heart, Lung, and Blood Institute
9000 Rockville Pike, Building 31,
  Room 4A21
Bethesda, MD 20892

National Institute on Aging
Information Office
Building 31, Room 5C35
Bethesda, MD 20205

Office of Cancer Communications
National Cancer Institute
Building 31, Room 10A18
90 Rockville Pike
Bethesda, MD 20205

USDA, Agricultural Research Service
6505 Belcrest Rd., Room 344
Hyattsville, MD 20782

USDA, Food Safety & Inspection Service
Room 1180 South, 14th and
  Independence Ave. S.W.
Washington, DC 20250

U.S. Government Printing Office
The Superintendent of Documents
Washington, DC 20402

Canada
Department of Community Health
1075 Ste-Foy Rd.
Quebec, Quebec G1S 2M1

Health and Welfare Canada
Canadian Government Publishing Center
Minister of Supply and Services
Ottawa, Ontario K1A 0S9

Home Economics Directorate
880 Portage Ave.
Second Floor
Winnipeg, Manitoba R3G 0P1

Nutrition Programs
446 Jeanne Mance Building
Tunney's Pasture
Ottawa, Ontario K1A 1B4

Nutrition Services
P.O. Box 488
Halifax, Nova Scotia B3J 3R8

Nutrition Services
P.O. Box 6000
Fredericton, New Brunswick E3B 5H1

Public Health Resource Service
15 Overlea Blvd.
Fifth Floor

Toronto, Ontario M4H 1A9
United Nations
Food and Agriculture Organization
   (FAO)
North American Regional Office
1001 22nd St. N.W.
Washington, DC 20437
or
Via della Terma di Caracella
0100 Rome, Italy

World Health Organization (WHO)
1211 Geneva 27
Switzerland

Trade organizations and companies that distribute nutrition information:

American Institute of Baking
P.O. Box 1148
Manhattan, KS 66502

American Meat Institute
P.O. Box 3556
Washington, DC 20007

Beech-Nut Nutrition Corporation
Booth 1414
Checkerboard Square
St. Louis, MO 63164

Best Foods
Consumer Service Department
Division of CPC International
International Plaza
Englewood Cliffs, NJ 07632

Campbell Soup Co.
Food Service Products Division
Campbell Plaza
Camden, NJ 08103

Continental Baking Company
Checkerboard Square
St. Louis, MO 63164

The Dannon Company, Inc.
120 White Plains Rd.
Tarrytown, NY 10591-5536

Del Monte Foods
One Market Plaza
San Francisco, CA 94105

Fleischman's Margarines
Standard Brands, Inc.
625 Madison Ave.
New York, NY 10022

General Foods Consumer Center
250 North St.
White Plains, NY 10625

General Mills
P.O. Box 1113
Minneapolis, MN 55440

Gerber Products Co.
445 State St.
Fremont, MI 49413

H.J. Heinz
Consumer Relations
P.O. Box 57
Pittsburgh, PA 15230

Idaho Potato Commission
P.O. Box 1968
Boise, ID 83701

Kellogg Co.
Department of Home Economics Services
Battle Creek, MI 49016

Kraft General Foods
Three Lakes Dr.
Northfield, IL 60093

Mead Johnson Nutritionals
2404 Pennsylvania Ave.
Evansville, IN 47721

National Dairy Council
10255 W. Higgins Rd.
Rosemont, IL 60018-4233

The NutraSweet Company
1751 Lake Cook Rd.
Deerfield, IL 60015

Pillsbury Co.
1177 Pillsbury Building
608 Second Ave. S.
Minneapolis, MN 55402

Rice Council
P.O. Box 740123
Houston, TX 77274

Ross Laboratories
Director of Professional Services
625 Cleveland Ave.
Columbus, OH 43216

Sunkist Growers, Inc.
14130 Riverside Dr.
Sherman Oaks, CA 91423

United Fresh Fruit and Vegetables
  Association
727 N. Washington St.
Alexandria, VA 22314

Vitamin Nutrition Information Service
  (VNIS)
Hoffmann-LaRoche
340 Kingsland Ave.
Nutley, NJ 07110

Answers to Nutrition Awareness Inventories

CHAPTER 1

1. *True*. Water is a large component of many foods, even meats.

2. *False*. Minerals cannot be further broken down or converted into other substances by ordinary chemical means.

3. *False*. Kilocalories (kcal) are 1000-calorie units. Although most people talk about energy units as calories, what they really mean is kilocalories (kcal). As a nutrition student, you need to be aware of the proper term.

4. *True*. One gram of protein yields 4 kcal, 1 g of carbohydrate 4 kcal, 1 g of fat 9 kcal, and 1 g of alcohol 7 kcal.

5. *False*. Vitamins provide no energy value in and of themselves. They merely aid in certain energy-yielding reactions.

6. *True*. When nutrient intake does not meet nutrient needs, nutrient stores can be used, such as calcium found in bones. However, as these stores are depleted, serious health problems can eventually result.

7. *False*. Many minerals, such as calcium and magnesium, are required in much larger amounts than vitamins, for example, grams versus milligrams.

8. *False*. Water has no capacity to yield a metabolizable energy source in the body. Do not confuse this fact with the definition of the heat measurement unit, the kcal, which uses water.

9. *False*. *Organic* refers to compounds containing carbon atoms bonded to hydrogen atoms. The term has nothing to do with organic gardening.

10. *False*. Malnutrition represents a poor nutrition state due to either an excess or an insufficient nutrient intake. Undernutrition represents an insufficient nutrient intake.

11. *True*. In a person severely deficient in iron, weakness is common and temperature control may be altered, causing the person to feel cold.

12. *True*. Five of the ten leading causes of death in our society are strongly linked to overnutrition—primarily kcal, fat, sodium, and alcohol.

13. *False*. Vitamins A and D and minerals such as iron and zinc can be harmful if taken in large amounts for long periods of time.

14. *True*. In fact, alcoholic beverages are the third leading contributor to energy intake for adults in the United States.

15. *False*. Food choices are most often determined by taste and habit. Nutrition knowledge is not scarce, but it sometimes seems that way in everyday life!

CHAPTER 2

1. *True*. These are the substances provided by foods that are necessary for life.

2. *False*. Children need to be in positive protein balance, in which intake exceeds output, in order to grow.

3. *False*. Few healthy people need vitamin and mineral supplements in order to meet nutrient needs set by RDAs (see Chapter 12 for details).

4. *False*. FDA now carefully regulates health claims appearing on food packages.

5. *False*. Most adults fail to meet the fruit and vegetable recommendations, for example.

6. *False*. RDA is the abbreviation for recommended *dietary* allowances.

7. *False*. No nutrient is absolutely required daily. You can maintain health for a few days on a diet free of water (fluid), and about 10 days on a diet free of the vitamin thiamin.

8. *True*. While nutrient recommendations are often similar, groups of scientists from different countries may disagree with each other. In addition, the type of diet consumed influences nutrient needs, such as higher vitamin B-6 needs arising from higher protein intake.

9. *False*. The RDAs form a recommendation only for group needs. They do not necessarily provide personal nutrient requirements, but provide a reasonable guide for diet construction.

10. *False*. Active people are likely to require closer to 2200 to 2800 kcal or more to meet energy needs.

11. *True*. Potatoes and bread have very similar carbohydrate:protein:fat ratios.

12. *True*. The Exchange System relieves us of having to memorize the composition of all foods: rather, it is a powerful tool for quickly and conveniently estimating the energy, protein, carbohydrate, and fat content of a food or meal.

13. *True*. Nutrient density is an important concept, especially for people on a low-kilocalorie diet. It refers to the ratio of a food's nutrient content to its energy content.

14. *True*. Nutrient content is expressed as a percentage of Daily Values (DVs). Daily Values are set by FDA for use on food labels, using the 1968 RDAs as a guideline.

15. *True*. No one food contains all the nutrients needed to maintain good health. Milk, for example, is low in iron, while eggs are low in calcium.

CHAPTER 3

1. *True*. Glucose combined with fructose forms sucrose, or table sugar.

2. *True*. Starch is the storage form of carbohydrate in plants. Glycogen is the storage form of carbohydrate in animals. The amount of glycogen present in meat that comes to the table is so small that it is not a food source of carbohydrate.

3. *False*. In comparison to fat, carbohydrate contains less energy per gram (4 kcal/g for carbohydrate versus 9 kcal/g for fat).

4. *True*. Carbohydrates are important energy-supplying nutrients.

5. *True*. Fiber is referred to as *roughage* or *bulk*, but *dietary fiber* is the preferred term.

6. *False*. There is no RDA for carbohydrate per se. However, we do need at least 50 to 100 g/day to prevent the body from breaking down its own protein to make glucose. About 55% of energy intake should come from carbohydrate.

7. *False*. Fiber mostly contributes to the health of the large intestine; it provides little energy for the body.

8. *True*. Sugars are fermented to acid in the mouth; the acid erodes the teeth. The frequency and form of the sugars eaten are especially important, more so than the total amount of sugars consumed.

9. *True*. When eaten in excess of energy needs, carbohydrates are stored to some extent as fat, but mostly as glycogen.

10. *False*. Almost all bread, including white bread, contains wheat flour, and so is wheat bread. It is whole-wheat flour that includes the fiber portion of the grain.

11. *True*. Sugar intake represents about 18% of total energy intake. Only 10% to 15% of energy intake should be from sugar, in order to allow for more healthful foods in the diet.

12. *True*. Honey may contain bacterial spores of *Clostridium botulinum*. These can grow in the infant's stomach and become fatal because an infant's stomach has yet to develop the strong acidic environment of an adult stomach. Acid reduces the harmful bacterium's growth.

13. *False*. Diabetes is a disorder of high blood glucose.

14. *False.* There is scant corroborating evidence for these theories. Sugars do have a low nutrient density, and energy intake from these may replace foods that contain essential nutrients. This is the main problem with foods rich in sugars in our diets, along with dental caries.

15. *True.* This was observed by Dr. Denis Burkitt, who attributes this phenomenon to the high dietary fiber intakes of Africans as compared with our society.

CHAPTER 4

1. *True.* Polyunsaturated fats are liquid at room temperature. Thus vegetable oils are liquid at room temperature.

2. *True.* Fats yield 9 kcal/g, while carbohydrates and proteins yield 4 kcal/g.

3. *False.* While serum cholesterol helps predict the risk of heart disease, knowing the LDL value and the ratio of total cholesterol to HDL cholesterol is more important.

4. *True.* Plants we eat do not produce cholesterol.

5. *True.* Animal fats are rich sources of the saturated fatty acids that raise serum cholesterol.

6. *True.* Triglyceride is the primary form of fat (lipid) in foods and in the body.

7. *False.* A small amount of certain types of fat in the diet is absolutely necessary for life because these supply essential fatty acids used to make vital body compounds.

8. *True.* By adding hydrogen to oils, the oils become solid at room temperature. In some cases this makes food production easier; hydrogenation also prevents the oils in many foods from turning rancid in transit and storage.

9. *True.* Most fruits and vegetables contain only traces of fat. Avocados and olives are exceptions.

10. *True.* BHA and BHT are examples of antioxidants found in salad dressings that reduce rancidity of fats. Vitamin E does the same in the body.

11. *True.* Vitamins A, E, D, and K are fat soluble, and their absorption is enhanced by dietary fat.

12. *False.* Everyone age 20 years or more should monitor and track his or her serum cholesterol. Some groups recommend that anyone over 2 years old who has a family history of early heart disease should do the same. Certain elevated blood lipoprotein values are risk factors for heart disease.

13. *True.* Butter and margarine contain the same number of kilocalories. Butter, however, contains more saturated fat than margarine, especially tub (soft) margarine.

14. *True.* The hydrogenated fats used in the fryers are rich in trans fatty acids. These raise serum cholesterol, as do most saturated fatty acids.

15. *True.* Dietary cholesterol has less of an effect on serum cholesterol than does saturated fat. Still, most health authorities suggest that we moderate intake of both.

CHAPTER 5

1. *False.* Most Americans eat such a varied assortment of food that if enough energy is consumed, it is difficult not to have a high-quality protein diet: a diet that contains enough of all nine essential amino acids.

2. *True.* Protein is particularly important for building new tissue during periods of rapid growth, such as in childhood.

3. *True.* Only a few enzymes are composed of other compounds.

4. *True.* Insulin, as an example, contains only amino acids in its structure.

5. *True.* Biological value represents the body's ability to retain the protein absorbed—a good measure of protein quality.

6. *True.* Milk proteins provide one of the highest possible biological values from foods. Egg white has the very highest biological value of any food.

7. *False.* More protein per pound of body weight is required during periods of growth, as in infancy.

8. *False.* All of us, including athletes, can meet our protein needs with basic foods, and rarely is an intake greater than twice the RDA necessary.

9. *True.* For this reason, trimming fat from meats and broiling them are good ideas to reduce saturated fat intake. Vegetable sources, such as legumes, provide protein without much fat, unless fat is added during preparation.

10. *True.* Although a lack of endurance can be caused by other things, it is a symptom of severe protein deficiency.

11. *False.* Gelatin is a low-quality protein; it lacks several of the essential amino acids, and thus cannot strengthen fingernails.

12. *True.* Starvation in infancy leads to marasmus, which means "to waste away." This is seen in famine conditions.

13. *False.* Plant proteins contain much dietary fiber and magnesium; in comparison, animal proteins supply the most absorbable form of iron and vitamin B-6.

14. *True.* Water-packed tuna contains about 85% of food energy as protein.

15. *True.* Fruits contain little protein; fruits are composed mostly of carbohydrate and water.

CHAPTER 6

1. *False.* For many foods, some digestion actually begins during cooking, when protein structures unfold, starch granules swell, and tough vegetable fibers are softened.

2. *True.* Water-soluble nutrients use a special portal vein that connects the intestinal tract to the liver. Many nutrients can enter the bloodstream only after passing through the liver; fats are the main exception.

3. *True.* A living person's small intestine is approximately 10 feet long; at autopsy it is approximately 23 feet long.

4. *False.* It is the acid produced by the stomach, not the mucus, that is responsible for killing most of the bacteria that enter the stomach.

5. *True.* The term *colon* also refers to the large intestine.

6. *False.* The digestive enzymes work efficiently no matter what combination of foods is eaten. Fruit and meat can be eaten together without fear of poor digestion.

7. *True.* Stomach enzymes require an acid pH for maximum activity, whereas the small intestine has a more neutral pH.

8. *False.* The cells that line the walls of the small intestine would be unable to effectively absorb nutrients through a thick mucus layer (like that of the stomach). The mechanism by which the small intestine is protected is the presence of the pyloric sphincter, which regulates the influx of stomach contents to the intestine. In addition, the pancreas secretes bicarbonate, a substance that neutralizes the stomach acid entering the small intestine.

9. *True.* Although bile is not required for the digestion of proteins and starches, it is absolutely essential for the efficient digestion, emulsification, and absorption of fats (especially long-chain fatty acids).

10. *False.* The liver, the pancreas, and the gallbladder all play key roles in digestion, but they are not part of the direct path taken by nutrients through the body.

11. *False.* The overwhelming amount of absorption (nearly 95%) takes place in the small intestine. The large intestine serves in only limited absorption of minerals, water, and bacterial by-products, such as vitamin K, the vitamin biotin, and short-chain fatty acids from fiber fermentation.

12. *True.* The sugar glucose is absorbed from the small intestine into the blood against a concentration gradient. Much glucose from the blood is present in the cells of the intestine. So energy must be expended if more glucose from the intestinal tract is to enter the intestinal cells. Conversely, the concentration of fat in the intestinal cells is low, allowing fat to be passively absorbed into them.

13. *True.* The peristaltic waves that propel food through the intestinal tract require a coordination of muscles, including both longitudinal muscles (which lie lengthwise down the intestinal tract) and circular muscles (which surround the intestinal tract).

14. *True.* Many undigested foods that enter the large intestine are nutrient sources for bacteria found there. The bacteria then make a variety of products, including various gases.

15. *False.* Only the large intestine contains much bacteria. In the stomach, bacterial growth is hampered by the gastric acids. The ileocecal sphincter that regulates the influx of contents from the small intestine into the large intestine also serves to prevent the prominent bacterial growth within the large intestine from moving into the small intestine. If these bacteria were able to enter the small intestine, they would compete for the nutrients and create problems with fat digestion.

CHAPTER 7

1. *True.* Carbohydrates provide both energy for the body and carbons that can be synthesized into fat.

2. *True.* Fat can be stored in adipose tissue for future energy needs or used for energy by cells, such as muscle cells.

3. *False.* The carbons in protein can become the carbons of fat; high-protein diets can be fattening.

4. *True.* The brain uses glucose primarily for energy. Ketone bodies can be used under special circumstances, such as in cases of semi-starvation.

5. *True.* Ketones increase in the blood during fasting, partly because the liver is engaged in gluconeogenesis and is prevented from metabolizing fat efficiently. Ketones are synthesized from breakdown products of fatty acids.

6. *False.* The carbons in alcohol can become the carbons of fat.

7. *True.* These vitamins form coenzymes used in metabolism, such as niacin forming NAD and riboflavin forming FAD.

8. *True.* The removal of amino groups from amino acids (deamination) requires vitamin B-6.

9. *True.* Both iron and copper participate in the electron transport chain. This is where most ATP is made in a cell.

10. *False.* Carnitine is used to shuttle fatty acids, not carbohydrates, into a cell's mitochondria for energy metabolism.

11. *False.* Ketones are primarily formed from acetyl-CoA, a breakdown product of fatty acids. Glycerol can form acetyl-CoA, but there is not enough glycerol in our diets to be of nutritional importance.

12. *True.* Mitochondria are the major sites of ATP production in the cell.

13. *True.* Carbons of carbohydrate, fat, protein, and alcohol molecules can all become the carbons of acetyl-CoA. This compound then has a pivotal role in energy metabolism. In essence, all roads can lead to acetyl-CoA.

14. *True.* Using photosynthesis, plants trap solar energy and store it in the chemical bonds of glucose and other organic compounds.

15. *True.* Once glycogen stores are depleted in fasting, body proteins are degraded to provide building blocks for glucose. The glycerol portion of the fat molecule can also be used in gluconeogenesis, but it represents only a small amount of the glucose produced.

CHAPTER 8

1. *True.* Signals that the liver is metabolizing absorbed nutrients contribute to the satiety signals sensed in the brain.

2. *True.* At the beginning of a meal, people usually choose a variety of foods. At the end of a meal, choices narrow and sweet food choices often predominate.

3. *False.* Adipose cell size may be involved with the regulation of eating week-to-week and month-to-month. It is only slightly involved in long-term hunger regulation, if at all.

4. *False.* The RDA represents an average energy need for a person performing light activity. The range given may or may not accurately estimate an individual's energy needs.

5. *True.* To keep a resting body alive, heart rate, respiration, body temperature, and other functions must be maintained. The energy used represents basal or resting metabolism, depending on the conditions in which it is measured.

6. *False.* Brown adipose tissue mostly disappears between infancy and adulthood. Its role in the average adult is unclear, but is likely of minor importance, whereas it is more important in infancy.

7. *False.* In general, obesity increases the risk for health problems and reduces life expectancy. The greater the obesity, the greater the effect it has on life expectancy. Occasionally a person may escape the health problems associated with obesity, but most people do not.

8. *True.* Your body weight may be greater than a desirable figure, as determined using the Metropolitan Life Insurance Table, but excess weight yields a health risk only if it is from excess body fat. Extra muscle mass poses no risk.

9. *False.* Women tend to store fat in the hip and thigh areas, whereas men tend to store fat in the abdominal area.

10. *True.* Health problems usually begin when a person exceeds a BMI of 25; the greater the increase, the greater the health risk.

11. *True.* Muscle tissue metabolizes energy at a high rate and thus has a great influence on resting metabolism.

12. *True.* The extra weight carried by an obese person raises the energy cost of physical activity.

13. *False.* There is little evidence that adult obesity in men is related to childhood obesity; conversely, there is a strong relationship between childhood obesity and adult obesity in women.

14. *False.* Probably less than 10% of all cases of obesity in the United States arise from diagnosed problems with the thyroid hormone status of the body.

15. *False.* Consuming only a few hundred extra kilocalories daily for a few years can create an obese state. Once an obese state is achieved, it takes little extra energy to maintain it.

CHAPTER 9

1. *False.* Although physical activity is helpful, controlling energy intake is equally important.

2. *True.* Diet relapse is a critical issue that is just now receiving focused attention.

3. *True.* A diet with fewer than 1000 kcal is likely to cause hunger and fatigue.

4. *False.* Most people regain much of the weight they lost within 1 year.

5. *True.* Much muscle tissue can be lost in rapid weight loss. Rapid weight loss is also impractical because of the high energy deficit required.

6. *True.* Changes in behavior are likely to both address bad habits and reduce the tendency to relapse into these habits.

7. *False.* There is no evidence that eating meat affects the body's ability to utilize milk.

8. *True.* High-carbohydrate foods generally contain less energy than high-fat foods.

9. *False.* Recent studies show that a low-fat diet is practical and can provide significant satiety if high in dietary fiber.

10. *True.* People who can change their habits are able to have more control over their food choices and behavior. This contributes to weight maintenance.

11. *True.* An example of stimulus control might be to avoid a candy machine that is on the way to class.

12. *False.* You must burn about 3000 extra kilocalories to lose 1 pound of fat stores.

13. *True.* This fact must be kept in mind as a plan for weight loss and later weight maintenance is developed.

14. *True.* Brisk walking burns about 4 to 5 kcal/min.

15. *True.* Weighing more than 100 pounds over desirable weight, or twice desirable body weight, is a measure of severe (morbid) obesity.

CHAPTER 10

1. *False.* A cell must first convert the energy stored in carbohydrate to ATP energy.

2. *False.* Carbohydrates and fats both provide energy for the body.

3. *False.* Only initial stages of carbohydrate metabolism do not require oxygen to function. Ultimate conversion of carbohydrate to carbon dioxide and water requires oxygen input.

4. *True.* Complete burning of all body fuels yields carbon dioxide as one of the by-products.

5. *False.* Evidence does not solidly support this assertion. Even if needs are elevated, vitamin and mineral intake beyond twice RDA standards provides no documented effect on performance.

6. *False.* Rapid weight loss, such as that practiced by wrestlers, can weaken the body. Long-term weight loss can reduce muscle mass and make it hard to keep glycogen stores adequate.

7. *False.* Given the high energy intakes of athletes, protein needs are easily met from typical food choices. Protein supplements are not needed.

8. *True.* Consuming carbohydrate soon after exercise is a key recommendation for endurance athletes and for carbohydrate-loading strategies.

9. *True.* The carbohydrate present can reduce glycogen use and the electrolytes can help maintain blood volume during endurance events, but sports drinks are not needed for routine athletic events.

10. *True.* Caffeine can enhance fat use by muscles, which may improve athletic performance in some endurance events.

11. *False.* The target heart rate range to promote general cardiovascular conditioning is 60% to 85% of maximum heart rate.

12. *False.* Cool-down exercises are just as important—if not more important—as warm-up exercises.

13. *False.* Thirst is not a good indicator of fluid replacement needs. A much better guide is weight loss: 2 cups (0.5 L) of water should eventually be consumed for every pound (0.5 kg) lost while exercising.

14. *False.* Loading up on carbohydrate will not be beneficial for short, sprint-type exercise; it mostly benefits exercise lasting longer than 1 hour.

15. *True.* Anabolic steroids are illegal substances used to encourage muscle development. Use can have dangerous health consequences.

CHAPTER 11

1. *False.* Women portrayed in the media often have body shapes and body fat content that most women would find hard to attain and maintain.

2. *True.* Maintaining a low weight to compete as a model or athlete can lead to an eating disorder in women.

3. *False.* They have an intense fear of gaining weight.

4. *True.* This vomiting is referred to as *purging.*

5. *False.* People with anorexia nervosa tend to be extremely competitive.

6. *True.* People with anorexia nervosa may find that their disorder can be used to control their lives, as well as the actions and emotions of others.

7. *True.* But they don't like to admit to bulimic practices.

8. *True.* This lean and angular look is reflected in advertisements.

9. *False.* People with bulimia often come from "chaotic" families.

10. *False.* Loss of regular menstrual periods results in bone loss as well, which is linked to changes in hormonal status.

11. *True.* Restrictive eating can create such hunger that binge eating is encouraged.

12. *True.* The damaging effect of late stages of these conditions increases the risk of permanent injury.

13. *True.* Bingeing and purging characterize bulimia nervosa.

14. *False.* Treatment of bulimia nervosa should emphasize informed choices as opposed to restriction.

15. *True.* Baryophobia should be suspected in children who exhibit lagging growth rates.

CHAPTER 12

1. *False.* No vitamin missing from a diet for less than a week leads to deficiency symptoms. Earliest evidence of deficiency appear with a thiamin-free diet after about 10 days. The first symptoms of a vitamin C deficiency are seen after 20 to 40 days.

2. *False.* Of the fat-soluble vitamins, vitamin K is most readily excreted from the body.

3. *True.* Sun exposure provides a source of vitamin D; this suffices for vitamin D needs for many children and adults.

4. *False.* Because fat-soluble vitamins do not dissolve rapidly in water, they are not leached out of foods during cooking to the same extent as most water-soluble vitamins.

5. *True.* There is a slight chance that one more vitamin remains to be discovered, but for the most part nutrition scientists feel they have isolated all the vitamins necessary for human health.

6. *True.* When in the active form, vitamin D, through a variety of mechanisms, improves calcium absorption from the small intestine.

7. *False.* Vitamin D is formed from a derivative of cholesterol, not beta carotene.

8. *True.* Vitamin A intake beyond about 5 times the RDA poses a high potential for toxicity, especially in pregnant women and in children.

9. *True.* Aided by the action of sunlight, the skin produces vitamin D, which can then be metabolized by the liver and kidneys to form the active vitamin D hormone. This compound is a hormone, since it is made in one part of the body and acts in another.

10. *True.* This can be done to milk to increase vitamin D content by changing some compounds in milk to vitamin D. However, for foods in general this is not possible; vitamin D itself is added to foods to supplement the product.

11. *False.* Instead, vitamin E stabilizes free radical compounds by donating an electron. This decreases free-radical attack on fatty acids and other electron-dense compounds.

12. *True.* Vitamin K adds carbon dioxide to the amino acid glutamate, in turn imparting calcium-binding properties to the blood-clotting proteins containing that amino acid.

13. *True.* Long-term antibiotic use can reduce the growth of bacteria in the small intestine and colon. These bacteria synthesize a form of vitamin K that we absorb and use.

14. *True.* Vegetables are a good source of vitamin K. This is just one reason why we should eat vegetables.

15. *False.* Currently there is little regulation of the production of nutrient supplements. FDA plans more scrutiny in the future; for now, look for a USP insignia as proof of quality and purity.

CHAPTER 13

1. *False.* Thiamin needs are more closely tied to carbohydrate intake because the conversion of pyruvate to acetyl-CoA requires thiamin. Carbohydrate metabolism generates pyruvate.

2. *True.* Pork is an excellent source of thiamin, as are sunflower seeds and dried beans.

3. *True.* Normally, highly processed grains, such as white rice, are stripped of much of their vitamin value. However, in the United States, grains are usually enriched and thus contain extra niacin, thiamin, riboflavin, and iron. Thus enriched white rice is a good source of niacin.

4. *True.* Milk is a good source of riboflavin for our diets.

5. *True.* A deficiency in a major B vitamin, such as riboflavin, suggests that other B vitamins are also deficient, since most are found in similar foods.

6. *True.* In the elderly years, cells in the stomach commonly decrease the synthesis of a factor (intrinsic factor) that is vital for vitamin B-12 absorption. The treatment is usually monthly injections of vitamin B-12.

7. *True.* The amino acid tryptophan is converted into niacin in the body. Niacin needs are then met by consuming both niacin-containing foods and protein in the diet.

8. *True.* A niacin deficiency causes severe dermatitis and skin redness, especially where the sun strikes, as well as diarrhea and dementia.

9. *True.* Nicotinic acid in pharmacological (high) doses can lower serum cholesterol. At the same time, it often causes redness of the skin and itching.

10. *True.* Alcohol decreases the absorption of folate, as well as vitamin B-6 and thiamin. Alcoholism is a major cause of B vitamin deficiencies.

11. *False.* Excessive supplementation of folate may mask a vitamin B-12 deficiency. One of the early effects of a vitamin B-12 deficiency is an impaired ability to recycle folate in cells. If excessive amounts of folate are available, this will not readily occur, so the resulting sign of megaloblastic anemia may not be apparent to the physician.

12. *True.* Vitamin B-12 is found only in foods of animal origin. It is not found in plants unless its presence is due to fermentation or contamination of the product from bits of soil or insects.

13. *True.* The formation of pinpoint hemorrhages in the skin near hair follicles is an early sign of scurvy. This occurs after 20 to 40 days of no vitamin C intake.

14. *True.* Vitamin C converts iron into a readily absorbable form.

15. *False.* High doses of vitamin C may moderately reduce the symptoms and duration of a cold; no food or medication can prevent colds.

CHAPTER 14

1. *False.* An electrolyte is a substance that dissociates into ions and thus is able to conduct electricity. Although in a water molecule the hydrogen atoms are slightly positive and the oxygen atom is slightly negative, each water molecule does not break down into individual ions.

2. *False.* The terms *major* and *trace* are not designations of nutritional importance. They are classifications referring only to the amount needed for daily functioning.

3. *True.* For example, the coenzyme for the vitamin thiamin requires magnesium to function efficiently.

4. *False.* Animal foods are often the best mineral sources, since animals concentrate the minerals they consume from plants. The exception is magnesium, which is most plentiful in green plants.

5. *True.* The body can conserve water, but some must be lost every day. Thus after only a few days, severe dehydration and death can result from lack of water intake. In comparison, death from starvation can take as long as 50 or more days in an adult.

6. *True.* Water evaporation from the skin requires heat energy. So when perspiration evaporates, heat energy is taken from the skin, leaving you feeling cooler.

7. *True.* This simple method of estimation (1 ml/kcal expended) yields results similar to those derived by totaling all typical water losses via lungs, skin, feces, and urine.

8. *False.* In cases of some mental disorders, such as schizophrenia, people may drink tremendous amounts of water in a short time. This can overwhelm the kidneys' excretion capacity and lead to headaches, blurred vision, and cramps.

9. *True.* About one half of the sodium consumed by American adults is supplied by processed foods. Sodium is found especially in foods such as frozen dinners, canned soups, convenience entrées, and salty snacks.

10. *False.* Many substances commonly found in dietary fiber, such as phytate in grain fibers, as well as oxalic acid in spinach and other vegetables, can actually bind minerals, inhibiting their absorption.

11. *True.* Although part of our preference for salt is related to the sodium receptors on the tongue, habit also has a role. If you grow up consuming salty foods, you are more likely to prefer salty foods. Preferences can be relearned by gradually decreasing added salt.

12. *False.* Cheese has added salt unless it is a "low salt" cheese. Milk does not have added salt and so is lower in sodium per kilocalorie.

13. *True.* Perspiration on the skin tastes salty, not because it has a higher sodium concentration than blood, but because once the water evaporates, concentrated sodium is left behind.

14. *False.* The effectiveness of dietary calcium in entirely preventing bone loss in adulthood has been disproved, but adequate dietary amounts can slow some bone loss in old age.

15. *False.* Alcohol intake is often not considered as a risk factor for hypertension, but it is. People with hypertension can benefit from restricting alcohol intake.

CHAPTER 15

1. *True.* The small amounts needed by the body make trace mineral deficiencies difficult to detect in humans. Laboratory techniques are not even available to adequately measure some trace elements in tissue, and there are gaps in our knowledge about metabolism and storage of many minerals. This hampers interpretation of laboratory results.

2. *True.* Trace minerals that have the same charge and are chemically similar or use the same carrier, such as zinc and copper, often compete with each other during absorption and metabolism. This must be considered when setting the RDA for a trace mineral and when using mineral supplements.

3. *True.* Eating a variety of foods will ensure an intake from a variety of soil conditions and help maximize the chances of consuming an adequate amount of trace minerals, such as selenium.

4. *True.* The refinement process strips food, such as flour, of many trace minerals. The enrichment process replaces only one: iron.

5. *True.* Women in their childbearing years have a greater need than men for iron due to their greater iron loss from menstruation.

6. *False.* The body has no efficient mechanism for eliminating excess iron. Excess iron intake can be very damaging. In response, iron absorption is regulated by the body; this helps prevent excess iron absorption.

7. *True.* A main function of zinc is promoting growth and development. A zinc deficiency can cause poor growth in children, whereas a zinc supplement can help increase the rate of weight gain in children recovering from undernutrition.

8. *False.* Hair analysis is not a reliable method for determining zinc or other mineral status at this time. Too many contaminating substances, such as shampoos, invalidate the results.

9. *True.* Megadose zinc supplements often disrupt the natural nutrient balance found in a good diet and thus can do more harm than good to immune function.

10. *True.* Copper is a component of the protein ceruloplasmin. This protein adds an electron to Fe^{2+} to form Fe^{3+}, the form of iron that can leave the mucosal cell and storage sites in the liver to bind with transferrin in the blood.

11. *True.* Copper and zinc compete with each other for absorption, so for this and other reasons, an excess intake of zinc can lead to a copper deficiency.

12. *False.* Most iodide in our diets comes from iodized salt added to foods during processing, cooking, or at the table.

13. *True.* Fluoride prevents dental caries in a variety of ways, one of which is to inhibit the growth and metabolism of bacteria present on teeth.

14. *False.* We know little about chromium metabolism, and it is likely that, as with other trace minerals, it is quite toxic even at moderate doses.

15. *False.* A prolonged iron deficiency can eventually lead to iron-deficiency anemia, but it takes years for most people with inadequate iron intake to develop symptoms if they remain untreated. In addition, some types of anemia are caused by conditions other than iron deficiency.

CHAPTER 16

1. *True.* Infants weighing less than 5.5 pounds (2.5 kg) at birth are considered to have low birthweight. The risk of sickness and death in the early months of life is much greater for these infants.

2. *False.* It is during the first trimester (13 weeks), when organs and body parts are forming, that the potential for birth defects is greatest.

3. *True.* The quality of the mother's diet and the amount of weight she gains during pregnancy are more important than genetic background in determining birthweight.

4. *True.* During pregnancy, an average increase of 300 kcal/day is needed during the second and third trimesters.

5. *True.* This range of weight gain normally allows optimal development of the fetus without an excessive increase of fat stores in the mother.

6. *True.* Gaining an excessive amount of weight from an overabundant energy intake is a problem for many pregnant women.

7. *False.* Eating a healthful diet requires learning to make wise food choices; instinct has little to do with it.

8. *True.* Many mineral needs, but particularly those for iron, calcium, and zinc, are increased. Iron requirements usually necessitate taking supplements in addition to changing the diet.

9. *True.* Symptoms of gestational diabetes will first occur during pregnancy and then disappear after birth. This happens more frequently in women who have a family history of diabetes.

10. *True.* Immune factors passed from mother to infant via human milk reduce the number of respiratory and intestinal infections.

11. *True.* Almost all women are capable of breastfeeding; the size of the breasts, and even the birth of twins, pose no major barrier. Lack of sufficient knowledge is the main barrier.

12. *True.* Many substances ingested by the mother, including medicines, are secreted into the milk, so physician approval of use is needed.

13. *True.* The placenta is a specialized organ of pregnancy that both secretes hormones and allows the transfer of oxygen, nutrients, and wastes between mother and fetus.

14. *True.* The risk of early spontaneous abortion means that good nutrition and health habits should be started in the months before pregnancy begins.

15. *False.* Unaltered cow's milk is too difficult for an infant to digest and safely consume until approximately 12 months of age.

CHAPTER 17

1. *True.* Although all nutrients and an adequate energy intake are needed for growth, protein is particularly important for reaching genetic potential.

2. *True.* Infancy is a period of very rapid growth in body length.

3. *False.* Brain growth rate is maximal at birth and continues at a fast pace through 12 to 15 months of age.

4. *False.* No evidence strongly links obesity in infancy to obesity in childhood or adulthood.

5. *False.* Infant energy needs are higher per pound compared with childhood.

6. *False.* Infants need relatively high-fat diets to support brain growth and supply enough energy for other body growth within a small volume of food.

7. *False.* Infants are not usually developmentally or nutritionally ready for solid food until 4 to 6 months of age.

8. *True.* It is not necessary to add salt, sugar, or spices to infant foods, as bland food is well accepted.

9. *True.* However, "heart healthy" diets are not recommended until 2 years of age, as younger children benefit from the concentrated energy source that fat supplies.

10. *True.* Cow's milk ideally should not be fed to a child until about 12 months of age.

11. *True.* Cow's milk is low in iron, and the protein is more difficult to digest than that in human milk. This latter characteristic may cause intestinal irritation that contributes to iron losses.

12. *False.* What is eaten is most important—not the meal schedule.

13. *True.* Anemia and obesity are the nutritional problems clinicians need to focus on with children.

14. *False.* Parents should control what food is available, but let children decide the amount to eat. With good foods available, children can reliably decide on serving size.

15. *False.* Scientific studies have never shown a very strong link between any dietary factor and acne.

CHAPTER 18

1. *False.* The average length of time Americans live has increased during the last century, but the age of the oldest people in the population has not increased significantly.

2. *True.* This amount of physical activity is the minimum advised by experts; even more is recommended to adequately stimulate the cardiovascular system and help reduce stress and obesity, once a pattern of 30 minutes per day is established.

3. *True.* Drug-nutrient interactions can be a problem at any age, but because the elderly generally take more and different combinations of drugs over a long period, nutritional status is more likely to be affected.

4. *True.* Overeating can lead to overweight. Being overweight contributes to almost all the chronic diseases common in our society.

5. *True.* In addition, because the elderly population is rapidly growing, society will need to continue dealing with this demand for health care.

6. *False.* Good nutrition can delay some effects of aging, but no diet can magically prevent aging; in fact, aging probably begins at conception.

7. *False.* The senses of smell and taste tend to decrease with age. Adding seasonings can enhance food appeal.

8. *True.* The sense of thirst may diminish with age, but not the need for fluids.

9. *True.* Stomach secretions that promote absorption of vitamin B-12 (acid and intrinsic factor) decrease with age.

10. *True.* Increasing fiber and fluid intakes can help reduce this constipation.

11. *True.* Excessive intake of vitamin A supplements results in many toxicity problems, and more so in the elderly.

12. *True.* Be aware of these nutrients if you are involved in the care of elderly people or have the chance to advise elderly relatives, as they are needed for wound healing.

13. *True.* Physical activity is an important part of body maintenance, including that of muscles and bones.

14. *False.* People differ in genetic background, ability to regulate cholesterol metabolism, and responsiveness to diets aimed at lowering serum cholesterol. There is, however, no way to know how much a diet will help lower cholesterol until a person tries it.

15. *False.* This age group, 65 years and older, varies more in physical ability than any other.

CHAPTER 19

1. *True.* We often do not realize that food-borne illness is so common because the symptoms mimic other disorders, such as certain viral infections.

2. *False.* Foods having the potential to cause food-borne illness often show no signs of it in taste, smell, or appearance.

3. *False.* Imported foods, such as soft cheeses from Mexico, have been implicated in food-borne illness. Although foods are inspected when they enter from foreign countries, there is not enough manpower to inspect all foods carefully.

4. *False.* Chemical structure—not origin—is the key to evaluating chemicals: whether a chemical is made in a laboratory or found in nature is irrelevant to its harmfulness to humans. Some naturally occurring toxins in foods, such as solanine in green potatoes, are

much more toxic than synthetic food additives.

5. *True.* When the pulp of an apple is exposed to oxygen, it turns brown. Antioxidants, such as the vitamin C found in lemon and orange juice, can prevent this browning.

6. *True.* The growth of bacteria and fungi in foods requires sufficient free water, that is, water not bound by other food compounds. If the water content of a food is reduced considerably, the lack of free water curtails growth of bacteria and fungi.

7. *False.* Only a few of the many bacteria, fungi, viruses, and other earthly microbes are known to cause food-borne illness.

8. *True.* And for this reason, foods generally should be kept cold (below 40° F or 4° C) or hot (above 140° F or 60° C).

9. *True.* The symptoms of food-borne illness are abdominal bloating, gas, diarrhea, vomiting, and headache, all of which can also be symptoms of certain viral infections.

10. *False.* One incident of food-borne illness provides no immunity against future attacks.

11. *True.* *Salmonella* bacteria are commonly associated with chickens, especially raw chicken carcasses. Raw chicken should be handled very carefully so that juices do not contaminate other foods, thereby spreading *Salmonella* bacteria.

12. *True.* The bacterium that produces the deadly botulism toxin is present in all soil.

13. *True.* *Clostridium botulinum* grows only in the absence of air. Thus it may be found in improperly canned foods and in thick foods where air is excluded from the center. Chili is an example of the latter.

14. *True.* Many viruses and parasites that may be present in raw fish are destroyed by cooking. Consuming raw fish poses a significant health risk for hepatitis, parasite infection, and other health problems, especially in people whose health is already compromised by cirrhosis, diabetes, cancer, or AIDS.

15. *False.* Aside from the alcohol present in high amounts (which over time can lead to cirrhosis of the liver), some alcoholic beverages contain urethanes, which FDA is now studying carefully to assess the degree of health risk these agents pose.

CHAPTER 20

1. *True.* But hunger is physiological as well, and can be described as an uneasiness, discomfort, weakness, or pain caused by lack of food.

2. *True.* This poverty can be caused by unemployment, homelessness, illiteracy, poor health, and other factors.

3. *False.* Diabetes is more common when food supplies are abundant.

4. *True.* Undernutrition is also the primary cause of many nutrient deficiency diseases, such as scurvy, pellagra, and anemia, among others.

5. *True.* No other social indicator shows a wider gap between the developing and industrialized world than the risk of death related to pregnancy.

6. *True.* The growing fetus needs a steady supply of energy, vitamins, protein, and minerals, provided by the mother's diet.

7. *True.* Failure of children to grow sufficiently is a common result of undernutrition.

8. *False.* Marginal iron deficiencies affect hundreds of millions of people worldwide.

9. *False.* Full recovery from undernutrition may never happen, and if it does, it is likely to take months or years.

10. *False.* The United States is in twenty-second place.

11. *True.* This homelessness is partly because the cost of housing has substantially increased and partly because federal support for subsidized housing and mental institutions was cut during the 1980s.

12. *False.* Economists estimate that world food production will continue to increase more rapidly than the world population in the near future, allowing the food/population ratio to increase through the year 2000. In the long run, however, food production will lag behind population growth.

13. *True.* There are many reasons for the greater number of child births. Among them is an economic imperative to have large families. Experts believe couples will choose to have fewer children only after each couple experiences an increased livelihood.

14. *True.* Most of these urban poor in the Third World live in overcrowded, self-made shelter, with inadequate public utilities.

15. *True.* WHO estimates that more than one billion people are without a safe and adequate water supply.

Answers to Critical Thinking Questions

CHAPTER 1

1. Supplements purchased in a store can provide vitamins and minerals. However, that is all they provide. Foods, on the other hand, not only supply vitamins and minerals, but also carbohydrates, proteins, fats, and fiber. These provide energy and bulk for a healthy digestive system.

2. Because vitamins act as coenzymes in metabolism, they are essential for health. However, high intakes of some vitamins can be toxic and thus detrimental to health. The potential for toxicity is greatest with the fat-soluble vitamins, which can be stored in large quantities in the liver, causing severe liver damage. Therefore consuming significantly more than the RDAs for the fat-soluble vitamins can be more dangerous than beneficial.

3. A diet consisting primarily of foods derived from animal sources contains mostly proteins and fats, with a high percentage of fats as saturated fats. Saturated fats are easily converted to cholesterol by the liver. High cholesterol levels are linked to increased risks of hypertension and cardiovascular disease. A diet high in fats is also related to increased rates of colon, breast, and prostate cancer.

Fruits and vegetables are rich in fibers, which help decrease cholesterol levels and increase the rate of peristalsis in the gastrointestinal tract. Fruits and vegetables, for the most part, contain low amounts of fats, if any, and are also low in kilocalories, thus helping to maintain normal body weight.

CHAPTER 2

1. Since the typical American diet consists of many foods high in fat and low in fiber, Devan should assess his diet with respect to these components. He should list all of the foods he eats, preferably for a whole week, and estimate how much fat and fiber he consumes. He then should change his eating habits to obtain recommended amounts of fat and fiber. Most likely, Devan will need to decrease fat intake as well as increase fiber in his diet.

2. The Food Guide Pyramid is designed to yield about 1600-1800 kcal/day. It provides the bulk of dietary energy intake from carbohydrates while limiting fat intake. Most foods are derived from the "base" of the pyramid, carbohydrates, with fruits and vegetables coming next, dairy and meats further up in the pyramid, and fats making up the "peak." The number of servings from each group depends on one's age and weight. The recommended servings can be proportioned for a person's age and weight as well. By choosing the minimum number of servings from foods from every group and varying the foods chosen, Joe could eat a variety of foods that would provide the necessary amounts of vitamins, minerals, and other essential nutrients for a healthy diet at a relatively low energy intake. A whole-grain breakfast cereal would be one excellent choice, as this provides dietary fiber and is moderately fortified with a number of vitamins and minerals.

3. A cup of skim milk provides 90 kcal, and a cup of whole milk provides 150 kcal. But both contain 8 g of protein and about 290 g of calcium. Skim milk delivers the same amount of protein and calcium as whole milk but with fewer kilocalories. Thus skim milk is more nutrient dense with respect to protein and calcium than whole milk. The difference in the energy content of skim and whole milk results from their fat contents: a cup of skim milk has only a trace of fat, whereas a cup of whole milk has 8 g of fat.

CHAPTER 3

1. Diverticulosis is a condition in which tiny pouches form in the wall of the colon. When foods are eaten that are not easily digestible, like nuts and seeds, undigested pieces may become trapped in the pouches. Bacteria then metabolize these particles into acids and gases that irritate the diverticula, causing them to swell; this condition is called *diverticulitis.* The acids and gases in the swollen pouches cause cramping and abdominal pain.

2. Diet pills, even over-the-counter ones, are expensive. The psyllium in Celia's diet pills is a fiber that produces bulk, which helps to make the dieter feel satiated. However, instead of buying expensive pills that make her feel full so that she will not eat as much, Celia should simply change her eating habits to include more fruits and vegetables. Not only do they contain dietary fiber, but they also supply vitamins and minerals. Beans, whole-wheat foods, oats, fruits, and vegetables all contain ample dietary fiber and are great low-energy sources of nutrients.

3. Foods that remain in the mouth, usually caught between the teeth, are a source of food that bacteria can metabolize. As a by-product of this metabolism, bacteria produce acids that can decay tooth enamel, causing caries. Chewing gum after meals decreases the risk of caries because chewing stimulates the secretion of saliva, which helps to dislodge foods that remain in the mouth. Sugar-free gums also contain sugar substitutes, which bacteria can't metabolize. In addition, saliva has a higher pH than the acids produced by bacterial metabolism. This helps to neutralize the acids.

CHAPTER 4

1. The general term *fats* refers to lipids in foods without reference to their structure. Only dietary fats with a high proportion of saturated fatty acids have been associated with cardiovascular disease. In the body, fat (primarily in the form of triglycerides) has many beneficial functions. Triglycerides form the main energy stores in the body and can release fatty acids, which serve as fuel for many cells, such as those in muscles at rest and during light activity. Stored fat insulates the body and protects vital organs. Absorption of fat-soluble vitamins from the intestine is aided by their association with dietary fats. In addition, the two essential fatty acids, linoleic acid and alpha-linolenic acid, are not synthesized by the body and must be in the diet to maintain health. Thus some fat is needed in the diet; moderation of intake, not elimination, is the goal.

2. In addition to ensuring good health by supplying essential fatty acids, triglycerides in foods promote satiety (i.e., a feeling of fullness). Triglycerides produce this effect by influencing certain hormonal responses, which in turn affect the rate of stomach emptying. After a nonfat meal, the stomach empties rapidly, so one feels hungry in a short time. In contrast, after a meal containing some fat, the rate of stomach emptying slows, so one feels satiated or satisfied for a longer period. If dieters with limited caloric intakes would include a small amount of fat in their meals, they would not feel hungry all the time. Increasing fiber intake provides the same benefit. As a result, dieters would be less likely to give up their diets quickly and would have a better chance of long-term success.

3. The amount of cholesterol carried in HDL (high-density lipoprotein) also indicates the risk of heart disease. If the serum HDL is greater than 60 mg/dl, the risk of heart disease is low. If it's less than 35 mg/dl, the risk is high. The ratio of total serum cholesterol to

HDL cholesterol is also a good indicator of one's risk. If the ratio exceeds 4.5 to 1, the risk is high. Since your total cholesterol was 210 mg/dl and your HDL cholesterol was 65 mg/dl, your ratio is 3.5 to 1 (210 mg/dl÷65 mg/dl), which means that you are not at risk for rapidly developing heart disease. Your LDL cholesterol, which is 125 mg/dl, is also not elevated (210 mg/dl-65 mg/dl-[100 mg/dl÷5]).

CHAPTER 5

1. From a nutritional standpoint, a high urea level indicates one of three problems:
(1) Excessive protein intake in the diet. Excess protein is deaminated in the liver, and fatty acid synthesis occurs. The amine portion becomes ammonia, which is then converted into urea by the liver.
(2) Increased protein breakdown caused by failure to maintain an appropriate protein balance while dieting.
(3) Too little carbohydrate in the diet, which forces the liver to deaminate amino acids in order to use the remaining carbon skeleton for glucose synthesis. In other words, proteins are used for energy rather than for the building and repair of structures.

2. *PKU* is the abbreviation for the disease *phenylketonuria*. The liver of a person with phenylketonuria cannot readily convert phenylalanine, an essential amino acid, to tyrosine. This defect is caused by insufficient enzyme action. Since phenylalanine cannot be sufficiently degraded, tyrosine must be considered an essential amino acid for people with PKU.

The inability to metabolize excess phenylalanine to tyrosine leads to the formation of abnormal products that arise from alternative metabolic pathways; these products can cause mental retardation. Thus it is vital to determine which infants have PKU, since the phenylalanine levels in their diets must be monitored. However, because it is an essential amino acid, some phenylalanine must be consumed.

3. Protein synthesis is a complex process by which a specific sequence and number of amino acids determine the primary structure of a protein. If a given amino acid is not present during protein synthesis, production will stop. In other words, protein is an all-or-none product: all of the amino acids necessary to make the protein must be available, or the protein will not be made at all.

CHAPTER 6

1. Although taste receptors for sweet, salty, sour, and bitter are located on the tongue, there are receptors associated with the nose that help us to taste various flavors. The olfactory receptor cells in the nose detect combinations of chemical molecules that, along with the taste receptors on the tongue, allow us to perceive the flavors in our foods. When you have a cold, the membranes in your nose secrete excess mucus, which prevents the molecules from exciting the olfactory receptors. Hence, your sense of taste is inhibited.

2. The small intestine is the most important absorption site in the digestive system because of its large surface area. Since much of the young girl's small intestine was removed, many of the nutrients she consumes are escaping absorption. It is likely that only a highly refined diet or intravenous therapy will succeed in keeping her adequately nourished.

3. A sphincter called the *lower esophageal sphincter* is located between the esophagus and the stomach. It opens up to allow food to enter the stomach, but otherwise remains closed to prevent reflux of food back into the esophagus. Because the stomach's environment is so acidic, regurgitation of stomach contents back into the esophagus would cause the burning sensation that we call heartburn.

Certain chemicals, such as caffeine, nicotine, and alcohol, can cause the lower esophageal sphincter to relax, allowing this to happen. Excessive eating can have the same effect, since a full stomach can cause backflow pressure on the sphincter. The hormonal changes that occur during pregnancy can encourage acid reflux as well. It is advisable for obese people to lose weight and eat only a moderate amount of food at each meal.

CHAPTER 7

1. Carnitine is a compound that shuttles fatty acids within the cell from the cytosol to the mitochondria. However, cells readily make all the carnitine they need. The use of supplements is pointless because they will not hasten the breakdown of fatty acids.

2. Mitochondria are the sites for cellular ATP synthesis—the powerhouses of the cell. Aerobic metabolism also takes place in the mitochondria. Wherever there is a need for the production of large amounts of ATP, such as in muscle cells, mitochondria will be found. The greater the need for energy, the greater the number of mitochondria.

3. Although osteoporosis is the decalcification of bone, vitamin D is converted to its usable form, calcitriol, by the liver. Vitamin D enhances calcium uptake by bone cells, which increases the mineralization of bone. Alcohol may not only cause bone cell dysfunction but may also cause the liver to decrease the rate of conversion of vitamin D to calcitriol.

CHAPTER 8

1. Energy intake must equal energy output in order for body weight to remain the same. Weight increases when energy intake is more than output. Since basal metabolism decreases by 2% for every decade over 30 years of age, either energy intake or energy output must be modified to maintain the same weight.

Energy balance can be attained by increasing physical activity, a facet of life that tends to decrease with aging. Taking up a sport, jogging, or even parking the car further away from a building to increase walking distance are all good methods. People tend to become less active and therefore expend less energy without reducing food intake as they age. By increasing physical activity, energy balance and desirable weight can be maintained.

2. Soluble fiber helps slow gastric emptying, so the stomach remains full for a longer time and the person feels satiated longer. If the stomach empties too quickly, the person may feel hunger again in a short time and eat again. Fiber keeps the person feeling satisfied, so he or she does not feel a need to overeat or eat again.

3. Fat-rich foods are very palatable. Many flavors that stimulate the senses of taste and smell are dissolved in lipids. Fat-rich foods also often have a pleasing texture, which enhances appetite. These energy-dense foods many times appear as small servings, such as cookies, brownies, and cake, which can easily be over-consumed. Given the choice of an apple or a cookie, most children as well as adults take the cookie.

CHAPTER 9

1. Low-carbohydrate diets, as well as "starvation diets," may lead to rapid reduction of body weight; however, they may also lead to problems. Most of the weight loss in a short time is due to loss of water and lean body tissue. Weight should be lost mostly from fat storage, not from muscle and other lean tissues. At the start of a diet, rapid weight loss also may be attributable to decreased salt intake and loss of glycogen from the liver and muscles. In addition, the liver is forced to undergo gluconeogenesis and ketogenesis to supply energy to "starving" cells. This type of diet, a quick-fix diet, yields only temporary results, with an eventual return to the higher weight.

2. Fad diets have certain common features. To spot a fad diet, Marie should look for the following:
- diets that guarantee quick fixes
- diets that restrict foods to only a few choices
- diets that seem too good to be true
- diets that have been used by famous people and are promoted as such
- diets that recommend the purchase of vitamins, minerals, or a particular manufacturer's foods
- diets that do not recommend a change in lifestyle or habits
- diets that claim to work for everyone

3. Although Hal has seen a steady decrease in his weight for the duration of his diet thus far, his body has built-in mechanisms that tend to fight weight loss. One of those factors is the basal metabolic rate. The BMR tends to decrease to conserve energy as the number of kilocalories in the diet decreases. Also, lipoprotein lipase activity increases in adipose cells, which increases lipid absorption. The increased activity of this enzyme allows the body to more efficiently take up fats from the blood after the dieting has stopped. It is essential for Hal to continue his diet and not give up at this point.

The body resists weight loss by physiological means; however, it may finally "surrender" to persistent dieting, and Hal will continue to lose weight as long as he continues to diet.

CHAPTER 10

1. Marty has enhanced his cardiovascular fitness, a laudable goal. In addition, after a period of training, muscle cells worked on a regular basis will make more mitochondria. Since mitochondria are the sites of aerobic metabolism, this means that more ATP can be generated. ATP is a necessary component for muscle contraction, so a greater amount of ATP production allows a greater amount of muscle contraction.

2. Many wrestlers and other athletes lose weight quickly by losing large amounts of water, usually by sweating. By doing so, an athlete can compete in a lower weight class and thus gain an advantage over an opponent. However, losing weight this way can significantly impede performance. Over time, repeated dehydration episodes can lead to serious complications, such as kidney failure. Athletes also risk becoming heat stressed during the event.

The loss of water before a competition is the quick method of losing weight. But if an athlete is serious about his or her sport, a gradual change in diet to create the best possible weight/muscle composition should be the goal.

3. A person's appropriate dietary intake of protein should be determined using the RDA for protein: 0.8 g/kg body weight. Athletes should increase their protein intake to 1.2 to 1.6 g/kg body weight to supply the amount of protein needed for muscle growth and development. Some athletes' needs may be even greater than that. Overall, about 15% of energy intake as protein is required. About 60% of energy intake should be supplied by carbohydrates, leaving about 25% of energy intake to be supplied by fat. The high carbohydrate intake is necessary to supply glucose for glycogen synthesis; glycogen is an important muscle fuel.

CHAPTER 11

1. Signs that could indicate an eating disorder include the following:
(1) Compulsive behavior patterns
(2) Obsession with being and looking thin
(3) Obsession with counting calories
(4) Not wanting to eat with others (e.g., refusing to go to a restaurant)
(5) Continually criticizing one's looks and comparing oneself to others, especially slender people
(6) Being convinced that one is fat

2. In addition to the detrimental social aspects of anorexia nervosa, such as alienation from others, there are serious physical consequences. Nutritional deficiencies may develop

that can cause an imbalance of the sex hormones. Jennifer has already stopped menstruating, reducing her fertility. The disease may also prevent her from gaining enough weight to support the developing fetus if she were to become pregnant later. Starvation leads to a loss of lean body tissue, such as muscle. The heart rate decreases as metabolism slows, which causes the person to become easily tired, increasing the need for sleep. Since tissue is lost from the heart muscle as well as from the rest of the body, heart function may also be impaired. Another potential problem is anemia caused by inadequate nutrient intake.

3. One of the most important topics Tom should discuss is proper nutrition. Using the concepts of adequacy, balance, and moderation, he can teach students about their diets. He should also present case studies of real people who have anorexia nervosa and bulimia nervosa so that his students can see firsthand the outcome of these diseases. Tom should also focus on increasing the self-esteem of young adults. The pre-puberty and teenage years are a time of self-evaluation and criticism. It is important for Tom to help his students feel good from within by emphasizing the importance of self-worth regardless of one's physical appearance. Finally, Tom can teach his students how to cope with difficult situations by showing them how to alleviate stress in positive and constructive ways.

CHAPTER 12

1. Vitamin A is associated with vision and night blindness but also has other important functions. Vitamin A exists in 3 different forms: retinol, retinoic acid, and retinaldehyde. The body uses each form for a different function: reproduction, growth and maturation of cells, and vision, respectively.

Insufficient amounts of vitamin A cause mucus-forming cells to deteriorate. Skin changes occur as well. In vitamin A deficiency, keratin replaces normal skin epithelium. Although keratin is a normal component of outer layers of skin, excess keratin is produced, which plugs hair follicles and gives skin a rough texture known as *hyperkeratosis*. Overall, it is a misconception to think that vitamin A's only function is that involved in vision.

2. A possible explanation for the lack of clot dissolution in Tim's leg is that he has been consuming many foods rich in vitamin K. This vitamin assists in clot formation and is antagonistic to oral anticoagulant medications. If the vitamin K is not reduced in Tim's diet, the therapy won't be very effective.

3. Many vitamins, such as the water-soluble ones, can often be excreted when taken in excess; however, the fat-soluble vitamins are not as readily excreted. Vitamins A and D, in particular, can accumulate in large amounts, causing toxic effects. These effects can occur at just five to ten times the Daily Values with regular usage of such excess quantities, espe-

cially in children. Excessive intakes of many water-soluble vitamins can also be toxic, but much higher doses are needed.

CHAPTER 13

1. People with alcoholism usually have unbalanced diets, which can impair absorption of vitamins and minerals from the GI tract. An associated problem is poor metabolism. The B vitamins are essential for metabolism: gluconeogenesis, lipogenesis, lipolysis, and overall carbohydrate metabolism. Alcohol consumption decreases the absorption of many B vitamins, such as thiamin, riboflavin, niacin, and folate. Vitamin C absorption is also decreased. All of these vitamins are important in maintaining proper metabolic and nervous system function.

2. Humans must obtain vitamin C from foods, because the body cannot synthesize it. An important function of this vitamin is to promote the formation of collagen, an important protein found in connective tissue. Collagen is an integral component of bone, skin, and blood vessels. Thus, a low intake of vitamin C will impair wound healing. Deficiency can also lead to scurvy, whose symptoms include bleeding gums and pinpoint hemorrhages on the skin.

Vitamin C is an antioxidant. It works with vitamin E against free radicals and helps "reactivate" vitamin E so that it can continue to function. Vitamin C also deters certain forms of cancer, enhances iron absorption, assists in carnitine production, and synthesizes norepinephrine, a neurotransmitter.

Finally, vitamin C is essential for lymphocytic activity within the immune system. Since it assists in the production of lymphocytes, maintaining appropriate vitamin C intake gives the body the building blocks it needs to fight off infections. However, vitamin C does *not* cure the common cold.

3. Many studies have shown that a nutritious diet, as well as specific environmental and lifestyle factors, reduces the risk of cancer initiation and promotion. In addition, obesity is associated with all major forms of cancer except lung cancer. Some evidence links excessive dietary fat with certain forms of cancer.

Some foods may contain carcinogenic substances, such as nitrites and nitrates. Vitamin C and vitamin E are anticarcinogenic in that they prevent the formation of nitrosamines, the carcinogenic compound made from nitrites and nitrates. Vitamin A and the mineral selenium are also anticarcinogenic. Fruits and vegetables can block cancer development because they are rich in fiber, vitamins A, C, and E, and selenium. Substances in broccoli, onions, and garlic also help block the action of carcinogens in the body.

In essence, a low-fat diet that includes many fruits and vegetables lowers the risk of cancer. Although many factors are involved in the initiation and promotion of cancer, there is strong scientific evidence that the incidence of cancer can be decreased through good nutrition.

CHAPTER 14

1. When doing physical work, such as mowing the lawn, one perspires. The degree of perspiration varies among people and also depends on the time of day. Muscle strength and endurance decline significantly when there is a 3% loss of body weight. Symptoms such as thirst may indicate a 2% loss of body weight caused by dehydration. With greater water loss, a headache and dizziness may develop. Even further water loss may induce a coma.

Any person who anticipates loss of body water through perspiration would benefit from hydrating before the activity, just as in preparation for an athletic event. Doing so will minimize dehydration. Drinking fluids during exertion is also helpful.

2. All foods contain sodium. Most of the sodium in our diets is added during cooking and at mealtimes. The American Heart Association recommends that all people limit their sodium intake to no more than 3 g/day. Still, sodium is essential to maintenance of normal fluid balance throughout the body and to normal nerve impulse conduction. Impulses are transmitted by the sodium ions that rush into nerve cells, which reverses the charge of the cell membrane. The resulting electrical current travels from nerve to nerve, from nerve to muscle, or from nerve to gland. This process allows "information" to be transmitted throughout the body. If sodium intake is inadequate, neuromuscular symptoms will appear, including muscle weakness, headache, irritability, and confusion.

3. Calcium is needed for normal bone growth and development. Bones serve as reservoirs of calcium for blood homeostasis. Regulation of blood calcium may necessitate the breakup of bone mineral deposits for the release of calcium from bone. Thus bone mineralization is vital before and during adolescence, when the greatest amount of bone development occurs. Manuela is already an adult, but she can still consume calcium in amounts sufficient to decrease the incidence of bone demineralization.

The best sources of calcium are milk and sardines, which Manuela, a vegan, will not eat. As an alternative, she should become aware of which vegetables contain calcium. She should also choose calcium-fortified foods, such as bread and some brands of orange juice. However, if she cannot meet her calcium needs by modifying her diet, based on a nutrient analysis of her current intake, calcium supplements are available.

CHAPTER 15

1. The doctor tells Tom that his participation in track could explain his anemia. "Runner's anemia" is a condition seen in new athletes. Iron deficiency, which contributes to anemia, occurs when iron needs greatly exceed normal intake. During physical activity, iron loss through perspiration increases. In addition, red blood cells are destroyed by trauma when they are flattened as they pass through the foot when it strikes the ground. Another factor that contributes to runner's anemia is the increase in blood volume associated with athletic fitness as physical activity increases. Finally, there is increased iron loss in the feces. Tom's age may also be a factor. He is likely in his pubertal growth spurt, which alone increases iron needs.

2. Vitamin C is important not only for collagen synthesis but also for treating iron-deficiency anemia, since it modestly enhances iron absorption in the GI tract. Nonheme iron is not absorbed as readily as heme iron; vitamin C increases absorption of nonheme iron by adding an electron to the ferric form of iron to create the ferrous form of iron, whch is absorbed better, and then chelating it as well.

3. The mineral selenium is a co-factor for the activity of the enzyme glutathione peroxidase. This enzyme participates in a system that metabolizes peroxides into less-toxic alcohol derivatives and water. Peroxides tend to become free radicals, which in turn can attack and break down cell membranes, causing cell damage. Selenium is considered to be important in protecting heart cells and other cells against oxidative damage. In addition, because it reduces the amount of free-radical damage to cells, selenium may be important in protecting against cancer.

CHAPTER 16

1. It is important to assess the nutritional and health status of the woman before pregnancy, not just while she is trying to become pregnant. The dietary habits of the mother can affect the health of the newborn. Good nutrition is critical during a woman's childbearing years. It has been shown that nutritional deficiencies can lead to improper fetal development. An adequate vitamin and mineral intake in the months before conception and during the pregnancy can help prevent fetal defects, such as with the vitamin folate. The time to focus on good nutrition and health is before the woman becomes pregnant, since many nutritional deficiencies can alter growth and development.

2. There are many changes that occur in a woman during pregnancy. Her uterus and breasts grow, and her total blood volume increases. The placenta develops, the heart and kidneys work harder, stores of body fat increase, and toward the latter part of the pregnancy, mammary glands prepare to produce milk. The nutrients needed to support these changes are listed below:

(1) Increased energy, about 300 more kilocalories per day, is necessary, especially during the second and third trimesters. This amount should allow adequate weight gain (25 to 35 pounds).

(2) Protein needs are also increased, by about 10 g/day for women over 24 years of age and about 15 g/day for women under 24. This amount should support adequate growth.

(3) Carbohydrate intake should be at least 100 g/day to prevent ketosis.

(4) Vitamin D should be increased to 10 μg/day by either increasing sunlight exposure or increasing vitamin-D fortified milk consumption. This amount will support fetal bone growth.

(5) Folate intake should increase to 400 μg/day to support red blood cell formation and DNA synthesis. This will also help prevent neural tube defects.

(6) Iron intake should increase to 30 mg/day. This will support hemoglobin synthesis.

(7) Calcium is needed to promote mineralization of fetal bones and teeth. Calcium intake should increase to 1200 to 1500 mg/day.

(8) Zinc is important for growth and development. Intake should increase to 12-15 mg/day to support this.

These nutrients should be obtained from foods. However, prenatal supplements can aid in supplying these nutrients to the pregnant woman, especially in circumstances that may prevent her from adequately consuming sufficient nutrients from foods.

3. As the pregnancy advances, the uterus will continue to grow to accommodate the growing fetus. As it does, it presses against the stomach as well as the intestines. Also, hormones produced in increased amounts during pregnancy relax muscles. This explains why heartburn may occur; the lower esophageal (cardiac) sphincter relaxes somewhat, allowing some foods and acid to regurgitate back into the esophagus; hence the heartburn. It is recommended that smaller quantities of foods be ingested and that the woman not recline after eating. High amounts of fats also decrease the rate of stomach emptying; therefore, decreasing the amounts of fats in the diet should also help. Since hormones relax muscles, the rate of peristalsis may also decrease and constipation may develop. It would be wise to gradually increase the amounts of fiber in Sandy's diet to improve her digestive system's peristaltic activity.

CHAPTER 17

1. Human milk is low in iron. Although it provides many essential nutrients to the baby, it doesn't meet all of a baby's needs after about 6 months, since iron stores are depleted by this time. This iron deficiency is called *anemia*. To prevent iron-deficiency anemia in infants, it is wise to begin feeding them iron-fortified cereal between 4 and 6 months of age. In addition, to prevent anemia, many pediatricians recommend giving iron supplements to breast-fed infants beginning shortly after birth.

2. Typical breakfast foods include cereal, eggs, toast, and pancakes, but any food can be

a breakfast, lunch, or dinner food as long as it is nutrient dense. If Tim doesn't like the traditional breakfast foods but enjoys a sandwich, macaroni and cheese, or yogurt, his parents can offer them. These nutritious foods are no more beneficial at lunchtime than they are at 7 A.M.

The depletion of carbohydrate stores that occurs during the night can cause children to be lethargic and inattentive in the morning. Eating early in the morning replenishes carbohydrate stores. Many but not all experts believe that the nutrients consumed stimulate attention in children, allowing them to perform better in school.

3. It usually takes a few days for signs of a food allergy to develop. Common allergic symptoms are diarrhea, vomiting, runny nose, wheezing, and swelling. An infection could produce the same symptoms, but it is usually accompanied by a fever. If Irene and Chris's baby is indeed having an allergic reaction, ceasing to feed the food to the baby should cause the symptoms to disappear. If they do disappear, it is likely that the food caused the allergy. The food can probably be reintroduced later, since babies outgrow most food allergies. Fortunately, the baby did not have the most generalized and severe kind of allergic reaction, an often fatal condition called *anaphylactic shock.*

CHAPTER 18

1. Science has established a considerable link between nutrition (diet) and health. For example, low-fat diets have been shown to reverse atherosclerosis and to improve diabetes control in some people by reducing body fat. Although body cells will age no matter what health practices are followed, morbidity can be decreased through diet and lifestyle. A consistently healthful diet and a regimen of regular physical activity has proved effective in maintaining a healthful body: muscles are firmer, bone fractures are less likely, and the person looks and feels better. The secret to enjoying "youth" throughout life is to establish a healthful physical, mental, and social framework.

2. Many elderly people have experienced the death of a lifelong companion. Men and women who have lived with another person for twenty, thirty, or sometimes over fifty years find the loss of their loved one to be traumatic. If they do not have an avenue to cope with this overwhelming loss, they may become depressed. It is common for depressed people to decrease the amount of food they eat, show little interest in meals, or stop eating altogether. In addition, many elderly people have depended on their loved ones for meal planning and food buying and preparation. The surviving partner may feel left behind and may not know about or care about these tasks.

As the body ages, the senses lose their acuity. People lose some taste receptors in the tongue and some smell receptors in the nose.

This loss of taste and smell contributes to apathy about eating (consider your appetite when you have a cold and can't smell or taste as well).

3. An increase in the RDA for calcium to 1500 mg/day would likely decrease the amount of calcium loss from bones, especially in the hip region. Since many elderly people, notably elderly women, have osteoporosis, it is important to ensure that they obtain an adequate amount of calcium. In addition, vitamin D is needed for calcium absorption. Finally, physical activity can also help elderly people by increasing the amount of mechanical stress the bones can bear, in turn reducing the loss of calcium from bone.

CHAPTER 19

1. The technique used to preserve the food must be analyzed individually. Any method mentioned is acceptable, provided that the food itself and the expected shelf life are taken into consideration.

Pasteurization, sterilization, refrigeration, freezing, canning, chemical preservation, and irradiation are the food-preservation techniques used today. Irradiation has been approved by FDA for the preservation of spices, potatoes, and grains. Irradiation prevents the growth of microorganisms by disrupting their cell membranes, breaking down the DNA and denaturing proteins. Irradiation can decrease the deterioration of the food; however, it can produce off flavors and off colors.

The traditional methods involve adding preservatives, such as BHT and vitamins C and E, as antioxidants. Pasteurization decreases milk contamination and is the best method for milk sterilization. Canning and curing foods are also effective methods. However, with any of these procedures, it should be noted that close observation and maintenance of rigid standards for the techniques used are necessary. If not, any of these methods can lead to food-borne illness by way of microbial contamination. Even traditional methods can cause trouble!

2. USDA recommends cutting boards with unmarred surfaces made from nonporous materials. These include plexiglass, plastic, and marble, which are easy to clean. Grooves or cuts on surfaces provide a "home" where bacteria can thrive. If Jon wants to buy a wooden cutting board, he should plan to clean it using hot, soapy water every time he cuts something. He should also try not to use the same board for both meats and vegetables or fruits. If he must use it for everything, he should cut the vegetables first, wash the board in hot, soapy water, and then cut the meats. Jon should also sanitize any board once a week in a solution of two teaspoons chlorine bleach per quart of water, to minimize any bacterial growth.

3. Bacteria thrive at room temperature, especially between 60° and 110° F. Some bacteria cause food-borne illness by releasing endotoxins and some by producing exotoxins.

Cooling by refrigeration slows down bacterial growth, but it does not stop it or destroy toxins already produced. Foods left at room temperature for 2 hours, or even 1 hour in hot weather, provide microorganisms with the opportunity to grow. Refrigeration after that time is too late. Diana is correct in wanting to discard the food.

CHAPTER 20

1. Undernourished children (and adults) often show apathy, muscular weakness, and decreased physical activity and work capability. Since undernutrition decreases resistance to disease, undernourished children are likely to have more frequent infections and to recover more slowly from illness than well-fed children.

2. Even when a sufficient supply of food energy is available and consumed, appropriate food choices and other aspects of a person's lifestyle are critical to nutritional status. Many of the soup kitchen recipients may select unwisely from the available food, obtaining enough energy but not enough protein, vitamins, and minerals. Undernutrition can be caused not just by insufficient energy intake, but also by an inadequate intake of essential nutrients, leading to symptoms of nutrient-deficiency diseases. Other characteristics of the recipients may contribute to their poor health. For example, they may be alcoholics or drug addicts, have poor personal hygiene, smoke excessively, or engage in little physical activity.

3. Where extreme food shortages exist, there is no choice but to supply hungry people with food—they are starving and dying. However, reliance on outside help is not a long-range solution. Rather, Third World countries need to develop their economies and infrastructures so that people are able to produce or buy sufficient amounts of nutritious food to meet their needs. Appropriate development includes many aspects: education, availability of machinery and other agricultural tools, and nonfarm employment opportunities. Small farms and businesses should be encouraged. As the overall economy expands, more people will be able to afford nutritious food. Agricultural production should focus on basic food crops to be consumed by a country's own citizens, rather than primarily on cash crops for export.

Medical Terminology to Aid in the Study of Nutrition

Term   Meaning

a-   Without, from
acyl   A carbon chain
aden-, adeno-   Gland
-algia   Pain
aliment   Food
-amine   Containing nitrogen
andr-, andro-   Man or male
apo-, ap-   Detached
arteri-, arterio-   Artery
arthr-, arthro-   Joint
-ase   Enzyme
-blast   Immature form, embryonic
brady-   Slow
buli-   Ox
canc-, carcino-   Malignancy
cardi-, cardio-   Heart
centi-   Divided into one hundred parts
chol-, chole-, cholo-   Bile, gall
cholecyst-   Gallbladder
chondr-, chondri-, chondro-   Cartilage
chrom-, chromo-   Color, colored
-clast   Something that breaks
col-, coli-, colo-   Colon
cyano-, cyan-   Blue
cyt-, cyto-   Cell
derm-, dermato-   Skin
dextr-, dextro-   Right, on or toward the right
duoden-, duodeno-   Duodenum
dys-   Difficult, painful
ect-, ecto-   Without, outside, external
ectomy   Excision of
-ein   A protein
em-   Blood
-emia   in blood
encephal-, encephalo-   Brain
endo-, ento-, end-, ent-   Within
enter-, entero-   Intestine
erythr-, erythro-   Red
esophag-, esophago-   Esophagus
eu-   Well, easy, good
gastr-, gastro-, gastri-   Stomach
gen-   To become or produce
gloss-, glosso-   Tongue
glyco-, glyc-   Sugar
gynec-, gyn-, gyne-   Woman or female (especially female reproductive organs)
hem-, hemat-   Blood
hepat-, hepato-   Liver
hexa-, hex-   Six

histo- hist-   Tissue
homeo-, homoeo, homoio   Sameness, similarity
hydr-, hydro-   Water
hyper-   Excessive, above, beyond
hypo-, hyp-   Under, beneath, deficient
hyster-, hystero-   Uterus
idio-   One's own, peculiar to, separate, distinct
ile-, ileo-   Ileum
inter-   Between, among
intra-   Within, during, between layers of
-itis   Inflammation of
jejun-, jejuno-   Jejunum
kilo-   One thousand
lact-, lacti-, lacto-   Milk
leuc-, leuk-   White, colorless
lev-, levo-   Left, levorot
lip-, lipo-   Fat, lipid
litho-, lith-   Stone
lymph-, lympho-   Waterlike
lysis   Destruction
mal-   Bad, badly
malac-, malaco-   Soft, a condition of abnormal softness
mega-, meg-   Large, great
meta-   After, later; change, exchange
metallo-   Containing metal
micro-   Divided into one million parts
milli-   Divided into one thousand parts
mono-   One
morph-, morpho-   Form, shape
my-, myo-   Muscle
myel-, myelo-   Marrow, spinal cord
nas-, naso-   Nose, nasal
necr-, necro-   Dead
nephr-, nephro-   Kidney
neur-, neuro-   Nerve
-oid   Formed like, resembling
-ol   Alcohol
olig-, oligo-   Few, scant
-oma   Tumor
ophthalmo-, ophthalm-   Eye, eyeball
-orex   Mouth
-orexis   Desire, appetite
-ose   Sugar, carbohydrate
-osis   Action, process, result, usually abnormal or diseased
ost-, osteo-, oste-   Bone
ot-   Ear
ovari-, ovario-   Ovary
ovo-, ovi   Eggs

pan-   All
pancreat-, pancreato-   Pancreas
para-   Beside
parieto-   Wall of a cavity, parietal bone
patho-, path-   Disease
ped-   Child, foot
-penia   Without, lack of
-phobia   Fear of
-plasm, -plasma   Formative, formed, cell or tissue substance
pneum-, pneumo-, pneumono-   Lung
-poiesis   Production, format
poly-   Many, much
post-   After
pre-   Before
prot-, proto-   First
pseud-, pseudo-   False
pulmo-, pulmon-, pulmono-   Lung
pyel-, pyelo-   Pelvis
pyr-   Fever, fire
rect-, recto-   Rectum
reni-, reno-   Kidney
rhin-, rhino-   Nose
-rrhagia   Rupture, excessive fluid discharge
-rrhea   Flow, discharge
sate   To fill
scler-, sclero-   Hard, hardness
-scopy   Viewing
seb-, sebi, sebo-   Hard fat sebum, sebaceous glands
semi-   Half
-soma, somat-, somato-   Body
-stasia, -stasis   Slowing or stopping of
stenosis   Narrowing of
stomat-, stomato-   Mouth, stoma
-stomy   Surgical opening
sub-   Under, below
super-   Over, above
tachy-   Swift, fast
thi-, thio-   Containing sulfur
thromb-, thrombo-   Blood clot
tox-, toxi-, toxo-   Poison
trache-, tracheo-   Trachea
-trophy   Growth or mutation
ure-, urea-, ureo-   Urine
uter-, utero-   Uterus
vas-, vaso-   Blood vessel
ven-, veni-, veno-   Vein
vita-   Life
xer-, xero-   Dry

Glossary Terms

absorption The process by which substances are taken up by the GI tract and enter the bloodstream.

absorptive cells A class of cells, also called *enterocytes,* that line the villi; fingerlike projections in the small intestine that participate in nutrient absorption.

acesulfame (ay-see-SUL-fame) An alternate sweetener that yields no energy to the body; it is 200 times sweeter than sucrose.

achlorhydria (ay-clor-HIGH-dre-ah) A state of reduced acid production by the stomach, primarily resulting from loss of the acid-producing cells in the stomach, which is associated with aging.

acid pH A pH less than 7. Lemon juice has an acid pH.

active absorption Absorption in which a carrier is used and ATP energy is expended. In this way the absorptive cell can absorb nutrients, such as glucose, against a concentration gradient.

adaptive thermogenesis Adaptive energy expended in heat production, due to exposure to cold environmental conditions or overfeeding.

adenosine triphosphate (ATP) (ah-DEN-o-sin try-FOS-fate) The main energy currency for cells. ATP energy is used to promote ion pumping, enzyme activity, and muscular contraction.

adipose (fat) cells (ADD-ih-pos) Fat-storing cells.

ad libitum (ad-LIB-itum) At one's desire or pleasure.

adult-onset obesity Obesity that develops in adulthood; characterized by a normal number of adipose cells, but each cell is enlarged because of fat storage.

aerobic (air-ROW-bic) Requiring oxygen; aerobic activities use large muscle groups at moderate intensities. This permits the body to use oxygen to supply energy and to maintain a steady rate for more than a few minutes.

alcohol Refers to ethyl alcohol or ethanol, CH_3CH_2OH.

alcohol dehydrogenase (dee-high-DRO-jen-ase) The enzyme used in alcohol (ethanol) breakdown; the major enzyme used in the liver when alcohol is in low concentration.

aldosterone (al-DOS-ter-own) A powerful hormone produced by the adrenal glands that acts on the kidneys to cause sodium reabsorption and, in turn, water conservation.

alimentary canal (al-ih-MEN-tah-ree) Gastrointestinal tract.

alkaline (basic) pH A pH greater than 7. Baking soda in water yields an alkaline pH.

allergy An immune response that occurs when antibodies react with a protein foreign to the body (antigen).

alpha bond A type of glycosidic bond that can be broken by human intestinal enzymes in digestion.

alpha-linolenic acid (AL-fah-lin-oh-LE-nik) An essential acid with 18 carbon atoms and 3 double bonds (omega-3).

alveoli (al-VE-o-lye) Small air sacs of the lung.

amenorrhea (A-men-or-ee-a) The absence of three to six consecutive menstrual cycles; the absence of menses in a female

amino acid (ah-MEE-noh) The building block for proteins containing a central carbon atom with a nitrogen atom and other atoms attached.

amniotic fluid (am-nee-OTT-ik) Fluid contained in a sac within the uterus. This fluid surrounds and protects the fetus during development.

amylase (AM-uh-lace) Starch-digesting enzyme from the salivary glands or pancreas.

amylopectin (am-ih-low-PEK-tin) A digestible branched-chain polysaccharide made of glucose units; component of starch.

amylose (AM-uh-los) A digestible straight-chain polysaccharide made of glucose units; component of starch.

anabolic/anabolism (an-AH-bol-iz-um) Building compounds.

anaerobic (AN-ah-ROW-bic) Not requiring oxygen; anaerobic activities use muscle groups at intensities that exceed the body's capacity to supply energy using only oxygen-requiring pathways.

analog A related substance, such as the derivative of vitamin A, 11-*cis* retinoic acid. Analogs generally contain extra or altered chemical groups compared with the native compound.

anaphylactic shock (an-ah-fih-LAK-tic) A severe allergic response that results in lowered blood pressure and respiratory and gastrointestinal distress. This can be fatal.

androgen (AN-dro-jen) A general term for hormones that stimulate development in male sex organs; for example, testosterone.

android obesity (AN-droyd) Obesity in which fat storage is located primarily in the abdominal area; defined as a waist-to-hip circumference ratio greater than 0.95 in men and 0.85 in women. Android obesity is closely associated with a high risk of heart disease, hypertension, and diabetes.

anergy (AN-er-jee) Lack of an immune response to foreign compounds entering the body.

angiotensin I (an-jee-oh-TEN-sin) An intermediary compound produced during the body's attempt to conserve water and sodium; it is converted in the lungs to angiotensin II.

angiotensin II A compound produced from angiotensin I, which increases blood vessel constriction and triggers production of the hormone aldosterone.

animal model Study of disease in animals that duplicates human disease. This can be used to understand more about human disease.

anorexia nervosa (an-oh-REX-ee-uh ner-VOH-sah) An eating disorder involving a psychological loss of appetite and self-starvation, resulting in part from a distorted body image and various social pressures; usually associated with puberty.

anthropometry (an-throw-po-MEH-tree) The measurement of weight, lengths, circumferences, and thicknesses of the body.

antibody (AN-tih-bod-ee) Blood protein that inactivates foreign proteins found in the body. This helps prevent infection.

antidiuretic hormone (ADH) (an-tie-dye-u-RET-ik) A hormone, secreted by the pituitary gland, that acts on the kidney to cause a decrease in water excretion.

antigen (AN-ti-jen) Any substance that induces a state of sensitivity and/or resistance to microbes or toxic substances after a latent period; substance that stimulates a specific arm of the immune system. Foreign antigens are introduced into the body. B-lymphocyte cells then begin to proliferate and secrete specific antibodies that bind to the antigen, labeling it as foreign and destined for destruction.

antioxidant A compound that prevents the oxidation of substances in food or the body, particularly lipids. Antioxidants are especially important in preventing the oxidation of polyunsaturated lipids in the membranes of cells. An antioxidant is able to donate electrons to electron-seeking compounds. This in turn reduces electron capture and thus breakdown of unsaturated fatty acids and other cell components by oxidizing agents. Vitamin E is one antioxidant cells use for protection.

apoferritin (ape-oh-FERR-ih-tin) A protein in the intestinal cell that binds with the ferric form of iron (Fe^{3+}) to form ferritin.

apolipoproteins (APE-oh-lip-oh-PRO-teens) Proteins imbedded in the outer shell of lipoproteins. They help other enzymes function, act as lipid transfer proteins, or help bind to a receptor.

appetite The external (psychological) influences that encourage us to find and eat food, often in the absence of obvious hunger.

arachidonic acid (ar-a-kih-DON-ik) A fatty acid with 20 carbon atoms and four double bonds (omega-6).

areola (ah-REE-oh-lah) The circular dark area of skin at the center of the breast.

ariboflavinosis (ah-rih-bo-flay-vih-NOH-sis) A condition resulting from a lack of riboflavin. The *a* means "without," and the *osis* stands for "a condition of."

arithmetic progression A series of numbers in which the difference between each number is the same.

aseptic processing (ah-SEP-tik) A method by which food and container are simultaneously sterilized; it allows manufacturers to produce boxes of milk that can be stored at room temperature. Variations of this process are also known as *ultra high temperature* (UHT) packaging.

aspartame (AH-spar-tame) An alternate sweetener made of two amino acids and methanol; it is 200 times sweeter than sucrose.

atherosclerosis (ath-e-roh-scle-ROH-sis) A buildup of fatty material in the arteries, including those surrounding the heart.

atom Smallest combining unit of an element.

autodigestion Literally, "self-digestion." The stomach limits autodigestion by covering itself with a thick layer of mucus and producing enzymes and acid only when needed for digestion of foodstuff.

autoimmune Immune reactions against normal body cells; self against self.

avidin (AV-ih-din) A protein found in raw egg whites that can bind biotin and inhibit its absorption. Avidin is destroyed by cooking.

baryophobia (bear-ee-oh-FO-bee-ah) A disorder associated with a poor rate of growth in children because the parents underfeed them in an attempt to prevent development of obesity and/or heart disease.

basal metabolism (BAY-sal) The minimum energy the body requires to support itself when resting and awake. To have basal metabolic rate (BMR) measured, a person must not have eaten in the previous 12 hours and be maintained in a warm, quiet environment during the measurement. It amounts to roughly 1 kcal/min, or about 1400 kcal per day.

beriberi (BEAR-ee-BEAR-ee) Thiamin deficiency disorder characterized by muscle weakness, loss of appetite, nerve degeneration, and sometimes edema.

beta (BEY-tuh) bond A type of glycosidic bond that is not digested by human intestinal enzymes when it is part of a long chain of glucose monosaccharides.

beta-oxidation The breakdown of a fatty acid into numerous acetyl-CoA molecules.

BHA and BHT (Butylated hydroxyanisole and butylated hydroxytoluene) Two common synthetic antioxidants added to foods.

bile A substance made in the liver and stored in the gallbladder; it is released into the small intestine to aid fat absorption by emulsifying it into micelles.

bile acids Emulsifiers synthesized by the liver and released by the gallbladder during digestion to aid in fat digestion.

binge-eating disorder A practice in which an abnormally large amount of food is eaten, in which there is a feeling of loss of control over eating. This eating pattern can be triggered by the experience of emotions such as frustration, anger, depression, or anxiety.

bioavailability The degree to which the amount of an ingested nutrient is absorbed and so is available to the body.

biochemical lesion (LEE-zhun) Nutritional deficiency symptoms observed in the blood or urine, such as low concentrations of nutrient byproducts or low enzyme activities, indicating reduced body function.

bioelectrical impedance (im-PEE-dance) A method to estimate total body fat that uses a low-energy electrical current. The more fat storage a person has, the more impedance (resistance) to electrical flow will be exhibited.

biological value (BV) of a protein A measurement of the body's ability to retain protein absorbed from a food.

biotechnology The use of advanced scientific techniques to alter and, ideally, improve characteristics of animals and plants.

bleaching process A process by which light depletes the rhodopsin concentration in the eye, which allows the eye to become adapted to bright light.

blood doping A technique by which an athlete's red blood cell count is increased. Blood is taken from the athlete, and the red blood cells are concentrated and then later reinjected into the athlete.

B-lymphocyte (LIM-fo-site) White blood cells processed by liver and spleen tissues that are responsible for antibody production. They are responsible for recognition of foreign substances (such as bacteria) in extracellular sites in the body.

body mass index Weight (in kilograms) divided by height squared (in meters). A value of 30 or greater shows obesity-related health risks.

bomb calorimeter (kal-oh-RIM-eh-ter) An instrument used to determine the kilocalorie content of a food.

bond A sharing of electrons, charges, or attractions linking two atoms.

bone mineral density Total mineral content of bone at a specific bone site divided by the width of the bone at that site.

bone remodeling A process by which bone is first resorbed by osteoclast cells and then reformed by osteoblast cells. This process allows the body to form bone where needed, such as in areas of high mechanical stress.

bone-resorbing cells Specialized bone cells that remove bone material, also called *osteoclasts*.

bound water Water that is attached to organic substances in foods. This is not available for microbial use.

brown adipose tissue (ADD-ih-pose) A specialized form of adipose tissue that produces large amounts of heat by metabolizing energy-yielding nutrients without synthesizing much ATP. The energy released simply forms heat.

buffer Compound that can take up or release hydrogen ions to maintain a certain pH value in a solution.

bulimia nervosa (boo-LEEM-ee-uh) An eating disorder in which large quantities of food are eaten at one time (bingeing) and then purged from the body by vomiting, use of laxatives, or other means.

cafeteria-fed animal A laboratory animal that is fed a high-fat, high-sugar diet to encourage it to overeat and become obese.

calcitriol (kal-sih-TRIH-ol) The active hormone form of vitamin D (1,25-dihydroxyvitamin D). It contains a derivative of cholesterol as part of its structure.

calmodulin (kal-MOD-you-lin) A cell protein that, once bound to calcium, can influence the activity of certain enzymes in the cell.

cancer A condition characterized by uncontrolled growth of abnormal body cells.

cancer initiation The step in the process of cancer development that begins with alterations in DNA, the genetic material in a cell. This may cause the cell to no longer respond to normal physiological controls.

cancer progression The final stage in the cancer process in which the cancer cell grows to a sufficient mass so it will significantly affect body metabolism.

cancer promotion The step in the cancer process when cell division increases, in turn decreasing the time available for repair enzymes to act on altered DNA, and encouraging cells with altered DNA to develop and grow. Anything that increases the rate of cell division decreases the chance that the repair enzymes will find the altered part of the DNA in time to do their work.

capillary bed Minute vessels one cell thick that create a junction between arterial and venous circulation. It is here where gas and nutrient exchange occurs between body cells and the bloodstream.

carbohydrate (kar-bow-HIGH-drate) A compound containing carbon, hydrogen, and oxygen atoms; most are known as *sugars, starches,* and *dietary fibers.*

carbohydrate-loading A process in which a 600-gram carbohydrate intake (or 70% of total energy, whichever is larger) is consumed for 3 days before an athletic event in an attempt to increase muscle glycogen stores.

cardiac input (CARD-ee-ack) The amount of blood pumped by the heart.

cardiovascular Referring to the heart and blood vessels.

cariogenic (CARE-ee-oh-jen-ik) Literally "caries producing"; a substance, often carbohydrate-rich (such as caramel), that promotes dental caries.

carnitine (CAR-nih-teen) A compound used to shuttle fatty acids from the cytosol of the cell into mitochondria.

carotenoids (kah-ROT-en-oyds) Plant pigments, some of which can yield vitamin A. Of the 600 or so carotenoids found in nature, about 50 yield vitamin A activity and thus are called provitamin A.

carpal tunnel syndrome (CAR-pull) (SIN-drom) A disease in which nerves that travel to the wrist are pinched as they pass through a narrow opening in a bone in the wrist.

casein (KAY-seen) Protein found in milk that forms curds when exposed to acid and is difficult for infants to digest.

cash crops Crops grown by a country specifically for export, in order to gain the ability to purchase goods from other countries, rather than to feed the country's citizens (e.g., coffee, tea, cocoa, and bananas).

catabolic/catabolism (cat-ah-BOL-ik) Breaking down compounds.

catalyst (CAT-ul-ist) A compound that speeds reaction rates but is not altered by the reaction.

celiac disease (SEA-lee-ak) Also known as *gluten-induced enteropathy.* It is caused by an allergy to protein found in wheat, rye, oats, and barley. If untreated, it causes severe flattening of the villi in the intestine, leading to severe malabsorption of nutrients.

cell A minute structure; the living basis of plant and animal organization. In animals it is bounded by a cell membrane. Cells contain both genetic material and systems for synthesizing energy-yielding compounds. Cells have the ability to take up compounds from and excrete compounds into their surroundings.

cellulose (SELL-you-los) A straight-chain polysaccharide of glucose molecules that is undigestible because of the presence of beta glycosidic bonds; part of insoluble fiber.

Celsius A centigrade measure of temperature. For conversion: (degrees in Fahrenheit − 32) × 5/9 = C°; (degrees in Celsius × 9/5) + 32 = F°.

cerebrovascular accident (CVA) (se-REE-bro-VAS-cue-lar) Death of part of the brain tissue due to a blood clot.

ceruloplasmin (se-RUE-low-PLAS-min) A blue, copper-containing protein component in the blood that can remove an electron from Fe^{2+} (the ferrous form) to yield Fe^{3+} (the ferric form). The Fe^{3+} form of iron can then bind with transport and storage proteins, such as transferrin.

chain-breaking Breaking the link between two or more actions that encourage problem behavior, such as snacking while watching television.

chelates (KEY-lates) Complexes formed between metal ions and substances with polar groups, such as proteins. The polar groups on the substance form two or more attachments with the metal ions, forming a ring structure. The metal ion is then firmly attached and sequestered.

chemical reaction An interaction between two compounds that changes both participants.

chemical score A ratio comparing the essential amino acid content of the protein in a food with the essential amino acid content in a reference protein, such as one established by the Food and Agriculture Organization. The lowest ratio for any essential amino acid is the chemical score.

cholecystokinin (CCK) (ko-la-sis-toe-KY-nin) A hormone that stimulates enzyme release from the pancreas and bile release from the gallbladder.

cholesterol (ko-LES-te-rol) A waxy lipid; it has a structure containing multiple chemical rings (steroid structure).

chronic (KRON-ik) Long-standing, developing over time; slow to develop or resolve. When referring to disease, this indicates that the disease progress, once developed, is slow and tends to remain; a good example is coronary heart disease.

chylomicrons (kye-lo-MY-krons) Dietary fat surrounded by a shell of cholesterol, phospholipids, and protein. These are made in the intestine after fat absorption and travel through the lymphatic system to the bloodstream.

chyme (KIME) A mixture of stomach secretions and partially digested food.

cirrhosis (see-ROH-sis) A loss of functioning liver cells, which are replaced by nonfunctioning connective tissue. Any substance that poisons liver cells can lead to cirrhosis. The most common cause is a chronic, excessive alcohol intake.

***cis* isomer (sis EYE-so-mer)** An isomer form seen in compounds with double bonds, such as fatty acids, in which the hydrogens on both ends of the double bond lie on the same side of the plane of that bond.

citric acid cycle A pathway that breaks down acetyl-CoA, yielding carbon dioxide, $FADH_2$, NADH, and GTP. The pathway can also be used to synthesize compounds.

clinical lesion (LEE-zhun) Nutritional deficiency sign seen on physical examination.

***Clostridium botulinum* (klo-STRID-ee-um BOT-you-LY-num)** A bacterium that can cause a fatal type of food-borne illness.

coenzymes Compounds made from certain vitamins that participate in many enzyme-catalyzed reactions. Coenzymes combine with an inactive protein called an *apoenzyme* to form an active compound called a *holoenzyme.*

cognitive restructuring Changing negative, self-defeating, or pessimistic thoughts that undermine weight control efforts to those that are positive, optimistic, and supportive of weight control.

colic (KOL-ik) Periodic, unconsolable crying in a healthy young infant.

colipase A protein secreted by the pancreas that in part acts to change the shape of pancreatic lipase, which facilitates its action.

colostrum (ko-LAHS-trum) The fluid secreted during late pregnancy and the first few days after birth. This thick fluid is rich in immune factors and protein.

comorbidity Disease conditions that are linked to a specific disease, such as heart disease and certain forms of cancer that are more common in people with obesity. Morbidity refers to disease.

complement A large group of blood proteins involved in immune responses, such as phagocytosis and the destruction of bacteria.

complementarity of proteins The ability of two food protein sources to make up for each other's insufficient contribution of specific essential amino acids, such that together they yield a high-quality protein diet.

complete proteins Proteins that contain ample amounts of all nine essential amino acids.

compound A group of different types of atoms bonded together in definite proportion (see **molecule**). Not all chemical compounds exist as molecules. Some compounds are made up of ions.

compression of morbidity Maintaining good health practices to delay the onset of disabilities caused by chronic disease.

conceptus That produced as a result of conception; embryo.

condensation reaction A reaction that forms a bond between two compounds by removing a water molecule.

conditioning The process through which an originally neutral stimulus repeatedly paired with a reinforcing agent elicits a predictable response.

congenital (con-JEN-i-tal) A term that means "present at birth." Thus a congenital abnormality is a defect that has been present since birth. These defects may be inherited from the parents, may occur as a result of damage or infection while in the uterus, or may occur at the time of birth.

conjugase (KON-ju-gase) Enzyme systems in the intestine that enhance folate absorption; they remove glutamate molecules from polyglutamate forms of folate.

connective tissue Protein tissue that holds different structures in the body together. Some structures are made up of connective tissue, notably tendons and cartilages. Connective tissue also forms part of bone and the nonmuscular structures of arteries and veins.

contingency management Forming a plan of action for responding to an environment in which overeating is likely, such as when snacks are within easy reach at a party.

control group Participants in an experiment whose habits or actions are not altered.

cortical bone (KORT-ih-kal) Dense, compact bone that comprises the outer surface and shafts of bone.

corticosteroid A steroid produced by the adrenal gland, an example of which is cortisol.

cortisol (KORT-ih-sol) A hormone made by the adrenal gland that, among other functions, stimulates the production of glucose from amino acids.

covalent bond (ko-VAY-lent) A union of two atoms formed by the sharing of electrons.

cretinism (KREET-in-ism) Stunting of body growth and mental development in infancy and later development that results from inadequate maternal intake of iodide during pregnancy.

Crohn's disease (Krown) A disease of unknown cause in which the small intestine becomes severely inflamed and its absorptive capacity limited.

crude fiber What remains of dietary fiber after acid and alkaline treatment. This consists primarily of cellulose and lignin.

cystic fibrosis (SIS-tik figh-BRO-sis) A disease that often leads to overproduction of mucus. Mucus can invade the pancreas, decreasing enzyme output. The lack of lipase enzyme then contributes to severe fat malabsorption.

cytochrome (SITE-o-krome) Electron-transfer agent that participates in the electron transport chain.

cytochrome P450 Enzymes in cells, also known as *mixed function oxidases*, that are designed to detoxify xenobiotics.

cytokines (SITE-o-kynes) Substances secreted by various white blood cells upon activation by antigen. Phagocytes release a variety of cytokines, such as various interleukins, which promote white blood cell activation, or may lead to toxic injury to foreign cells. Cytokines produced by monocytes and macrophages are called *monokines,* and those produced by lymphocytes are called *lymphokines.*

cytotoxic test (SITE-o-TOX-ik) An unreliable test to define food allergies that involves mixing whole blood with food proteins.

Daily Reference Values (DRV) Standards of intake for certain components of a diet (such as carbohydrate, fat, saturated fat, cholesterol, sodium, potassium, and dietary fiber) set by FDA for which no RDAs exist. These values are intended to be used for comparing intakes of these factors to desirable (or maximum) intakes. DRVs help consumers evaluate individual food choices and determine how they fit into a total diet as they form part of the Daily Values.

Daily Values Standards for expressing nutrient content on nutrition labels. FDA uses the Daily Values as a single list of reference values for showing nutrition information on food labels.

dark adaptation A process by which the rhodopsin concentration in the eye increases in dark conditions, allowing improved vision in the dark.

deamination (dee-am-ih-NA-shun) The removal of an amino group from an amino acid.

Delaney clause A clause to the 1958 Food Additives Amendment of the Pure Food and Drug Act in the United States that prevents the intentional (direct) addition to foods of a compound that has been shown to cause cancer in animals or man.

dementia (de-MEN-sha) General persistent loss or decrease in mental function.

denature (dee-NAY-ture) Alteration of the tertiary structure of a protein, usually as a result of treatment by heat, acid, base, or agitation.

dental caries (KARE-ees) Erosions in the surface of a tooth caused by acids made by bacteria as they metabolize sugars.

depolarize Reversal of membrane potential from production of action potential in nerve and muscle cells.

dextrin Partial breakdown product of starch that contains few to many glucose molecules. These appear when starch is being digested into many units of maltose by salivary and pancreatic amylase.

diabetes (DYE-uh-BEET-eez) A disease characterized by high blood glucose (hyperglycemia), resulting from either insufficient insulin release by the pancreas or general inability of insulin to act on certain body cells, such as adipose cells (see **insulin-dependent diabetes** and **noninsulin-dependent diabetes**).

diastolic blood pressure (dye-ah-STOL-ik) The pressure in the arterial blood vessels when the heart is between beats.

dietary fiber Substances in food (essentially from plants) that are not digested by the processes that take place in the stomach or small intestine. These add bulk to feces.

Dietary Goals Specific goals for nutrient intakes set in 1977 by a committee of the U.S. Senate.

Dietary Guidelines General goals for nutrient intake and diet composition set by government agencies—USDA and DHHS.

dietitian See **Registered Dietitian.**

digestibility (dye-JES-tih-bil-it-ee) The proportion of food substances eaten that can be broken down in the intestinal tract for absorption into the bloodstream.

digestion The process by which large ingested molecules are mechanically and chemically broken down to produce smaller forms that can be absorbed across the wall of the GI tract.

diphosphoglycerate (dye-foss-foe-GLISS-er-ate) A compound used in the red blood cells that is involved in the release of oxygen from hemoglobin.

direct calorimetry (kal-oh-RIM-eh-tree) A method to determine energy use by the body by measuring heat that emanates from the body, usually using an insulated chamber.

disaccharides (dye-SACK-uh-rides) Class of sugars formed by the chemical bonding of two monosaccharides.

diuretic (dye-u-RET-ik) A substance that, when ingested, increases the flow of urine.

diverticula (DYE-ver-TIK-you-luh) Pouches that protrude through the wall of the large intestine to the outside of the intestine.

diverticulitis (DYE-ver-tik-you-LITE-us) An inflammation of the diverticula caused by acids produced by bacterial metabolism inside them.

diverticulosis (DYE-ver-tik-you-LOH-sis) The condition of having many diverticula in the large inestine.

docosahexaenoic acid (DHA) (DOE-co-sa-hex-a-ee-no-ik) An omega-3 fatty acid with 22 carbons and six carbon-carbon double bonds. DHA is present in fish oils and also may be synthesized from alpha-linolenic acid.

double-blind study An experiment in which the subjects and researchers are unaware of the subject's assignment (test or placebo) or the outcome of the study until it is completed. An independent third party holds the code and the data until the study is completed.

duodenum (doo-oh-DEE-num, or doo-ODD-num) The first 12 inches (30 cm) of the small intestine.

ecosystem A "community" in nature that includes plants and animals and the environment associated with them.

ectomorph (EK-tuh-morf) A body type associated with very long, thin bones and very long, thin fingers.

edema (uh-DEE-muh) The build-up of excess fluid in extracellular spaces.

eicosanoids (eye-KOH-san-oyds) Hormonelike compounds synthesized from polyunsaturated fatty acids. Within this class of compounds are prostaglandins, thromboxanes, and leukotrienes.

eicosapentaenoic acid (EPA) (eye-KOH-sah-pen-tah-ee-NO-ik) An omega-3 fatty acid with 20 carbon atoms and five double bonds; present in fish oils and may be synthesized from alpha-linolenic acid.

electrolytes (ih-LEK-tro-lites) Substances that break down into ions in water and, in turn, are able to conduct an electrical current. These include sodium, chloride, and potassium.

electron A part of an atom that is negatively charged. Electrons orbit the nucleus.

electron transport chain A series of reactions using oxygen that convert NADH and $FADH_2$ into free NAD and FAD, yielding water and ATP.

elements Substances that cannot be broken down further by using ordinary chemical procedures.

elimination diet A restrictive diet that systematically tests foods that may cause an allergic response by first eliminating them for 1 to 2 weeks and then adding them back, one at a time.

embryo (EM-bree-oh) The developing human life form during the second to eighth week after conception.

emulsify (ee-MULL-sih-fye) To suspend fat in water by isolating individual fat drops using sheets of water molecules or other substances to prevent the fat from coalescing.

endocrine-onset obesity (EN-doh-krin) Obesity caused by rare hormonal abnormalities or rare genetic disorders. This is the cause of less than 10% of obesity cases in America.

endocytosis (phagocytosis/pinocytosis) Forms of active absorption in which the absorptive cell forms an indentation in its membrane and particles (phagocytosis) or fluids (pinocytosis) entering the indentation are then engulfed by the cell.

endometrium (en-doh-ME-tree-um) The membrane that lines the inside of the uterus. It increases in thickness during the menstrual cycle until ovulation occurs. The surface layers are shed during menstruation if conception does not take place.

endomorph (EN-doh-morf) A body type characterized by short, stubby bones, a short trunk, and short fingers.

endorphins (en-DOR-fins) Natural body tranquilizers that may be involved in the feeding response and function in pain reduction.

endotoxin A toxin made by bacteria that is released by bacteria as they die and their cell walls are broken.

energy balance A state in which the energy intake, in the form of food or alcohol, matches the energy expended, primarily through basal metabolism and physical activity.

enriched A term generally meaning that the vitamins thiamin, niacin, and riboflavin and the mineral iron have been added to a grain product to improve nutritional quality.

enterohepatic circulation (EN-ter-oh-heh-PAT-ik) Recycling of compounds between the small intestine and the liver over and over again, as happens with bile acids.

enzyme (EN-zime) A compound that speeds the rate of a chemical reaction but is not altered by the chemical reaction. Almost all enzymes are proteins.

epidemiology (ep-uh-dee-me-OLL-uh-gee) The study of how disease rates vary between different population groups, such as the rate of stomach cancer in Japan compared with that in Canada.

epigenetic carcinogens (promoters) (ep-ih-je-NET-ik car-SIN-oh-jens) Compounds that increase cell division and thereby increase the chance that a cell with altered DNA will develop into cancer.

epinephrine (ep-ih-NEF-rin) Also known as *adrenaline*. This hormone is released by the adrenal gland. A related form, norepinephrine, is released from various nerve endings in the body. Both hormones act to increase glycogen breakdown in the liver, among other functions.

epiphyses (ep-a-FEE-seas) End of a long bone. The epiphyseal plate is made of cartilage and allows growth of bone to occur. This is sometimes referred to as a *growth plate*. During childhood the cartilage cells multiply and absorb calcium to develop into bone.

epithelial cells (ep-ih-THEE-lee-ul) The surface cells that line the outside of the body and all external passages within it.

equilibrium (ee-kwih-LIB-ree-um) In nutrition, a state in which nutrient intake equals nutrient losses. Thus the body maintains a stable condition.

ergogenic (ur-go-JEN-ic) Work producing. An ergogenic aid is a physical, mechanical, nutritional, psychological, or pharmacological substance or treatment that is intended to directly improve exercise performance.

erythropoietin (eh-REE-throw-POY-eh-tin) A hormone secreted mostly by the kidneys that enhances red blood cell synthesis and stimulates red blood cell release from bone marrow.

essential (indispensable) amino acids Amino acids not efficiently synthesized by humans that must therefore be included in the diet. There are nine essential amino acids.

essential fatty acids Fatty acids that must be present in the diet to maintain health. These are linoleic acid and alpha-linolenic acid.

essential nutrient In nutritional terms, this represents a substance that, when left out of a diet, leads to signs of poor health. The body either can't produce these nutrients or can't produce them fast enough to meet its needs. Then, if added back to a diet before permanent damage occurs, the affected aspects of health are restored.

esterification (e-ster-ih-fih-KAY-shun) With regard to fats, the process of attaching fatty acids to a glycerol molecule, creating an ester bond and releasing water. Removing a fatty acid is called deesterification; reattaching a fatty acid is called reesterification.

estimated safe and adequate daily dietary intake (ESADDI) Nutrient intake recommendations first made by the Food and Nutrition Board in 1980. A range for intake for these nutrients is given, as not enough information is available to set a more specific RDA.

eustachian tubes (you-STAY-shun) Thin tubes connected to the middle ear that open into the throat.

exchange The serving size of a food on a specific exchange list.

Exchange System A system for classifying foods into numerous lists based on their macronutrient composition and establishing serving sizes so that one serving of each food on a list contains the same amount of carbohydrate, protein, fat, and energy (kilocalories).

exotoxin A toxin made by bacteria that is excreted into its surrounding medium as the toxin is made.

experiment A test made to examine the validity of a hypothesis.

extracellular fluid Fluid present outside the cells; this includes intravascular and interstitial fluids.

extracellular space The space between cells.

facilitated absorption Absorption where a carrier is used to shuttle substances into the absorptive cells, but no energy is expended. A concentration gradient higher in the intestinal contents than in the absorptive cell drives the absorption.

failure to thrive Inadequate gains in height and weight in infancy, often due to an inadequate food intake.

famine A time of massive starvation, often associated with crop failures, war, and political strife.

fasting hypoglycemia (HIGH-po-gligh-SEE-me-ah) Low blood glucose that follows about a day or so of fasting.

fatty acids Acids found in lipids, composed of carbon atoms and hydrogen atoms with an acid group ($—\overset{O}{\overset{\|}{C}}—$) at one end and a methyl group ($—CH_3$) at the other.

feces (FEE-seas) Substances discharged from the bowel during defecation, consisting of the undigested residue of food, dead GI tract cells, mucus, bacteria, and other waste material. Another term for feces is *stool*.

feeding center A group of cells in the hypothalamus that, when stimulated, causes hunger.

fermentation The conversion, without use of oxygen, of carbohydrates to alcohols, acids, and carbon dioxide.

ferritin (FERR-ih-tin) A protein compound that serves as the storage form of iron in the blood and tissues.

fetal alcohol syndrome (FAS) (FEET-al) A group of physical and mental abnormalities in the infant that result from the mother consuming alcohol during pregnancy.

fetus (FEET-us) The developing life form from 8 weeks until birth.

flavin adenine dinucleotide (FAD) (FLAY-vin ADD-en-neen dye-NUK-lee-oh-tide) A hydrogen carrier in the cell; synthesized from the vitamin riboflavin.

fluoroapatite (fleur-oh-APP-uh-tite) A tooth crystal containing fluoride ions. Presence of this crystal makes the tooth relatively acid resistant.

follicular hyperkeratosis (HI-per-care-a-TOE-sis) A condition in which keratin, a protein, accumulates around hair follicles.

food-borne illness sickness caused by ingestion of foods containing toxic substances produced by microorganisms.

food intolerance An adverse reaction to food that does not involve an allergic reaction.

food sensitivity A mild reaction to a substance in a food that might be expressed as slight itching or redness of the skin.

fore milk The first breast milk delivered in the nursing session.

fortified A term generally meaning that vitamins, minerals, or both have been added to a food product in excess of what was originally found in the product.

fraternal twins Fetuses that develop from two separate ova and sperm and therefore have separate genetic identities, although they develop simultaneously in the mother.

free erythrocyte protoporphyrins (FEP) (eh-RITH-row-sight pro-tow-POR-fy-rins) Immature red blood cells released from the bone marrow. An increased FEP in the blood reflects a decreased ability to make red blood cells and suggests iron-deficiency anemia. Lead poisoning also raises the blood concentration of FEP.

free radical Short-lived form of compounds that exist with an unpaired electron in the outer electron shell. This causes an electron-seeking nature, which can be very destructive to electron-dense areas of a cell, such as DNA and cell membranes.

free water The water not bound to the compounds in a food. This is available for microbial use.

fructose (FROOK-tose) A monosaccharide with six carbons that form a five-membered or six-membered ring with oxygen in the ring; found in fruits and honey.

fruitarian (froot-AIR-een-un) A person who eats primarily fruits, nuts, honey, and vegetable oils.

galactose (gah-LAK-tose) A six-carbon monosaccharide; an isomer of glucose.

galactosemia (gah-LAK-toh-SEE-mee-ah) A rare, genetic disease characterized by the buildup of the monosaccharide galactose in the bloodstream resulting from the inability of the liver to metabolize it. If present at birth and left untreated, this disease causes severe mental and growth retardation in the infant.

gastric inhibitory peptide (GIP) (GAS-trik in-HIB-ih-tor-ee PEP-tide) A hormone that slows gastric motility and stimulates insulin release from the pancreas.

gastrin (GAS-trin) A hormone that stimulates enzyme and acid secretion in the stomach.

gastrointestinal distention (GAS-troh-in-TES-tin-al) Expansion of the walls of the stomach or intestines due to pressure caused by the presence of gases, food, drink, or other factors.

gastrointestinal (GI) tract The main sites in the body used for digestion and absorption of nutrients. It consists of the mouth, esophagus, stomach, small intestine, large intestine, rectum, and anus.

gastroplasty (GAS-troh-plas-tee) Surgery performed on the stomach to limit its volume to approximately 50 ml, the size of a shot glass

gene (JEAN) The genetic material on chromosomes that makes up DNA. Genes provide the blueprint for the production of cell proteins.

generally recognized as safe (GRAS) A list of food additives that in 1958 were considered safe for consumption. Manufacturers were allowed to continue to use these additives, without special clearance, when needed for food products. FDA bears responsibility for proving they are not safe, but can remove unsafe products from the list.

genetic engineering Alteration of genetic material in plants or animals with the intent of improving growth, disease resistance, or other characteristics.

genotoxic carcinogen (initiator) (JEH-no-TOK-sik car-SIN-oh-jen) A compound that alters DNA in a cell, providing the potential for cancer to develop.

geometric progression A large group of numbers in which the division of each number by its immediate predecessor yields the same answer (e.g., 3, 9, 27, 81).

gestation (jes-TAY-shun) The time of fetal growth from conception to birth; a period of about 40 weeks after the woman's last menstrual period.

gestational diabetes (jes-TAY-shun-al) Elevated blood glucose that develops during pregnancy but returns to normal after birth; one cause is placental production of hormones that antagonize blood glucose regulation.

glucagon (GLOO-kuh-gon) A hormone made by the alpha cells of the pancreas that stimulates the breakdown of glycogen in the liver into glucose; this raises blood glucose. Glucagon also performs other functions.

gluconeogenesis (gloo-ko-nee-oh-JEN-uh-sis) The production of new glucose molecules by metabolic pathways in the cell. The source of the carbon atoms for these new glucose molecules is usually amino acids.

glucose (GLOO-kos) A six-carbon atom carbohydrate found in blood and in table sugar bound to fructose; also known as *dextrose*, it is one of the simple sugars.

glucose polymer A carbohydrate source used in some sports drinks that consists of a few glucose molecules bonded together.

glutathione peroxidase (gloo-tah-THIGH-own per-OX-ih-dase) A selenium-containing enzyme that can break down peroxides. It acts in conjunction with vitamin E to reduce free-radical damage to cells.

glycemic index (gligh-SEE-mik) A ratio used to measure the relative ability of a carbohydrate to raise blood glucose compared with the ability of white bread (or glucose) to raise blood glucose.

glycerol (GLISS-er-ol) An alcohol containing three hydroxyl groups (— OH); used to help form the "backbone" of triglyceride molecules.

glycocalyx (gly-co-KAY-licks) Hairlike projections that cover the microvilli of the absorptive cells.

glycogen (GLIGH-ko-jen) A carbohydrate made of multiple units of glucose; exhibits a highly branched structure; the storage form of carbohydrate for muscle and liver; sometimes known as *animal starch.*

glycolysis (gligh-COLL-ih-sis) The pathway that results in the breakdown of glucose into two pyruvate (or lactate) molecules.

glycosidic bond (gligh-coh-SID-ik) The covalent bond formed between two monosaccharides when a water molecule is lost.

goiter (GOY-ter) An enlargement of the thyroid gland; this can be caused by a lack of iodide in the diet.

goitrogen (GOY-troh-jen) Substance in food and water that interferes with thyroid gland metabolism and so may cause goiter if consumed in large amounts.

gram Measure of weight in the metric system. One gram equals 1/28 of an ounce.

green revolution A period in the 1960s when much emphasis was placed on improving strains and cultivation practices of cereal grains, such as rice, wheat, and corn.

growth hormone A pituitary hormone that causes body growth and the release of fat from storage, among other effects.

gum A dietary fiber containing chains of galactose, glucuronic acid, and other monosaccharides; characteristically found in exudates from plant stems.

gynecoid obesity (GIGH-nih-coyd) Obesity in which fat storage is located primarily in the buttocks and thigh area.

H2 blockers Medications, such as cimetidine (Tagamet), that block the stimulation of stomach acid production caused by histamine.

Harris-Benedict equation An equation that predicts resting metabolic rate based on a person's weight, height, and age.

heartburn A pain emanating from the esophagus, caused by stomach acid backing up into the esophagus and irritating the esophageal tissue.

heart disease Disease usually caused by the deposition of fatty material in the blood vessels in the heart. This in turn reduces blood flow to the heart, thereby reducing heart function, which can lead to death.

heat-labile (LAY-bile) A structure or activity that is changed by heating.

hematocrit (hee-MAT-oh-krit) The percentage of total blood volume occupied by red blood cells.

heme iron (HEEM) Iron provided from animal tissues as hemoglobin and myoglobin. Approximately 40% of the iron in meat is heme iron; it is readily absorbed.

hemicellulose (hem-ih-SELL-you-los) A dietary fiber containing xylose, galactose, glucose, and other monosaccharides bonded together.

hemochromatosis (heem-oh-krom-ah-TOE-sis) A disorder of iron metabolism characterized by increased absorption, saturation of iron-binding proteins, and deposition of hemosiderin in the liver tissue.

hemoglobin (HEEM-oh-glow-bin) The iron-containing part of the red blood cell that carries oxygen to the cells and some carbon dioxide away from the cells. It is also responsible for the red color of blood.

hemolysis (hee-MOL-ih-sis) A breakdown of red blood cells caused by the destruction of the red blood cell membranes.

hemorrhagic stroke (hem-or-AJ-ic) A stroke refers to damage to part of the brain caused by interruption of its blood supply or leakage of blood outside of vessel walls. A hemorrhagic stroke specifically refers to the latter cause and results from rupture of a blood vessel and subsequent bleeding within or over the surface of the brain.

hemorrhoid (HEM-or-oyd) A pronounced swelling in a large vein, particularly veins found in the anal region.

hemosiderin (heem-oh-SID-er-in) An insoluble iron-protein compound found in the liver. Hemosiderin stores iron when the amount of iron in the body exceeds the storage capacity of ferritin.

herbicide (ERB-ih-side) A compound that reduces the growth and reproduction of plants.

hexose (HEK-sos) A general term describing a carbohydrate containing six carbon atoms.

high-density lipoprotein (HDL) The lipoprotein synthesized primarily by the liver and small intestine that picks up cholesterol from dying cells and other sources and transfers it to the other lipoproteins in the bloodstream as well as directly to the liver. A low blood HDL value increases the risk for heart disease.

high-fructose corn syrup A corn syrup that has been manufactured to contain between 40% and 90% fructose.

high-quality proteins Dietary proteins that contain ample amounts of all nine amino acids.

hind milk (HYND) The milk secreted at the end of a nursing session; it is higher in fat than fore milk.

histamine (HISS-tuh-meen) A breakdown product of the amino acid histidine that stimulates acid secretion by the stomach and has other effects on the body, such as contraction of smooth muscles, increased nasal secretions, relaxation of blood vessels, and changes in relaxation of airways. It appears to decrease hunger and food intake.

homeostasis A series of adjustments that act to prevent change in the internal environment in the body.

hormone A compound secreted into the bloodstream that acts to control the function of target organ cells. Hormones can be either proteinlike or fatlike, such as insulin or estrogen.

hospice (HAHS-pis) Hospital care that emphasizes comfort and dignity in death.

hunger The internal or physiological drive to find and eat food.

hydrogenation (high-dro-jen-AY-shun) The addition of hydrogen atoms to the double bonds of polyunsaturated and monounsaturated fatty acids to reduce the extent of unsaturation. This process turns liquid vegetable oils into solid fats and is used to make margarine and shortening. *Trans* fatty acids are also produced by this process.

hydrolysis (high-DROL-ih-sis) A chemical reaction in which a compound is broken down by the addition of water to the products. One product receives the hydrogen ion (H^+) while the other product receives the hydroxyl ion (OH^-). Hydrolytic enzymes break down compounds using water in the manner just described.

hydrophilic (high-dro-FILL-ik) Attracts water (literally, "water loving").

hydrophobic (high-dro-FO-bik) Repels water (literally, "water fearing").

hydroxyapatite (high-drox-ee-APP-uh-tite) A compound, composed primarily of calcium and phosphate, that is deposited into the bone protein matrix to give bone strength and rigidity ($Ca_{10}[PO_4]_6OH_2$).

hyperactivity A poorly defined term generally used to label inattention, irritability, and excessively active behavior in children.

hypercalcemia (high-per-kal-SEE-mee-ah) A high concentration of calcium in the bloodstream. This can lead to loss of appetite, calcium deposits in organs, and other health problems.

hypercarotenemia (high-per-car-oh-teh-NEEM-ee-ah) High concentration of carotene in the bloodstream, usually caused by a diet high in carrots or other yellow-orange vegetables.

hyperglycemia (HIGH-per-gligh-SEE-me-uh) High blood glucose, above 140 mg/100 ml of blood.

hypergymnasia Exercising beyond that amount required for good physical fitness or maximum performance in a sport; excessive exercise.

hyperplasia (high-per-PLAY-zee-uh) An increase in cell number.

hypertension (high-per-TEN-shun) A condition in which blood pressure remains persistently elevated, especially when the heart is between beats.

hypertrophy (high-PURR-tro-fee) An increase in cell size.

hypochromic (high-po-KROME-ik) Pale red blood cells lacking sufficient hemoglobin as a result of an iron deficiency. Hypochromic cells have a reduced oxygen-carrying ability.

hypoglycemia (HIGH-po-gligh-SEE-mee-uh) Low blood glucose, below 40 to 50 mg/100 ml of blood.

hypothalamus (high-po-THALL-uh-mus) A part of the brain that contains cells that play a role in the regulation of hunger, respiration, body temperature, and other body functions.

hypothesis (high-POTH-eh-sis) An "educated guess" by a scientist to explain a phenomenon.

identical twins Two fetuses that develop from a single ovum and sperm and, consequently, have the same genetic makeup.

ileum (ILL-ee-um) The terminal segment of the small intestine.

immunoglobulins Proteins found in the blood that are responsible for antibody-mediated immunity, and bind specifically to antigen. Also called *antibodies*. Immunoglobulins are produced by B-lymphocytes in response to a foreign substance (antigen) in the bloodstream.

incidental food additives Additives that gain access to food products indirectly from environmental contamination of food ingredients, or during the manufacturing process.

incomplete (low-quality) protein Food protein that lacks ample amount of one or more of the essential amino acids needed to support human protein needs.

indirect calorimetry (kal-oh-RIM-eh-tree) A method to measure the energy output by the body by measuring oxygen uptake and/or carbon dioxide output. Formulas are then used to convert these gas exchange values into kilocalorie use.

infectious disease (in-FEK-shus) Any disease caused by an invasion of the body by microorganisms, such as bacteria, fungi, or viruses.

infrastructure The basic framework of a system or organization. For society, this includes roads, bridges, telephones, and other basic technologies.

inorganic Free of carbon atoms bonded to hydrogen atoms.

insensible losses Fluid losses that are not perceptible to the senses, such as losses through lungs, feces, and skin (an exception is heavy perspiration).

insoluble fibers (in-SOL-you-bul) Fibers that, for the most part, do not dissolve in water nor are digested by bacteria in the large intestine. These include cellulose, some hemicelluloses, and lignin.

insulin (IN-suh-lin) A hormone produced by the beta cells of the pancreas. Insulin increases the synthesis of glycogen in the liver and the movement of glucose from the bloodstream into muscle and adipose cells, among other processes.

insulin-dependent diabetes A form of diabetes prone to ketosis and that requires insulin therapy.

intentional food additives Additives knowingly (directly) incorporated into food products by manufacturers.

interferon (in-ter-FEAR-on) A group of proteins (α, β, γ) released by virus-infected cells that bind to other cells and stimulate them to produce antiviral proteins that in turn inhibit viral multiplication.

intermediate A chemical compound formed in one of the many steps in a metabolic pathway. For example, pyruvic acid is an intermediate in the glycolysis pathway.

intermediate-density lipoprotein (IDL) (lip-oh-PRO-teen) The product formed after a very-low-density lipoprotein (VLDL) has most of its triglyceride removed.

international unit (IU) A crude measure of vitamin activity, often based on the growth rate of animals. Today these units have been replaced by more precise microgram quantities.

interstitial fluid (in-ter-STISH-ul) Fluid between cells.

intracellular fluid Fluid contained within a cell.

intrauterine Within the uterus.

intravascular fluid Fluid within the bloodstream (that is, in the arteries, veins, and capillaries).

intravenous (in-tra-VEEN-us) Introduced directly into the bloodstream.

intrinsic factor A proteinlike compound produced by the stomach that enhances vitamin B-12 absorption.

in utero (in YOU-ter-oh) "In the uterus" or, during pregnancy.

ion An atom with an unequal number of electrons and protons. Negative ions have more electrons than protons; positive ions have more protons than electrons.

ionic bond (eye-ON-ik) A union between two atoms formed by an attraction of a positive ion to a negative ion, as seen in table salt (Na^+Cl^-).

irradiation (ir-RAY-dee-AY-shun) A process whereby radiation energy is applied to foods, creating compounds (free radicals) within the food that destroy cell membranes, break down DNA, link proteins together, limit enzyme activity, and alter a variety of other proteins and cell functions that would otherwise lead to food spoilage.

isomers (EYE-so-mers) Different chemical structures for compounds that share the same chemical formula.

isotope (EYE-so-towp) An alternate form of a chemical element. It differs from other atoms of the same element in the number of neutrons in its nucleus.

jaundice (JAWN-diss) A yellow staining of the skin and sclera (white of the eye) resulting from a buildup of bile pigments in the bloodstream. Liver or gallbladder disease is often the cause.

jejunem (je-JOON-um) The first half of the small intestine (minus the first 12 inches, which is the duodenum).

juvenile-onset obesity Obesity that develops in childhood; often characterized by an excess number of adipose cells that are also very large because of abundant fat storage.

ketogenic A name often given to diets that lead to the abundant production of ketones by the liver. This can be caused by a low carbohydrate intake.

ketones (KEE-tones) Incomplete breakdown products of fat containing three or four carbons and a ketone functional group, hence the name. An example is acetoacetic acid.

ketosis (kee-TOE-sis) The condition of having a high concentration of ketones in the bloodstream.

kidney nephrons (NEF-rons) Unit of kidney cells that filter wastes from the bloodstream.

kilocalorie (kill-oh-KAL-oh-ree) (kcal) The heat needed to raise the temperature of 1000 g (1 L) of water 1 degree Celsius.

kilojoule (KIL-oh-jool) (kJ) A measure of work in which 1 kJ equals the work needed to move 1 kg a distance of 1 meter with the force of 1 newton. One kcal equals 4.18 kJ.

kwashiorkor (kwash-ee-OR-core) A disease seen primarily in young children who have an existing disease and who consume a marginal amount of energy and considerably insufficient protein in the face of high needs. The child suffers from infection and exhibits edema, poor growth, weakness, and an increased susceptibility to further illness.

lactic acid (LAK-tik) A three-carbon acid; also called *lactate,* formed during anaerobic cell metabolism; a partial breakdown product of glucose.

lactobacillus bifidus factor (lak-toe-bah-SIL-us BIFF-id-us) A protective factor secreted in colostrum that encourages growth of beneficial bacteria in the newborn's intestines.

lacto-ovo vegetarian A person who consumes only plant products, dairy products, and eggs.

lacto-ovo-peso vegetarian A person who consumes only plant products, dairy products, eggs, and fish.

lactose (LAK-tose) A sugar made up of glucose linked to galactose.

lactose intolerance (primary and secondary) Primary lactose intolerance occurs when lactase production declines for no apparent reason. Secondary lactose intolerance occurs when a specific cause, like long-standing diarrhea, results in a decline in lactase production.

lactovegetarian (lak-toe-vej-eh-TEAR-ree-an) A person who consumes only plant products and dairy products.

lanugo (lah-NEW-go) Downlike hair that appears on a person who has lost much body fat during semistarvation. The hair stands erect and traps air, which acts as insulation to the body, replacing that usually supplied by body fat. Fetuses also have lanugo.

larva (LAR-va) An early developmental stage in the life history of some microorganisms, such as parasites.

laxative A medication or other substance that stimulates evacuation of the intestinal tract.

lean body mass The part of the human body that is free of all but essential body fat. About 2% of body weight as fat is essential. The rest of the fat in the body represents storage and so is not part of lean body mass. Lean body mass includes muscle, bone, organs, connective tissue, skin, and other body parts.

lecithin (LESS-uh-thin) Any of several phospholipids containing two fatty acids, a phosphate group, and a choline molecule.

"let-down reflex" A reflex stimulated by infant suckling that causes the release (ejection) of milk from milk ducts in the mother's breast.

leukotriene (loo-ko-TRY-een) An important mediator of many diseases involving inflammatory or hypersensitivity reactions, such as asthma; it is derived from fatty acids.

life expectancy The average length of life for a given group of people.

life span The potential oldest age to which a person can survive.

lignin (LIG-nin) An insoluble fiber made up of a multiringed alcohol (noncarbohydrate) structure.

limiting amino acid The essential amino acid in the lowest concentration in a food in comparison with the body's needs.

linoleic acid (lin-oh-LEE-ik) An essential fatty acid with 18 carbon atoms and two carbon-carbon double bonds; omega-6.

lipase (LYE-pase) Fat-digesting enzyme; gastric lipase is produced by the stomach and pancreatic lipase by the pancreas.

lipid (LIP-id) A compound containing much carbon and hydrogen, little oxygen, and sometimes other atoms. Lipids dissolve in ether or benzene and include fats, oils, and cholesterol.

lipid peroxidation Production of unstable lipids containing more than the normal amount of oxygen. In the formation of a fatty acid of this type first a carbon-carbon double bond is broken. The resulting breakdown products react with oxygen to form peroxides (—C—C—O—O—H) or free radicals (—C—C—O—O).

lipofuscin (ceroid pigments) (lip-oh-FEW-shun) (SER-oyd) Lipid breakdown products in cells. These compounds have fluorescence, and in that way can be detected in aged cells, such as those in the eye, the heart, and the brain.

lipogenesis (lye-poh-JEN-eh-sis) The building of fatty acids using derivatives of acetyl-CoA molecules.

lipogenic (lye-poh-JEN-ik) Means creating lipid. The liver is the major organ with lipogenic potential in the human body.

lipolysis (lye-POL-ih-sis) The breakdown of triglycerides to glycerol and fatty acids.

lipoprotein (lye-poh-PRO-teen) A compound found in the bloodstream containing a core of lipids with a shell of protein, phospholipid, and cholesterol.

lipoprotein lipase (lye-poh-PRO-teen LYE-pase) An enzyme attached to the outside of some cells that line the bloodstream; it breaks down triglycerides into free fatty acids and glycerol.

liter (LEE-ter) (L) A measure of volume in the metric system. One liter equals 0.96 quarts.

lobules (LOB-you-els) Saclike structures in the breast that store milk.

long-chain fatty acids Fatty acids that contain more than 12 carbon atoms.

low birth weight (LBW) Infant weight at birth of less than 2.5 kg (5.5 pounds); usually caused by preterm birth; these infants are at higher risk for health problems.

low-density lipoprotein (LDL) The product of the intermediate-density lipoprotein (IDL) containing primarily cholesterol. An elevated value is strongly linked to heart disease risk.

low input sustainable agriculture (LISA) A form of farming that attempts to limit use of purchased materials, such as manufactured fertilizers and pesticides. Use of manure and crop rotation are typical substitutes.

low-quality (incomplete) proteins Food proteins that lack an ample amount of one or more amino acids essential for human protein needs.

lumen (LOO-men) The inside cavity of a tube, such as the GI tract.

lymphatic system (lim-FAT-ick) A system of vessels in the body that can convey lymph particles, such as chylomicrons, from tissues into the bloodstream.

lymphocyte A class of white blood cells involved in the immune system, generally composing about 25% of all white blood cells. There are several types of lymphocytes with diverse functions, including antibody production, allergic reactions, graft rejections, tumor control, and regulation of the immune system.

lysosome (LYE-so-som) A cellular organelle that contains digestive enzymes for use inside the cell for turnover of cell parts.

lysozyme (LYE-so-zime) A set of enzyme substances produced by a variety of cells in the body that can destroy bacteria by rupturing their cell membranes.

macrocyte (MAC-row-site) An abnormally enlarged mature red blood cell with a short life span.

macrophage Any large mononuclear, phagocytic cell that is able to engulf and digest cellular debris and invading bacteria.

macular degeneration (MACK-u-lure) A cause of failing visual acuity and blindness because of degeneration of the macula, a small area of the retina of the eye that distinguishes fine detail. Consumption of foods rich in carotenoids, in particular dark green, leafy vegetables, decreases the risk of developing macular degeneration.

major mineral A mineral vital to health that is required in the diet in amounts greater than 100 mg per day.

malnutrition Failing health that results from a long-standing dietary intake that is insufficient to meet, or greatly exceeds, nutritional needs

maltose (MAWL-tose) Glucose bonded to glucose; a simple sugar.

mannitol (MAN-it-tol) An alcohol derivative of fructose.

marasmus (mah-RAZ-mus) A disease that results from insufficient consumption of protein and energy; usually seen in infancy. It is the equivalent of protein-energy malnutrition in adults. The person with marasmus has little or no fat stores and shows muscle wasting. Death from infection is common.

marginal Noticeable but not severe.

mass movement A peristaltic wave that simultaneously coordinates contraction over a large area of the colon. Mass movements move material from one portion of the colon to another and from the colon into the rectum.

mast cells Cells that contain histamine and are responsible for some aspects of allergic and inflammatory reactions.

maximum volume of oxygen consumption (Vo_{2max}) The maximum oxygen consumption a person can achieve during exercise, such as when riding a bicycle or running on a treadmill.

meconium (mee-KOH-nee-um) The first thick, mucuslike stool passed after birth.

medium-chain fatty acids Fatty acids that contain 8 to 10 carbon atoms.

megadose Intake of nutrient in excess of 10 times human needs.

megaloblast (MEG-ah-low-blast) A large, nucleated, immature red blood cell that results from an inability for cell division during red blood cell development.

memory cells Lymphocytes derived from B-cells or T-cells that have been exposed to an antigen; when exposed to the same antigen a second time, memory cells rapidly respond to provide immunity.

menaquinones (men-AH-kwih-nones) Forms of vitamin K that come from animal food sources or bacterial synthesis.

menarche (men-AR-kee) The onset of menstruation. Menarche usually occurs around age 13, two or three years after the first signs of puberty start to appear.

menopause (MEN-oh-paws) The cessation of menses in women, usually beginning at about 50 years of age.

mesomorph (MEZ-oh-morf) A body type associated with average bone size, trunk size, and finger length.

metabolism (meh-TAB-oh-lizm) Chemical reactions that occur in the body, enabling cells to release energy from foods, convert one substance into another, and prepare end products for excretion.

metallothionein (meh-TAL-oh-THIGH-oh-neen) A protein that binds and regulates the release of zinc and copper in intestinal and liver cells.

meter A measure of length in the metric system. One meter equals 39.4 inches.

MHC molecules Major Histocompatibility Complex (MHC) molecules are a large group of cell surface antigens unique to each individual.

micelle (MY-sell) An emulsification product in which individual emulsifiers organize with their hydrophobic parts to the center of the micelle and their hydrophilic parts to the outside. Lipids are attracted to the center area, and water is attracted to the outside periphery.

microcytic (my-kro-SIT-ik) Literally means "small cell." Microcytic red blood cells are smaller than normal.

microcytic hypochromic anemia An anemia exhibiting small, pale red blood cells lacking sufficient hemoglobin (often caused by an iron deficiency); these red blood cells have reduced oxygen-carrying ability.

microfractures Small fractures, undetectable by x-rays or other bone scans, that may develop constantly in bones.

microsomal ethanol oxidizing system (my-kro-SO-mol) An alternative pathway for alcohol metabolism when alcohol is in high concentration in the liver; uses rather than yields energy for the body, in comparison to alcohol dehydrogenase activity.

minerals Elements used in the body to promote chemical reactions and help form body structures.

miscarriage Termination of pregnancy that occurs before the fetus can survive; also called *spontaneous abortion.*

mitochondria Organelles inside most cells, including muscle cells. These are the main sites of energy production in a cell. Mitochondria also contain the pathway for burning fat for fuel, among other metabolic pathways.

modified food starch Starch molecules that have been chemically linked together to increase stability.

molecule A group of atoms chemically bonded together; that is, tightly connected by attractive forces (see **compound**).

monocyte A type of white blood cell that transforms to become a macrophage after moving into tissue; constitutes about 3% to 7% of all white blood cells.

monoglyceride (mon-oh-GLIS-er-ide) A breakdown product of a triglyceride consisting of one fatty acid bonded to a glycerol backbone.

monosaccharide (mon-oh-SACK-uh-ride) A class of simple sugars, such as glucose, that is not broken down further during digestion.

monounsaturated fatty acid A fatty acid containing one carbon-carbon double bond.

mortality This represents a population's death rate. The term *morbidity* refers to the amount of sickness present.

mottling (MOT-ling) Discoloration or marking of the surface of teeth from fluorosis.

mucilage (MYOU-sih-laj) A dietary fiber consisting of chains of galactose, mannose, and other monosaccharides; characteristically found in seaweed.

mucopolysaccharide (MYOO-ko-POL-ee-SAK-ah-ride) Substance containing protein and carbohydrate parts; found in bone and other organs.

mucosa (MYOO-co-saw) Mucous membrane consisting of cells and supporting connective tissue. In the digestive tract there is also a layer of smooth muscle supporting the mucosa. Mucosa lines cavities that open to the outside of the body such as the stomach and intestine and generally contains glands that secrete mucus.

mucus (MYOO-cuss) A thick fluid secreted by glands throughout the body. It contains a compound that has both carbohydrate and protein parts (glycoprotein). It acts as a lubricant and means of protection for cells.

mycotoxin (MY-ko-tok-sin) A group of toxic compounds produced by molds, such as aflatoxin B-1 found on moldy grains.

myocardial infarction (MY-oh-CARD-ee-ahl in-FARK-shun) Death of part of the heart muscle.

myoglobin (my-oh-GLOW-bin) Iron-containing compound that binds oxygen (O_2) in muscle.

negative energy balance The state in which the energy intake is less than the energy expended. The result of this is a decrease in body mass.

net protein utilization Biological value of a protein multiplied by digestibility of that protein.

neural tube defect A defect in the formation of the neural tube occurring during early fetal development. These are seen in about 2500 infants per year in the United States. The defect results in various nervous system disorders, such as spina bifida. Folate deficiency in the pregnant woman increases the risk of the fetus developing this disorder.

neuroendocrine Substances or functions linked to combined action of both endocrine glands and the nervous system. Examples include substances released from glands in response to nerve stimulation.

neuromuscular junction The junction between nerve and muscle.

neutron (NEW-tron) The part of an atom that has no charge.

neutrophil (NEW-tro-fil) The major form for white blood cells, comprising 55% to 65% of their total number. These take up microbes and destroy them.

nicotinamide adenine dinucleotide (NAD) (nik-oh-TIN-ah-mide AD-en-een dye-NUK-lee-oh-tide) A hydrogen carrier that represents a potential form of energy; made from the vitamin niacin.

nonessential (dispensable) amino acids Amino acids that can be readily made by the body. There are 11 nonessential amino acids.

nonheme iron Iron provided from plant sources and animal tissues other than hemoglobin and myoglobin. Nonheme iron is less efficiently absorbed than heme iron, as absorption is also more closely dependent on body needs.

non–insulin-dependent diabetes A form of diabetes in which ketosis is not commonly seen. Insulin therapy can be used, but often is not required.

nonpolar A neutral compound; no positive or negative poles present.

no observable effect level (NOEL) This corresponds to the highest dose of an additive that produces no deleterious health effect in animals.

nuclear receptor A site on the DNA in a cell where compounds (such as hormones) bind. Cells that contain DNA receptors for a specific compound are affected by that compound.

nucleus (NEW-klee-us) In chemistry, the core of an atom; it contains protons and neutrons.

nutrient density The ratio formed by dividing a food's contribution to the needs for a nutrient by its contribution to energy needs. When the contribution to nutrient needs exceeds that to energy needs, the food is considered to have a favorable nutrient density for that nutrient.

nutrient receptor Proposed site in the small intestine that is a mechanism to elicit a feeling of satiety.

nutrients Chemical substances in food that nourish the body by providing energy, building materials, and factors to regulate needed chemical reactions in the body.

nutrition The Council on Food and Nutrition of the American Medical Association defines nutrition as "the science of food; the nutrients and the substances therein; their action, interaction, and balance in relation to health and disease; and the process by which the organism (i.e., body) ingests, digests, absorbs, transports, utilizes, and excretes food substances."

nutrition label A label that must be included on most foods. It depicts nutrient content in comparison to the Daily Values set by FDA.

nutritional status The nutritional health of a person as determined by **a**nthropometric measures (height, weight, circumferences, and so on), **b**iochemical measures of nutrients or their by-products in blood and urine, a **c**linical (physical) examination, and a **d**ietary analysis (ABCD).

nutritionist A person who advises about nutrition and/or works in the field of food and nutrition. In many states in the United States a person does not need formal training to use this title. Some states reserve this title for Registered Dietitians.

obesity (oh-BEES-ih-tee) A condition characterized by excess body fat, often defined as 20% above desirable weight or a body mass index above 27-30.

oleic acid A fatty acid with 18 carbons and one carbon-carbon double bond; omega-9.

olfactory receptor cells Cells in the nasal region that discriminate numerous chemical molecules and transmit that information to the brain. This information represents one of the components of what we describe as flavor.

oligosaccharides (ol-ih-go-SAK-ah-rides) Carbohydrates containing three to ten monosaccharide units.

omega-3 (ω-3) fatty acid An unsaturated fatty acid with its first double bond at the third carbon atom from the methyl end ($—CH_3$).

omega-6 (ω-6) fatty acid An unsaturated fatty acid with its first double bond at the sixth carbon atom from the methyl end (—CH₃).

omnivore (AHM-nih-voor) A person who consumes foods from both plant and animal sources.

oncogene (AHN-ko-jeen) Gene that codes for a protein that in turn leads to cellular growth and development.

oncotic force (ahn-KAH-tik) The osmotic potential exerted by blood proteins in the bloodstream.

organ A group of tissues designed to perform a specific function; for example, the heart. It contains muscle tissue, nerve tissue, and so on.

organic A compound that contains carbon atoms bonded to hydrogen atoms.

organism A living thing. The human body is an organism consisting of many organs that act in a coordinated manner to support life.

osmosis Passive diffusion of solvent (water) through a semipermeable membrane from a less concentrated solution to a more concentrated solution.

osmotic potential (oz-MOT-ik) The tendency to attract water across a semipermeable membrane, usually to dilute some constituent in a fluid.

osmotic pressure The exerted pressure needed to keep particles in a solution from drawing liquid across a semipermeable membrane.

osteomalacia (OS-tee-oh-mal-AY-shuh) Adult rickets. A vitamin D deficiency disease that causes weak bones and increases fracture risk.

osteopenia (os-tee-oh-PEE-nee-ah) Decreased bone mass, resulting from cancer, hyperthyroidism, or other causes.

osteoporosis (os-tee-oh-po-ROH-sis) A bone disease that develops primarily after menopause in women and is characterized by a decrease in bone density.

ostomy (OSS-toh-mee) A surgically created "short circuit" in intestinal flow where the end point usually opens from the abdominal cavity, rather than the anus, as is the case with a colostomy.

outpatient A person treated by medical personnel outside the hospital setting; for example, in a clinic or a physician's office.

overnutrition A state in which nutritional intake exceeds the body's needs.

oxidation Loss of an electron by an atom or molecule. In metabolism, often associated with a gain of oxygen or loss of hydrogen. Oxidation (loss of an electron) and reduction (gain of an electron) take place simultaneously in metabolism, because an electron that is lost by one atom is accepted by another.

oxidize (OX-ih-dize) To lose an electron or gain an oxygen atom.

oxidizing agent In one sense, a substance capable of capturing an electron from another compound. A compound is "oxidized" when it loses an electron.

p53 gene Tumor suppressor gene; it can be subject to mutations.

palatable (PAL-it-ah-bull) Pleasing to taste.

paresthesia An abnormal spontaneous sensation, such as of burning, pricking, numbness, etc.

passive absorption Absorption that uses no energy. It requires permeability for the substance through the wall of the small intestine and a concentration gradient higher in the lumen of the intestine than in the absorptive cell.

pasteurization (pas-tur-ih-ZAY-shun) The process of heating food products to kill pathogenic microorganisms. One method heats milk at 161°F for at least 20 seconds.

pathway A metabolic progression of individual steps from starting materials to ending products, like C₆H₁₂O₆ (glucose) + O₂ yielding CO₂ + H₂O.

pectin (PEK-tin) A dietary fiber containing chains of galacturonic acid and other monosaccharides; characteristically found between plant cell walls.

peer-reviewed journal A journal that publishes research only after two or three scientists who were not part of the study agree it was well conducted and the results are fairly represented. Thus the research has been approved by peers of the research team.

pellagra (peh-LAHG-rah) A disease characterized by inflammation of the skin, diarrhea, and eventual mental incapacity; results from the lack of the vitamin niacin in the diet.

pepsin (PEP-sin) A protein-digesting enzyme produced by the stomach.

peptide bond A chemical bond formed by the reaction of an amino group with an acid group while splitting off a water molecule. This is the main bond that links amino acids in a protein.

peptide A few amino acids chemically bonded together; often two to four.

peptone A partial breakdown product of proteins.

percentile Classification of a measurement of a unit into divisions of 100 units.

peristalsis (per-ih-STALL-sis) A coordinated muscular contraction that is used to propel food down the gastrointestinal tract.

pernicious anemia (per-NISH-us ah-NEE-mee-ah) The anemia that results from a lack of vitamin B-12 absorption. It is pernicious (deadly) because of the associated nerve degeneration that can result in eventual paralysis and death.

pH A measure of the hydrogen ion concentration in a solution.

phagocytic cells (fag-oh-SIT-ick) Cells that engulf substances; these cells include neutrophils and macrophages.

phagocytosis/pinocytosis (FAG-oh-sigh-TOW-sis/PIN-oh-sigh-TOW-sis) A form of active absorption in which the absorptive

cell forms an indentation, and particles or fluids entering the indentation are then engulfed by the cell.

phenylalanine An amino acid.

phenylketonuria (PKU) (fen-ihl-kee-toh-NEW-ree-ah) A disease caused by a defect in the ability of the liver to metabolize the amino acid phenylalanine into the amino acid tyrosine.

phenylpropanolamine (fen-ihl-pro-pan-OL-ah-meen) An over-the-counter decongestant that has a mild appetite-reducing effect.

phosphocreatine (PCr) (fos-fo-CREE-a-tin) A high-energy compound that can be used to form adenosine triphosphate (ATP) from adenosine diphosphate (ADP).

photosynthesis (foto-sin-tha-sis) The process by which plants use energy from the sun to produce energy-yielding compounds, such as glucose.

phylloquinone (fil-oh-KWIN-own) A form of vitamin K that comes from plants.

physiological anemia The normal increase in blood volume in pregnancy that dilutes the concentration of red blood cells, resulting in anemia; also called *hemodilution.*

phytic acid (phytate) (FY-tick, FY-tate) A constituent of plant fibers that binds positive ions to its multiple phosphate groups.

phytobezoar (fy-tow-BEE-zor) A pellet of fiber characteristically found in the stomach.

phytochemical A chemical found in plants. Some phytochemicals may contribute to a reduced risk of cancer or heart disease in people who consume them regularly.

pica (PIE-kah) The practice of eating non-food items such as dirt, laundry starch, or clay.

placebo (plah-SEE-bo) A fake medicine used to disguise the roles of participants in an experiment; if fake surgery is performed, that is called a *sham operation.*

placenta (plah-SEN-tah) An organ formed in a woman only during pregnancy that secretes hormones and makes possible the transfer of oxygen and nutrients from the mother's blood to the fetus, as well as removal of fetal wastes.

plaque (PLACK) In terms of heart disease, a cholesterol-rich substance deposited in the blood vessels. It also contains various white blood cells and smooth muscle cells, cholesterol and other lipids, and eventually calcium.

plasma cell Antibody-producing cell resulting from the multiplication and differentiation of a B-lymphocyte that has interacted with an antigen; a mature plasma cell can produce from 3000 to 30,000 antibody molecules per second.

polar A compound with distinct positive and negative charges (poles) on it. These charges act like poles on a magnet.

polyglutamate form (POL-ee-GLOO-tah-mate) Folate with more than one glutamate molecule attached.

polypeptide (POL-ee-PEP-tide) Fifty to 100 amino acids bonded together.

polysaccharide (POL-ee-SACK-uh-ride) Carbohydrate containing many glucose units, up to 3000 or more.

polyunsaturated fatty acid A fatty acid containing two or more carbon-carbon double bonds.

pool The amount of a nutrient stored within the body that can be easily mobilized when needed.

portal vein A large vein that distributes blood from the intestine to the liver through capillaries.

positive balance A state in which nutrient intake exceeds losses. This causes a net gain of the nutrient in the body, such as when tissue protein is gained during growth. The opposite of this is negative balance, where losses exceed intake, as in cases of starvation.

precursor A compound that comes before; to precede.

pregnancy-induced hypertension A serious disorder that can include high blood pressure, kidney failure, convulsion, and even death of the mother and the fetus. Although the exact cause is not known, good nutrition, especially calcium intake, and prenatal care may prevent or limit its severity. Mild cases are known as *preeclampsia;* more severe cases are called *eclampsia* (formally called *toxemia*).

premenstrual syndrome A disorder (also referred to as *PMS*) found in some women a few days before the onset of menses and characterized by depression, headache, bloating, and mood swings.

preservatives Compounds that extend the shelf life of foods by inhibiting microbial growth or minimizing the destructive effect of oxygen and metals.

preterm An infant born before 38 weeks of gestation.

prevalence The number of people at any one time that have a specific disease, such as obesity or cancer.

primary disease A disease process that is not simply caused by another disease process.

primary structure of a protein The order of amino acids in the protein molecule.

progestins (pro-JES-tins) Hormones, including progesterone, that are necessary for maintaining pregnancy and lactation.

prognosis (prog-NO-sis) A forecast of the course and end of a disease.

prohormone Precursor of a hormone.

prolactin (pro-LACK-tin) A hormone secreted by the mother that stimulates the synthesis of milk.

prostacyclin (prost-tah-SIGH-klin) A prostaglandin made by the blood vessel walls that is a potent inhibitor of blood clotting.

prostaglandin (pros-tah-GLAN-din) One of several potent hormonelike compounds made of polyunsaturated fatty acids that produce diverse effects in the body.

prostaglandin I2 An inhibitor of blood clotting made by blood vessel cells.

prostate gland A solid, chestnut-shaped organ surrounding the first part of the urethra in the male. The prostate gland is situated immediately under the bladder and in front of the rectum. The prostate gland secretes substances into the semen as the fluid passes through ducts leading from the seminal vesicles into the urethra.

proteins Compounds made of amino acids; contain carbon, hydrogen, oxygen, nitrogen, and sometimes other atoms, in a specific configuration.

protein digestibility corrected amino acid score (PDCAAS) A measure of protein quality that has recently been accepted by FDA. This replaces PER evaluations for foods intended for children over 4 years of age and nonpregnant adults. PDCAAS of a protein is based on its chemical score multiplied by digestibility.

protein efficiency ratio (PER) A measure of protein quality determined by the ability of a protein to support the growth of a young animal.

protein-energy malnutrition (PEM) A condition resulting from regularly consuming insufficient amounts of energy and protein. The deficiency eventually results in body wasting and an increased susceptibility to infection.

prothrombin (pro-THROM-bin) A blood protein needed for blood clotting that requires vitamin K for its synthesis.

proton (PRO-ton) The part of an atom that is positively charged.

proto-oncogene (PRO-tow-AHN-ko-jeen) Growth-promoting gene found naturally in human cells.

psyllium (SIL-ee-um) A mostly soluble type of dietary fiber found in the seeds of the plantain plant.

raffinose (RAF-ih-nos) An indigestible oligosaccharide containing three monosaccharide units (galactose-glucose-fructose).

rancid (RAN-sid) Containing products of decomposed fatty acids; these yield off-flavors and odors.

rationalization The process of mentally distorting information and denying facts in an attempt to hold onto a certain opinion.

reactive hypoglycemia (HIGH-po-gligh-SEE-mee-uh) Low blood glucose that may follow a meal high in simple sugars, with corresponding symptoms of irritability, headache, nervousness, and sweating. The actual prevalence of this disease is low.

receptive framework for learning The process by which a person opens up to learning more about a problem; it usually involves seeking more information about the issue from books and people. In the case of seeking behavior changes, it involves examining background experiences to evaluate whether a behavior change is feasible.

receptor A site in a cell at which compounds (such as hormones) bind. Cells that contain receptors for a specific compound are partially controlled by that compound.

receptor pathway for cholesterol uptake A process by which LDL molecules (cholesterol-containing) are bound by cell receptors, with the incorporation of the LDL molecule into the cell.

Recommended Dietary Allowances (RDAs) Recommended intakes of nutrients that meet the needs of almost all healthy people of similar age and gender. These are established by the Food and Nutrition Board of the National Academy of Sciences.

Recommended Nutrient Intake (RNI) The Canadian version of RDA.

redox agents Chemicals that can readily undergo both oxidation (loss of an electron) and reduction (gain of an electron).

reducing agent In one sense, a compound capable of donating electrons (also hydrogen ions) to another compound (see Appendix B).

reduction The gain of an electron by an atom; takes place simultaneously with oxidation (loss of an electron by an atom) in metabolism because an electron that is lost by one atom is accepted by another. In metabolism reduction is often associated with the gain of hydrogen.

Reference Daily Intake (RDI) Standards established by FDA for expressing nutrient content on nutrition labels. RDIs are generally based on the maximum 1968 RDA values set for a nutrient that span a particular age range, such as children over 4 years through adults. *RDI* replaced the term *U.S. RDA.*

Registered Dietitian (RD) (dye-eh-TISH-shun) A person who has completed a baccalaureate degree program approved by The American Dietetic Association, performed at least 900 hours of supervised professional practice, and passed a registration examination.

relapse prevention A set of strategies used by people to help prevent and cope with weight control lapses, such as recognizing high-risk situations and deciding beforehand on appropriate responses.

renin (REN-in) An enzyme formed in the kidney in response to low blood pressure; it acts on a blood protein to produce angiotensin I.

requirement The amount of a nutrient required by one person to maintain health. This varies between individuals. We do not know our individual requirements for each nutrient.

reserve capacity The extent to which an organ can preserve essentially normal function despite decreasing cell number or cell activity.

respiration The utilization of oxygen; in the human organism, the inhalation of oxygen and the exhalation of carbon dioxide; in cells, the oxidation (electron removal) of food molecules, particularly in the citric acid cycle, to obtain energy.

resting metabolic rate The amount of energy used during rest, without stringently controlling recent physical activity. Essentially the same as the basal metabolic rate, but the subject does not need to meet the strict conditions used for a basal metabolic rate determination. Today, both terms are often used interchangeably.

restraint A feeling that occurs as a result of restricted food intake, often associated with the belief that there are good and bad foods.

retinoids (RET-ih-noyds) Various forms of preformed vitamin A; one source is animal foods, like liver. Forms include retinol, retinal, and retinoic acid.

reverse transport of cholesterol The process by which cholesterol is picked up by HDL molecules and transferred to the liver or to other lipoproteins that can dispose of it in the liver.

rhodopsin (row-DOP-sin) A protein involved in vision; it is made in the eye and incorporates a protein called *opsin* and a form of vitamin A; especially important in night vision.

ribose (RIGH-bos) A five-carbon sugar found in genetic material, specifically RNA.

rickets A disease characterized by softening of the bones because of poor calcium deposition. This deficiency disease arises in infancy and childhood from lack of vitamin D activity in the body.

risk factor A characteristic or a behavior that contributes to the chances of developing an illness.

R-protein A protein produced by the salivary glands that enhances vitamin B-12 absorption, possibly by protecting it during its passage through the GI tract.

runner's anemia (ah-NEE-me-ah) A decrease in the blood's ability to carry oxygen, found in athletes, which may be caused by iron loss through perspiration and feces, red blood cell destruction due to the impact of exercise as the foot strikes the ground, or increased blood volume.

saccharin (SACK-ah-rin) An alternative sweetener that yields no energy to the body; it is 300 times sweeter than sucrose.

saliva (sah-LIGH-vah) A watery fluid produced by the salivary glands in the mouth that contains lubricants, enzymes, and other substances.

salt Generally refers to a compound of sodium and chloride in a 40:60 ratio.

satiety (suh-TIE-uh-tee) A state in which there is no longer a desire to eat; a feeling of satisfaction.

saturated fatty acid A fatty acid containing no carbon-carbon double bonds.

scavenger pathway for cholesterol uptake A process by which LDL molecules (cholesterol-containing) are taken up by scavenger cells embedded in the blood vessels.

scurvy (SKER-vee) The deficiency disease that results after a few weeks of consuming a diet free of vitamin C; pinpoint hemorrhages on the skin are an early sign.

sebaceous glands (seh-BAY-shus) Sebaceous glands surround hair follicles on the face, ears, chest, eyelid, back, and elsewhere. Blockage of a duct in a gland can lead to an infection and local pressure, resulting in an acne lesion.

sebum (SEE-bum) Secretion of the sebaceous gland, consisting of waxes and various triglycerides.

secondary deficiency A deficiency caused not by lack of the nutrient in question, but by lack of a substance that is needed for that nutrient to function.

secondary disease A disease process that develops as a result of another disease.

secondary structure of a protein The interactions (bonds) formed between amino acids placed close together in the primary structure.

secretin (SEE-kreh-tin) A hormone that causes bicarbonate ion release from the pancreas.

segmentation Contractions of the circular muscles in the intestines that lead to a dividing and mixing of the intestinal contents. This action aids digestion and absorption of nutrients.

self-monitoring A process of tracking foods eaten and conditions affecting eating; actions are usually recorded in a diary, along with location, time, and state of mind. This is a tool to help a person understand more about his or her eating habits.

self-talk The internal dialogue that each one of us carries on in our heads as we sort out beliefs, feelings, attitudes, and events happening in our lives.

semiessential amino acids Amino acids that, when consumed, spare the need to use an essential amino acid for their synthesis. Tyrosine in the diet, for example, spares the need to use phenylalanine for its synthesis.

sequesterant (see-KWES-ter-ant) Compound that binds free metal ions. By so doing, it reduces the ability of ions to cause rancidity in compounds containing fat.

serotonin (ser-oh-TONE-in) A neurotransmitter synthesized from the amino acid tryptophan that appears to both decrease the desire to eat carbohydrates and induce sleep.

serum The portion of the blood fluid remaining after (1) the blood is allowed to clot and (2) the red and white blood cells are removed by centrifugation.

set point Often refers to the close regulation of body weight. It is not known what cells control this set point nor how it actually functions in weight regulation. There is no doubt, however, that there are mechanisms that help regulate weight.

short-chain fatty acids Fatty acids that contain fewer than eight carbon atoms.

sickle cell anemia (ah-NEE-me-ah) An anemia that results from a malformation of the red blood cell because of an incorrect primary structure in part of its hemoglobin protein chains. The disease can lead to episodes of severe bone and joint pain, abdominal pain, headache, convulsions, paralysis, and even death.

sign A change in health status that is apparent on physical examination.

small-for-gestational age (SGA) (jes-TAY-shun-al) Infants who weigh less than the expected weight for their length of gestation. This corresponds to less than 2.5 kg (5.5 pounds) at term.

sodium bicarbonate An alkaline substance made basically of sodium and carbon dioxide ($NaHCO_3$).

soluble fibers (SOL-you-bull) Fibers that either dissolve or swell when put into water or are metabolized (fermented) by bacteria in the large intestine. These include pectins, gums, mucilages, and some hemicelluloses.

solvent A substance that other substances dissolve in.

sorbitol (SOR-bih-tol) An alcohol derivative of glucose.

specific heat Heat required to raise the temperature of 1 g of a substance 1°C. Water has a high specific heat, meaning that a relatively large amount of heat is required to raise its temperature; therefore it tends to resist large temperature fluctuations.

sphincter (SFINK-ter) A muscular valve that controls flow of foodstuff in the GI tract.

spontaneous abortion Loss of pregnancy, also called *miscarriage,* that occurs within 28 weeks of conception.

stable isotope (I-so-tope) An isotope is an alternate form of a chemical element. It differs from other atoms of the same element in the number of neutrons in its nucleus. Being stable means that the isotope does not emit radioactivity, as some isotope forms do.

stachyose (STAK-ee-os) An indigestible oligosaccharide with four monosaccharide units (galactose-galactose-glucose-fructose).

starch A carbohydrate made of multiple units of glucose attached together in a form the body can digest; also known as *complex carbohydrate.*

steroids (STARE-oyds) A group of hormones and related compounds that are derivatives of cholesterol.

sterol A compound containing a multiring (steroid) structure and a hydroxyl group (—OH).

stimulus control Altering the environment to minimize the stimuli for eating; for example, removing foods from sight and storing them in kitchen cabinets.

stress fracture A fracture that occurs from repeated jarring of a bone. Common sites include bones of the foot.

stroke The loss of body function that results from a blood clot in the brain, which in turn causes the death of brain tissue.

subclinical Not seen on a clinical (physical) examination.

subclinical disease Disease or disorder that is present but not severe enough to produce symptoms that can be detected or diagnosed.

subjects Participants in an experiment.

sucrose (SOO-kros) Fructose bonded to glucose; table sugar.

sugar Simple carbohydrate form with a chemical composition of CH_2O. Most sugars form ringed structures when in solution.

superoxide dismutase (soo-per-OX-ide DISS-myoo-tase) An enzyme that can quench (deactivate) a superoxide free radical. This can contain the minerals manganese, copper, or zinc.

sympathetic nervous system Part of the nervous system that regulates involuntary vital functions, including the activity of the heart, smooth muscles, and adrenal glands. The sympathetic nervous system specifically accelerates heart rate, constricts blood vessels, and raises blood pressure. The parasympathetic nervous system slows heart rate, increases intestinal peristalsis and gland activity, and relaxes sphincters.

symptom A change in health status noted by the person with the problem, such as a stomach pain.

synapse (SIN-aps) Space between nerve cells. One nerve cell stimulates other nearby cells, including other nerve cells, by releasing chemicals that cross the synapse. These chemicals excite neighboring cells.

systolic blood pressure (sis-TOL-lik) The pressure in the arterial blood vessels associated with the pumping of blood from the heart.

teratogen (ter-A-toe-jen) An agent that causes physical defects in a developing fetus.

tertiary structure of a protein (TER-she-air-ee) The three-dimensional structure of a protein, formed by interactions of amino acids placed far apart in the primary structure.

tetany (TET-ah-nee) A state marked by sharp contraction of muscles with failure to relax afterward; usually caused by abnormal calcium metabolism.

theory An explanation for a phenomenon that has numerous lines of evidence to support it.

thermic effect of food The increase in energy use that occurs during the digestion, absorption, and metabolism of energy-yielding nutrients. This represents about 10% of energy consumed.

"thrifty" metabolism A metabolism that characteristically uses less energy than normal, such that the risk of weight gain and obesity is enhanced.

thromboxane A stimulant of blood clotting made in the blood from polyunsaturated fatty acids.

thyroid-stimulating hormone A hormone that regulates the uptake of iodide by the thyroid gland and is secreted in response to a low concentration of circulating thyroxine.

tissue A group of cells designed to perform a specific function; nerve tissue is an example.

t-lymphocyte (tee-LYMF-oh-site) White blood cell processed by the thymus gland and responsible for recognition of foreign substances (such as viruses) in intracellular sites in the body.

tocopherol (tuh-KOFF-er-all) The chemical name for some forms of vitamin E.

tocotrienol (toe-co-TRY-en-ol) Compound related to tocopherol, but differs in the fatty acid side chain on the molecules, in that they contain more carbon-carbon double bonds.

trabecular bone (trah-BEK-you-lar) The spongy, inner matrix of bone, found primarily in the spine, pelvis, and ends of bones.

trace mineral A mineral vital to health that is required in the diet in amounts less than 100 mg per day.

transamination (trans-am-ih-NAY-shun) The transfer of an amino group from an amino acid to a carbon skeleton to form a new amino acid.

trans **fatty acids** An isomer form of unsaturated fatty acids. The hydrogens of both carbons forming the double bond lie on opposite sides of the plane of that bond.

transferrin A blood protein that transports iron in the blood.

trans **isomer (EYE-so-mer)** An isomer form found in compounds with double bonds, such as fatty acids, where the hydrogens of both carbon atoms forming the double bond lie on opposite sides of the plane of that bond.

triglyceride (try-GLISS-uh-ride) The major form of lipid in the body and in food. It is composed of three fatty acids bonded to glycerol, an alcohol.

trimester The normal pregnancy of 38 to 42 weeks is divided into three 13- to 14-week periods called *trimesters.*

trypsin (TRIP-sin) A protein-digesting enzyme secreted by the pancreas (in a zymogen form) that acts in the small intestine.

ulcer (UL-sir) Erosion of the tissue lining usually in the stomach (gastric ulcer) or the upper small intestine (duodenal ulcer). These are generally referred to as *peptic ulcers.*

umami A brothy, meaty, savory flavor in some foods. Monosodium glutamate enhances this flavor when added to foods.

uncoupling The dissociation between the liberation of energy from energy-yielding substances and the formation of ATP.

undernutrition Failing health that results from a longstanding dietary intake that regularly fails to meet nutritional needs.

underwater weighing A method to estimate total body fat by weighing the individual first normally and then when submerged in

water. The loss of weight when submerged in water is used to estimate total body fat.

underweight Body weight for height about 15% to 20% below desirable weight, or a body mass index below about 19. These cut-offs are less precise than for obesity because less study of this condition has been undertaken.

vagus nerves Nerves arising from the brain that branch off to other organs and are essential for control of speech, swallowing, and gastrointestinal function.

variability In a nutritional sense, the variation expected in nutrient requirements in a group of individuals.

vegan (VEE-gun) A person who eats only plant foods.

very-low-calorie diet (VLCD) Known also as *protein-sparing modified fast* (PSMF), this diet allows a person 400 to 700 kcal/day, often in liquid form. Of this, 30 to 120 g is carbohydrate, while the rest is high–biological value protein.

very-low-density lipoprotein (VLDL) The lipoprotein that initially leaves the liver. It carries both the cholesterol and lipid newly synthesized by the liver.

villi (VIL-eye) Fingerlike protrusions into the small intestine that participate in digestion and absorption of foodstuff.

vitamins Organic compounds needed in very small amounts in the diet to help regulate and support chemical reactions in the body.

VO_2max Maximum volume of oxygen consumed per unit of time during exercise.

water activity A measure of the amount of free water in a food. Most bacteria need a water activity greater than 0.9 to grow, but molds can grow in water activity as low as 0.6.

whey (WAY) Proteins, such as lactalbumin, that are found in great amounts in human milk and are easy to digest.

white blood cells One of the formed elements of the circulating blood system also called *leukocytes.* Five types of leukocytes are lymphocytes, monocytes, neutrophils, basophils, and eosinophils. White blood cells are able to squeeze through intracellular spaces and migrate. Leukocytes phagocytize bacteria, fungi, and viruses, as well as detoxify proteins that may result from allergic reactions, cellular injury, and other immune system cells.

whole grains Grains containing the entire seed of the plant, including the bran, germ, and endosperm (starchy interior).

xanthine dehydrogenase (ZAN-thin de-HY-droj-eh-nase) An enzyme containing molybdenum and iron that functions in the formation of uric acid and the mobilization of iron from liver ferritin stores.

xenobiotic (ZEE-no-bye-OT-ic) Compound that is foreign to the body. The principal classes are drugs, chemical carcinogens, and environmental substances such as pesticides.

xerophthalmia (zer-of-THAL-mee-uh) Literally "dry eye." A cause of blindness that results from infection of the eye secondary to a vitamin A deficiency. The specific cause is a lack of mucus production by the eye, which then leaves it more vulnerable to surface dirt and bacterial infection.

xylitol (ZIGH-lih-tol) An alcohol derivative of the five-carbon monosaccharide, xylose.

yo-yo dieting The practice of losing weight and then regaining it, only to lose it and regain it again. This practice has been shown to lead to an increased risk for heart disease in some studies.

zymogen (zigh-MO-gin) An inactive form of an enzyme that requires the removal of some minor part of the chemical structure in order for it to work. The zymogen is converted into an active enzyme at the appropriate time, such as when released into the stomach or small intestine.

Credits

Index